Oxford Textbook of

Neurocritical Care

Free personal online access for 12 months

Individual purchasers of this book are also entitled to free personal access to the online edition for 12 months on *Oxford Medicine Online* (www.oxfordmedicine.com). Please refer to the access token card for instructions on token redemption and access.

Online ancillary materials, where available, are noted at the end of the respective chapters in this book. Additionally, *Oxford Medicine Online* allows you to print, save, cite, email, and share content; download high-resolution figures as PowerPoint® slides; save often-used books, chapters, or searches; annotate; and quickly jump to other chapters or related material on a mobile-optimized platform.

We encourage you to take advantage of these features. If you are interested in ongoing access after the 12-month gift period, please consider an individual subscription or consult with your librarian.

Oxford Textbook of

Neurocritical Care

Edited by

Martin Smith MBBS, FRCA, FFICM

Consultant and Honorary Professor in Neurocritical Care, The National Hospital for Neurology and Neurosurgery, University College London Hospitals, London, UK

National Institute for Health Research, University College London Hospitals, Biomedical Research Centre, London, UK

Giuseppe Citerio MD

Professor in Anaesthesia and Critical Care, School of Medicine and Surgery, University of Milano-Bicocca, Italy

Director of Neurocritical Care and Neuroanaesthesia, Department of Anaesthesiology and Critical Care, San Gerardo Hospital, Monza, Italy

W. Andrew Kofke MD, MBA, FCCM, FNCS

Professor and Director of Neuroscience in Anaesthesiology and Critical Care Program; Co-Director of Neurocritical Care, Department of Anaesthesiology and Critical Care, University of Pennsylvania, Philadelphia, USA

Professor in Department of Neurosurgery, University of Pennsylvania, Philadelphia, USA

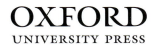

OXFORD
UNIVERSITY PRESS

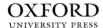

UNIVERSITY PRESS

Great Clarendon Street, Oxford, OX2 6DP,
United Kingdom

Oxford University Press is a department of the University of Oxford.
It furthers the University's objective of excellence in research, scholarship,
and education by publishing worldwide. Oxford is a registered trade mark of
Oxford University Press in the UK and in certain other countries

First Edition published in 2016
Impression: 1

Published in the United States of America by Oxford University Press
198 Madison Avenue, New York, NY 10016, United States of America

British Library Cataloguing in Publication Data
Data available

Library of Congress Control Number: 2015949015

ISBN 978–0–19–873955–5

Printed in Great Britain by
Bell & Bain Ltd., Glasgow

Foreword

The emergence of intensive care from the dark ages after World War II was the result of a combination of factors. The experience gained in the polio epidemics of the 1940s and 1950s had left a legacy of theoretical and practical knowledge of managing patients with inadequate respiration and airway protection. The frequency that respiratory failure often accompanied a terminal decline made it an obvious target for intervention. General intensive care, for respiratory support irrespective of aetiology, evolved then but in the context of more specialized approaches for specific pathologies, such as acute brain damage. The importance of brain injury as a major cause of death and disability became clear and the pessimistic view that these outcomes were largely inevitable was challenged.

But what was not appreciated at the beginning was the complexity of the processes involved, how they are compounded by the interactions between intracranial and extracranial events, with possible benefits of powerful treatments (such as barbiturates or hypothermia) offset by contrary adverse effects. The *Oxford Textbook of Neurocritical Care* shows just how the specialty has now advanced to meet these challenges.

The editors have brought together an impressive group of more than 60 experts in general critical care, respiratory medicine, specialized neurocritical care, neurology, neurosurgery, and radiology. Their work has been well orchestrated, reducing redundancies and overlaps to an unavoidable minimum.

The structure of the book properly reflects what intensive care should be about: grounded on physiopathology and mechanisms (part 1 is devoted to basic principles), based on continuous and sophisticated measurements (part 2 covers a range of monitoring modalities), and fine-tuned to specific pathological conditions (part 3), from post-operative care to neuromuscular disorders.

The evidentiary basis of practice is reviewed extensively and synthesized clearly. There is an average of 122 citations per chapter, leading to an impressive total of 3789 references. Each topic includes investigations of disease mechanisms, and how these can be modified in experimental models and in patients, together with results from rigorous clinical studies. The quality of tables and figures is excellent, with schematic drawings of anatomical features, down to microscopic details, and clear definitions of terms. Chapters on neuropathophysiology and blood flow regulation are exemplary, with useful schematic illustrations of histology, anatomy, and neurophysiology. This effective educational style is expressed in several topics: for example, when fluid management is addressed, water homeostasis and compartmentalization are carefully described, and illustrated in diagrams. When possible, as in the case of sedation, a practical approach is proposed, with a logical algorithm presenting the various options faced in everyday clinical practice.

Inevitably in several areas there are educated opinions rather than strong evidence. This honest admission doesn't leave the reader in a limbo of uncertainty, but clearly separates what is proven from what is not; options, in these cases, are still presented with clinical wisdom and experience.

Brain damage may be fatal, or have lifelong consequences. The social implications of acute brain injury, for survivors and their families, are acknowledged. The last chapter is devoted to outcome and prognosis, with specific data on risk adjustment and prognostic models in different pathologies. Survival rates, and quality of survival, are addressed. Ethical implications are wide, both for grading intensity of care and for withdrawing futile therapies. These issues are covered in a precise chapter which reports legal and ethical implications, and in a further chapter focused on organ donation.

Neurointensive care is rapidly evolving and expanding. Several features are changing, new competencies are required, and keeping up to date may appear to favour rapid access to the latest online information. Nevertheless, clinicians still need a clear, comprehensive, and credible source of the core of information upon which the speciality is based. This textbook, in a quickly moving scenario, provides the necessary account of the foundations of neurocritical care. We believe it will be valued by both the diligent student and the more experienced practitioner.

Professor Graham M. Teasdale, DSc
Mental Health and Wellbeing,
University of Glasgow
Gartnavel Royal Hospital
Glasgow, United Kingdom

Professor Nino Stocchetti
Department of Physiopathology and Transplantation
Milan University
Neuro ICU Fondazione IRCCS Cà Granda
Ospedale Maggiore Policlinico
Milan, Italy

Preface

Neurocritical care has evolved rapidly in the last two decades from its initial focus on the management of postoperative neurosurgical patients to a multidisciplinary specialty that provides comprehensive management for all life-threatening disorders of the central nervous system (CNS) and their complications. Managing the complex interaction between the injured brain and systemic organ systems is the cornerstone of neurocritical care which, in parallel with increased understanding of the pathophysiology of CNS disease and advances in monitoring and imaging techniques, has led to the introduction of more effective and individualized treatment strategies that have translated into improved outcomes for critically ill neurological patients.

The cornerstone of neurocritical care is the identification of individuals at risk of developing secondary brain injury and the delivery of targeted interventions to provide the optimal conditions to minimize such injury and maximize the chances of good neurological outcome. A major challenge for the neurointensivist is balancing the risks and benefits of various treatment options, being mindful that brain injury and brain-directed therapies can have potentially adverse effects on systemic organ systems and management of failing systemic organ systems can similarly have adverse effects on the injured brain. Thus the delivery of effective neurocritical care requires an understanding of underlying physiological and pathophysiological processes and interpretation of subtle clinical changes in association with neuromonitoring and neuroimaging data. Possibly more than any other branch of intensive care medicine, neurocritical care also requires collaboration and cooperation between clinicians from multiple disciplines. Whilst the neurointensivist and their teams coordinate and direct the management of patients on the neurocritical care unit, input from other disciplines, including neurology, neurosurgery, neuroradiology, trauma, and stroke physicians, is of crucial importance.

The *Oxford Textbook of Neurocritical Care* recognizes the common knowledge base and skills that are required for the management of critically ill neurological patients and has gathered together a group of international experts from multiple disciplines to provide a comprehensive global overview of the specialty. Each chapter of this book highlights advances in the respective areas but also emphasizes the importance of getting the basics right. Management of systemic and cerebral physiology is as important as interventions targeted to a specific neurological pathology or disease state, and this textbook quite rightly emphasizes throughout the importance of doing lots of little things consistently well. In this way, we hope that it will provide a framework for developing the meticulous attention to detail that underlies the clinical practice of neurocritical care.

Although primarily aimed at those working in neurocritical care, we anticipate that this textbook will also be of interest to those from other disciplines who have regular or occasional contact with patients with acute neurological disease. We particularly hope that it will be a useful educational resource for trainees from many disciplines and that it might stimulate their interest in neurocritical care.

We would like to thank our colleagues who have contributed to this book, our families for their forbearance during its preparation, and of course our patients from whom we have learned so much.

Martin Smith
Giuseppe Citerio
W. Andrew Kofke

Contents

Abbreviations

3D	three-dimensional		CIM	critical illness myopathy
AAN	American Academy of Neurology		CIP	critical illness polyneuropathy
ABI	acute brain injury		CK	creatine kinase
ABP	arterial blood pressure		CMR	cerebral metabolic rate
ACTH	adrenocorticotropic hormone		$CMRO_2$	cerebral metabolic rate of oxygen
ADC	apparent diffusion coefficient		CNS	central nervous system
ADEM	acute disseminated encephalomyelitis		CO_2	carbon dioxide
ADH	antidiuretic hormone		CoCBF	cortical cerebral blood flow
AED	antiepileptic drug		CPAP	continuous positive airway pressure
AF	atrial fibrillation		CPP	cerebral perfusion pressure
AHA	American Heart Association		CRS-R	Coma Recovery Scale—Revised
AIS	acute ischaemic stroke		CSF	cerebrospinal fluid
AKI	acute kidney injury		CSW	cerebral salt wasting
ALI	acute lung injury		CT	computed tomography
AMPA	α-amino-3-hydroxy-5-methyl-4-i soxazolepropionic acid		CTA	computed tomography angiography
			CTP	computed tomography perfusion
ANS	autonomic nervous system		DAG	diacylglycerol
APACHE	Acute Physiology And Chronic Health Evaluation		DBP	diastolic blood pressure
			DCD	donation after cardiac death
AQP	aquaporin		DCI	delayed cerebral ischaemia
ARDS	acute respiratory distress syndrome		DCS	diffuse correlation spectroscopy
ASA	American Stroke Association		DI	diabetes insipidus
aSAH	aneurysmal subarachnoid haemorrhage		DND	donation after neurological death
ASL	arterial spin labelling		DSA	digital subtraction angiography
ASPECTS	Alberta Stroke Programme Early CT Score		DTI	diffusion tensor imaging
ATLS	Advanced Trauma Life Support		DWI	diffusion-weighted imaging
ATP	adenosine triphosphate		EAAT	excitatory amino acid transporter
AVM	arteriovenous malformation		ECF	extracellular fluid
BAO	basilar artery occlusion		ECG	electrocardiogram
BBB	blood–brain barrier		ED	emergency department
BFV	blood flow velocity		EDH	extradural haematoma
BI	Barthel Index		EDHF	endothelial-derived hyperpolarization factor
BNP	brain natriuretic peptide		EEG	electroencephalogram
BOLD	blood oxygen level-dependent		EF	ejection fraction
BP	blood pressure		EGL	endothelial glycocalyx layer
BTF	Brain Trauma Foundation		EMG	electromyogram
CBF	cerebral blood flow		EP	evoked potential
CBV	cerebral blood volume		EPO	erythropoietin
CCP	critical closing pressure		EPOR	erythropoietin receptor
CEA	carotid endarterectomy		ET	endothelin
cEEG	continuous electroencephalogram		EVD	external ventricular drain
CFU	colony forming unit		FFP	fresh frozen plasma
CI	confidence interval			

FLAIR	fluid-attenuated inversion recovery	NMDA	*N*-methyl-D-aspartate
fMRI	functional magnetic resonance imaging	NO	nitric oxide
FOUR	Full Outline of UnResponsiveness	NSAID	non-steroidal anti-inflammatory drug
FV	flow velocity	NSE	neuron-specific enolase
FVC	forced vital capacity	O_2	oxygen
GABA	gamma-aminobutyric acid	OEF	oxygen extraction fraction
GCS	Glasgow Coma Scale	OHCA	out-of-hospital cardiac arrest
GH	growth hormone	OR	odds ratio
GOS	Glasgow outcome score	$PaCO_2$	partial pressure of arterial carbon dioxide
GRE	gradient-echo	PAF	platelet-activating factor
HFO	high-frequency oscillation	PaO_2	partial pressure of arterial oxygen
HMPAO	hexamethylpropyleneamine oxime	PCAS	post-cardiac arrest syndrome
HPA	hypothalamic–pituitary–adrenal	PCI	primary percutaneous intervention
HR	heart rate	PCT	perfusion computed tomography
HSP	heat shock protein	PCV	pressure control ventilation
HSV	herpes simplex virus	PED	periodic epileptiform discharge
IA	intra-arterial	PEEP	positive end-expiratory pressure
ICAM	intercellular adhesion molecule	PET	positron emission tomography
ICH	intracerebral haemorrhage	PKC	protein kinase C
ICP	intracranial pressure	PLED	periodic lateralized epileptiform discharge
ICU	intensive care unit	PP	periodic paralysis
IHCA	in-hospital cardiac arrest	PRx	pressure reactivity index
IL	interleukin	PSH	paroxysmal sympathetic hyperactivity
IP3	inositol 1,4,5-triphosphate	$PtiO_2$	brain tissue oxygen tension
IPC	intermittent pneumatic compression	PTT	partial thromboplastin time
ITP	intrathoracic pressure	PVS	persistent vegetative state
ITT	intensive insulin therapy	PWI	perfusion-weighted imaging
LDF	laser Doppler flowmetry	qEEG	quantitative electroencephalogram
LEMS	Lambert–Eaton myasthenic syndrome	QOL	quality of life
LLA	lower limit of autoregulation	RAA	renin–angiotensin–aldosterone
LMWH	low-molecular-weight heparin	ROS	reactive oxygen species
LOS	length of stay	ROSC	return of spontaneous return circulation
LV	left ventricular	RR	respiratory rate
MABP	mean arterial blood pressure	rtPA	recombinant tissue plasminogen activator
MAC	minimal alveolar concentration	RV	right ventricular
MAP	mean arterial pressure	RWMA	regional wall motion abnormality
MCS	minimally conscious state	SAH	subarachnoid haemorrhage
MD	microdialysis	SaO_2	arterial oxygen saturation
MDCT	multidetector-row computed tomography	SAPS	Severity of Illness And Physiology Score
MEP	maximal expiratory pressure	SBP	systolic blood pressure
MG	myasthenia gravis	SCI	spinal cord injury
MIP	maximal inspiratory pressure	SDH	subdural haematoma
MODS	Multiple Organ Dysfunction Score	SE	status epilepticus
MPM	Mortality Prediction Model	SG	specific gravity
MRA	magnetic resonance angiography	SIADH	syndrome of inappropriate antidiuretic hormone secretion
MRC	Medical Research Council		
MRI	magnetic resonance imaging	sICH	symptomatic intracerebral haemorrhage
MRP	magnetic resonance perfusion	$SjvO2$	jugular venous oxygen saturation
MTT	mean transit time	SOFA	Sequential Organ Failure Score
MUAP	motor unit action potential	SPECT	single-photon emission computed tomography
NCCT	non-contrast computed tomography	SpO_2	peripheral oxygen saturation
NCCU	neurocritical care unit	SSEP	somatosensory evoked potential
NCSE	non-convulsive status epilepticus	STEMI	ST-segment elevation myocardial infarction
NCSz	non-convulsive seizures	TAI	traumatic axonal injury
NDD	neurological determination of death	TBI	traumatic brain injury
NF-κB	nuclear factor kappa B	TCD	transcranial Doppler
NICU	neurointensive care unit	TDF	thermal diffusion flowmetry
NIHSS	National Institutes for Health Stroke Scale	TIA	transient ischaemic attack
NIRS	near-infrared spectroscopy	TNF	tumour necrosis factor

TOF	time-of-flight		VC	vital capacity
tPA	tissue plasminogen activator		VCAM	vascular cell adhesion protein
TRP	transient receptor potential		VEGF	vascular endothelial growth factor
UCNS	United Council of Neurological Subspecialties		VILI	ventilator-induced lung injury
UFH	unfractionated heparin		VTE	venous thromboembolism
UNOS	United Network for Organ Sharing		VZV	varicella zoster virus
UTI	urinary tract infection		WFNS	World Federation of Neurological Surgeons
UWS	unresponsive wakefulness syndrome		WLST	withdrawal of life-sustaining therapy
VAP	ventilator-associated pneumonia			

Contributors

Imoigele Aisiku Assistant Professor, Harvard Medical School, Brigham and Women's Hospital, Boston, MA, USA

Craig Anderson Professor of Stroke Medicine and Clinical Neuroscience, The George Institute for Global Health, University of Sydney, Australia, Head of Neurology, Royal Prince Alfred Hospital, Sydney, Australia

Jonathan Ball Consultant and Honorary Senior Lecturer in General and Neuro Intensive Care, St George's Hospital, London, UK

Ronny Beer Assistant Professor, Department of Neurology, Neuro-ICU, Medical University of Innsbruck, Innsbruck, Austria

Antonio Belli Professor of Trauma Neurosurgery, University of Birmingham, Queen Elizabeth Hospital and NIHR Surgical Reconstruction and Microbiology Research Centre, Birmingham, UK

Olivier Bodart Research Fellow in Neurology, Coma Science Group, University and University Hospital of Liège, Liège, Belgium

Nicolas Bruder Professor, Aix-Marseille Université, CHU Timone, Marseille, France

Iole Brunetti Department of Surgical Sciences and Integrated Diagnostics IRCCS AOU San Martino—IST, Genoa, Italy

Jayaram Chelluri Critical Care Fellow, University of Pittsburgh, Presbyterian Hospital, Pittsburgh, PA, USA

Lakshmi P. Chelluri Professor, University of Pittsburgh School of Medicine, Pittsburgh, PA, USA

Newton Cho Division of Neurosurgery and Spinal Program, Toronto Western Hospital, Toronto, Canada

Chandril Chugh Fellow in Endovascular Surgical Neuroradiology, Texas Stroke Institute, Plano, TX, USA

Jan Claassen Associate Professor of Neurology, Columbia University College of Physicians & Surgeons, New York, NY, USA

Giuseppe Citerio Professor in Anaesthesia and Critical Care, School of Medicine and Surgery, University of Milano-Bicocca, Italy
Director of Neurocritical Care and Neuroanaesthesia, Department of Anaesthesiology and Critical Care, San Gerardo Hospital, Monza, Italy

David W. Crippen Professor, University of Pittsburgh Medical Center, Pittsburgh, PA, USA

Barry M. Czeisler Assistant Professor of Neurology, Division of Neurocritical Care, New York University School of Medicine, New York, NY, USA

Neha S. Dangayach Assistant Professor, Mount Sinai Hospital, New York, NY, USA

Candice Delcourt Clinical Research Fellow, The George Institute for Global Health, University of Sydney, Royal Prince Alfred Hospital, Camperdown, Australia

Michael N. Diringer Professor of Neurology, Neurosurgery and Anaesthesiology, Washington University School of Medicine, St. Louis, MO, USA

Nazzareno Fagoni Consultant, Department of Anaesthesia, Critical Care and Emergency, Spedali Civili University Hospital, Brescia, Italy

Michael G. Fehlings Professor of Neurosurgery, University of Toronto, Toronto, Canada; Medical Director Krembil Neuroscience Center, Toronto Western Hospital, Toronto, Canada

Jennifer A. Frontera Associate Professor of Neurology, Cleveland Clinic Lerner College of Medicine and Case Western Reserve University, Cleveland, OH, USA

Olivia Gosseries Post-Doctoral Researcher, Coma Science Group, University and University Hospital of Liège, Liège, Belgium

Raimund Helbok Assistant Professor, Department of Neurology, Neuro-ICU, Medical University of Innsbruck, Innsbruck, Austria

J. Claude Hemphill III Professor of Neurology and Neurological Surgery, University of California, San Francisco, CA, USA

Hooman Kamel Assistant Professor of Neurology, Weill Cornell Medical College, New York, NY, USA

Matthew A. Kirkman Specialty Trainee in Neurosurgery and Honorary Fellow in Neurocritical Care, The National Hospital for Neurology and Neurosurgery, University College London Hospitals, London, UK

W. Andrew Kofke Professor and Director of Neuroscience in Anaesthesiology and Critical Care Program; Co-Director of Neurocritical Care, Department of Anaesthesiology and Critical Care, University of Pennsylvania, Philadelphia, USA
Professor in Department of Neurosurgery, University of Pennsylvania, Philadelphia, USA

Peter Komlosi Department of Radiology, Neuroradiology Division, University of Pittsburgh Medical Center, Pittsburgh, PA, USA

Nicola Latronico Director, University Division of Anesthesia and Critical Care Medicine and School of Speciality in Anesthesia and Critical Care Medicine, University of Brescia at Spedali Civili, Piazzale Ospedali Civili, Brescia, Italy

Steven Laureys Director, Coma Science Group, University and University Hospital of Liège, Liège, Belgium

Andrea Lavinio Director, Neurosciences and Trauma Critical Care Unit, Consultant, Department of Anaesthesia, Cambridge University Hospitals NHS Foundation Trust, Cambridge, UK

Stephan A. Mayer Director, Neurocritical Care, Mount Sinai Health System, Professor of Neurology and Neurosurgery, Icahn School of Medicine at Mount Sinai, New York, NY, USA

RajaNandini Muralidharan Division of Neurocritical Care, Department of Neurology, University of Pennsylvania, Philadelphia, PA, USA

Jerry P. Nolan Honorary Professor of Resuscitation Medicine, University of Bristol, UK, Consultant in Anaesthesia and Intensive Care Medicine, Royal United Hospital, Bath, UK

Jan Novy Consultant Neurologist, Centre Hospitalier Universitaire Vaudois, Lausanne, Switzerland

Mauro Oddo Staff Physician, Department of Intensive Care Medicine, Centre Hospitalier Universitaire Vaudois, Lausanne, Switzerland

Paolo Pelosi Dipartimento Scienze Chirurgiche e Diagnostiche Integrate (DISC), Università degli Studi di Genova, AOU IRCCS San Martino IST, Genova, Italy

Bettina Pfausler Assistant Professor, Department of Neurology, Neuro-ICU, Innsbruck Medical University, Innsbruck, Austria

Derek J. Roberts Surgery and Clinician Investigator Program Resident, Foothills Medical Centre, Alberta, Canada

Claudia Robertson Professor, Baylor College of Medicine, Houston, TX, USA

Andrea O. Rossetti Director of the Epilepsy Unit, Centre Hospitalier Universitaire Vaudois, Lausanne, Switzerland

Daniel Sahlein Assistant Professor of Clinical Radiology, Columbia University Medical Centre, New York, NY, USA

Erich Schmutzhard Professor of Neurology and Critical Care Medicine, Department of Neurology, Neuro-ICU, Medical University Innsbruck, Innsbruck, Austria

Sam Shemie Professor, Division of Critical Care, Montreal Children's Hospital, McGill University Health Centre, Montreal, Canada

Ivan Rocha Ferreira da Silva Director, Neurocritical Care Department, Americas Medical City, Rio de Janeiro, Brazil

Adikarige Haritha Dulanka Silva Specialist Registrar in Neurosurgery, Queen Elizabeth University Hospital, Birmingham, UK

Martin Smith Consultant and Honorary Professor in Neurocritical Care, The National Hospital for Neurology and Neurosurgery, University College London Hospitals, London, UK
National Institute for Health Research, University College London Hospitals, Biomedical Research Centre, London, UK

Luzius A. Steiner Professor and Chairman, Department of Anaesthesia, University Hospital Basel, Basel, Switzerland

Pouya Tahsili-Fahadan Neurocritical Care Section, Department of Neurology, Washington University in St. Louis, St. Louis, MO, USA

Jeanne Teitelbaum Associate Professor, Neurology, Neurosurgery and Critical Care, Montreal Neurological Institute, McGill University, Montreal, Canada

Aurore Thibaut Research Fellow, Coma Science Group, University and University Hospital of Liège, Liège, Belgium

Maria Vargas Dipartimento Scienze Chirurgiche e Diagnostiche Integrate (DISC), Università degli Studi di Genova, AOU IRCCS San Martino IST, Genova, Italy

Lionel Velly Associate Professor in Anaesthesiology, Centre Hospitalier Universitaire Timone, Marseille, France

Bala Venkatesh Professor of Intensive Care, University of Queensland, Brisbane, Australia

Federico Villa San Gerardo Hospital, Monza, Italy

Leslie M. Whetstine Associate Professor, Walsh University, North Canton, OH, USA

Hayden White Associate Professor and Director, Logan Hospital Meadowbrook, Australia

Jefferson R. Wilson Department of Surgery, University of Toronto, Toronto, Canada

Max Wintermark Department of Radiology, Neuroradiology Division, Stanford University, Stanford, CA, USA

Mingxing Xie Department of Ultrasound, Union Hospital, Tongji Medical College, Huazhong University of Science and Technology, Wuhan, China

Yanrong Zhang, Department of Ultrasound, Union Hospital, Tongji Medical College, Huazhong University of Science and Technology, Wuhan, China

David A. Zygun Division of Critical Care Medicine, University of Alberta and the University of Alberta Hospital, Alberta, Canada

PART 1

General principles

CHAPTER 1

Introduction to neurocritical care

Martin Smith

Critical care medicine has evolved rapidly in recent decades as therapeutic and technological advances have led to improved outcomes in a wide variety of life-threatening conditions. This is particularly the case in traumatic, haemorrhagic, and ischaemic brain injury where improved understanding of pathophysiology and advances in monitoring and imaging techniques have led to the introduction of more effective and individualized treatment strategies that have translated into improved outcomes for patients. In parallel, neurocritical care has developed as a subspecialty of intensive care medicine dedicated to the treatment of critically ill neurological patients (1).

History of neurocritical care

The origins of modern critical care lie in the poliomyelitis epidemics of the 1940s and 1950s when the principles of mechanical ventilation and high-intensity nursing in dedicated wards were established. During the 1970s and 1980s, developments in neuroanaesthesia and neurosurgical techniques allowed more complex operative interventions that required higher levels of care in the early postoperative period. Patients were managed in dedicated areas of neurosurgical wards where a team of skilled nursing staff provided close monitoring to detect neurological deterioration. In association with immediate access to neurosurgical support in the event of such deterioration, the earliest neurosurgical critical care units were established. In the United States, Allan Ropper (neurologist), Sean Kennedy (neuroanaesthetist), and Nicholas Zervas (neurosurgeon) developed the first combined neurological and neurosurgical intensive care unit (ICU) at the Massachusetts General Hospital in Boston, and their collaboration led to the publication of the first textbook of neurocritical care in 1983 (2).

Subsequently, neurocritical care has broadened to provide comprehensive management for all life-threatening disorders of the central nervous system (CNS) and their complications. Managing the complex interaction between the injured brain and systemic organ systems is the cornerstone of neurocritical care which has evolved from its original focus on the CNS into a speciality providing all aspects of a critically ill neurological patient's care.

Neurocritical care gained formal recognition by the United Council of Neurological Subspecialties (UCNS) in October 2005 and this led to the accreditation of neurocritical care training programmes and certification of neurointensivists in the United States (3). Although there is no similar recognition in Europe and many other countries, the UCNS neurocritical care curriculum is comprehensive and has broad relevance.

Principles of neurointensive care

Critically ill neurological patients require meticulous general intensive care support as well as interventions targeted to their neurological disorder. The management of acute brain injury (ABI) is particularly complex. In addition to brain-targeted therapy, general intensive care principles including optimization of cardiorespiratory variables, glycaemic control, management of pyrexia, and early enteral nutrition are of key importance (Table 1.1). Therapeutic targets in neurocritical care are often different from those on the general ICU. For example, cardiovascular management in the context of ABI is quite different from that after acute myocardial infarction. After ABI, therapeutic efforts are aimed towards providing the optimal conditions to minimize secondary brain injury and optimize neurological outcome. In some cases, brain-directed therapy can have potentially adverse effects on systemic organ systems and vice versa.

Management protocols have evolved with international consensus and provide guidelines that assist clinicians in delivering optimal care, although many do not focus on the critical care aspects of patient management (4–7). Recent developments have changed the way in which acute disorders of the CNS are treated. In particular, the critical care management of ABI has undergone extensive revision following evidence that longstanding and established practices are not as efficacious or innocuous as previously believed (8). Traditional therapies such as routine fluid restriction and hyperventilation are no longer recommended, and newer or 're-invented' therapies, such as targeted temperature management and decompressive craniectomy, remain controversial. The sole goal of identifying and treating intracranial hypertension has been superseded by a focus on the prevention of secondary brain insults using a systematic, stepwise approach to maintenance of adequate cerebral perfusion and oxygenation (9). Further, the substantial temporal and regional pathophysiological heterogeneity after ABI means that some interventions may be ineffective, unnecessary, or even harmful in certain patients at certain times, emphasizing the importance of monitor-guided individualized therapy.

Neuromonitoring

The monitoring of critically ill neurological patients has become increasingly complex. Along with the close monitoring and

4 PART 1 GENERAL PRINCIPLES

Table 1.1 Summary of neurocritical care management of patients with acute brain injury

Respiratory	◆ PaO_2 > 13 kPa and $PaCO_2$ 4.5–5.0 kPa
	◆ Positive end-expiratory pressure (≤15 cmH_2O) to maintain oxygenation
	◆ Protective ventilatory strategies with low tidal volume as $PaCO_2$ permits
	◆ Ventilator care bundle to minimize risk of pneumonia
Cardiovascular	◆ Mean arterial pressure > 90 mmHg
	◆ Euvolaemia
	◆ Vasopressors/inotropes
ICP and CPP management (for TBI)	◆ ICP < 20 mmHg and CPP 50–70 mmHg
	◆ Sedation/analgesia
	◆ 20–30° head-up tilt
	◆ Volume expansion plus norepinephrine (noradrenaline) to maintain CPP
Treatment of intracranial hypertension	◆ Cerebrospinal fluid drainage
	◆ Sedation
	◆ Osmotic therapy (mannitol or hypertonic saline)
	◆ CPP optimization
	◆ Moderate hyperventilation
	◆ Moderate hypothermia
	◆ Barbiturates
	◆ Decompressive craniectomy
Miscellaneous	◆ Normoglycaemia
	◆ Normothermia
	◆ Early enteral nutrition
	◆ Thromboembolic prophylaxis
	◆ Seizure control

assessment of cardiac and respiratory variables relevant to all critically ill patients, neurocritical care utilizes a range of neuromonitoring techniques to identify or predict secondary brain insults and guide therapeutic interventions (10,11).

Fundamental to neurological monitoring is the serial clinical assessment of neurological status by a trained nurse at the bedside. The Glasgow Coma Scale (GCS) provides a standardized, internationally recognized method for evaluating a patient's global neurological status by recording best eye opening, motor, and verbal responses to physical and verbal stimuli (see Chapter 26). In association with identification and documentation of localizing signs such as pupil responses and limb weaknesses, the GCS remains the mainstay of clinical assessment 50 years since its first description (12). Clinical assessment is limited in sedated patients or those with decreased conscious level and several techniques are available for global and regional brain monitoring which provide assessment of cerebral perfusion, oxygenation, and metabolic status, and early warning of impending brain hypoxia and ischaemia (13). These techniques are discussed in detail elsewhere in this book (see Chapters 9–12).

While intracranial pressure (ICP) and cerebral perfusion pressure (CPP) are crucially important and routinely monitored variables after ABI, they provide no assessment of the adequacy of cerebral perfusion and therefore of the risk of brain ischaemia (9). Multiple

studies have demonstrated that secondary brain ischaemic/hypoxic insults may go unnoticed when therapy is guided by ICP/CPP monitoring alone, and that brain hypoxia can occur despite ICP and CPP being within accepted thresholds for normality (14,15). Measurement of ICP and CPP in association with monitors of the *adequacy* of cerebral perfusion, such as brain tissue oxygenation and biochemistry, provide a more complete picture of the injured brain and its response to treatment (10,13). Therapeutic targets and choice of therapy are therefore best determined by monitoring more than one variable (multimodal monitoring). In current clinical practice this most commonly involves the simultaneous measurement of ICP/CPP and brain tissue oxygen tension, possibly in combination with other modalities such as cerebral blood flow and microdialysis.

Multimodal monitoring allows cross validation between different monitoring variables and guides individually tailored, patient-specific management. Apart from being used to guide treatment interventions, multimodal monitoring also gives clinicians confidence to withhold potentially dangerous therapy in those with no evidence of brain ischaemia/hypoxia or metabolic disturbance (13). Multimodal monitoring generates large and complex datasets, and systems that analyse and present information in a user-friendly format at the bedside are essential to maximize its clinical relevance (see Chapter 13) (16).

Case mix

As neurocritical care has evolved, so has its case mix broadened. Although traumatic brain injury (TBI), subarachnoid haemorrhage (SAH), and intracerebral haemorrhage (ICH) continue to make up a large proportion of cases, the admission of patients with other diagnoses, such as acute ischaemic stroke (AIS), neuromuscular disorders, status epilepticus, and CNS infection, is becoming increasingly common. Patients with severe ABI that would previously have been considered unsalvageable are now being admitted to the neurocritical care unit (NCCU) and there is evidence that early aggressive intervention can result in excellent outcomes in some patients (17).

Acute brain injury

The intensive care management of severe TBI requires a coordinated and comprehensive approach to treatment, including strategies to prevent secondary brain injury by avoidance of systemic physiological disturbances, such as hypotension, hypoxaemia, hypo- and hyperglycaemia, and hyperthermia, and maintenance of adequate cerebral perfusion and oxygenation. Management protocols have evolved with international consensus, providing evidence-based guidelines that assist clinicians in delivering optimal care (4). Improved diagnostic and monitoring modalities are improving the understanding of the pathophysiology of head injury and allowing the delivery of individualized therapy (9).

Less invasive interventions for securing a ruptured aneurysm have allowed treatment of more unstable patients and, as a result, greater numbers of poor-grade SAH patients are being admitted to the NCCU (18). Aggressive cardiopulmonary and neurological resuscitation, early aneurysm control, and advanced monitoring and management in a NCCU delivers good outcomes for such patients despite their substantial co-morbidities and high risk of intracranial and systemic complications (17,18). ICH is the most devastating form of stroke, with high rates of mortality and morbidity, but aggressive treatment, including meticulous blood pressure, fluid balance, and glycaemic control, and management of intracranial complications, is associated with improved outcome (19). Early studies confirmed that patients cared for by dedicated stroke teams in stroke units have better outcomes, and integrated multidisciplinary services for stroke patients are now commonplace (20). An increasing proportion of patients with severe AIS now require admission to an ICU for neurological monitoring and management of post-stroke complications (21).

Neurological disease

Neurocritical care is also concerned with the management of primary neurological illness and its consequences. Patients with myasthenia gravis, Guillain–Barré syndrome, encephalopathies, status epilepticus, and CNS infections require treatment of the underlying condition as well as management of ensuing complications such as ventilatory failure and autonomic disturbances (see Chapter 22). Many patients remain dependent on ventilatory support for considerable periods of time, resulting in substantial psychological problems for the patient and their carers.

Systemic complications

Brain injury and brain-directed therapies can lead to non-neurological organ system dysfunction and failure, and systemic organ system dysfunction and failure can also adversely affect the injured brain (22,23). Non-neurological organ dysfunction and failure are independent contributors to morbidity and mortality after ABI and therefore represent potentially modifiable risk factors (see Chapter 27). However, their management presents significant challenges because the optimum treatment for the failing systemic organ system may conflict with brain-directed therapies.

Benefits of neurocritical care units

There is accumulating evidence that treatment in a dedicated NCCU is beneficial for patients with neurological disease generally and for those with ABI in particular. In an early study, data collected prospectively by Project Impact, the national critical care data system of the Society of Critical Care Medicine, from 42 participating ICUs over a 3-year period demonstrated that not being in an NCCU was associated with an increased hospital mortality rate (odds ratio (OR) 3.4) after acute ICH (24). A recent systematic review and meta-analysis including 18 studies and more than 40,000 patients confirmed that the management of critically ill patients with ABI in an NCCU is associated with a lower risk of mortality (OR 0.72) and poor neurological outcome (OR 0.7) when compared to management in a general ICU (25). The potential benefits of neurocritical care are likely to be multifactorial (Box 1.1) (26,27).

Damian and colleagues used the UK Intensive Care National Audit and Research Centre database to assess mortality in critically ill neurological patients (including more than 10,300 patients with primary ICH) over time and to determine whether the type of ICU in which the patients were treated affected mortality (28). There was a statistically significant decrease in ICH-related mortality between 1996 and 2009, and hospital mortality was lower in patients treated in an NCCU compared to a general ICU even after adjusting for multiple confounders including surgery. There was a greater reduction in mortality over time in patients treated in an NCCU, but a longer ICU and hospital length of stay. A population-based study

---

Box 1.1 Aspects of neurocritical care that contribute to improved outcome

- Delivery of individualized, protocol-guided care
- Multimodal monitoring-guided treatment strategies
- Dedicated, specialist multidisciplinary team including specialist neuroscience critical care nurses and therapists
- Supervision of management by dedicated neurointensivists
- Rapid access to neurosurgical services
- Increased expertise from higher caseload
- Awareness of the interplay between the injured brain and systemic organ systems:
  - improved control of systemic physiology
  - greater understanding of the causes and treatment of non-neurologic organ system dysfunction and failure.

---

of more than 4000 patients admitted to four Canadian ICUs over an 11-year period also demonstrated that mortality decreased and outcome in survivors improved over time, and in this study these effects were most pronounced in patients with TBI and SAH (29). Multiple practice modifications, including the introduction of neurointensivists, implementation of a TBI management protocol, and improved management of systemic physiological variables, are likely to have contributed to the improved outcomes identified in this study. However, temporal improvements in outcome can also occur in the absence of a defined change in the model of care. In a study of patients with ICH, mortality was 19% in those admitted to hospital between 2005 and 2009 compared to 62% in those admitted between 1990 to 1994 despite similar baseline characteristics and management in a specialist NCCU in both periods (30).

Despite multiple studies examining its impact there is no agreement on what exactly constitutes neurocritical care, and different models of care delivery predominate in different countries. In some, neurocritical care is delivered by neurointensivists in a specialist unit admitting only critically ill neurological patients. This is the most common model in the United States and increasingly in Europe. Neurocritical care can also be provided by neurointensivists in dedicated areas of a mixed ICU, whereas in other centres critically ill neurological patients are managed in a mixed ICU without specialty-specific arrangements. In addition to different care delivery locations, the availability of full-time neurointensivists and protocol-driven care also varies between centres. Thus when examining the evidence of benefits from neurocritical care, it is important that the context of care delivery and who provides it is understood. It is also uncertain whether the potential outcome benefits of neurocritical care apply to all neurological diseases equally, or primarily to ABI (25).

Caseload

Specialization attracts a greater caseload and with it increased expertise. Higher caseloads have been associated with improved outcome after TBI (31), SAH (32), ICH (24), and AIS (33). In an Austrian study of 1856 patients with severe TBI, those admitted to large centres treating more than 30 cases per year had lower mortality compared to those admitted to medium (10–30 cases/year) and small (< 10 cases/year) centres (31). Multiple studies have confirmed that mortality after SAH is also significantly reduced in high-volume centres that provide access to specialized multidisciplinary neurocritical care, and the Neurocritical Care Society has recently recommended that all patients should be managed in centres treating more than 60 cases per year (34).

The neurocritical care team

The benefits of a multidisciplinary critical care team and the presence of a full-time intensivist are well established in general intensive care (35), and similar findings have recently been confirmed in neurocritical care. In one study, the presence of a full-time neurointensivist was associated with a 51% reduction in NCCU mortality, a 12% shorter length of stay in hospital, and 57% greater odds of being discharged to home or a rehabilitation unit compared to a long-term care facility (36). More recently, the introduction of a multidisciplinary neurocritical care team has been shown to be associated with decreased ICU and hospital lengths of stay and a greater proportion of patients with haemorrhagic and ischaemic stroke being discharged home (37).

The presence of a neurocritical care team has been shown to be an independent predictor of decreased hospital mortality (OR 0.7) and is associated with reduced NCCU and hospital lengths of stay without increasing ICU readmission rates (38). The 24/7 provision of experienced neurocritical care staff ensures that the application of individualized therapies aimed at preventing secondary brain injury by optimization of intracranial and systemic physiological variables are applied in a timely and consistent fashion (39). Neurocritical care teams are familiar with the unique aspects of CNS disease processes and the effects of interventions on the injured brain, and integrate all aspects of neurological and medical management into a single care plan (1). Systemic physiological derangements have specific consequences in the context of ABI and require different management strategies than in the general ICU setting (40). Neurocritical care teams have the experience to identify and appropriately manage such derangements and are mindful of the complex interactions between the injured brain and systemic physiological disturbances (26).

Neurocritical care nurses require excellent general ICU skills and in addition must be proficient at neurological examination to a greater degree of sophistication and precision than their general ICU counterparts (39). Not only is the neurocritical care nurse the most important bedside neurological monitor, he/she is also in a unique position to make sure that local management protocols are delivered. Acute rehabilitation plays a major role in securing improved long-term neurological outcomes after ABI, and intervention from neurophysiotherapists, including early patient mobilization, is likely to occur more reliably in a specialist than a general unit (41).

Management protocols

Most neurocritical care treatments are directed by consensus guidance rather than a clear evidence base (42). Very few specific interventions have been shown to improve outcome in large randomized controlled trials and, with the possible exception of avoidance of hypotension and hypoxaemia (43), most are based on observational studies or analysis of physiology and pathophysiology. There is a focus on preventing or rapidly correcting even minor abnormalities in physiological variables such as arterial blood pressure, arterial blood gases, blood glucose, sodium, and temperature. Given the complex pathophysiology of ABI it is unlikely that any one of these interventions in isolation will affect outcome, but their combination into a management protocol designed to avoid secondary brain injury can have a powerful effect (44,45). Compliance with standard protocols has been shown to be associated with improved outcome (46). A recent study demonstrated that increased adherence to Brain Trauma Foundation guidelines for ICP and CPP management was associated with a pronounced reduction in severe TBI mortality, suggesting a causal relationship (47).

Length of stay and cost-effectiveness

Although some early single-centre studies suggested that management in an NCCU was associated with a shorter length of stay and lower resource usage compared to a general ICU (48), most data indicate the contrary (24,28,49). In a population-based study, ICU length of stay increased as outcome improved over time (29). This might be related to more aggressive and longer duration therapy, or be the result of delayed decisions about withdrawal of life-sustaining interventions arising from an increased appreciation of satisfactory outcome after initially severe ABI. In a recent UK study, management of patients with severe TBI in an NCCU was associated with a higher 6-month cost but higher quality of life and lower long-term health and social care costs compared to management in a general ICU, suggesting that management in an NCCU may be cost-effective (50).

Therapeutic nihilism

Patients with severe brain injury that would previously have been considered unsalvageable are increasingly being offered treatment, with excellent results in many cases (17). Other patients will have a poor outcome despite maximal intervention and it is essential that aggressive early treatment is linked to compassionate end-of-life care if a satisfactory degree of clinical improvement does not occur within an appropriate timescale (51). The confidence to withdraw treatment after a failed trial of early maximal intervention means that the usual justification for withholding treatment in the acute phase (survival with a devastating neurological injury) becomes irrelevant. In this way, patients have access to care that might allow them to recover beyond initial expectations.

Therapeutic nihilism is a major factor adversely affecting outcome after ABI. Too early an assessment of poor prognosis and subsequent withdrawal of care or do-not-resuscitate orders leads to a self-fulfilling prophecy (52). Tools to predict long-term prognosis in severe ABI are imperfect (53), but those who work regularly with critically ill brain-injured patients develop a deeper understanding of the factors that influence recovery, including the effects of brain plasticity and neurological rehabilitation, and apply more robust assessments of outcome as well as more realistic time frames for recovery (54).

Research

There are limited data to guide the majority of interventions during neurocritical care and management guidelines are often developed based on expert consensus (42). Numerous drugs with promising neuroprotective effects in preclinical studies have failed to translate into outcome benefits for patients in large clinical studies, and the effectiveness of many treatment algorithms and physiological interventions that are routinely applied during neurocritical care has not been evaluated in large studies. While there might be reluctance to subject long-standing clinical practices to rigorous investigation, there is an urgent need for well-conducted studies to determine optimal strategies for many neurocritical care interventions. Patient registry or large observational cohorts are important in disease surveillance or to understand the pathophysiology of specific disease states, while adequately designed and well-conducted phase I and II studies are required to assess the safety profile and efficacy of established and novel pharmaceuticals so that only agents with a reasonable chance of success enter phase III. The establishment of the Neurocritical Care Research Network, under the auspices of the Neurocritical Care Society, will facilitate multicentre, international collaboration and patient enrolment into neurocritical care clinical trials (55). In this way it is anticipated that future research will determine which of the many interventions that are currently provided on an empirical basis are of particular benefit and which might possibly be causing harm.

References

1. Rincon F, Mayer SA. Neurocritical care: a distinct discipline? *Curr Opin Crit Care.* 2007;13:115–21.
2. Bleck TP. Historical aspects of critical care and the nervous system. *Crit Care Clin.* 2009;25:153–64.
3. Mayer SA, Coplin WM, Chang C, Suarez J, Gress D, Diringer MN, *et al.* Core curriculum and competencies for advanced training in neurological intensive care: United Council for Neurologic Subspecialties guidelines. *Neurocrit Care.* 2006;5:159–65.
4. The Brain Trauma Foundation. The American Association of Neurological Surgeons. The Joint Section on Neurotrauma and Critical Care. *J Neurotrauma.* 2007;24:S1–S106.
5. Diringer MN, Bleck TP, Claude HJ, III, Menon D, Shutter L, Vespa P, *et al.* Critical care management of patients following aneurysmal subarachnoid hemorrhage: recommendations from the Neurocritical Care Society's Multidisciplinary Consensus Conference. *Neurocrit Care.* 2011;15:211–40.
6. Jauch EC, Saver JL, Adams HP, Jr, Bruno A, Connors JJ, Demaerschalk BM, *et al.* Guidelines for the early management of patients with acute ischemic stroke: a guideline for healthcare professionals from the American Heart Association/American Stroke Association. *Stroke.* 2013;44:870–947.
7. Morgenstern LB, Hemphill JC, III, Anderson C, Becker K, Broderick JP, Connolly ES Jr, *et al.* Guidelines for the management of spontaneous intracerebral hemorrhage: a guideline for healthcare professionals from the American Heart Association/American Stroke Association. *Stroke.* 2010;41:2108–29.
8. Roberts I, Schierhout G, Alderson P. Absence of evidence for the effectiveness of five interventions routinely used in the intensive care management of severe head injury: a systematic review. *J Neurol Neurosurg Psychiatry.* 1998;65:729–33.
9. Kirkman MA, Smith M. Intracranial pressure monitoring, cerebral perfusion pressure estimation, and ICP/CPP-guided therapy: a standard of care or optional extra after brain injury? *Br J Anaesth.* 2014;112:35–46.
10. Oddo M, Villa F, Citerio G. Brain multimodality monitoring: an update. *Curr Opin Crit Care.* 2012;18:111–18.
11. Tisdall MM, Smith M. Multimodal monitoring in traumatic brain injury: current status and future directions. *Br J Anaesth.* 2007;99:61–7.
12. Barlow P. A practical review of the Glasgow Coma Scale and Score. *Surgeon.* 2012;10:114–19.
13. Kirkman MA, Smith M. Multimodal intracranial monitoring: implications for clinical practice. *Anesthesiol Clin.* 2012;30:269–87.
14. Chang JJ, Youn TS, Benson D, Mattick H, Andrade N, Harper CR, *et al.* Physiologic and functional outcome correlates of brain tissue hypoxia in traumatic brain injury. *Crit Care Med.* 2009;37:283–90.
15. Oddo M, Levine JM, Mackenzie L, Frangos S, Feihl F, Kasner SE, *et al.* Brain hypoxia is associated with short-term outcome after severe traumatic brain injury independently of intracranial hypertension and low cerebral perfusion pressure. *Neurosurgery.* 2011;69:1037–45.
16. Hemphill JC, Andrews P, De Georgia M. Multimodal monitoring and neurocritical care bioinformatics. *Nat Rev Neurol.* 2011;7:451–60.
17. Komotar RJ, Schmidt JM, Starke RM, Claassen J, Wartenberg KE, Lee K, *et al.* Resuscitation and critical care of poor-grade subarachnoid hemorrhage. *Neurosurgery.* 2009;64:397–410.
18. Lerch C, Yonekawa Y, Muroi C, Bjeljac M, Keller E. Specialized neurocritical care, severity grade, and outcome of patients with aneurysmal subarachnoid hemorrhage. *Neurocrit Care.* 2006;5:85–92.
19. Flower O, Smith M. The acute management of intracerebral hemorrhage. *Curr Opin Crit Care.* 2011;17:106–14.
20. Stroke Unit Trialists' Collaboration. Organised inpatient (stroke unit) care for stroke. *Cochrane Database Syst Rev.* 2013;9:CD000197.
21. Kirkman MA, Citerio G, Smith M. The intensive care management of acute ischemic stroke: an overview. *Intensive Care Med.* 2014;40:640–53.
22. Wartenberg KE, Mayer SA. Medical complications after subarachnoid hemorrhage. *Neurosurg Clin N Am.* 2010;21:325–38.
23. Zygun DA, Kortbeek JB, Fick GH, Laupland KB, Doig CJ. Non-neurologic organ dysfunction in severe traumatic brain injury. *Crit Care Med.* 2005;33:654–60.
24. Diringer MN, Edwards DF. Admission to a neurologic/neurosurgical intensive care unit is associated with reduced mortality rate after intracerebral hemorrhage. *Crit Care Med.* 2001;29:635–40.
25. Kramer AH, Zygun DA. Neurocritical care: why does it make a difference? *Curr Opin Crit Care.* 2014;20:174–81.
26. Suarez JI. Outcome in neurocritical care: advances in monitoring and treatment and effect of a specialized neurocritical care team. *Crit Care Med.* 2006;34:S232–S238.
27. Teig M, Smith M. Where should patients with severe traumatic brain injury be managed? All patients should be managed in a neurocritical care unit. *J Neurosurg Anesthesiol.* 2010;22:357–9.
28. Damian MS, Ben-Shlomo Y, Howard R, Bellotti T, Harrison D, Griggs K, *et al.* The effect of secular trends and specialist neurocritical care on mortality for patients with intracerebral haemorrhage, myasthenia gravis and Guillain–Barré syndrome admitted to critical care: an analysis of the Intensive Care National Audit & Research Centre (ICNARC) national United Kingdom database. *Intensive Care Med.* 2013;39:1405–12.
29. Kramer AH, Zygun DA. Declining mortality in neurocritical care patients: a cohort study in Southern Alberta over eleven years. *Can J Anaesth.* 2013;60:966–75.
30. Tsitsopoulos PP, Enblad P, Wanhainen A, Tobieson L, Hårdemark HG, Marklund N. Improved outcome of patients with severe thalamic hemorrhage treated with cerebrospinal fluid drainage and neurocritical care during 1990–1994 and 2005–2009. *Acta Neurochir (Wien).* 2013;155:2105–13.
31. Mauritz W, Steltzer H, Bauer P, Dolanski-Aghamanoukjan L, Metnitz P. Monitoring of intracranial pressure in patients with severe traumatic brain injury: an Austrian prospective multicenter study. *Intensive Care Med.* 2008;34:1208–15.
32. Cross DT, III, Tirschwell DL, Clark MA, Tuden D, Derdeyn CP, Moran CJ, *et al.* Mortality rates after subarachnoid hemorrhage: variations according to hospital case volume in 18 states. *J Neurosurg.* 2003;99:810–17.
33. Saposnik G, Baibergenova A, O'Donnell M, Hill MD, Kapral MK, Hachinski V, *et al.* Hospital volume and stroke outcome: does it matter? *Neurology.* 2007;69:1142–51.
34. Vespa P, Diringer MN. High-volume centers. *Neurocrit Care.* 2011;15:369–72.
35. Pronovost PJ, Angus DC, Dorman T, Robinson KA, Dremsizov TT, Young TL. Physician staffing patterns and clinical outcomes in critically ill patients: a systematic review. *JAMA.* 2002;288:2151–62.

36. Varelas PN, Eastwood D, Yun HJ, Spanaki MV, Hacein Bey L, Kessaris C, *et al.* Impact of a neurointensivist on outcomes in patients with head trauma treated in a neurosciences intensive care unit. *J Neurosurg.* 2006;104:713–19.

37. Varelas PN, Schultz L, Conti M, Spanaki M, Genarrelli T, Hacein-Bey L. The impact of a neuro-intensivist on patients with stroke admitted to a neurosciences intensive care unit. *Neurocrit Care.* 2008;9:293–9.

38. Suarez JI, Zaidat OO, Suri MF, Feen ES, Lynch G, Hickman J, *et al.* Length of stay and mortality in neurocritically ill patients: impact of a specialized neurocritical care team. *Crit Care Med.* 2004;32:2311–17.

39. Bleck TP. The impact of specialized neurocritical care. *J Neurosurg.* 2006;104:709–10.

40. Wartenberg KE, Mayer SA. Medical complications after subarachnoid hemorrhage: new strategies for prevention and management. *Curr Opin Crit Care.* 2006;12:78–84.

41. Smith M. Neurocritical care: has it come of age? *Br J Anaesth.* 2004;93:753–5.

42. English SW, Turgeon AF, Owen E, Doucette S, Pagliarello G, McIntyre L. Protocol management of severe traumatic brain injury in intensive care units: a systematic review. *Neurocrit Care.* 2013;18:131–42.

43. McHugh GS, Engel DC, Butcher I, Steyerberg EW, Lu J, Mushkudiani N, *et al.* Prognostic value of secondary insults in traumatic brain injury: results from the IMPACT study. *J Neurotrauma.* 2007;24:287–93.

44. Elf K, Nilsson P, Enblad P. Outcome after traumatic brain injury improved by an organized secondary insult program and standardized neurointensive care. *Crit Care Med.* 2002;30:2129–34.

45. Patel HC, Menon DK, Tebbs S, Hawker R, Hutchinson PJ, Kirkpatrick PJ. Specialist neurocritical care and outcome from head injury. *Intensive Care Med.* 2002;28:547–53.

46. Talving P, Karamanos E, Teixeira PG, Skiada D, Lam L, Belzberg H, *et al.* Intracranial pressure monitoring in severe head injury: compliance with Brain Trauma Foundation guidelines and effect on outcomes: a prospective study. *J Neurosurg.* 2013;119:1248–54.

47. Gerber LM, Chiu YL, Carney N, Hartl R, Ghajar J. Marked reduction in mortality in patients with severe traumatic brain injury. *J Neurosurg.* 2013;119:1583–90.

48. Mirski MA, Chang CW, Cowan R. Impact of a neuroscience intensive care unit on neurosurgical patient outcomes and cost of care: evidence-based support for an intensivist-directed specialty ICU model of care. *J Neurosurg Anesthesiol.* 2001;13:83–92.

49. Kurtz P, Fitts V, Sumer Z, Jalon H, Cooke J, Kvetan V, *et al.* How does care differ for neurological patients admitted to a neurocritical care unit versus a general ICU? *Neurocrit Care.* 2011;15:477–80.

50. Harrison DA, Prabhu G, Grieve R, Harvey SE, Sadique MZ, Gomes M, *et al.* Risk Adjustment In Neurocritical care (RAIN)—prospective validation of risk prediction models for adult patients with acute traumatic brain injury to use to evaluate the optimum location and comparative costs of neurocritical care: a cohort study. *Health Technol Assess.* 2013;17:vii–viii, 1–350.

51. Smith M. Treatment withdrawal and acute brain injury: an integral part of care. *Anaesthesia.* 2012;67:941–5.

52. Becker KJ, Baxter AB, Cohen WA, Bybee HM, Tirschwell DL, Newell DW, *et al.* Withdrawal of support in intracerebral hemorrhage may lead to self-fulfilling prophecies. *Neurology.* 2001;56:766–72.

53. Stevens RD, Sutter R. Prognosis in severe brain injury. *Crit Care Med.* 2013;41:1104–23.

54. Mayer SA, Kossoff SB. Withdrawal of life support in the neurological intensive care unit. *Neurology.* 1999;52:1602–9.

55. Suarez JI, Geocadin R, Hall C, Le Roux PD, Smirnakis S, Wijman CA, *et al.* The neurocritical care research network: NCRN. *Neurocrit Care.* 2012;16:29–34.

CHAPTER 2

Applied neuropathophysiology and neuropharmacology

RajaNandini Muralidharan and W. Andrew Kofke

Neural function is essential to human existence and the loss of any neural element represents a major loss to the individual. Thus the primary aim of the management of critically ill neurological patients is the preservation of neural function. The brain is the most vulnerable organ in the human body for several reasons. It is has a high energy requirement but very limited ability to store substrate so is dependent on a continued blood supply to deliver oxygen and essential nutrients to support aerobic metabolism. It is also unable to expand physically because of its containment in the rigid skull and therefore has limited ability to compensate for insults such as haemorrhage, oedema, and inflammation.

In brain injury, neurons or their supporting elements may be lost in a small, virtually unnoticeable manner or there may be widespread neuronal loss and tissue infarction. Based on the notion that maintenance of some level of neural function is the essence of acceptable survival, it is crucial to consider neural viability and the impact and interactions of primary disease processes and therapeutic interventions on the central nervous system (CNS) during the critical care management of brain injury. Mature neurons cannot proliferate except possibly in a few brain areas or under special circumstances (1), but they can undergo adaptive change in response to injury. However, beyond a certain threshold adaptive mechanisms fail and subsequent neuronal loss translates into loss of function for the individual. In a general sense, brain injury involves one or more of ischaemia, trauma, neuroinflammation, and neuroexcitation, all of which have distinct yet interrelated pathways that ultimately result in neuronal death if unchecked.

Neurophysiology

This section will review the important overarching concepts of neurophysiology and pathophysiology relevant to neurocritical care and the reader is referred elsewhere in this book for detailed discussions of pathology-specific issues.

Cells of the central nervous system

Despite the nervous system's wide distribution and complexity, it contains only two principal categories of cells—neurons and glia. There are an estimated 100 billion neurons and ten times as many glial cells in the nervous system (2), although the actual number and distribution is uncertain (3). Neurons are the most important structural and functional cells of the nervous system and sustain moment-to-moment neurological function by the transmission of electrical and chemical information.

Once thought to be detrimental to neuronal recovery after injury, glial cells such as astrocytes provide metabolic and reparative support to neurons. Glia are spatially arranged throughout the brain and in contact with tens of thousands of synapses and each other via a network of gap junctions known as the astrocytic syncytium. This allows the rapid diffusion of molecules, particularly calcium, in response to glutaminergic synaptic transmission and facilitates local and long-distance synaptic modulation of the composition and concentration of multiple molecules in the extracellular milieu via uptake or release of multiple neurotransmitters, ions, and neuromodulators. These connections also allow intimate coupling with neuronal metabolism and, via astrocytic foot process, with neurovascular coupling (4). Under a myriad of pathological conditions, including hypoxia, ischaemia, and excitotoxicity, astrocytes are able to interact and modulate their environments in concert with neurons. Understanding the role of astrocytes in response to brain injury is crucial as they may serve as viable future targets for manipulation and treatment.

Other cell types in the CNS include microglia. These are derived from mesoderm and enter the CNS via white matter tracts and blood vessels early during development. Microglia are in a 'resting' state in the mature brain until a pathological event triggers microglial activation when they transform into amoeboid phagocytic cells that rapidly proliferate and migrate in response to injury (5).

Cerebrospinal fluid

Cerebrospinal fluid (CSF) is produced in the choroid plexus at a rate of 0.2–0.4 mL/min or 500–600 mL a day (6). It circulates through the ventricular system into the subarachnoid space and is absorbed into the venous system via arachnoid granulations that line the convexity of the brain. Equilibrium normally exists between CSF production and absorption, and disruption of this can lead to hydrocephalus and raised intracranial pressure (ICP). Hydrocephalus is generally categorized as communicating or non-communicating. In communicating hydrocephalus, CSF circulation between the site of production and absorption is intact but abnormally decreased absorption (e.g. secondary to inflammation or infection) or increased production (e.g. choroid plexus papilloma) results in CSF accumulation. In non-communicating hydrocephalus, CSF pathways are blocked such that CSF cannot circulate to the convexity of the brain to be absorbed.

CSF circulation has many roles. It transports hormones, cofactors, and chemical messengers which aide various processes including neuronal metabolism and behaviour (6). It has a mechanically supportive role as a hydraulic cushion for the brain and spinal cord within their rigid enclosures and also can act as a compensatory mechanism as its volume decreases to maintain ICP in the presence of space occupying lesions (see Chapter 7). CSF absorption is driven by the hydrostatic differences in the CSF and venous compartments and is directly proportional to ICP. Hence increases in ICP lead to increased rate of CSF clearance (7) and CSF diversion plays a vital role in ameliorating increased ICP.

The choroid plexus is the primary site of CSF production and comprises a capillary network that lacks tight junctions intertwined with ependymal cells. CSF was previously thought to be an ultrafiltrate of blood but its ionic composition differs from that of plasma. It has higher chloride and magnesium concentrations and a slightly lower pH due to lack of buffering capacity because of its low protein content compared to plasma (6). CSF production is an energy-dependent process utilizing adenosine triphosphate (ATP) and various transporters including sodium-potassium and other ATPase membrane pumps. The production of hydrogen (H^+) and bicarbonate (HCO_3^-) ions required for these processes depends on the activity of the enzyme carbonic anhydrase which catalyses the formation of carbonic acid from water and CO_2, a process that is inhibited by acetazolamide (6).

CSF pH is tightly coupled to minute-to-minute control of breathing. Central chemoreceptors located in the ventral medulla are extremely sensitive and respond directly to changes in CSF pH and indirectly to $PaCO_2$. For example, a rise in $PaCO_2$ leads to a rapid increase in CSF H^+ concentration. Carbon dioxide is carried in the blood as H^+ and HCO_3^- but readily converts into CO_2 in the brain when it can cross the blood–brain barrier (BBB) into the CSF and be converted back to H^+ and HCO_3^-. The cerebral vasodilatation that accompanies increased $PaCO_2$ further enhances this diffusion. Liberated H^+ acts on central chemoreceptors to stimulate respiration, which in turn reduces both arterial and CSF CO_2 (6).

Another, newer concept, of CSF dynamics is the so-called glymphatics system. Ilkiff et al. described this intricate network of paravascular pathways by which CSF and solutes can pass and eventually be cleared along paravenous routes (8). Aquaporin-dependent astrocytic water transport appears to be involved in this mechanism. Moreover, beta-amyloid and possibly other 'waste product' substances may be cleared from the brain by the glymphatic system, with a notable link of these processes to sleep (9).

Blood–brain barrier

The BBB has several roles including:

- promoting entry of nutrients into the brain and egress of waste products, and preventing entry of harmful molecules

- maintenance of an optimal milieu for neuron function by control of brain ionic homeostasis

- protecting the brain from fluctuations in systemic ionic composition which may inappropriately alter neuronal function

- separating neuroactive substances between central and peripheral compartments, allowing the same molecule to be used between compartments without crosstalk (4).

The BBB is formed by endothelial cells joined by tight junctions, pericytes, basal lamina, and astrocytic foot processes (Figure 2.1) which together form the functional 'neurovascular unit' that maintains the chemical composition of cerebral extracellular fluid (ECF) relatively independent of changes in the blood (4). The astrocytic foot processes serve as conduits for water, nutrients, and ions between the ECF and capillaries, whereas tight junctions prevent movement of hydrophilic compounds and proteins (4). The BBB contains several channels and luminal and abluminal transport systems which move ions, glucose, proteins, vitamins, and drugs. The barrier is maintained by active transport using receptor-based and less specific adaptive transcytosis (4), and facilitated diffusion along ion gradients created by energy-dependent sodium-potassium pumps. It is thus unsurprising that virtually any insult to the brain, be it trauma, ischaemia, or seizures, leads to breakdown of the BBB with resultant brain oedema, oxidative stress, toxin accumulation, and neuroinflammation. The permeability of the BBB may also be increased by vasoactive substances such as histamine and thrombin through increased expression of cell adhesive molecules via cytokines released in response to inflammation and growth factors, such as vascular endothelial growth factor (VEGF), in tumourigenesis (10,11). The importance of BBB function cannot be over-emphasized as it carries a myriad of clinical implications and offers potential targets in neuronal repair. The major elements and functions of the BBB are summarized in Table 2.1.

Cerebral energy metabolism

Although the brain comprises approximately 2% of body weight it utilizes 20% of total energy consumption and receives 15% of total cardiac output (12). This reflects its critical dependence on a constant supply of glucose (and/or lactate from astrocytes) and oxygen to maintain metabolic function. The primary source of the brain's energy is ATP via oxidative metabolism in the Krebs cycle and mitochondrial respiratory chain, and the vast majority of its energy requirement is to support the sodium-potassium ATPase pumps which maintain and restore ionic gradients and membrane potentials during excitatory neural transmission (12,13). ATP-dependent pumps also facilitate uptake of glutamate from the synaptic cleft and thus prevent inappropriate activation of excitatory postsynaptic receptors that would lead to massive calcium influx into cells and trigger cell death cascades (14).

An increase in neuronal metabolic demand is first met with an increase in local tissue oxygen extraction followed by an increase in cerebral blood flow (CBF) (5). Astrocytes are key players in regulating blood flow to neurons via their foot processes that line cerebral arterioles and capillaries. Metabolism-related changes in CBF arise from local vasodilatory mediators such as nitric oxide (NO), arachidonic acid, potassium, and adenosine which are believed to be released from neurons and glia following excitatory glutaminergic transmission during synaptic activity rather than as a direct effect of the energy deficit (5). This reinforces the important concept that although energy utilization and local CBF operate in parallel they are not causally related. This is relevant in functional magnetic resonance imaging where blood oxygen level-dependent (BOLD) signals should be interpreted as a reflection of neuronal signalling and not necessarily as a locus of increased energy utilization (15).

Glycogen can also support brain metabolism in conditions of low glucose supply or energy failure. Astrocytes play a key role in this process and therefore in neuronal metabolism and coupling of CBF to energy demand. As noted, neuronal activity releases chemical factors such as potassium, glutamate, and glucose that reach astrocytes through the ECF and trigger changes in astrocytic function

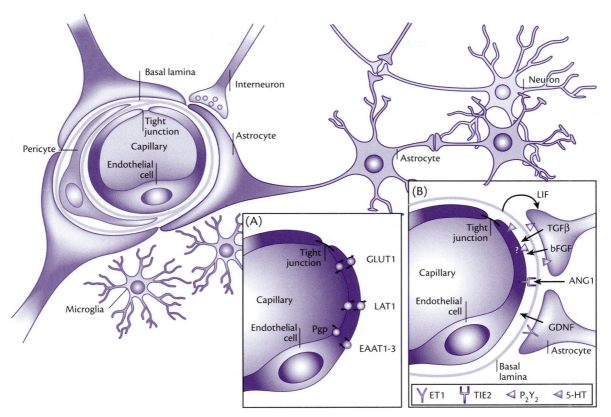

Fig. 2.1 The blood–brain barrier. The blood–brain barrier is formed by capillary endothelial cells, surrounded by basal lamina and astrocytic perivascular endfeet. Astrocytes provide the cellular link to the neurons. The figure also shows pericytes and microglial cells.

(A) Brain endothelial cell features observed in cell culture. The cells express a number of transporters and receptors, some of which are shown.

EAAT1–3, excitatory amino acid transporters 1–3; GLUT1, glucose transporter 1; LAT1, L-system for large neutral amino acids; Pgp, P-glycoprotein.

(B) Examples of bidirectional astroglial–endothelial induction necessary to establish and maintain the BBB. Some endothelial cell characteristics (receptors and transporters) are shown.

5-HT, 5-hydroxytryptamine (serotonin); ANG1, angiopoietin 1; bFGF, basic fibroblast growth factor; ET1, endothelin 1; GDNF, glial cell line-derived neurotrophic factor; LIF, leukaemia inhibitory factor; P_2Y_2, purinergic receptor; TGFβ, transforming growth factor-β; TIE2, endothelium-specific receptor tyrosine kinase 2. Data obtained from astroglial–endothelial co-cultures and the use of conditioned medium.

Reprinted by permission from Macmillan Publishers Ltd: *Nature Reviews Neuroscience*, 7, 1, Abbott NJ *et al.*, 'Astrocyte–endothelial interactions at the blood–brain barrier', pp. 41–53, copyright 2006.

Table 2.1 Elements of the blood–brain barrier

BBB element	Definition
Tight junction	A belt-like region of adhesion between adjacent cells. Tight junctions regulate paracellular flux, and contribute to the maintenance of cell polarity by stopping molecules from diffusing within the plane of the membrane
Abluminal membrane	The endothelial cell membrane that faces away from the vessel lumen, towards the brain
Meninges	The complex arrangement of three protective membranes surrounding the brain, with a thick outer connective tissue layer (dura) overlying the barrier layer (arachnoid), and finally the thin layer covering the glia limitans (pia). The subarachnoid layer has a sponge-like structure filled with CSF
Circumventricular organs (CVOs)	Brain regions that have a rich vascular plexus with a specialized arrangement of blood vessels. The junctions between the capillary endothelial cells are not tight in the blood vessels of these regions, which allow the diffusion of large molecules. These organs include the organum vasculosum of the lamina terminalis, the subfornical organ, the median eminence, and the area postrema
Receptor-mediated transcytosis	The mechanism for vesicle mediated transfer of substances across the cell, the first step of which requires specific binding of the ligand to a membrane receptor, followed by internalization (endocytosis)
Adsorptive-mediated transcytosis	The mechanism for vesicle-mediated transfer of substances across the cell, the first step of which involves non-specific binding of the ligand to membrane surface charges, followed by internalization (endocytosis)

Adapted by permission from Macmillan Publishers Ltd: *Nature Reviews Neuroscience*, 7, 1, Abbott NJ *et al.*, 'Astrocyte–endothelial interactions at the blood–brain barrier', pp. 41–53, copyright 2006.

including activation of glucose metabolism. Glycogen is stored in astrocytes where it is converted to lactate and then shuttled to neurons to sustain their oxidative metabolism: the astrocyte–neuron lactate shuttle model of energy production (16). Glutamate uptake from the synaptic space into astrocytes occurs via the excitatory amino acid transporter (EAAT)-1 and EAAT-2. This process is sodium dependent and triggers ATP consumption and, through a series of events, stimulates glycolysis which produces the lactate that is released to neurons for utilization as an energy source (Figure 2.2) (16,17). The stoichiometry of this process is such that for each glutamate molecule that is taken up (with three sodium ions), one molecule of glucose enters an astrocyte resulting in the production of two ATP molecules through aerobic glycolysis and release of two molecules of lactate. The lactate is then taken up by neurons and, under aerobic conditions, converted to pyruvate which yields 17 ATP molecules per lactate molecule in the Krebs cycle and mitochondrial respiratory chain (17).

Although often associated with anaerobic conditions, lactate can also be generated in the non-anaerobic states as previously described and this situation can be identified by a rise in the microdialysis-monitored lactate pyruvate ratio in the presence of normal brain tissue oxygen tension (18). The now accepted role of lactate as an alternate cerebral energy source means that it can be neuroprotective in the context of glucose deprivation (19)

and there is also some evidence to support a role for exogenous administration of lactate in several types of ischaemic insults (19,20). Some support for this derives from work of Smith and colleagues who used 2-fluoro-2-deoxy-D-glucose positron emission tomography to demonstrate a decrement in brain glucose utilization associated with elevations in blood lactate levels during exercise (21). A clinical study by Bouzat et al. reported that hypertonic lactate administration decreased ICP and glutamate and spared brain glucose utilization (19). Lactate also has a signalling role in vascular regulation, memory, and axonal regeneration (20,22,23). An excellent foundational overview of brain energy metabolism relevant to several pathologies encountered on the neurocritical care unit (NCCU) can be found in Siesjö's textbook (24).

Clinical syndromes leading to brain injury

There are many clinical syndromes that may result in brain injury. The important unifying concepts are reviewed in the following sections and pathology-specific issues discussed in detail elsewhere in this book.

Ischaemia

Ischaemia is defined as a decrement in blood flow sufficient to induce anaerobic metabolism and is seen in a variety of neurological

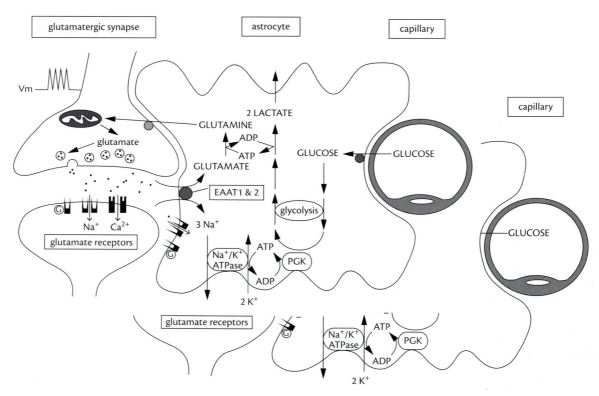

Fig. 2.2 Schematic representation of the mechanism for glutamate-induced glycolysis in astrocytes during physiologic activation *in vitro*.
At glutaminergic synapses, presynaptically released glutamate depolarizes postsynaptic neurons by acting at specific receptor subtypes. The action of glutamate is terminated by Na+ coupled glutamate uptake system located primarily in astrocytes. The resulting increase in intracellular Na+ in astrocytes activates Na+/K+ ATPase, which in turn stimulates glycolysis with resultant glucose use and lactate production. Lactate, after release from astrocytes, is taken up by local neurons as an energy substrate.
Reproduced from Magistretti PJ and Pellerin L, 'Cellular mechanisms of brain energy metabolism and their relevance to functional brain imaging', *Philosophical Transactions of the Royal Society B: Biological Sciences* , 1999, 354, 1387, pp. 1155–1163, by permission of the Royal Society.

disorders. Regional and global brain ischaemia are the primary pathophysiological processes in acute ischaemic stroke (AIS) and post-cardiac arrest respectively. Ischaemia and its resultant energy failure is associated with a massive increase in the levels of extracellular excitatory neurotransmitters, particularly glutamate, and intracellular calcium (25,26). Metabotropic glutamate receptors and agonist-gated ionotropic receptors activate phospholipase C which in turn results in production of phospholipid-derived second messengers such as inositol 1,4,5-triphosphate (IP3) and diacylglycerol (DAG) (27,28). DAG stimulates protein kinase C (PKC) (29) and IP3 (30) leading to a further increase in intracellular calcium released from smooth endoplasmic reticulum via action on ryanodine receptors (25).

Activation of the α-amino-3-hydroxy-5-methyl-4-isoxazolepropionic acid (AMPA) subset of glutamate receptors induces intracellular influx of sodium and calcium, and promotes intracellular hyperosmolarity and cellular swelling (31). Increases in intracellular calcium occur because of both exogenous and endogenous (e.g. endoplasmic reticulum) entry and activate calcium-dependent protein kinase (32) and a variety of other enzyme systems with multiple responses including alterations in gene expression involved with cell death (33). Gene expression takes several hours to develop and likely accounts for the delay in observable injury, particularly to vulnerable neurons (34), supporting the notion of delayed maturation of ischaemic neuronal injury (5,34,35) but with selective vulnerability of different neuron types (36). If the burden of ischaemia (in terms of duration and/or decrement in blood flow) is sufficiently substantial, cells die acutely and maturation of injury becomes irrelevant.

Cerebral oedema

Brain oedema can occur as a result of a primary increase in brain water content or an increase in intracellular osmoles such as sodium and subsequent movement of water into the cell along the osmotic gradient. There are two main types of oedema—cytotoxic and vasogenic (37). In the context of ischaemia there can be progression from cytotoxic to vasogenic of oedema and, subsequently, to haemorrhagic conversion (38). Notably, progression to vasogenic oedema requires an element of perfusion to add fluid to the tissue and produce swelling which in turn reduces perfusion and function of adjacent tissue (Figure 2.3).

Vasogenic brain oedema occurs with breakdown of the BBB in the presence of continued perfusion and arises mainly in association with tumours and mass lesions. It can also be related to trauma, inflammation, infection and can develop several hours after AIS in those brain regions with residual perfusion. The compromise of regional perfusion and worsening of ischaemia by vasogenic oedema occurs because of direct compressive effects and also movement of fluid from the vasculature into tissue (37). Tumours such as high-grade gliomas express VEGF which increase angiogenesis and vascular permeability with the new vessels promoting increased cellular oedema.

Cytotoxic oedema is the result of intracellular fluid accumulation because of failure of ion pumps, primarily sodium-potassium ATPase, or osmotic disturbances in the presence of an intact BBB. It is primarily seen in ischaemia, hypoxia, metabolic derangements, and after traumatic injury brain injury (TBI) (37). It can be a primary driver leading to post-ischaemia vasogenic oedema (Figure 2.3) (38). Astrocytes are the cells primarily affected and

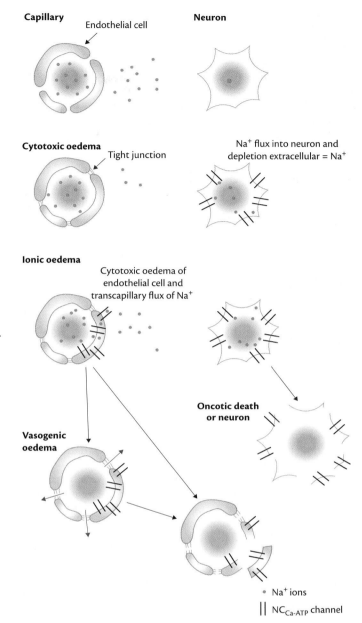

Fig. 2.3 Schematic representation of oedema and its progression. Normally, Na$^+$ concentrations in serum and in extracellular space are the same, and much higher than inside the neuron. Cytotoxic oedema of neurons is due to entry of Na$^+$ into ischaemic neurons via pathways such as NC$_{Ca-ATP}$ channels, depleting extracellular Na$^+$ and thereby setting up a concentration gradient between intravascular and extracellular compartments. Ionic oedema results from cytotoxic oedema of endothelial cells, due to expression of cation channels on both the luminal and abluminal side, allowing Na$^+$ from the intravascular compartment to traverse the capillary wall and replenish Na$^+$ in the extracellular space. Vasogenic oedema results from degradation of tight junctions between endothelial cells, transforming capillaries into 'fenestrated' capillaries that allow extravasation (outward filtration) of proteinaceous fluid. Oncotic death of neurons is the ultimate consequence of cytotoxic oedema. Oncotic death of endothelial cells results in complete loss of capillary integrity and in extravasation of blood, that is, haemorrhagic conversion.

Reprinted from *The Lancet Neurology*, 6, 3, Simard JM *et al.*, 'Brain oedema in focal ischaemia: molecular pathophysiology and theoretical implications', pp. 258–268, Copyright 2007, with permission from Elsevier.

swell early because of the presence of aquaporin 4 (AQP4) receptors in their cell membranes which promote intracellular influx of water. Continued cellular swelling compromises capillary perfusion because of swollen astrocytic foot processes and leads to local mass effect (39). After AIS, increased transport of sodium across an intact BBB contributes to oedema formation in the early hours after stroke onset, and the AQP4 inhibitor, bumetanide, has been shown to reduce brain oedema in rodent models of stroke (39,40).

Brain trauma

The initial impact of TBI can result in widespread abnormalities including structural disruption, mass effect, and perfusion disturbances. At the cellular level there is loss of cellular integrity with failure of neuronal and astrocytic energy metabolism and ion channel dysfunction that leads to metabolic derangements from the moment of the initial impact but also related to secondary phenomena that cause further (secondary) injury (see Chapter 17) (41). Though cellular membranes are quite resistant to mechanical deformation, including those encountered with high-force sheer injury, ion channels are not so resistant (42). Damaged neurons release excitatory neurotransmitters, chiefly glutamate, which lead to calcium-mediated cellular injury and activation of multiple cell death cascades (41,42). There is also evidence that glutamate transporter levels in astrocytes decrease acutely following TBI, further decreasing synaptic cleft glutamate uptake and potentiating excitotoxicity (43). This leads to an increase in glucose metabolism to restore cellular integrity, membrane potentials, and clear toxic neurotransmitters from the synaptic space (41,44). However, in the presence of inadequate oxygen supply, anaerobic glycolysis ensues and leads to lactate production and tissue acidosis. Finally, local blood flow becomes dysregulated due to BBB disruption, compression of microvasculature due to oedema, and failure of local autoregulation, and this leads to secondary ischaemia because of insufficient supply of glucose and oxygen (41). These processes cumulatively result in cellular oedema and fluid and blood extravasation into the extracellular space leading to increases in brain tissue and intracranial blood volumes respectively. The resultant increases in ICP feed into the vicious cycles of further reductions in CBF, worsening oedema, and additional ischaemic brain injury (see Chapter 7) (42).

Seizures

Seizures are caused by abnormal, hypersynchronous discharges from a group of cortical neurons in response to systemic or neurological insults (45). At a cellular level, neuronal excitability is normally supported by the electrochemical gradients maintained by sodium-potassium ATPases, and disruption of these membrane potentials may occur because of excitatory transmission and dysfunctional ion channels. Seizures themselves produce massive extracellular potassium shifts that increase neuron excitability and depolarize other nearby neurons (45). Glutamate is the major excitatory neurotransmitter in the CNS and acts via various receptors including AMPA, kainate, and N-methyl-D-aspartate (NMDA) which facilitate depolarization at synapses. Gamma-aminobutyric acid (GABA) is the major inhibitory neurotransmitter and it acts via two major receptor subtypes—postsynaptic chloride channel $GABA_A$ and presynaptic second messenger-mediated channel $GABA_B$ receptors (46). Enhanced NMDA receptor function and alteration in GABA receptor efficacy play important roles in seizure propagation and termination respectively (47).

Though cellular excitation occurs because of these underlying mechanisms, neurons must also form a synchronized network in order to generate a seizure. Gap junctions and glutaminergic synapses generate rapid and effective synchronization (45), resulting in paroxysmal depolarizing shift or sustained neuronal depolarization that leads to a burst of action potentials followed by rapid GABA-mediated repolarization and hyperpolarization. Seizure propagation occurs because of facilitation of the first phase of this response and failure of the second in specific macrocircuits (45,46). Animal (48–50) and human studies (51) confirm that seizures result in substantial brain injury. One animal study confirmed electron microscopic evidence of neuronal injury within 20–32 minutes of continuous seizure activity and potential for post-seizure maturation of brain injury (49). Notably, animal models of status epilepticus indicate increased cerebral metabolic rate (CMR) (52,53) with substantial decrements in glycogen, glucose and phosphocreatine but a relatively small decrement in ATP and other markers of energy availability (54). Excessive excitatory amino acid release appears to be the primary underlying driver of seizure-related brain damage (55,56).

Neuroinflammation

The brain is an immunologically privileged site with the exception of microglia and endothelial cells which take part in immune responses via microglial activation and facilitation of the passage of mediating cells respectively. Multiple ion channels in microglia detect disturbances in the neuronal milieu and become activated and proliferate in response to neuronal injury (57). After activation, microglia take on an amoeboid appearance and produce receptors for many inflammatory mediators including histamine, bradykinin, platelet-activating factor (PAF), and complement, and release a number of proinflammatory substances such as tumour necrosis factor (TNF)-α, interleukin (IL)-6, and NO that attract more inflammatory cells to the injured tissue. They are ultimately involved in destroying invading organisms via phagocytosis, T-cell activation, and upregulation of cell adhesion molecules (57).

Proinflammatory cytokines and chemokines also play a role in inflammation and immune mediated disorders. Cytokines such as IL-1, TNF-α and interferon-γ increase expression of vascular endothelium adhesion molecules including vascular cell adhesion protein 1 (VCAM-1), also known as vascular cell adhesion molecule 1, and intercellular adhesion molecule 1 (ICAM-1). They also increase the activity of matrix metalloproteinases that promote the uptake of circulating leucocytes. These inflammatory mediators activate microglia and astrocytes and indirectly lead to the production of free radicals, proteases, and complement, all of which potentiate the inflammatory response (5,58–60).

Biochemical pathways to brain injury

The survival of neurons depends on several factors including adequate supply of oxygen, glucose, and other substrates (particularly lactate and ketones), maintained mitochondrial metabolism and processing, and transport of proteins and growth trophic factors (5). All pathological processes affecting the CNS produce a loss of neurons and other cell types chiefly through one of two morphologically distinguishable, but not mutually exclusive, processes—necrosis and apoptosis (5,25,61,62). Though a steep rise in intracellular calcium is a key initiator of cell death in both mechanisms, the contribution of each to a cell's ultimate fate is determined by the severity and abruptness of the insult. In general terms, more profound changes initiate necrosis whereas less severe ones induce apoptosis (62).

Necrosis occurs after an abrupt cessation of oxygen and/or glucose supply leading to failure of ATP production and cell breakdown and inflammatory infiltration. It is associated with TBI, ischaemia/hypoxia, hypo- and hyperglycaemia, hyperthermia, and prolonged seizures. Acute failure of ATP production leads to neuronal cell depolarization following failure of sodium-potassium membrane pumps, and loss of neuronal excitability with massive release of glutamate. Neuronal injury stems from the accumulation of glutamate, whose uptake is an ATP-dependent process in both neurons and astrocytes (25,61–63). This leads to activation of post-synaptic AMPA, kainate, and, most importantly, NMDA glutamate receptors, resulting in massive calcium influx into cells (25) and, in turn, cell membrane degradation via action of calpains and caspases. Subsequent calcium entry into the mitochondria causes distortion of DNA, the production of oxygen free radicals, and failure of the mitochondrial respiratory chain. This process is collectively known as excitotoxicity (25,62).

Mitochondrial failure is a critical component of cell necrosis and is induced primarily by NMDA glutamate receptor-mediated toxicity (64). Intracellular calcium influx leads to subsequent uptake into the mitochondria via the mitochondrial membrane calcium uniporter, mitochondrial membrane depolarization, and release of cytochrome c into the cytosol. It is believed that this change in mitochondrial membrane permeability is an important milestone in a cell's transition to death (65,66) and therefore a potential target for neuroprotection (65). However, the cell does not become committed to death by this initial sequence of events but by subsequent calcium dysregulation as a result of downregulation of ion exchangers following calpain activation that occurs hours after the initial insult (64,67).

Apoptosis on the other hand results in selective cell death orchestrated by various genes following DNA damage and low energy supply. Although apoptosis plays a role in the pathological response to brain injury, it is also essential for normal brain development and cellular homeostasis (5,35,63). Even with apparently satisfactory return of blood flow and energy supply after transient global or focal ischaemia, delayed cell death may occur because of ischaemic apoptosis as well as acute necrosis, even in the absence of immediate structural damage (35,62,63,67). The apoptotic cascade involves three main steps—activation of death receptors (68), release of cytochrome c from the inner mitochondrial membrane as a result of interactions between proapoptotic and antiapoptotic proteins (25,35,62,64,68,69), and activation of proteolytic enzymes called caspases (35,68). Cells subsequently shrink and break into dense spheres called apoptotic bodies, and are subsequently absorbed by other cells without initiation of inflammatory cascades (63).

Mediators of brain injury

Different brain injury types have a similar underling pathophysiological process associated with secondary injury. This is essentially a cascade of seemingly disparate and multiple biochemical reactions and their consequent mediators that each contributes to the death of neural tissue. The specific biochemical mediators involved in neuronal injury are discussed in the following sections and summarized in Figure 2.4 (70).

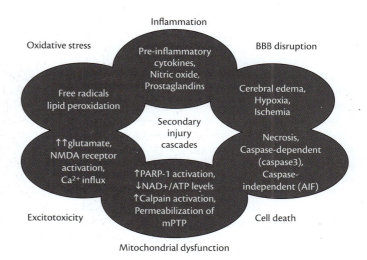

Fig. 2.4 Mediators of neuronal injury. The multiple pathways contributing to neuronal death.

Reprinted from *Trends in Pharmacological Sciences*, 31, 12, Loane DJ and Faden AI, 'Neuroprotection for traumatic brain injury: translational challenges and emerging therapeutic strategies', pp. 596–604, Copyright 2010, with permission from Elsevier.

Calcium

Calcium plays a key role in secondary brain injury and subsequent neuronal death. It accumulates intracellularly as a direct result of glutaminergic activation in neuronal injury via several pathways (64,67,68). AMPA receptors, though thought to be primarily permeable to sodium and potassium, are now believed to be also permeable to calcium and, following upregulation in response to ischaemia, are likely responsible for the resultant increases in intracellular calcium concentration (25). Increased intracellular calcium also occurs via NMDA and kainate receptors through overstimulation and impaired reuptake of glutaminergic excitotoxic neurotransmitters, and other ion channels and transporters such as transient receptor potential (TRP) channels, Na^+/Ca^{2+} exchanger channels (NCX), acid-sensing ion channels (ASICs), L-type voltage-dependent Ca^{2+} channels, and hemichannels. In addition, malfunctions in internal calcium storage systems, especially in the endoplasmic reticulum and mitochondria, also contribute to elevated intracellular calcium concentration secondary to breakdown of membranes or dysfunction of the ryanodine receptor (71).

There are numerous signalling pathway consequences of excitotoxin-mediated calcium dysautoregulation leading to apoptotic or necrotic cell death. Intracellular calcium becomes sequestered into the mitochondria, particularly during prolonged endoplasmic reticulum stress (71), leading to failure of respiratory chain function and formation of reactive oxygen species (ROS) that deplete ATP and cause further cell damage (64). This then triggers several catabolic enzymatic reactions that lead to further cell damage and death (Figure 2.4) (67). Moreover, calcium effects can be mediated via phospholipase A2 which acts on membrane phospholipids to release arachidonic acid. This is then metabolized to form several inflammatory and thrombogenic mediators, including prostaglandins and leukotrienes. Calcium also activates calpains, caspases, endonucleases, and kinases which lead to increased free radical production, damaged mitochondria and endoplasmic reticulum, acidosis, cellular oedema, cytoskeletal breakdown, loss of integrity of cell, and fragmented DNA. Together these several pathways kill the cell (25,61).

Reactive oxygen species

ROS are highly unstable free radicals because of an unpaired electron in their outer electron shell. If not deactivated, they lead to neuronal destruction (5,41). Enzymes such as super oxide dismutase (SOD), glutathione peroxidase, and catalase scavenge free radicals, and astrocytes protect neurons against oxidative damage by providing precursors for glutathione synthesis and an array of antioxidant enzymes (72). The mitochondrial respiratory chain contains the chief source of electrons required to reduce molecular oxygen to form ROS which include hydrogen peroxide (H_2O_2) and the hydroxyl (HO^-) and superoxide (O_2^-) radicals (5,73,74). Interestingly, NO which has neuroprotective actions in ischaemia and TBI (75,76) may exert a double effect of membrane peroxidation and DNA destruction after reacting with superoxide radicals to form peroxynitrite ($ONOO^-$) (72,74). Free radicals are produced following mitochondrial energy failure, glutamate-mediated influx of calcium (which activates NO synthase), activation of the phospholipase A2–cyclooxygenase pathway, and in the presence of free ferrous iron which serves as a catalyst for ROS generation (41,72,73). In addition, neutrophils yield a significant proportion of ROS through oxidation of nicotinamide adenine dinucleotide phosphate (NADPH) (73,74) which results in peroxidation of cell membranes (5,41,72–74).

Stress proteins

Several heat shock proteins (HSPs) are transcriptionally activated in response to cellular injury. HSP70 is the most abundant in normal cells and induced by denatured proteins (77). It mitigates cell damage by binding to denatured proteins in an attempt to salvage their enzymatic activity. HSP70 is upregulated and produced in massive quantities in response to ischaemic tissue damage, particularly in neurons and glia in penumbral regions of infarcts, resulting in ischaemia-induced tolerance and promotion of cell survival (77).

HSP32, also known as haem-oxygenase-1 (HO1), is primarily synthesized in glia and regulates haem turnover and iron metabolism. It is upregulated in subarachnoid haemorrhage and may play a role in protection against oxidative stress (78). Nuclear factor kappa B (NF-κB) is a transcriptional factor that functions as a 'stress sensor' and is believed to play a dual role (79). It has neuroprotective actions during brief periods of ischaemia but prolonged proapoptotic actions. In unstimulated cells, NF-κB exists in a latent form complexed to an inhibitory protein called inhibitor of κB (IκB). It is activated by multiple stimuli including oxidative stress, bacterial and viral by-products, and proinflammatory cytokines such as IL-1 and TNF. This leads to the dissociation of IκB and translocation of NF-κB into the cell nucleus where it up-regulates mRNA transcription of several protective genes, including *SOD* (5,79).

Caspases

Like calpains, caspases are cysteine proteases which when active form tetramers that induce apoptosis (35,68). Caspase activation is regulated by interactions between proapoptotic and antiapoptotic proteins (68). Apoptotic signals trigger 'initiator' caspases such as caspase-2 (also -8, -9, and -10) which recruit 'effector' caspases, such as caspase-3 (also -4, -5, -6, -7, -11, -12, and -13), which carry out cell destruction (35,68,80). Caspase-3, and to a lesser extent caspase-8, inactivates polyadenosine diphosphate (ADP)-ribose polymerase (PARP), thus inhibiting DNA repair (35,80). Other caspases have a range of actions including destruction of nuclear lamina, inactivation of antiapoptotic proteins, and destruction of cytoskeletal structure. Caspases also induce cell death via proteolytic inactivation of effector molecules (68).

There are several pathways that converge on caspase activation. The death receptor pathway includes transmembrane receptors such as TNF-α and cell death 95 (CD95), both of which have intracellular death domains. Binding of specific ligands to these receptors triggers activation of Fas-activated death domain and subsequent apoptosis via activation of caspases (68). The ceramide pathway involves cleavage of sphingomyelin in response to cellular stress with the production of membrane-bound ceramide and activation of ceramide-dependent protein kinase which promotes apoptosis via multiple mechanisms. The mitochondrial pathway involves release of cytochrome c and subsequent activation of caspase-8 which commits the cell to death (68).

Cell adhesion molecules

Cerebral ischaemia precipitates adhesion and transendothelial migration of leucocytes with the potential for exacerbation of neuronal injury. Three families of leucocyte adhesion molecules have been identified—the immunoglobulin gene superfamily, integrins, and selectins such as P-selectin (81). The immunoglobulin gene superfamily includes ICAM-1 and VCAM-1. These are cell surface glycoproteins expressed on the vascular endothelium which facilitate leucocyte adhesion (81). Their expression is increased following transient and permanent ischaemia (81,82).

Proapoptotic and antiapoptotic factors

Apoptosis is regulated by the balance of activity of pro- and antiapoptotic proteins. B-cell lymphoma-2 (Bcl-2), B-cell lymphoma-extra large (Bcl-xL), and inhibitor of apoptosis (IAP) proteins are pro-survival (35,77), while BAX, BAK, and proteins from the BcL-2 homology 3 (BH3) subfamily, such as BAD, promote cell death (5,35,62,74,83). All form heterodimers which control opening of the mitochondrial permeability transition pore and allow dissipation of mitochondrial H^+ and uncoupling of the respiratory chain. Antiapoptotic proteins prevent the transition pore from opening whereas proapoptotic proteins promote opening (35). Opening of the pore results in loss of the proton gradient across the inner mitochondrial membrane (the transmembrane potential) leading to intracellular influx of water and rupture of the outer mitochondrial membrane with subsequent release of cytochrome c into the cytosol (25,35,62,64,68,69,74). Proapoptotic proteins such as BAX polymerize to form pores in the outer mitochondrial membrane through which cytochrome c can also escape. Cytochrome c then binds with apoptotic protease-activating factor 1 (APAF-1) to form the apoptosome which recruits and activates caspase-9, triggering several cascades that ultimately lead to cell death (35,74).

Platelet-activating factor

PAF is a potent phospholipid and mediator of neuronal injury. It causes free radical-associated damage and upregulation of gene expression of TNF-α and COX-2 which participate in inflammation and apoptosis (84). PAF antagonists such as LAU-0901 and the free radical scavenger alpha-phenyl-N-tertiary-butyl nitrone (PBN) reduce PAF-triggered inflammation and neurodegeneration in PAF-stressed neural cells (85). PBN most efficiently represses COX-2 and TNF-α, suggesting that a significant component of

PAF-induced neuronal injury is related to oxidative stress and free radial damage.

Toll-like receptors

Toll-like receptors (TLRs) are cell surface proteins that recognize foreign cell constituents such as lipids and proteins. They play a key role in immune surveillance (86). Once believed to be present only in leucocytes, TLRs are now known to be associated with different tissue types including cortical neurons and glial cells (86). Activation of TLRs initiates signal cascades primarily involving NF-κb which in turn induces expression of cytokines and pro-inflammatory molecules such as IL-6, IL-1β, and TNF-α, triggering neuronal apoptosis (86,87). In mice cortical neurons, TLR-2 and TLR-4 promote neuronal death in the setting of glucose deprivation and elimination of TLRs protects neurons from cell death (87).

Erythropoietin

Erythropoietin (EPO) is a member of the haematopoietic cytokine 1 superfamily whose expression is induced by the hypoxia-inducible factor (HIF) family of transcription factors in response to hypoxia (88). Activation of the EPO receptor (EPOR) by low oxygen conditions inhibits apoptosis in the bone marrow and leads to erythropoiesis and angiogenesis thereby increasing erythrocyte circulation (88). EPOR forms homodimers after binding to EPO, triggering autophosphorylation of EPOR-associated Janus-tyrosine kinase-2 (JAK-2) (89) which in turn leads to the phosphorylation of multiple protein kinases and transcription factors including NF-κB (89). These in turn upregulate the prosurvival protein Bcl-xL (88).

In the brain, both EPO and EPOR play a critical role in neuronal survival, particularly after hypoxic/ischaemic injury. They are typically found in low concentrations in brain tissue but become upregulated in many conditions including AIS where there is particular expression in penumbral regions (90). EPO has additional neuroprotective effects including reduction of synaptic release of glutamate and amelioration of glutamate-induced excitotoxicity (90).

Aquaporins

Aquaporins are transmembrane water-channel proteins that regulate cellular water balance. AQP4 is the most abundant aquaporin in the brain and chiefly located in the astrocytic foot processes. Water transport through AQP4 is driven by the osmotic gradient across the cell and regulated by receptor–ligand interactions. Activation of these receptors leads to phosphorylation of AQP4 with resultant activation of calcium and/or protein kinases, and either up- or downregulation of AQP4 with variable effects on cellular oedema (39). Though AQP4 modulation might appear to offer a straightforward treatment option for cerebral oedema, inhibition of AQP4 has opposing roles in cytotoxic and vasogenic oedema making a simple targeted approach challenging (39,91). Hypertonic saline and bumetanide have been shown to reduce cerebral oedema via AQP4 modulation in clinical conditions such as AIS (40).

Sex hormones

Progesterone is a steroid hormone synthesized in glial cells that has been shown to confer neuroprotective effects in a variety of neurological conditions (92). It has been particularly well studied in TBI in which the effects of progesterone were first identified when female rats were observed to recover better than male rats after brain trauma. Subsequent animal models have shown numerous protective effects for progesterone including reduction in cerebral oedema (93), decreased neuronal loss (94), anti-inflammatory effects via inhibition cytokine release (95), antioxidant effects (95), and improved cognitive outcomes (94).

The multifactorial nature of brain injury

The impetus for elucidating the pathophysiological basis of brain injury is to allow rational development of neuroprotective strategies. The multiple pathways involved in the genesis of brain injury underscores the significant physiological and biochemical complexity involved in neuronal demise from various types of neurological insult. With this in mind, it is unsurprising that success in the development of neuroprotective strategies based on amelioration of one pathway has been elusive. At the time of writing, there are more than 23,000 publications dealing with stroke and its treatment in various animal models, and more than 2310 completed clinical trials listed on the Stroke Trials Registry. Despite the large volume of encouraging preclinical data, few neuroprotective therapies have translated into clinical effectiveness, illustrating the problems of dealing with complex pathophysiological processes. Donnan, in the 2007 Feinberg lecture, made this remarkable statement about neuroprotection research: 'We have reached a stage at which research in this area should stop altogether or radical new approaches adopted' (96). Various causes for the apparent futility in pathophysiologically based neuroprotection research have been suggested and these have been reviewed elsewhere by Kofke who promoted a multimodal therapy paradigm as the optimal solution (97).

Neuropharmacology

Pharmaceuticals are central to the practice of neurocritical care. An overview of basic concepts can be found in most standard textbooks of pharmacology and this chapter will provide an overview of neuropharmacology relevant to neurocritical care. More detailed information about neuropharmacological issues relevant to specific disease states or situations is also available elsewhere in this book.

Antiepileptic drugs

First-generation antiepileptic drugs (AEDs), such as phenytoin, phenobarbital, primidone, benzodiazepines, ethosuximide, carbamazepine, and valproate, have multiple drug interactions and adverse effects related to enzyme induction and/or inhibition. Second-generation AEDs have been developed since the early 1990s and include felbamate, vigabatrin, lamotrigine, gabapentin, topiramate, tiagabine, oxcarbazepine, levetiracetam, pregabalin, and zonisamide. The newer drugs offer advantages of fewer drug interactions, greater safety, unique mechanisms of action, and broader spectrum of activity, although most still do have significant adverse side effects and potential for drug interactions (98). AEDs act on diverse molecular targets through effects on multiple receptors and neurotransmitters, although their mechanisms of action can generally be categorized into modulation of voltage-dependent ion channels, inhibition of synaptic excitation, and enhancement of synaptic inhibition (98,99). Efficacy is related to the degree of modification of the excitability of neurons such that seizure activity is attenuated without disturbing normal (non-epileptic) neuronal activity. The major mechanisms of AEDs are summarized in Figure 2.5 (99–101).

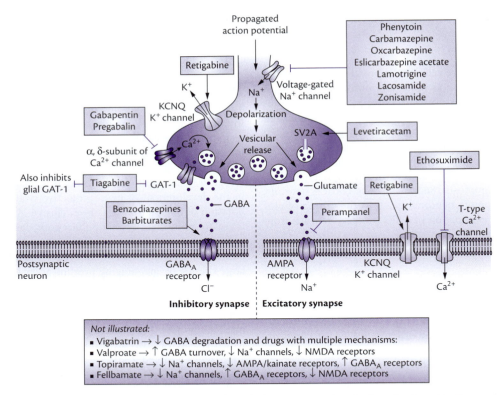

Fig. 2.5 Principal mechanisms of action of antiepileptic drugs. Antiepileptic drugs display a spectrum of mechanisms of action, with effects on both inhibitory (left-hand side) and excitatory (right-hand side) nerve terminals.
AMPA, α-amino-3-hydroxy-5-methyl-4-isoxazole propionic acid; GABA, γ-aminobutyric acid; GAT-1, sodium- and chloride-dependent GABA transporter 1; SV2A, synaptic vesicle glycoprotein 2A.
Reproduced with permission from Macmillan Publishers Ltd: *Nature Reviews Neurology*, 8, 12, Wolfgang Loscher and Dieter Schmidt, 'Epilepsy: Perampanel-new promise for refractory epilepsy?', pp. 661–662 © 2012. Originally adapted by permission from Macmillan Publishers Ltd: *Nature Reviews Drug Discovery*, 9, 1, Bialer M and White HS, 'Key factors in the discovery and development of new antiepileptic drugs', pp. 68–82 © 2010.

Anaesthetic and sedative agents

Several factors are important when designing a therapeutic paradigm that leads to a safe and comfortable patient in the NCCU (see also Chapter 6).

Hypnosis, anxiolysis, and amnesia

The GABA receptor and its various subclasses play a central role in the action of many hypnotic agents (102). Stimulation of the GABA receptor leads to increase in cell membrane chloride conductance and hyperpolarization of the neuron such that the effects of neuroexcitatory neurotransmitters, which ordinarily cause depolarization, are neutralized. This leads to a dose-dependent decrement in the level of consciousness, on a continuum from minimal depression with disinhibition and electroencephalogram (EEG) activation to deep anaesthesia with significant metabolic suppression and an isoelectric EEG (103). In general, GABAergic drugs, such as barbiturates (103,104), benzodiazepines, propofol, and etomidate (103), produce a decrease in CMR and a coupled decrease in CBF (103) and therefore reduce ICP in a normally reactive brain (105).

Non-GABergic hypnotic drugs include dexmedetomidine and ketamine. Dexmedetomidine is an alpha-2 adrenergic agonist thought to exert its effects primarily in the locus coeruleus (106) which produces mild analgesia and a reduced level of consciousness from which the patient can easily be aroused (107). It is associated with a small coupled decrease in CMR and CBF (108). Dexmedetomidine also has a role in the treatment of delirium

(109). Ketamine acts by blocking NMDA receptors (110) and produces hypnosis and analgesia associated with a concomitant array of neuroexcitatory phenomena and increased CMR and ICP (103).

Analgesics

The brain is richly supplied with opiate receptors and corresponding endogenous opiate ligands (111). There are multiple pain pathways and nerve fibre types. Peripheral receptors and their proteins (e.g. substance P) transduce pain through fast somatic fibres and smaller and slower visceral and sympathetic pain fibres. Pain pathways meet in the thalamus from which there is further transmission to multiple cortical areas (112). Interruption of these pathways by disease processes can lead to pain syndromes (113). Moreover, chronic exposure to opioids leads to downregulation of opioid receptors and upregulation of cAMP pathway associated with many chronic pain syndromes. Thus patients in the NCCU may have pre-existing pain syndromes, pathological alterations of pain pathways, or both (114,115), in addition to acute pain related to surgery, trauma, or prolonged immobility. The underlying taxonomy of pain describes nociceptive, inflammatory, neuropathic, and dysfunctional pain types. The mainstay of analgesia in the NCCU is centred on the use of mu opioid agonists, adjunct agents such as gabapentin, and occasionally nerve blocks.

Mu opioids are agonists at endogenous mu opioid receptors which mediate analgesics via G-protein-linked increased inward potassium flux and decreased outward sodium flux (103,115).

The attenuation of pain involves a significant element of thalamic depression among other mechanisms (53). At usual doses, mu opioids produce only modest decreases or minimal direct effects on global CMR and CBF (116), and all can cause respiratory depression, hypotension, and nausea and vomiting (117). Gabapentin is a useful adjunct in the management of acute (118) and neuropathic pain syndromes (119) and may have a role in the prevention of chronic neuropathic pain after surgery (119). Multiple putative mechanisms for the antinociceptive effect of gabapentin have been described including (but not limited to) upregulation of N-type calcium channels in the spinal cord (120), inhibition of catecholamine release from adrenal chromaffin cells (121), interference with development of opioid tolerance (122), inhibition of GABA release from the locus coeruleus cells (123), and increased concentration of cortical GABA (124).

Immobility and shivering control

Immobility can usually be achieved by producing a comfortable patient but additional pharmacological methods may be required to reduce the risk of injury during uncontrolled movements in delirious or agitated patients, or those with involuntary movements including shivering. All antipsychotic drugs that interfere with dopaminergic transmission may induce an element of hypokinesis (125).There are a multitude of antishivering drugs but the most commonly used are meperidine, dexmedetomidine, clonidine, and buspirone. Meperidine potently decreases shivering (126) although there is concern about potential proconvulsant effects of its metabolite normeperidine (127). Buspirone, a serotonin (5-HT_{1A}) partial agonist with minimal intrinsic sedative actions, is unimpressive in isolation but synergistically augments the antishivering effects of meperidine (126). Neuromuscular blockade may also be needed to effect control of shivering under certain circumstances.

Neuromuscular blocking agents

Neuromuscular blocking drugs include depolarizing and non-depolarizing types. The depolarizing neuromuscular blocking agent suxamethonium produce an excessive nicotinic cholinergic stimulation that causes sodium channels adjacent to the endplate to remain in an inactivated state with consequent intense but short-lived neuromuscular blockade (128). Succinylcholine increases CBF and ICP briefly (129), likely related to the massive stimulus associated with fasciculations (129). It should be avoided in patients with ICU-acquired or pre-existing myopathy, recent lower motor neuron denervation, or after prolonged immobilization in whom it can lead to a precipitous and life-threatening increase in serum potassium.

Non-depolarizing agents such as vecuronium and rocuronium directly and competitively block the nicotinic neuromuscular junction (128) and provide varying degrees of neuromuscular blockade which can be monitored by peripheral electromyography monitoring (128). Non-depolarizing neuromuscular blockade is reversed with an anticholinesterase agent such as neostigmine, edrophonium, or pyridostigmine in association with a muscarinic anticholinergic agent to prevent muscarinic acetylcholine-mediated bradycardia, bronchoconstriction, bronchorrhoea, and alimentary hyperperistalsis. Thus common problems associated with reversal of neuromuscular blockade include tachycardia and bradycardia which can confuse the evaluation, postoperative tachycardia, and bradycardia (128). Vecuronium and its congeners have minimal cerebrovascular effects (130).

Sympathetic hyperactivity

Many syndromes are associated with 'autonomic storms', more accurately referred to as paroxysmal sympathetic hyperactivity (131), and this is likely to represent a lack of cortical inhibitory modulation of nociceptive inputs (132). Controlling sympathetic hyperactivity is an important element of management in some patient groups in the NCCU. After adequate sedation and analgesia is ensured, centrally acting sympatholytic drugs, such as dexmedetomidine, clonidine, and propranolol (131), may be effective. Dexmedetomidine and clonidine are central alpha-2 agonists that act predominantly at the locus coeruleus to diminish central adrenergic activity (106). Propranolol is a beta-adrenergic antagonist which crosses the BBB (133) and has been reported to be effective in controlling symptoms of sympathetic hyperactivity (131). Other possible therapeutic modalities include centrally (134) or peripherally administered baclofen (131).

Antipsychotic drugs

Antipsychotic drugs including phenothiazines and structurally similar compounds such as butyrophenones, diphenylbutylpiperidines and indolones were developed for use in schizophrenia and other psychotic disorders. However, they also have a role in the management of delirium, amphetamine intoxication, paranoias, mania, and Alzheimer's-associated agitation (135). Although there is chemical dissimilarity between different antipsychotic drugs, there are many pharmacological similarities. They are classified into typical and atypical subtypes (Table 2.2). Atypical antipsychotics have varied mechanisms compared to typical antipsychotics, are associated with a substantially lower risk of extrapyramidal side effects, and have become the preferred antipsychotic agents in the NCCU (135). Typical antipsychotic drugs include haloperidol and droperidol and primarily act as D_2 dopamine receptor antagonists (135). They are characterized as neuroleptic agents. In contrast, atypical antipsychotics provide a broader range of selective neurochemical effects including (to varying extents) antiserotonergic (5-HT_{2A} and 5-HT_{1A}), antidopaminergic (D_1 and D_2), antiadrenergic, and antihistaminic (H_1) actions with lower anticholinergic activity. The disparate receptor effects of various antipsychotic drugs are summarized in Table 2.3.

Nausea and vomiting

Nausea and vomiting is a common symptom in the NCCU, particularly after surgery when it occurs in up to one-third of patients overall (136–138). It has been reported in one-half of patients after supratentorial craniotomy with an even higher incidence after infratentorial craniotomy (139,140). Vomiting is particularly unwelcome after neurosurgery when retching and associated systemic hypertension and increased venous pressure may predispose to postoperative intracranial bleeding. First-line treatment of nausea and emesis is typically with a single agent such as ondansetron, although multimodal therapy with agents with different mechanisms of action is required in many cases (see Chapter 16) (141).

Ondansetron is a 5HT_3 receptor antagonist (142) with reliable antiemetic actions after intracranial neurosurgery (139,140). It has no effect on cerebral haemodynamics or ICP (143) and causes minimal sedation (139,140), although headache, dizziness (137), and dystonic/encephalopathic reactions (144) have been reported. Low-dose droperidol is also an effective antiemetic after

Table 2.2 Antipsychotic drugs

Typical antipsychotics		Atypical antipsychotics
Phenothiazine	**Non-phenothiazine**	
Acetophenazine	Haloperidol (butyrophenone)	Aripiprazole
Chlorpromazine	Iloperidone	Clozapine
Fluphenazine	Loxapine (tricyclic)	Fluoxetine
Promethazine	Molindone	Olanzapine
Mesoridazine	Pimozide (butyrophenone)	Olanzapine
Perphenazine	Sertindole	Paliperidone
Perphenazine;	Thiothixene	Quetiapine
Prochlorperazine	Xanomeline	Risperidone
Promazine	Zotepine	Ziprasidone
Promethazine		
Thiethylperazine		
Thioridazine		
Trifluoperazine		

Data from Brunton LL *et al.* (eds), *Goodman & Gilman's The Pharmacological Basis of Therapeutics*, 11th Edition: McGrawHill, 2006.

craniotomy (145). Droperidol is a butyrophenone with D_2 receptor antagonist activity (146) and minimal cerebral haemodynamic, ICP, and sedative affects (147), although it causes a small decrease in systemic blood pressure (145). It is associated with extrapyramidal side effects (137) and can produce dysphoria when used without other sedative agents (148). Phenothiazines such as chlorpromazine, promethazine, prochlorperazine, and perphenazine are also D_2 antagonists (146) but with additional moderate antihistamine and anticholinergic actions (137). They are effective in controlling postoperative nausea and vomiting but can also produce extrapyramidal reactions. Trimethobenzamide is believed to work by inhibiting the chemoreceptor trigger zone (149). It has less potential to cause extrapyramidal side effects than some other agents because it is only a weak D_2 antagonist (146). It causes minimal sedation. Scopolamine is a centrally acting anticholinergic which blocks impulses from vestibular nuclei to higher areas in the CNS to reduce vomiting (137). Its central cholinergic antagonism can lead to delirium which is reversible with physostigmine, a centrally acting cholinesterase inhibitor (150). Scopolamine produces mild sedation. Metoclopramide is an effective postoperative antiemetic (151) with both D_2 and $5HT_3$ antagonist effects (146). It also increases gastric motility (152) but has the potential to produce dystonic reactions which can lead to life-threatening respiratory compromise (153). Hydroxyzine is an antihistamine and anticholinergic drug which blocks acetylcholine in the vestibular apparatus and histamine H_1 receptors in the nucleus of the solitary tract (137). Although an effective antiemetic, it is sedative (137).

Two drugs primarily used for other indications in the NCCU also have antiemetic actions. Propofol in small doses has similar efficacy to established antiemetic drugs after surgery (154), although its antiemetic mechanism of action is unknown (137). Dexamethasone and other glucocorticoids are also effective antiemetics (141,151) with unclear mechanisms of action (137).

Catecholamines

Dopamine, epinephrine, and norepinephrine are endogenous central neurotransmitters and as such have a role in normal neural function (155). However, catecholamines can also act as toxic neurotransmitters in multiple brain pathologies (156) and this has substantial implications during the use of exogenous catecholamines to maintain blood pressure in the NCCU.

Catecholamines are centrally acting neurotransmitters whose synthesis is tightly regulated, largely through tyrosine hydroxylase (155). Following release into synaptic vesicles, catecholamines are either degraded by catechol-*O*-methyl transferase or monoamine oxidase, or taken up by the presynaptic membrane to be repackaged into new synaptic vesicles (155). Synthetic adrenergic analogue drugs such as phenylephrine, methoxamine, dobutamine, and isoproterenol can also be taken up and repackaged into presynaptic vesicles, thus theoretically becoming false neurotransmitters with effects on their quantal potency (157). Exogenous catecholamines also undergo synaptic cleft degradation by the same enzymatic pathways as endogenous counterparts. Uptake of adrenergic compounds and their precursors from the blood is a regulated process involving transport proteins in the BBB (158,159). Notably, variations in blood concentration of catecholamines have a direct effect on their uptake and synthesis (159). Nonetheless, simple diffusion is a minor to absent element of transport of adrenergic compounds and their precursors into the brain with an intact BBB.

The normal function of catecholamine neurotransmitters is to activate neural processes, generally enhancing cognitive processing (160). The net result is increased CMR and, in uninjured brain, a coupled increase in CBF (161). Notably the brain is sparsely populated with endothelial adrenergic receptors, although they are not absent (157). With these considerations in mind, adrenergic drug infusions have only a small, but not absent, effect on CBF in the normal brain with intact BBB (162,163). Further, any CBF effects are primarily believed to be indirect, occurring as a consequence of peripheral effects on systemic blood pressure. However, in the injured brain with a disrupted BBB, peripheral administration of adrenergic agents can have multiple CNS effects. Entry of the drugs into brain parenchyma via the disrupted BBB allows them to act in a similar manner to an endogenous neurotransmitter and cause neural activation and increases in CMR and CBF (Figure 2.6)

Table 2.3 Potencies of standard and experimental antipsychotic agents at neurotransmitter receptors[a,b]

Drugs	Receptor								
	Dopamine D_2	Serotonin 5-HT_2	5-HT_{2A}/D_2 ratio	Dopamine		Muscarinic cholinergic	Adrenergic		Histamine H_1
				D_1	D_4		1	2	
Ziprasidone	×	×	1.0	4×	×××	5×	3×	4×	3×
cis-Thiothixene	×	4×	289	4×	3×	5×	3×	4×	2×
Sertindole	×	×	0.8	3×	3×	6×	×	5×	4×
Fluphenazine	×	3×	24	3×	2×	5×	2×	5×	3×
Zotepine	2×	×	0.6	3×	2×	4×	2×	4×	2×
Perphenazine	2×	2×	24	—	—	4×	3×	4×	—
Thioridazine	2×	3×	18	3×	3×	3×	3×	—	—
Pimozide	2×	3×	5.2	—	3×	—	—	—	—
Risperidone	2×	×	0.05	4×	3×	> 6×	2×	3×	3×
Aripiprazole	2×	2×	1.0	4×	3×	> 6×	3×	—	3×
Haloperidol	2×	3×	9.0	3×	3×	> 6×	2×	5×	5×
Ziprasidone	2×	×	0.09	4×	3×	6×	3×	—	3×
Mesoridazine	2×	2×	1.26	—	3×	—	—	—	—
Sulpiride	2×	5×	135	5×	3×	4×	5×	—	—
Olanzapine	3×	2×	0.36	3×	2×	2×	3×	4×	2×
Chlorpromazine	3×	2×	0.07	3×	3×	3×	×	4×	2×
Loxapine	3×	2×	0.02	—	3×	3×	3×	5×	2×
Pipamperone	3×	2×	0.01	5×	—	5×	3×	4×	5×
Molindone	4×	5×	40	—	—	—	5×	4×	>6×
Amperozide	4×	3×	0.14	4×	—	5×	4×	4×	4×
Quetiapine	4×	4×	1.84	4×	5×	4×	3×	5×	3×
Clozapine	4×	2×	0.01	3×	2×	2×	2×	4×	3×
Melperone	4×	3×	0.16	—	4×	—	—	—	—
Remoxipride	4×	6×	36	6×	5×	6×	6×	5×	6×

[a] Data summarize approximate relative K_i values (nM) determined by competition with radioligands for binding to the indicated receptors. Data indicate on an approximate logarithmic scale K_i values from 0–0.99 (×), 1.0–9.9 (2×), 10–99 (3×), 100–999 (4×), 1000–9999 (5×), and 10,000–99,000 (6×).

Compounds are in rank-order of dopamine D_2 receptor affinity; 5-HT_{2A}/D_2 ratio indicates relative preference for D_2 vs serotonin 5-HT_{2A} receptors. Compounds include clinically used and experimental agents.

[b] Muscarinic cholinergic receptor K_i values are pooled results obtained with radioligands that are non-selective for muscarinic receptor subtypes or that are selective for the M_1 subtype.

Data from Brunton LL et al. (eds), *Goodman & Gilman's The Pharmacological Basis of Therapeutics*, 11th Edition: McGrawHill, 2006.

(161,164). However, Dhar and colleagues reported no increase in CBF or CMR during administration of unidentified vasopressors to patients with SAH (165), presumably a group with disrupted BBB function (166). The role of the BBB in mediating the central effects of systemic catecholamines is summarized in Figure 2.6. Whilst the exact relevance to clinical practice in the NCCU is unsettled, it seems reasonable to maintain concern about potential deleterious effects of exogenous catecholamine administration on CMR and CBF pending more definitive information.

Multiple studies also support the notion of catecholamine-related neurotoxicity in the injured brain. Serum catecholamine levels increase dramatically after SAH, peak simultaneously with the peak incidence of SAH-related vasospasm, and high serum catecholamine levels correlate with the development of symptoms of delayed cerebral ischaemia (DCI) (167,168). Such observations support the hypothesis tested in laboratory models (169,170) that catecholamine-related hypothalamic injury may be an important factor in the genesis of DCI and cerebral infarction after SAH. Confirmation also comes from clinical reports that treatment with beta- and alpha-adrenergic antagonists is associated with an improvement in neurological outcome (171) and electrocardiographic abnormalities (167) after SAH. Data describing adrenergic neurotoxicity in human studies of SAH

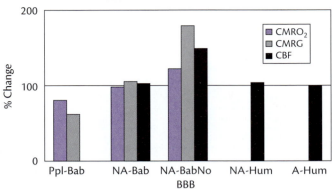

Adrenergic Effects on CBF and CMR in Human and SubHuman Primates: Role of BBB

Fig. 2.6 Effects of adrenergic drugs on cerebral blood flow and metabolism. This chart depicts the effects of intracarotid infusion of propranolol, noradrenaline (norepinephrine), and adrenaline (epinephrine) to subhuman and human primates. Baboon studies indicate that propranolol, which crosses the BBB acts to depress CMR. Noradrenaline infusion to baboons has minimal effect on CMR and CBF with an intact BBB. However, prior disruption of the BBB with urea results in noradrenaline increasing CMR and CBF. Comparable findings were reported in humans with intact BBB undergoing intracarotid infusion of adrenaline or noradrenaline during cerebral angiography. These observations indicate that CBF and CMR are activated by adrenergic influences and that the BBB has an important role in mediating the effects of systemic administration of catecholamines.

A, adrenaline; Bab, baboon; BBB, blood–brain barrier; CBF, cerebral blood flow; CMRG, cerebral metabolic rate for glucose; CMRO$_2$, cerebral metabolic rate for oxygen; Hum, human; NA, noradrenaline; Ppl, propranolol.

Data from MacKenzie E *et al.*, 'Influence of endogenous norepinephrine on CBF and metabolism', *The American Journal of Physiology*, 1976, 231, p. 489; Olesen J, 'The effect of intracarotid epinephrine, norepinephrine, and angiotensin on the regional CBF in man', *Neurology*, 1972, 22, pp. 978–987; MacKenzie ET *et al.*, 'Cerebral circulation and norepinephrine: relevance of the blood brain barrier', *American Journal of Physiology*, 1976, 231, 2, pp. 483–488.

provide strong support for the use of sympatholytic drugs as preferred antihypertensive agents in the NCCU. In addition, beta-adrenergic blocking drugs have not been reported to cause cerebral vasodilatation or increase ICP (172,173).

Calcium channel blockers

The dihydropyridine calcium channel antagonists nimodipine and nicardipine bind to the α1 subunit of the calcium channel and antagonize the slow and L-type voltage-sensitive calcium channels (174). These receptors mediate calcium entry into vascular smooth muscle cells and their blockade prevents increased cytosolic calcium and the consequent cascade of events leading to actin–myosin coupling resulting in arteriolar relaxation (174).

Nimodipine is used routinely after SAH (see Chapter 18) (174,175), where its putative neuroprotectant actions may outweigh any actions to diminish vasospasm directly (176). Nicardipine is a systemic arteriolar vasodilator (including coronary arteries) which has been used as an intra-arterial dilator during interventional neuroradiology procedures for cerebral vasospasm (177,178). It has also been delivered intrathecally with encouraging early reports of efficacy against vasospasm after SAH (179,180). Intra-arterial infusions of nimodipine (181) and verapamil (182) have also been reported as treatment for cerebral vasospasm.

Calcium channel blockers may also be reasonable choices for antihypertensive therapy in SAH based solely on the observations of their potential neuroprotective actions. However, as they are vasodilators they can modestly increase ICP (183). Nicardipine is a particularly useful antihypertensive drug in the acute phase after SAH (184) as its pharmacokinetics allow for convenient bolus administration (185).

Vasodilators

Peripheral vasodilators such as nitroprusside, nitroglycerine, and hydralazine all have potential to induce cerebral vasodilatation and cause hyperaemic intracranial hypertension (186–188). Moreover they are associated with a compensatory increase in peripheral catecholamines and renin (189), factors which theoretically may worsen ischaemic brain injury (169,170). However, the lack of bradycardia and bronchoconstriction associated with their use may make them a useful option in some patient groups.

Apart from direct cerebrovascular effects, there is concern that any antihypertensive agent may increase ICP in a normally reactive brain because of secondary cerebral vasodilation in response to reduction in systemic and cerebral perfusion pressure below relevant thresholds (190).

References

1. Mitchell BD, Emsley JG, Magavi SSP, Arlotta P, Macklis JD. Constitutive and induced neurogenesis in the adult mammalian brain: manipulation of endogenous precursors toward CNS repair. *Dev Neurosci.* 2004;26(2–4):101–17.
2. Noctor SC, Martínez-Cerdeño V, Kriegstein AR. Contribution of intermediate progenitor cells to cortical histogenesis. *Arch Neurol.* 2007;64(5):639–42.
3. Lent R, Azevedo FAC, Andrade-Moraes CH, Pinto AVO. How many neurons do you have? Some dogmas of quantitative neuroscience under revision. *Eur J Neurosci.* 2011;35(1):1–9.
4. Abbott NJ, Rönnback L, Hansson E. Astrocyte-endothelial interactions at the blood-brain barrier. *Nat Rev Neurosci.* 2006;7(1):41–53.
5. Benarroch EE. *Basic Neurosciences with Clinical Applications.* Edinburgh: Butterworth Heinemann/Elsevier; 2006.
6. Brown PD, Davies SL, Speake T, Millar ID. Molecular mechanisms of cerebrospinal fluid production. *Neuroscience.* 2004;129(4):957–70.
7. Boulton M, Armstrong D, Flessner M, Hay J, Szalai JP, Johnston M. Raised intracranial pressure increases CSF drainage through arachnoid villi and extracranial lymphatics. *Am J Physiol.* 1998;275(3 44–3):R889–R96.
8. Iliff JJ, Wang M, Liao Y, Plogg BA, Peng W, Gundersen GA, et al. A paravascular pathway facilitates CSF flow through the brain parenchyma and the clearance of interstitial solutes, including amyloid beta. *Sci Transl Med.* 2012;4(147):147ra11.
9. Xie L, Kang H, Xu Q, Chen MJ, Liao Y, Thiyagarajan M, et al. Sleep drives metabolite clearance from the adult brain. *Science.* 2013;342:373–7.
10. Nag S, Kapadia A, Stewart DJ. Review: Molecular pathogenesis of blood-brain barrier breakdown in acute brain injury. *Neuropathol Appl Neurobiol.* 2011;37(1):3–23.
11. Yang Y, Rosenberg GA. Blood-brain barrier breakdown in acute and chronic cerebrovascular disease. *Stroke.* 2011;42(11):3323–8.
12. Attwell D, Laughlin SB. An energy budget for signaling in the grey matter of the brain. *J Cereb Blood Flow Metab.* 2001;21(10):1133–45.
13. Rolfe DFS, Brown GC. Cellular energy utilization and molecular origin of standard metabolic rate in mammals. *Physiol Rev.* 1997;77(3):731–58.
14. Haydon PG, Carmignoto G. Astrocyte control of synaptic transmission and neurovascular coupling. *Physiol Rev.* 2006;86(3):1009–31.

15. Attwell D, Iadecola C. The neural basis of functional brain imaging signals. *Trends Neurosci.* 2002;25(12):621–5.
16. Chi CP, Roberts EL Jr. Energy substrates for neurons during neural activity: a critical review of the astrocyte-neuron lactate shuttle hypothesis. *J Cereb Blood Flow Metab.* 2003;23(11):1263–81.
17. Magistretti PJ, Pellerin L. Cellular mechanisms of brain energy metabolism and their relevance to functional brain imaging. *Philos Trans R Soc Lond B Biol Sci.* 1999;354(1387):1155–63.
18. Larach DB, Kofke WA, Le Roux P. Potential non-hypoxic/ischemic causes of increased cerebral interstitial fluid lactate/pyruvate ratio: a review of available literature. *Neurocrit Care.* 2011;15(3):609–22.
19. Bouzat P, Sala N, Suys T, Zerlauth JB, Marques-Vidal P, Feihl F, et al. Cerebral metabolic effects of exogenous lactate supplementation on the injured human brain. *Intensive Care Med.* 2014;40(3):412–21.
20. Bouzat P, Oddo M. Lactate and the injured brain: friend or foe? *Curr Opin Crit Care.* 2014;20(2):133–40.
21. Smith D, Pernet A, Hallett WA, Bingham E, Marsden PK, Amiel SA. Lactate: a preferred fuel for human brain metabolism in vivo. *J Cereb Blood Flow Metab.* 2003;23(6):658–64.
22. Leybaert L. Neurobarrier coupling in the brain: a partner of neurovascular and neurometabolic coupling? *J Cereb Blood Flow Metab.* 2005;25(1):2–16.
23. Pellerin L. Lactate as a pivotal element in neuron-glia metabolic cooperation. *Neurochem Int.* 2003;43(4-5):331–8.
24. Siesjö B. *Brain Energy Metabolism.* New York: John Wiley & Sons; 1978.
25. Szydlowska K, Tymianski M. Calcium, ischemia and excitotoxicity. *Cell Calcium.* 2010;47(2):122–9.
26. Benveniste H. The excitotoxin hypothesis in relation to cerebral ischemia. *Cerebrovasc Brain Metab Rev.* 1991;3:213–45.
27. Alexander SPH, Peters JA. Receptor and ion channel nomenclature supplement. *Trends Pharmacol Sci.* 1997;Suppl:1–84.
28. Gilman AG. G proteins: transducers of receptor-generated signals. *Annu Rev Biochem.* 1987;56:615–49.
29. Nishizuka Y. The role of protein kinase C in cell surface signal transduction and tumour promotion. *Nature.* 1984;308(5961):693–8.
30. Bell RM. Protein kinase C activation by diacylglycerol second messengers. *Cell.* 1986;45(5):631–2.
31. Matsuoka Y, Hossmann KA. Brain tissue osmolality after middle cerebral artery occlusion in cats. *Exp Neurol.* 1982;77(3):599–611.
32. Schulman H, Lou LL. Multifunctional Ca2+/calmodulin-dependent protein kinase: domain structure and regulation. *Trends Biochem Sci.* 1989;14(2):62–6.
33. Sheng M, McFadden G, Greenberg ME. Membrane depolarization and calcium induce c-fos transcription via phosphorylation of transcription factor CREB. *Neuron.* 1990;4(4):571–82.
34. Pulsinelli WA, Brierley JB, Plum F. Temporal profile of neuronal damage in a model of transient forebrain ischemia. *Ann Neurol.* 1982;11(5):491–8.
35. Bratton SB, Cohen GM. Apoptotic death sensor: an organelle's alter ego? *Trends Pharmacol Sci.* 2001;22(6):306–15.
36. Araki T, Kato H, Kogure K. Selective neuronal vulnerability following transient cerebral ischemia in the gerbil: distribution and time course. *Acta Neurol Scand.* 1989;80:548–53.
37. Klatzo I. Evolution of brain edema concepts. *Acta Neruochir.* 1994;60:3–6.
38. Simard JM, Kent TA, Chen M, Tarasov KV, Gerzanich V. Brain oedema in focal ischaemia: molecular pathophysiology and theoretical implications. *Lancet Neurol.* 2007;6(3):258–68.
39. Iacovetta C, Rudloff E, Kirby R. The role of aquaporin 4 in the brain. *Vet Clin Pathol.* 2012;41(1):32–44.
40. Migliati ER, Amiry-Moghaddam M, Froehner SC, Adams ME, Ottersen OP, Bhardwaj A. Na(+)-K (+)-2Cl (-) cotransport inhibitor attenuates cerebral edema following experimental stroke via the perivascular pool of aquaporin-4. *Neurocrit Care.* 2010;13(1):123–31.
41. Bullock R. Injury and cell function. In Reilly P, Bullock R (eds) *Head Injury: Pathophysiology and Management of Severe Closed Injury.* London: Chapman & Hall; 1997:121–41.
42. Tavalin SJ, Ellis EF, Satin LS. Mechanical perturbation of cultured cortical neurons reveals a stretch- induced delayed depolarization. *J Neurophysiol.* 1995;74(6):2767–73.
43. Van Landeghem FKH, Weiss T, Oehmichen M, Von Deimling A. Decreased expression of glutamate transporters in astrocytes after human traumatic brain injury. *J Neurotrauma.* 2006;23(10):1518–28.
44. Palmer A, Marion D, Botscheller M, Swedlow P, Styren S, DeKosky S. Traumatic brain injury-induced excitotoxicity assessed in a controlled cortical impact mode. *J Neurochem.* 1993;61:2015–24.
45. Scharfman HE. The neurobiology of epilepsy. *Curr Neurol Neurosci Rep.* 2007;7(4):348–54.
46. Fisher R, Pedley T, Moody WJ Jr, Prince DA. The role of extracellular potassium in hippocampal epilepsy. *Arch Neurol.* 1976;33:76–83.
47. McDonald J, Garofalo E, Hood T, Sackellares JC, Gilman S, McKeever P. Altered excitatory and inhibitory amino acid receptor binding in hippocampus of patients with temporal lobe epilepsy. *Ann Neurol.* 1991;29:529–41.
48. O'Connell B, Towfighi J, Kofke W, Hawkins R. Neuronal lesions in mercaptopropionic acid-induced status epilepticus. *Acta Neuropathol.* 1988;77:47–54.
49. Towfighi J, Kofke W, O'Connell B. Substantia nigra lesions in mercaptopropionic acid induced status epilepticus: a light and electron microscopic study. *Acta Neuropathol.* 1989;77:612–20.
50. Lothman EW, Collins RC. Kainic acid induced limbic seizures: metabolic, behavioral, electroencephalographic and neuropathological correlates. *Brain Res.* 1981;218(1–2):299–318.
51. Teitelbaum JS, Zatorre RJ, Carpenter S, Gendron D, Evans AC, Gjedde A, et al. Neurologic sequelae of domoid acid intoxication due to the ingestion of contaminated mussels. *N Engl J Med.* 1990;322(25):1781–7.
52. Plum F, Posner JB, Troy B. Cerebral metabolic and circulatory responses to induced convulsions in animals. Arch *Neurol.* 1968;18(1):1–13.
53. Kofke W, Garman R, Tom W, Rose M, Hawkins R. Alfentanil-induced hypermetabolism, seizure, and neuropathology in rats. *Anesth Analg.* 1992;75:953–64.
54. Chapman AG, Meldrum BS, Siesjö BK. Cerebral metabolic changes during prolonged epileptic seizures in rats. *J Neurochem.* 1977;28(5):1025–35.
55. Cendes F, Andermann F, Carpenter S, Zatorre RJ, Cashman NR. Temporal lobe epilepsy caused by domoic acid intoxication: evidence for glutamate receptor-mediated excitotoxicity in humans. *Ann Neurol.* 1995;37(1):123–6.
56. Ueda Y, Yokoyama H, Nakajima A, Tokumaru J, Doi T, Mitsuyama Y. Glutamate excess and free radical formation during and following kainic acid-induced status epilepticus. *Exp Brain Res.* 2002;147(2):219–26.
57. Kettenmann H, Hanisch UK, Noda M, Verkhratsky A. Physiology of microglia. *Physiol Rev.* 2010;91(2):461–553.
58. Benarroch EE. Blood-brain barrier: recent developments and clinical correlations. *Neurology.* 2012;78(16):1268–76.
59. Devinsky O, Vezzani A, Najjar S, De Lanerolle NC, Rogawski MA. Glia and epilepsy: excitability and inflammation. Trends Neurosci. 2013;36(3):174–84.
60. Lakhan SE, Kirchgessner A, Hofer M. Inflammatory mechanisms in ischemic stroke: therapeutic approaches. *J Transl Med.* 2009;7:97.
61. Czogalla A, Sikorski A. Spectrin and calpain: a 'target' and a 'sniper' in the pathology of neuronal cells. *Cell Mol Life Sci.* 2005;62(197):1913–24.
62. Martin LJ, Al-Abdulla NA, Brambrink AM, Kirsch JR, Sieber FE, Portera-Cailliau C. Neurodegeneration in excitotoxicity, global cerebral ischemia, and target deprivation: a perspective on the contributions of apoptosis and necrosis. *Brain Res Bull.* 1998;46(4):281–309.
63. Syntichaki P, Tavernarakis N. The biochemistry of neuronal necrosis: rogue biology? *Nat Rev.* 2003;4(8):672–84.
64. Celsi F, Pizzo P, Brini M, Leo S, Fotino C, Pinton P, et al. Mitochondria, calcium and cell death: a deadly triad in neurodegeneration. *Biochim Biophys Acta.* 2009;1787(5):335–44.

65. Akdemir G, Ergungor MF, Sezer M, Albayrak L, Daglioglu E, Kilinc K, et al. Therapeutic efficacy of intraventricular cyclosporine A and methylprednisolone on a global cerebral ischemia model in rats. *Neurol Res.* 2005;27(8):827–34.

66. Schinder AF, Olson EC, Spitzer NC, Montal M. Mitochondrial dysfunction is a primary event in glutamate neurotoxicity. *J Neurosci.* 1996;16(19):6125–33.

67. Sattler R, Tymianski M. Molecular mechanisms of calcium-dependent excitotoxicity. *J Mol Med (Berl).* 2000;78(1):3–13.

68. Chan SL, Mattson MP. Caspase and calpain substrates: roles in synaptic plasticity and cell death. *J Neurosci Res.* 1999;58(1):167–90.

69. Duchen MR. Mitochondria and calcium: from cell signalling to cell death. *J Physiol.* 2000;529 Pt 1:57–68.

70. Loane DJ, Faden AI. Neuroprotection for traumatic brain injury: translational challenges and emerging therapeutic strategies. *Trends Pharmacol Sci.* 2010;31(12):596–604.

71. Sokka AL, Putkonen N, Mudo G, Pryazhnikov E, Reijonen S, Khiroug L, et al. Endoplasmic reticulum stress inhibition protects against excitotoxic neuronal injury in the rat brain. *J Neurosci.* 2007;27(4):901–8.

72. Fernandez-Fernandez S, Almeida A, Bolanos JP. Antioxidant and bioenergetic coupling between neurons and astrocytes. *Biochem J.* 2012;443(1):3–11.

73. Lewen A, Matz P, Chan PH. Free radical pathways in CNS injury. *J Neurotrauma.* 2000;17(10):871–90.

74. Bolanos JP, Moro MA, Lizasoain I, Almeida A. Mitochondria and reactive oxygen and nitrogen species in neurological disorders and stroke: therapeutic implications. *Adv Drug Deliv Rev.* 2009;61(14):1299–315.

75. Terpolilli NA, Kim SW, Thal SC, Kuebler WM, Plesnila N. Inhaled nitric oxide reduces secondary brain damage after traumatic brain injury in mice. *J Cereb Blood Flow Metab.* 2013;33(2):311–18.

76. Charriaut-Marlangue C, Bonnin P, Gharib A, Leger PL, Villapol S, Pocard M, et al. Inhaled nitric oxide reduces brain damage by collateral recruitment in a neonatal stroke model. *Stroke.* 2012;43(11):3078–84.

77. Sharp FR, Massa SM, Swanson RA. Heat-shock protein protection. *Trends Neurosci.* 1999;22(3):97–9.

78. Fukuda K, Panter SS, Sharp FR, Noble LJ. Induction of heme oxygenase-1 (HO-1) after traumatic brain injury in the rat. *Neurosci Lett.* 1995;199(2):127–30.

79. O'Neill LA, Kaltschmidt C. NF-kappa B: a crucial transcription factor for glial and neuronal cell function. *Trends Neurosci.* 1997;20(6):252–8.

80. Le DA, Wu Y, Huang Z, Matsushita K, Plesnila N, Augustinack JC, et al. Caspase activation and neuroprotection in caspase-3- deficient mice after in vivo cerebral ischemia and in vitro oxygen glucose deprivation. *Proc Natl Acad Sci U S A.* 2002;99(23):15188–93.

81. Frijns CJ, Kappelle LJ. Inflammatory cell adhesion molecules in ischemic cerebrovascular disease. *Stroke.* 2002;33(8):2115–22.

82. Zhang RL, Chopp M, Zaloga C, Zhang ZG, Jiang N, Gautam SC, et al. The temporal profiles of ICAM-1 protein and mRNA expression after transient MCA occlusion in the rat. *Brain Res.* 1995;682(1-2):182–8.

83. Bergeron L, Yuan J. Sealing one's fate: control of cell death in neurons. *Curr Opin Neurobiol.* 1998;8(1):55–63.

84. Zhu P, DeCoster MA, Bazan NG. Interplay among platelet-activating factor, oxidative stress, and group I metabotropic glutamate receptors modulates neuronal survival. *J Neurosci Res.* 2004;77(4):525–31.

85. Boetkjaer A, Boedker M, Cui JG, Zhao Y, Lukiw WJ. Synergism in the repression of COX-2- and TNF-α-induction in platelet activating factor-stressed human neural cells. *Neurosci Lett.* 2007;426(1):59–63.

86. Tang SC, Arumugam TV, Xu X, Cheng A, Mughal MR, Dong GJ, et al. Pivotal role for neuronal Toll-like receptors in ischemic brain injury and functional deficits. *Proc Natl Acad Sci U S A.* 2007;104(34):13798–803.

87. Tang SC, Lathia JD, Selvaraj PK, Jo DG, Mughal MR, Cheng A, et al. Toll-like receptor-4 mediates neuronal apoptosis induced by amyloid Î2-peptide and the membrane lipid peroxidation product 4-hydroxynonenal. *Exp Neurol.* 2008;213(1):114–21.

88. Siren A, Ehrenreich H. Erythropoietin—a novel concept for neuroprotection. *Eur Arch Psych Clin Neurosci.* 2001;251(4):179–84.

89. Dawson TM. Preconditioning-mediated neuroprotection through erythropoietin? *Lancet.* 2002;359(9301):96–7.

90. Siren AL, Knerlich F, Poser W, Gleiter CH, Brück W, Ehrenreich H. Erythropoietin and erythropoietin receptor in human ischemic/hypoxic brain. *Acta Neuropathol.* 2001;101(3):271–6.

91. Klatzo I. Pathophysiological aspects of brain edema. *Acta Neuropathol.* 1987;72(3):236–9.

92. Stein DG. Brain damage, sex hormones and recovery: a new role for progesterone and estrogen? *Trends Neurosci.* 2001;24(7):386–91.

93. Wright DW, Bauer ME, Hoffman SW, Stein DG. Serum progesterone levels correlate with decreased cerebral edema after traumatic brain injury in male rats. *J Neurotrauma.* 2001;18(9):901–9.

94. Roof RL, Duvdevani R, Braswell L, Stein DG. Progesterone facilitates cognitive recovery an reduces secondary neuronal loss caused by cortical contusion injury in male rats. *Exp Neurol.* 1994;129(1):64–9.

95. Chao TC, Van Alten PJ, Walter RJ. Steroid sex hormones and macrophage function: modulation of reactive oxygen intermediates and nitrite release. *Am J Reprod Immunol.* 1994;32(1):43–52.

96. Donnan GA. The 2007 Feinberg lecture: a new road map for neuroprotection. *Stroke.* 2008;39(1):242–8.

97. Kofke WA. Incrementally applied multifaceted therapeutic bundles in neuroprotection clinical trials … time for change. *Neurocrit Care.* 2010;12(3):438–44.

98. Stefan H, Feuerstein TJ, Stefan H, Feuerstein TJ. Novel anticonvulsant drugs. *Pharmacol Therapeut.* 2007;113(1):165–83.

99. LaRoche SM, Helmers SL, LaRoche SM, Helmers SL. The new antiepileptic drugs: scientific review. *JAMA.* 2004;291(5):605–14.

100. Bialer M, White HS. Key factors in the discovery and development of new antiepileptic drugs. *Nat Rev Drug Discov.* 2010;9(1):68–82.

101. Loscher W, Schmidt D. Epilepsy: perampanel—new promise for refractory epilepsy? *Nat Rev Neurol.* 2012;8(12):661–2.

102. Hemmings HC, Jr., Akabas MH, Goldstein PA, Trudell JR, Orser BA, Harrison NL. Emerging molecular mechanisms of general anesthetic action. *Trends Pharmacol Sci.* 2005;26(10):503–10.

103. Sloan TB. Anesthetics and the brain. *Anesthesiol Clin North America.* 2002;20(2):265–92.

104. Smith AL, Wollman H. Cerebral blood flow and metabolism: effects of anesthetic drugs and techniques. *Anesthesiology.* 1972;36(4):378–400.

105. Shapiro HM, Galindo A, Wyte SR, Harris AB, Shapiro HM, Galindo A, et al. Rapid intraoperative reduction of intracranial pressure with thiopentone. *Br J Anaesth.* 1973;45(10):1057–62.

106. Mizobe T, Maghsoudi K, Sitwala K, Tianzhi G, Ou J, Maze M. Antisense technology reveals the alpha(2A) adrenoceptor to be the subtype mediating the hypnotic response to the highly selective agonist, dexmedetomidine, in the locus coeruleus of the rat. *J Clin Invest.* 1996;98(5):1076–80.

107. Bekker AY, Basile J, Gold M, Riles T, Adelman M, Cuff G, et al. Dexmedetomidine for awake carotid endarterectomy: efficacy, hemodynamic profile, and side effects. *J Neurosurg Anesthesiol.* 2004;16(2):126–35.

108. Drummond JC, Dao AV, Roth DM, Cheng C-R, Atwater BI, Minokadeh A, et al. Effect of dexmedetomidine on cerebral blood flow velocity, cerebral metabolic rate, and carbon dioxide response in normal humans. *Anesthesiology.* 2008;108(2):225–32.

109. Mirski MA, Lewin JJ, 3rd, Ledroux S, Thompson C, Murakami P, Zink EK, et al. Cognitive improvement during continuous sedation in critically ill, awake and responsive patients: the Acute Neurological ICU Sedation Trial (ANIST). *Intensive Care Med.* 2010;36(9):1505–13.

110. Anis N, Berry S, Burton N, Lodge D. The dissociative anesthetics, ketamine and phencyclidine, selectively reduce excitation of central mammalian neurones by N-methyl-aspartate. *Br J Pharmacol.* 1983;79:565–75.

111. Henriksen G, Willoch F. Imaging of opioid receptors in the central nervous system. *Brain.* 2008;131(Pt 5):1171–96.

112. Wainger B, Brenner G. Mechanisms of chronic pain. In Longnecker D, Brown D, Newman M, Zapol WM (eds) *Anesthesiology* (2nd edn). New York: McGraw Hill; 2012:1516–32.

113. Fornasari D. Pain mechanisms in patients with chronic pain. *Clin Drug Invest*. 2012;32 Suppl 1:45–52.

114. Apkarian AV, Bushnell MC, Treede R-D, Zubieta J-K. Human brain mechanisms of pain perception and regulation in health and disease. *Eur J Pain*. 2005;9(4):463–84.

115. Nestler EJ, Aghajanian GK. Molecular and cellular basis of addiction. *Science*. 1997;278(5335):58–63.

116. Hoffman WE, Cunningham F, James MK, Baughman VL, Albrecht RF. Effects of remifentanil, a new short-acting opioid, on cerebral blood flow, brain electrical activity, and intracranial pressure in dogs anesthetized with isoflurane and nitrous oxide. *Anesthesiology*. 1993;79(1):107–13.

117. Rosow C, Dershwitz M. Pharmacology of opioid analgesics. In Longnecker D, Brown D, Newman M, Zapol WM (eds) *Anesthesiology* (2nd edn). New York: McGraw Hill; 2012:869–96.

118. Ajori L, Nazari L, Mazloomfard MM, Amiri Z. Effects of gabapentin on postoperative pain, nausea and vomiting after abdominal hysterectomy: a double blind randomized clinical trial. *Arch Gynecol Obstet*. 2012;285(3):677–82.

119. Clarke H, Bonin RP, Orser BA, Englesakis M, Wijeysundera DN, Katz J. The prevention of chronic postsurgical pain using gabapentin and pregabalin: a combined systematic review and meta-analysis. *Anesth Analg*. 2012;115(2):428–42.

120. Morimoto S-i, Ito M, Oda S, Sugiyama A, Kuroda M, Adachi-Akahane S. Spinal mechanism underlying the antiallodynic effect of gabapentin studied in the mouse spinal nerve ligation model. *J Pharmacol Sci*. 2012;118(4):455–66.

121. Todd RD, McDavid SM, Brindley RL, Jewell ML, Currie KPM. Gabapentin inhibits catecholamine release from adrenal chromaffin cells. *Anesthesiology*. 2012;116(5):1013–24.

122. Wei X, Wei W. Role of gabapentin in preventing fentanyl- and morphine-withdrawal-induced hyperalgesia in rats. *J Anesth*. 2012;26(2):236–41.

123. Yoshizumi M, Parker RA, Eisenach JC, Hayashida K-i. Gabapentin inhibits γ-amino butyric acid release in the locus coeruleus but not in the spinal dorsal horn after peripheral nerve injury in rats. *Anesthesiology*. 2012;116(6):1347–53.

124. Cai K, Nanga RP, Lamprou L, Schinstine C, Elliott M, Hariharan H, *et al*. The impact of gabapentin administration on brain GABA and glutamate concentrations: a 7T (1)H-MRS study. *Neuropsychopharmacology*. 2012;37(13):2764–71.

125. Matsui-Sakata A, Ohtani H, Sawada Y. Pharmacokinetic-pharmacodynamic analysis of antipsychotics-induced extrapyramidal symptoms based on receptor occupancy theory incorporating endogenous dopamine release. *Drug Metab Pharmacokinet*. 2005;20(3):187–99.

126. Mokhtarani M, Mahgoub AN, Morioka N, Doufas AG, Dae M, Shaughnessy TE, *et al*. Buspirone and meperidine synergistically reduce the shivering threshold. *Anesth Analg*. 2001;93(5):1233–9.

127. Simopoulos TT, Smith HS, Peeters-Asdourian C, Stevens DS. Use of meperidine in patient-controlled analgesia and the development of a normeperidine toxic reaction. *Arch Surg*. 2002;137(1):84–8.

128. Pino R, Ali A. Monitoring and managing neuromuscular blockade. In Longnecker D, Brown D, Newman M, Zapol WM (eds) *Anesthesiology* (2nd edn). New York: McGraw Hill; 2012:619–38.

129. Lanier WL, Iaizzo PA, Milde JH. Cerebral function and muscle afferent activity following intravenous succinylcholine in dogs anesthetized with halothane: the effects of pretreatment with a defasciculating dose of pancuronium. *Anesthesiology*. 1989;71(1):87–95.

130. Kofke W, Shaheen N, McWhorter J, Sinz E, Hobbs G. Transcranial Doppler ultrasonography with induction of anesthesia and neuromuscular blockade in surgical patients. *J Clin Anesth*. 2001;13:335–8.

131. Rabinstein AA, Benarroch EE. Treatment of paroxysmal sympathetic hyperactivity. *Curr Treat Options Neurol*. 2008;10(2):151–7.

132. Baguley IJ, Heriseanu RE, Cameron ID, Nott MT, Slewa-Younan S, Baguley IJ, *et al*. A critical review of the pathophysiology of dysautonomia following traumatic brain injury. *Neurocrit Care*. 2008;8(2):293–300.

133. Olesen J, Hougard K, Hertz M. Isoproterenol and propranolol: ability to cross the blood-brain barrier and effects on cerebral circulation in man. *Stroke*. 1978;9(4):344–9.

134. Becker R, Benes L, Sure U, Hellwig D, Bertalanffy H. Intrathecal baclofen alleviates autonomic dysfunction in severe brain injury. *J Clin Neurosci*. 2000;7(4):316–19.

135. Baldessarini RJ, Tarazi FI. Pharmacotherapy of psychosis and mania and accompanying on line drug monographs. In Brunton LL, Lazo JS, Parker KL, Buxton IO, Blumenthal DK (eds) *Goodman & Gilman's The Pharmacological Basis of Therapeutics* (11th edn). New York: McGrawHill; 2006:461–500.

136. Gan TJ. Postoperative nausea and vomiting—can it be eliminated? *JAMA*. 2002;287(10):1233–6.

137. Kovac AL. Prevention and treatment of postoperative nausea and vomiting. *Drugs*. 2000;59(2):213–43.

138. Watcha MF. Postoperative nausea and emesis. *Anesthesiol Clin North America*. 2002;20(3):709–22.

139. Fabling JM, Gan TJ, Guy J, Borel CO, el-Moalem HE, Warner DS. Postoperative nausea and vomiting. A retrospective analysis in patients undergoing elective craniotomy. *J Neurosurg Anesthesiol* 1997;9(4):308–12.

140. Fabling JM, Gan TJ, El-Moalem HE, Warner DS, Borel CO. A randomized, double-blind comparison of ondansetron versus placebo for prevention of nausea and vomiting after infratentorial craniotomy. *J Neurosurg Anesth*. 2002;14(2):102–7.

141. Apfel CC, Korttila K, Abdalla M, Kerger H, Turan A, Vedder I, *et al*. A factorial trial of six interventions for the prevention of postoperative nausea and vomiting. *N Engl J Med*. 2004;350(24):2441–51.

142. Seynaeve C, Verweij J, de Mulder PH. 5-HT3 receptor antagonists, a new approach in emesis: a review of ondansetron, granisetron and tropisetron. *Anticancer Drugs*. 1991;2(4):343–55.

143. Jacot A, Bissonnette B, Favre J, Ravussin P. The effect of ondansetron on intracranial pressure and cerebral perfusion pressure in neurosurgical patients. *Ann Fr Anesth Reanim*. 1998;17(3):220–6.

144. Ritter MJ, Goodman BP, Sprung J, Wijdicks EF. Ondansetron-induced multifocal encephalopathy. *Mayo Clin Proc*. 2003;78(9):1150–2.

145. Fabling JM, Gan TJ, El-Moalem HE, Warner DS, Borel CO. A randomized, double-blinded comparison of ondansetron, droperidol, and placebo for prevention of postoperative nausea and vomiting after supratentorial craniotomy. *Anesth Analg*. 2000;91(2):358–61.

146. Hamik A, Peroutka SJ. Differential interactions of traditional and novel antiemetics with dopamine D2 and 5-hydroxytryptamine3 receptors. *Cancer Chemother Pharmacol*. 1989;24(5):307–10.

147. Misfeldt BB, Jorgensen PB, Spotoft H, Ronde F. The effects of droperidol and fentanyl on intracranial pressure and cerebral perfusion pressure in neurosurgical patients. *Br J Anaesth*. 1976;48(10):963–8.

148. Lim BS, Pavy TJ, Lumsden G. The antiemetic and dysphoric effects of droperidol in the day surgery patient. *Anaesth Intensive Care*. 1999;27(4):371–4.

149. Coppolino CA, Wallace G. Trimethobenzamide antiemetic in immediate postoperative period. Double-blind study in 2,000 cases. *JAMA*. 1962;180:326–8.

150. Crowell EB, Jr., Ketchum JS. The treatment of scopolamine-induced delirium with physostigmine. *Clin Pharmacol Ther*. 1967;8(3):409–14.

151. Contreras-Dominguez V, Carbonell-Bellolio P. Prophylactic antiemetic therapy for acute abdominal surgery. A comparative study of droperidol, metoclopramide, tropisetron, granisetron and dexamethasone. *Rev Bras Anestesiol*. 2008;58(1):35–44.

152. MacLaren R, Kiser TH, Fish DN, Wischmeyer PE. Erythromycin vs metoclopramide for facilitating gastric emptying and tolerance to intragastric nutrition in critically ill patients. *JPEN J Parenter Enteral Nutr*. 2008;32(4):412–19.

153. Newton-John H. Acute upper airway obstruction due to supraglottic dystonia induced by a neuroleptic. *BMJ*. 1988;297(6654):964–5.

154. Unlugenc H, Guler T, Gunes Y, Isik G. Comparative study of the antiemetic efficacy of ondansetron, propofol and midazolam in the early postoperative period. *Eur J Anaesthesiol*. 2004;21(1):60–5.

155. Cooper JR, Bloom FER, Robert H. *The Biochemical Basis of Neuropharmacology* (8th edn). New York: Oxford University Press; 2002.

156. Buisson A, Callebert J, Mathieu E, Plotkine M, Boulu RG. Striatal protection induced by lesioning the substantia nigra of rats subjected to focal ischemia. *J Neurochem*. 1992;59(3):1153–7.

157. Westfall T, Westfall D. Adrenergic agonists and antagonists. In Brunton L, Chabner B, Knollmann B (eds) *Goodman & Gilman's The Pharmacological Basis of Therapeutics* (12th edn). New York: McGraw-Hill; 2011:277–333.

158. Pardridge WM, Oldendorf WH. Transport of metabolic substrates through the blood-brain barrier. *J Neurochem*. 1977;28(1):5–12.

159. Fernstrom JD, Fernstrom MH. Tyrosine, phenylalanine, and catecholamine synthesis and function in the brain. *J Nutr*. 2007;137(6 Suppl 1):1539S–47S.

160. Berridge CW, Devilbiss DM. Psychostimulants as cognitive enhancers: the prefrontal cortex, catecholamines, and attention-deficit/hyperactivity disorder. *Biol Psychiatry*. 2011;69(12):e101–11.

161. MacKenzie E, McCulloch J, Harper A. Influence of endogenous norepinephrine on CBF and metabolism. *Am J Physiol*. 1976;231:489–94.

162. Olesen J. The effect of intracarotid epinephrine, norepinephrine, and angiotensin on the regional CBF in man. *Neurology*. 1972;22:978–87.

163. Greenfield Jr JC, Tindall GT. Effect of norepinephrine, epinephrine, and angiotensin on blood flow in the internal carotid artery of man. *J Clin Invest*. 1968;47(7):1672–84.

164. MacKenzie ET, McCulloch J, O'Keane M, Pickard JD, Harper AM. Cerebral circulation and norepinephrine: relevance of the blood brain barrier. *Am J Physiol*. 1976;231(2):483–8.

165. Dhar R, Scalfani MT, Zazulia AR, Videen TO, Derdeyn CP, Diringer MN. Comparison of induced hypertension, fluid bolus, and blood transfusion to augment cerebral oxygen delivery after subarachnoid hemorrhage. *J Neurosurg*. 2012;116(3):648–56.

166. Germano A, D'Avella D, Cicciarello R, Hayes RL, Tomasello F, Doczi T, *et al*. Blood-brain barrier permeability changes after experimental subarachnoid hemorrhage. *Neurosurgery*. 1992;30(6):882–6.

167. Cruickshank J, Neil-Dwyer G, Lane J. The effect of oral propranolol upon the ECG changes occurring in subarachnoid hemorrhage. *Cardiovasc Res*. 1975;9:236–45.

168. Svengaard N, Brismar J, Delgado T, Rosengren E. Subarachnoid haemorrhage in the rat: effect on the development of vasospasm of selective lesions of the catecholamine systems in the lower brain stem. *Stroke*. 1985;16:602–8.

169. Werner C, Hoffman W, Thomas C, Miletich D, Albrecht R. Ganglionic blockade improves neurologic outcome from incomplete ischemia in rats: partial reversal by exogenous catecholamines. *Anesthesiology*. 1990;73:923–9.

170. Busto R, Harik S, Yoshida S, Scheinberg P, Ginsberg M. Cerebral norepinephrine depletion enhances recovery after brain ischemia. *Ann Neurol*. 1985;18:329–36.

171. Neil-Dwyer G, Walter P, Cruickshank J. Beta-blockade benefits patients following a subarachnoid hemorrhage. *Eur J Clin Pharmacol*. 1985;28:25–9.

172. Schroeder T, Schierbeck J, Howardy P, Knudsen L, Skafte-Holm P, Gefke K. Effect of labetalol on CBF and middle cerebral arterial flow velocity in healthy volunteers. *Neurol Res*. 1991;13:10–12.

173. Van Aken H, Puchstein C, Schweppe M-L, Heinecke A. Effect of labetalol on intracranial pressure in dogs with and without intracranial hypertension. *Acta Anaesth Scand*. 1982;26:615–19.

174. Michel T, Hoffman B. Treatment of myocardial ischemia and hypertension. In Brunton L, Chabner B, Knollmann B (eds) *Goodman & Gilman's The Pharmacological Basis of Therapeutics* (12th edn). New York: McGraw-Hill; 2011:745–88.

175. Pickard J, Murray G, Illingworth R, Shaw M, Teasdale G, Foy P, *et al*. Effect of oral nimodipine on cerebral infarction and outcome after subarachnoid haemorrhage: British aneurysm nimodipine trial. *BMJ*. 1989;298:636–42.

176. Laskowitz DT, Kolls BJ. Neuroprotection in subarachnoid hemorrhage. *Stroke*. 2010;41(10 Suppl):S79–84.

177. Badjatia N, Topcuoglu MA, Pryor JC, Rabinov JD, Ogilvy CS, Carter BS, *et al*. Preliminary experience with intra-arterial nicardipine as a treatment for cerebral vasospasm. *AJNR Am J Neuroradiol*. 2004;25(5):819–26.

178. Nogueira RG, Lev MH, Roccatagliata L, Hirsch JA, Gonzalez RG, Ogilvy CS, *et al*. Intra-arterial nicardipine infusion improves CT perfusion-measured cerebral blood flow in patients with subarachnoid hemorrhage-induced vasospasm. *AJNR Am J Neuroradiol*. 2009;30(1):160–4.

179. Barth M, Capelle H-H, Weidauer S, Weiss C, Munch E, Thome C, *et al*. Effect of nicardipine prolonged-release implants on cerebral vasospasm and clinical outcome after severe aneurysmal subarachnoid hemorrhage: a prospective, randomized, double-blind phase IIa study. *Stroke*. 2007;38(2):330–6.

180. Ehtisham A, Taylor S, Bayless L, Samuels OB, Klein MW, Janzen JM. Use of intrathecal nicardipine for aneurysmal subarachnoid hemorrhage-induced cerebral vasospasm. *South Med J*. 2009;102:150–3.

181. Wolf S, Martin H, Landscheidt JF, Rodiek SO, Schurer L, Lumenta CB. Continuous selective intraarterial infusion of nimodipine for therapy of refractory cerebral vasospasm. *Neurocrit Care*. 2010;12(3):346–51.

182. Albanese E, Russo A, Quiroga M, Willis RN, Jr., Mericle RA, Ulm AJ. Ultrahigh-dose intraarterial infusion of verapamil through an indwelling microcatheter for medically refractory severe vasospasm: initial experience. *J Neurosurg*. 2010;113:913–22.

183. Hayashi M, Kobayashi H, Kawano H, Handa Y, Hirose S. Treatment of systemic hypertension and intracranial hypertension and intracranial hypertension in cases of brain hemorrhage. *Stroke*. 1988;19:314–21.

184. Flamm E, Adams HJ, Beck DW, Pinto RS, Marler JR, Walker MD, *et al*. Dose-escalation study of intravenous nicardipine in patients with aneurysmal subarachnoid hemorrhage. *J Neurosurg*. 1988;68:393–400.

185. Cheung AT, Guvakov DV, Weiss SJ, Savino JS, Salgo IS, Meng QC. Nicardipine intravenous bolus dosing for acutely decreasing arterial blood pressure during general anesthesia for cardiac operations: pharmacokinetics, pharmacodynamics, and associated effects on left ventricular function. *Anesth Analg*. 1999;89(5):1116–23.

186. Overgaard J, Skinhoj E. A paradoxical cerebral hemodynamic effect of hydralazine. *Stroke*. 1975;6(4):402–10.

187. Griswold W, Reznik V, Mendoza S. Nitroprusside induced intracranial hypertension. *JAMA*. 1981;246:2679–80.

188. Dohi S, Matsumoto M, Takahashi K. The effects of nitroglycerin on cerebrospinal fluid pressure in awake and anesthetized humans. *Anesthesiology*. 1981;54:511–14.

189. Stanek B, Zimpfer M, Fitzal S, Raberger G. Plasma catecholamines, plasma renin activity and haemodynamics during sodium nitroprusside-induced hypotension and additional beta-blockage with bunitrolol. *Eur J Clin Pharmacol*. 1981;19:317–22.

190. Rosner M, Becker D. Origin and evolution of plateau waves. Experimental observations and a theoretical model. *J Neurosurg*. 1984;50:312–24.

CHAPTER 3

Cerebral blood flow physiology, pharmacology, and pathophysiology

Chandril Chugh and W. Andrew Kofke

Cerebral blood flow (CBF) is defined as the amount of blood received by the brain in a given time, and expressed in millilitres per 100 g of brain per minute. The adult brain receives around 15% of the resting cardiac output, approximately 700 mL of blood every minute, and accounts for 20% of basal oxygen consumption. Blood flow to the grey and white matter is around 50 mL/100 g/min and 20 mL/100 g/min respectively (1,2). CBF is very tightly regulated and understanding the physiological basis of this regulation is very important in the management of patients with brain injury.

Anatomy of cerebral vasculature

The aortic arch gives rise to three arterial vessels which provide macrovascular arterial inflow to the brain as depicted in Figure 3.1. Unlike in other major organs, this anatomical arrangement provides the brain with inherent cerebrovascular reserve and collateral flow based on redundant inflow paths via the circle of Willis, thereby providing a first level of protection against conductance vessel obstruction. The cerebral microvasculature is a complex array of small arterioles supplying a hexagonal column of cortical tissue, with intervening boundary zones (1). This arrangement, with its extrinsic neural innervations (see 'Neural Control of Cerebral Blood Flow'), prevents brain tissue from being exposed to surges in systemic blood pressure. Histologically, cerebral arteries and arterioles have only a single elastic lamina and this influences their response to alteration in luminal pressure. They are also lacking a vasa vasorum (3) and were believed to derive their nutrition from the cerebrospinal fluid (CSF) via adventitial hollow channels (4). However, it is tempting to speculate that the recently described glymphatic system of perivascular CSF flow is the primary mechanism by which CSF provides the endothelial nutritive source throughout the brain as well as being a functional waste clearance pathway (5).

Cerebral microvessels are notably different from systemic vessels through their intimate relation to perivascular astrocytic foot processes which, together, constitute the blood–brain barrier (BBB). The BBB and the vascular endothelium lack the fenestrations seen in systemic vessels and have fewer pinocytic vesicles but five to six times more mitochondria. Together these form the microvascular unit which exerts significant control on nutrient and metabolite ingress and egress, and regulation of the cerebral circulation (6). Taken together, the neurons, astrocytes and other glia, vascular endothelium as a constituent of the BBB, and vascular elements comprise a functional neurovascular unit which controls neurovascular, neurometabolic, and neurobarrier coupling and integration (7). This concept is illustrated in Figure 3.2, and its physiological consequences are reviewed subsequently in this chapter.

Pial veins do not follow the same routes as pial arteries and do not significantly change in diameter with changes in CBF. The venous endothelium is part of the BBB and is the most frequent site of BBB breakdown (6). The venous drainage of the brain is via parenchymal venules and veins which, after traversing CSF-containing spaces, continue via endothelialized channels and sinuses embedded within the dura (Figure 3.3A). These ultimately drain into the jugular veins. Elevations in intracranial pressure (ICP) can obstruct venous outflow, thus creating a venous vascular 'waterfall' effect wherein intracranial venous pressure is effectively isolated from extracranial venous pressure (Figure 3.3B) (8–11). This might account for the notion that increases in venous pressure, for example, from positive end-expiratory pressure during mechanical ventilation, are not transmitted to the brain if ICP exceeds venous pressure (12). Increased ICP can increase intracranial venous pressure and thereby predispose to tissue oedema (13). It was previously believed that blood from the supratentorial compartment drained exclusively into the right internal jugular vein, and that from infratentorial brain tissue into the left internal jugular vein, but recent studies have shown that there is considerable variation between individuals (14).

Physiology of the regulation of cerebral blood flow

CBF is regulated via complex mechanisms involving neural, humoral, and myogenic processes (15–17) that together are responsible for cerebral autoregulation, flow–metabolism coupling, and neurogenic CBF regulation.

Pressure autoregulation

Cerebral pressure autoregulation is the process by which constant blood flow to the brain is maintained in the face of changes in mean arterial (MAP) and cerebral perfusion (CPP) pressures. CBF is maintained at a relatively constant level when MAP is between 50 and

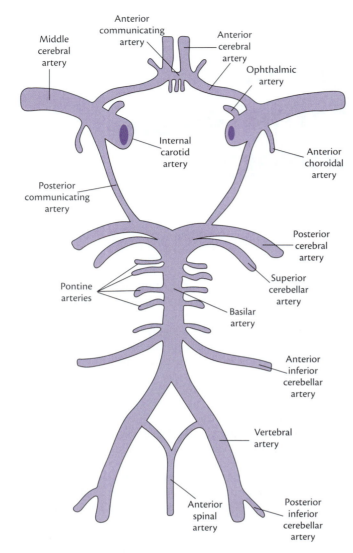

Fig. 3.1 Arterial supply to the brain. Schematic representation of the circle of Willis, arteries of the brain, and brainstem. Blood enters and flows up to the brain through the vertebral arteries and through the internal carotid arteries.
Figure reproduced with permission from http://commons.wikimedia.org/wiki/File:Circle_of_Willis_en.svg. Adapted from: This figure was originally published in *Gray's Anatomy*, Twentieth edition, thoroughly revised and re-edited by Warren H. Lewis, plate 722, Elsevier. Copyright the editors, 1918.

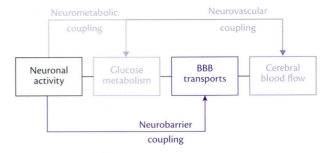

Fig. 3.2 The neurovascular unit and neurovascular coupling. Neuronal activity triggers various responses that act together to adapt the delivery of energy substrate to the local neuronal needs. Neurovascular coupling involves the dilation of blood vessels to increase the local blood flow as needed, while neurometabolic coupling involves the stimulation of energy metabolism in line with cellular ATP consumption. It is proposed that neuronal activity brings about changes at the level of the blood–brain barrier (BBB), establishing neurobarrier coupling that acts to increase the transport of energy substrate, mainly glucose, across the barrier.

demonstrate that the LLA for individual non-anaesthetized patients occurs at a MAP level approximately 25% lower than basal MAP, and that symptoms of cerebral hypoperfusion arise when MAP reaches 40–50% of the basal value. Nonetheless, no studies have validated the existence (or the specific value) of a LLA above 50 mmHg in normal humans, although there is some inferential evidence that it might be higher in the context of traumatic brain injury (TBI) (23). In a study utilizing the pressure reactivity index (PRx) as a measure of autoregulatory function (see Chapter 10), Steiner and colleagues demonstrated that cerebral autoregulation was maintained in many TBI patients within a narrow MAP window (10–20 mmHg versus the conventionally accepted 100 mmHg range) that is unique to each patient, but generally in the 70–90 mmHg range of CPP (24). Overall we consider the LLA to be an unsettled issue and likely to be individual specific in pathological conditions.

The detailed mechanisms underlying cerebral pressure autoregulation are not fully elucidated, but vascular endothelium, vascular smooth muscle, and nerves appear to be directly involved. Endothelium is a mechanoreceptor that is very sensitive to changes in blood pressure and mechanical forces. Increased blood flow velocity (FV), shear stress, and transmural pressure are the strongest vasoconstrictor stimuli to the endothelium (25). Vascular smooth muscle is directly responsible for arteriolar vasoconstriction, and the presence of endothelial-derived vasoconstrictors in arteries exposed to high blood pressure has been demonstrated (26–28). In response to mechanical stress the endothelium responds by reflex vasoconstriction, the so-called Bayliss effect (26), via activation of endothelial mediators (Figure 3.5). The Bayliss effect underlies the myogenic hypothesis of cerebral autoregulation which caters to continuous constriction of vascular smooth muscle in the presence of mechanical stress (29). Myogenic tone thus develops and adjusts to blood pressure and underlies the notion of a cerebral critical closing pressure (CCP), which is defined as that acutely changed decrease in systemic blood pressure at which CBF falls to zero (30,31). Based on variations in basal myogenic tone in response to basal luminal pressure, CCP increases and decreases commensurate with changes in blood pressure. The net effect is to maintain a constant relationship between MAP and CCP and an alternate, physiological, definition of CPP is MAP-CCP (30–32). It has been

150 mmHg, but above and below these values varies directly with MAP (Figure 3.4). Although the MAP range of 50–150 mmHg has become a key part of traditional physiological teaching, questions have been raised about the validity of 50 mmHg as the lower limit of autoregulation (LLA). Presuppositions about the LLA underlie many clinical decisions but, in an editorial, Drummond argues that a higher pressure of around 70 mmHg might be a more appropriate LLA in many circumstances (18). His scepticism partly arises from the original value of 50 mmHg being derived from a 1959 study in which blood pressure was lowered in pregnant volunteers using a cerebral vasodilator (hydralazine) (19). Many subsequent studies have suggested that the LLA is likely to be higher than 50 mmHg, but this value has persisted in the literature. Of note, the investigations of Finnerty and colleagues (20), and Strandgaard (21,22),

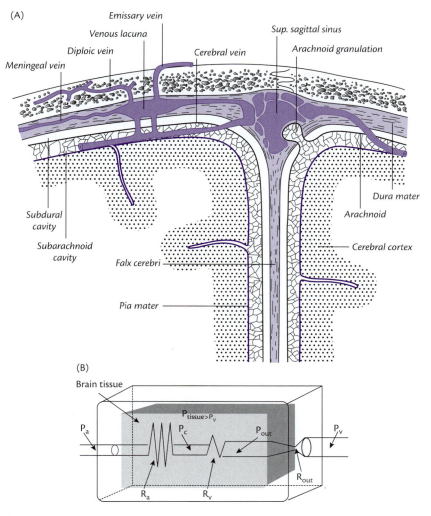

Fig. 3.3 Cerebral venous drainage.
(A) Cerebral veins and sinuses. The cerebral veins traverse the skull and the cerebrospinal fluid space as blood flows out of the brain. The sagittal sinus is depicted. Note the arachnoid granulations from which CSF is transported from brain to blood and the cerebral vein traversing from brain, across CSF to the sagittal sinus.
http://www.netterimages.com/image/1369.htm.
(B) Schematic illustration of the brain and its surroundings being enclosed in a rigid shell. When pressure in the CSF space exceeds pressure in the traversing veins a vascular waterfall condition can be established with increased P_{out} which encourages brain oedema and further increases in ICP.

P_a, intra-arterial hydrostatic pressure; P_c, intracapillary hydrostatic pressure; P_{out}, hydrostatic pressure in large cerebral veins; P_{tissue}, hydrostatic pressure in brain tissue; P_v, hydrostatic pressure in extracranial veins; R_a, precapillary flow resistance; R_{out}, venous outflow resistance which is affected by C pressure as the vein transits from brain to skull or sinus; R_v, venous flow resistance.
Reproduced from Grände P-O et al., 'Volume-targeted therapy of increased intracranial pressure: the Lund concept unifies surgical and non-surgical treatments', *Acta Anaesthesiologica Scandinavia*, 46, 8, pp. 929–941, Copyright 2002, with permission from John Wiley & Sons and The Acta Anaesthesiologica Scandinavica Foundation.

suggested that CCP can also be defined clinically at the bedside by a combined extrapolation of transcranial Doppler and arterial waveforms to zero blood FV (Figure 3.6) (33–40).

Flow–metabolism coupling

In addition to the aforementioned myogenic processes which maintain appropriate flow with varying blood pressure independent of metabolic needs, blood flow to the brain also varies according to metabolic requirements (Figure 3.7). In this way regional blood flow and metabolism are tightly coupled. Action potential generation as well as interneuron interactions are potent stimuli of multiple mediators of neurovascular coupling (41,42), including potassium and hydrogen ions which relax vascular smooth muscles and cause

cerebral vasodilatation (43). Cerebral metabolites also play an important role in regulation of CBF. The concentration of adenosine increases during neuronal transmission and in its turn causes vasodilation. Elevation of excitatory neurotransmitters such as glutamate also leads to increases in the concentration of adenosine and subsequent vasodilation (44). Nitric oxide (NO) has been known for some time to cause cerebral vasodilation but recent research suggests that it may primarily act as a second messenger supplying cGMP for other compounds to act on vascular smooth muscle (45).

An important element of flow–metabolism coupling is the CBF response to physiological and metabolic abnormalities, including changes in carbon dioxide, oxygenation, and glucose, to maintain adequate nutritive flow.

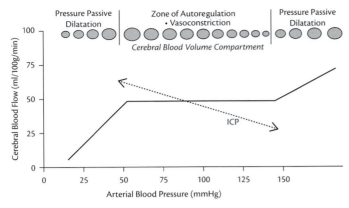

Fig. 3.4 Cerebral autoregulation. Within the autoregulatory range between 50 and 150 mmHg MAP (x-axis), CBF (y-axis) remains stable. Over this range there is no correlation between pressure and flow, whereas above and below the autoregulatory range there is a degree of correlation of CBF with MAP. Note also that changes in CBV arise secondary to normal autoregulation and that this can be important in the context of elevated ICP. This diagram indicates the potential for CBV changes in normally autoregulating brain areas to affect ICP in the context of reduced intracranial compliance (dashed line). Note that this neglects considerations of blood pressure effects on CBV on injured, poorly regulating brain areas, which can display pressure passive dilatation with increased pressure, rather than vasoconstriction that arises with normal autoregulation.
CBF, cerebral blood flow; CBV, cerebral blood volume; ICP, intracranial pressure; MAP, mean arterial blood pressure.
Reprinted from *Journal of Clinical Neuroscience*, 12, 6, Yam AT et al., 'Cerebral autoregulation and ageing', pp. 643–646, Copyright 2005, with permission from Elsevier.

Carbon dioxide

Tissue acidosis, indicating anaerobic metabolism, causes an increase in CBF. Hydrogen ions have been implicated in mediating the vasodilatory effects of metabolically produced carbon dioxide and lactic acid, although NO may be the preferred mediator for hypercapnia-induced vasodilation as NO inhibition prevents carbon dioxide-induced vasodilation (46,47). Hypercapnia produces acidosis and leads to hyperaemia, whereas hypocapnia produces significant decrements in CBF (Figure 3.8) (48,49). Notably, hyperventilation can decrease CBF enough to lead to increased lactate production (49–52), brain tissue hypoxia (49), and related electroencephalogram changes (51), although it has never been shown to produce histologically verifiable tissue damage. Nonetheless, the routine application of hyperventilation has been associated with worse outcome after TBI (53).

Oxygen

Hypoxaemia is a potent cerebral vasodilator, producing significant hyperaemia when PaO_2 decreases below 6.7 kPa (50.25 mmHg) (Figure 3.8) (54), likely secondary to brain tissue lactic acidosis (55). Conversely hyperoxia produces mild vasoconstriction (53).

Anaemia

CBF responds to changes in haematocrit according to oxygen delivery, such that anaemia produces increases in flow (56). Animal studies (57) and theoretical analysis (58) suggest that, with progressive decrement in haematocrit, CBF is initially increased due to anaemia-related reduction in viscosity. Subsequent active

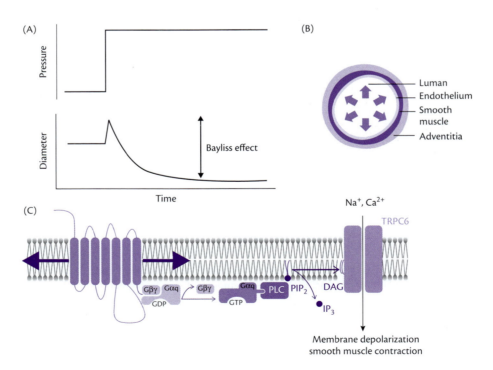

Fig. 3.5 The Bayliss effect.
(A) Increasing pressure in certain blood vessels causes vasoconstriction, a phenomenon known as the Bayliss effect.
(B) The Bayliss effect is mediated by the smooth muscle layer of the vessel, independent of the inner layer of endothelial cells.
(C) Proposed mechanism for stretch-induced activation of the transient receptor potential cation channel, subfamily C, member 6 (TRPC6), in vascular smooth muscle membranes.

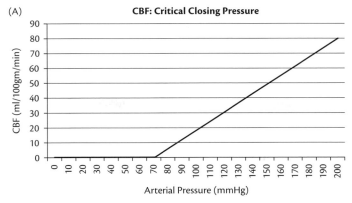

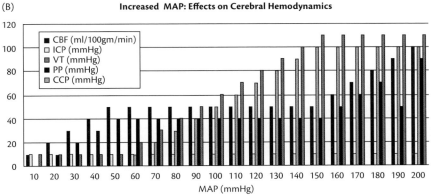

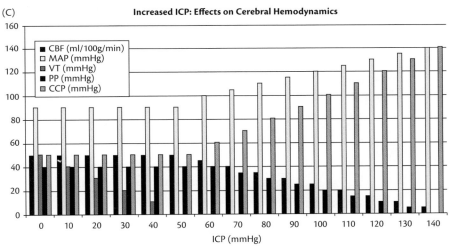

Fig. 3.6 Critical closing pressure (CCP).

(A) Dynamic pressure–flow relationships (DPFRs) for the cerebral vascular bed in subhuman primates. Data were obtained by oscillating aortic pressures between 230 and 105 mmHg. All data points are obtained within a 4-second period. Closed squares represent averaged values for each heartbeat during the entire pump cycle. Open triangles represent data obtained during a prolonged diastole occurring during the run. The overall mean arterial pressure (MAP) is shown by the large closed circle. The CCP in this case is 70 mmHg. The perfusion pressure at any point along this line is the observed pressure – CCP. At the operating point, the perfusion pressure is MAP – CCP.

(B) Conceptual relationship between mean arterial pressure (MAP) and cerebral blood flow (CBF) with ICP held constant. CBF is noted to follow the classic pattern, being constant within but pressure passive below and above the autoregulatory range, in this example 50–150 mmHg. Vasomotor tone (VT) adjusts across the autoregulatory range, increasing with higher MAP within the autoregulatory range. This results in critical closing pressure (CCP = VT + ICP) adjusting such that at higher MAP the CCP will be higher and the dynamic perfusion pressure (PP), MAP – CCP remains constant within the autoregulatory range.

(C) Conceptual relationship between ICP and CBF reflecting the effects of increasing ICP on CBF, VT, CCP, and PP. ICP is raised continuously, as shown on the horizontal axis. Vasomotor tone compensates for this by decreasing to zero but is exhausted by the time ICP is 40 mmHg. The net effect is that critical closing pressure (CCP = VT + ICP) increases but with very high ICP the CCP eventually equals MAP with a coincident gradual decrement in PP, MAP – CCP.

Panels A–C from Dewey R, Pieper H, Hunt W, 'Experimental cerebral hemodynamics. Vasomotor tone, critical closing pressure, and vascular bed resistance', *J Neurosurg*, 1974, 41, pp. 597–606.

(D) Pressure–blood flow velocity relationships for 1-minute steady-state segments at rest and during exercise in humans demonstrating a method of evaluating zero flow pressure using transcranial Doppler ultrasonography. Representative data are presented for calculating CCP from systolic and diastolic values of arterial blood pressure from an arterial cannula and middle cerebral artery blood velocity (MCA *V*) at rest (filled circles) and during heavy exercise (open circles). In this case CCP appears to increase commensurate with increased MAP suggesting maintenance of constant perfusion pressure (MAP – CCP).

Panel D reproduced from Ogoh S *et al.*, 'Estimation of cerebral vascular tone during exercise; Evaluation by critical closing pressure in humans', *Experimental Physiology*, 95, 6, pp. 678–685, John Wiley & Sons, © 2010 The Authors. Journal compilation © 2010 The Physiological Society.

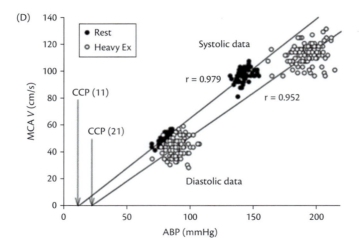

Fig. 3.6 (Continued)

vasodilation increases CBF in a 'dose-dependent' manner as haematocrit is reduced to below 30%.

Glucose

In humans, significant hypoglycaemia is associated with cerebral hyperaemia (59), whereas laboratory studies indicate variable CBF responses, that is, no change, hyperaemia, and post-hypoglycaemic

hypoperfusion (60–62). Conversely, CBF decreases with hyperglycaemia (63–65), possibly related to hyperosmolarity or viscosity effects (65).

Cerebrovascular reserve

An important concept in understanding CBF physiology is the notion of cerebrovascular reserve. The above-described physiology of autoregulation indicates that the brain is normally actively vasodilating and vasoconstricting to maintain a constant nutritive blood flow. Such changes arise not only in the context of varying perfusion pressure (due to systemic blood pressure changes or proximal vessel occlusion) but also in the context of limitations in nutrient supply as may arise with vasodilatation due to anaemia (57,58), hypoglycaemia (59), and hypoxaemia (54,66,67). This means that CBF may be entirely normal but associated with a state of maximal vasodilatation compensating for a physiological stress. Under such circumstances, when the limit of cerebrovascular reserve is reached, there is no possibility for further vasodilatation in response to additional challenges to nutrient supply. Such considerations underlie

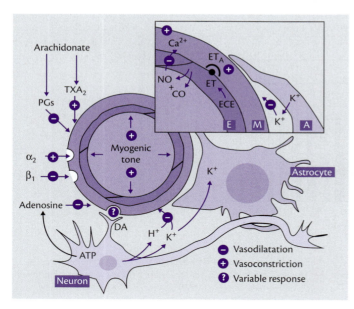

Fig. 3.7 Mechanisms involved in the regulation of regional cerebral blood flow in health and disease. The figure shows a neurovascular unit comprised of a cerebral resistance vessel in the vicinity of a neuron and an astrocyte illustrating many of the competing factors which regulate cerebral vascular tone. Arachidonate metabolism can produce prostanoids that are either vasodilators (e.g. prostacyclin) or vasoconstrictors (e.g. thromboxane A2). Endothelin (ET), produced by endothelin-converting enzyme in endothelial cells, balances the vasodilator effects of nitric oxide in a tonic manner by exerting its influences at ET_A receptors in the vascular smooth muscle.

A, astrocyte; CO, carbon monoxide; DA, dopamine; E, endothelium; ECE, endothelin-converting enzyme; ET, endothelin; ET_A, ET_A receptor; M, muscular layer; NO, nitric oxide; PGs, prostaglandins; TXA_2, thromboxane A_2.

Reprinted from *Anaesthesia & Intensive Care Medicine*, 5, 10, Nortje J and Menon DK, 'Applied cerebrovascular physiology', pp. 325–331, Copyright 2004, with permission from Elsevier.

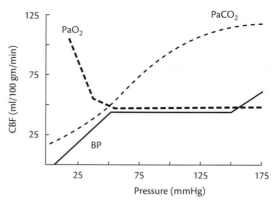

Fig. 3.8 Factors affecting cerebral blood flow. Changes in cerebral blood flow due to alterations in $PaCO_2$ (dashed line), PaO_2 (parallelogram dashes), and blood pressure (solid line) are shown.

This figure was published in *Anesthesia*, Miller RD, Chapter: Anesthesia effects upon cerebral blood flow, cerebral metabolism, and the electroencephalogram, pp. 795–798, Churchill-Livingstone, Copyright Elsevier 1981.

the concept of haemodynamic stroke, wherein a maximally vasodilated brain develops a stroke related to a physiological challenge that would otherwise be well tolerated (68,69). This is supported by observations that patients with impaired cerebrovascular reserve are at increased risk for stroke (70,71), early deterioration after stroke onset (72), and anaemia- (73) and hypoxaemia-induced (74) stroke. Thus many clinical decisions in critically ill brain-injured patients, such as transfusion triggers or goals for blood pressure, PaO_2, and $PaCO_2$, must take into consideration the patient's likely current cerebrovascular reserve.

Endothelium and astrocytes

As described earlier, cerebrovascular endothelium plays a central role in controlling CBF by secreting various vasoactive molecules, including NO, endothelins, eicosanoids, and endothelial-derived hyperpolarization factor (EDHF). Although NO plays a central role in cerebral vasodilation, inhibition of the NO pathway does not prevent vasodilation, suggesting that other pathways must also exist. EDHF is one factor responsible for non-NO-mediated vasodilatation (75,76), likely through hyperpolarization of membranes as its action is inhibited by potassium channel blockers (77). Eicosanoids are derived from the arachidonic acid pathway mediated by cyclooxygenase, epoxygenase, and lipoxygenase enzymes. Metabolites of the cyclooxygenase pathway, particularly prostaglandins (PGE2 and PGI2), are potent vasodilators but, under physiological conditions, do not have a prominent role. The cyclooxygenase pathway also produces poorly characterized vasoconstrictor molecules known as endothelium-derived contracting factors, and these may play an important role after TBI and subarachnoid haemorrhage (SAH) (78,79). Endothelins are vasoactive modulators secreted by the endothelium. There are two endothelin receptors (ET_A and ET_B) and three ligands (ET_1, ET_2, and ET_3). The ET_A receptor causes vasoconstriction and ET_B vasodilatation. Endothelins have only a minor role under physiological conditions, but are important in pathological states such as cerebral ischaemia and vasospasm (80).

Astrocytes as an integral element of the neurovascular unit link neuronal activity to blood vessels. Astrocytes are potassium ion buffers and facilitate cell-to-cell communications through gap junctions. They take up extracellular potassium and transport it to the foot processes which are in direct contact with the arterioles, and this process forms the basis of neuronal activity causing vasodilatation (see later) (81).

Neural control of cerebral blood flow

Neural control of CBF occurs at intrinsic and extrinsic levels, and the intrinsic system is comprised of local and distal elements. Local intrinsic regulation arises from the cortex and interneurons projecting to nearby arterioles, and controls the micro-environmental concentrations of vasoactive metabolites such as CO_2, NO, vasoactive intestinal peptide, gamma-aminobutyric acid (GABA), and PGE2. Distal intrinsic CBF regulation arises when a distant brain nucleus affects CBF in other area, for example, the functions of the cerebellar fastigial nucleus, the locus coeruleus, raphe nuclei, and nucleus basalis magnocellularis in controlling supratentorial CBF (6,82), and when injury to one area of the brain affects CBF in another, uninjured, brain structure (83).

Extrinsic neural control of CBF is primarily exerted by perivascular sympathetic and parasympathetic innervation of cerebral vessels. This is thought to have a neuroprotective effect in the context of hypertension in that associated vasoconstriction of innervated vessels protects the parenchyma from haemorrhage-inducing pressure surges (6). Such effects are limited to conductance vessels because smaller vessels have minimal innervation.

Effects of drugs on cerebral blood flow

Control of CBF is the cornerstone of the clinical management of ICP, primarily through secondary effects on cerebral blood volume (CBV). CBV itself is difficult to measure so CBF is more often monitored and used as a therapeutic goal during neurointensive care unit (see Chapter 10). In the normal brain, CBV is approximately 5 mL/100 g of brain, and, over a $PaCO_2$ range of approximately 3.3–9.3 kPa (25–70 mmHg), changes by about 0.49 mL/100 g for each 1.3 kPa (10 mmHg) change in $PaCO_2$ (Figure 3.8) (84).

Anaesthetic agents

Anaesthetic agents cause dose-related changes in many aspects of cerebral physiology and play an important role in managing CBF and cerebral metabolism in disease states, particularly after brain injury. They are used to manipulate cerebral physiology to maintain an optimal environment for brain recovery and function. Intravenous GABAergic anaesthetic agents, such as thiopental and propofol, reduce cerebral metabolic rate (CMR) and, via vascular coupling, CBF (85). Anaesthetics which are N-methyl-D-aspartic acid receptor antagonists, such as ketamine, tend to produce neuroexcitation with an accompanying increase in CBF. Volatile anaesthetic agents, although decreasing CMR, have some inherent vasoactive properties which affect the CBF accordingly (Table 3.1) (85).

Muscle relaxants

Cisatracurium and rocuronium are reported to have no cerebrovascular effects based on transcranial Doppler FV measurements (86).

Table 3.1 Effects of drugs on cerebral blood flow and metabolism

Drug	CBF	CMR
Barbiturates	↓	↓
Propofol	↓	↓
Etomidate	↓	↓
Narcotics	↓↑	↑↓
Benzodiazepines	↓	↓
Ketamine	↑	↑
Lidocaine	↓	≈↓
Volatile anaesthetics	↑↓	↓
Nitrous oxide	↑	↑
Xenon	↑	↑
Muscle relaxants	≈	≈
Vasodilators (hydralazine, nitroprusside)	−↑	≈
Non vasodilators (high-dose beta blockers)	↓	↓
Vasopressors (BBB injury)	↑	↑

BBB, blood–brain barrier; CBF, cerebral blood flow; CMR, cerebral metabolic rate.

Depolarizing muscle relaxants, such as succinylcholine, cause slight increases in ICP most likely due to cerebral activation caused by afferent activity of muscle spindle apparatus (87). However, a study in neurosurgical patients suggests that succinylcholine does not cause a clinically relevant increase in ICP (88).

Vasoactive drugs

Vasoactive drugs have direct and indirect effects on CBF and these must be taken into account during their use in brain-injured patients.

Vasodilators

Multiple studies report increases in ICP secondary to systemic administration of systemic vasodilators, presumed to be due to associated cerebral vasodilatation. However, it is seldom clear whether the cerebral vasodilation is related to a direct action of the drug on the cerebral vasculature or because of an autoregulatory response to the induced reduction in systemic blood pressure. Marsh and colleagues reported an increase in ICP in humans associated with the use of nitroprusside (89) and nitroglycerine (90), although another study found no CBF increase with nitroprusside (91). Intracarotid injection of either agent has not been found to increase CBF in humans (92,93), suggesting that the increases in ICP are due to indirect cerebral vasodilation arising in compensation for a decrease in systemic blood pressure. Nonetheless, nitroglycerine, long appreciated as a drug which induces headache, does have potential for direct large cerebral vessel dilation (94). Hydralazine has also been reported to increase ICP (95), in association with modest increases in CBF (96).

Non-vasodilator antihypertensive agents

Angiotensin-converting enzyme inhibitors have little effect on CBF (97) or autoregulation (98). Beta blockers also have little effect on CBF and CMR at usual clinical doses (99), although they may attenuate the CBF response to hypercapnia and neuroexcitation (100). At higher doses, beta blockers such as propranolol, which can cross the BBB (101,102), may decrease CMR and CBF (103). Calcium channel antagonists, such as nimodipine and nicardipine, are dihydropyridines which bind to the $\alpha 1$ subunit and antagonize voltage-sensitive calcium channels (L-type or slow channels) (104). These receptors mediate entry of calcium into vascular smooth muscle cells and their blockade by calcium channel blockers produces arteriolar relaxation by preventing increased cytosolic calcium and the consequent cascade of events leading to actin–myosin coupling (104). Both nimodipine and nicardipine have been used to reverse or prevent cerebral vasospasm after SAH (105–107). Intravenous nimodipine infusion has little effect on CBF in the uninjured primate, but a vasodilator effect following intra-arterial infusion or in the context of BBB disruption (108). In contrast, when given intravenously to hypertensive patients with unilateral carotid artery occlusion, nicardipine increases CBF in the non-occluded side (109). Thus calcium channel antagonists appear to dilate vasospastic cerebral arteries and thereby have a context-sensitive potential to increase CBF (106,110).

Vasopressors

In the normal brain, adrenergic drug infusions have only a small, but not absent, effect on CBF. The effects of catecholamine vasopressors on CBF and cerebral vascular resistance are thought to be indirect, occurring as a consequence of their effects on systemic blood pressure. Moreover, given the impermeability of the BBB to these drugs they also have little effect on CMR (111). However, in the injured brain with a disrupted BBB, systemic administration of adrenergic drugs can have multiple cerebral effects. Entry of the drug into the brain parenchyma presumably allows it to act like an endogenous neurotransmitter and cause neural activation, and increases in CMR and CBF (112). In addition, if there is concomitant cerebral dysautoregulation, the systemic blood pressure effects of adrenergic agents will result in secondary increases in CBF. Both these effects to increase CBF may cause secondary increases in ICP (see Chapter 2).

Cerebral blood flow in pathological states

The important pathophysiological changes in CBF and CMR in various neurological conditions are discussed below and their clinical implications reviewed in subsequent, disease-specific, chapters.

Cerebral ischaemia

Ischaemia by definition indicates a critical reduction in CBF below that required to meet metabolic demands. Depending on the extent of the CBF decrement there is a continuum of changes that lead ultimately to cell death. The critical CBF threshold for the development of irreversible tissue damage is 10–15 mL/100 g/min (113), and studies using xenon-enhanced computed tomography CBF measurement suggest that infarction ensues when CBF decreases to below 10 mL/100 g/min (114). The changes leading to irreversible cellular damage are multiple, including the development of acidosis, reduction in protein synthesis and the eventual loss of energy-requiring osmotic regulation and the Donnan equilibrium (115) consequent to failure of the energy-requiring reactions that maintain cellular ionic homeostasis. Cell death ensures. Clinical ischaemic stroke is associated with a core of very low blood flow and a penumbra of low flow with 'at risk' but potentially salvageable tissue (116,117).

Traumatic brain injury

Brain tissue damage due to TBI is attributed to the primary insult and ensuing secondary pathological alterations. There is substantial temporal and regional heterogeneity in CBF that is significantly impacted by other pathophysiological changes as well as by the presence of an associated mass lesion (118). A contusion which is initially benign may mature days later to produce malignant intracranial hypertension, with associated dysautoregulation and wide variations in CBF (119). Conversely an initially hyperaemic state can change to one of persistent pathologically low CBF (118,120). This contrasts with pure shear injury with potentially limited ICP effects, and devastating diffuse axonal injury with early hyperaemia (121). A lower Glasgow Coma Scale score tends to correlate with reduced CBF in the first 24 hours after injury, and portends a poor outcome (118,121). In addition, TBI produces varying degrees of normal to depressed CO_2 response (120) as well as pressure dysautoregulation (24,122,123).

Mechanisms which contribute to CBF abnormalities after TBI include mechanical vessel injury, systemic hypotension, impaired autoregulation, inadequate NO production, release of endothelial vasoconstrictive factors, and local biochemical abnormalities (124). Thus, TBI can produce ischaemia, hyperaemia, or both, with substantial regional and temporal variation. Cerebral ischaemia is one of the most important determinants of outcome after TBI, and both focal and global ischaemia are very common (125). This might in part be related to vasospasm which has been reported to occur in up to 45% of patients (126). Smooth muscle depolarization, release of vasoactive factors, such as endothelins and prostaglandins, paucity of NO, and free radical damage may all be implicated in the pathogenesis of vasospasm in this context. However, hyperaemia also occurs commonly after TBI (118,120) and is associated with increases in CBV and ICP (120), and worsened outcome (127). Taken together, these findings suggest that CBF and metabolic demand are often uncoupled after TBI.

When autoregulation is intact, changes in MAP produce no or small changes in CBF, blood FV, brain tissue oxygenation, and ICP but, when autoregulation is disrupted, changes in MAP result in a continuum of changes in all these variables. Correlation of slow wave changes in MAP with multiple neuromonitoring variables have been used as non-invasive assessments of cerebral autoregulatory reserve, and this is discussed in more detail in Chapters 9 and 10.

Subarachnoid haemorrhage

SAH is a neurological emergency with high rates of morbidity and mortality (128). In the hyperacute phase there is a rapid increase in ICP and reduction in CPP (129–131) that can be so severe that a period of intracranial circulatory arrest is induced (132). A state of hypoperfusion may remain even after CPP normalizes (133). This period of hypoperfusion resembles that seen after global brain ischaemia (134) and suggests that the initial period of intracranial circulatory arrest may be a physiological analogue to that situation. Other abnormal responses, including loss of CO_2 reactivity (135), uncoupling of flow and metabolism (136), release of inflammatory mediators (137), and disruption of BBB function (138–141), have also been reported during this early phase after SAH. Moreover, endothelial injury leads to loss of collagen IV and activation of matrix metallopeptidase 9, resulting in vasoconstriction and cellular swelling (142). An intense prothrombotic response is exhibited by platelets and this can lead to mechanical blockage of cerebral vessels causing further decreases in CBF (143). Notably, CBF in the first few days after SAH is related to clinical grade and outcome: poor grade is associated with lower CBF and worse outcome. In the worst-case scenario this early period of low blood flow progresses to cerebral infarction, increased ICP, and, in extreme cases, brain death. In less severe cases there may be a return to more normal cerebrovascular physiology and functional recovery.

Later stages of SAH may be marked by the development of cerebral vasospasm in 40–70% of patients, which is symptomatic in 17–40% of them (144). Although vasospasm is classically demonstrated angiographically, ischaemia can also arise in the absence of angiographic vasospasm suggesting the presence of microvascular spasm or other occlusive processes (see Chapter 18) (145). ET_1 has been cited as the most important mediator of delayed vasospasm and may also be related to the early vasoconstriction that can lead to global hypoperfusion after SAH. ET_1 antagonists are being evaluated for their potential to prevent or treat cerebral vasospasm (146). Another mediator of CBF is 20-hydroxyeicosatetraenoic acid (20-HETE) which activates rho-kinase and protein kinase C to sensitize the vascular endothelium to calcium. 20-HETE may play a role in vasodilation and vasoconstriction equally, although studies have shown that increased CSF levels are associated with decreased CBF after SAH (147). Moreover, inhibiting 20-HETE improves hypoperfusion and chronic vasospasm (148).

Another important aspect of delayed vasospasm is inadequate supply of NO. Oxyhaemoglobin, which spills into the subarachnoid space after SAH, scavenges NO stores and also triggers ischaemia by initiating spreading depolarization and releasing excitatory neurotransmitters. Unopposed vasoconstriction in the absence of NO can cause global hypoperfusion (149), and application of an NO donor reverses the vasoconstriction (150). The same principle applies in the use of statins which stimulate NO synthase, thereby increasing NO production (151).

Intracerebral haemorrhage

In intracranial haemorrhage (ICH), three phases of CBF alteration have been described in the perihaematoma tissue (see Chapter 19) (152). The 'hibernation' phase, in the first 48 hours, is marked by perilesional hypoperfusion that is associated with decreased metabolism in excess of the decrease in CBF. Thus, although CBF is low it is usually sufficient to support the reduced metabolic demand. Although the duration of reduced CBF may be prolonged in some patients, depending on haematoma expansion and other contributing insults, a 'reperfusion' phase of variable CBF response usually follows after 48 hours. Despite persistence in some patients of a lower than normal perilesional CBF, the tissue may remain or become hyperaemic relative to metabolic demand because of impaired autoregulation and local release of inflammatory mediators. In the final 'normalization' phase, normal metabolism and CBF are restored as the haematoma resolves. However, low blood flow may persist in the centre of the haematoma because of the presence of non-viable tissue.

Fainardi et al. (153) and Zhou et al. (154) evaluated CBF in lesional and perilesional tissue in the hyperacute (< 6 hours) and acute (7–24 hours) phases after ICH in humans. A clear gradient of blood flow, from near zero at the centre of the haematoma to progressive increase through the perihaematoma areas, was observed. Perihaematoma tissue with zero flow did not recover whereas some regions of 'at-risk' tissue (CBF of 10–20 mL/100 g/min) survived but others did not. Further, the extent of CBF compromise was related to the size of the ICH, with a larger haematoma associated with lower perilesional blood flow. Notably these authors reported hyperaemia in the contralateral hemisphere. Another study has also reported a relationship between CBF and ICH size, with diffuse hypoperfusion associated with haematomas greater than 4.5 cm in diameter (155). Importantly there was a greater decrement in perilesional tissue CMR than CBF, resulting in no significant decrease in oxygen extraction fraction (156). As in previous studies, this strongly suggests that the risk of perilesional ischaemia is somewhat less than might be expected from the degree of CBF reduction (156). Mayer et al. observed the development of perilesional oedema and suggested that restoration of flow in damaged tissue might be the cause of this (157).

Reperfusion injury after ischaemic stroke and carotid endarterectomy

Hyperperfusion injury has been reported after large arteriovenous malformation (AVM) resection, thrombolysis after acute ischaemic stroke, and carotid endarterectomy (CEA). It may also be a contributor to the encephalopathy of hepatic failure.

Although thrombolysis after acute ischaemic stroke improves outcome in selected patient populations, it can lead to reperfusion injury which can manifest as either ischaemia or hyperperfusion. Ischaemia can paradoxically develop when blood flow is restored after thrombolysis because of an influx of leucocytes which have been sensitized to adhesion molecules on the endothelium as a result of the original tissue ischaemia (158,159). The leucocytes attach themselves to the endothelium and plug the capillaries leading to mechanical obstruction to blood flow (160,161). In a similar way platelets may also attach to the endothelium leading to microthrombi formation and capillary occlusion. Hyperperfusion can also occur after thrombolysis, and may be associated with oedema and haemorrhage. The physiological response to acute ischaemic stroke is to maintain blood flow to the ischaemic penumbra by increasing blood pressure. However, in the setting of ischaemia the BBB is also disrupted leading to highly permeable capillaries. Once blood flow is restored, these injured capillaries are unable to withstand the high systemic pressures and the endothelium is damaged leading to reperfusion injury and haemorrhagic transformation (162). Cerebral autoregulation normally protects the brain from changes in systemic blood pressure but autoregulation is also impaired in ischaemic brain, and there is therefore no check on transmission of systemic pressures to brain capillaries.

After CEA, similar pathophysiology may apply in those with high-grade stenosis and chronic low-grade ischaemia (22). The endothelium secretes vasodilatory molecules to maintain CBF and hence capillaries are maximally dilated. Previously low, with chronic vasodilation and intracranial hypotension, CBF is restored after CEA but, in the context of the previous chronic compensatory shift of the cerebral autoregulation curve, capillary dilatation persists and leads to increased CBF resulting in hyperperfusion injury and a risk of postoperative ICH (163). In one study, 6.6% of 76 patients with bilateral CEA developed hyperperfusion syndrome, compared to 1.1% of 379 with unilateral CEA (164). Risk factors for post-ischaemic reperfusion injury after CEA include post-reperfusion hypertension, high-grade stenosis with poor collateral flow, decreased cerebral vasoreactivity, recent contralateral CEA (< 3 months), and intraoperative distal carotid pressure of less than 40 mmHg (162,165).

Fulminant hepatic failure

The extensive effects of liver failure on brain physiology and function have recently been reviewed in detail (166). Fulminant hepatic failure is frequently complicated by cerebral oedema and increased ICP (167), but there are conflicting data regarding its effects on CBF. Aggarwal and colleagues reported variable changes in CBF and CMR and linked these to the temporal progression of worsening severity of hepatic encephalopathy (168,169) although, in general, fulminant liver failure is a hyperdynamic state. Similar to laboratory models of hepatic encephalopathy (170), Wendon and Harrison demonstrated that CMR falls drastically in patients with severe hepatic failure but, despite this, cerebral lactate production increases suggesting that the increased flow does not meet demand (171).

References

1. Shirahata N, Henriksen L, Vorstrup S, Holm S, Lauritzen M, Paulson OB, *et al*. Regional cerebral blood flow assessed by 133Xe inhalation and emission tomography: normal values. *J Comput Assist Tomo*. 1985;9(5):861–6.

2. Lassen NA. Normal average value of cerebral blood flow in younger adults is 50 ml/100 g/min. *J Cereb Blood Flow Metab*. 1985;5(3):347–9.

3. Stehbens WE. Focal intimal proliferation in the cerebral arteries. *Am J Pathol*. 1960;36:289–301.

4. Aydin F. Do human intracranial arteries lack vasa vasorum? A comparative immunohistochemical study of intracranial and systemic arteries. *Acta Neuropathol*. 1998;96(1):22–8.

5. Iliff JJ, Wang M, Liao Y, Plogg BA, Peng W, Gundersen GA, *et al*. A paravascular pathway facilitates CSF flow through the brain parenchyma and the clearance of interstitial solutes, including amyloid beta. *Sci Transl Med*. 2012;4(147):147ra11.

6. Kulik T, Kusano Y, Aronhime S, Sandler AL, Winn HR. Regulation of cerebral vasculature in normal and ischemic brain. *Neuropharmacology*. 2008;55(3):281–8.

7. Leybaert L. Neurobarrier coupling in the brain: A partner of neurovascular and neurometabolic coupling? *J Cereb Blood Flow Metab*. 2005;25(1):2–16.

8. McPherson RW, Koehler RC, Traystman RJ. Effect of jugular venous pressure on cerebral autoregulation in dogs. *Am J Physiol*. 1988;255(6 Pt 2):1516–24.

9. Nemoto EM. Dynamics of cerebral venous and intracranial pressures. *Acta Neurochir Suppl*. 2006;96:435–7.

10. Nakagawa Y, Tsuru M, Yada K. Site and mechanism for compression of the venous system during experimental intracranial hypertension. *J Neurosurg*. 1974;41(4):427–34.

11. Piechnik SK, Czosnyka M, Richards HK, Whitfield PC, Pickard JD. Cerebral venous blood outflow: a theoretical model based on laboratory simulation. *Neurosurgery*. 2001;49(5):1214–22.

12. Huseby J, Luce J, Cary J, Pavlin E, Butler J. Effects of positive end-expiratory pressure on intracranial pressure in dogs with intracranial hypertension. *J Neurosurg*. 1981;55(5):704–5.

13. Grände P, Asgeirsson B, Nordstrom C. Volume-targeted therapy of increased intracranial pressure: the Lund concept unifies surgical and non-surgical treatments. *Acta Anaesth Scand*. 2002;46(8):929–41.

14. Beards SC, Yule S, Kassner A, Jackson A. Anatomical variation of cerebral venous drainage: the theoretical effect on jugular bulb blood samples. *Anaesthesia*. 1998;53(7):627–33.

15. Ursino M. Mechanisms of cerebral blood flow regulation. *Crit Rev Biomed Eng*. 1991;18(4):255–88.

16. Kuschinsky W. Coupling of blood flow and metabolism in the brain. *J Basic Clin Physiol Pharmacol*. 1990;1(1–4):191–201.

17. Meyer JS, Shimazu K, Okamoto S, Koto A, Ouchi T, Sari A, *et al*. Effects of alpha adrenergic blockade on autoregulation and chemical vasomotor control of CBF in stroke. *Stroke*. 1973;4(2):187–200.

18. Drummond JC. The lower limit of autoregulation: time to revise our thinking? *Anesthesiology*. 1997;86(6):1431–3.

19. Lassen NA. Cerebral blood flow and oxygen consumption in man. *Physiol Rev*. 1959;39(2):183–238.

20. Finnerty FA, Jr., Witkin L, Fazekas JF. Cerebral hemodynamics during cerebral ischemia induced by acute hypotension. *J Clin Invest*. 1954;33(9):1227–32.

21. Strandgaard S. Autoregulation of cerebral blood flow in hypertensive patients. The modifying influence of prolonged antihypertensive treatment on the tolerance to acute, drug-induced hypotension. *Circulation*. 1976;53(4):720–7.

22. Strandgaard S, Paulson OB. Cerebral autoregulation. *Stroke*. 1984;15(3):413–16.

23. Brady KM, Lee JK, Kibler KK, Easley RB, Koehler RC, Czosnyka M, *et al*. The lower limit of cerebral blood flow autoregulation is increased with elevated intracranial pressure. *Anesth Analg*. 2009;108(4):1278–83.

24. Steiner LA, Czosnyka M, Piechnik SK, Smielewski P, Chatfield D, Menon DK, *et al*. Continuous monitoring of cerebrovascular pressure reactivity allows determination of optimal cerebral perfusion pressure in patients with traumatic brain injury. *Crit Care Med*. 2002;30(4):733–8.

25. Edvinsson L, MacKenzie E, McCulloch J. *Cerebral Blood Flow and Metabolism*. New York: Raven Press; 1993.

26. Voets T, Nilius B. TRPCs, GPCRs and the Bayliss effect. *EMBO J*. 2009;28(1):4–5.

27. Harder DR. Pressure-induced myogenic activation of cat cerebral arteries is dependent on intact endothelium. *Circ Res*. 1987;60(1):102–7.

28. Rubanyi GM, Freay AD, Kauser K, Johns A, Harder DR. Mechanoreception by the endothelium: Mediators and mechanisms of pressure- and flow-induced vascular responses. *Blood Vessels*. 1990;27(2-5):246–57.

29. Bayliss WM. On the local reactions of the arterial wall to changes of internal pressure. *J Physiol*. 1902;28(3):220–31.

30. Dewey R, Pieper H, Hunt W. Experimental cerebral hemodynamics. Vasomotor tone, critical closing pressure, and vascular bed resistance. *J Neurosurg*. 1974;41:597–606.

31. Early C, Dewey R, Peiper H, Hunt W. Dynamic pressure-flow relationships in the monkey. *J Neurosurg*. 1974;41:590–6.

32. Czosnyka M, Smielewski P, Piechnik S, Al-Rawi PG, Kirkpatrick PJ, Matta BF, *et al*. Critical closing pressure in cerebrovascular circulation. *J Neurol Neurosurg Psychiatry*. 1999;66(5):606–11.

33. Marzban C, Illian PR, Morison D, Moore A, Kliot M, Czosnyka M, *et al*. A method for estimating zero-flow pressure and intracranial pressure. *J Neurosurg Anesthesiol*. 2013:25–32.

34. Whittaker SR, Winton FR. The apparent viscosity of blood flowing in the isolated hindlimb of the dog, and its variation with corpuscular concentration. *J Physiol*. 1933;78(4):339–69.

35. Weyland A, Buhre W, Grund S, Ludwig H, Kazmaier S, Weyland W, *et al*. Cerebrovascular tone rather than intracranial pressure determines the effective downstream pressure of the cerebral circulation in the absence of intracranial hypertension. *J Neurosurg Anesthesiol*. 2000;12(3):210–16.

36. Athanassiou L, Hancock SM, Mahajan RP. Doppler estimation of zero flow pressure during changes in downstream pressure in a bench model of a circulation using pulsatile flow. *Anaesthesia*. 2005;60(2):133–8.

37. Hancock SM, Mahajan RP, Athanassiou L. Noninvasive estimation of cerebral perfusion pressure and zero flow pressure in healthy volunteers: the effects of changes in end-tidal carbon dioxide. *Anesth Analg*. 2003;96(3):847–51.

38. Marzban C, Illian PR, Morison D, Moore A, Kliot M, Czosnyka M, *et al*. A method for estimating zero-flow pressure and intracranial pressure. *J Neurosurg Anesthesiol*. 2012;25(1):25–32.

39. Athanassiou L, Hancock SM, Mahajan RP. Doppler estimation of zero flow pressure during changes in downstream pressure in a bench model of a circulation using pulsatile flow. *Anaesthesia*. 2005;60(2):133–8.

40. Buhre W, Heinzel FR, Grund S, Sonntag H, Weyland A. Extrapolation to zero-flow pressure in cerebral arteries to estimate intracranial pressure. *Br J Anaesth*. 2003;90(3):291–5.

41. Logothetis NK, Pauls J, Augath M, Trinath T, Oeltermann A. Neurophysiological investigation of the basis of the fMRI signal. *Nature*. 2001;412(6843):150–7.

42. Mathiesen C, Caesar K, Akgören N, Lauritzen M. Modification of activity-dependent increases of cerebral blood flow by excitatory synaptic activity and spikes in rat cerebellar cortex. *J Physiol*. 1998;512(2):555–66.

43. Quayle JM, Nelson MT, Standen NB. ATP-sensitive and inwardly rectifying potassium channels in smooth muscle. *Physiol Rev*. 1997;77(4):1165–232.

44. Hoehn K, White TD. Role of excitatory amino acid receptors in K^+- and glutamate-evoked release of endogenous adenosine from rat cortical slices. *J Neurochem*. 1990;54(1):256–65.

45. Iliff JJ, D'Ambrosio R, Ngai AC, Winn HR. Adenosine receptors mediate glutamate-evoked arteriolar dilation in the rat cerebral cortex. *Am J Physiol Heart Circ Physiol*. 2003;284(5 53-5):H1631–H7.

46. Iadecola C. Does nitric oxide mediate the increases in cerebral blood flow elicited by hypercapnia? *Proc Natl Acad Sci U S A*. 1992;89(9):3913–16.

47. Persson PB. Modulation of cardiovascular control mechanisms and their interaction. *Physiol Rev*. 1996;76(1):193–244.

48. McHenry Jr LC, Slocum HC, Bivens HE, Mayes HA, Hayes GJ. Hyperventilation in awake and anesthetized man. effects on cerebral blood flow and cerebral metabolism. *Arch Neurol*. 1965;12:270–7.

49. Clausen T, Scharf A, Menzel M, Soukup J, Holz C, Rieger A, *et al*. Influence of moderate and profound hyperventilation on cerebral blood flow, oxygenation and metabolism. *Brain Res*. 2004;1019(1-2):113–23.

50. Alexander SC, Smith TC, Strobel G, Stephen GW, Wollman H. Cerebral carbohydrate metabolism of man during respiratory and etabolic alkalosis. *J Appl Physiol*. 1968;24(1):66–72.

51. Alexander SC, Cohen PJ, Wollman H, Smith TC, Reivich M, Vandermolen RA. Cerebral carbohydrate metabolism during hypocarbia in man: studies. *Anesthesiology*. 1965;26:624–32.

52. Cohen PJ, Wollman H, Alexander SC, Chase PE, Behar MG. Cerebral carbohydrate metabolism in man during halothane anesthesia: effects of $PaCO_2$ on some aspects of carbohydrate utilization. *Anesthesiology*. 1964;25:185–91.

53. Muizelaar J, Marmarou A, Ward J, Kontos H, Choi S, Becker D, *et al*. Adverse effects of prolonged hyperventilation in patients with severe head injury: a randomized clinical trial. *J Neurosurg*. 1991;75:731–9.

54. Kogure K, Scheinberg P, Reinmuth OM, Fujishima M, Busto R. Mechanisms of cerebral vasodilatation in hypoxia. *J Appl Physiol*. 1970;29(2):223–9.

55. Floyd T, Clark J, Gelfand R, Detre J, Ratcliffe S, Guvakov D, *et al*. Independent cerebral vasoconstrictive effects of hyperoxia and accompanying arterial hypocapnia at 1 ATA. *J App Physiol*. 2003;95(6):2453–61.

56. Brown MM, Wade JPH, Marshall J. Fundamental importance of arterial oxygen content in the regulation of cerebral blood flow in man. *Brain*. 1985;108(1):81–93.

57. Borgstrom L, Johannsson H, Siesjo B. The influence of acute normovolemic anemia on cerebral blood flow and oxygen consumption of anesthetized rats. *Acta Physiol Scand*. 1975;93(40):505–14.

58. Dexter F, Hindman BJ. Effect of haemoglobin concentration on brain oxygenation in focal stroke: a mathematical modelling study. *Br J Anaesth*. 1997;79(3):346–51.

59. Porta PD, Maiolo AT, Negri VU, Rossella E. Cerebral blood flow and metabolism in therapeutic insulin coma. *Metabolism*. 1964;13(2):131–40.

60. Nilsson B, Agardh CD, Ingvar M, Siesjo BK. Cerebrovascular response during and following severe insulin-induced hypoglycemia: CO2-sensitivity, autoregulation, and influence of prostaglandin synthesis inhibition. *Acta Physiol Scand*. 1981;111(4):455–63.

61. Ghajar JBG, Plum F, Duffy TE. Cerebral oxidative metabolism and blood flow during acute hypoglycemia and recovery in unanesthetized rats. *J Neurochem*. 1982;38(2):397–409.

62. Cilluffo JM, Anderson RE, Michenfelder JD, Sundt Jr TM. Cerebral blood flow, brain pH, and oxidative metabolism in the cat during severe insulin-induced hypoglycemia. *J Cereb Blood Flow Metab*. 1982;2(3):337–46.

63. Duckrow RB, Beard DC, Brennan RW. Regional cerebral blood flow decreases during hyperglycemia. *Ann Neurol*. 1985;17(3):267–72.

64. Duckrow RB, Beard DC, Brennan RW. Regional cerebral blood flow decreases during chronic and acute hyperglycemia. *Stroke*. 1987;18(1):52–8.

65. Duckrow RB. Decreased cerebral blood flow during acute hyperglycemia. *Brain Res*. 1995;703(1-2):145–50.

66. Ainslie PN, Barach A, Murrell C, Hamlin M, Hellemans J, Ogoh S. Alterations in cerebral autoregulation and cerebral blood flow velocity during acute hypoxia: rest and exercise. *Am J Physiol Heart Circ Physiol*. 2007;292(2):H976–H83.

67. Shimojyo S, Scheinberg P, Kogure K, Reinmuth O. The effects of graded hypoxia upon transient CBF and oxygen consumption. *Neurology*. 1968;18(2):127–33.

68. Siemund R, Cronqvist M, Andsberg G, Ramgren B, Knutsson L, Holtås S. Cerebral perfusion imaging in hemodynamic stroke: be aware of the pattern. *Interv Neuroradiol*. 2009;15(4):385–94.

69. Bladin CF, Chambers BR. Frequency and pathogenesis of hemodynamic stroke. *Stroke*. 1994;25(11):2179–82.

70. Vernieri F, Pasqualetti P, Passarelli F, Rossini PM, Silvestrini M. Outcome of carotid artery occlusion is predicted by cerebrovascular reactivity. *Stroke*. 1999;30(3):593–8.

71. Silvestrini M, Vernieri F, Pasqualetti P, Matteis M, Passarelli F, Troisi E, *et al.* Impaired cerebral vasoreactivity and risk of stroke in patients with asymptomatic carotid artery stenosis. *JAMA*. 2000;283 (16):2122–7.

72. Alvarez FJ, Segura T, Castellanos M, Leira R, Blanco M, Castillo J, *et al.* Cerebral hemodynamic reserve and early neurologic deterioration in acute ischemic stroke. *J Cereb Blood Flow Metab*. 2004;24(11):1267–71.

73. Bosel J, Ruscher K, Ploner CJ, Valdueza JM. Delayed neurological deterioration in a stroke patient with postoperative acute anemia. *Eur Neurol*. 2005;53(1):36–8.

74. Baumgartner RW, Siegel AM, Hackett PH. Going high with preexisting neurological conditions. *High Alt Med Biol*. 2007;8(2):108–16.

75. Hutcheson IR, Chaytor AT, Evans WH, Griffith TM. Nitric oxide-independent relaxations to acetylcholine and A23187 involve different routes of heterocellular communication: role of gap junctions and phospholipase A 2. *Circ Res*. 1999;84(1):53–63.

76. You J, Johnson TD, Marrelli SP, Bryan Jr RM. Functional heterogeneity of endothelial P2 purinoceptors in the cerebrovascular tree of the rat. *Am J Physiol Heart Circ Physiol*. 1999;277(3, 46-3):H893–H900.

77. Golding EM, Marrelli SP, You J, Bryan Jr RM. Endothelium-derived hyperpolarizing factor in the brain: a new regulator of cerebral blood flow? *Stroke*. 2002;33(3):661–3.

78. You J, Golding EM, Bryan Jr RM. Arachidonic acid metabolites, hydrogen peroxide, and EDHF in cerebral arteries. *Am J Physiol Heart Circ Physiol*. 2005;289(3, 58-3):H1077–H83.

79. Kontos HA, Wei EP. Endothelium-dependent responses after experimental brain injury. *J Neurotrauma*. 1992;9(4):349–54.

80. Vatter H, Konczalla J, Seifert V. Endothelin related pathophysiology in cerebral vasospasm: what happens to the cerebral vessels? *Acta Neurochir Suppl*. 110(Pt 1):177–80.

81. Newman EA, Frambach DA, Odette LL. Control of extracellular potassium levels by retinal glial cell K^+ siphoning. *Science*. 1984;225(4667):1174–5.

82. Nakai M, Iadecola C, Ruggiero DA, Tucker LW, Reis DJ. Electrical stimulation of cerebellar fastigial nucleus increases cerebral cortical blood flow without change in local metabolism: evidence for an intrinsic system in brain for primary vasodilation. *Brain Res*. 1983;260(1):35–49.

83. Mountz JM, Liu H-G, Deutsch G. Neuroimaging in cerebrovascular disorders: measurement of cerebral physiology after stroke and assessment of stroke recovery. *Semin Nucl Med*. 2003;33(1):56–76.

84. Powers WJ, Raichle ME. Positron emission tomography and its application to the study of cerebrovascular disease in man. *Stroke*. 1985;16(3):361–76.

85. Sloan TB. Anesthetics and the brain. *Anesthesiol Clin North America*. 2002;20(2):265–92.

86. Kofke W, Shaheen N, McWhorter J, Sinz E, Hobbs G. Transcranial Doppler ultrasonography with induction of anesthesia and neuromuscular blockade in surgical patients. *J Clin Anesth*. 2001;13:335–8.

87. Lanier WL, Iaizzo PA, Milde JH, Sharbrough FW. The cerebral and systemic effects of movement in response to a noxious stimulus in lightly anesthetized dogs: possible modulation of cerebral function by muscle afferents. *Anesthesiology*. 1994;80(2):392–401.

88. Kovarik WD, Mayberg TS, Lam AM, Mathisen TL, Winn HR. Succinylcholine does not change intracranial pressure, cerebral blood flow velocity, or the electroencephalogram in patients with neurologic injury. *Anesth Analg*. 1994;78(3):469–73.

89. Marsh M, Shapiro H, Smith R, Marshall LF. Changes in neurologic status and intracranial pressure associated with sodium nitroprusside administration. *Anesthesiology*. 1979;51:336–8.

90. Dohi S, Matsumoto M, Takahashi K. The effects of nitroglycerin on cerebrospinal fluid pressure in awake and anesthetized humans. *Anesthesiology*. 1981;54:511–14.

91. Pinaud M, Souron R, Lelausque JN, Gazeau MF, Lajat Y, Dixneuf B, *et al.* Cerebral blood flow and cerebral oxygen consumption during nitroprusside-induced hypotension to less than 50 mmHg. *Anesthesiology*. 1989;70(2):255–60.

92. Joshi S, Young WL, Duong H, Aagaard BA, Ostapkovich ND, Connolly ES, *et al.* Intracarotid nitroprusside does not augment cerebral blood flow in human subjects. *Anesthesiology*. 2002;96(1):60–6.

93. Joshi S, Young WL, Pile-Spellman J, Fogarty-Mack P, Sciacca RR, Hacein-Bey L, *et al.* Intra-arterial nitrovasodilators do not increase cerebral blood flow in angiographically normal territories of arteriovenous malformation patients. *Stroke*. 1997;28(6):1115–22.

94. Dahl A, Russell D, Nyberg-Hansen R, Rootwelt K. Effect of nitroglycerin on cerebral circulation measured by transcranial Doppler and SPECT. *Stroke*. 1989;20(12):1733–6.

95. Robertson CS, Clifton GL, Taylor AA, Grossman RG. Treatment of hypertension associated with head injury. *J Neurosurg*. 1983;59(3):455–60.

96. Overgaard J, Skinhoj E. A paradoxical cerebral hemodynamic effect of hydralazine. *Stroke*. 1975;6 (4):402.

97. Waldemar G, Schmidt JF, Andersen AR, Vorstrup S, Ibsen H, Paulson OB. Angiotensin converting enzyme inhibition and cerebral blood flow autoregulation in normotensive and hypertensive man. *J Hypertens*. 1989;7(3):229–35.

98. Britton K, Grnowska M, Nimmon CC, Horne T. CBF in hypertensive patients with cerebrovascular disease: technique for measurement and effect of captopril. *Nucl Med Commun*. 1985;6(5):251–61.

99. Globus M, Keren A, Eldad M, Granot C, Tzivoni D, Levy S, *et al.* The effect of chronic propranolol therapy on regional CBF in hypertensive patients. *Stroke*. 1983;14(6):964.

100. Schmalbruch IK, Linde R, Paulson OB, Madsen PL. Activation-induced resetting of cerebral metabolism and flow is abolished by beta-adrenergic blockade with propranolol. *Stroke*. 2002;33(1):251–5.

101. Pardridge WM, Sakiyama R, Fierer G. Blood-brain barrier transport and brain sequestration of propranolol and lidocaine. *Am J Physiol*. 1984;247(3 Pt 2):R582–8.

102. Olesen J, Hougard K, Hertz M. Isoproterenol and propranolol: ability to cross the blood-brain barrier and effects on cerebral circulation in man. *Stroke*. 1978;9(4):344.

103. Aqyagi M, Deshmukh VD, Meyer JS, Kawamura Y, Tagashira Y. Effect of beta-adrenergic blockade with propranolol on cerebral blood flow, autoregulation and CO2 responsiveness. *Stroke*. 1976;7(3):291–5.

104. Michel T, Hoffman B. Treatment of myocardial ischemia and hypertension. In Brunton L, Chabner B, Knollmann B (eds) *Goodman & Gilman's The Pharmacological Basis of Therapeutics* (12th edn). New York: McGraw-Hill; 2011:745–88.

105. Flamm E, Adams HJ, Beck D, Pinto RS, Marler JR, Walker MD, *et al.* Dose-escalation study of intravenous nicardipine in patients with aneurysmal subarachnoid hemorrhage. *J Neurosurg*. 1988;68:393–400.

106. Badjatia N, Topcuoglu MA, Pryor JC, Rabinov JD, Ogilvy CS, Carter BS, *et al.* Preliminary experience with intra-arterial nicardipine as a treatment for cerebral vasospasm. *AJNR: Am J Neuroradiol*. 2004;25(5):819–26.

107. Allen G, Ahn H, Presiosi T, Battye R, Boone SC, Boone SC, *et al.* Cerebral arterial spasm: a controlled trial of nimodipine in patients with subarachnoid hemorrhage. *N Engl J Med*. 1983;308:619–24.

108. Harper AM, Craigen L, Kazda S. Effect of the calcium antagonist, nimodipine, on cerebral blood flow and metabolism in the primate. *J Cereb Blood Flow Metab*. 1981;1(3):349–56.

109. Nagahama Y, Fukuyama H, Yamauchi H, Katsumi Y, Dong Y, Konishi J, *et al.* Effect of nicardipine on cerebral blood flow in hypertensive patients with internal carotid artery occlusion: a PET study. *J Stroke Cerebrovasc Dis*. 1997;6(5):325–31.

110. Barth M, Capelle H-H, Weidauer S, Weiss C, Munch E, Thome C, *et al.* Effect of nicardipine prolonged-release implants on cerebral vasospasm and clinical outcome after severe aneurysmal

subarachnoid hemorrhage: a prospective, randomized, double-blind phase IIa study. *Stroke.* 2007;38(2):330–6.

111. Olesen J. The effect of intracarotid epinephrine, norepinephrine, and angiotensin on the regional CBF in man. *Neurology.* 1972;22:978–87.

112. MacKenzie E, McCulloch J, Harper A. Influence of endogenous norepinephrine on CBF and metabolism. *Am J Physiol.* 1976;231:489–94.

113. Cunningham AS, Salvador R, Coles JP, Chatfield DA, Bradley PG, Johnston AJ, et al. Physiological thresholds for irreversible tissue damage in contusional regions following traumatic brain injury. *Brain.* 2005;128(8):1931–42.

114. Kaufmann AM, Firlik AD, Fukui MB, Wechsler LR, Jungries CA, Yonas H. Ischemic core and penumbra in human stroke. *Stroke.* 1999;30(1):93–9.

115. Hill TL. Osmotic pressure, protein solutions and active transport. II. *J Am Chem Soc.* 1958;80(12):2923–6.

116. Firlik AD, Kaufmann AM, Wechsler LR, Firlik KS, Fukui MB, Yonas H. Quantitative cerebral blood flow determinations in acute ischemic stroke: relationship to computed tomography and angiography. *Stroke.* 1997;28(11):2208–13.

117. Firlik AD, Rubin G, Yonas H, Wechsler LR. Relation between cerebral blood flow and neurologic deficit resolution in acute ischemic stroke. *Neurology.* 1998;51(1):177–82.

118. Marion DW, Darby J, Yonas H. Acute regional cerebral blood flow changes caused by severe head injuries. *J Neurosurg.* 1991;74(3):407–14.

119. Katayama Y, Tsubokawa T, Miyazaki S, Kawamata T, Yoshino A. Oedema fluid formation within contused brain tissue as a cause of medically uncontrollable elevation of intracranial pressure: the role of surgical therapy. *Acta Neurochir Suppl.* 1990;51:308–10.

120. Obrist W, Langfitt T, Jaggi J, Cruz J, Gennarelli TA. CBF and metabolism in comatose patients with acute head injury. Relationship to intracranial hypertension. *J Neurosurg.* 1984;61:241–53.

121. Raggueneau JL, Bellec C, Jarrige B. Cerebral blood flow (CBF) in head injuries. *Agressologie.* 1988;29(4):237–40.

122. Czosnyka M, Smielewski P, Piechnik S, Steiner LA, Pickard JD. Cerebral autoregulation following head injury. *J Neurosurg.* 2001;95(5):756–63.

123. Jaeger M, Schuhmann MU, Soehle M, Meixensberger J. Continuous assessment of cerebrovascular autoregulation after traumatic brain injury using brain tissue oxygen pressure reactivity. *Crit Care Med.* 2006;34(6):1783–8.

124. McIntosh TK, Smith DH, Meaney DF, Kotapka MJ, Gennarelli TA, Graham DI. Neuropathological sequelae of traumatic brain injury: relationship to neurochemical and biomechanical mechanisms. *Lab Invest.* 1996;74(2):315–42.

125. Coles JP, Fryer TD, Smielewski P, Rice K, Clark JC, Pickard JD, et al. Defining ischemic burden after traumatic brain injury using 15O PET imaging of cerebral physiology. *J Cereb Blood Flow Metab.* 2004;24(2):191–201.

126. Martin NA, Doberstein C, Zane C, Caron MJ, Thomas K, Becker DP. Posttraumatic cerebral arterial spasm: Transcranial Doppler ultrasound, cerebral blood flow, and angiographic findings. *J Neurosurg.* 1992;77(4):575–83.

127. Kelly DF, Kordestani RK, Martin NA, Nguyen T, Hovda DA, Bergsneider M, et al. Hyperemia following traumatic brain injury: relationship to intracranial hypertension and outcome. *J Neurosurg.* 1996;85(5):762–71.

128. Beseoglu K, Holtkamp K, Steiger HJ, Hänggi D. Fatal aneurysmal subarachnoid haemorrhage: causes of 30-day in-hospital case fatalities in a large single-centre historical patient cohort. *Clin Neurol Neurosurg.* 2012;115(1):77–81.

129. Rabinstein AA, Pichelmann MA, Friedman JA, Piepgras DG, Nichols DA, McIver JI, et al. Symptomatic vasospasm and outcomes following aneurysmal subarachnoid hemorrhage: a comparison between surgical repair and endovascular coil occlusion. *J Neurosurg.* 2003;98(2):319–25.

130. Handa Y, Kubota T, Kaneko M, Tsuchida A, Kobayashi H, Kawano H, et al. Expression of intercellular adhesion molecule 1 (ICAM-1) on the cerebral artery following subarachnoid haemorrhage in rats. *Acta Neurochir.* 1995;132(1–3):92–7.

131. Lanzino G, Juvela S. Plasma glucose levels and outcome after aneurysmal subarachnoid hemorrhage. *J Neurosurg.* 2005;102(6):974–6.

132. Eng C, Lam A, Byrd S, Newell D. The diagnosis and management of a perianesthetic cerebral aneurysmal rupture aided with transcranial Doppler ultrasonography. *Anesthesiology.* 1993;78(1):191–4.

133. Bederson JB, Germano IM, Guarino L, Muizelaar JP. Cortical blood flow and cerebral perfusion pressure in a new noncraniotomy model of subarachnoid hemorrhage in the rat. *Stroke.* 1995;26(6):1086–92.

134. Kofke W, Nemoto E, Hossman K, Taylor F, Kessler P, Stezoski S. Brain blood flow and metabolism after global brain ischemia and post insult thiopental therapy in monkeys. *Stroke.* 1979;10:554–60.

135. Prunell GF, Mathiesen T, Svendgaard NA, Dempsey RJ, Selman WR, Connolly Jr ES, et al. Experimental subarachnoid hemorrhage: cerebral blood flow and brain metabolism during the acute phase in three different models in the rat. *Neurosurgery.* 2004;54(2):426–37.

136. Busch E, Beaulieu C, De Crespigny A, Moseley ME. Diffusion MR imaging during acute subarachnoid hemorrhage in rats. *Stroke.* 1998;29(10):2155–61.

137. Kusaka G, Ishikawa M, Nanda A, Granger DN, Zhang JH. Signaling pathways for early brain injury after subarachnoid hemorrhage. *J Cereb Blood Flow Metab.* 2004;24(8):916–25.

138. Xie ZY, Shen WW, Ma Y, Cheng Y. Identification of blood-brain barrier function following subarachnoid hemorrhage in rats at different stages. *Neural Regen Res.* 2008;3(4):444–8.

139. Zhang JH, Gules I, Satoh M, Nanda A. Apoptosis, blood-brain barrier, and subarachnoid hemorrhage. *Acta Neurochirurgica, Supplementum* 2003:483–7.

140. Germano A, D'Avella D, Cicciarello R, Hayes RL, Tomasello F, Doczi T, et al. Blood-brain barrier permeability changes after experimental subarachnoid hemorrhage. *Neurosurgery.* 1992;30(6):882–6.

141. Germano A, D'Avella D, Imperatore C, Caruso G, Tomasello F. Time-course of blood-brain barrier permeability changes after experimental subarachnoid haemorrhage. *Acta Neurochir.* 2000;142(5):575–81.

142. Sehba FA, Mostafa G, Knopman J, Friedrich Jr V, Bederson JB. Acute alterations in microvascular basal lamina after subarachnoid hemorrhage. *J Neurosurg.* 2004;101(4):633–40.

143. Sehba FA, Mostafa G, Friedrich Jr V, Bederson JB. Acute microvascular platelet aggregation after subarachnoid hemorrhage. *J Neurosurg.* 2005;102(6):1094–100.

144. Zipfel GJ, Dacey RG. Cerebral vasospasm. *Neurosurg Focus.* 2006;21(3):E14.

145. Dhar R, Scalfani MT, Blackburn S, Zazulia AR, Videen T, Diringer M. Relationship between angiographic vasospasm and regional hypoperfusion in aneurysmal subarachnoid hemorrhage. *Stroke.* 2012;43(7):1788–94.

146. Schubert GA, Schilling L, Schmiedek P, Thomé C. *Clazosentan, a Novel Selective Endothelin A Antagonist, Prevents Cerebral Hypoperfusion During the Acute Phase of Massive Experimental SAH: A Laser-Doppler-Flowmetry Study in Rats.* Strasbourg: Jahrestagung der Deutschen Gesellschaft für Neurochirurgie e.V. (DGNC); 2005.

147. Poloyac SM, Reynolds RB, Yonas H, Kerr ME. Identification and quantification of the hydroxyeicosatetraenoic acids, 20-HETE and 12-HETE, in the cerebrospinal fluid after subarachnoid hemorrhage. *J Neurosci Methods.* 2005;144(2):257–63.

148. Takeuchi K, Renic M, Bohman QC, Harder DR, Miyata N, Roman RJ. Reversal of delayed vasospasm by an inhibitor of the synthesis of 20-HETE. *Am J Physiol Heart Circ Physiol.* 2005;289(5 58-5):H2203–H11.

149. Schwartz AY, Sehba FA, Bederson JB, Dacey RG, Dietrich H. Decreased nitric oxide availability contributes to acute

cerebral ischemia after subarachnoid hemorrhage. *Neurosurgery.* 2000;47(1):208–15.

150. Agrawal A, Patir R, Kato Y, Chopra S, Sano H, Kanno T. Role of intraventricular sodium nitroprusside in vasospasm secondary to aneurysmal subarachnoid haemorrhage: a 5-year prospective study with review of the literature. *Minim Invasive Neurosurg.* 2009;52(1):5–8.

151. Yamada M, Huang Z, Dalkara T, Endres M, Laufs U, Waeber C, et al. Endothelial nitric oxide synthase-dependent cerebral blood flow augmentation by L-arginine after chronic statin treatment. *J Cereb Blood Flow Metab.* 2000;20(4):709–17.

152. Qureshi AI, Hanel RA, Kirmani JF, Yahia AM, Hopkins LN. Cerebral blood flow changes associated with intracerebral hemorrhage. *Neurosurg Clin N Am.* 2002;13(3):355–70.

153. Fainardi E, Borrelli M, Saletti A, Schivalocchi R, Azzini C, Cavallo M, et al. CT perfusion mapping of hemodynamic disturbances associated to acute spontaneous intracerebral hemorrhage. *Neuroradiology.* 2008;50(8):729–40.

154. Zhou J, Zhang H, Gao P, Lin Y, Li X. Assessment of perihematomal hypoperfusion injury in subacute and chronic intracerebral hemorrhage by CT perfusion imaging. *Neurol Res.* 2010;32(6):642–9.

155. Uemura K, Shishido F, Higano S, Inugami A, Kanno I, Takahashi K, et al. Positron emission tomography in patients with a primary intracerebral hematoma. *Acta Radiol Suppl.* 1986;369:426–8.

156. Zazulia AR, Diringer MN, Videen TO, Adams RE, Yundt K, Aiyagari V, et al. Hypoperfusion without ischemia surrounding acute intracerebral hemorrhage. *J Cereb Blood Flow Metab.* 2001;21(7):804–10.

157. Mayer SA, Lignelli A, Fink ME, Kessler DB, Thomas CE, Swarup R, et al. Perilesional blood flow and edema formation in acute intracerebral hemorrhage: a SPECT study. *Stroke.* 1998;29(9):1791–8.

158. Dietrich WD. Morphological manifestations of reperfusion injury in brain. *Ann N Y Acad Sci.* 1994;723:15–24.

159. Kuroda S, Siesjö BK. Reperfusion damage following focal ischemia: pathophysiology and therapeutic windows. *Clin Neurosci.* 1997;4(4):199–212.

160. Hallenbeck JM, Dutka AJ, Tanishima T, Kochanek PM, Kumaroo KK, Thompson CB, et al. Polymorphonuclear leukocyte accumulation in brain regions with low blood flow during the early postischemic period. *Stroke.* 1986;17(2):246–53.

161. Janoff A, Schaefer S, Scherer J, Bean MA. Mediators of inflammation in leukocyte lysosomes. II. Mechanism of action of lysosomal cationic protein upon vascular permeability in the rat. *J Exp Med.* 1965;122(5):841–51.

162. McCabe DJH, Brown MM, Clifton A. Fatal cerebral reperfusion hemorrhage after carotid stenting. *Stroke.* 1999;30(11):2483–6.

163. Hosoda K, Kawaguchi T, Shibata Y, Kamei M, Kidoguchi K, Koyama J, et al. Cerebral vasoreactivity and internal carotid artery flow help to identify patients at risk for hyperperfusion after carotid endarterectomy. *Stroke.* 2001;32(7):1567–73.

164. Ascher E, Markevich N, Schutzer RW, Kallakuri S, Jacob T, Hingorani AP. Cerebral hyperperfusion syndrome after carotid endarterectomy: predictive factors and hemodynamic changes. *J Vasc Surg.* 2003;37(4):769–77.

165. Adhiyaman V, Alexander S. Cerebral hyperperfusion syndrome following carotid endarterectomy. *QJM.* 2007;100(4):239–44.

166. Felipo V. Hepatic encephalopathy: effects of liver failure on brain function. *Nat Rev.* 2013;14(12):851–8.

167. Ede RJ, Gimson AES, Bihari D, Williams R. Controlled hyperventilation in the prevention of cerebral oedema in fulminant hepatic failure. *J Hepatol.* 1986;2(1):43–51.

168. Aggarwal S, Kramer D, Yonas H, Obrist W, Kang Y, Martin M, et al. Cerebral hemodynamic and metabolic changes in fulminant hepatic failure: a retrospective study. *Hepatology.* 1994;19:80–7.

169. Aggarwal S, Obrist W, Yonas H, Kramer D, Kang Y, Scott V, et al. Cerebral hemodynamic and metabolic profiles in fulminant hepatic failure: relationship to outcome. *Liver Transpl.* 2005;11(11):1353–60.

170. Mans AM, DeJoseph MR, Hawkins RA. Metabolic abnormalities and grade of encephalopathy in acute hepatic failure. *J Neurochem.* 1994;63(5):1829–38.

171. Wendon JA, Harrison PM. Cerebral blood flow and metabolism in fulminant liver failure *Hepatology.* 1994;19(6):1407–13.

CHAPTER 4

Cardiorespiratory support in critically ill neurological patients

Maria Vargas, Iole Brunetti, and Paolo Pelosi

Critically ill neurological patients present a complex management challenge. The injured brain may cross-talk with other organ systems via complex pathways that lead to non-neurological organ dysfunction, particularly involving the heart and lungs (1). Patients admitted to the neurocritical care unit (NCCU) may therefore have cardiopulmonary abnormalities that may be related to their underlying neurological pathology or occur incidentally. In a recent analysis by the Ventilia Study Group, 26.5% and 23.0% of mechanically ventilated patients with neurological disease developed cardiovascular and pulmonary complications respectively (2).

This chapter will review the management of cardiorespiratory variables in critically ill neurological patients and highlight the management challenges.

Cardiovascular system

The cardiovascular and central nervous (CNS) systems are intimately related by the same disease processes and their risk factors. For example, age, gender, smoking, diabetes, hypertension, and dyslipidaemia are risk factors for both coronary artery disease and ischaemic and haemorrhagic stroke. Moreover, the CNS regulates cardiovascular function via complex neural pathways and mediators, and these processes may be deranged after brain and spinal cord injury leading to cardiovascular dysfunction (3). Conversely, cardiac and respiratory dysfunction adversely affects the injured brain and spinal cord (see Chapter 27).

The brainstem is responsible for control of cardiovascular function. The nucleus of the tractus solitarius receives afferent information from peripheral arteries, cardiopulmonary chemoreceptors, and baroreceptors via the glossopharyngeal and vagus nerves, and the brainstem responds via parasympathetic and sympathetic efferent pathways. Parasympathetic cholinergic responses control heart rate and contractility as well as many gastrointestinal processes via the vagus nerve while sympathetic responses act on blood vessels, the heart, kidneys, and adrenal medulla in response to barosensitive, thermosensitive, and glucosensitive efferents (4).

Cardiovascular manifestations of central nervous system disease

Acute brain injury (ABI) is associated with a profound and varied catecholamine response. Catecholamines act on receptors located in intracerebral and pial vessels and an excess may lead to systemic cardiovascular dysfunction, including effects on blood vessels and heart rhythm and contractility. The usual response to acute ischaemic or haemorrhagic stroke is hypertension, but blood pressure (BP) control can be challenging because of the substantial heterogeneity between stroke subtypes and an incomplete understanding of the cause of BP changes that occur with each subtype (5). Spinal cord injury may be associated with peripheral vasodilation, bradycardia, and hypotension because of interruption of peripheral sympathetic tone with unopposed vagal effects (6).

Cardiac arrhythmias are also associated with ABI. Sinus bradycardia may occur if the brainstem is compressed by direct pressure or intracranial hypertension, whereas sinus tachycardia and atrial and ventricular arrhythmias are catecholamine related and associated with a poor prognosis. In addition, several acute intracranial disorders can have direct effects on the coronary circulation and/or contractile function of the heart, manifesting as myocardial ischaemia (7) and neurogenic stress cardiomyopathy respectively (8). These issues are discussed in detail in Chapter 27.

Blood pressure management

BP is closely related to cerebral perfusion pressure (CPP), which is the difference between mean arterial pressure (MAP) and intracranial pressure (ICP). In physiological conditions, ICP is small compared to MAP, so MAP essentially determines CPP. Constant cerebral blood flow (CBF) is maintained over a wide range of MAP (60–150 mmHg in normotensive patients) because of cerebral autoregulatory mechanisms (see Chapter 3) (9). When MAP decreases below the lower limit of autoregulation, cerebral vessels dilate in an attempt to maintain CBF. When a critical MAP threshold (for an individual) is reached as autoregulatory mechanisms become exhausted, brain perfusion is compromised. If MAP increases above the upper limit of autoregulation, CBF is pressure passive and increases with MAP, leading to increases in intraluminal pressure, blood–brain barrier (BBB) disruption, and cerebral oedema.

Blood pressure management in specific disease states

Several acute neurological conditions such as subarachnoid (SAH) and intracerebral (ICH) haemorrhage, acute ischaemic stroke (AIS), and traumatic brain injury (TBI) are associated with hypertension as a physiological response to maintain adequate CPP in the context of an acutely injured brain. On the other hand, excessive hypertension may itself exacerbate oedema in injured brain regions or lead to further CNS dysfunction, as is the case in hypertensive encephalopathy and posterior reversible encephalopathy syndrome.

The aim of cardiovascular support in critically ill neurological patients is to stabilize MAP and CPP, and thereby optimize cerebral perfusion and metabolism. There is little evidence to guide cardiovascular management after ABI and therapy should be guided by systemic and cerebral haemodynamic responses assessed by monitoring arterial BP, CPP, and ICP.

Acute ischaemic stroke
More than 75% of patients with AIS have elevated BP (10), but the optimal level of BP control in an individual patient is unknown (5). The American Heart Association (AHA) and American Stroke Association (ASA) recommend that treatment should be instituted only if systolic blood pressure (SBP) is ≥ 220 mmHg and diastolic blood pressure (DBP) is ≥ 120 mmHg (11). It might be reasonable to lower BP by 15% during the first 24 hours after AIS in some patients (see Chapter 20) but a large decrease in BP should be avoided as this is associated with early neurological deterioration, increase in infarct volume, worse neurological outcome, and death (12). Although a degree of hypertension may be beneficial because of its effects to increase CBF (13), BP should be maintained lower than 180/105 mmHg in patients receiving thrombolysis to minimize the risk of haemorrhagic conversion (14). The first step in the pharmacological management of hypertension is intermittent intravenous boluses of a non-vasodilatory antihypertensive agent such as labetalol, although nicardipine is widely used in the USA. If BP is not controlled within 30 minutes, a continuous intravenous infusion should be used (15) in which case labetalol is also the preferred agent (16).

Intracerebral haemorrhage
The ASA/AHA guidelines for the management of spontaneous ICH recommend reduction in BP if SBP and DBP are ≥ 200 mmHg and ≥ 150 mmHg respectively (17). The non-inferiority Antihypertensive Treatment of Acute Cerebral Hemorrhage (ATACH) and Intensive Blood Pressure Reduction in Acute Cerebral Haemorrhage (INTERACT) trials confirmed that lowering of SBP to 140 mmHg decreases the rate of haematoma expansion without causing neurological deterioration, but these studies were not powered to detect beneficial outcome effects (18,19). The subsequent INTERACT 2 trial, published in 2013, provides the best data to date on acute BP management after spontaneous ICH (20). In this large study, early intensive BP lowering (target SBP 140 mmHg within 1 hour) did not result in a significant reduction in the rate of death or major disability at 90 days compared to standard treatment (SBP < 180 mmHg) as most expected it would, although secondary outcome analysis suggested that intensive BP lowering improved functional outcomes in survivors. Intensive BP lowering was not associated with an increased rate of serious adverse events, so BP control might be a reasonable option after spontaneous ICH. BP control after ICH is discussed in more detail in Chapter 19.

Traumatic brain injury
Reductions in BP compromise cerebral perfusion and haemodynamics after TBI so it is crucially important to optimize BP to maintain adequate CPP and minimize the risk of secondary ischaemic brain injury (see Chapter 17). The Brain Trauma Foundation

recommends that CPP should be maintained between 50 and 70 mmHg (21). In the absence of ICP monitoring, SBP should be maintained greater than 90 mmHg because systolic hypotension is the most powerful predictor of poor outcome after TBI (22).

Spinal cord injury
Primary and secondary spinal cord injury (SCI) lead to haemodynamic dysfunction, including decreased heart rate, systemic vascular resistance, and BP (23). A stepwise treatment approach incorporating volume resuscitation and pharmacological support with vasopressors controls BP in most patients after acute SCI (6). Occasionally pacemaker support is required for refractory bradycardia.

Principles of blood pressure management
Fluid resuscitation to euvolaemia is a prerequisite for optimal cardiovascular support after ABI and SCI. Fluid management is covered in detail in Chapter 5 and also in the pathology-specific chapters elsewhere in this book; it will not be consider further here.

Although a hyperdynamic circulation is the acute response to ABI, this is often followed by a period of relative hypotension that can be aggravated by the negative cardiovascular effects of sedation. Many factors affect the ability to control CBF and CPP by manipulation of systemic cardiovascular variables including attenuation or loss of cerebral autoregulation (24) and variations in the arterial partial pressure of oxygen (PaO_2) and carbon dioxide ($PaCO_2$) (25). BBB integrity, which is essential for optimal control of CPP by systemic interventions, may also be compromised after ABI (26).

Despite these issues, inotropes or vasopressors are often the only realistic option to maintain and manage BP and CPP, particularly in the presence of sedation-related hypotension. Different inotropes and vasopressors have varying effects on cerebral haemodynamics and there is little evidence to support the use of one over another (see Chapter 2). In animal models of cortical injury, norepinephrine and dopamine increase MAP to similar degrees, whereas CPP is more effectively sustained by norepinephrine (27). However, in animal models of hypoxic hypotensive cerebral injury norepinephrine and dopamine are unable to increase CPP in the presence of severe acidosis (28,29). A study evaluating the effects of norepinephrine and dopamine on CPP in adult human TBI demonstrated that CBF velocity measured by transcranial Doppler ultrasonography was improved by norepinephrine but not dopamine (30). In another study, dopamine was associated with higher levels of ICP compared to norepinephrine at similar levels of MAP, but the two agents had similar effects on CBF presumably because of intact cerebral autoregulation (31). Another study in patients with severe TBI used positron emission tomography to evaluate the effect of increasing CPP from 70 to 90 mmHg with norepinephrine in ischaemic brain (32). An increase in CPP led to small increases in CBF in all regions of interest except the ischaemic core. Although pericontusional oedematous tissue was associated with lower absolute values of CBF and cerebral blood volume compared to non-oedematous tissue, there was no difference in their relative response to CPP elevation suggesting that the ischaemic core may be unaffected by CPP augmentation. In a retrospective study of patients with severe TBI, phenylephrine produced a greater increase in MAP and CPP compared to norepinephrine and dopamine, although the effects on ICP were similar (33). In brain-injured patients, vasopressors can be associated with side effects such as increased ICP and they may therefore not effectively increase CPP even if they have positive haemodynamic effects (29).

Respiratory system

Respiratory abnormalities, including pneumonia, neurogenic pulmonary oedema, acute respiratory distress syndrome (ARDS), and acute lung injury (ALI), are frequently encountered in critically ill neurological patients (34). Although pulmonary complications have long been related to brain injury-induced increases in sympathetic activity (35), recent evidence also indicates a major role for inflammation (1). Local effects, such as pulmonary aspiration and trauma, also contribute to pulmonary dysfunction in neurological patients (see Chapter 27).

Although ABI and ARDS/ALI are independent pathological entities they can interact, worsen, and trigger each other (1). A study in pigs confirmed the reciprocal and synergistic effects of ABI and ARDS on neuronal and pulmonary damage, and demonstrated that extravascular lung water was higher in animals with ARDS than in those with intracranial hypertension in isolation but highest in those with ARDS and raised ICP in combination (36). The lowest PaO_2 in this study was seen in animals with intracranial hypertension and ARDS, and this was associated with the greatest degree of tissue damage in the hippocampus.

The overarching aim of ventilation after ABI is to maintain oxygenation and normal $PaCO_2$ in order to optimize cerebral perfusion, but care must be taken to minimize its adverse effects, particularly ventilator-induced lung injury (VILI). VILI is a syndrome triggered by over-distension of the lung during mechanical ventilation, recruitment–derecruitment of collapsed alveoli, and activation of inflammatory processes. It can be minimized by the application of protective ventilation strategies (Figure 4.1) (37).

Endotracheal intubation

Endotracheal intubation is one of the most common interventions on the NCCU. Patients with acute neurological problems usually require intubation and ventilation for reasons other than primary pulmonary pathology (34). In a study of more than 2000 patients with ABI admitted to a NCCU, almost 90% required mechanical ventilation at some stage and the primary neurological disease was the indication for intubation and ventilation in two-thirds (38). There are both neurological and respiratory indications for intubation and ventilation in critically ill neurological patients (Box 4.1).

Patients with decreased consciousness have reduced oropharyngeal muscle tone which allows the tongue to be displaced posteriorly and cause varying degrees of airway obstruction. Furthermore, impaired swallow and poor cough and gag reflexes lead to a high risk of pulmonary aspiration and impaired clearance of secretions (39). Patients in whom these states are unlikely to be rapidly reversible require endotracheal intubation, and in such circumstances intubation can be a matter of life and death (40). With lesser degrees of compromise it may be sufficient to monitor a patient closely in a critical care unit where they can be rapidly intubated should their condition worsen. In some circumstances it is prudent to institute intubation and mechanical ventilation in anticipation of neurological and secondarily pulmonary deterioration.

Brain injury also causes respiratory dysrhythmias. Normal control of breathing requires both conscious and automatic neural inputs as well as input from central and peripheral chemoreceptors. The centres for the automatic control of breathing are located in the pons and medulla and these regulate respiration via homeostatic mechanisms to maintain oxygenation and acid–base status. The conscious input to breathing which is beyond awareness interacts with automatic inputs via descending pathways from the cortex. In comatose patients, input from the cortex is absent and breathing is controlled by brainstem centres triggered primarily by changes in $PaCO_2$. The most common breathing patterns in patients with brain injury are tachypnoea and hyperventilation, and these are most commonly associated with cortical and subcortical injury (34). There are also classic respiratory patterns associated with lesions in specific brain regions, often in association with increased ICP. Cheyne–Stokes respiration is characterized by cyclical increases and decreases in respiratory rate and tidal volume and associated with disruption of inter-hemispheric connections and dysfunction of the medial forebrain. Apneustic breathing occurs with lesions of the lower tegmentum and pons and is characterized by prolonged inspiratory pauses. Cluster breathing, seen in lesions of the lower pons or upper medulla, manifests as irregular rapid breaths interposed with long pauses. Ataxic breathing is similar except that there is complete loss of rhythmicity of breathing. Apnoea indicates total loss of brainstem inputs to breathing.

Although endotracheal intubation can be life-saving, if poorly performed it may itself result in secondary brain injury because of hypoxaemia, large swings in BP, and increased ICP (41). This is more likely during rapid sequence induction. Airway manipulation, including laryngoscopy and endotracheal intubation, increases catecholamine levels and activates systemic and intracranial haemodynamic responses resulting in tachycardia, hypertension, and increases in ICP. This can provoke brain herniation in

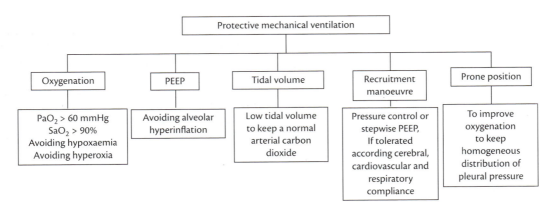

Fig. 4.1 Beneficial effects of different mechanical ventilation variables in neurocritical care.

Box 4.1 Indications for intubation and mechanical ventilation

Neurological

◆ Coma

◆ Decreasing conscious level

◆ Predicted neurological deterioration

◆ Inability to protect the airway and clear secretions

◆ Intracranial hypertension

◆ Severe neuromuscular weakness.

Respiratory

◆ Pulmonary aspiration

◆ Pneumonia

◆ Acute respiratory distress syndrome/acute lung injury

◆ Pulmonary embolism

◆ Neurogenic pulmonary oedema

◆ Inability to handle and clear secretions.

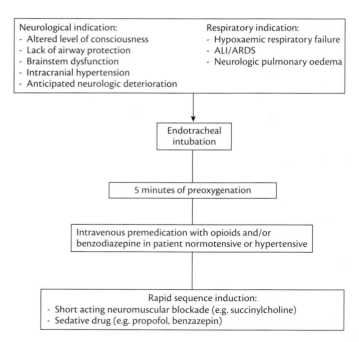

Fig. 4.2 Algorithm for endotracheal intubation in critically ill brain-injured patients. Note: life-threatening contraindications, including concomitant crush injury, long-standing immobilization, myopathy, spinal cord injury with paraplegia, and a history of malignant hyperthermia, must be excluded prior to the use of succinylcholine. If any of these possibilities exist, an alternate form of neuromuscular blockade (or intubation without it) needs to be planned.

the presence of a critical mass lesion. Sedation is a prerequisite for successful endotracheal intubation to minimize the hyperdynamic responses to laryngoscopy but care must be taken to minimize sedation-related hypotension, particularly after the institution of positive pressure ventilation which diminishes venous return and therefore cardiac output. Sedation also obscures clinical neurological examination during the early and often most critical period of neurological and neurosurgical decision-making. Rapid patient stabilization must occur concurrently with well-documented and detailed neurological assessment which should ideally take place prior to the administration of sedative and paralysing medications in order to provide a baseline assessment (40). A recommended protocol for endotracheal intubation in brain-injured patients designed to minimize these adverse effects is shown in Figure 4.2.

The exact timing of endotracheal intubation in TBI patients has been a topic of considerable interest and research. Studies investigating the benefits of pre-hospital intubation are conflicting with some showing benefits and others harm possibly related to longer field times, misplaced tracheal tubes, and overly aggressive hyperventilation (42). In a retrospective study, 23% of almost 11,000 TBI patients with a Glasgow Coma Scale (GCS) score of 3 were intubated in a pre-hospital setting and the mortality rate was higher compared to those who were intubated in hospital (62% vs 35%) (43). A more recent study randomly allocated patients with severe TBI to paramedic rapid sequence intubation or transport to hospital for intubation by physicians and found that pre-hospital intubation significantly increased the rate of favourable neurological outcome at 6 months (44). However, a meta-analysis of 13 largely observational studies including more than 15,000 patients reported that the adjusted odds of in-hospital mortality for patients who underwent pre-hospital intubation and mechanical ventilation ranged from 0.24 to 1.42, suggesting that inadequate evidence exists to support a benefit of early advanced airway placement (42).

Mechanical ventilation

Mechanical ventilation is often necessary in critically ill brain-injured patients, providing essential life support in many cases. However, no large studies have systematically investigated the impact of different ventilator strategies on cerebral oxygenation.

The ARDSNet protocol has been shown to reduce mortality in the setting of ARDS and advocates the use of low tidal volumes, relatively high levels of positive end-expiratory pressure (PEEP), and permissive hypercapnia to reduce VILI (45). Such protective ventilator strategies can be achieved in many patients with ABI and ALI without threatening cerebral perfusion. However, this can be less straightforward in patients with poor intracranial compliance and refractory intracranial hypertension, and the optimal balance between brain-directed and protective ventilator strategies is uncertain (37). In the Ventilia Study Group analysis, volume-cycled assist controlled ventilation was the most common ventilator mode applied in neurological patients, similar to that in the general ICU population (2). However, the majority of patients in this study were ventilated with tidal volumes between 6 and 12 mL/kg predicted body weight and more than 80% with PEEP equal to or less than 5 cmH$_2$O in the presence of adequate arterial oxygenation, suggesting that clinicians were (possibly inappropriately) focused on the injured brain at the expense of the lungs. This is a cause for concern as ARDS/ALI are frequently seen in critically ill neurological patients (34). Up to 35% of patients with TBI and SAH develop ARDS/ALI and this is associated with poor outcome (46–49).

The optimal ventilator strategy to manage respiratory failure after ABI has not been determined with certainty and the following commentary represents the authors' recommendations for the management of respiratory complication in critically ill neurological patients, based on current evidence.

Arterial oxygenation and carbon dioxide tension

Hypoxaemia is a major cause of secondary brain injury and poor outcome after ABI. In animal models of focal brain injury, hypoxaemia results in neuronal death in vulnerable brain regions and is associated with functional motor deficits (50). Similarly after traumatic axonal injury, hypoxaemia is associated with greater degrees of axonal damage and macrophage infiltration, enhanced astrogliosis in the corpus callosum and brainstem, and delayed recovery compared to normoxic animals, suggesting that secondary brain injury in the context of hypoxaemia may be induced by enhanced neuroinflammation and a prolonged period of metabolic dysfunction (51).

Hypoxaemia is also associated with a poor outcome in human TBI (52). In a meta-analysis of seven phase III randomized clinical trials and three TBI population-based series in the IMPACT database, hypoxaemia and hypotension were strongly associated with a poorer outcome (odds ratios 2.1 and 2.7 respectively) in moderate or severe TBI (22). Patients with both hypoxaemia and hypotension had worse outcomes than those with either insult alone. The occurrence of secondary systemic physiological insults prior to or on admission to hospital in TBI is strongly related to worse outcome and their prevention or immediate treatment is therefore a priority. The adverse effects of systemic hypoxaemia are unsurprising given that it has two effects—it decreases cerebral oxygen delivery and dilates the cerebral vasculature. A reduction in brain tissue oxygenation has well-known effects on cerebral metabolism, and the resultant hypoxic cerebral vasodilation increases ICP and reduces CPP, further reducing cerebral oxygen delivery (see Chapters 2 and 7). Although the avoidance of hypoxaemia is a priority, hyperoxaemia can also be deleterious after ABI particularly in the first 24 hours after injury when it has been associated with a higher mortality and worse functional outcome (53). High oxygen levels increase lipid peroxidation in the cerebral cortex and induce oxidative brain damage (54). In its guidance, the Brain Trauma Foundation recommends avoiding hypoxaemia, defined as PaO_2 lower than 8.0 kPa (60 mmHg) or oxygen saturation less than 90% (55). Ideally PaO_2 should be maintained between 10.7 and 13.3 kPa (80–100 mmHg), using appropriate nontoxic (as able) FiO_2 and levels of PEEP, to ensure adequate cerebral oxygenation (56).

Although the primary ventilation goal after ABI is normocapnia, permissive hypercapnia is frequently incorporated into ventilation strategies on the NCCU to allow lower tidal volume and PEEP to minimize the risk of VILI, and has not been shown to induce brain injury (34). However, in patients with intact cerebral haemodynamic responses to $PaCO_2$, careful monitoring including ICP monitoring is required to minimize adverse effects of hypercapnia on the injured brain, including the potential for herniation syndromes.

Positive end-expiratory pressure

A moderate level of PEEP avoids progressive alveolar collapse and pulmonary consolidation during mechanical ventilation and thereby improves arterial oxygenation and reduces the elastance of the respiratory system (56). PEEP is a key component of the ARDSNet protocol but the use of PEEP is controversial in the critical care management of brain-injured patients.

PEEP has been reported to increase ICP and this has been thought to be related to reduced venous return from the intracranial compartment as a result of increased intrathoracic pressure (ITP) (57,58). However, other studies have reported no such association, and the influence of PEEP on ICP therefore remains controversial (59,60). It has been suggested that only patients with compliant lungs will experience cerebral venous outflow compromise and increases in ICP with higher levels of PEEP. Non-compliant lungs, such as may occur in pneumonia or ALI/ARDS, are incapable of transmitting the pressure associated with PEEP to the central venous system and thus there is little effect on systemic or cerebral venous return. Moreover, increased venous pressure from PEEP (via compliant lungs) needs to approach or exceed the level of ICP in order to affect cerebral venous outflow. It therefore seems likely that in some patients at least the predominant mechanism by which elevated ICP is increased further by PEEP is via decreased systemic BP and reflex cerebral vasodilation, rather than a direct effect to reduce cerebral venous outflow. In a study of ABI patients with poor pulmonary compliance, varying levels of PEEP had no significant effect on cerebral and systemic haemodynamics but did improve systemic oxygenation (59). This study and theoretical considerations suggest that PEEP may be safe in brain-injured patients and that it might also have beneficial effects on the brain if it improves systemic and therefore cerebral oxygenation. Certainly allowing hypoxaemia because of concerns about PEEP is inappropriate after ABI.

Venous blood flow from the brain is related to the balance between ICP driving in out of the cranium and jugular venous pressure impeding the exit of blood from the brain. It therefore seems likely that PEEP may be safe when it does not exceed ICP (58,60). The effect of PEEP on cerebral haemodynamics also depends on whether it results in recruitment or hyperinflation of alveolar units because of their different effects on $PaCO_2$ and therefore brain perfusion (36).

In addition to potential adverse effects on ICP, PEEP can also decrease venous return, cardiac output, MAP, and thereby CPP. However, the use of appropriate levels of PEEP during mechanical ventilation appears to have limited effect on CPP and MAP in many patients (61).

Overall, PEEP is a useful adjunct to improve pulmonary compliance and increase alveolar oxygenation and oxygen saturation in the setting of ABI and pulmonary dysfunction, but close monitoring of haemodynamic variables, pulmonary compliance, gas exchange, and ICP are mandatory to quantify the risks and benefits of its use.

Tidal volume

Low tidal volumes (6 mL/kg ideal body weight) reduce ventilator days and mortality in patients with ARDS (45), whereas high tidal volume ventilation exacerbates the pulmonary and systemic inflammatory response of ARDS and leads to VILI (62). High tidal volume and respiratory rate are the most powerful independent predictors of early ARDS after TBI, with a dose response between tidal volume and risk of developing ARDS (62). Tidal volume should therefore be chosen to balance the adverse cerebral haemodynamic effects of low or high $PaCO_2$ secondary to over- or under-ventilation against the risk of ARDS.

Recruitment manoeuvres

A recruitment manoeuvre is a strategy to increase transpulmonary pressure transiently with the aim of reopening unventilated or poorly aerated alveolar units in patients with ARDS. Recruitment manoeuvres can be performed using an increase in airway pressure with an appropriate level of PEEP or by transiently increasing tidal volume. Both have potential adverse effects including increased ITP and ICP, and decreased preload, cardiac output, and CPP. In a study in patients with coexistent acute brain and lung injury, an increase in P_{max} from baseline to 60 cmH_2O over 30 seconds, and maintained for 30 seconds, decreased MAP and increased ICP, leading to a critical reduction in CPP and a decrease in jugular venous oxygen saturation (63). In another study comparing 35 cmH_2O of continuous positive airway pressure (CPAP) for 40 seconds to pressure control ventilation (PCV) with 15 cmH_2O of PEEP and 35 cmH_2O of pressure control above PEEP in patients with SAH and ARDS, the CPAP recruitment manoeuvre significantly increased ICP and decreased MAP and CPP whilst the PCV manoeuvre had no or little effect on ICP or cerebral haemodynamics (64). The effect of PEEP-induced recruitment manoeuvres on cerebral haemodynamics in brain-injured patients is related to baseline respiratory system compliance and haemodynamic status, and such manoeuvres should only be performed with close monitoring of MAP, ICP, and CPP (65).

Prone positioning

The prone position is an established rescue measure in patients with ARDS. It has been reported to increase oxygenation in up to 80% of patients (66). Likely mechanisms include alterations in thoracoabdominal compliance coupled with changes in regional ventilation and improvements in end-expiratory lung volume and ventilation–perfusion matching (67). However, concerns exist over use of the prone position in brain-injured patients (56,68). Transitioning into the prone position or maintaining prone ventilation may result in inadvertent removal or displacement of intracranial monitoring devices and invasive vascular catheters (56). Facial and truncal ulcers have also been reported in comatose patients managed in the prone position. A randomized controlled trial of 51 comatose patients found that prone position ventilation for 4 hours daily was associated with improved pulmonary function compared to ventilation in supine position, although this resulted in an increase in ICP from 11 mmHg to 24 mmHg by 1 hour after turning prone (68). The prone position had to be abandoned in two patients in this study because ICP increased above 30 mmHg. However, some recent studies have reported potential beneficial effects of the prone position in patients with ABI and ARDS. In a study in critically ill neurological patients with pulmonary complications, the prone position was associated with improved oxygenation compared with supine (69). Although there was a slight increase ICP in the prone position, there was improvement in CPP because of an increase in cardiac output and MAP.

Prone positioning should be considered an option to prevent and ameliorate pulmonary complications during neurocritical care, but should only be used in association with comprehensive haemodynamic and cerebral monitoring to identify potential complications early.

Other rescue strategies

Although many patients with ABI may be managed with the earlier mentioned strategies, some may require additional rescue procedures for failing oxygenation. As repetitive over-distension of lung units may exacerbate ALI and ARDS there has been recent interest in novel ventilatory strategies, such as high-frequency oscillation (HFO), which may be associated with less risk of barotrauma. HFO delivers extremely small tidal volumes (1–2 mL/kg) at very high respiratory rates (3–15 breaths/second). Although several randomized controlled trials suggested a benefit of HFO in non-neurological patients with ARDS (70), a recent systematic review of HFO in brain-injured patients concluded that its effect on patient outcome as well as on systemic and cerebral haemodynamics are largely uncertain (71).

The use of extracorporeal membrane oxygenation has been described in patients with TBI and severe ARDS or neurogenic pulmonary oedema (72) and it has been suggested that nitric oxide may also be of benefit (70). However, the role of these interventions in brain-injured patients remains largely unknown.

Weaning from mechanical ventilation

Weaning from mechanical ventilation is classified according to temporal criteria as simple, difficult, or prolonged (68). Weaning is considered to be simple when patients are extubated on the first attempt, difficult when up to three spontaneous breathing trials (SBT) are required, but extubation is successful in less than 7 days from the first trial, and prolonged when a patient fails the first three SBTs or requires more than 7 days to be weaned from the ventilator.

Critically ill neurological patients with brain injury or neuromuscular disease are more difficult to wean from ventilation than other ICU patients because of the contribution of their neurological illness to respiratory function and the high rate of associated pulmonary dysfunction (73). As a consequence, extubation is often delayed and this is associated with an increased risk of ventilator-associated pneumonia (VAP) and ICU length of stay (74). Furthermore, delayed extubation is relatively common in neurological patients who are otherwise ready to wean by conventional respiratory and haemodynamic criteria because of factors related to their neurological disease (75). In a retrospective review of 1265 patients who were intubated for neurological reasons, 844 (67%) were successfully extubated and only 129 (10%) required reintubation during their hospital stay (41). The most common reasons for reintubation in this study were ARDS associated with altered mental state, followed by pneumonia. A prospective clinical trial demonstrated that it is the presence of a cough associated with effective secretion clearance and not neurological status per se that is predictive of successful extubation in critically ill neurological patients (76). In this study, substantial numbers of patients meeting standard readiness criteria had extubation delayed because of concerns with neurological status (depressed level of consciousness), but this delay was associated with a higher incidence of VAP and longer ICU and hospital lengths of stay. In a randomized clinical trial, a protocol-driven strategy using general cardiorespiratory readiness criteria for extubation, GCS score higher than 8, the presence of an effective cough, and tolerance of a 1-hour SBT was compared to physician-driven discontinuation of mechanical ventilation (77). The reintubation rate was lower in the protocol-driven group but there was no difference in mortality, rate of tracheostomy, and duration of mechanical ventilation between the groups. Patients with infratentorial pathology deserve special mention because of the relatively high rates of bulbar dysfunction and conscious level disturbance. In a retrospective study, 18% of patients with an infratentorial lesion required elective tracheostomy because of extubation failure, and GCS score lower than 8 was a good predictor of the need for tracheostomy (78).

A practical strategy for weaning from mechanical ventilation in neurocritical care includes ongoing assessment of neurological status, including level of consciousness, presence of protective airway reflexes, and effective secretion clearance, in addition to standard respiratory and cardiovascular readiness criteria. Overall the evidence suggests that there is often little justification for delaying extubation in patients who meet standard readiness criteria if the only indication for continued intubation is a depressed level of consciousness. An optimal level of oxygenation, BP, ICP, and CPP should be assured during the weaning process which should only be considered when ICP is stable.

Tracheostomy

Tracheostomy is indicated in patients requiring prolonged mechanical ventilation and/or those who are difficult to wean from ventilation. It offers many advantages over translaryngeal intubation including reduced work of breathing, lower incidence of pneumonia, and better tolerance by the patient resulting in reduced sedation requirements. Tracheostomy may also reduce the length of ICU stay and overall pulmonary complication rate in brain-injured patients (79). The largest randomized clinical trial investigating the timing of tracheostomy in a heterogeneous cohort of critically ill patients was performed in Italian ICUs, and early tracheostomy (performed after 6–8 days of mechanical ventilation) was associated with a reduction in ventilator-free days but not with the incidence of VAP, mortality, or length of hospital stay compared to late tracheostomy (performed after 13–15 days of ventilation) (80).

The timing of tracheostomy in critically ill neurological patients remains a matter of intense debate. In a prospective randomized trial in patients with TBI, early tracheostomy was associated with fewer days of mechanical ventilation compared with prolonged endotracheal intubation but it did not reduce mortality, incidence of VAP, or ICU length of stay (81). In another study, 66 (2.7%) of 2481 patients with severe TBI required a tracheostomy and 16 of these were performed early and 50 late (82). The ICU length of stay was significantly shorter, the incidence of nosocomial pneumonia lower, and duration of antibiotic use shorter in the early tracheostomy group. However, a recent meta-analysis demonstrated that although the duration of mechanical ventilation decreases with early tracheostomy after severe TBI, the risk of hospital death increases (83). An important consideration when deciding on the timing of tracheostomy is the physiological stability of a patient in the early phase after ABI. The need to place the patient supine with the attendant risk of increased ICP, and the risk of interruption of oxygenation are important factors that can mitigate against early tracheostomy in such patients. Thus, routine early tracheostomy does not appear to be a prudent policy in many patients with severe brain injury.

Based on limited evidence, physiologically stable patients with a GCS score lower than 8 at 1 week after admission to the NCCU, those with brainstem pathology with a reasonable prospect of survival, and those severely affected with neuromuscular syndromes with anticipation of prolonged mechanical ventilation should be considered for early tracheostomy (84).

Ventilator-associated pneumonia

The incidence of VAP in neurocritical care patients is between 30% and 50%, depending on the definition used (85), and the development of VAP adversely affects outcome (see Chapter 27). In a case–control study, patients with severe brain injury and VAP had an increased duration of mechanical ventilation and ICU and hospital lengths of stay (86). Early-onset VAP was primarily related to infection with *Staphylococcus aureus*, whereas *Haemophilus influenza* and *Pseudomonas aeruginosa* were the most common pathogens in late-onset VAP. More severe injury, GCS score lower than 6, and/or the presence of cervical fracture with neurological deficit had a specificity of 97% for the prediction of VAP. Severity of injury has also been associated with the development of VAP after TBI (87). In a case–control series of 144 patients with severe TBI, approximately one-half developed VAP, of which 42% was early onset and 58% late onset (88). The development of VAP was associated with a higher mortality rate (20.8% vs 15.3%), increased duration of mechanical ventilation, and increased ICU length of stay.

The diagnosis of VAP is based on the presence of new or progressive pulmonary infiltrates and at least two of fever or hypothermia (temperature $\geq$ 38°C or $\leq$ 36°C), leucocytosis or leucopoenia (> 12×10^9/L or < 3.5×10^9/L), purulent respiratory secretions, and clinical pulmonary infectious score higher than 6. Microbiological confirmation relies on the isolation of at least one potentially pathogenic organism in tracheobronchial aspirates (> 10^5 CFU/mL), blind bronchoalveolar lavage fluid (> 10^4 CFU/mL), and/or bronchoscopic protected brush specimens (> 10^3 CFU/mL) (87).

According to consensus guidelines (89), strategies to prevent VAP should include:

- an oral hygiene programme for all intubated patients
- a programme to minimize aspiration of microbiologically contaminated secretions, including:
  - elevation of the patient's head greater than 30° above horizontal
  - suctioning of pooled secretion in the oropharynx
  - avoidance of gastric distension
  - avoidance of medications to increase gastric pH
  - ventilator tubes clear of condensation
- frequent hand washing, use of gloves when in direct patient contact, and alcohol gel at every bedside
- standardized ventilator weaning protocols.

In cases of suspected VAP, empirical antibiotic treatment directed against likely pathogens should be instituted as soon as possible after respiratory samples have been obtained, with de-escalation of treatment based on culture results and/or sensitivities. The duration of antibiotic treatment should be directed by the clinical response, avoiding predetermined lengths of treatments. In most cases, an appropriate clinical response will be noted and antibiotics can be stopped within 8 days.

References

1. Pelosi P, Rocco PR. The lung and the brain: a dangerous cross-talk. *Crit Care*. 2011;15:168.
2. Pelosi P, Ferguson ND, Frutos-Vivar F, Anzueto A, Putensen C, Raymondos K, *et al*. Management and outcome of mechanically ventilated neurologic patients. *Crit Care Med*. 2011;39:1482–92.
3. Zygun DA, Kortbeek JB, Fick GH, Laupland KB, Doig CJ. Non-neurologic organ dysfunction in severe traumatic brain injury. *Crit Care Med*. 2005;33:654–60.
4. Green AL, Paterson DJ. Identification of neurocircuitry controlling cardiovascular function in humans using functional neurosurgery: implications for exercise control. *Exp Physiol*. 2008;93:1022–8.

5. Grise EM, Adeoye O. Blood pressure control for acute ischemic and hemorrhagic stroke. *Curr Opin Crit Care*. 2012;18:132–8.

6. Stevens RD, Bhardwaj A, Kirsch JR, Mirski MA. Critical care and perioperative management in traumatic spinal cord injury. *J Neurosurg Anesthesiol*. 2003;15:215–29.

7. Marion DW, Segal R, Thompson ME. Subarachnoid hemorrhage and the heart. *Neurosurgery*. 1986;18:101–6.

8. Nguyen H, Zaroff JG. Neurogenic stunned myocardium. *Curr Neurol Neurosci Rep*. 2009;9:486–91.

9. Strandgaard S, Olesen J, Skinhoj E, Lassen NA. Autoregulation of brain circulation in severe arterial hypertension. *Br Med J*. 1973;1:507–10.

10. Oppenheimer S, Hachinski V. Complications of acute stroke. *Lancet*. 1992;339:721–4.

11. Adams HP, Jr., del Zoppo G, Alberts MJ, Bhatt DL, Brass L, Furlan A, *et al*. Guidelines for the early management of adults with ischemic stroke: a guideline from the American Heart Association/ American Stroke Association Stroke Council, Clinical Cardiology Council, Cardiovascular Radiology and Intervention Council, and the Atherosclerotic Peripheral Vascular Disease and Quality of Care Outcomes in Research Interdisciplinary Working Groups: The American Academy of Neurology affirms the value of this guideline as an educational tool for neurologists. *Circulation*. 2007;115:e478–e534.

12. Castillo J, Leira R, Garcia MM, Serena J, Blanco M, Davalos A. Blood pressure decrease during the acute phase of ischemic stroke is associated with brain injury and poor stroke outcome. *Stroke*. 2004;35:520–6.

13. Hillis AE, Ulatowski JA, Barker PB, Torbey M, Ziai W, Beauchamp NJ, *et al*. A pilot randomized trial of induced blood pressure elevation: effects on function and focal perfusion in acute and subacute stroke. *Cerebrovasc Dis*. 2003;16:236–46.

14. Burns JD, Green DM, Metivier K, DeFusco C. Intensive care management of acute ischemic stroke. *Emerg Med Clin North Am*. 2012;30:713–44.

15. Qureshi AI. Acute hypertensive response in patients with stroke: pathophysiology and management. *Circulation*. 2008;118:176–87.

16. Barer DH, Cruickshank JM, Ebrahim SB, Mitchell JR. Low dose beta blockade in acute stroke ("BEST" trial): an evaluation. *Br Med J (Clin Res Ed)*. 1988;296:737–41.

17. Broderick J, Connolly S, Feldmann E, Hanley D, Kase C, Krieger D, *et al*. Guidelines for the management of spontaneous intracerebral hemorrhage in adults: 2007 update: a guideline from the American Heart Association/American Stroke Association Stroke Council, High Blood Pressure Research Council, and the Quality of Care and Outcomes in Research Interdisciplinary Working Group. *Stroke*. 2007;38:2001–23.

18. Anderson CS, Huang Y, Wang JG, Arima H, Neal B, Peng B, *et al*. Intensive blood pressure reduction in acute cerebral haemorrhage trial (INTERACT): a randomised pilot trial. *Lancet Neurol*. 2008;7:391–9.

19. Qureshi AI. Antihypertensive Treatment of Acute Cerebral Hemorrhage (ATACH): rationale and design. *Neurocrit Care*. 2007;6:56–66.

20. Anderson CS, Heeley E, Huang Y, Wang J, Stapf C, Delcourt C, *et al*. Rapid blood-pressure lowering in patients with acute intracerebral hemorrhage. *N Engl J Med*. 2013;368:2355–65.

21. The Brain Trauma Foundation. The American Association of Neurological Surgeons. The Joint Section on Neurotrauma and Critical Care. Cerebral perfusion pressure thresholds. *J Neurotrauma*. 2007;24:S59–S64.

22. McHugh GS, Engel DC, Butcher I, Steyerberg EW, Lu J, Mushkudiani N, *et al*. Prognostic value of secondary insults in traumatic brain injury: results from the IMPACT study. *J Neurotrauma*. 2007;24:287–93.

23. Chittiboina P, Cuellar-Saenz H, Notarianni C, Cardenas R, Guthikonda B. Head and spinal cord injury: diagnosis and management. *Neurol Clin*. 2012;30:241–76.

24. Mascia L, Andrews PJ, McKeating EG, Souter MJ, Merrick MV, Piper IR. Cerebral blood flow and metabolism in severe brain injury: the role of pressure autoregulation during cerebral perfusion pressure management. *Intensive Care Med*. 2000;26:202–5.

25. Hurn PD, Traystman RJ. Changes in arterial gas tension. In Edvinsson L, Krause DN (eds) *Cerebral Blood Flow and Metabolism*. Philadelphia, PA: Lippincott Williams & Wilkins; 2002:384–94.

26. Edvinsson L, Krause DN. Catecholamines. In Edvinsson L, Krause DN (eds) *Cerebral Blood Flow and Metabolism*. Philadelphia, PA: Lippincott, Williams & Wilkins; 2002:191–211.

27. Kroppenstedt SN, Sakowitz OW, Thomale UW, Unterberg AW, Stover JF. Norepinephrine is superior to dopamine in increasing cortical perfusion following controlled cortical impact injury in rats. *Acta Neurochir Suppl*. 2002;81:225–7.

28. Ract C, Vigue B, Bodjarian N, Mazoit JX, Samii K, Tadie M. Comparison of dopamine and norepinephrine after traumatic brain injury and hypoxic-hypotensive insult. *J Neurotrauma*. 2001;18:1247–54.

29. Stubbe HD, Greiner C, Westphal M, Rickert CH, Aken HV, Eichel V, *et al*. Cerebral response to norepinephrine compared with fluid resuscitation in ovine traumatic brain injury and systemic inflammation. *Crit Care Med*. 2006;34:2651–7.

30. Steiner LA, Johnston AJ, Czosnyka M, Chatfield DA, Salvador R, Coles JP, *et al*. Direct comparison of cerebrovascular effects of norepinephrine and dopamine in head-injured patients. *Crit Care Med*. 2004;32:1049–54.

31. Ract C, Vigue B. Comparison of the cerebral effects of dopamine and norepinephrine in severely head-injured patients. *Intensive Care Med*. 2001;27:101–6.

32. Steiner LA, Coles JP, Johnston AJ, Czosnyka M, Fryer TD, Smielewski P, *et al*. Responses of posttraumatic pericontusional cerebral blood flow and blood volume to an increase in cerebral perfusion pressure. *J Cereb Blood Flow Metab*. 2003;23:1371–7.

33. Sookplung P, Siriussawakul A, Malakouti A, Sharma D, Wang J, Souter MJ, *et al*. Vasopressor use and effect on blood pressure after severe adult traumatic brain injury. *Neurocrit Care*. 2011;15:46–54.

34. Chang WT, Nyquist PA. Strategies for the use of mechanical ventilation in the neurologic intensive care unit. *Neurosurg Clin N Am*. 2013;24:407–16.

35. Touho H, Karasawa J, Shishido H, Yamada K, Yamazaki Y. Neurogenic pulmonary edema in the acute stage of hemorrhagic cerebrovascular disease. *Neurosurgery*. 1989, 25:762–8.

36. Heuer JF, Pelosi P, Hermann P, Perske C, Crozier TA, Bruck W, *et al*. Acute effects of intracranial hypertension and ARDS on pulmonary and neuronal damage: a randomized experimental study in pigs. *Intensive Care Med*. 2011;37:1182–91.

37. Lowe GJ, Ferguson ND. Lung-protective ventilation in neurosurgical patients. *Curr Opin Crit Care*. 2006;12:3–7.

38. Karanjia N, Nordquist D, Stevens R, Nyquist P. A clinical description of extubation failure in patients with primary brain injury. *Neurocrit Care*. 2011;15:4–12.

39. Wijdicks EF, Borel CO. Respiratory management in acute neurologic illness. *Neurology* 1998;50:11–20.

40. Seder DB, Riker RR, Jagoda A, Smith WS, Weingart SD. Emergency neurological life support: airway, ventilation, and sedation. *Neurocrit Care*. 2012;17 Suppl 1:S4–20.

41. Stevens RD, Lazaridis C, Chalela JA. The role of mechanical ventilation in acute brain injury. *Neurol Clin*. 2008;26:543–63.

42. von Elm E, Schoettker P, Henzi I, Osterwalder J, Walder B. Pre-hospital tracheal intubation in patients with traumatic brain injury: systematic review of current evidence. *Br J Anaesth*. 2009;103:371–86.

43. Irvin CB, Szpunar S, Cindrich LA, Walters J, Sills R. Should trauma patients with a Glasgow Coma Scale score of 3 be intubated prior to hospital arrival? *Prehosp Disaster Med*. 2010;25:541–6.

44. Bernard SA, Nguyen V, Cameron P, Masci K, Fitzgerald M, Cooper DJ, *et al*. Prehospital rapid sequence intubation improves functional outcome for patients with severe traumatic brain injury: a randomized controlled trial. *Ann Surg*. 2010;252:959–65.

45. The Acute Respiratory Distress Syndrome Network. Ventilation with lower tidal volumes as compared with traditional tidal volumes for acute lung injury and the acute respiratory distress syndrome. *N Engl J Med.* 2000;342:1301–8.

46. Bratton SL, Davis RL. Acute lung injury in isolated traumatic brain injury. *Neurosurgery.* 1997;40:707–12.

47. Holland MC, Mackersie RC, Morabito D, Campbell AR, Kivett VA, Patel R, et al. The development of acute lung injury is associated with worse neurologic outcome in patients with severe traumatic brain injury. *J Trauma.* 2003;55:106–11.

48. Kahn JM, Caldwell EC, Deem S, Newell DW, Heckbert SR, Rubenfeld GD. Acute lung injury in patients with subarachnoid hemorrhage: incidence, risk factors, and outcome. *Crit Care Med.* 2006;34:196–202.

49. Robertson CS, Valadka AB, Hannay HJ, Contant CF, Gopinath SP, Cormio M, et al. Prevention of secondary ischemic insults after severe head injury. *Crit Care Med.* 1999;27:2086–95.

50. Clark RS, Kochanek PM, Dixon CE, Chen M, Marion DW, Heineman S, et al. Early neuropathologic effects of mild or moderate hypoxemia after controlled cortical impact injury in rats. *J Neurotrauma.* 1997;14:179–89.

51. Yan EB, Hellewell SC, Bellander BM, Agyapomaa DA, Morganti-Kossmann MC. Post-traumatic hypoxia exacerbates neurological deficit, neuroinflammation and cerebral metabolism in rats with diffuse traumatic brain injury. *J Neuroinflammation.* 2011;8:147.

52. Chi JH, Knudson MM, Vassar MJ, McCarthy MC, Shapiro MB, Mallet S, et al. Prehospital hypoxia affects outcome in patients with traumatic brain injury: a prospective multicenter study. *J Trauma.* 2006;61:1134–41.

53. Brenner M, Stein D, Hu P, Kufera J, Wooford M, Scalea T. Association between early hyperoxia and worse outcomes after traumatic brain injury. *Arch Surg.* 2012;147:1042–6.

54. Solberg R, Longini M, Proietti F, Vezzosi P, Saugstad OD, Buonocore G. Resuscitation with supplementary oxygen induces oxidative injury in the cerebral cortex. *Free Radic Biol Med.* 2012;53:1061–7.

55. The Brain Trauma Foundation. The American Association of Neurological Surgeons. The Joint Section on Neurotrauma and Critical Care. Blood pressure and oxygenation. *J Neurotrauma.* 2007;24:S7–S13.

56. Young N, Rhodes JK, Mascia L, Andrews PJ. Ventilatory strategies for patients with acute brain injury. *Curr Opin Crit Care.* 2010;16:45–52.

57. Huynh T, Messer M, Sing RF, Miles W, Jacobs DG, Thomason MH. Positive end-expiratory pressure alters intracranial and cerebral perfusion pressure in severe traumatic brain injury. *J Trauma.* 2002;53:488–92.

58. McGuire G, Crossley D, Richards J, Wong D. Effects of varying levels of positive end-expiratory pressure on intracranial pressure and cerebral perfusion pressure. *Crit Care Med.* 1997;25:1059–62.

59. Caricato A, Conti G, Della CF, Mancino A, Santilli F, Sandroni C, et al. Effects of PEEP on the intracranial system of patients with head injury and subarachnoid hemorrhage: the role of respiratory system compliance. *J Trauma.* 2005;58:571–6.

60. Johnson VE, Huang JH, Pilcher WH. Special cases: mechanical ventilation of neurosurgical patients. *Crit Care Clin.* 2007;23:275–90.

61. Mascia L, Grasso S, Fiore T, Bruno F, Berardino M, Ducati A. Cerebro-pulmonary interactions during the application of low levels of positive end-expiratory pressure. *Intensive Care Med.* 2005;31:373–9.

62. Mascia L, Zavala E, Bosma K, Pasero D, Decaroli D, Andrews P, et al. High tidal volume is associated with the development of acute lung injury after severe brain injury: an international observational study. *Crit Care Med.* 2007;35:1815–20.

63. Bein T, Kuhr LP, Bele S, Ploner F, Keyl C, Taeger K. Lung recruitment maneuver in patients with cerebral injury: effects on intracranial pressure and cerebral metabolism. *Intensive Care Med.* 2002;28:554–8.

64. Nemer SN, Caldeira JB, Azeredo LM, Garcia JM, Silva RT, Prado D, et al. Alveolar recruitment maneuver in patients with subarachnoid hemorrhage and acute respiratory distress syndrome: a comparison of 2 approaches. *J Crit Care.* 2011;26:22–7.

65. Zhang XY, Yang ZJ, Wang QX, Fan HR. Impact of positive end-expiratory pressure on cerebral injury patients with hypoxemia. *Am J Emerg Med.* 2011;29:699–703.

66. Gattinoni L, Tognoni G, Pesenti A, Taccone P, Mascheroni D, Labarta V, et al. Effect of prone positioning on the survival of patients with acute respiratory failure. *N Engl J Med.* 2001;345:568–73.

67. Abroug F, Ouanes-Besbes L, Dachraoui F, Ouanes I, Brochard L. An updated study-level meta-analysis of randomised controlled trials on proning in ARDS and acute lung injury. *Crit Care.* 2011;15:R6.

68. Beuret P, Carton MJ, Nourdine K, Kaaki M, Tramoni G, Ducreux JC. Prone position as prevention of lung injury in comatose patients: a prospective, randomized, controlled study. *Intensive Care Med.* 2002;28:564–9.

69. Nekludov M, Bellander BM, Mure M. Oxygenation and cerebral perfusion pressure improved in the prone position. *Acta Anaesthesiol Scand.* 2006;50:932–6.

70. Papadimos TJ. The beneficial effects of inhaled nitric oxide in patients with severe traumatic brain injury complicated by acute respiratory distress syndrome: a hypothesis. *J Trauma Manag Outcomes.* 2008;2:1.

71. Young NH, Andrews PJ. High-frequency oscillation as a rescue strategy for brain-injured adult patients with acute lung injury and acute respiratory distress syndrome. *Neurocrit Care.* 2011;15:623–33.

72. Szerlip NJ, Bholat O, McCunn MM, Aarabi B, Scalea TM. Extracorporeal life support as a treatment for neurogenic pulmonary edema and cardiac failure secondary to intractable intracranial hypertension: a case report and review of the literature. *J Trauma.* 2009;67:E69–E71.

73. Boles JM, Bion J, Connors A, Herridge M, Marsh B, Melot C, et al. Weaning from mechanical ventilation. *Eur Respir J.* 2007;29:1033–56.

74. Brochard L, Thille AW. What is the proper approach to liberating the weak from mechanical ventilation? *Crit Care Med.* 2009;37:S410–S415.

75. Lapinsky SE, Posadas-Calleja JG, McCullagh I. Clinical review: ventilatory strategies for obstetric, brain-injured and obese patients. *Crit Care.* 2009;13:206.

76. Coplin WM, Pierson DJ, Cooley KD, Newell DW, Rubenfeld GD. Implications of extubation delay in brain-injured patients meeting standard weaning criteria. *Am J Respir Crit Care Med.* 2000;161:1530–6.

77. Navalesi P, Frigerio P, Moretti MP, Sommariva M, Vesconi S, Baiardi P, et al. Rate of reintubation in mechanically ventilated neurosurgical and neurologic patients: evaluation of a systematic approach to weaning and extubation. *Crit Care Med.* 2008;36:2986–92.

78. Qureshi AI, Suarez JI, Parekh PD, Bhardwaj A. Prediction and timing of tracheostomy in patients with infratentorial lesions requiring mechanical ventilatory support. *Crit Care Med.* 2000;28:1383–7.

79. Mascia L, Corno E, Terragni PP, Stather D, Ferguson ND. Pro/con clinical debate: tracheostomy is ideal for withdrawal of mechanical ventilation in severe neurological impairment. *Crit Care.* 2004;8:327–30.

80. Terragni PP, Antonelli M, Fumagalli R, Faggiano C, Berardino M, Pallavicini FB, et al. Early vs late tracheotomy for prevention of pneumonia in mechanically ventilated adult ICU patients: a randomized controlled trial. *JAMA.* 2010;303:1483–9.

81. Bouderka MA, Fakhir B, Bouaggad A, Hmamouchi B, Hamoudi D, Harti A. Early tracheostomy versus prolonged endotracheal intubation in severe head injury. *J Trauma.* 2004;57:251–4.

82. Wang HK, Lu K, Liliang PC, Wang KW, Chen HJ, Chen TB, et al. The impact of tracheostomy timing in patients with severe head injury: an observational cohort study. *Injury.* 2012;43:1432–6.

83. Dunham CM, Cutrona AF, Gruber BS, Calderon JE, Ransom KJ, Flowers LL. Early tracheostomy in severe traumatic brain injury: evidence for decreased mechanical ventilation and increased hospital mortality. *Int J Burns Trauma.* 2014;4:14–24.

84. Lazaridis C, DeSantis SM, McLawhorn M, Krishna V. Liberation of neurosurgical patients from mechanical ventilation and tracheostomy in neurocritical care. *J Crit Care.* 2012;27:417–18.

85. Pelosi P, Barassi A, Severgnini P, Gomiero B, Finazzi S, Merlini G, et al. Prognostic role of clinical and laboratory criteria to

identify early ventilator-associated pneumonia in brain injury. *Chest.* 2008;134:101–8.

86. Cavalcanti M, Ferrer M, Ferrer R, Morforte R, Garnacho A, Torres A. Risk and prognostic factors of ventilator-associated pneumonia in trauma patients. *Crit Care Med.* 2006;34:1067–72.

87. Zygun DA, Zuege DJ, Boiteau PJ, Laupland KB, Henderson EA, Kortbeek JB, *et al.* Ventilator-associated pneumonia in severe traumatic brain injury. *Neurocrit Care.* 2006;5:108–14.

88. Rincon-Ferrari MD, Flores-Cordero JM, Leal-Noval SR, Murillo-Cabezas F, Cayuelas A, Munoz-Sanchez MA, *et al.* Impact of ventilator-associated pneumonia in patients with severe head injury. *J Trauma.* 2004;57:1234–40.

89. Minei JP, Nathens AB, West M, Harbrecht BG, Moore EE, Shapiro MB, *et al.* Inflammation and the Host Response to Injury, a Large-Scale Collaborative Project: patient-oriented research core—standard operating procedures for clinical care. II. Guidelines for prevention, diagnosis and treatment of ventilator-associated pneumonia (VAP) in the trauma patient. *J Trauma.* 2006;60:1106–13.

CHAPTER 5

Fluid management

Jonathan Ball

This chapter identifies and discusses the general issues surrounding the fluid management of critically ill patients. These are universal, regardless of whether or not there is significant brain or spinal cord pathology. Issues related to specific neurological conditions are covered in the relevant chapters elsewhere in this book.

By way of introduction, a fluid is defined as a substance that continually deforms under an applied shear stress. This physical property lends itself to many biological processes, in particular as the medium for convective and diffusive transport.

Water homeostasis

Water is the predominant and essential fluid in human biology but its biophysical properties are still incompletely understood and remain the focus of much research (1–5).

Total body water

Healthy humans comprise approximately 60% water overall (~ 42 L in a 70 kg adult). With the exception of fat, which is 10% water, all tissues, including the brain (6), are 70–80% water. Thus, the proportion of fat, which increases with age and in obesity, determines the percentage of body mass that is made up of water.

Water is distributed between two compartments—intracellular and extracellular. The latter is subdivided into the extravascular, or interstitial, space and the intravascular space (see Figure 5.1).

Brain water

The average intracranial volume is approximately 1700 mL of which about 1400 mL is brain, 150 mL blood, and 150 mL cerebrospinal fluid (CSF). The average adult human brain weighs approximately 1350 g, and comprises about 77% water (70% of white matter is water and 80% of grey matter).

CSF is 99% water and formed at a fairly constant rate of 0.2–0.4 mL/min or 400–600 mL/day. Production occurs via diffusion, filtration, pinocytosis, and active transfer by the choroid plexus (~ 50%), with the remainder forming around cerebral vessels and along the ventricular walls. CSF is passively absorbed through the arachnoid villi into the venous sinuses, and also drains directly into lymphatic vessels. The rate of absorption is primarily dependent on the CSF to venous hydrostatic pressure gradient. There is no feedback system between production and absorption of CSF so, if the latter is impaired, CSF accumulates leading to hydrocephalus. For a review of the different types of hydrocephalus and their management please refer to Chapter 7, or the article by Bergsneider et al. (7).

Homeostasis of total body water

Table 5.1 details the organs involved in the control of total body water. Water is lost as a consequence of thermoregulation (heat loss via evaporation of sweat), ventilation (expiration of 100% humidified gas), digestion, and excretion. For a 70 kg, healthy human adult in a temperate climate undertaking normal levels of activity and eating a standard (mixed) diet, the total daily water loss is in the order of 2500 mL. Approximately 300 mL of water is produced as a metabolic by-product, leaving about 2200 mL to be replaced by enteral intake.

Assuming normal losses in a healthy adult, physiological adaption to changing circumstances can accommodate reductions in water intake to a minimum of approximately 1000 mL per day. Reductions beyond this threshold, and/or excessive losses of water with or without sodium or other osmolytes, result in progressive dehydration and adverse, but initially reversible, effects on all organ systems. The brain, skeletal muscle, and skin (heat loss) are the organs most affected initially, followed by cardiovascular decompensation. Both the rate of loss and cumulative deficit of water determine the point of irreversible organ injury. Acute deficits of greater than 15% of total body water may be fatal.

Physiological adaptation to excess fluid intake is considerable and dependent not merely on the amount, but also the composition and rate of administration/ingestion. The limit of physiological renal excretion of ingested water is around 600 mL per hour for a 70 kg adult, beyond which water intoxication occurs.

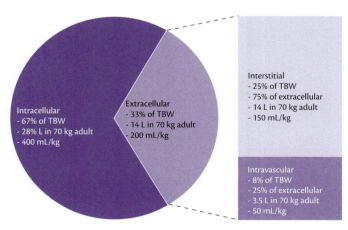

Fig. 5.1 The distribution of water between body compartments. TBW, total body water.

Table 5.1 Daily water homeostasis for a 70 kg, healthy human adult, in a temperate climate, undertaking normal levels of activity, eating a standard (mixed) diet

Tissue	Net contribution	Components/dependent upon	Physiological process
Skin	Loss ~ 250–500 mL	Ambient temperature and humidity Heat production from activity: ♦ Minimum ~ 100 mL ♦ Maximum ~ 8000 mL	Thermoregulation—heat loss through evaporation
Respiratory tract	Loss ~ 500–750 mL	Temperature and humidity of inspired gas Upper airway anatomy Ratio of nasal to oral breathing Minute ventilation Core temperature	As part of the conditioning process of inspired gas, it is filtered, becomes heated to core body temperature and takes up water to become ~ 100% humidified
Kidney	Loss ~ 1500 mL	Cardiac output Systemic blood pressure Glomerular filtration rate Renal tubular function Plasma osmolarity: ♦ Maximum concentration ~ 1400 mOsm/L ♦ Minimum concentration ~ 50 mOsm/L ♦ Assuming a daily clearance of 700 mOsm this equates to urine volumes of ~ 500–14,000 mL	Excretion and principal organ of water balance. Water retention (resorption) mediated by aldosterone (in response to systemic hypotension) and vasopressin (in response to plasma hyperosmolarity). Water loss mediated by the absence of the above hormones and enhanced by the natriuretic peptides (in response to cardiac stretch)
Total loss	**~ 2500 mL**		
Gastrointestinal tract	Gain ~ 2200 mL	Intake: ♦ Water in food ~ 1500 mL ♦ Water in beverages ~ 2000 mL Total ~ 3500 mL Output: ♦ Saliva ~ 1500 mL ♦ Stomach ~ 1500 mL ♦ Biliary system ~ 750 mL ♦ Pancreas ~ 1500 mL ♦ Small bowel secretions ~ 1500 mL Total ~ 6750 mL Absorption: ♦ Small bowel ~ 9000 mL ♦ Large bowel ~ 1000 mL but capacity to increase up to 4500 mL principally under the control of aldosterone (systemic hypotension) Total ~ 10,000–14,500 mL Losses: ♦ Large bowel stool ~ 200 mL	Volitional intake ± stimulated thirst Digestion Absorption Excretion
Metabolic production of water	Gain ~ 300 mL	♦ Basal metabolic rate ♦ Level of activity	By-product of enzymatic conversion of fuels to energy
Total gain	**~ 2500 mL**		

Water passes freely between the body compartments through a variety of semipermeable cellular membranes, extracellular matrices, and intercellular junctions. The permeability of these barriers varies with tissue type and is affected by physiological and pathological processes. Water flux between compartments is principally passive and determined by hydrostatic and osmotic forces (8). However, active co-transport of water against these gradients (uphill) does occur and there is increasing evidence of the importance of this mechanism (9).

The critical intracellular and extracellular osmolytes are potassium and sodium respectively. Maintenance of this compartmental gradient, via plasma membrane-bound sodium/potassium adenosine triphosphatase (Na^+/K^+-ATPase), consumes around 20% of cellular energy expenditure. Exceptionally, this activity may account for

60–70% of energy expenditure in neurons, making them particularly vulnerable to sodium and water influx. The osmotic gradient between the extra- and intravascular compartments is the result of colloids, principally albumin. Thus any discussion of fluid management cannot be dissociated from issues affecting electrolytes and colloids.

The physiology of the intravascular compartment volume and composition

The intravascular space has a number of homeostatic mechanisms that maintain effective convective transportation despite significant changes in intravascular volume. The circulation is designed such that 60–70% of the circulating volume is contained within the venules and veins which act as a rapidly responsive reservoir to respond to both volume losses and gains.

Volume changes in the intravascular space result in changes in venous, atrial, ventricular, and arterial pressures, which are detected by baroreceptors. The changes in the firing rates of these receptors result in changes in the autonomic output to the various components of the cardiovascular system, and compensatory changes aimed at preserving cardiac output and perfusion pressure. Thus, fluid loss triggers venoconstriction, tachycardia, positive inotropy, and arterial vasoconstriction. Failure of the vasoconstrictor response is commonly seen in acute severe illnesses, including the more severe forms of the systemic inflammatory response syndrome (SIRS). In addition to the cardiovascular compensatory responses, hormonally driven renal (and colonic) sodium and water retention, mediated by increased secretion of aldosterone (sodium and water, kidney and colon) and vasopressin (water, kidney) is triggered. By contrast, intravascular volume gains are initially absorbed by the reserve capacity of the compliant venous circulation. If isotonic volume gains continue, venous pressure and hence cardiac filling pressures rise, leading to increased cardiac output with a consequent diuresis. This is mediated by a combination of increased renal filtration and hormonally permitted (passive) renal sodium losses, generated to a greater extent by the absence of aldosterone and vasopressin than by the secretion of natriuretic peptides derived from increased cardiac stretch. From an evolutionary perspective, humans possess extensive, rapid (minutes), and effective physiological adaptations to limited water availability, moderate free water excess, and a paucity of sodium. By contrast, the response to sodium excess is very limited and slow, occurring over hours and days.

The volume of blood in the microcirculation is locally controlled within tissues by rapidly responsive changes in vessel calibre in response to local oxygen tension and carbon dioxide and other waste acid concentrations. Of note, the effectiveness and efficiency of microcirculatory convective transportation is principally determined by blood viscosity (10), which in turn is determined by the haematocrit and concentrations of plasma proteins.

The microcirculation has variable permeability in different tissues and in response to physiological and pathological processes, allowing a proportion of plasma to pass into the interstitial space. The driving force for this movement is the hydrostatic pressure gradient between the intravascular and interstitial spaces, but a number of factors limit the flow of water, solutes, and macromolecules down this pressure gradient. The Starling principle of microvascular downstream resorption of interstitial fluid back into the vascular space because of the colloid osmotic pressure of whole blood has repeatedly proven to be false, and recently been replaced

by the glycocalyx model of transvascular fluid exchange (11). The differences between the old and new theories are summarized in Table 5.2. The glycocalyx model is based on the discovery of the endothelial glycocalyx layer (EGL), a web of membrane-bound glycoproteins and proteoglycans on the luminal side of the vascular endothelial cells. It is associated with various glycosaminoglycans which contribute to the volume of the layer and is the active interface between blood and vessel wall, functioning as a filter. The EGL varies in thickness from 0.2 μm in capillaries to 8 μm in larger vessels, and is semipermeable with respect to anionic macromolecules such as albumin and other plasma proteins, whose size and structure determine their ability to penetrate the layer.

Four microvascular phenotypes have been described in different tissues (see Figure 5.2). Each exhibits specialist structural features affecting the EGL, the presence or absence of cellular fenestrations, variations in intercellular junctions, and basement membranes. In health, the EGL acts to maintain the colloid osmotic pressure, limiting the hydrostatically driven filtration of plasma such that net fluid movement only occurs when the hydrostatic pressure gradient exceeds the plasma colloid osmotic pressure. Understanding the physiology and pathophysiology of the EGL is thus essential to allow a rational choice of intravenous fluid therapy (11).

Plasma and interstitial fluid sodium concentration is regulated by vasopressin and aldosterone (see above and below). In health, plasma colloid osmotic pressure is principally determined by plasma albumin concentration. Albumin is synthesized exclusively by hepatocytes, and immediately released into the circulation. The rate of production is dependent on substrate availability, hormonal status (principally insulin), and, most importantly, the colloid osmotic pressure of the interstitial fluid around hepatocytes (12). Thus, any increase in plasma colloid osmotic pressure, from either an endogenous or exogenous source, results in decreased albumin production and a resultant fall in plasma albumin concentration to maintain normal colloid osmotic pressure. By contrast, a fall in plasma colloid osmotic pressure results in increased albumin production, a response that is inhibited by inflammatory cytokines (12,13). An albumin molecule lasts about 30 days in healthy individuals. Around 10% of the body's albumin is catabolized daily, with increased catabolism in response to protein and/or calorie deprivation, and acute systemic illness injury. The utility of monitoring plasma albumin concentration and the value of exogenous supplementation are discussed in the relevant sections below.

The physiology of the interstitial compartment volume and composition

The interstitial space is very plastic. The volume (water content) of healthy tissues is kept to a minimum to facilitate rapid diffusion between the convective transport of the intravascular space and the intracellular environment. This is achieved by drainage of interstitial fluid into the intravascular space via the lymphatic system, a process driven by gravity, skeletal muscle contraction, and negative intrathoracic pressure during breathing. In response to injury or inflammation, effectors of the innate immune system, principally toll-like receptors and integrins, modulate the structure of the extracellular matrix which results in an acute fall in compartment hydrostatic pressure. This can be sufficient to cause (up to) a 20-fold increase in transendothelial fluid flux as well as the compositional changes described below (11). Accumulation of excess fluid in the interstitial space is termed oedema, and originates principally

Table 5.2 Comparison of the old and the new paradigms that govern net fluid movement between the microvascular and interstitial spaces

Original Starling principle	The glycocalyx model of transvascular fluid exchange
Intravascular volume consists of plasma and cellular elements	Intravascular volume consists of glycocalyx volume, plasma volume, and red cell distribution volume
Capillaries separate plasma with high protein concentration from ISF with low protein concentration	Sinusoidal tissues (marrow, spleen, and liver) have discontinuous capillaries and their ISF is essentially part of the plasma volume Open fenestrated capillaries produce the renal glomerular filtrate Diaphragm fenestrated capillaries in specialized tissues can absorb ISF to plasma Continuous capillaries exhibit 'no absorption' The EGL is semi-permeable to anionic proteins and their concentration in the intercellular clefts below the glycocalyx is very low
The important Starling forces are the transendothelial pressure difference and the plasma–interstitial COP difference	The important Starling forces are the transendothelial pressure difference and the plasma–subglycocalyx COP difference. ISF COP is not a direct determinant of J_v
Fluid is filtered from the arterial end of capillaries and absorbed from the venous end. Small proportion returns to the circulation as lymph	J_v is much less than predicted by Starling's principle, and the major route for return to the circulation is as lymph
Raising plasma COP enhances absorption and shifts fluid from ISF to plasma	Raising plasma COP reduces J_v but does not cause absorption
At subnormal capillary pressure, net absorption increases plasma volume	At subnormal capillary pressure, J_v approaches zero. Auto transfusion is acute, transient, and limited to about 500 mL
At supranormal capillary pressure, net filtration increases ISF volume	At supranormal capillary pressure, when the COP difference is maximal, J_v is proportional to transendothelial pressure difference
Infused colloid solution is distributed through the plasma volume, and infused ISS through the extracellular volume	Infused colloid solution is initially distributed through the plasma volume, and infused ISS through the intravascular volume At supranormal capillary pressure, infusion of colloid solution preserves plasma COP, raises capillary pressure, and increases J_v At supranormal capillary pressure, infusion of ISS also raises capillary pressure, but it lowers COP and so increases J_v more than the same colloid solution volume At subnormal capillary pressure, infusion of colloid solution increases plasma volume and infusion of ISS increases intravascular volume, but Jv remains close to zero in both cases

COP, colloid osmotic pressure; EGL, endothelial glycocalyx layer; ISF, interstitial fluid; ISS, isotonic salt solution; J_v, the net fluid movement between the intravascular and interstitial spaces.

Reproduced from Woodcock TE and Woodcock TM, 'Revised Starling equation and the glycocalyx model of transvascular fluid exchange: an improved paradigm for prescribing intravenous fluid therapy', *British Journal of Anaesthesia*, 2012, 108, 3, pp. 384–394, by permission of Oxford University Press and the Board of Management and Trustees of the *British Journal of Anaesthesia*.

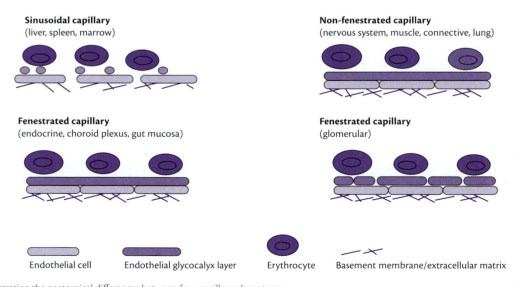

Fig. 5.2 A figure illustrating the anatomical differences between four capillary phenotypes.
Reproduced from Woodcock TE and Woodcock TM, 'Revised Starling equation and the glycocalyx model of transvascular fluid exchange: an improved paradigm for prescribing intravenous fluid therapy', *British Journal of Anaesthesia*, 2012, 108, 3, pp. 384–394, by permission of Oxford University Press and the Board of Management and Trustees of the *British Journal of Anaesthesia*.

from the vascular compartment. Not only does this limit diffusional transport but, as fluid accumulation continues, extravascular hydrostatic pressure exceeds venous and then microvascular pressure, resulting in tissue ischaemia.

Extracellular fluid osmolarity is tightly controlled, principally by hypothalamic osmoreceptors that regulate the secretion of vasopressin from the posterior pituitary. Increases in osmolarity of more than 1% stimulate thirst and release of vasopressin which in turn increases the permeability of the renal collecting ducts to water. This results in increased water resorption from filtered plasma back into the circulation (14), thereby normalizing plasma osmolarity. Decreases in osmolarity have the opposite effects. Acute and chronic changes in osmolarity that exceed the limits of this homeostatic process, or are a consequence of its failure, have profound effects on brain function and can lead to permanent injury and even death. The brain's physiological adaptation to osmotic challenges has been reviewed in detail by Verbalis (15).

The colloid osmotic pressure of interstitial fluid, like that of blood, is principally determined by albumin concentration. It is worth noting that in healthy subjects around 60% of total body albumin is contained in the interstitial space, although at only 40% of its concentration in plasma (12). However, this albumin pool is not static. Five per cent of intravascular albumin crosses into the interstitial space each hour with an equivalent amount returning to the circulation via the lymphatic system. In response to injury and inflammation there is a small, acute, and transient efflux of albumin from the vascular to the interstitial space (16), although this is insufficient to explain the hypoalbuminaemia observed (17). Albumin has a circulation half-life of approximately 16 hours.

The physiology of the intracellular compartment volume and composition

Cells must actively manage their volume (water content) to avoid lethal injury. In association with the central role of plasma membrane-bound Na^+/K^+-ATPase, the family of water channel proteins, the aquaporins (18), and the large variety of uphill co-transporters are pivotal in this regard (9). The complexity and regulation of cellular volume homeostasis remains incompletely understood but is an area of active research and rapid development (19). Much of this research has focused on brain tissue as these processes are central to acute and chronic brain pathologies (see Chapter 3). Cellular injury, regardless of pathology, frequently results in failure of water content homeostasis and an intracellular influx of water (20). As our understanding of these processes evolves, it is hoped that effective therapies will emerge (21).

In contrast, adaptation to cellular dehydration as a consequence of hyperosmolar extracellular milieu (global water losses) is a highly conserved, fundamental stress response (22). Cells initially adapt to the osmotic efflux of water by active influx of inorganic solutes, in particular potassium, sodium, and chloride ions (23). However, these ions inhibit and/or become toxic to intracellular processes and cells start to synthesize heat shock proteins and accumulate non-toxic osmolytes, including neutral amino acids or their derivatives, polyols such as sorbitol and myo-inositol, and methylamines such as betaine. Although the precise detection and regulation of this process is not fully elucidated, the endoplasmic reticulum appears to play a key role by responding to cytoplasmic un- or misfolded proteins that accumulate as a direct consequence of critical water loss (24). Acute pathologies that may result in acute cellular

dehydration include gastrointestinal infections and hyperglycaemic, diabetic emergencies. The natural histories and responses to therapy of these conditions is testament to the effectiveness of the cellular dehydration response. Maladaptation or failure of this response may be a central driver in many chronic degenerative diseases (24).

Assessment and management of fluid status

Although fluid management is a fundamental component of the care of critically ill patients, including those with neurological disease, our ability to assess patients' needs for, and responses to, fluid therapy and titrate it accordingly remains surprisingly haphazard. Both inadequate and excessive fluid replacement is harmful and not infrequently adds a significant iatrogenic insult to the burden of the underlying disease process. Given the long history of fluid management, the gaps in our knowledge are both surprising and regrettable. Indeed, in an attempt to address these deficiencies there has been a resurgence of both basic science and clinical trial data published on these topics in recent years.

To mimic a patient's journey, this chapter will first consider fluid resuscitation before discussing maintenance therapy and the active management of daily fluid balance.

Fluid resuscitation: cardiovascular optimization versus iatrogenic injury

The primary role of the cardiovascular system is the convectional delivery of substrates (in particular oxygen) to within, and removal of wastes from, a diffusional distance of cells. There are two related components to this delivery—flow and pressure—although the latter cannot be used as a reliable surrogate for the former. There are many methods to assess the adequacy of single-organ and global perfusion, all of which have limitations (25,26). It is also important to remember that intravascular volume is but one of four physiological variables—heart rate and rhythm, myocardial contractility and relaxation, and vascular tone—that determine cardiac output and perfusion pressure. In addition to these variables, oxygen and other vital substrate delivery is affected by blood composition (viscosity and oxygen carrying capacity) and microcirculatory variables (functional capillary density and flow rate). Hence cardiovascular/oxygen delivery optimization requires at least consideration, if not direct measurement, of all six of these variables.

All patients with acute severe illness or trauma, or undergoing major surgery, require cardiovascular monitoring and support, a major component of which is resuscitation and maintenance of an adequate intravascular volume using intravenous fluid and/or blood component products. Failure to provide such support results in tissue injury through hypoperfusion, the extent and duration of which adversely affect outcome (27). Fluid therapy in excess of restoration of adequate volume also leads to significant tissue injury through oedema formation, primarily affecting the lungs, brain, kidneys, bowel, and soft tissues, and is responsible for delays in the return of normal organ function, organ failure, prolonged hospital stay, and excess mortality.

The following questions are a useful guide when assessing the amount and timing of fluid resuscitation.

1. How much of what fluid has been lost and/or redistributed, and over what time period?

2. What is the cause of the fluid loss, is it still ongoing, and what can be done to minimize further losses?

3. How compromised is the cardiovascular system or, more importantly, is there any evidence of one or more hypoperfused organs?

4. How much of what fluid should be administered and how quickly? By what means can the response to fluid therapy be judged?

5. Having established that a patient is no longer fluid responsive, how long should one wait before re-challenging the patient's physiology?

Assessment of fluid loss and/or redistribution

Clinical history, physical examination, and routine blood tests (discussed later) should enable a reasonable estimation of fluid losses. The clinical signs of acute hypovolaemia are non-specific and include sinus tachycardia, atrial fibrillation, normotension, hypotension, absent jugular venous pulsation, tachypnoea, normal mentation, altered mentation, poor peripheral perfusion, reduced skin turgor, and dry mucous membranes.

Historically, the gold standard physiological measure of intravascular volume status has been a static measure of central venous pressure, but this has repeatedly been shown to be no better than tossing a coin in predicting the stroke volume and cardiac output response to an intravenous fluid bolus (28,29). The same can also be said of the measurement of pulmonary artery occlusion pressure. There are a myriad of better static markers but all are derived from stroke volume/cardiac output monitors, and all demonstrate lower reliability than clinical care demands. Dynamic measures, in which the percentage change in a measured variable in response to the respiratory cycle or a vascular manoeuvre is used to predict volume responsiveness, are significantly better than static markers, although also subject to limitations (28).

Assessment of the cause of fluid loss

Initial fluid resuscitation should be guided by the working diagnosis of the degree of hypovolaemia and its cause. There are broadly three clinical scenarios that result in hypovolaemia:

1. Excess fluid losses—most commonly renal or gastrointestinal losses secondary to diabetic ketoacidosis, hyperosmolar hyperglycaemic states, or norovirus infection.

2. SIRS/sepsis—increased losses due to pyrexia and tachypnoea, reduced intake, vasodilatation, and fluid shifts out of the intravascular space.

3. Haemorrhage—gastrointestinal tract, trauma, obstetric, ruptured aortic aneurysm, or surgical.

Determining the likely aetiology is crucial because resuscitating patients following haemorrhage requires a significantly different approach to the hypovolaemia of water (± electrolyte) loss and SIRS/sepsis. There are substantial risks of significant iatrogenic secondary injury if aggressive fluid resuscitation is delivered before effective control of a bleeding source. Such resuscitation disrupts clots already formed, dilutes the coagulation system and accentuates both hypothermia and acidosis, thereby precipitating further blood loss and worsening of any coagulopathy (30). In short, if haemorrhage is known or suspected as the cause of hypovolaemia, don't delay haemostasis especially to deliver fluid resuscitation.

Intravenous fluids should of course be administered, but in the minimum volume necessary to achieve clearly defined and measurable endpoints. The optimal choice of fluid in this setting is discussed below. By contrast, the rapid correction of hypovolaemia in the scenarios of excess fluid loss or SIRS/sepsis is strongly advocated.

Assessment of the cardiovascular system and adequacy of organ perfusion

Heart rate and blood pressure, except at extremes, are poor guides to cardiovascular adequacy. Normal mentation confirms adequate brain perfusion but altered mentation has multiple causes, only one of which is brain hypoperfusion. Poor peripheral perfusion can be chronic as well as acute and doesn't necessarily reflect vital organ perfusion. Good peripheral perfusion may also occur in distributive shock. Urine output is an unreliable marker of renal perfusion (31). A diagnosis of oliguria can only be made by hourly observations for 4–6 hours and is the physiological response to stress hormones (catecholamines, aldosterone, and vasopressin) regardless of intravascular volume status and renal perfusion.

Hence, the use of trend data of multiple variables, in particular stroke volume and cardiac output, arterial and central venous lactate and base deficit, central and mixed venous oxygen saturations, and central venous-to-arterial carbon dioxide difference, and their response to dynamic manoeuvres, is strongly recommended (25,26,32). Collectively these variables are surrogates for the ideal variables, namely the kinetics of global and organ-specific oxygen supply–demand balance (27).

Assessment of volume replacement and the responsiveness to fluid therapy

For a hypovolaemic or shocked adult, 250 mL aliquots of the most appropriate (least harmful) fluid should be administered as rapidly as possible (< 5 minutes), and the response assessed by continuous measurement of stroke volume/cardiac output. All available monitoring methods have their limitations and can only reliably detect changes in excess of 15%, though increases of 10% or more are often considered a positive response. Repeat boluses of fluid should be administered until the monitored response is less than 10–15%. Arterial/central venous lactate and base deficit, central/mixed venous oxygen saturations, and central venous-to-arterial carbon dioxide difference after 15–30 minutes (the plasma half-life of lactate is ~ 20 minutes) should be reassessed.

On the basis of the extent of change in all cardiovascular parameters, titration of vasoactive drugs should next be considered. The value of targeting fluid and vasoactive drug therapy to an oxygen delivery index of 600 mL/min/m² has biological plausibility but remains contentious (33), although it is certainly a reliable marker of prognosis. Adequately powered trials targeting this parameter in specific patient groups are currently underway and will hopefully clarify the utility of this target.

In the absence of invasive monitoring, the response to fluid boluses can be judged against changes in heart rate, blood pressure, and mentation. This applies especially in the pre-hospital and acute admission setting. In the context of haemorrhagic hypovolaemia, the pragmatic advice is to aim for a palpable radial pulse, roughly equivalent to a systolic blood pressure of 80 mmHg. However, in the presence of significant brain or spinal cord injury current consensus opinion recommends targeting a systolic blood pressure of 100–110 mmHg.

Fluid unresponsiveness

In the absence of fluid responsiveness, the optimal length of time before re-challenging the patient's physiology depends on the clinical circumstances. If fluid losses continue, if vasodilatation occurs, and as fluid shifts between body compartments ensues, the trends in cardiovascular parameters, in particular stroke volume/cardiac output, will decline. Given the limits of detectability, a greater than 10–15% decrease should prompt consideration of a further fluid bolus. A lack of response in this setting should trigger a systemic review of the cause of the hypovolaemia, and of the other five previously noted physiological variables that determine adequate perfusion.

Post resuscitation: doing the simple things well—daily fluid balance

The resuscitated patient will commonly have received a water, sodium, and chloride load that exceeds their needs. This is in part the consequence of fluid shifts from the intravascular to the interstitial space, but also the result of (over-) enthusiastic fluid replacement. As explained previously, the physiological response to acute severe illness, injury, and major surgery, sometimes exacerbated by significant renal injury, is active retention of sodium and water and a limitation of the rate at which the kidneys can excrete excess fluid (31). Thus, although there is a theoretical minimum amount of water, sodium, and potassium that a patient requires each day, this must take into account the cumulative picture and make allowances for any predictable further losses together with unavoidable gains, in particular from intravenous therapies.

Any calculated maintenance requirement is best delivered, along with nutritional support, via the enteral route. As a starting point, a euvolaemic patient with no excess fluid loading requires 25–35 mL/kg of water, 1–1.5 mmol/kg of sodium, and 1 mmol/kg of potassium each day. Beyond this, it would be ideal to measure all water and sodium losses and gains, thereby titrating the maintenance regimen to the patient's requirements.

It is standard practice in critical care to record hourly fluid inputs, enteral and intravenous, and outputs, urinary, nasogastric, surgical drains, and so on. From these hourly measurements, a cumulative balance is calculated for a 24-hour period together with a daily reckoning of the cumulative balance since admission. Although estimates can be made of the additional unmeasured losses from the skin, respiratory tract, and gastrointestinal tract (based on the data in Table 5.1), this is inconsistently performed and may not take into account factors such as the patient's temperature or presence of respiratory gas humidification. A simple, although somewhat unreliable, method to confirm cumulative fluid balance calculations is change in the patient's daily weight, and some modern intensive care unit (ICU) beds have a built-in weighing facility. Alternatively, bed and patient weighing devices have been developed. Despite these simple technologies, concerns regarding the imprecision of daily weight results in it being rarely performed. Whether trend data of daily weight is sufficiently useful to guide daily fluid balance targets remains uncertain, not least because there is a paucity of published data on the subject.

Daily clinical examination should attempt to estimate the degree of oedema, or perhaps more importantly any change in the degree of oedema, particularly in the dependant peripheries/soft tissues, lungs, gastrointestinal tract, and brain. The extent and change in lung oedema can be inferred from trends in derived variables of the efficiency of oxygenation, such as oxygenation index, and standardized dynamic lung compliance, but not reliably from plain chest X-ray series. Gastrointestinal oedema may result in ileus and/or intra-abdominal hypertension and trending regular, standardized measurements of intra-abdominal pressure may alert clinicians to the development of this complication of a positive cumulative fluid balance. In brain-injured patients, trending measures of intracranial compliance, and correlation of these to local and/or global measures of the adequacy of brain perfusion, may influence decisions regarding the active management of cumulative fluid balance.

Additional insights into cumulative fluid balance can be gained from trends in routine haematological and plasma biochemical parameters, specifically haematocrit, sodium, urea, creatinine, and total protein, but not albumin. However, all are affected by multiple variables in addition to changes in intravascular and total body water. Haematocrit falls as a consequence of intravascular dilution and rises in response to intravascular water depletion. However, loss of red blood cells through bleeding and blood sampling on the ICU, and shortened red cell lifespan and inhibition of red cell production by acute severe illness confounds this relationship. Plasma sodium concentration is determined by multiple factors reflecting hydration and hormonal status, renal function, and sodium losses and gains. Unlike fluid balance, hourly/daily sodium balance is not routinely measured or used to titrate daily fluid administration. Critical care commonly results in significant sodium (and chloride) loading from intravenous drug therapies and other routine practices (34), and a positive cumulative sodium balance is probably detrimental and should be minimized. An increase in the plasma urea to creatinine ratio is often used as a marker of dehydration. Both are freely filtered by the kidney but only urea is passively reabsorbed; the degree of resorption is proportional to that of water and hence is increased in dehydrated patients with good renal function. However, similar patterns of change are also seen following upper gastrointestinal haemorrhage, in hypercatabolic states, and in urinary tract outflow obstruction.

Plasma total protein (TP) measurements can be used to estimate colloid osmotic pressure using the following formula (35):

$$\text{Colloid osmotic pressure} = \left(2.1 \times TP\right) + \left(0.16 \times TP^2\right) + \left(0.009 \times TP^3\right)$$

This doesn't account for the effect of administered synthetic colloids, so measuring colloid osmotic pressure using a relatively simple, quick, and reliable laboratory technique is preferred (36). However, given the controversies surrounding all colloid therapies, the value of knowing the colloid osmotic pressure and its trends is arguably no longer likely to influence fluid therapy (11).

In summary, trend data and clinical acumen are required to interpret each of the relevant elements contributing to fluid status, and to reach a conclusion in setting daily fluid and electrolyte balance targets. This should take account of essential therapies such as nutrition and intravenous medication, and may necessitate the use of diuretics or renal replacement therapy to control fluid volume. It is vital to review these goals regularly and, if necessary, revise them. Dynamic challenges with fluid boluses or fluid removal may also be helpful in determining both fluid status and optimal strategy.

Choice of intravenous fluid therapy

Intravenous salt solutions (crystalloids) have been used since the 1830s. Sydney Ringer first described his physiological salt solution in the early 1880s, and Alexis Hartmann modified Ringer's recipe in the 1930s. Despite their work, 0.9% sodium chloride, misnamed 'normal' saline, went on to become, and remains, the most commonly administered intravenous fluid. The first gelatin-based colloids were developed in 1915 and the first reported use of albumin infusion is ascribed to the American military in 1941. Yet, despite hundreds of clinical trials and countless meta-analyses, consensus statements, and evidence-based guidelines, the controversies and uncertainties surrounding the correct choice of intravenous fluid therapy remain. However, publication of the SAFE study in 2004 (37) and the subsequent large-scale trials it spawned, the paradigm shift in trauma resuscitation accelerated by the conflicts in Iraq and Afghanistan (30), the evolution of the glycocalyx model of transvascular fluid exchange (11), and the retractions of publications and inquiry into the work of Joachim Boldt (38) have resulted in significant recent advances in fluid management after years of stagnation.

The questions that must be answered, most especially in the context of a vulnerable brain, are:

◆ Are the more physiological ('balanced') solutions less harmful than unphysiological 0.9% sodium chloride?

◆ Do any colloids provide outcome benefits over crystalloids, or over each other?

Balanced solutions versus 0.9% sodium chloride

Table 5.3 details the composition, osmolarity, and pH of commonly prescribed crystalloid solutions using plasma as the reference solution. As 0.9% sodium chloride is mildly hyperosmotic and contains 50% more chloride ions per litre than plasma, infusion of

significant volumes results in hyperchloraemic acidosis. Although the acidosis is rapidly buffered, the effects of hyperchloraemia are several and include impaired mental function, nausea, gastrointestinal dysfunction, renal vasoconstriction, hyperkalaemia, impaired coagulation, and a pro-inflammatory response (39). What is less clear is whether these effects are clinically important.

Yunos and colleagues examined the renal effects of iatrogenic hyperchloraemia in a prospective, open-label, sequential period pilot study in 1533 ICU patients (40). They found that a 30% mean reduction in chloride loading resulted in a 50% reduction in both the incidence of acute kidney injury (AKI) and acute renal replacement therapy but no difference in hospital mortality, hospital or ICU length of stay, or the need for renal replacement therapy after hospital discharge. Shaw and colleagues examined the effects of iatrogenic hyperchloraemia in an observational study of adult patients undergoing major open abdominal surgery, comparing the outcomes of 30,994 patients who received 0.9% sodium chloride with 926 patients who received a balanced crystalloid on the day of surgery (41). For the entire cohort, the in-hospital mortality was 5.6% in the saline group and 2.9% in the balanced crystalloid group (P < 0.001). One or more major complications occurred in 33.7% of patients in the saline group and 23% in the balanced group (P < 0.001). The authors performed a 3:1 propensity-matched comparison and confirmed that treatment with the balanced fluid was associated with fewer major complications (odds ratio 0.79; 95% confidence interval 0.66–0.97) and less resource utilization. In particular, patients receiving 0.9% sodium chloride had a 4.8 times greater need for dialysis (P < 0.001) and a 40% higher incidence of major infection. The Cochrane group has undertaken a systematic review of trials comparing balanced solutions with 0.9% sodium chloride, and 13 randomized trials that together enrolled 706 very heterogeneous patients were identified (42). Clinically important outcomes were reported in only a minority of the trials, with most being assessed in fewer than 300 patients, and no

Table 5.3 Comparison of plasma to commonly available intravenous crystalloid solutions

[Electrolyte] in mmol/L	Plasma	0.9% NaCl	5% Dextrose	4% Dextrose 0.18% NaCl	Hartmann's	Ringer's	1.26% NaHCO₃
Cations							
Na⁺	135–145	154	0	30	131	130	150
K⁺	3.5–5.2	0	0	0	5.0	4.0	0
Mg²⁺	0.7–1.0	0	0	0	0	0	0
Ca²⁺	2.2–2.6	0	0	0	2.0	2.5	0
Anions							
Cl⁻	98–105	154	0	30	111	109	0
PO₄³⁻	0.8–1.4	0	0	0	0	0	0
Lactate	0.5–2.0	0	0	0	29	28	0
HCO₃⁻	18–24	0	0	0	0	0	150
Others	Significant	0	0	0	0	0	0
Osmolarity mOsm/L	275–295	308	252	262	275	273	300
pH @ 37°C	7.35–7.45	5.0	4.0	4.0	6.5	6.5	8.6
Calories kcal/L			170	136			

significant differences between the fluid replacement groups were detected. However, this systematic review is based on inadequate data and the studies by Yunos et al. and Shaw et al. (40,41), though non-randomized, do suggest that iatrogenic hyperchloraemia may cause significant harm and should be avoided. A large, multicentre, randomized controlled trial, analogous to the SAFE study, is required to confirm this conclusion.

A largely uninvestigated option to limit chloride loading is the use of 1.26–1.4% sodium bicarbonate. The traditional role of intravenous bicarbonate has been the reversal of severe acidosis and, although it increases pH, it has never been shown to positively affect outcome (43). This is perhaps unsurprising given that it can be argued that acidosis per se is never the cause of the problem, but merely a marker of the severity of illness or injury (39,44,45). Human cells are very resistant to extracellular acidosis and, analogous with dehydration, cellular adaptation to, and recovery from, it is a highly conserved fundamental stress response. On the other hand, sodium bicarbonate has never been shown to be harmful and is recommended in the management of rhabdomyolysis (46), overdose of certain drugs (47), prevention of contrast-induced renal injury (48), and as the basis of replacement fluid in renal replacement therapies.

To date, only two small studies, both in patients undergoing cardiac surgery, have compared routine sodium bicarbonate administration with 0.9% sodium chloride. In the first, a double-blind, randomized controlled trial enrolling 100 patients at high risk of postoperative AKI, the groups were well matched and there was a significantly lower incidence of AKI in the bicarbonate group (49). In the second trial, a retrospective cohort analysis of all patients treated during two sequential time periods in a single centre was undertaken (50). There was no outcome difference between 280 patients who received bicarbonate and 304 historical controls who received 0.9% sodium chloride. As this study has obvious methodological weaknesses, the only conclusion that can be drawn is that bicarbonate may benefit selected patients, probably those at high risk of AKI.

Sodium bicarbonate may yet prove to be an important addition to fluid management regimens and a logical next step would be to include bicarbonate therapy in a chloride restrictive fluid strategy, perhaps based on that employed by Yunos and colleagues (40), and compare this to a standard, liberal chloride fluid strategy. From a neurointensive care perspective, 8.4% sodium bicarbonate has been shown to be as effective and as safe as 5% sodium chloride in the management of raised intracranial pressure following traumatic brain injury (TBI) (51).

Colloids

Talk of the colloid verses crystalloid debate is akin to a fruit verses vegetable debate. Whilst there is the obvious distinction of colloid osmotic pressure, there are as many differences between the various colloids and crystalloids, as there are between fruit and vegetables. Table 5.4 sets out a summary and comparison of different colloid types. The discussion that follows has been dramatically simplified by the results of several recent landmark trials.

Albumin

There is an appealing logic to the argument that if any colloid is going to be beneficial it should be the predominant endogenous colloid, albumin. Importantly, albumin performs a myriad of vital molecular binding functions in addition to providing intravascular colloid osmotic pressure (12), and should therefore be considered a drug with distinct pharmacodynamic and kinetic properties.

However, its binding properties make it vulnerable to chemical damage, in particular oxidation. Consequently, intravenous formulations exhibit a high degree of variability in binding potential (52), and this heterogeneity might be responsible for some of the inconsistency in clinical trial outcomes.

Hypoalbuminaemia is a near ubiquitous consequence of acute severe illness, although the precise mechanisms contributing to its development remain obscure (17). The consequences are also widely debated as are the safety, timing, and efficacy of maintenance and replacement strategies, sometimes coupled with aggressive fluid restriction and active diuresis (53). The SAFE study (37) was the first large-scale, pragmatic fluid trial of the current era of ICU trials and set a new standard for such studies. It put an end to the protracted and acrimonious debate about the safety of intravenous albumin that had resulted from a series of meta-analyses reaching diametrically opposing conclusions using the same flawed data. SAFE randomized 7000 ICU patients, covering the whole spectrum of severity of illness and diagnoses, to receive either 4% albumin in 0.9% sodium chloride or 0.9% sodium chloride, as resuscitation fluid during the first 28 days of ICU admission. There were no statistically significant differences in 28-day mortality or in any of a myriad of secondary endpoints. In short, 4% albumin is safe but, in the doses given to a deliberately heterogeneous ICU patient population, of no benefit. Of note, patients in the albumin group received, on average, 40% less resuscitation fluid than those receiving 0.9% sodium chloride. Further, subgroup analysis on the basis of admission diagnosis suggested that there might be benefit in patients with severe sepsis and that there was harm in those with TBI (54). Although there remains controversy in some quarters regarding the latter conclusion (55,56), this subgroup analysis of the SAFE study represents the largest fluid trial in TBI to date. There is some evidence to support the early use of a bolus of 25% albumin following acute stroke (57) and subarachnoid haemorrhage (58), with further trials in progress. A number of trials of albumin in patients with severe sepsis are also underway (59).

In summary, albumin appears to be safe and may be efficacious in specific conditions. It should be avoided in patients with TBI, although a well-designed randomized controlled trial in this group could be justified. If a clear therapeutic role emerges, a cost–benefit analysis will be required.

Dextrans

The dextrans were developed in the 1950s and have all but been consigned to history, with a few geographical exceptions. Their purported utility in peripheral and microvascular surgery (60) has been superseded by superior and safer fluid and antithrombotic strategies (61).

In the only recently published study, a retrospective, historical, cohort analysis of 332 patients with septic shock treated in a single institution demonstrated no benefit of dextrans over Ringer's solution (62). However, two additional findings of this study are noteworthy. First, the doses of dextran were large and perhaps not surprisingly associated with a significantly higher incidence of major bleeding—51/171 (30%) in the dextran cohort versus 31/161 (19%) in the Ringer's cohort. Second, there was no difference in the total volume of fluid required for resuscitation, demonstrating that the claimed volume-sparing effect of dextrans appears to be false. The only other recent trials using dextrans have been in the pre-hospital resuscitation of shocked trauma patients, and these will be addressed in the trauma resuscitation section below.

Table 5.4 A comparison of albumin solutions and synthetic colloid solutions

	Human albumin	Dextrans	Starches	Gelatins
Chemistry	Single polypeptide chain of 585 amino acids with a molecular weight of 69 kDa. Derived from donated, pooled human plasma	Highly branched polysaccharide with average molecular weights of 40–70 kDa	Chemically modified hydrolysed amylopectin fragments with various mean molecular weights from 130 to 200 kDa	Chemically modified hydrolysed collagen fragments with molecular weights of 5–50 kDa
Metabolism and excretion	Lost into the gastrointestinal tract and catabolized to amino acids in a variety of organs	Smaller molecules excreted unchanged in urine. Larger molecules hydrolysed (days)	Smaller molecules excreted unchanged in urine. Larger molecules hydrolysed by amylase, excreted into bile or sequestrated in reticuloendothelial system	Excreted unchanged in urine
Common formulations	4–5% albumin in 0.9% sodium chloride. 20–25% in hypotonic NaCl	10% solution with an average molecular weight of 40 kDa in 0.9% sodium chloride. 6% solution with an average molecular weight of 70 kDa in 0.9% sodium chloride	6–10% solutions of varying composition, mostly 0.9% NaCl but some in balanced crystalloids	3–5% solutions of varying composition. Na 145–155 mmol/L, Cl 105–145 mmol/L, Some with K/Ca/Mg, All pH 7.4
Claimed advantages	Physiological. Myriad of therapeutic binding properties	Anticoagulation. Enhance microvascular flow	Efficacy in expanding the intravascular volume thereby reducing cumulative volume required when compared to crystalloids and gelatins. Proven not to be true (64,65)	Least expensive colloid
Known problems	Cost. Risk of transmission of blood-borne pathogens	Anaphylaxis. Anticoagulation. RBC opsonization and rouleaux formation—interferes with cross-matching. Acute kidney injury	Cost. Anaphylaxis. Unpredictable anticoagulation. Acute kidney injury. Accumulation in all tissues, especially skin causing pruritus	Anaphylaxis. Unpredictable anticoagulation. ? Acute kidney injury
Comments				Shortest intravascular half-life of all the colloids

In summary, a resurgence of interest in the use of dextrans would appear both unlikely and unjustifiable.

Starches

Due in no small part to the marketing by the manufacturers, the use of starches worldwide has grown exponentially over the last decade (63). However, increasing concerns about their safety and efficacy, coupled with the retraction of a number of studies supporting their use, led to two large-scale randomized control trials.

The 6S study randomized ICU patients with severe sepsis to receive either starch (6% 130/0.42 in Ringer's) or Ringer's for resuscitation, with the primary outcome of the study being death or dependence on dialysis at 90 days (64). A total of 1211 patients were screened, 804 randomized, and complete data sets are available for 798. There was no demonstrable volume-sparing effect in the starch group, which had a 20% higher relative risk for receiving blood products. The primary outcome occurred in 51% of patients in the starch group but in only 43% in the Ringer's group (P = 0.03), and Kaplan–Meier survival curve analysis demonstrates separation between days 10 and 50. Renal replacement therapy was required in 22% of patients in the starch group compared to 16% in the Ringer's group (P = 0.04). In summary, the use of starch in this study conferred no benefits over Ringer's solution and was associated with a higher mortality and incidence of renal failure.

The Hydroxyethyl Starch or Saline for Fluid Resuscitation in Intensive Care (CHEST) study randomized ICU patients who required intravenous fluid resuscitation to receive either starch (6% 130/0.4 in 0.9% sodium chloride) or 0.9% sodium chloride (65). The primary and secondary outcomes were death at 90 days and renal failure within 90 days respectively. A total of 19,475 patients were screened, 8863 were eligible, and 7000 were randomized. There was no clinically significant volume-sparing effect and no difference in death at any time point in the 90 days between the two fluid regimens. There was also no difference in days receiving mechanical ventilation or renal replacement therapy, or ICU and hospital length of stay. There was, however, a significantly higher incidence of renal injury and pruritus in the starch group.

In summary, use of starches confers no demonstrable benefit over crystalloids and may cause significant harm, most especially in the sickest patients. In association with the very high comparative costs, these recent clinical trials should result in the cessation of the use of starches.

Gelatins

As a consequence of non-medical factors (63), gelatins have been geographically confined to Europe and their use has yet to benefit from the spotlight of a clinical trial akin to SAFE. In the inadequate and largely outdated trials comparing gelatins to crystalloids and other colloids, they appear to offer no benefits, and have a better safety profile than starches but a worse safety profile than crystalloids. Two systematic reviews are also worthy of note. An expert panel commissioned by the European Society of Intensive Care Medicine reviewed all data from published trials up to May 2011 and concluded that synthetic colloids should not be used outside clinical trials (66), and the Cochrane group also independently reached the same conclusion (67).

Although they are the cheapest colloid, gelatins are still significantly more expensive than crystalloids. In short, it is increasingly difficult to justify the use of gelatins outside of a well-conducted clinical trial.

Resuscitation following major haemorrhage and haemorrhagic shock

Regardless of the cause of haemorrhage, a large body of data, mostly from military and civilian trauma settings, supports minimal, delayed, titrated, and hypotensive fluid resuscitation until control of active bleeding and/or minimization of the risk of re-bleeding has been achieved (30). These data also support the concept of minimizing the volume of administered crystalloids or colloids, and, in their place, the early use of blood component products

(uncross-matched if necessary) in a near physiological ratio. Initial resuscitation should use 1:1–2 packed red blood cells to fresh frozen plasma (FFP), supplied together in a 'shock pack' and administered simultaneously. The need for ongoing resuscitation beyond 2–4 units of red cells and FFP should include platelets, again in a physiological ratio (68). The volumes administered should be titrated to pragmatic cardiovascular endpoints, haematocrit (target 0.30) and normalization of thromboelastography parameters (69). This resuscitation paradigm encapsulates the early and simultaneous treatment of hypovolaemia, coagulopathy, and endothelial dysfunction (70). A high dose of FFP is critical in correcting fibrinogen concentration, which is the first and most important factor deficiency in haemorrhagic coagulopathy (71–73). In addition to clotting factors, FFP contains hundreds of other proteins, including immunoglobulins and albumin, and, as such, acts as a volume expander with physiological colloid osmotic pressures. Data from animal models also suggest that FFP, in contradistinction to synthetic colloids and Ringer's, has restorative effects on endothelial permeability and vascular stability (see Figure 5.3) (70). A final word of caution regarding this approach is warranted. Transfused blood products have myriad negative effects as well as positive benefits (74), and they are also an expensive and limited resource. Thus

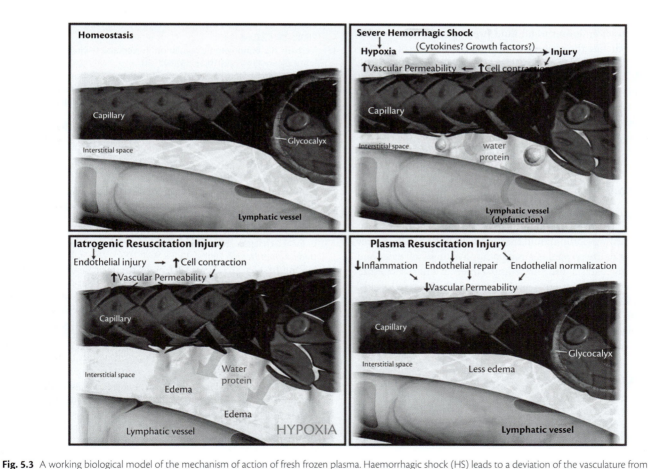

Fig. 5.3 A working biological model of the mechanism of action of fresh frozen plasma. Haemorrhagic shock (HS) leads to a deviation of the vasculature from homeostasis. HS induces hypoxia, endothelial cell tight junction breakdown, inflammation, and leucocyte diapedesis. Fresh frozen plasma repairs and 'normalizes' the vascular endothelium by restoring tight junctions, re-building the glycocalyx, and inhibiting inflammation and oedema, all detrimental processes that are exacerbated by iatrogenic injury with synthetic colloid and crystalloids.

Reproduced from Pati S et al., 'Protective Effects of Fresh Frozen Plasma on Vascular Endothelial Permeability, Coagulation, and Resuscitation After Hemorrhagic Shock Are Time Dependent and Diminish Between Days 0 and 5 After Thaw', Journal of Trauma and Acute Care Surgery, 69, 1, pp. 55–63, copyright 2010, with permission from Wolters Kluwer.

titration to predefined cardiovascular and haemostatic endpoints, using the minimum of these resources, should be applied.

So compelling is the evidence to support this approach to resuscitation that many pre-hospital services are now equipped with uncross-matched packed red blood cells and FFP for use in haemorrhagic shock. However, this is neither a universal nor necessarily practical option, nor one proven to be beneficial. What then are the best, or least worst, alternatives?

There has been a longstanding enthusiasm for administering small volumes of hypertonic fluid for pre-hospital resuscitation of both haemorrhagic shock with or without presumed significant TBI. Both hypertonic and hyperoncotic (dextrans) fluids have been studied, but independent, systematic review of these options has found no evidence of benefit or harm when compared to either the mildly hypertonic 0.9% sodium chloride or the mildly hypotonic Ringer's/Hartmann's solution (67,75). The optimal strategy for resuscitating a patient with haemorrhagic shock and significant TBI remains a clinical paradox in which the risk of inducing further bleeding has to be weighed against the secondary brain injury associated with hypotension.

Maintaining hydration *not* maintenance fluids

The anachronistic dogma of giving x mL/kg/hour of 'maintenance' intravenous crystalloid solutions to all critically ill patients should be consigned to history. There must be a clear rationale and a measurable target endpoint to all fluid prescriptions. The desired endpoint will dictate the rational fluid choice and route of administration for the particular circumstances of an individual patient. For example, a haemodynamically stable patient with a significant positive fluid balance following resuscitation may develop large nasogastric aspirates. However, if as a consequence of this loss the patient achieves their daily fluid balance target (whilst any electrolyte derangement is avoided), the losses should be considered therapeutic.

Conclusion

Fluid management is a core task in critical care, including neuro-intensive care. Historically, there have been diametrically opposing views regarding optimal fluid management but a much clearer understanding of the physiology and pathophysiology of water and electrolyte homeostasis and intercompartmental fluxes, together with the effects of the various components of administered fluids, has recently emerged. Fluid therapy should be titrated to an individual patient's needs and circumstances, avoiding fluids for which there is no evidence of benefit, at least some evidence of harm, and those with a cost that significantly exceeds a safer alternative.

References

1. Finney JL. Water? What's so special about it? *Philos Trans R Soc Lond B Biol Sci.* 2004;359(1448):1145–63.
2. Finney JL, Bowron DT. Experimental configurational landscapes in aqueous solutions. *Philos Transact A Math Phys Eng Sci.* 2005;363 (1827):469–90.
3. Knight C, Voth GA. The curious case of the hydrated proton. *Acc Chem Res.* 2012;45(1):101–9.
4. Winter R, Dzwolak W. Exploring the temperature-pressure configurational landscape of biomolecules: from lipid membranes to proteins. *Philos Transact A Math Phys Eng Sci.* 2005;363(1827):537–62.
5. Stanley HE, Buldyrev SV, Franzese G, Giovambattista N, Starr FW. Static and dynamic heterogeneities in water. *Philos Transact A Math Phys Eng Sci.* 2005;363(1827):509–23.
6. Neeb H, Zilles K, Shah NJ. Fully-automated detection of cerebral water content changes: study of age- and gender-related H2O patterns with quantitative MRI. *Neuroimage.* 2006;29(3):910–22.
7. Bergsneider M, Miller C, Vespa PM, Hu X. Surgical management of adult hydrocephalus. *Neurosurgery.* 2008;62 Supplement(2):643–60.
8. Nave CR. *Osmosis.* [Online] http://hyperphysics.phy-astr.gsu.edu/hbase/kinetic/diffus.html
9. MacAulay N, Zeuthen T. Water transport between CNS compartments: contributions of aquaporins and cotransporters. *Neuroscience.* 2010;168(4):941–56.
10. Salazar Vazquez BY, Martini J, Chavez Negrete A, Cabrales P, Tsai AG, Intaglietta M. Microvascular benefits of increasing plasma viscosity and maintaining blood viscosity: counterintuitive experimental findings. *Biorheology.* 2009;46(3):167–79.
11. Woodcock TE, Woodcock TM. Revised Starling equation and the glycocalyx model of transvascular fluid exchange: an improved paradigm for prescribing intravenous fluid therapy. *Br J Anaesth.* 2012;108(3):384–94.
12. Fanali G, di Masi A, Trezza V, Marino M, Fasano M, Ascenzi P. Human serum albumin: from bench to bedside. *Mol Aspects Med.* 2012;33(3):209–90.
13. Ruot B, Bechereau F, Bayle G, Breuille D, Obled C. The response of liver albumin synthesis to infection in rats varies with the phase of the inflammatory process. *Clin Sci (Lond).* 2002;102(1):107–14.
14. Boone M, Deen PM. Physiology and pathophysiology of the vasopressin-regulated renal water reabsorption. *Pflugers Arch.* 2008;456(6):1005–24.
15. Verbalis JG. Brain volume regulation in response to changes in osmolality. *Neuroscience.* 2010;168(4):862–70.
16. Ruot B, Papet I, Bechereau F, Denis P, Buffiere C, Gimonet J, et al. Increased albumin plasma efflux contributes to hypoalbuminemia only during early phase of sepsis in rats. *Am J Physiol Regul Integr Comp Physiol.* 2003;284(3):R707–13.
17. Redelmeier D. New thinking about postoperative hypoalbuminemia: a hypothesis of occult protein-losing enteropathy. *Open Med.* 2009;3(4):E215–19.
18. Benga O, Huber VJ. Brain water channel proteins in health and disease. *Mol Aspects Med.* 2012;33(5–6):562–78.
19. Benfenati V, Ferroni S. Water transport between CNS compartments: functional and molecular interactions between aquaporins and ion channels. *Neuroscience.* 2010;168(4):926–40.
20. Simard JM, Kent TA, Chen M, Tarasov KV, Gerzanich V. Brain oedema in focal ischaemia: molecular pathophysiology and theoretical implications. *Lancet Neurol.* 2007;6(3):258–68.
21. Walcott BP, Kahle KT, Simard JM. Novel treatment targets for cerebral edema. *Neurotherapeutics.* 2012;9(1):65–72.
22. Caramelo JJ, Iusem ND. When cells lose water: Lessons from biophysics and molecular biology. *Prog Biophys Mol Biol.* 2009;99(1):1–6.
23. Alfieri RR, Petronini PG. Hyperosmotic stress response: comparison with other cellular stresses. *Pflugers Arch.* 2007;454(2):173–85.
24. Prahlad V, Morimoto RI. Integrating the stress response: lessons for neurodegenerative diseases from C. elegans. *Trends Cell Biol.* 2009;19(2):52–61.
25. Holley A, Lukin W, Paratz J, Hawkins T, Boots R, Lipman J. Review article: Part two: Goal-directed resuscitation—which goals? Perfusion targets. *Emerg Med Australas.* 2012;24(2):127–35.
26. Vallee F, Vallet B, Mathe O, Parraguette J, Mari A, Silva S, et al. Central venous-to-arterial carbon dioxide difference: an additional target for goal-directed therapy in septic shock? *Intensive Care Med.* 2008;34(12):2218–25.
27. Barbee RW, Reynolds PS, Ward KR. Assessing shock resuscitation strategies by oxygen debt repayment. *Shock.* 2010;33(2):113–22.
28. Durairaj L, Schmidt GA. Fluid therapy in resuscitated sepsis: less is more. *Chest.* 2008;133(1):252–63.

29. Marik PE. Techniques for assessment of intervascular volume in critically ill patients. *J Intensive Care Med.* 2009;24(5):329–37.

30. Bonanno FG. Hemorrhagic shock: the "physiology approach". *J Emerg Trauma Shock.* 2012;5(4):285–95.

31. Powell-Tuck J, Gosling P, Lobo DN, Allison SP, Carlson GL, Gore M, *et al. British Consensus Guidelines on Intravenous Fluid Therapy for Adult Surgical Patients.* GIFTASUP; 2008. [Online] http://www.bapen. org.uk/pdfs/bapen_pubs/giftasup.pdf

32. Rixen D, Siegel JH. Bench-to-bedside review: oxygen debt and its metabolic correlates as quantifiers of the severity of hemorrhagic and post-traumatic shock. *Crit Care.* 2005;9(5):441–53.

33. Rampal T, Jhanji S, Pearse RM. Using oxygen delivery targets to optimize resuscitation in critically ill patients. *Curr Opin Crit Care.* 2010;16(3):244–9.

34. Bihari S, Ou J, Holt AW, Bersten AD. Inadvertent sodium loading in critically ill patients. *Crit Care Resusc.* 2012;14(1):33–7.

35. Haynes GR, Conroy JM, Baker JD, 3rd, Cooke JE. Colloid oncotic pressure as a guide for the anesthesiologist in directing fluid therapy. *South Med J.* 1989;82(5):618–23.

36. Bisera J, Weil MH, Michaels S, Bernardo A, Stein B. An "oncometer" of clinical measurement of colloid osmotic pressure of plasma. *Clin Chem.* 1978;24(9):1586–9.

37. The SAFE Study Investigators. A comparison of albumin and saline for fluid resuscitation in the intensive care unit. *N Engl J Med.* 2004;350(22):2247–56.

38. Retraction Watch. *Boldt Inquiry Concludes: False Findings in at Least 10 Studies, But No Harm to Patients.* 2012 [Online] http://retractionwatch. wordpress.com/2012/08/10/boldt-inquiry-concludes-false-findings-in-at-least-10-studies-but-no-harm-to-patients/#more-9197

39. Handy JM, Soni N. Physiological effects of hyperchloraemia and acidosis. *Br J Anaesth.* 2008;101(2):141–50.

40. Yunos N, Bellomo R, Hegarty C, Story D, Ho L, Bailey M. Association between a chloride-liberal vs chloride-restrictive intravenous fluid administration strategy and kidney injury in critically ill adults. *JAMA.* 2012;308(15):1566–72.

41. Shaw AD, Bagshaw SM, Goldstein SL, Scherer LA, Duan M, Schermer CR, *et al.* Major complications, mortality, and resource utilization after open abdominal surgery: 0.9% saline compared to Plasma-Lyte. *Ann Surg.* 2012;255(5):821–9.

42. Burdett E, Dushianthan A, Bennett-Guerrero E, Cro S, Gan TJ, Grocott MP, *et al.* Perioperative buffered versus non-buffered fluid administration for surgery in adults. *Cochrane Database Syst Rev.* 2012;12:CD004089.

43. Jung B, Rimmele T, Le Goff C, Chanques G, Corne P, Jonquet O, *et al.* Severe metabolic or mixed acidemia on intensive care unit admission: incidence, prognosis and administration of buffer therapy. A prospective, multiple-center study. *Crit Care.* 2011;15(5):R238.

44. Ijland MM, Heunks LM, van der Hoeven JG. Bench-to-bedside review: hypercapnic acidosis in lung injury—from 'permissive' to 'therapeutic'. *Crit Care.* 2010;14(6):237.

45. Forsythe SM, Schmidt GA. Sodium bicarbonate for the treatment of lactic acidosis. *Chest.* 2000;117(1):260–7.

46. Khan FY. Rhabdomyolysis: a review of the literature. *Neth J Med.* 2009;67(9):272–83.

47. Smith SW. Drugs and pharmaceuticals: management of intoxication and antidotes. *EXS.* 2010;100:397–460.

48. Kwok CS, Pang CL, Yeong JK, Loke YK. Measures used to treat contrast-induced nephropathy: overview of reviews. *Br J Radiol.* 2013;86(1021):20120272.

49. Haase M, Haase-Fielitz A, Bellomo R, Devarajan P, Story D, Matalanis G, *et al.* Sodium bicarbonate to prevent increases in serum creatinine after cardiac surgery: a pilot double-blind, randomized controlled trial. *Crit Care Med.* 2009;37(1):39–47.

50. Heringlake M, Heinze H, Schubert M, Nowak Y, Guder J, Kleinebrahm M, *et al.* A perioperative infusion of sodium bicarbonate does not improve renal function in cardiac surgery patients: a prospective observational cohort study. *Crit Care.* 2012;16(4):R156.

51. Bourdeaux CP, Brown JM. Randomized controlled trial comparing the effect of 8.4% sodium bicarbonate and 5% sodium chloride on raised intracranial pressure after traumatic brain injury. *Neurocrit Care.* 2011;15(1):42–5.

52. Bar-Or D, Bar-Or R, Rael LT, Gardner DK, Slone DS, Craun ML. Heterogeneity and oxidation status of commercial human albumin preparations in clinical use. *Crit Care Med.* 2005;33(7):1638–41.

53. Cordemans C, De Laet I, Van Regenmortel N, Schoonheydt K, Dits H, Martin G, *et al.* Aiming for a negative fluid balance in patients with acute lung injury and increased intra-abdominal pressure: a pilot study looking at the effects of PAL-treatment. *Ann Intensive Care.* 2012;2 Suppl 1:S15.

54. The SAFE Study Investigators. Saline or albumin for fluid resuscitation in patients with traumatic brain injury. *N Engl J Med.* 2007;357(9):874–84.

55. Rodling Wahlström M, Olivecrona M, Nyström F, Koskinen LO, Naredi S. Fluid therapy and the use of albumin in the treatment of severe traumatic brain injury. *Acta Anaesthesiol Scand.* 2009;53(1):18–25.

56. Ginsberg MD. Fluid resuscitation in traumatic brain injury. *Crit Care Med.* 2008;36(2):661–2.

57. Hill MD, Martin RH, Palesch YY, Tamariz D, Waldman BD, Ryckborst KJ, *et al.* The Albumin in Acute Stroke Part 1 Trial: an exploratory efficacy analysis. *Stroke.* 2011;42(6):1621–5.

58. Suarez JI, Martin RH, Calvillo E, Dillon C, Bershad EM, Macdonald RL, *et al.* The Albumin in Subarachnoid Hemorrhage (ALISAH) multicenter pilot clinical trial: safety and neurologic outcomes. *Stroke.* 2012;43(3):683–90.

59. Delaney AP, Dan A, McCaffrey J, Finfer S. The role of albumin as a resuscitation fluid for patients with sepsis: a systematic review and meta-analysis. *Crit Care Med.* 2011;39(2):386–91.

60. Abir F, Barkhordarian S, Sumpio BE. Efficacy of dextran solutions in vascular surgery. *Vasc Endovascular Surg.* 2004;38(6):483–91.

61. Roderick P, Ferris G, Wilson K, Halls H, Jackson D, Collins R, *et al.* Towards evidence-based guidelines for the prevention of venous thromboembolism: systematic reviews of mechanical methods, oral anticoagulation, dextran and regional anaesthesia as thromboprophylaxis. *Health Technol Assess.* 2005;9(49):iii–iv, ix–x, 1–78.

62. Hvidt LN, Perner A. High dosage of dextran 70 is associated with severe bleeding in patients admitted to the intensive care unit for septic shock. *Dan Med J.* 2012;59(11):A4531.

63. Singer M. Management of fluid balance: a European perspective. *Curr Opin Anaesthesiol.* 2012;25(1):96–101.

64. Perner A, Haase N, Guttormsen AB, Tenhunen J, Klemenzson G, Aneman A, *et al.* Hydroxyethyl starch 130/0.42 versus Ringer's acetate in severe sepsis. *N Engl J Med.* 2012;367(2):124–34.

65. Myburgh JA, Finfer S, Bellomo R, Billot L, Cass A, Gattas D, *et al.* Hydroxyethyl starch or saline for fluid resuscitation in intensive care. *N Engl J Med.* 2012;367(20):1901–11.

66. Reinhart K, Perner A, Sprung CL, Jaeschke R, Schortgen F, Johan Groeneveld AB, *et al.* Consensus statement of the ESICM task force on colloid volume therapy in critically ill patients. *Intensive Care Med.* 2012;38(3):368–83.

67. Perel P, Roberts I. Colloids versus crystalloids for fluid resuscitation in critically ill patients. *Cochrane Database Syst Rev.* 2012;6:CD000567.

68. Godier A, Samama CM, Susen S. Plasma/platelets/red blood cell ratio in the management of the bleeding traumatized patient: does it matter? *Curr Opin Anaesthesiol.* 2012;25(2):242–7.

69. Bolliger D, Seeberger MD, Tanaka KA. Principles And Practice Of Thromboelastography In Clinical Coagulation Management And Transfusion Practice. *Transfus Med Rev.* 2012;26(1):1–13.

70. Pati S, Matijevic N, Doursout M-Fo, Ko T, Cao Y, Deng X, *et al.* Protective effects of fresh frozen plasma on vascular endothelial permeability, coagulation, and resuscitation after hemorrhagic shock are time dependent and diminish between days 0 and 5 after thaw. *J Trauma.* 2010;69 Suppl 1:S55–63.

71. Davenport R, Manson J, De'Ath H, Platton S, Coates A, Allard S, *et al.* Functional definition and characterization of acute traumatic coagulopathy. *Crit Care Med.* 2011;39(12):2652–8.

72. Frith D, Goslings JC, Gaarder C, Maegele M, Cohen MJ, Allard S, *et al.* Definition and drivers of acute traumatic coagulopathy: clinical and experimental investigations. *J Thromb Haemost.* 2010;8(9):1919–25.

73. Lance MD, Ninivaggi M, Schols SE, Feijge MA, Oehrl SK, Kuiper GJ, *et al.* Perioperative dilutional coagulopathy treated with fresh frozen plasma and fibrinogen concentrate: a prospective randomized intervention trial. *Vox Sang.* 2012;103(1):25–34.

74. Sihler KC, Napolitano LM. Complications of massive transfusion. *Chest.* 2010;137(1):209–20.

75. Tan PG, Cincotta M, Clavisi O, Bragge P, Wasiak J, Pattuwage L, *et al.* Review article: Prehospital fluid management in traumatic brain injury. *Emerg Med Australas.* 2011;23(6):665–76.

CHAPTER 6

Sedation and analgesia in the neurocritical care unit

Mauro Oddo and Luzius A. Steiner

Sedation and analgesia play key roles in the management of critically ill patients to improve tolerance of intubation and mechanical ventilation, and generally facilitate patient management. Sedation has additional specific functions in the management of acute brain injury (ABI) during neurocritical care. It reduces the cerebral metabolic rate of oxygen ($CMRO_2$), cerebral blood flow (CBF), and cerebral blood volume (CBV) and thereby increases the tolerance of the brain to potential ischaemic insults, as well as playing a key role in the prevention of intracranial hypertension and the management of elevated intracranial pressure (ICP).

Indications for sedation

There are general and neurological-specific indications for sedation in patients with ABI.

General indications

Sedative agents are routinely administered to critically ill patients to reduce anxiety, pain, and discomfort, to prevent agitation, and facilitate mechanical ventilation. They prevent surges of systemic blood pressure and ICP in response to interventions, thereby protecting the injured brain against secondary insults. Critically ill adult patients have historically been deeply sedated to ensure comfort and facilitate ventilator management, but prolonged and high-dose sedation is associated with intensive care unit (ICU)-acquired encephalopathy, weakness, and delirium. It is becoming increasingly clear that ventilator management with less or even no sedation (as tolerated) is associated with improved patient outcome. Limiting the dose of sedation using the ABCDE care bundle (awake and breathing coordination, delirium monitoring, early mobility, and exercise) has been associated with improvements in the management of mechanically ventilated patients (1,2). While a more conservative approach to sedation management in patients in general ICU is now widespread, a blanket extension of such a strategy to patients with severe ABI is questionable and should only be applied when ICP and cerebral perfusion pressure (CPP) are normalized.

Brain-specific indications

During the early phase after ABI, the imbalance between increased cerebral metabolic demand and limited energy reserve exposes the brain to a risk of secondary (ischaemic) insults. Sedative agents reduce $CMRO_2$ and improve the brain's tolerance to ischaemia and energy dysfunction. In a normally reactive brain, sedative agents also decrease CBF thereby inducing a proportional reduction in CBV and ICP.

Sedation titrated to patient needs reduces cerebral metabolic demand related to agitation, pain, motor hyperactivity, cough, patient–ventilator asynchrony, tracheal suctioning, shivering, and transportation, which may all increase ICP. Standard sedation is therefore part of the first-line management of elevated ICP. Deep sedation, titrated to maintain ICP below a predetermined level (usually < 20–25 mmHg) or to electroencephalogram (EEG)-monitored burst suppression, may be required in some cases. A combination of several sedatives agents, including propofol, midazolam, and barbiturates, may be required to manage intracranial hypertension refractory to first-line therapies (see Chapter 7). Many sedatives, including benzodiazepines, propofol, and barbiturates, have intrinsic antiepileptic properties and are also used in the management of refractory status epilepticus (see Chapter 23).

Sedative and analgesic agents

The following section reviews the pharmacological profile of the drugs available for sedation and analgesia in the neurocritical care unit (NCCU), emphasizing their cerebral haemodynamic and side effects (Table 6.1).

Propofol

Propofol (2,6-diisopropyl phenol) is the most widely used sedative agent in the NCCU. It is insoluble in water and presented as a soybean oil-based emulsion with glycerol and egg lecithin emulsifiers. Two concentrations of propofol, 1% and 2%, are currently available.

Propofol enhances gamma-aminobutyric acid (GABA) neurotransmission and is an *N*-methyl-D-aspartate (NMDA) antagonist. Although it has neuroprotective actions in animal studies, human data confirming neuroprotection are lacking (3).

Continuous infusion of propofol induces sedation in a dose-dependent manner. Despite elimination from poorly perfused tissues being slow, the volume of distribution of propofol is very large thereby guaranteeing rapid awakening even after prolonged infusion. Propofol is primarily eliminated in the liver. Renal and pulmonary clearance also occurs but renal dysfunction does not prolong propofol elimination.

Cerebral haemodynamic actions

Propofol lowers ICP in patients with and without intracranial hypertension. However, it also decreases mean arterial pressure

Table 6.1 Cerebral haemodynamic and side effects of commonly used sedative and analgesic agents

	Mechanism of action	Effect on brain haemodynamics	Side effects	Comments
Propofol	GABAergic agonist NMDA antagonist	↓ ICP, ↓ MAP (particularly in hypovolaemic patients), thus may ↓ CPP; ↓ $CMRO_2$ and CBF, preserved CO_2 reactivity and cerebral autoregulation; ↓ cerebral electrical activity, can be used to induce burst suppression and treat status epilepticus (at high dose)	↑ triglycerides, ↓ MAP, peripheral vasodilation (venous > arterial), myocardial depression, propofol-infusion syndrome (↓ HR, ↑ pH, ↑ lactate, ↑ CPK, myocardial failure)	Relatively rapid awakening even with prolonged infusions; only drug that is recommended by the Brain Trauma Foundation guidelines to treat elevated ICP
Midazolam	GABAergic agonist	↓ $CMRO_2$ and CBF; mild ↓ of ICP, preserved CO_2 reactivity and cerebral autoregulation; antiepileptic effect	Protracted coma, particularly during prolonged administration and if kidney/liver function impaired; prolonged use can cause tachyphylaxis and withdrawal	
Lorazepam	GABAergic agonist	↓ $CMRO_2$ and CBF; antiepileptic effects	Exacerbation of ICU delirium; continuous infusion can cause ethylene glycol-induced metabolic acidosis	Long half-life (15 h); not suitable for continuous intravenous sedation in brain-injured patients
Morphine	μ-opioid receptor agonist	↑ ICP via ↓ cerebrovascular resistance, ↑ CBF or ↑ $PaCO_2$; disturbed cerebral autoregulation; opiate-related increase in ICP is mainly due to a decrease in MAP	Prolonged duration of MV, particularly in patients with kidney/liver failure; withdrawal symptoms in patients who received long-term sedation; opiate-induced hyperalgesia	The dose needed to produce analgesia is very variable
Fentanyl, sufentanil	μ-opioid receptor agonist	↑ ICP via ↓cerebrovascular resistance, ↑ CBF or ↑ $PaCO_2$; disturbed cerebral autoregulation; opiate-related increase in ICP is mainly due to a decrease in MAP	Same as for morphine	Rapid onset of action
Remifentanil	μ-opioid receptor agonist	The effects of remifentanil on ICP, CPP, and CBF are overall comparable to those of other opiates, and are modest if MAP is kept stable	Bradycardia	Rapid clearance and highly predictable onset and offset of effect; terminal half-life of ~ 10–20 min
Barbiturates	GABAergic agonist, via the inhibition of intracellular Ca^{2+} influx and the blockade of glutamate receptors	↓↓ CBF that is proportional to the ↓↓ of $CMRO_2$; during burst suppression, the ↓ of cerebral metabolism can be of about 60% compared to baseline; by ↓ CBF and CBV, barbiturates have a strong effect on ICP	↓ MAP/CPP; increased risk of infection; adrenal dysfunction	Barbiturates should be limited to the treatment of refractory ICP and refractory SE, in combination with other sedatives and titrated to the lowest effective dose; EEG may be helpful to titrate barbiturate therapy
Alpha-2 agonists (clonidine, dexmedetomidine, DEX)	Alpha-2 adrenoreceptor agonists	↓ CBF by DEX may be mainly related to a reduction in $CMRO_2$ rather than to a direct cerebral vasoconstrictive effect; α_2/α_1 adrenal-receptor ratio of DEX is approximately 7–8 times higher than clonidine; DEX elimination half-life is 2 h vs 8 h for clonidine	Hypotension Bradycardia	No respiratory depression; clonidine can be particularly useful to treat delirium, especially in patients with symptoms of benzodiazepine or alcohol withdrawal
Etomidate	GABA-like effects	↓ ICP, ↓ CBF, and ↓ $CMRO_2$ ↓ MAP and CPP	Adrenal insufficiency; increased susceptibility to infections	Not recommended as the first choice agent for rapid-sequence intubation of NCCU patients; propofol is preferred to etomidate

(continued)

Table 6.1 (Continued)

	Mechanism of action	Effect on brain haemodynamics	Side effects	Comments
Haloperidol	Dopamine antagonist	↑ CBF	Prolongation of the QT interval; torsades de pointes; may lower seizure threshold and increase epileptic activity; neuroleptic malignant syndrome	
Ketamine	NMDA antagonist	No significant negative effects on ICP and cerebral haemodynamics; may be used as adjunct for the management of refractory SE	Hallucinations, dysphoria, blurred vision, nystagmus, diplopia	
Inhaled anaesthetics	Not fully established: may act at several sites (reduction in junctional conductance; activation of Ca^{2+}-dependent ATPase; binding to the GABA receptor, the large conductance Ca^{2+} activated K^+ channel, the glutamate receptor, and the glycine receptor)	Dose-related suppression of cerebral electrical activity and hence cerebral metabolism, which leads to ↓ in CBF; dose-dependent direct cerebral vasodilator effect that might ↑ CBF, CBV, and ↑ ICP; the net effect results from the balance between these two mechanisms; ↓ CBF at low concentrations, ↑ CBF and CBV at high concentrations; sevoflurane is the inhaled anaesthetic with the least vasodilator properties	In patients with decreased intracranial compliance, may ↑ ICP; myocardial depression; malignant hyperthermia	

CBF, cerebral blood flow; CBV, cerebral blood volume; $CMRO_2$, cerebral metabolic rate of oxygen; CPP, cerebral perfusion pressure; EEG, electroencephalography; GABA, gamma-aminobutyric acid; ICP, intracranial pressure; ICU intensive care unit; LOS, length of stay; MAP, mean arterial pressure; MV, mechanical ventilation; NCCU, neurocritical care unit; NMDA, N-methyl D-aspartate; SAH, subarachnoid haemorrhage; SE, status epilepticus.

(MAP) and may therefore reduce CPP despite its ICP-lowering actions. Propofol is as effective as fentanyl or pentobarbital plus morphine at controlling ICP, but more effective than morphine alone or morphine plus midazolam (3). It is currently the only drug recommended in the Brain Trauma Foundation guidelines for the control of ICP (level II recommendation), except for high-dose barbiturates to control refractory intracranial hypertension (4).

Propofol lowers $CMRO_2$ and CBF but flow–metabolism coupling, CO_2 reactivity, and autoregulation are typically preserved in the normal brain. However, there are reports that propofol has a cerebral vasoconstrictor effect which has been associated with a decrease in jugular venous saturation and also deterioration in static autoregulation at higher doses (5). High-dose propofol effectively suppresses cerebral electrical activity and is often used to induce burst suppression in the management of seizures and status epilepticus (see Chapter 23). Propofol may have pro-convulsive actions at low doses but this phenomenon is not observed at higher doses (6). Nevertheless, caution has been advised when repeated small boluses of propofol are used during procedural sedation in patients with known seizure disorders. Despite its beneficial effects on cerebral haemodynamics, there are no clinical studies showing that propofol sedation is associated with improved outcome in critically ill neurological patients.

Side effects

The main side effects of propofol are dose-dependent cardiovascular depression necessitating more frequent use and higher doses of vasopressors to maintain CPP. This is related to several mechanisms. Peripheral vasodilatation, more pronounced in the venous than in the arterial bed, myocardial depression, and interference with baroreceptor function have all been reported. This is a particular concern in older patients with diastolic dysfunction and in hypovolaemic patients susceptible to the preload reduction induced by propofol.

Propofol infusion syndrome

A major concern regarding the use of propofol for sedation in the NCCU is the development of the propofol infusion syndrome (PRIS) (7,8). This was initially described in children but there have also been a large number of reports of PRIS in adults, particularly in critically ill neurological patients. It is characterized by metabolic lactic acidosis, elevated creatine kinase, myocardial failure, and death. Bradycardia is described in children but, in adults, tachyarrhythmias, including ventricular tachycardia, are more common (8). The underlying mechanism of PRIS is believed to be specific disruption of fatty-acid oxidation because of impairment of entry of long-chain acylcarnitine esters into the mitochondria, and subsequent failure of the mitochondrial respiratory chain (9). Because of the concerns regarding the development of PRIS, propofol is contraindicated for sedation in paediatric patients and doses exceeding 5 mg/kg/h should not be used for longer than 48 hours in adults. Propofol should also be avoided in patients with inborn errors of fatty acid metabolism and mitochondrial disorders (10).

Because of the obligatory lipid load during propofol infusion it is also recommended that propofol should not be used for sedation in hypothermic patients, when metabolism of fatty acids is reduced, or when triglyceride levels exceed 4 mmol/L. The 2% solution was developed specifically to reduce exposure to the lipid vehicle, but it can still result in a significant increase in serum triglycerides. This suggests that triglyceridaemia during propofol infusion is not simply caused by the lipid vehicle, but also by pharmacodynamic effects consistent with the postulated mechanism of PRIS (11).

Benzodiazepines

Benzodiazepines are GABA agonists with sedative, anxiolytic, amnesic, and antiepileptic actions. They are frequently used as sedative agents on the NCCU, often in association with an opioid such as morphine.

Midazolam is a short-acting benzodiazepine with a relatively short (1-hour) half-life and is often used for continuous intravenous sedation in the NCCU. It has a stable haemodynamic profile and fewer cardiovascular side effects than propofol. Lorazepam has a much longer half-life (15 hours) and is not suitable for continuous intravenous sedation. However, when administered as intermittent intravenous boluses, lorazepam may have a place as an alternative to midazolam during weaning of agitated patients from ventilation, particularly those at risk of benzodiazepine or alcohol withdrawal (12).

Cerebral haemodynamic actions

Benzodiazepines reduce CBF and increase cerebrovascular resistance proportional to the decrease in $CMRO_2$ (13). Midazolam causes no or only a mild reduction in ICP, but preserves cerebrovascular autoregulation and CO_2 reactivity (14). Three randomized controlled trials comparing propofol to midazolam reported similar effects on ICP and CPP (11,15,16).

Side effects

Benzodiazepines have few haemodynamic side effects. The main concern with midazolam is delayed awakening, particularly after prolonged administration or when kidney and/or liver function are impaired (17), but there is large inter-individual variability in this effect (18). Tachyphylaxis is common during prolonged use of midazolam, as are symptoms of withdrawal when the drug is stopped. Continuous infusion of lorazepam can lead to ethylene glycol-induced metabolic acidosis and is not recommended. All benzodiazepines, but particularly lorazepam, have been linked to the development of delirium in ICU patients (19).

Opioids

Pain may occur as a consequence of surgery, trauma, or inflammation and, in ICU patients, because of the presence of an endotracheal tube, full bladder or bowel, chest drains, or immobility. Sedative agents do treat pain and analgesics are indicated.

Opioids reinforce the effects of sedatives, and the combination of an opioid and a sedative is the general rule in the NCCU. Recent data suggest that ICU patients often suffer from inadequate pain management, and daily pain assessment and optimization of analgesia has been associated with reduced duration of mechanical ventilation and ICU length of stay (LOS) (20). As well as being part of general patient management, adequate analgesia is mandatory in patients with elevated ICP. Boluses of analgesia before potentially painful manoeuvres may attenuate unwanted increases in ICP.

The morphine dose required to produce effective analgesia is variable and depends on factors such as opioid tolerance, metabolism, and excretion. The usual adult dose of morphine for a patient receiving mechanical ventilation is a continuous infusion at a rate of 1–10 mg/h, or 2–5 mg intermittent boluses. Morphine may accumulate in patients with renal failure and dose adjustment is required. Fentanyl is a synthetic opioid that is 75–200 times more potent than morphine. It penetrates membranes quickly and thus has a rapid onset of action. Its duration of action is relatively short, but prolonged infusion leads to accumulation. In patients requiring

mechanical ventilation, fentanyl is infused at a rate of 100–200 mcg/h, or as 50–100 mcg boluses. Sufentanil is also a synthetic opioid, usually administered as a continuous intravenous infusion at a rate of 0.3–0.9 mcg/kg/h, or as bolus doses of 1–2 mcg/kg.

Morphine, fentanyl, and sufentanil undergo hepatic metabolism, and continuous infusion can lead to accumulation and prolonged effects, including delayed recovery and respiratory depression. This is especially the case in critically ill patients in whom drug clearance may be substantially reduced. Agents with a shorter half-life, such as sufentanil, are often preferred.

Remifentanil is a potent selective μ-opioid receptor agonist and an ultra-short acting agent originally designed for use in anaesthesia. It differs from other opioids in being metabolized by esterases which are widely distributed in all body tissues. Even during the anhepatic period of liver transplantation there is little change in remifentanil pharmacokinetics, highlighting its independence from the usual routes of metabolism. Because of its unique pharmacokinetic profile, remifentanil is characterized by a rapid and uniform clearance and a highly predictable onset and offset of effect. It has an effective biological half-life of 3–10 minutes (21), which offers potential advantage when weaning patients from sedation and analgesia (22). Remifentanil is metabolized to remifentanil acid which has very weak opioid actions but even in renal failure remifentanil acid is unlikely to exert a clinically significant effect. The ability to provide intense analgesia with remifentanil means that lower doses of co-administered sedative agents are required.

Cerebral haemodynamic actions

Morphine, fentanyl, and sufentanil are associated with increases in ICP and CBF, and disturbed cerebral autoregulation (23–26). Three randomized controlled trials have demonstrated that boluses or short infusions of opioids result in clinically and statistically significant increases in ICP, and decreases in systemic blood pressure and CPP (23,24,27). These effects are usually transient but, in one study, persisted for some hours (23). The ICP effects are likely to be related to reductions in blood pressure and consequent cerebral vasodilation leading to increased ICP (28). Thus, the ICP and CPP effects of opioids can be minimized by the prevention of hypotension with volume resuscitation and vasopressors. One trial found that morphine was associated with higher requirements for ICP-lowering interventions and poorer ICP control after 3 days of infusion compared to propofol (29). Remifentanil has similar effects on ICP, CPP, and CBF to other opioids, which are also modest if systemic blood pressure is maintained.

Side effects

The main side effects of opioids are respiratory depression in self-ventilating patients and prolonged duration of mechanical ventilation, particularly in patients with kidney or liver dysfunction. Withdrawal symptoms in those who have received long-term sedation/analgesia and opiate-induced hyperalgesia are also reported. Remifentanil can cause a significant reduction in heart rate and chest wall rigidity at high doses.

Other analgesics

Paracetamol (acetaminophen) is a non-opioid analgesic that can be administered enterally, rectally, and intravenously in divided doses of 500–1000 mg. The maximum daily dose is 4 g.

Non-steroidal anti-inflammatory drugs (NSAIDs) have several potentially adverse effects including antiplatelet actions, acute kidney injury, and gastrointestinal bleeding. Despite these risks, NSAIDs are often used as analgesics in neurological patients. The more commonly used NSAIDs include ketorolac (10 mg 6-hourly) and ibuprofen (400–600 mg 8-hourly).

Barbiturates

Barbiturates act at multiple sites in the brain by increasing GABAergic activity, inhibiting the intracellular influx of calcium and blocking glutamate receptors (30). Given their numerous side effects, the indications for barbiturates are limited to the treatment of refractory elevated ICP and status epilepticus, when they are usually administered in combination with other sedative agents (4).

Cerebral haemodynamic actions

Barbiturates decrease $CMRO_2$ with a proportional reduction in CBF. At EEG burst suppression, cerebral metabolism is reduced by 60% compared to baseline. Barbiturates have a strong ICP reducing action secondary to their effects to reduce CBF and CBV (31,32). CBF and $CMRO_2$ coupling, cerebrovascular autoregulation, and CO_2 reactivity are unaffected by barbiturate infusion.

Because of the ICP lowering effects, barbiturate coma is a therapeutic option for refractory intracranial hypertension (4). In a small randomized controlled trial of 44 patients with severe traumatic brain injury (TBI) and elevated ICP, thiopental was more effective than pentobarbital in reducing the period of time with ICP greater than 20 mmHg (33). Although barbiturate therapy is usually titrated to the desired ICP, there is a weak correlation between barbiturate concentrations and ICP response (34) and EEG should be used to guide barbiturate therapy and minimize side effects (35,36).

Side effects

Barbiturates result in leucopoenia and immune suppression and therefore increase the susceptibility to infection (33). They also cause significant reductions in systemic blood pressure and CPP (33,37), and have been associated with adrenal dysfunction (38). These adverse effects often offset the beneficial effects of barbiturates on ICP reduction, and might explain why pentobarbital is less effective than mannitol in the management of intracranial hypertension (39).

Alpha-2 agonists

Clonidine and dexmedetomidine are the two clinically available α_2-agonists. Although there is considerable interest in the use of these drugs in the general ICU, there are few studies in critically ill neurological patients. Both produce dose-dependent sedation, anxiolysis, and analgesia through actions at spinal and supra-spinal sites, without respiratory depression.

Dexmedetomidine is a highly selective α_2-adrenoreceptor agonist with an α_2/α_1 adrenoreceptor ratio approximately seven to eight times higher than that of clonidine. The elimination half-life of dexmedetomidine is 2 hours compared to 8 hours for clonidine, and the α-half-life is 6 minutes. This makes dexmedetomidine very suitable for intravenous titration and more suitable than clonidine as an ICU sedative.

Cerebral haemodynamic actions

In a study in rabbits with and without intracerebral lesions, dexmedetomidine did not increase ICP over a wide dose range (40). It also had no effect on lumbar cerebrospinal fluid pressure in a study in 16 postoperative patients (41). There has been some concern about a dexmedetomidine-induced reduction in CBF and, in one study in healthy human volunteers, sedation with dexmedetomidine was associated with a 33% decrease in CBF (42). It was unclear whether this effect was related to direct α_2-receptor-dependent vasoconstriction or to compensatory CBF changes as a result of dexmedetomidine-induced decreases in $CMRO_2$. However, in another human volunteer study, the $CBF/CMRO_2$ ratio was unchanged by dexmedetomidine (43). Dexmedetomidine impairs cerebrovascular pressure autoregulation in the healthy brain (44). Overall, these data suggest that dexmedetomidine-induced decreases in CBF are mainly coupled with a reduction in $CMRO_2$ rather than related to direct cerebral vasoconstrictive actions (45).

In animal models of drug-induced epilepsy, pro- and anticonvulsant effects of α_2-agonists have been reported. This is in contrast to findings in humans where no proconvulsant activity has been identified. Although dexmedetomidine did not reduce epileptiform discharges in one study of adult patients with epilepsy (46), there are no reports of dexmedetomidine-induced seizures in humans. Unlike other sedative drugs, dexmedetomidine does not adversely affect the recording of sensory and motor evoked potentials (47).

Comparison with other sedative agents

In a pilot study, dexmedetomidine and propofol were equally effective for sedation in brain-injured patients and neither was associated with adverse cerebral physiological effects as assessed by multimodal monitoring (48). The potential for dexmedetomidine to prevent or treat delirium has been extensively studied in general ICU patients. A recent meta-analysis demonstrated that the incidence of delirium is not significantly different with dexmedetomidine compared to other sedative drugs (49). However, dexmedetomidine appears to preserve cognitive function, with specific preservation of focus and attention, in comparison to propofol (50).

Data relating to the effect of dexmedetomidine on the duration of mechanical ventilation and ICU LOS are controversial, and there are none specific to critically ill neurological patients. After cardiac surgery, dexmedetomidine infusion (0.4 mcg/kg/h during the procedure and 0.2 mcg/kg/h in the ICU) reduced the time to extubation and ICU LOS (51). In a study comparing dexmedetomidine to haloperidol in agitated mechanically ventilated general ICU patients, those receiving dexmedetomidine were also extubated earlier (52). However, in a retrospective analysis comparing two doses of dexmedetomidine with propofol in trauma patients, those in the higher-dose dexmedetomidine group (> 0.7 mcg/kg/h) had higher rates of hypotension, longer duration of mechanical ventilation, and longer ICU and hospital LOS (53). There are no data on neurological outcome and mortality in patients sedated with α_2-agonists.

Although α_2-agonists, particularly dexmedetomidine, are promising sedative agents in neurological patients, further studies are needed to identify their exact role and utility in the management of sedation in the NCCU.

Side effects

The haemodynamic effects of clonidine and dexmedetomidine are well described. An initial phase of hypertension is often seen, but the major side effects are (mild) hypotension and bradycardia. This has led to some controversy regarding the ideal loading dose and maximum infusion rate of dexmedetomidine. Typically a bolus of 1 mcg/kg is administered, followed by a 0.2–0.7 mcg/kg/h continuous intravenous infusion. As there appears to be a link between cardiovascular side effects and loading dose, some clinicians prefer to omit this and start with an infusion.

Apart from these cardiovascular effects, no other relevant side effects of α_2-agonists have been described. In contrast to other commonly used sedative and analgesic agents, they do not cause respiratory depression.

Etomidate

Etomidate has a rapid-onset effect and short duration of action, and has historically been used as part of a rapid-sequence induction technique. It reduces ICP, CBF, and $CMRO_2$ (54,55) and, although it may cause hypotension and reduce CPP (55), etomidate is less hypotensive than barbiturates or propofol during induction of anaesthesia. However, it has potentially serious side effects, specifically acute adrenal insufficiency, and is therefore not recommended as the first choice for rapid sequence induction in the NCCU. Further, it does not adequately control the hypertensive (and therefore ICP) response to laryngoscopy, and propofol or barbiturates are preferable induction agents in cases of suspected or confirmed intracranial hypertension, providing blood pressure is maintained.

Side effects

Etomidate increases the susceptibility to pneumonia in trauma patients (56) and is associated with increased acute adrenal insufficiency and higher mortality (57). Adrenal suppression can occur after only a single 0.3 mg/kg dose of etomidate (58). These effects are potentiated by severe sepsis (57,59).

Antipsychotic drugs for agitation

Agitation and delirium are everyday challenges in the NCCU, but the distinction between agitation and delirium is often difficult. Agitation may be related to an underlying brain injury, while delirium is primarily related to the consequence of prolonged sedation and ICU interventions. Although therapeutic strategies differ, both agitation and delirium often require administration of antipsychotic agents.

Haloperidol, a dopamine agonist of the typical class of antipsychotics, is the standard of care for treatment of agitation and delirium (60). However, it may cause prolongation of the QT interval and lead to the development of torsades de pointes. Atypical antipsychotics, such as risperidone, quetiapine, and olanzapine, are enteral agents acting on dopaminergic and serotonergic systems that have recently been introduced into the NCCU as alternatives to haloperidol. Although none of these drugs is licensed for use in agitated ICU patients, several studies have found that atypical antipsychotics have acceptable safety profiles (61–63). However, caution should be exercised during prolonged utilization of these agents given the FDA warning regarding mortality when they are used to treat agitation in elderly patients with dementia (64). Antipsychotic agents may also lower the seizure threshold and induce or increase the risk of epileptic activity.

Cerebral haemodynamic actions

There are few data on the effects of antipsychotics on cerebral haemodynamics. Studies have typically been carried out in patients with schizophrenia, and are predominantly limited to haloperidol and risperidone. Haloperidol increases global (65) and regional (66) CBF compared to risperidone, but whether these differences are clinically relevant, or translate into effects on ICP, is unclear.

In general, antipsychotics decrease the severity of symptoms of agitation by 43–70%, and 50–100% of patients respond to such treatment (67). Whether this is also the case in critically ill neurological patients is unknown. Quetiapine resolves several symptoms of ICU-related delirium more rapidly than placebo (61), but in a study in general ICU patients there was no difference in clinical improvement between olanzapine and haloperidol (63). There are no data comparing any of these drugs in the NCCU, and no studies have examined the effect of the treatment of delirium with antipsychotic agents on outcome.

Alternative drugs to treat agitation

Potential alternatives to antipsychotic drugs warrant mention. As dysfunction of cholinergic transmission is one of the hypothetical causes of agitation, cholinesterase inhibitors such as rivastigmine may be a potential treatment option. However, a recent randomized controlled trial exploring the utility of rivastigmine as an adjunct to haloperidol was stopped prematurely because of an increased mortality in the rivastigmine group (68). Benzodiazepines have historically been used to treat agitation but, apart from their use in alcohol withdrawal-related delirium where they are clearly indicated (12), data suggest that they actually increase the risk of delirium and should be avoided (19). Alpha-2 agonists have also been used to treat agitation in the ICU, and clonidine can be particularly useful in patients with symptoms of benzodiazepine or alcohol withdrawal.

Side effects

Haloperidol, risperidone, olanzapine, and quetiapine are all weak α-antagonists and hence peripheral vasodilators. Blood pressure changes are generally mild but profound hypotension following a single dose has been reported (69). The main concerns are prolongation of the QT interval and risk of development of torsades de pointes, and reduction in the seizure threshold. This is less pronounced in the more potent typical antipsychotics, so haloperidol has the least marked effect on seizure threshold. Atypical antipsychotics have a better safety profile in this regard. All antipsychotic agents might cause dyskinesia.

Typical antipsychotics are contraindicated in Parkinson's disease. Despite atypical antipsychotics also having dopamine antagonist actions, they have been used safely in patients with Parkinson's disease, and olanzapine is recommended (70). The neuroleptic malignant syndrome is a rare but serious adverse reaction to antipsychotic drugs and has been associated with therapeutic doses of typical and atypical antipsychotics (71). The essential features of neuroleptic malignant syndrome are muscle rigidity and hyperpyrexia that may be associated, autonomic instability, mental state changes, and muscle catabolism. The suspected mechanism is dopaminergic blockade-related muscle rigidity that contributes to impaired heat dissipation and hyperthermia. Therapy is mostly symptomatic but intravenous dantrolene has been used successfully.

Comparative studies of sedative agents

Three randomized controlled trials have compared maintenance doses of propofol (1.5–5 mg/kg/h) with midazolam (0.1–0.3 mg/kg/h) and found no difference in ICP control (11,15,16). In two of these, there was also no difference in ICU LOS or quality of sedation between propofol and midazolam (11,16). However, there was a higher rate of therapeutic failure with propofol when sedation was continued for more than 2 days (6–9 days), characterized by elevated triglyceride levels and the need for high doses greater than 6 mg/kg/h (11). Weaning and extubation occur earlier with propofol compared to midazolam (6,72) but, in the context of nurse-led, protocol-directed sedation, propofol and midazolam provide similar quality of sedation (73). A systematic review including 13 studies in 384 patients with TBI concluded that propofol and midazolam sedation have comparable effects on mortality, duration of mechanical ventilation, ICU LOS, and quality and depth of sedation (74). Of note, no data are available comparing propofol to midazolam for other types of brain injury. In a study comparing propofol with morphine, less adjunctive ICP therapy but increased vasopressor use was required in the propofol group (41).

There are limited data comparing propofol with barbiturates during neurocritical care. In a small trial of ten patients with TBI, propofol was equally effective at controlling ICP when compared to fentanyl (75) or pentobarbital plus morphine (3). Two studies suggest that remifentanil might reduce the duration of mechanical ventilation compared to morphine (76) or fentanyl (77) in NCCU patients.

In conclusion, propofol and midazolam are used interchangeably as first-line sedative agents after ABI, and there is no evidence that one is superior to the other. Practice varies between clinicians and countries, and is likely driven by individual clinician experience and cost. When choosing a sedative agent in brain-injured patients, some practical issues must be kept in mind:

- Propofol and midazolam are equally effective in controlling ICP.
- Sedative agents may cause hypotension and a reduction in CPP-maintenance of normovolaemia and MAP is essential.
- ICP control with midazolam may require increasingly high doses because of tachyphylaxis, with ensuing prolonged duration of coma, mechanical ventilation, and ICU LOS.
- Despite its ICP-lowering actions, propofol (particularly at high doses) may not guarantee an adequate CPP because of associated hypotension.
- Propofol is more costly than midazolam.

Adjunct agents

Several adjunct agents have been described in the management of sedation on the NCCU.

Ketamine

Ketamine is an NMDA antagonist that is categorized as a dissociative agent because it causes brain functional and electrophysiological dissociation rather than true sedation. It creates a trance-like cataleptic state resulting in profound analgesia and amnesia, with retention of protective airway reflexes and maintenance of spontaneous respiration and cardiopulmonary stability. Ketamine is marketed as a racemic mixture but also as the (S)-ketamine form which has a threefold superior analgesic and anaesthetic potency but comparable pharmacokinetics to (R)-ketamine. It has been used as an adjunct to other sedative drugs in the NCCU.

Cerebral haemodynamic actions
Early work found that ketamine has stimulating properties on the brain leading to an increase in CBF, CBV, $CMRO_2$, and ICP.

However, more recent studies examining ketamine as an adjunct to other sedatives or analgesic drugs found no significant negative effects on ICP or cerebral haemodynamics (78,79). Given its effect at the NMDA receptor, ketamine is used as an adjunct in chronic pain management and after painful surgery (e.g. complex spine surgery with instrumentation), as well as for the management of refractory status epilepticus (see Chapter 23) (80).

Side effects
The main side effects of ketamine, particularly when large doses are used, are neuropsychiatric, including hallucinations, unpleasant dreams, dysphoria, blurred vision, nystagmus, and diplopia. However, when ketamine is used in combination with midazolam or propofol these side effects are rare. Hypersalivation is a further unwanted effect. The bronchodilator activity of ketamine may be beneficial, although there is considerable tachyphylaxis when ketamine is used as a continuous infusion for the treatment of severe bronchospasm.

Inhaled anaesthetic agents

Until recently, inhaled anaesthetics were only exceptionally used for sedation in the ICU because of difficulty in their delivery. The introduction of the AnaConDa™ device has allowed administration of isoflurane and sevoflurane via a syringe pump, that is, not via a vaporizer, allowing compatibility with ICU ventilators (81). Although environmental contamination with volatile anaesthetics is a concern with the AnaConDa™ device, in practice the measured atmospheric concentrations are very low (82). There is therefore increasing interest in the use of these drugs in the NCCU (see below) (83).

Cerebral effects
Inhaled anaesthetics produce a dose-related suppression of cerebral electrical activity and cerebral metabolism leading to a secondary reduction in CBF because of preserved flow–metabolism coupling. However, all inhaled anaesthetics also have a dose-dependent direct cerebral vasodilator action that increases CBF, CBV and therefore ICP at higher doses (> 1 minimal alveolar concentration (MAC)). The net effect results from the balance between these two mechanisms, with a decrease in CBF at low inspired concentrations and an increase in CBF and CBV at higher concentrations.

Sevoflurane is the inhaled anaesthetic with the least vasodilator properties and, at concentrations below 1 MAC, has almost no effect on CBV and CBF. Although sevoflurane has not been shown to increase ICP, most studies have been performed in patients with preserved intracranial compensatory reserve, that is, normal brain compliance. In patients with decreased intracranial compliance, the effects of inhaled anaesthetics on ICP may be different and there is a risk that they may precipitate intracranial hypertension at higher doses. However, the inspired concentrations used for sedation in the ICU are typically lower than those used intraoperatively, so these effects are possibly less likely (84).

Inhaled anaesthetics also have a dose-dependent depressive effect on cerebral autoregulation. Low-dose isoflurane (0.5 MAC) delays but does not reduce the autoregulatory response, whereas higher concentrations (1.5 MAC) significantly impair cerebral autoregulation. Sevoflurane is generally reported to have minimal impact on cerebral autoregulation at concentrations less than 1.5 MAC, although some studies demonstrate a deterioration of dynamic autoregulation (85). Carbon dioxide reactivity is preserved with inhaled anaesthetics in the normal brain, and at clinically used concentrations (84).

All volatile anaesthetics suppress cerebral electrical activity and hence cerebral metabolism in a dose-related but non-linear manner. One MAC of sevoflurane reduces $CMRO_2$ by 47–74% and the cerebral metabolic rate for glucose by about 40%. Volatile agents also influence EEG activity in a dose-related manner, with agent-specific effects. Sevoflurane and isoflurane have similar EEG effects and MAC equivalent administration is associated with equipotent EEG suppression. With increasing concentrations the EEG evolves from a low-voltage, fast-wave to a high-voltage, slow-wave pattern, and finally to burst suppression. There are however concerns regarding epileptogenic effects of sevoflurane at higher concentrations (> 1.5 MAC) (86).

Comparative studies

There are limited data on the use of volatile anaesthetics in the NCCU. In a small group of patients suffering from ischaemic stroke and intracranial haemorrhage it was possible to maintain therapeutic sedation levels with isoflurane for an average of 3.5 days without clinically relevant increases in ICP in patients in whom baseline

Table 6.2 Advantages and disadvantages of commonly used sedatives and analgesics in the neurocritical care unit

	Advantages	**Disadvantages**
Propofol	Rapid onset and short duration of action Clearance independent of renal or hepatic function No significant drug interactions	No amnesia, especially at low doses No analgesic effect ↓ MAP, ↓ CPP (particularly in hypovolaemic patients) ↑ Triglycerides Propofol-infusion syndrome (↓ HR, ↑ pH, ↑ lactate, ↑ CK, myocardial failure)
Midazolam	Amnesia and analgesia Rapid onset of effect in acutely agitated patient Haemodynamic stability (may prevent CPP reductions)	Tolerance and tachyphylaxis Hepatic metabolism to active metabolite May accumulate in renal dysfunction May prolong the duration of MV May increase ICU delirium
Barbiturates	By ↓↓ CBF and CBV, barbiturates have a strong effect on ↓↓ ICP Indications of barbiturates are limited to the treatment of refractory ICP, titrated to the lowest effective dose. EEG may help with the titration of barbiturate therapy	Hypotension, ↓↓ MAP/CPP Immune suppression, ↑ risk of infections (pneumonia) Adrenal dysfunction
Morphine	Low cost In relay of long-term infusions of sedation/analgesia	Low predictability to control ICP Histamine release Accumulation with hepatic/renal impairment
Fentanyl and sufentanil	More potent opioids than morphine	Accumulation with hepatic impairment May prolong the duration of MV
Remifentanil	More potent opioid than morphine Rapid onset and short duration of action to permit neurological assessment Clearance independent of renal or hepatic function	Hyperalgesia at the cessation of drug infusion Limited effect to control ICP during painful procedures Tachyphylaxis High cost
Dexmedetomidine	Sedative, analgesic, and anxiolytic Short acting, no accumulation, patient may be frequently assessed neurologically Minimal respiratory depression May reduce incidence/severity of delirium	Limited clinical experience in the NCCU In non-neurointensive care population: Hypotension, bradycardia Arrhythmias including atrial fibrillation Hyperglycaemia May require high doses; deep sedation may not be possible High cost
Ketamine	Short acting, rapid onset of action Induces sedation, analgesia, and anaesthesia No respiratory depression Haemodynamic stability, preserves MAP May be used as an adjunct for refractory seizures No withdrawal symptoms	Hallucinations and emergence phenomena

CK, creatine kinase; CPP, cerebral perfusion pressure; HR, heart rate; ICP, intracranial pressure; MAP, mean arterial pressure; MV, mechanical ventilation.

ICP was low or only moderately elevated (87). However, a decrease in MAP and CPP was reported in this study. In a recent cross-over trial in 13 patients with aneurysmal subarachnoid haemorrhage, regional CBF was almost doubled (from about 20 to about 40 mL/100 g/min) with 0.8% isoflurane sedation compared to propofol, but there were no significant difference in ICP and CPP (88).

Whether volatile anaesthetics allow more rapid weaning from mechanical ventilation or faster awakening when compared to intravenous sedation is controversial (84,89), and most studies have investigated only short-term sedation. Furthermore, concerns regarding neurotoxicity advise caution for their use in the NCCU.

Side effects

All inhaled anaesthetics have similar depressive effects on the cardiovascular system. Cardiac index declines, systemic vascular resistance decreases, and heart rate increases in a dose-dependent manner. Sevoflurane is better at preserving myocardial function than propofol and, in patients without cardiovascular disease, is superior to propofol in preserving left ventricular relaxation and maintaining targeted CPP. Inhaled anaesthetics may trigger malignant hyperthermia.

Inhaled anaesthetics have both protective (90) and toxic effects (91) on the central nervous system mediated by different mechanisms that are dependent on exposure time and concentration. Almost all data on neurotoxicity are based on *in vitro* or animal models and it is often difficult to compare studies because of the different models, methods, and outcomes. There are no clinical data currently available that allow definitive conclusions to be drawn on the important topic of neurotoxicity.

Monitoring sedation

Sedatives may obscure or prevent neurological examination and can prolong the length of mechanical ventilation and ICU LOS. A recent review of sedation assessment tools in the NCCU concluded that the Sedation Analgesia Scale (SAS) and the Richmond Agitation Sedation Scale (RASS) are valid and useful (92–94).

Bispectral index monitoring

The bispectral index (BIS) was developed for monitoring the depth of general anaesthesia in patients without brain pathology. Intracranial pathology may influence the BIS algorithm because of EEG changes related to the pathology itself rather than to the sedative state so its role in sedation monitoring in the NCCU is not defined. In a randomized clinical trial of 67 patients, BIS in addition to subjective scale clinical assessment reduced the amount of propofol sedation and the time to awakening compared to routine clinical sedation monitoring alone (95). However, three other studies did not confirm these findings, demonstrating only a weak relationship between BIS and level of consciousness in general ICU patients (96–98). Given the available data, BIS monitoring cannot currently be recommended for monitoring depth of sedation in the NCCU. However, in critically ill brain-injured patients BIS may be a potential alternative to standard EEG for monitoring the induction and maintenance of burst suppression in patients treated with barbiturate coma for refractory intracranial hypertension (99,100).

Sedation holds

Studies conducted in the early 2000s demonstrated that daily interruption of sedation and awakening (sedation hold) reduces the

duration of mechanical ventilation and LOS in general ICU patients (1,101). These studies focused attention on the importance of strict sedation management in the ICU and led to the widespread introduction of protocolized sedation management strategies which have subsequently been shown to be more important in modulating outcome than sedation holds. In one study, the addition of daily sedation holds to a sedation protocol tool using validated sedation and analgesia scores did not provide additional benefits in terms of duration of mechanical ventilation or ICU LOS (102).

Daily sedation holds might be appropriate in NCCU patients to allow neurological assessment, as well as for their general benefits of reducing duration of mechanical ventilation and the need for tracheostomy. However, these potential benefits are counter-balanced by the deleterious effects of sedation holds on cerebral haemodynamics, particularly in the early stages after brain injury. Interruption of sedation has been associated with increases in ICP and reductions in CPP (103). While there was a large variability in the ICP response to sedation hold in this study, it rose to dangerous levels (> 40 mmHg) in some patients with concomitant reductions in CPP. ICP elevations were greatest

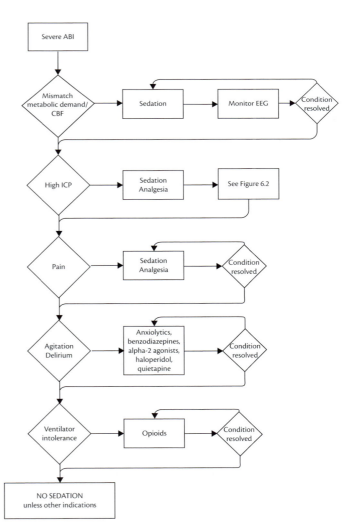

Fig. 6.1 Suggested algorithm for managing sedation in the neurocritical care unit. CBF, cerebral blood flow; EEG, electroencephalogram.
Reproduced with permission from G. Citerio.

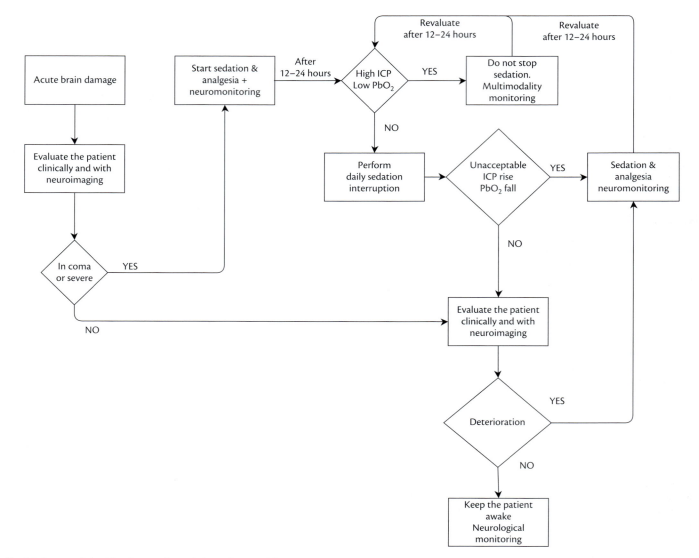

Fig. 6.2 Suggested algorithm for targeting sedation to intracranial pressure.
ICP, intracranial pressure; PbO₂, brain tissue oxygen tension.
Reproduced with permission from G. Citerio.

in the first few days after ABI, and sedation withdrawal after 4–5 days had modest ICP effects. Sedation holds are associated with increases in the level of several stress hormones such as cortisol and catecholamines (104). Helbok and colleagues showed that 34% of sedation interruption trials had to be aborted because of a significant increase in ICP and associated reduction in CPP, and 20% were associated with a significant decrease in brain tissue PO_2 below the critical thresholds of cerebral hypoxia (105). In addition, new neurological deficits were observed in a small minority of wake-up tests in this study.

Another important role of sedation after ABI is the prevention of shivering during targeted temperature management (106). In this setting, interruption of sedation must be postponed until normothermia is restored.

In conclusion, daily interruption and weaning of sedation should be considered in all patients on the NCCU but only when ICP and brain tissue PO_2 are no longer therapeutic targets, or when cerebral physiology has normalized. This is generally after 5–7 days.

A practical approach to sedation management

The application of a structured approach to sedation management, including the use of guidelines, protocols, and algorithms, reduces the likelihood of excessive and/or prolonged sedation. Many sedation protocols have been tested in clinical trials and are associated with shorter duration of mechanical ventilation, reduced ICU LOS, and superior sedation management compared to non-protocolized care (107). The advantages and disadvantages of different sedative agents are shown in Table 6.2. Practical algorithms for sedation and analgesia management in patients with ABI are illustrated in Figures 6.1 and 6.2.

The following is a recommended approach to sedation and analgesia management on the NCCU:

1. Critically ill brain-injured patients require sedation and analgesia in the acute phase.

2. When choosing a sedative it is preferable to use an agent with a short half-life, such as propofol, sufentanil/remifentanil, administered by continuous infusions, with the avoidance of bolus administration.

3. Sedation should be titrated to the desired effect (e.g. ICP control) using the lowest dose in order to avoid unwanted effects, particularly hypotension.

4. When cerebral physiology has stabilized, and there is no further risk of elevated ICP or reduction of CPP or brain tissue PO_2, daily sedation holds should be instituted and consideration given to reducing or stopping sedation.

References

1. Girard TD, Kress JP, Fuchs BD, Thomason JW, Schweickert WD, Pun BT, et al. Efficacy and safety of a paired sedation and ventilator weaning protocol for mechanically ventilated patients in intensive care (Awakening and Breathing Controlled trial): a randomised controlled trial. Lancet. 2008;371(9607):126–34.

2. Morandi A, Brummel NE, Ely EW. Sedation, delirium and mechanical ventilation: the 'ABCDE' approach. Curr Opin Crit Care. 2011;17(1):43–9.

3. McKeage K, Perry CM. Propofol: a review of its use in intensive care sedation of adults. CNS Drugs. 2003;17(4):235–72.

4. Brain Trauma Foundation, American Association of Neurological Surgeons, Congress of Neurological Surgeons, AANS/ CNS Joint Section on Neurotrauma and Critical Care, Bratton SL, Chestnut RM, et al. Guidelines for the management of severe traumatic brain injury. XI. Anesthetics, analgesics, and sedatives. J Neurotrauma. 2007;24 Suppl 1:S71–6.

5. Steiner LA, Johnston AJ, Chatfield DA, Czosnyka M, Coleman MR, Coles JP, et al. The effects of large-dose propofol on cerebrovascular pressure autoregulation in head-injured patients. Anesth Analg. 2003;97(2):572–6.

6. Hutchens MP, Memtsoudis S, Sadovnikoff N. Propofol for sedation in neuro-intensive care. Neurocrit Care. 2006;4(1):54–62.

7. Iyer VN, Hoel R, Rabinstein AA. Propofol infusion syndrome in patients with refractory status epilepticus: an 11-year clinical experience. Crit Care Med. 2009;37(12):3024–30.

8. Kang TM. Propofol infusion syndrome in critically ill patients. Ann Pharmacother. 2002;36(9):1453–6.

9. Wolf A, Weir P, Segar P, Stone J, Shield J. Impaired fatty acid oxidation in propofol infusion syndrome. Lancet. 2001;357(9256):606–7.

10. Steiner LA, Studer W, Baumgartner ER, Frei FJ. Perioperative management of a child with very-long-chain acyl-coenzyme A dehydrogenase deficiency. Paediatr Anaesth. 2002;12(2):187–91.

11. Sandiumenge Camps A, Sanchez-Izquierdo Riera JA, Toral Vazquez D, Sa Borges M, Peinado Rodriguez J, Alted Lopez E. Midazolam and 2% propofol in long-term sedation of traumatized critically ill patients: efficacy and safety comparison. Crit Care Med. 2000;28(11):3612–19.

12. Mayo-Smith MF, Beecher LH, Fischer TL, Gorelick DA, Guillaume JL, Hill A, et al. Management of alcohol withdrawal delirium. An evidence-based practice guideline. Arch Intern Med. 2004;164(13):1405–12.

13. Cheng MA, Hoffman WE, Baughman VL, Albrecht RF. The effects of midazolam and sufentanil sedation on middle cerebral artery blood flow velocity in awake patients. J Neurosurg Anesthesiol. 1993;5(4):232–6.

14. Leone M, Visintini P, Alliez JR, Albanese J. [What sedation for prevention and treatment secondary brain insult?]. Ann Fr Anesth Reanim. 2006;25(8):852–7.

15. Ghori KA, Harmon DC, Elashaal A, Butler M, Walsh F, O'Sullivan MG, et al. Effect of midazolam versus propofol sedation on markers of neurological injury and outcome after isolated severe head injury: a pilot study. Crit Care Resusc. 2007;9(2):166–71.

16. Sanchez-Izquierdo-Riera JA, Caballero-Cubedo RE, Perez-Vela JL, Ambros-Checa A, Cantalapiedra-Santiago JA, Alted-Lopez E. Propofol versus midazolam: safety and efficacy for sedating the severe trauma patient. Anesth Analg. 1998;86(6):1219–24.

17. Pohlman AS, Simpson KP, Hall JB. Continuous intravenous infusions of lorazepam versus midazolam for sedation during mechanical ventilatory support: a prospective, randomized study. Crit Care Med. 1994;22(8):1241–7.

18. Swart EL, Zuideveld KP, de Jongh J, Danhof M, Thijs LG, Strack van Schijndel RM. Comparative population pharmacokinetics of lorazepam and midazolam during long-term continuous infusion in critically ill patients. Br J Clin Pharmacol. 2004;57(2):135–45.

19. Pandharipande P, Shintani A, Peterson J, Pun BT, Wilkinson GR, Dittus RS, et al. Lorazepam is an independent risk factor for transitioning to delirium in intensive care unit patients. Anesthesiology. 2006;104(1):21–6.

20. Payen JF, Bosson JL, Chanques G, Mantz J, Labarere J, DOLOREA Investigators. Pain assessment is associated with decreased duration of mechanical ventilation in the intensive care unit: a post Hoc analysis of the DOLOREA study. Anesthesiology. 2009;111(6):1308–16.

21. Wilhelm W, Kreuer S. The place for short-acting opioids: special emphasis on remifentanil. Crit Care. 2008;12 Suppl 3:S5.

22. Baillard C, Cohen Y, Le Toumelin P, Karoubi P, Hoang P, Ait Kaci F, et al. [Remifentanil-midazolam compared to sufentanil-midazolam for ICU long-term sedation]. Ann Fr Anesth Reanim. 2005;24(5):480–6.

23. Albanese J, Viviand X, Potie F, Rey M, Alliez B, Martin C. Sufentanil, fentanyl, and alfentanil in head trauma patients: a study on cerebral hemodynamics. Crit Care Med. 1999;27(2):407–11.

24. Sperry RJ, Bailey PL, Reichman MV, Peterson JC, Petersen PB, Pace NL. Fentanyl and sufentanil increase intracranial pressure in head trauma patients. Anesthesiology. 1992;77(3):416–20.

25. Urwin SC, Menon DK. Comparative tolerability of sedative agents in head-injured adults. Drug Safe. 2004;27(2):107–33.

26. Werner C, Kochs E, Bause H, Hoffman WE, Schulte am Esch J. Effects of sufentanil on cerebral hemodynamics and intracranial pressure in patients with brain injury. Anesthesiology. 1995;83(4):721–6.

27. de Nadal M, Munar F, Poca MA, Sahuquillo J, Garnacho A, Rossello J. Cerebral hemodynamic effects of morphine and fentanyl in patients with severe head injury: absence of correlation to cerebral autoregulation. Anesthesiology. 2000;92(1):11–19.

28. Kofke WA, Tempelhoff R, Dasheiff RM. Anesthetic implications of epilepsy, status epilepticus, and epilepsy surgery. J Neurosurg Anesthesiol. 1997;9(4):349–72.

29. Kelly DF, Goodale DB, Williams J, Herr DL, Chappell ET, Rosner MJ, et al. Propofol in the treatment of moderate and severe head injury: a randomized, prospective double-blinded pilot trial. J Neurosurg. 1999;90(6):1042–52.

30. Kawaguchi M, Furuya H, Patel PM. Neuroprotective effects of anesthetic agents. J Anesth. 2005;19(2):150–6.

31. Eisenberg HM, Frankowski RF, Contant CF, Marshall LF, Walker MD. High-dose barbiturate control of elevated intracranial pressure in patients with severe head injury. J Neurosurg. 1988;69(1):15–23.

32. Schreckinger M, Marion DW. Contemporary management of traumatic intracranial hypertension: is there a role for therapeutic hypothermia? Neurocrit Care. 2009;11(3):427–36.

33. Perez-Barcena J, Llompart-Pou JA, Homar J, Abadal JM, Raurich JM, Frontera G, et al. Pentobarbital versus thiopental in the treatment of refractory intracranial hypertension in patients with traumatic brain injury: a randomized controlled trial. Crit Care. 2008;12(4):R112.

34. Huynh F, Mabasa VH, Ensom MH. A critical review: does thiopental continuous infusion warrant therapeutic drug monitoring in the critical care population? Therapeutic drug monitoring. 2009;31(2):153–69.

35. Ramesh VJ, Umamaheswara Rao GS. Quantification of burst suppression and bispectral index with 2 different bolus doses of thiopentone sodium. J Neurosurg Anesthesiol. 2007;19(3):179–82.

36. Winer JW, Rosenwasser RH, Jimenez F. Electroencephalographic activity and serum and cerebrospinal fluid pentobarbital levels in determining the therapeutic end point during barbiturate coma. *Neurosurgery.* 1991;29(5):739–41.

37. Roberts I. Barbiturates for acute traumatic brain injury. *Cochrane Database Syst Rev.* 2000;2:CD000033.

38. Llompart-Pou JA, Perez-Barcena J, Raurich JM, Burguera B, Ayestaran JI, Abadal JM, et al. Effect of barbiturate coma on adrenal response in patients with traumatic brain injury. *J Endocrinol Invest.* 2007;30(5):393–8.

39. Schwartz ML, Tator CH, Rowed DW, Reid SR, Meguro K, Andrews DF. The University of Toronto head injury treatment study: a prospective, randomized comparison of pentobarbital and mannitol. *Can J Neurol Sci.* 1984;11(4):434–40.

40. Zornow MH, Scheller MS, Sheehan PB, Strnat MA, Matsumoto M. Intracranial pressure effects of dexmedetomidine in rabbits. *Anesth Analg.* 1992;75(2):232–7.

41. Talke P, Tong C, Lee HW, Caldwell J, Eisenach JC, Richardson CA. Effect of dexmedetomidine on lumbar cerebrospinal fluid pressure in humans. *Anesth Analg.* 1997;85(2):358–64.

42. Prielipp RC, Wall MH, Tobin JR, Groban L, Cannon MA, Fahey FH, et al. Dexmedetomidine-induced sedation in volunteers decreases regional and global cerebral blood flow. *Anesth Analg.* 2002;95(4):1052–9.

43. Drummond JC, Dao AV, Roth DM, Cheng CR, Atwater BI, Minokadeh A, et al. Effect of dexmedetomidine on cerebral blood flow velocity, cerebral metabolic rate, and carbon dioxide response in normal humans. *Anesthesiology.* 2008;108(2):225–32.

44. Ogawa Y, Iwasaki K, Aoki K, Kojima W, Kato J, Ogawa S. Dexmedetomidine weakens dynamic cerebral autoregulation as assessed by transfer function analysis and the thigh cuff method. *Anesthesiology.* 2008;109(4):642–50.

45. Drummond JC, Sturaitis MK. Brain tissue oxygenation during dexmedetomidine administration in surgical patients with neurovascular injuries. *J Neurosurg Anesthesiol.* 2010;22(4):336–41.

46. Talke P, Stapelfeldt C, Garcia P. Dexmedetomidine does not reduce epileptiform discharges in adults with epilepsy. *J Neurosurg Anesthesiol.* 2007;19(3):195–9.

47. Bala E, Sessler DI, Nair DR, McLain R, Dalton JE, Farag E. Motor and somatosensory evoked potentials are well maintained in patients given dexmedetomidine during spine surgery. *Anesthesiology.* 2008;109(3):417–25.

48. James ML, Olson DM, Graffagnino C. A pilot study of cerebral and haemodynamic physiological changes during sedation with dexmedetomidine or propofol in patients with acute brain injury. *Anaesth Intensive Care.* 2012;40(6):949–57.

49. Tan JA, Ho KM. Use of dexmedetomidine as a sedative and analgesic agent in critically ill adult patients: a meta-analysis. *Intensive Care Med.* 2010;36(6):926–39.

50. Goodwin HE, Gill RS, Murakami PN, Thompson CB, Lewin JJ, 3rd, Mirski MA. Dexmedetomidine preserves attention/calculation when used for cooperative and short-term intensive care unit sedation. *J Crit Care.* 2013;28(6):1113 e7–e10.

51. Carollo DS, Nossaman BD, Ramadhyani U. Dexmedetomidine: a review of clinical applications. *Curr Opin Anaesthesiol.* 2008;21(4):457–61.

52. Reade MC, O'Sullivan K, Bates S, Goldsmith D, Ainslie WR, Bellomo R. Dexmedetomidine vs. haloperidol in delirious, agitated, intubated patients: a randomised open-label trial. *Crit Care.* 2009;13(3):R75.

53. Devabhakthuni S, Pajoumand M, Williams C, Kufera JA, Watson K, Stein DM. Evaluation of dexmedetomidine: safety and clinical outcomes in critically ill trauma patients. *J Trauma.* 2011;71(5):1164–71.

54. Dearden NM, McDowall DG. Comparison of etomidate and althesin in the reduction of increased intracranial pressure after head injury. *Br J Anaesth.* 1985;57(4):361–8.

55. Prior JG, Hinds CJ, Williams J, Prior PF. The use of etomidate in the management of severe head injury. *Intensive Care Med.* 1983;9(6):313–20.

56. Asehnoune K, Mahe PJ, Seguin P, Jaber S, Jung B, Guitton C, et al. Etomidate increases susceptibility to pneumonia in trauma patients. *Intensive Care Med.* 2012;38(10):1673–82.

57. Chan CM, Mitchell AL, Shorr AF. Etomidate is associated with mortality and adrenal insufficiency in sepsis: a meta-analysis. *Crit Care Med.* 2012;40(11):2945–53.

58. Hildreth AN, Mejia VA, Maxwell RA, Smith PW, Dart BW, Barker DE. Adrenal suppression following a single dose of etomidate for rapid sequence induction: a prospective randomized study. *J Trauma.* 2008;65(3):573–9.

59. Cherfan AJ, Arabi YM, Al-Dorzi HM, Kenny LP. Advantages and disadvantages of etomidate use for intubation of patients with sepsis. *Pharmacotherapy.* 2012;32(5):475–82.

60. Jacobi J, Fraser GL, Coursin DB, Riker RR, Fontaine D, Wittbrodt ET, et al. Clinical practice guidelines for the sustained use of sedatives and analgesics in the critically ill adult. *Crit Care Med.* 2002;30(1):119–41.

61. Devlin JW, Skrobik Y, Riker RR, Hinderleider E, Roberts RJ, Fong JJ, et al. Impact of quetiapine on resolution of individual delirium symptoms in critically ill patients with delirium: a post-hoc analysis of a double-blind, randomized, placebo-controlled study. *Crit Care.* 2011;15(5):R215.

62. Hakim SM, Othman AI, Naoum DO. Early treatment with risperidone for subsyndromal delirium after on-pump cardiac surgery in the elderly: a randomized trial. *Anesthesiology.* 2012;116(5):987–97.

63. Skrobik YK, Bergeron N, Dumont M, Gottfried SB. Olanzapine vs haloperidol: treating delirium in a critical care setting. *Intensive Care Med.* 2004;30(3):444–9.

64. Food and Drug Administration. *Atypical Antipsychotic Drugs.* Washington, DC: Food and Drug Administration; 2005.

65. Lee SM, Chou YH, Li MH, Wan FJ, Yen MH. Effects of haloperidol and risperidone on cerebrohemodynamics in drug-naive schizophrenic patients. *J Psychiatr Res.* 2008;42(4):328–35.

66. Miller DD, Andreasen NC, O'Leary DS, Watkins GL, Boles Ponto LL, Hichwa RD. Comparison of the effects of risperidone and haloperidol on regional cerebral blood flow in schizophrenia. *Biol Psychiatry.* 2001;49(8):704–15.

67. Seitz DP, Gill SS, van Zyl LT. Antipsychotics in the treatment of delirium: a systematic review. *J Clin Psychiatry.* 2007;68(1):11–21.

68. van Eijk MM, Roes KC, Honing ML, Kuiper MA, Karakus A, van der Jagt M, et al. Effect of rivastigmine as an adjunct to usual care with haloperidol on duration of delirium and mortality in critically ill patients: a multicentre, double-blind, placebo-controlled randomised trial. *Lancet.* 2010;376(9755):1829–37.

69. Markowitz JS, DeVane CL, Boulton DW, Liston HL, Risch SC. Hypotension and bradycardia in a healthy volunteer following a single 5 mg dose of olanzapine. *J Clin Pharmacol.* 2002;42(1):104–6.

70. Kuzuhara S. Drug-induced psychotic symptoms in Parkinson's disease. Problems, management and dilemma. *J Neurol.* 2001;248 Suppl 3:III28–31.

71. Gortney JS, Fagan A, Kissack JC. Neuroleptic malignant syndrome secondary to quetiapine. *Ann Pharmacother.* 2009;43(4):785–91.

72. Ostermann ME, Keenan SP, Seiferling RA, Sibbald WJ. Sedation in the intensive care unit: a systematic review. *JAMA.* 2000;283(11):1451–9.

73. Huey-Ling L, Chun-Che S, Jen-Jen T, Shau-Ting L, Hsing IC. Comparison of the effect of protocol-directed sedation with propofol vs. midazolam by nurses in intensive care: efficacy, haemodynamic stability and patient satisfaction. *J Clin Nurs.* 2008;17(11):1510–17.

74. Roberts DJ, Hall RI, Kramer AH, Robertson HL, Gallagher CN, Zygun DA. Sedation for critically ill adults with severe traumatic brain injury: a systematic review of randomized controlled trials. *Crit Care Med.* 2011;39(12):2743–51.

75. Farling PA, Johnston JR, Coppel DL. Propofol infusion for sedation of patients with head injury in intensive care. A preliminary report. *Anaesthesia.* 1989;44(3):222–6.

76. Karabinis A, Mandragos K, Stergiopoulos S, Komnos A, Soukup J, Speelberg B, et al. Safety and efficacy of analgesia-based sedation with remifentanil versus standard hypnotic-based regimens in intensive

care unit patients with brain injuries: a randomised, controlled trial [ISRCTN50308308]. *Crit Care.* 2004;8(4):R268–80.

77. Bauer C, Kreuer S, Ketter R, Grundmann U, Wilhelm W. [Remifentanil-propofol versus fentanyl-midazolam combinations for intracranial surgery: influence of anaesthesia technique and intensive sedation on ventilation times and duration of stay in the ICU]. *Der Anaesthesist.* 2007;56(2):128–32.

78. Bourgoin A, Albanese J, Leone M, Sampol-Manos E, Viviand X, Martin C. Effects of sufentanil or ketamine administered in target-controlled infusion on the cerebral hemodynamics of severely brain-injured patients. *Crit Care Med.* 2005;33(5):1109–13.

79. Bourgoin A, Albanese J, Wereszczynski N, Charbit M, Vialet R, Martin C. Safety of sedation with ketamine in severe head injury patients: comparison with sufentanil. *Crit Care Med.* 2003;31(3):711–17.

80. Rossetti AO, Lowenstein DH. Management of refractory status epilepticus in adults: still more questions than answers. *Lancet Neurol.* 2011;10(10):922–30.

81. Meiser A, Laubenthal H. Inhalational anaesthetics in the ICU: theory and practice of inhalational sedation in the ICU, economics, risk-benefit. *Best Pract Res Clin Anaesthesiol.* 2005;19(3):523–38.

82. Pickworth T, Jerath A, Devine R, Kherani N, Wasowicz M. The scavenging of volatile anesthetic agents in the cardiovascular intensive care unit environment: a technical report. *Can J Anaesth.* 60(1):38–43.

83. Villa F, Citerio G. Surpassing boundaries: volatile sedation in the NeuroICU. *Intensive Care Med.* 2012;38(12):1914–16.

84. Soukup J, Scharff K, Kubosch K, Pohl C, Bomplitz M, Kompardt J. State of the art: sedation concepts with volatile anesthetics in critically Ill patients. *J Crit Care.* 2009;24(4):535–44.

85. Ogawa Y, Iwasaki K, Shibata S, Kato J, Ogawa S, Oi Y. The effect of sevoflurane on dynamic cerebral blood flow autoregulation assessed by spectral and transfer function analysis. *Anesth Analg.* 2006;102(2):552–9.

86. Jaaskelainen SK, Kaisti K, Suni L, Hinkka S, Scheinin H. Sevoflurane is epileptogenic in healthy subjects at surgical levels of anesthesia. *Neurology.* 2003;61(8):1073–8.

87. Bosel J, Purrucker JC, Nowak F, Renzland J, Schiller P, Perez EB, *et al.* Volatile isoflurane sedation in cerebrovascular intensive care patients using AnaConDa((R)): effects on cerebral oxygenation, circulation, and pressure. *Intensive Care Med.* 2012;38(12):1955–64.

88. Villa F, Iacca C, Molinari AF, Giussani C, Aletti G, Pesenti A, *et al.* Inhalation versus endovenous sedation in subarachnoid hemorrhage patients: effects on regional cerebral blood flow. *Crit Care Med.* 2012;40(10):2797–804.

89. Migliari M, Bellani G, Rona R, Isgro S, Vergnano B, Mauri T, *et al.* Short-term evaluation of sedation with sevoflurane administered by the anesthetic conserving device in critically ill patients. *Intensive Care Med.* 2009;35(7):1240–6.

90. Head BP, Patel P. Anesthetics and brain protection. *Curr Opin Anaesthesiol.* 2007;20(5):395–9.

91. Perouansky M, Hemmings HC, Jr. Neurotoxicity of general anesthetics: cause for concern? *Anesthesiology.* 2009;111(6):1365–71.

92. Riker RR, Picard JT, Fraser GL. Prospective evaluation of the Sedation-Agitation Scale for adult critically ill patients. *Crit Care Med.* 1999;27(7):1325–9.

93. Sessler CN, Gosnell MS, Grap MJ, Brophy GM, O'Neal PV, Keane KA, *et al.* The Richmond Agitation-Sedation Scale: validity and reliability in adult intensive care unit patients. *Am J Resp Crit Care Med.* 2002;166(10):1338–44.

94. Teitelbaum JS, Ayoub O, Skrobik Y. A critical appraisal of sedation, analgesia and delirium in neurocritical care. *Can J Neurol Sci.* 2011;38(6):815–25.

95. Olson DM, Thoyre SM, Peterson ED, Graffagnino C. A randomized evaluation of bispectral index-augmented sedation assessment in neurological patients. *Neurocrit Care.* 2009;11(1):20–7.

96. De Deyne C, Struys M, Decruyenaere J, Creupelandt J, Hoste E, Colardyn F. Use of continuous bispectral EEG monitoring to assess depth of sedation in ICU patients. *Intensive Care Med.* 1998;24(12):1294–8.

97. Frenzel D, Greim CA, Sommer C, Bauerle K, Roewer N. Is the bispectral index appropriate for monitoring the sedation level of mechanically ventilated surgical ICU patients? *Intensive Care Med.* 2002;28(2):178–83.

98. Nasraway SS, Jr., Wu EC, Kelleher RM, Yasuda CM, Donnelly AM. How reliable is the bispectral index in critically ill patients? A prospective, comparative, single-blinded observer study. *Crit Care Med.* 2002;30(7):1483–7.

99. Jaggi P, Schwabe MJ, Gill K, Horowitz IN. Use of an anesthesia cerebral monitor bispectral index to assess burst-suppression in pentobarbital coma. *Pediatr Neurol.* 2003;28(3):219–22.

100. Riker RR, Fraser GL, Wilkins ML. Comparing the bispectral index and suppression ratio with burst suppression of the electroencephalogram during pentobarbital infusions in adult intensive care patients. *Pharmacotherapy.* 2003;23(9):1087–93.

101. Kress JP, Pohlman AS, O'Connor MF, Hall JB. Daily interruption of sedative infusions in critically ill patients undergoing mechanical ventilation. *N Engl J Med.* 2000;342(20):1471–7.

102. Mehta S, Burry L, Cook D, Fergusson D, Steinberg M, Granton J, *et al.* Daily sedation interruption in mechanically ventilated critically ill patients cared for with a sedation protocol: a randomized controlled trial. *JAMA.* 2012;308(19):1985–92.

103. Skoglund K, Enblad P, Marklund N. Effects of the neurological wake-up test on intracranial pressure and cerebral perfusion pressure in brain-injured patients. *Neurocrit Care.* 2009;11(2):135–42.

104. Skoglund K, Enblad P, Hillered L, Marklund N. The neurological wake-up test increases stress hormone levels in patients with severe traumatic brain injury. *Crit Care Med.* 2012;40(1):216–22.

105. Helbok R, Kurtz P, Schmidt MJ, Stuart MR, Fernandez L, Connolly SE, *et al.* Effects of the neurological wake-up test on clinical examination, intracranial pressure, brain metabolism and brain tissue oxygenation in severely brain-injured patients. *Crit Care.* 2012;16(6):R226.

106. Oddo M, Frangos S, Maloney-Wilensky E, Andrew Kofke W, Le Roux PD, Levine JM. Effect of shivering on brain tissue oxygenation during induced normothermia in patients with severe brain injury. *Neurocrit Care.* 2010;12(1):10–16.

107. Sessler CN, Pedram S. Protocolized and target-based sedation and analgesia in the ICU. *Crit Care Clin.* 2009;25(3):489–513.

CHAPTER 7

Intracranial hypertension

Andrea Lavinio

Raised intracranial pressure (ICP), or intracranial hypertension, may occur as the consequence of numerous conditions including traumatic brain injury (TBI), subarachnoid haemorrhage (SAH), intracerebral haemorrhage (ICH), brain tumours, and hydrocephalus. Elevated ICP can precipitate cerebral hypoperfusion and herniation, resulting in secondary brain injury and death. This chapter will review the underlying pathophysiology of intracranial hypertension and outline a rational approach to its treatment.

Pathophysiology

ICP is the pressure inside the skull and thus in the brain tissue, and is synonymous with the cerebrospinal fluid (CSF) pressure in the lateral ventricles. Normal ICP varies with age and body position. In healthy, resting supine adults, normal mean ICP is lower than 10 mmHg (1).

In the presence of intracranial space-occupying lesions or cerebral oedema, a finite amount of CSF and venous blood can be displaced from the intracranial compartment into the extracranial subarachnoid space to maintain a constant ICP. When this compensatory reserve becomes exhausted, further volume increments in one of the intracranial contents lead to intracranial hypertension. The relationship between the relative volumes of the intracranial constituents and ICP is described by the Monro–Kellie doctrine and this is discussed in detail in Chapter 9. The pathophysiology of intracranial hypertension is summarized in Table 7.1.

The largest body of clinical evidence relating to ICP and its management comes from severe TBI. ICP in excess of 20–25 mmHg is associated with poor functional outcome and death after TBI in a time-dependent fashion (2). For this reason, ICP thresholds of 20 and 25 mmHg have pragmatically been adopted to define intracranial hypertension in adults, and to trigger the administration of ICP-lowering therapies. Thresholds vary in the paediatric population in which it is recommended that treatment should be initiated when ICP exceeds 15 mmHg in infants, 18 mmHg in children up to 8 year of age, and 20 mm Hg in older children and teenagers (3).

Following severe TBI, intracranial hypertension can develop immediately or over a period of hours and days. Although the majority of patients suffer maximum ICP elevation in the first 3 days post injury, around one-quarter develop profound intracranial hypertension after the fifth day (4). Aside from large haemorrhagic contusions and haematomas amenable to surgical evacuation, the main cause of sustained intracranial hypertension after severe TBI is cytotoxic brain oedema, that is, intracellular fluid accumulation (mostly into astrocytes) because of the failure of ion pumps and osmotic disturbances. This is followed by a period of vasogenic brain oedema related to disruption of the blood–brain barrier (BBB)

and extracellular fluid extravasation (5). Thrombosis of the cerebral venous sinuses is a relatively rare but potentially treatable cause of delayed intracranial hypertension following severe TBI (6).

The contribution of intracranial hypertension to secondary brain injury and poor functional outcome is not restricted to TBI. Large ICH compounded by perihematomal oedema (7,8) is also associated with intracranial hypertensive crises requiring ICP-lowering treatments and consideration of surgical decompression. The rupture of a cerebral arterial aneurysm into the subarachnoid space during SAH results in a hyperacute increase in ICP to values close to that of mean arterial blood pressure (MAP) leading to global cerebral ischaemia and, in severe cases, transitory cerebral circulatory arrest (9). This can result in significant irreversible neurological damage and is frequently accompanied by a transitory Cushing response with associated neurogenic cardiomyopathy and pulmonary oedema (see Chapter 27) (10). Intraventricular blood can lead to acute obstructive hydrocephalus and increased ICP requiring immediate ventricular drainage (11).

The general pathophysiology and treatment of intracranial hypertension is best considered by differentiating the effects of elevated ICP on cerebral haemodynamics from the mechanical effects on brain parenchyma, that is, between intracranial hypertension-related cerebral hypoperfusion and herniation. The disease-specific aspects of intracranial hypertension are discussed in the relevant chapters elsewhere in this book.

Intracranial hypertension as a cause of cerebral hypoperfusion

Bridging veins in the subdural and subarachnoid spaces drain venous blood from the cerebral cortex into venous sinuses. When ICP exceeds venous pressure, these bridging veins collapse thereby reducing cerebral venous outflow and hence cerebral perfusion. Abnormally elevated ICP can therefore result in inadequate cerebral perfusion even in the presence of normal systemic blood pressure. Cerebral circulatory arrest occurs when ICP approaches MAP and cerebral perfusion pressure (CPP) approaches zero.

Intracranial hypertension as a cause of cerebral herniation

Elevated ICP can also cause death and disability because of the development of pressure gradients across dural folds or the foramen magnum. When space-occupying lesions or brain oedema obliterate the subarachnoid space and impede free circulation of CSF, intracranial hypertension and the development of intracranial or craniospinal pressure gradients may lead to herniation of the brain across the falx cerebri (subfalcine herniation), the

Table 7.1 The pathophysiology of intracranial hypertension. The incompressible contents of the cranial cavity—brain, blood, and cerebrospinal fluid (CSF)—are bounded by a rigid skull with a fixed capacity. Unless the volume of one of the other constituents is displaced out of the cranium, an increase in volume of CSF, cerebral blood volume or brain parenchyma, or the presence of a space-occupying lesion will result in raised intracranial pressure. This table provides an overview of its pathogenesis of intracranial hypertension. The classification is arbitrary and artificial as, in many instances, different mechanisms coexist and contribute synchronously or in a sequential manner to the development of intracranial hypertension. For example, vasogenic and cytotoxic oedema coexist in traumatic brain injury and ischaemic stroke, and obstructive hydrocephalus complicates subarachnoid haemorrhage

Pathogenesis	Subtype	Mechanism	Examples
CSF dynamics	Obstructive hydrocephalus	Impaired CSF outflow	Aqueduct stenosis (congenital or acquired) Intraventricular haemorrhage
	Communicating hydrocephalus	Impaired CSF absorption at the arachnoid granulation	Post-traumatic hydrocephalus Post-infective hydrocephalus
	Excess CSF production	Tumours of the choroid plexus	Ependymoma
Cerebral oedema	Cytotoxic oedema	Cellular swelling due to ischaemic energy depletion and rise in intracellular Na^+ and water	Ischaemic stroke Hypoxia Trauma Acute liver failure
	Vasogenic oedema	Expansion of the extracellular compartment due to increased permeability of the blood–brain barrier	Malignancy High-altitude cerebral oedema Inflammatory/infective malignant hypertension
	Osmotic oedema	Rapid reduction in plasma osmolarity resulting in a reversal of the brain–plasma water gradient	Dialysis disequilibrium syndrome Acute hyponatraemia (SIADH)
	Interstitial oedema	Increased CSF pressure results in permeation of CSF in the adjacent brain	Obstructive hydrocephalus with periventricular 'lucency'
Cerebrovascular	Subarachnoid haemorrhage	Hyperacute increase in CSF pressure due to free communication between arterial blood and subarachnoid space	Ruptured cerebral aneurysm
	Cerebral venous sinus thrombosis	Impaired cerebral venous outflow	Thrombophilia Meningitis Homocystinuria
	Cerebral venous sinus stenosis	Impaired cerebral venous outflow	Idiopathic intracranial hypertension
	Increased central venous pressure	Impaired cerebral venous outflow	Superior vena cava syndrome Jugular vein thrombosis
Space-occupying lesions	Haematomas (extradural, subdural, intraparenchymal)		
	Tumours		
	Abscess		
	Foreign bodies		

tentorium cerebelli (ascending and descending transtentorial herniation), and foramen magnum (tonsillar herniation) as shown in Figure 7.1. Herniation syndromes result in catastrophic focal necrosis from direct mechanical injury and vascular compression, and lead to potentially lethal ischaemic brain damage, including brain death (12).

Principles of treatment

ICP-lowering treatments are aimed at maintaining adequate cerebral perfusion and preventing cerebral herniation. Mortality is dramatically increased in severely brain-injured patients that do not respond to ICP-reducing therapy. The odds ratio for death in ICP unresponsive patients is 114 (95% confidence interval 40.5–322.3) compared to those in whom ICP is responsive (13).

While ICP control is a cornerstone of neurocritical care, it is important to note that treatment itself is not devoid of potentially serious adverse effects and that ICP greater than 25 mmHg doesn't (in isolation) always warrant treatment (14). The decision to initiate ICP lowering therapy should be determined for each patient individually after consideration of three factors:

1. The pathophysiological burden of the intracranial hypertension, that is, its duration, magnitude, and clinical context.

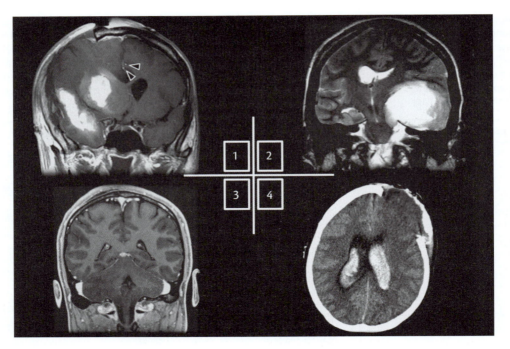

Fig. 7.1 Cranial imaging showing brain herniation states
1. *Subfalcine (cingulate) herniation*—is the most common herniation state. Compression of the pericallosal arteries (arrowheads) may result in infarction of the distal anterior cerebral artery territory.
2. *Transtentorial (uncal) herniation*—the temporal lobe herniates downwardly across the tentorium cerebelli, compressing the midbrain and pons (leading to Duret's haemorrhage), the III cranial nerve (causing ipsilateral fixed mydriasis), the posterior cerebral artery causing (ipsilateral occipital and thalamic infarction), and the aqueduct (causing obstructive hydrocephalus).
3. *Transforaminal (tonsillar) herniation*—herniation of the cerebellar tonsils through the foramen magnum compresses the medulla oblongata (causing respiratory arrest and haemodynamic instability) and the posterior inferior cerebellar arteries (causing brainstem and upper cervical spinal cord infarction).
4. *Transcalvarial herniation*—herniation through a craniectomy defect may lead to compression of cortical vessels and result in ischaemic necrosis of the portion of the herniated brain.

2. The risk–benefit ratio of potential treatment options.

3. The reliability of the ICP monitoring device, that is, exclusion of artefactual elevations of ICP.

Pathophysiological burden of intracranial hypertension

The pathophysiological burden of intracranial hypertension is context sensitive, and ICP elevations that require aggressive treatment in the acute phase after TBI may be tolerated when physiological compensatory mechanisms are preserved. Clinical experience acquired during CSF infusion studies in patients with hydrocephalus provides an illuminating example. In such diagnostic studies an isotonic solution is infused at a constant rate into the cerebral ventricles or lumbar subarachnoid space of awake, self-ventilating patients. CSF pressure is continuously monitored and an estimate of CSF dynamics obtained by analysis of the CSF pressure waveforms. During the infusion ICP can exceed 40 mmHg for several minutes with negligible effects on cerebral blood flow (CBF) and no neurological symptoms (15). These very same levels of ICP are strongly associated with death and disability following severe TBI. The explanation for this differential response lies in the presence (in the case of hydrocephalic patients undergoing infusion studies) or absence (in the case of severe TBI) of two key compensatory mechanisms—free circulation of CSF and cerebral pressure autoregulation (16). Circulation of CSF between intracranial and

spinal subarachnoid spaces neutralizes regional pressure gradients and nullifies the risk of cerebral herniation irrespective of absolute ICP. At the same time, pressure-flow autoregulation maintains CBF over a wide range of CPP. It would therefore seem reasonable to assume that TBI patients with open basal cisterns and preserved pressure autoregulation may tolerate ICP exceeding the 20–25 mmHg thresholds without negative consequences. This is clinically relevant during short-lived ICP spikes caused by coughing and desynchronization from mechanical ventilation during sedation holds in the subacute phase after severe TBI. In this case, the ICP spikes are probably similar to those experienced by healthy subjects during a Valsalva manoeuvre (17). Thus, in the presence of radiological appearances suggestive of preserved intracranial volume-buffering reserve (i.e. open basal cisterns, normal appearances of ventricles, and cortical sulci), short-lived episodes of ICP exceeding the 25 mmHg threshold should not necessarily prompt immediate ICP-lowering treatment. In this situation, re-establishing sedation is likely to result in unnecessarily prolonged duration of sedation and mechanical ventilation whilst providing no benefit to the injured brain. At the opposite end of the spectrum are patients with large space-occupying lesions or severe cerebral oedema resulting in compressed cortical sulci and basal cisterns, and midline shift. These radiological features suggest that CSF pathways are obliterated and that there is a high risk for the development of intracranial pressure gradients and cerebral herniation. In this context, intracranial hypertension can be rapidly fatal and ICP should be aggressively controlled. Further, ICP-lowering treatments should only be de-escalated after careful review of clinical status and other brain monitoring variables in patients with radiological evidence of exhausted intracranial volume-buffering reserve. Normal ICP values in the presence of radiological evidence of impending cerebral herniation may be falsely reassuring and should always prompt review for ICP probe malfunction.

Reliability of ICP monitoring techniques

Commercially available ICP monitors are robust and provide reliable clinical data, although they are not completely immune to measurement bias. The possibility of over-estimation of ICP should always be considered before applying ICP-lowering treatments with potentially significant side effects, and ICP probe malfunction should be excluded in patients with persistently elevated measured ICP and normal brain radiographic appearances. The reliability of ICP monitoring technologies is discussed in detail in Chapter 9.

Treatment

ICP-lowering strategies have distinct risk–benefit profiles, ranging from relatively safe to extremely dangerous. Relatively safe measures include head-up positioning, sedation, seizure management, and controlled normothermia, whereas hyperventilation, barbiturate-induced burst suppression, therapeutic hypothermia, and surgical decompression are associated with significant complications.

ICP-lowering therapies should be administered in a stepwise fashion, starting with first-line, safe interventions (Figure 7.2). Higher-risk treatment options should be reserved for patients at immediate risk of cerebral herniation or those with multimodality brain monitoring evidence of critically reduced brain tissue oxygenation or cerebral metabolic derangement, such as increased lactate/pyruvate ratio.

Basic measures

First-line treatments are directed towards the maintenance of cerebral physiological homeostasis and prompt diagnosis and correction of a remediable underlying intracranial abnormality. Intracranial lesions exerting mass effect should be evacuated, hydrocephalus drained, and oedema associated with intracranial tumours treated with high-dose steroids (18). ICP-lowering treatments can provide a life-saving bridge to these definitive treatments.

Blood pressure

Haemodynamic stability is crucial because of the direct effects of arterial hypotension on CPP and also because an acute reduction in MAP can precipitate intracranial hypertension via the vasodilatory cascade. In patients with decreased intracranial compliance but preserved cerebrovascular reactivity, systemic hypotension is followed by compensatory cerebral vasodilation, increased cerebral blood volume (CBV), a further increase in ICP, and reduction in CPP (19). Further compensatory vasodilation results in sustained ICP plateau waves as intracranial volume-buffering reserve becomes exhausted (Figure 7.3).

Arterial blood pressure should be maintained within age-appropriate normal values. In young adults, systolic blood pressure should be supported above 100 mmHg (20) whereas in patients with a history of uncontrolled hypertension, in whom the

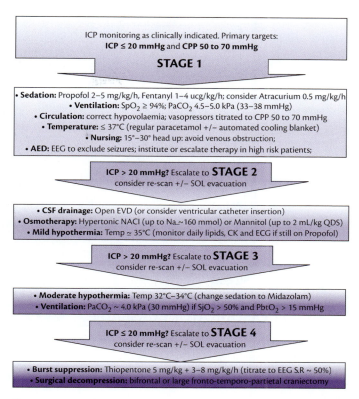

Fig. 7.2 Intracranial management protocol. A rational approach to the treatment of intracranial hypertension consists of a stepwise escalation of ICP-lowering therapies.

AED, antiepileptic drugs; CK, creatine kinase; EEG S.R, electroencephalographic suppression ratio; EVD, external ventricular drainage; PbtO₂, brain tissue oxygen tension; SjO₂, jugular venous oxygen saturation; SOL, space-occupying lesion.

autoregulatory curve is shifted to the right, adequate cerebral perfusion might require significantly higher MAP and CPP targets (21). On the other hand, uncontrolled arterial hypertension can cause or accelerate intracranial haemorrhage and should be avoided, especially in patients with haemorrhagic contusions. Malignant arterial hypertension, defined as MAP exceeding the upper limit of cerebral autoregulation (> 140 mmHg), can cause endothelial dysfunction and cerebral oedema, leading to intracranial hypertension in the absence of haemorrhage. If antihypertensive therapy is required, short-acting agents with no direct cerebral dilatory actions such as labetalol are preferred to vasodilators such as nitrates (22,23).

Airway and ventilation

Comatose patients and those unable to protect their airway require prompt endotracheal intubation. Careful administration of opioids, sedatives, and muscle relaxants facilitates laryngoscopy and prevents coughing and increases in ICP during tracheal intubation. Central vasomotor depression should be anticipated and short-acting vasopressors used to treat haemodynamic instability (24). Hypoxaemia defined as PaO_2 less than 8.0 kPa (< 60 mmHg) or SpO_2 less than 90%, and hypercapnia defined as $PaCO_2$ greater than 6.0 kPa (> 45 mmHg), are major causes of secondary brain injury and should be avoided (20). Their adverse effects are related to the direct detrimental effects of low PaO_2 on the injured brain as well as increases in ICP consequent to hypoxic and hypercapnic cerebral vasodilation. There is a strong correlation between

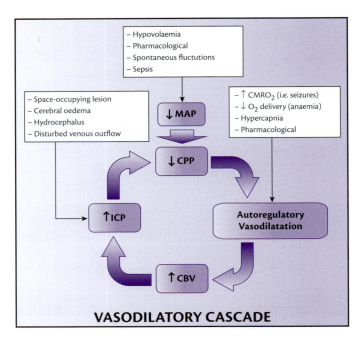

Fig. 7.3 The vasodilatory cascade. The vasodilatory cascade illustrates how a reduction in mean arterial pressure (MAP) and cerebral perfusion pressure (CPP) is followed by cerebral autoregulatory vasodilation and increased cerebral blood volume (CBV). In patients with exhausted intracranial volume-buffering reserve, the increase in CBV results in an increase in ICP. If MAP remains unchanged, CPP will further decrease feeding the vicious cycle until exhaustion of autoregulatory reserve and ICP plateau waves. Note that the cascade may be initiated at different points of the cycle by pathophysiological stimuli causing an increase in ICP, direct cerebral vasodilation, or a reduction in MAP. Conversely, augmentation of MAP can interrupt the vicious cycle and terminate the ICP plateau wave. $CMRO_2$, cerebral metabolic rate of oxygen.

hypoxaemia and poor outcome after TBI, and intubation and mechanical ventilation may be required to optimize cerebral physiology even in conscious patients. However, care should be taken to avoid hyperventilation and hypocapnia as the consequent cerebral vasoconstriction and reduced CBF may precipitate or worsen cerebral ischaemia (25). Despite previous enthusiasm for the potential benefits of normobaric hyperoxia, a convincing body of clinical and experimental evidence confirms that it can be detrimental following TBI, stroke, and hypoxic-ischaemic neurological injury (26–28). Standard clinical practice is therefore directed towards controlled re-oxygenation (maintaining $SpO_2 \geq 94\%$). Therapeutic hyperoxia ($PaO_2 > 300$ mmHg) should be restricted to experimental studies.

Fluid resuscitation

Fluid resuscitation is directed towards maintenance of euvolaemia and plasma osmolarity. Hypo-osmotic solutions such as 0.45% NaCl or 5% dextrose worsen brain oedema and should be avoided in all patients at risk of intracranial hypertension (29).

Transfusion strategies

The precise haemoglobin concentration to optimize oxygen delivery to the injured brain is undefined. While there is widespread consensus in support of restrictive transfusion strategies in critically ill patients without neurological injury, there is a body of evidence suggesting that brain-injured patients are susceptible to anaemia-related secondary brain insults. Cerebral vasodilation

proportional to the reduction in blood oxygen content during haemodilution is described in both experimental and clinical studies (30,31), and this can be sufficient to trigger the vasodilatory cascade and precipitate intracranial hypertension. Recent clinical studies suggest that a haemoglobin concentration lower than 9 g/dL is associated with an increased incidence of brain hypoxia and cellular energy dysfunction after SAH, and increased mortality after TBI (32,33). In 67 patients with moderate to severe TBI, a 'restrictive' transfusion strategy (haemoglobin 7–9 g/dL) was associated with a non-significant higher mortality (17% versus 13%) compared to a 'liberal' strategy (haemoglobin 10–12 g/dL) (34). A haemoglobin target of 9 g/dL or higher seems reasonable in patients with increased ICP, especially if multimodal monitoring confirms cerebral hypoxia and metabolic failure at lower haemoglobin levels.

Seizures

Seizures increase cerebral metabolic rate, dramatically increase ICP, and adversely affect outcome (35). They should be treated promptly in all patients but particularly those at risk of intracranial hypertension. Current TBI management guidelines recommend prophylactic anticonvulsants for 7 days post injury in those at high risk of seizure development (20), including patients with a depressed skull fracture, penetrating wound, subdural, epidural, or intraparenchymal haematomas, cortical contusions, or previous seizures. Phenytoin has historically been used to prevent early post-traumatic seizures after TBI, but it has significant side effects including multiple drug interactions (see Chapter 2). Levetiracetam has equal efficacy and is rapidly becoming the anticonvulsant of choice in many centres although its superiority over phenytoin remains unproven. Levetiracetam has a superior safety profile compared to phenytoin, is available for intravenous administration, and does not require regular measurement of plasma levels because of its wider therapeutic index (36,37).

The prophylactic use of anticonvulsants is not recommended after aneurysmal SAH because of the low risk of seizures and high rate of antiepileptic drug-related complications (38,39). Adverse drug effects have been reported in 23% of patients after SAH (40), in which prophylactic phenytoin is independently associated with worse cognitive outcome (41).

Fever management

Fever is a frequent event following TBI and SAH and worsens ischaemic neurological damage (42). Current consensus supports controlled normothermia to maintain core temperature around 36.5°C in critically ill neurological patients (43,44). Paracetamol is used widely. Non-steroidal anti-inflammatory drugs also effectively reduce body temperature (by ~ 0.6°C) but should be used with caution because of the increased risk of bleeding. Automated non-invasive cooling devices are effective and should be utilized as part of a multimodal approach for the maintenance of normothermia in patients with TBI (45–47).

Head elevation

Brain-injured patients are traditionally nursed with the head of the bed elevated to 30°. This lowers ICP by a hydrostatic effect and improved jugular venous drainage. Head elevation is also associated with a similar hydrostatic reduction in carotid blood pressure but without significant changes in CPP or CBF (48). In hypovolaemic patients, head elevation can result in a significant reduction in venous return, and subsequent reduction in MAP, CPP, and CBF, but systemic hypotension can be prevented by adequate fluid resuscitation and judicious use of vasopressors.

Special care must be taken when positioning the arterial pressure transducer in semi-recumbent patients. The definition of CPP as the difference between MAP and ICP relies on blood pressure measured at the level of the brain, that is, with the transducer sited and 'zeroed' at the level external acoustic meatus. If the transducer is positioned at the level of the heart, as is common practice in general intensive care units, calculated 'CPP' overestimates actual CPP by approximately 10 mmHg in the 30° head-up position (49). Thus, the blood pressure transducer should always be sited at the level of the external acoustic meatus in critically ill brain-injured patients.

Sedation and analgesia

Sedation and analgesia are required to provide endotracheal tube tolerance and facilitate mechanical ventilation. In addition, sedation is used to reduce cerebral metabolic rate, lower ICP, and control seizures after TBI (24). Appropriate levels of sedation and analgesia are therefore key components of the management of patients at risk of intracranial hypertension. Muscle relaxants should be restricted to patients who require escalation of treatment of intracranial hypertension (50). There is limited evidence to guide the choice of sedative agent in patients with ABI, with each agent having specific advantages and disadvantages (see Chapter 6) (51). Propofol and midazolam are the most commonly used sedatives in clinical practice, with barbiturates reserved for management of ultra-refractory intracranial hypertension (Figure 7.2) (52).

Propofol

Propofol is a gamma-aminobutyric acid type A ($GABA_A$) receptor agonist with rapid onset and offset of action. Its context-sensitive half-life compares favourably with other commonly used sedatives, allowing rapid wake-up and reliable neurological examination even after prolonged infusion (53). Compared to midazolam, propofol provides improved quality of sedation and a faster recovery of consciousness, making it the preferred sedative for haemodynamically stable neurological patients (54). It reduces ICP and cerebral metabolic rate, and can maintain electroencephalographic (EEG) burst suppression without affecting cerebrovascular CO_2 reactivity or pressure autoregulation (55,56). Propofol reduces MAP in a dose-dependent manner through centrally mediated suppression of sympathetic tone and it is therefore relatively contraindicated in haemodynamically unstable patients (57). Prolonged infusion at doses exceeding 4 mg/kg/h can be associated with the relatively rare but sometimes fatal propofol infusion syndrome (see Chapter 6) (58,59), which is particularly common in brain-injured patients (60).

Sedation can be guided by monitoring the EEG suppression ratio (SR), although any potential benefits of propofol sedation targeted to SR are unproven (61). A SR of 50% is indicative of EEG burst suppression and 100% of electrical 'silence' (isoelectric EEG). Propofol-induced burst suppression does not necessarily protect the brain from secondary injury. It is not associated with a decrease in the number of jugular desaturation episodes during cardiopulmonary bypass or in the ischaemic burden in brain-injured patients with normal ICP (62,63). Thus, targeting propofol sedation to burst suppression should be restricted to patients with refractory intracranial hypertension and multimodal monitoring evidence of brain

hypoxia or cerebral metabolic failure. There is limited theoretical benefit by deepening sedation from burst suppression to electrical silence and the author proposes that the target SR should be no higher than 50%. Additional increments in plasma propofol concentration cannot cause further electrophysiological benefits if the SR is already 100%, so using this as a sedation target risks inadvertent overdose of propofol. Special concerns are raised by the use of propofol in hypothermic patients because a temperature lower than 34°C can impair propofol metabolism and result in significant increases in plasma concentration (64).

Midazolam

Midazolam has a stable haemodynamic profile and no temperature-related effects on metabolism so is the preferred sedative in unstable and hypothermic neurological patients (65). Another reason that midazolam is preferable to propofol in hypothermic patients is that hypothermia itself can induce reversible ECG changes (66) thereby limiting ECG as a monitoring tool for the propofol infusion syndrome.

Midazolam has a relatively short context-sensitive half-life of 2–2.5 hours (67) but has a number of active metabolites that can accumulate during prolonged infusion and lead to delayed wake-up times, particularly in the elderly and those with hepatic impairment. Benzodiazepines are associated with an increased incidence of delirium (68) and withdrawal symptoms (69) compared to propofol. Midazolam reduces cerebral metabolic rate, CBF, and ICP but does not affect cerebral autoregulation and CO_2 reactivity. However, the level of metabolic suppression that can be achieved with midazolam is less profound than with propofol and barbiturates, and even large doses of midazolam do not induce an isoelectric EEG or burst suppression in normothermic patients (70,71). Burst suppression can be induced if high-dose midazolam is used in conjunction with other central nervous system depressants such as anticonvulsants (72).

Barbiturates

Prior to the introduction of propofol, oxybarbiturates (pentobarbitone) and thiobarbiturates (thiopental) were used extensively for sedation and ICP reduction in brain-injured patients (73,74). Barbiturates have sedative, anaesthetic, and antiepileptic properties via allosteric modulation of $GABA_A$ chloride ion channels that leads to neuronal hyperpolarization and inhibition of the action potential. They also inhibit excitatory L-glutamate AMPA receptors and reduce the flow of calcium through several types of voltage-gated calcium channels on neurons (75) suggesting that they may have neuroprotective effects that are independent of metabolic suppression. The potential neuroprotective effects of barbiturates include inhibition of excitotoxicity and free radical-mediated lipid peroxidation (76,77) and are used to justify their role as potential third-line treatment for refractory intracranial hypertension. Burst suppression is not required to elicit maximal neuroprotective efficacy of barbiturates in animal models of brain ischaemia (78).

Barbiturates have many side effects that significantly limit their clinical use. They cause direct myocardial and central vasomotor depression leading to profound haemodynamic instability, and also accumulate during intravenous infusion. Barbiturates have a long context-sensitive half-life (thiopental 6–46 hours, pentobarbitone 15–48 hours) and elimination kinetics that change from first-order to zero-order at plasma levels required to achieve EEG burst suppression (24). This means that there is only a weak correlation between rate of infusion, plasma concentration, and clinical effect of barbiturates, a situation that is aggravated by their numerous active metabolites. Barbiturates should therefore be administered in incremental doses titrated to an EEG SR of 50%.

Studies investigating the use of high-dose barbiturates for the treatment of intracranial hypertension were performed in an era when high-dose steroids, prophylactic hyperventilation, and fluid restriction were routine (20), and their applicability to current practice is debatable at best. A 2012 Cochrane review concluded that barbiturates are no longer indicated for maintenance sedation after TBI (79), and they should restricted to patients with refractory intracranial hypertension who have not responded to other treatments and then only when the likely risks and potential benefits have been assessed.

Osmotic agents

Brain volume is extremely responsive to changes in water content. If plasma osmolarity is rapidly increased by solutes that do not easily diffuse across the BBB, the brain–plasma osmotic gradient that develops results in net water diffusion from brain parenchyma into the circulating volume. Vice versa, when plasma osmolarity decreases, free water diffuses across the BBB from the circulation into brain parenchyma, leading to cerebral oedema (80).

The effects of the rapid infusion of hyper- and hypo-osmolar solutions on CSF pressure were first described in 1919. During an experiment designed to determine whether intravenously administered sodium would diffuse into the CSF space of anaesthetized cats, Weed and McKibben serendipitously observed that hypertonic sodium solution resulted in a rapid reduction in CSF pressure and, conversely, that intravenous administration of water and dextrose solutions caused a protracted increase in CSF pressure (81). Substances that generate clinically relevant osmotic gradients across the BBB include mannitol and sodium.

Urea

Concentrated urea was the first osmotic agent used in the treatment of intracranial hypertension in humans but is now only of historic interest (82). Its clinical effectiveness is hindered by diffusibility across cell membranes and it is no longer used clinically. However, it is important to note the effects on the central nervous system of rapid reductions in plasma urea concentration because this situation can arise in patients undergoing haemodialysis. In chronically uraemic patients, cerebral osmolality tends to equilibrate over time with the higher plasma osmolality. Haemodialysis can result in a rapid reduction of plasma urea and osmolality and an acute reversal of the brain–plasma water gradient leading to water diffusion across the BBB and cerebral oedema. This is called the dialysis disequilibrium syndrome which is characterized by nausea, tremor, disturbed consciousness, and seizures. In rare cases, significant brain oedema has resulted in cerebral herniation and death (83).

Mannitol

Mannitol has been used for decades to treat intracranial hypertension (84–86). It is a sugar alcohol with osmotic diuretic properties. In contrast to concentrated urea, mannitol does not diffuse easily across cell membranes and the resulting lower volume of distribution, coupled with its ability to dehydrate erythrocytes, makes it a vastly superior osmotic agent. Mannitol reduces ICP through three different mechanisms:

1. Haemodynamic and antiviscosity effects: mannitol dehydrates erythrocytes, reducing their volume, rigidity, and cohesiveness. The subsequent reduction in blood viscosity, along with a mild positive inotropic effect and reduction of systemic vascular resistance, leads to increased cardiac output and improved cerebral perfusion and oxygenation. Due to metabolic coupling, the CBF increase is accompanied by rapid cerebral vasoconstriction with subsequent reduction in ICP and further improvements in brain perfusion (87). This accounts for the rapid onset of action of mannitol.

2. Osmotic effects: mannitol creates an osmotic gradient across the BBB resulting in osmotic mobilization of water from brain parenchyma into the circulating volume. The reflection coefficient is a measure of how well solutes cross a membrane, and the reflection coefficient of mannitol is 0.9. This means that 90% of the drug remains in the capillaries and exerts an osmotic gradient across the intact BBB. Clinically relevant doses of mannitol generate substantial blood–brain osmotic gradients and direct removal of water from brain parenchyma. This accounts for the more prolonged effects of mannitol.

3. Diuretic effects: mannitol can theoretically cause systemic dehydration and a sustained increase in plasma osmolality which, if not corrected, results in a long-lasting brain dehydrating effect. This effect is of little clinical relevance as the diuretic actions of mannitol are compensated by proportionate volume resuscitation to maintain euvolaemia (88).

Mannitol is usually given as bolus doses of 0.25–2.0 g/kg, over 30–60 minutes, repeated as required. It is available as 10% and 20% solutions and both can be administered through central or peripheral venous catheters. The 20% solution tends to precipitate and a 15-micron in-line filter should be used. Care should be taken to avoid extravasation which is associated with painful thrombophlebitis. Following TBI, a single dose of 20% mannitol reduces ICP within 10–15 minutes, with a maximal effect within 20–60 minutes (89).

Hypertonic saline

Hypertonic saline (HS) solutions have gained popularity for the treatment of intracranial hypertension since the 1990s (85,90). Like mannitol, sodium does not cross the BBB. Its reflection coefficient is 1, meaning that 100% remains in the capillaries and exerts an osmotic gradient across the intact BBB. Like mannitol, the ICP-lowering effects of HS depend on a direct increase in plasma osmolality and a net flow of water from brain parenchyma into the circulating volume, and also on dehydration of erythrocytes with reduced blood viscosity, improved CBF, and compensatory reductions in CBV and ICP (91).

There are important difference between mannitol and HS. Mannitol causes an osmotic diuresis and volume depletion whereas HS results in sustained intravascular volume expansion. Although this can precipitate congestive heart failure in susceptible patients, volume expansion is generally helpful in the management of critically ill patients, especially in the context of trauma. Boluses of HS cause a short-lived and generally clinically irrelevant hyperchloraemic acidosis (92). Several cases of central pontine myelinolysis have been reported during rapid sodium correction in patients with chronic hyponatraemia. For this reason, HS is not considered safe in the context of chronic hyponatraemia, although central pontine myelinolysis has never been reported in normonatraemic TBI patients treated with HS (20).

HS is available as 3%, 7.5%, and 23.4% solutions, and is typically administered in 150 mL, 75 mL, and 30 mL boluses respectively. A 3% HS solution can be administered peripherally but 7.5% and 23.4% solutions must be infused via a central venous catheter. Some experts recommend administration of HS as a continuous infusion titrated to a plasma sodium concentration of 145–155 mmol/L. No significant side effects or significant rebounds in ICP on discontinuation of therapy have been reported with such a regimen (93). Plasma sodium levels should be routinely measured at the bedside and, if serum sodium concentration exceeds 160 mmol/L, additional doses of HS are unlikely to have further beneficial effects on ICP (80). At the time of writing there is no definitive evidence to guide the optimal method of administration (bolus versus continuous infusion) of HS, duration of therapy, or plasma sodium targets.

Compared to mannitol, equiosmolar boluses of HS achieve similar reductions in ICP after TBI (94) and equal or superior brain relaxation during elective brain surgery (95). A recent meta-analysis argued that HS may be superior to mannitol in terms of safety and efficacy (96), but the choice between an osmotic diuretic and a volume-expanding agent should always be based on individual assessment of volume status and renal, cardiac, and respiratory function.

Complications of hyperosmolar therapy

The ICP effects of hyperosmolar therapy are primarily exerted by dehydration of normal brain tissue, and in injured brain regions the free diffusion of solutes across the BBB negates its dehydrating effects. Although such considerations might seem to indicate that osmotic agents can worsen ICP gradients and precipitate brain herniation in patients with large focal injuries, this theoretical concern appears largely unfounded. Osmotic therapy has negligible effects on midline shift even in patients with hemispheric infarcts (97,98).

Acute kidney injury (AKI) is a clinically relevant risk of high-dose mannitol but not HS because of renal vasoconstriction and intravascular volume depletion. This risk is higher if more than 200 g of mannitol are administered each day, or if plasma osmolality exceeds 400 mOsm. A previously proposed upper limit of plasma osmolality of 320 mOsm during hyperosmolar treatment is arbitrary and this threshold is often exceeded in clinical practice without significant repercussions on renal function (88).

In response to prolonged brain dehydration, astrocytes and neurons produce polyols, amino acids, and other osmotically active molecules that contribute to gradual re-equilibration of the osmotic gradient between the extracellular space and brain parenchyma. When a state of serum hyperosmolarity has been maintained over a number of days, care should therefore be taken to prevent a rapid reversal of the brain–plasma water gradient on discontinuation of therapy as this can lead to rebound brain oedema similar to that previously described in the dialysis disequilibrium syndrome.

Arterial carbon dioxide tension

Carbon dioxide is a potent dilator of pial arterioles (99). Hypercapnia increases CBV and can precipitate intracranial hypertension in patients with exhausted volume-buffering reserve. Controlled normocapnia is crucial to minimize the risk of secondary brain injury and, in this regard at least, pre-hospital intubation and controlled ventilation guided by continuous end-tidal CO_2 monitoring has been shown to improve functional outcome when compared to delayed, in-hospital intubation (100).

Hyperventilation reduces $PaCO_2$ and lowers ICP within seconds as a result of cerebral vasoconstriction. The induction of hypocapnia by hyperventilation can be life-saving in patients at risk of imminent cerebral herniation because of its fast onset of action, but prolonged hyperventilation risks cerebral vasoconstriction sufficient to reduce CBF below critical thresholds and can precipitate or worsen cerebral ischaemia (101). This is particularly relevant in the first 24 hours after severe TBI when CBF may already be critically reduced. Positron emission tomography (PET) studies have demonstrated that hyperventilation to a target $PaCO_2$ of 4.0 kPa (30 mmHg) in patients with moderately increased ICP can result in significant regional ischaemia in the first 10 days after TBI (102). Notably, PET-confirmed regional ischaemia is undetected by jugular venous oxygen saturation monitoring suggesting that the ischaemic burden associated with modest hyperventilation is not always detected by global monitors of cerebral oxygenation.

As is the case with other ICP-lowering strategies, $PaCO_2$ targets should be determined on an individual basis. Ventilation is routinely targeted to normocapnia, that is, $PaCO_2$ 4.5–5.0 kPa (33–38 mmHg), and modest hyperventilation to $PaCO_2$ 4.0 kPa (30 mmHg) should be considered only in patients in whom ICP remains elevated despite first- and second-line treatments. Cerebral oxygenation and microdialysis monitoring can provide some degree of reassurance regarding the adequacy of cerebral perfusion during hyperventilation, and to fine-tune $PaCO_2$ and CPP targets in an individual patient (101,103,104). More aggressive hyperventilation to $PaCO_2$ less than 4.0 kPa (< 30 mmHg) provides limited additional benefits in terms of ICP control and should be avoided (105). Current guidance from the Brain Trauma Foundation recommends that prophylactic hypocapnia ($PaCO_2$ < 4.0 kPa (< 30 mmHg)) should be avoided, and that hyperventilation should only be used as a temporizing measure for the reduction of elevated ICP in patients at imminent risk of herniation (20).

Hypothermia

Although there is a wealth of experimental data describing beneficial effects of hypothermia on the brain, at the time of writing, perinatal asphyxia is the only indication supported by level 1 evidence (106). There is some evidence supporting targeted temperature management to 36°C for anoxic-ischaemic encephalopathy following out-of-hospital cardiac arrest (see Chapter 25) (107–110). The outcome effect of therapeutic hypothermia in patients with refractory intracranial hypertension after TBI is currently being addressed in the Eurotherm3235 Trial (111).

The potential benefits of therapeutic hypothermia are best understood by distinguishing between its ICP-lowering effects which are primarily mediated via a temperature-dependent reduction in cerebral metabolic rate and CBV, and its ICP-independent neuroprotective effects via inhibition of excitotoxicity and neuronal apoptosis (112,113), suppression of the inflammatory cascade (114,115), reduction of BBB disruption (116), and reduced cytotoxic oedema (117). As intracranial hypertension plays only a minor role in secondary brain injury following perinatal asphyxia and cardiac arrest, it could be argued that the neuroprotective effects of hypothermia that are independent from its ICP-lowering properties are likely to be the most clinically relevant in these contexts. On the other hand, hypothermia-induced improvements in outcome in conditions such as TBI where intracranial hypertension is a determining factor remain unproven (118). It has long been argued that a delayed initiation of hypothermia has contributed to the inconsistent findings in clinical studies but a recent study confirmed that even early hypothermia does not improve outcome after TBI (119).

Although there is no evidence to support the use of hypothermia as a primary neuroprotective strategy following severe TBI, there is evidence for its use as an ICP-lowering strategy in patients with intracranial hypertension refractory to first-line medical treatment (89). Sedative agents lower the cerebral metabolic rate associated with neuronal function whereas hypothermia reduces cellular metabolism associated with the maintenance of transmembrane ion gradients and brain tissue viability (120). Thus moderate hypothermia can reduce brain metabolism irrespective of the depth of sedation, and also generate significant ICP reductions in patients with sedation-induced EEG burst suppression (109). Therapeutic hypothermia should be titrated to ICP response with depth and duration determined by an individualized risk–benefit assessment. Preliminary data suggest that hypothermia should be maintained for at least 48 hours and that rewarming should be slow (1°C every 4 hours) to prevent rebound increases in ICP and followed by controlled normothermia (121,122).

Deep hypothermia to a core temperature of 16°C is associated with profound metabolic suppression and can be used to extend the 'safe' brain ischaemic time during major vascular procedures requiring circulatory arrest. Despite theoretical neuroprotective advantages, there is no evidence to support the use of deep hypothermia following TBI (123). Further, life-threatening cardiac arrhythmias and profound haemodynamic instability prevent its clinical use during neurocritical care (124). In the context of intracranial hypertension, the depth of hypothermia should not exceed 32°C but even higher temperatures are associated with coagulopathy, immunological suppression, and electrolyte disturbances (125). Such complications are time and temperature dependent, are usually treatable, and rarely life-threatening.

Safe, rapid, and inexpensive induction of hypothermia can be achieved by intravenous infusion of ice-cold fluids. In combination with surface cooling, the infusion of 30 mL/kg 4°C saline reduces core temperature by 4.0 ± 0.3°C within 60 minutes without adverse effects on haemodynamic stability (126). Cooling devices with automated temperature feedback minimize the risk of under- or over-cooling that can be associated with ice packs and cold air blankets (106). A number of intravascular cooling catheters are commercially available and reported to deliver shorter time-to-target-temperature and maintenance of more stable temperature compared to surface cooling methods (127). Endovascular cooling devices are associated with potentially severe complications such as deep venous thrombosis (DVT) and catheter-related infections. The reported incidence of asymptomatic DVT is around 50% and a sixfold increase in the incidence of bloodstream infections has been reported with endovascular-cooling devices compared to surface cooling (128,129). The clinical superiority of endovascular devices remain to be proven and surface cooling technologies may offer a superior safety profile when hypothermia needs to be continued for more than 24 hours as is often the case in the management of intracranial hypertension.

Surgery

Surgical management of intracranial hypertension includes evacuation of space-occupying lesions, drainage of CSF, and decompressive craniectomy.

Space-occupying lesions

Immediate surgical evacuation is indicated for extradural and acute subdural haematomas if there is clinical or radiological evidence of mass effect (130). The surgical management of intraparenchymal haemorrhages and contusions remains controversial, with indications for surgery being related to the size, number, and location of haematomas, and presence or absence of intraventricular haemorrhage extension. Patients with large lobar spontaneous haemorrhagic lesions causing intracranial hypertension benefit from prompt surgical evacuation (131,132), but the role of surgery for traumatic haemorrhagic contusions remains a matter of controversy. The issue has been investigated in the Surgical Trial in Traumatic Intracerebral Haemorrhage (133) unfortunately terminated earlier than planned.

Cerebrospinal fluid drainage

Placement of an external ventricular drain (EVD) allows therapeutic drainage of CSF to control intracranial hypertension as well as monitoring of ICP (20). ICP monitored via an EVD can be grossly underestimated during CSF drainage and should not be measured via an open drain (see Chapter 9) (135). CSF drainage is a second-tier option for the treatment of intracranial hypertension. In patients with compressed ventricles, placement of an EVD can be technically difficult and the effects of CSF drainage on ICP marginal and short lived. The major complications associated with EVDs are discussed in detail in Chapters 9 and 24.

Decompressive craniectomy

Decompressive craniectomy involves removal of a large skull segment and opening of the underlying dura. It rapidly controls ICP in patients with intracranial hypertension refractory to maximal medical treatment, hypothermia, and CSF drainage. A number of different techniques of decompressive craniectomy have been described related to the location (frontal, temporal, parietal, or occipital), laterality (unilateral or bilateral), and dural technique (opened in wide surgical flaps or 'stabbed'). Surgical closure can include suturing of the dural flaps or only scalp closure. Unilateral decompression is indicated in patients with unilateral lesions or brain swelling resulting in a midline shift, whereas a large bifrontal decompression is indicated in patients with diffuse cerebral oedema (136).

Despite the publication of a single, small trial supporting the use of decompressive craniectomy in the paediatric population (137), the impact of decompressive craniectomy on outcome following TBI in adults remains controversial. There is little doubt that decompressive surgery is effective in controlling intracranial hypertension but concern remains that it might result in increased rates of disability in survivors. A randomized trial evaluating the role of early decompressive craniectomy in patients with intracranial hypertension following severe TBI (DECRA) demonstrated worse 6-month outcome in patients undergoing decompression (138). The clinical relevance of DECRA is limited because the differences in outcome between the groups were no longer significant after adjustment for pupil reactivity at baseline; 27% of patients randomized to surgical decompression had bilaterally fixed and dilated pupils before randomization compared to 12% in the medical management group.

Another limitation of the DECRA study is the relatively low ICP burden that triggered surgical decompression. Patients underwent surgery when ICP exceeded 20 mmHg for 15 minutes despite first-tier interventions, and this is considered too early by many experts (139). The surgical technique in this study involved cruciate opening of the dura without sectioning the falx cerebri and the effectiveness of this has also been questioned by some experts. DECRA has increased rather than resolved the controversy about the indications, technique, timing, and selection of patients for decompressive craniectomy and it is hoped that RESCUEicp, a UK-based, international randomized trial evaluating surgical decompression compared to best medical management after severe TBI, will answer some of these outstanding questions (140).

There is limited value in routine ICP monitoring or placement of a ventriculostomy in patients with a large supratentorial hemispheric stroke (141). However, in malignant middle cerebral artery (MCA) infarction and decreased level of consciousness, surgical decompression with dural expansion reduces mortality and increases favourable outcomes, irrespective of ICP or whether the infarction is in the dominant or non-dominant hemisphere (142). The benefit of surgical decompression in patients older than 60 years of age with malignant MCA syndrome is uncertain as the overall prognosis in this age group is poor. For all these reasons, the indications for surgical decompression following malignant MCA infarction should be considered carefully on an individual basis taking into account age, comorbidities, and the patient's wishes (143).

Suboccipital craniectomy with dural opening can be life-saving in patients with posterior fossa stroke and brainstem compression. As in supratentorial stroke, neurological deterioration rather than ICP monitoring should guide surgical intervention. If ventriculostomy is indicated to relieve obstructive hydrocephalus after a cerebellar infarct, it should be accompanied by a posterior fossa craniectomy to prevent upward cerebellar displacement. In the absence of established brainstem infarcts, surgery after a cerebellar infarct is associated with acceptable functional outcomes in most patients (144).

Significant brain swelling and intracranial hypertension can occur in patients with encephalitis, and the term 'fulminant' encephalitis refers to infectious encephalitis associated with clinical or radiological evidence of brainstem compression. In this context, the limited evidence available suggests that surgical decompression results in excellent recovery of functional independence in both children and adults, even in the presence of early signs of brainstem dysfunction (145,146).

References

1. Bradley KC. Cerebrospinal fluid pressure. *J Neurol Neurosurg Psychiatry*. 1970;33(3):387–97.
2. Marmarou A, Eisenberg HM, Foulkes M, Marshall LF, Jane JA. Impact of ICP instability and hypotension on outcome in patients with severe head trauma. *J Neurosurg*. 1991;75:S159–S66.
3. Mazzola CA, Adelson PD. Critical care management of head trauma in children. *Crit Care Med*. 2002;30(11 Suppl):S393–401.
4. Stocchetti N, Colombo A, Ortolano F, Videtta W, Marchesi R, Longhi L, et al. Time course of intracranial hypertension after traumatic brain injury. *J Neurotrauma*. 2007;24(8):1339–46.
5. Marmarou A, Fatouros PP, Barzo P, Portella G, Yoshihara M, Tsuji O, et al. Contribution of edema and cerebral blood volume to traumatic brain swelling in head-injured patients. *J Neurosurg*. 2000;93(2):183–93.
6. Matsushige T, Nakaoka M, Kiya K, Takeda T, Kurisu K. Cerebral sinovenous thrombosis after closed head injury. *J Trauma*. 2009;66(6):1599–604.
7. Heuts SG, Bruce SS, Zacharia BE, Hickman ZL, Kellner CP, Sussman ES, et al. Decompressive hemicraniectomy without clot evacuation in dominant-sided intracerebral hemorrhage with ICP crisis. *Neurosurg Focus*. 2013;34(5):E4.
8. Rincon F, Mayer SA. Clinical review: critical care management of spontaneous intracerebral hemorrhage. *Crit Care*. 2008;12(6):237.
9. Su CF, Yang YL, Lee MC, Chen HI. A severe vicious cycle in uncontrolled subarachnoid hemorrhage: the effects on cerebral blood flow and hemodynamic responses upon intracranial hypertension. *Chin J Physiol*. 2006;49(1):56–63.
10. Lee VH, Connolly HM, Fulgham JR, Manno EM, Brown RD, Jr., Wijdicks EF. Tako-tsubo cardiomyopathy in aneurysmal subarachnoid hemorrhage: an underappreciated ventricular dysfunction. *J Neurosurg*. 2006;105(2):264–70.
11. Germanwala AV, Huang J, Tamargo RJ. Hydrocephalus after aneurysmal subarachnoid hemorrhage. *Neurosurg Clin N Am*. 2010;21(2):263–70.
12. Mayer SA, Coplin WM, Raps EC. Cerebral edema, intracranial pressure, and herniation syndromes. *J Stroke Cerebrovasc Dis*. 1999;8(3):183–91.
13. Treggiari MM, Schutz N, Yanez ND, Romand JA. Role of intracranial pressure values and patterns in predicting outcome in traumatic brain injury: a systematic review. *Neurocrit Care*. 2007;6(2):104–12.
14. Badri S, Chen J, Barber J, Temkin NR, Dikmen SS, Chesnut RM, et al. Mortality and long-term functional outcome associated with intracranial pressure after traumatic brain injury. *Intensive Care Med*. 2012;38(11):1800–9.
15. Lavinio A, Czosnyka Z, Czosnyka M. Cerebrospinal fluid dynamics: disturbances and diagnostics. *Eur J Anaesthesiol Suppl*. 2008;42:137–41.
16. Lavinio A, Menon DK. Intracranial pressure: why we monitor it, how to monitor it, what to do with the number and what's the future? *Curr Opin Anaesthesiol*. 2011;24(2):117–23.
17. Goyal V, Srinivasan M. Don't hold your breath. *J Gen Intern Med*. 2011;26(3):345.
18. Dunn LT. Raised intracranial pressure. *J Neurol Neurosurg Psychiatry*. 2002;73 Suppl 1:i23–7.
19. Rosner MJ, Rosner SD, Johnson AH. Cerebral perfusion pressure: management protocol and clinical results. *J Neurosurg*. 1995;83(6):949–62.
20. Bratton SL, Chestnut RM, Ghajar J, McConnell Hammond FF, Harris OA, Hartl R, et al. Guidelines for the management of severe traumatic brain injury. *J Neurotrauma*. 2007;24 Suppl 1:S1–S106.
21. Paulson OB, Strandgaard S, Edvinsson L. Cerebral autoregulation. *Cerebrovasc Brain Metab Rev*. 1990;2(2):161–92.
22. Moppett IK, Sherman RW, Wild MJ, Latter JA, Mahajan RP. Effects of norepinephrine and glyceryl trinitrate on cerebral haemodynamics: transcranial Doppler study in healthy volunteers. *Br J Anaesth*. 2008;100(2):240–4.
23. Burt DE, Verniquet AJ, Homi J. The response of canine intracranial pressure to systemic hypotension induced with nitroglycerine. *Br J Anaesth*. 1982;54(6):665–71.
24. Flower O, Hellings S. Sedation in traumatic brain injury. *Emerg Med Int*. 2012;2012:637171.
25. Muizelaar JP, Marmarou A, Ward JD, Kontos HA, Choi SC, Becker DP, et al. Adverse effects of prolonged hyperventilation in patients with severe head injury: a randomized clinical trial. *J Neurosurg*. 1991;75(5):731–9.
26. Davis DP, Meade W, Sise MJ, Kennedy F, Simon F, Tominaga G, et al. Both hypoxemia and extreme hyperoxemia may be detrimental in patients with severe traumatic brain injury. *J Neurotrauma*. 2009;26(12):2217–23.
27. Balan IS, Fiskum G, Hazelton J, Cotto-Cumba C, Rosenthal RE. Oximetry-guided reoxygenation improves neurological outcome after experimental cardiac arrest. *Stroke*. 2006;37(12):3008–13.

28. Kilgannon JH, Jones AE, Shapiro NI, Angelos MG, Milcarek B, Hunter K, et al. Association between arterial hyperoxia following resuscitation from cardiac arrest and in-hospital mortality. *JAMA.* 2010;303(21):2165–71.

29. Talmor D, Shapira Y, Artru AA, Gurevich B, Merkind V, Katchko L, et al. 0.45% saline and 5% dextrose in water, but not 0.9% saline or 5% dextrose in 0.9% saline, worsen brain edema two hours after closed head trauma in rats. *Anesth Analg.* 1998;86(6):1225–9.

30. Hare GM, Tsui AK, McLaren AT, Ragoonanan TE, Yu J, Mazer CD. Anemia and cerebral outcomes: many questions, fewer answers. *Anesth Analg.* 2008;107(4):1356–70.

31. Biousse V, Rucker JC, Vignal C, Crassard I, Katz BJ, Newman NJ. Anemia and papilledema. *Am J Ophthalmol.* 2003;135(4):437–46.

32. Oddo M, Milby A, Chen I, Frangos S, MacMurtrie E, Maloney-Wilensky E, et al. Hemoglobin concentration and cerebral metabolism in patients with aneurysmal subarachnoid hemorrhage. *Stroke.* 2009;40(4):1275–81.

33. Sekhon MS, McLean N, Henderson WR, Chittock DR, Griesdale DE. Association of hemoglobin concentration and mortality in critically ill patients with severe traumatic brain injury. *Crit Care.* 2012;16(4):R128.

34. McIntyre LA, Fergusson DA, Hutchison JS, Pagliarello G, Marshall JC, Yetisir E, et al. Effect of a liberal versus restrictive transfusion strategy on mortality in patients with moderate to severe head injury. *Neurocrit Care.* 2006;5(1):4–9.

35. Solheim O, Vik A, Gulati S, Eide PK. Rapid and severe rise in static and pulsatile intracranial pressures during a generalized epileptic seizure. *Seizure.* 2008;17(8):740–3.

36. Zafar SN, Khan AA, Ghauri AA, Shamim MS. Phenytoin versus levetiracetam for seizure prophylaxis after brain injury—a meta analysis. *BMC Neurol.* 2012;12:30.

37. Inaba K, Menaker J, Branco BC, Gooch J, Okoye OT, Herrold J, et al. A prospective multicenter comparison of levetiracetam versus phenytoin for early posttraumatic seizure prophylaxis. *J Trauma Acute Care Surg.* 2013;74(3):766–71.

38. Lanzino G, D'Urso PI, Suarez J, Participants in the International Multi-Disciplinary Consensus Conference on the Critical Care Management of Subarachnoid H. Seizures and anticonvulsants after aneurysmal subarachnoid hemorrhage. *Neurocrit Care.* 2011;15(2):247–56.

39. Steiner T, Juvela S, Unterberg A, Jung C, Forsting M, Rinkel G, et al. European Stroke Organization guidelines for the management of intracranial aneurysms and subarachnoid haemorrhage. *Cerebrovasc Dis.* 2013;35(2):93–112.

40. Choi KS, Chun HJ, Yi HJ, Ko Y, Kim YS, Kim JM. Seizures and epilepsy following aneurysmal subarachnoid hemorrhage: incidence and risk factors. *J Korean Neurosurg Soc.* 2009;46(2):93–8.

41. Naidech AM, Kreiter KT, Janjua N, Ostapkovich N, Parra A, Commichau C, et al. Phenytoin exposure is associated with functional and cognitive disability after subarachnoid hemorrhage. *Stroke.* 2005;36(3):583–7.

42. Childs C, Vail A, Protheroe R, King AT, Dark PM. Differences between brain and rectal temperatures during routine critical care of patients with severe traumatic brain injury. *Anaesthesia.* 2005;60(8):759–65.

43. Marion DW. Controlled normothermia in neurologic intensive care. *Crit Care Med.* 2004;32(2 Suppl):S43–5.

44. Greer DM, Funk SE, Reaven NL, Ouzounelli M, Uman GC. Impact of fever on outcome in patients with stroke and neurologic injury: a comprehensive meta-analysis. *Stroke.* 2008;39(11):3029–35.

45. Douds GL, Tadzong B, Agarwal AD, Krishnamurthy S, Lehman EB, Cockroft KM. Influence of fever and hospital-acquired infection on the incidence of delayed neurological deficit and poor outcome after aneurysmal subarachnoid hemorrhage. *Neurol Res Int.* 2012;2012:479865.

46. Stocchetti N, Rossi S, Zanier ER, Colombo A, Beretta L, Citerio G. Pyrexia in head-injured patients admitted to intensive care. *Intensive Care Med.* 2002;28(11):1555–62.

47. Puccio AM, Fischer MR, Jankowitz BT, Yonas H, Darby JM, Okonkwo DO. Induced normothermia attenuates intracranial hypertension and reduces fever burden after severe traumatic brain injury. *Neurocrit Care.* 2009;11(1):82–7.

48. Feldman Z, Kanter MJ, Robertson CS, Contant CF, Hayes C, Sheinberg MA, et al. Effect of head elevation on intracranial pressure, cerebral perfusion pressure, and cerebral blood flow in head-injured patients. *J Neurosurg.* 1992;76(2):207–11.

49. Sykes M, Vickers M, Hull C. *Principles of Measurement and Monitoring in Anaesthesia* (3rd edn). Oxford: Blackwell Science Publications; 1991.

50. Hsiang JK, Chesnut RM, Crisp CB, Klauber MR, Blunt BA, Marshall LF. Early, routine paralysis for intracranial pressure control in severe head injury: is it necessary? *Crit Care Med.* 1994;22(9):1471–6.

51. Roberts DJ, Hall RI, Kramer AH, Robertson HL, Gallagher CN, Zygun DA. Sedation for critically ill adults with severe traumatic brain injury: a systematic review of randomized controlled trials. *Crit Care Med.* 2011;39(12):2743–51.

52. Patel HC, Menon DK, Tebbs S, Hawker R, Hutchinson PJ, Kirkpatrick PJ. Specialist neurocritical care and outcome from head injury. *Intensive Care Med.* 2002;28(5):547–53.

53. Hutchens MP, Memtsoudis S, Sadovnikoff N. Propofol for sedation in neuro-intensive care. *Neurocrit Care.* 2006;4(1):54–62.

54. Ronan KP, Gallagher TJ, George B, Hamby B. Comparison of propofol and midazolam for sedation in intensive care unit patients. *Crit Care Med.* 1995;23(2):286–93.

55. Illievich UM, Petricek W, Schramm W, Weindlmayr-Goettel M, Czech T, Spiss CK. Electroencephalographic burst suppression by propofol infusion in humans: hemodynamic consequences. *Anesth Analg.* 1993;77(1):155–60.

56. Matta BF, Lam AM, Strebel S, Mayberg TS. Cerebral pressure autoregulation and carbon dioxide reactivity during propofol-induced EEG suppression. *Br J Anaesth.* 1995;74(2):159–63.

57. Robinson BJ, Ebert TJ, O'Brien TJ, Colinco MD, Muzi M. Mechanisms whereby propofol mediates peripheral vasodilation in humans. Sympathoinhibition or direct vascular relaxation? *Anesthesiology.* 1997;86(1):64–72.

58. Cremer OL. The propofol infusion syndrome: more puzzling evidence on a complex and poorly characterized disorder. *Crit Care.* 2009;13(6):1012.

59. Junttila MJ, Gonzalez M, Lizotte E, Benito B, Vernooy K, Sarkozy A, et al. Induced Brugada-type electrocardiogram, a sign for imminent malignant arrhythmias. *Circulation.* 2008;117(14):1890–3.

60. Otterspoor LC, Kalkman CJ, Cremer OL. Update on the propofol infusion syndrome in ICU management of patients with head injury. *Curr Opin Anaesthesiol.* 2008;21(5):544–51.

61. Doyle PW, Matta BF. Burst suppression or isoelectric encephalogram for cerebral protection: evidence from metabolic suppression studies. *Br J Anaesth.* 1999;83(4):580–4.

62. Johnston AJ, Steiner LA, Chatfield DA, Coleman MR, Coles JP, Al-Rawi PG, et al. Effects of propofol on cerebral oxygenation and metabolism after head injury. *Br J Anaesth.* 2003;91(6):781–6.

63. Souter MJ, Andrews PJ, Alston RP. Propofol does not ameliorate cerebral venous oxyhemoglobin desaturation during hypothermic cardiopulmonary bypass. *Anesth Analg.* 1998;86(5):926–31.

64. Leslie K, Sessler DI, Bjorksten AR, Moayeri A. Mild hypothermia alters propofol pharmacokinetics and increases the duration of action of atracurium. *Anesth Analg.* 1995;80(5):1007–14.

65. Jakob SM, Ruokonen E, Grounds RM, Sarapohja T, Garratt C, Pocock SJ, et al. Dexmedetomidine vs midazolam or propofol for sedation during prolonged mechanical ventilation: two randomized controlled trials. *JAMA.* 2012;307(11):1151–60.

66. Ortega-Carnicer J, Benezet J, Calderon-Jimenez P, Yanes-Martin J. Hypothermia-induced Brugada-like electrocardiogram pattern. *J Electrocardiol.* 2008;41(6):690–2.

67. Urwin SC, Menon DK. Comparative tolerability of sedative agents in head-injured adults. *Drug Saf.* 2004;27(2):107–33.

68. Clegg A, Young JB. Which medications to avoid in people at risk of delirium: a systematic review. *Age Ageing.* 2011;40(1):23–9.

69. Korak-Leiter M, Likar R, Oher M, Trampitsch E, Ziervogel G, Levy JV, et al. Withdrawal following sufentanil/propofol and sufentanil/midazolam. Sedation in surgical ICU patients: correlation with central nervous parameters and endogenous opioids. Intensive Care Med. 2005;31(3):380–7.

70. Menon DK. Cerebral protection in severe brain injury: physiological determinants of outcome and their optimisation. Br Med Bull. 1999;55(1):226–58.

71. Fleischer JE, Milde JH, Moyer TP, Michenfelder JD. Cerebral effects of high-dose midazolam and subsequent reversal with Ro 15-1788 in dogs. Anesthesiology. 1988;68(2):234–42.

72. ter Horst HJ, Brouwer OF, Bos AF. Burst suppression on amplitude-integrated electroencephalogram may be induced by midazolam: a report on three cases. Acta Paediatr. 2004;93(4):559–63.

73. Jeevaratnam DR, Menon DK. Survey of intensive care of severely head injured patients in the United Kingdom. BMJ. 1996;312(7036):944–7.

74. Perez-Barcena J, Llompart-Pou JA, Homar J, Abadal JM, Raurich JM, Frontera G, et al. Pentobarbital versus thiopental in the treatment of refractory intracranial hypertension in patients with traumatic brain injury: a randomized controlled trial. Crit Care. 2008;12(4):R112.

75. Werz MA, Macdonald RL. Barbiturates decrease voltage-dependent calcium conductance of mouse neurons in dissociated cell culture. Mol Pharmacol. 1985;28(3):269–77.

76. Goodman JC, Valadka AB, Gopinath SP, Cormio M, Robertson CS. Lactate and excitatory amino acids measured by microdialysis are decreased by pentobarbital coma in head-injured patients. J Neurotrauma. 1996;13(10):549–56.

77. Kassell NF, Hitchon PW, Gerk MK, Sokoll MD, Hill TR. Alterations in cerebral blood flow, oxygen metabolism, and electrical activity produced by high dose sodium thiopental. Neurosurgery. 1980;7(6):598–603.

78. Warner DS, Takaoka S, Wu B, Ludwig PS, Pearlstein RD, Brinkhous AD, et al. Electroencephalographic burst suppression is not required to elicit maximal neuroprotection from pentobarbital in a rat model of focal cerebral ischemia. Anesthesiology. 1996;84(6):1475–84.

79. Roberts I, Sydenham E. Barbiturates for acute traumatic brain injury. Cochrane Database Syst Rev. 2012;12:CD000033.

80. Ropper AH. Hyperosmolar therapy for raised intracranial pressure. N Engl J Med. 2012;367(8):746–52.

81. Weed LH, McKibben PS. Pressure changes in the cerebrospinal fluid following intravenous injection of solutions of various concentrations. Am J Physiol. 1919;48:512–30.

82. Javid M, Settlage P. Effect of urea on cerebrospinal fluid pressure in human subjects; preliminary report. JAMA. 1956;160(11):943–9.

83. Patel N, Dalal P, Panesar M. Dialysis disequilibrium syndrome: a narrative review. Semin Dial. 2008;21(5):493–8.

84. Wakai A, McCabe A, Roberts I, Schierhout G. Mannitol for acute traumatic brain injury. Cochrane Database Syst Rev. 2013;8:CD001049.

85. Meyer MJ, Megyesi J, Meythaler J, Murie-Fernandez M, Aubut JA, Foley N, et al. Acute management of acquired brain injury part II: an evidence-based review of pharmacological interventions. Brain Inj. 2010;24(5):706–21.

86. Grande PO, Romner B. Osmotherapy in brain edema: a questionable therapy. J Neurosurg Anesthesiol. 2012;24(4):407–12.

87. Scalfani MT, Dhar R, Zazulia AR, Videen TO, Diringer MN. Effect of osmotic agents on regional cerebral blood flow in traumatic brain injury. J Crit Care. 2012;27(5):526 e7–12.

88. Diringer MN, Zazulia AR. Osmotic therapy: fact and fiction. Neurocrit Care. 2004;1(2):219–33.

89. Rangel-Castilla L, Gopinath S, Robertson CS. Management of intracranial hypertension. Neurol Clin. 2008;26(2):521–41.

90. Hartl R, Ghajar J, Hochleuthner H, Mauritz W. Hypertonic/hyperoncotic saline reliably reduces ICP in severely head-injured patients with intracranial hypertension. Acta Neurochir Suppl. 1997;70:126–9.

91. Mortazavi MM, Romeo AK, Deep A, Griessenauer CJ, Shoja MM, Tubbs RS, et al. Hypertonic saline for treating raised intracranial pressure: literature review with meta-analysis. J Neurosurg. 2012;116(1):210–21.

92. Schwarz S, Georgiadis D, Aschoff A, Schwab S. Effects of hypertonic (10%) saline in patients with raised intracranial pressure after stroke. Stroke. 2002;33(1):136–40.

93. Roquilly A, Mahe PJ, Latte DD, Loutrel O, Champin P, Di Falco C, et al. Continuous controlled-infusion of hypertonic saline solution in traumatic brain-injured patients: a 9-year retrospective study. Crit Care. 2011;15(5):R260.

94. Francony G, Fauvage B, Falcon D, Canet C, Dilou H, Lavagne P, et al. Equimolar doses of mannitol and hypertonic saline in the treatment of increased intracranial pressure. Crit Care Med. 2008;36(3):795–800.

95. Wu CT, Chen LC, Kuo CP, Ju DT, Borel CO, Cherng CH, et al. A comparison of 3% hypertonic saline and mannitol for brain relaxation during elective supratentorial brain tumor surgery. Anesth Analg. 2010;110(3):903–7.

96. Kamel H, Navi BB, Nakagawa K, Hemphill JC, 3rd, Ko NU. Hypertonic saline versus mannitol for the treatment of elevated intracranial pressure: a meta-analysis of randomized clinical trials. Crit Care Med. 2011;39(3):554–9.

97. Frank JI. Large hemispheric infarction, deterioration, and intracranial pressure. Neurology. 1995;45(7):1286–90.

98. Manno EM, Adams RE, Derdeyn CP, Powers WJ, Diringer MN. The effects of mannitol on cerebral edema after large hemispheric cerebral infarct. Neurology. 1999;52(3):583–7.

99. Muizelaar JP, van der Poel HG, Li ZC, Kontos HA, Levasseur JE. Pial arteriolar vessel diameter and CO2 reactivity during prolonged hyperventilation in the rabbit. J Neurosurg. 1988;69(6):923–7.

100. Bernard SA, Nguyen V, Cameron P, Masci K, Fitzgerald M, Cooper DJ, et al. Prehospital rapid sequence intubation improves functional outcome for patients with severe traumatic brain injury: a randomized controlled trial. Ann Surg. 2010;252(6):959–65.

101. Stocchetti N, Maas AI, Chieregato A, van der Plas AA. Hyperventilation in head injury: a review. Chest. 2005;127(5):1812–27.

102. Coles JP, Fryer TD, Coleman MR, Smielewski P, Gupta AK, Minhas PS, et al. Hyperventilation following head injury: effect on ischemic burden and cerebral oxidative metabolism. Crit Care Med. 2007;35(2):568–78.

103. Gupta AK, Hutchinson PJ, Al-Rawi P, Gupta S, Swart M, Kirkpatrick PJ, et al. Measuring brain tissue oxygenation compared with jugular venous oxygen saturation for monitoring cerebral oxygenation after traumatic brain injury. Anesth Analg. 1999;88(3):549–53.

104. Marion DW, Puccio A, Wisniewski SR, Kochanek P, Dixon CE, Bullian L, et al. Effect of hyperventilation on extracellular concentrations of glutamate, lactate, pyruvate, and local cerebral blood flow in patients with severe traumatic brain injury. Crit Care Med. 2002;30(12):2619–25.

105. Wei EP, Kontos HA, Patterson JL, Jr. Dependence of pial arteriolar response to hypercapnia on vessel size. Am J Physiol. 1980;238(5):697–703.

106. Edwards AD, Brocklehurst P, Gunn AJ, Halliday H, Juszczak E, Levene M, et al. Neurological outcomes at 18 months of age after moderate hypothermia for perinatal hypoxic ischaemic encephalopathy: synthesis and meta-analysis of trial data. BMJ. 2010;340:c363.

107. Rivera-Lara L, Zhang J, Muehlschlegel S. Therapeutic hypothermia for acute neurological injuries. Neurotherapeutics. 2012;9(1):73–86.

108. Peberdy MA, Callaway CW, Neumar RW, Geocadin RG, Zimmerman JL, Donnino M, et al. Part 9: post-cardiac arrest care: 2010 American Heart Association Guidelines for Cardiopulmonary Resuscitation and Emergency Cardiovascular Care. Circulation. 2010;122(18 Suppl 3):S768–86.

109. Schreckinger M, Marion DW. Contemporary management of traumatic intracranial hypertension: is there a role for therapeutic hypothermia? Neurocrit Care. 2009;11(3):427–36.

110. Nielsen N, Wetterslev J, Cronberg T, Erlinge D, Gasche Y, Hassager C, et al. Targeted temperature management at 33 degrees C versus 36 degrees C after cardiac arrest. N Engl J Med. 2013;369(23):2197–206.

111. Andrews PJ, Sinclair HL, Battison CG, Polderman KH, Citerio G, Mascia L, et al. European society of intensive care medicine study of therapeutic hypothermia (32–35 degrees C) for intracranial pressure reduction after traumatic brain injury (the Eurotherm3235Trial). *Trials*. 2011;12:8.

112. Suehiro E, Fujisawa H, Ito H, Ishikawa T, Maekawa T. Brain temperature modifies glutamate neurotoxicity in vivo. *J Neurotrauma*. 1999;16(4):285–97.

113. Globus MY, Alonso O, Dietrich WD, Busto R, Ginsberg MD. Glutamate release and free radical production following brain injury: effects of posttraumatic hypothermia. *J Neurochem*. 1995;65(4):1704–11.

114. Kimura A, Sakurada S, Ohkuni H, Todome Y, Kurata K. Moderate hypothermia delays proinflammatory cytokine production of human peripheral blood mononuclear cells. *Crit Care Med*. 2002;30(7):1499–502.

115. Aibiki M, Maekawa S, Ogura S, Kinoshita Y, Kawai N, Yokono S. Effect of moderate hypothermia on systemic and internal jugular plasma IL-6 levels after traumatic brain injury in humans. *J Neurotrauma*. 1999;16(3):225–32.

116. Smith SL, Hall ED. Mild pre- and posttraumatic hypothermia attenuates blood-brain barrier damage following controlled cortical impact injury in the rat. *J Neurotrauma*. 1996;13(1):1–9.

117. Jurkovich GJ, Pitt RM, Curreri PW, Granger DN. Hypothermia prevents increased capillary permeability following ischemia-reperfusion injury. *J Surg Res*. 1988;44(5):514–21.

118. Sydenham E, Roberts I, Alderson P. Hypothermia for traumatic head injury. *Cochrane Database Syst Rev*. 2009;2:CD001048.

119. Clifton GL, Valadka A, Zygun D, Coffey CS, Drever P, Fourwinds S, et al. Very early hypothermia induction in patients with severe brain injury (the National Acute Brain Injury Study: Hypothermia II): a randomised trial. *Lancet Neurol*. 2011;10(2):131–9.

120. Nemoto EM, Klementavicius R, Melick JA, Yonas H. Suppression of cerebral metabolic rate for oxygen (CMRO2) by mild hypothermia compared with thiopental. *J Neurosurg Anesthesiol*. 1996;8(1):52–9.

121. Peterson K, Carson S, Carney N. Hypothermia treatment for traumatic brain injury: a systematic review and meta-analysis. *J Neurotrauma*. 2008;25(1):62–71.

122. Lavinio A, Timofeev I, Nortje J, Outtrim J, Smielewski P, Gupta A, et al. Cerebrovascular reactivity during hypothermia and rewarming. *Br J Anaesth*. 2007;99(2):237–44.

123. Svyatets M, Tolani K, Zhang M, Tulman G, Charchaflieh J. Perioperative management of deep hypothermic circulatory arrest. *J Cardiothorac Vasc Anesth*. 2010;24(4):644–55.

124. Erecinska M, Thoresen M, Silver IA. Effects of hypothermia on energy metabolism in Mammalian central nervous system. *J Cereb Blood Flow Metab*. 2003;23(5):513–30.

125. Polderman KH, Herold I. Therapeutic hypothermia and controlled normothermia in the intensive care unit: practical considerations, side effects, and cooling methods. *Crit Care Med*. 2009;37(3):1101–20.

126. Polderman KH, Rijnsburger ER, Peerdeman SM, Girbes AR. Induction of hypothermia in patients with various types of neurologic injury with use of large volumes of ice-cold intravenous fluid. *Crit Care Med*. 2005;33(12):2744–51.

127. Finley Caulfield A, Rachabattula S, Eyngorn I, Hamilton SA, Kalimuthu R, Hsia AW, et al. A comparison of cooling techniques to treat cardiac arrest patients with hypothermia. *Stroke Res Treat*. 2011;2011:690506.

128. Simosa HF, Petersen DJ, Agarwal SK, Burke PA, Hirsch EF. Increased risk of deep venous thrombosis with endovascular cooling in patients with traumatic head injury. *Am Surg*. 2007;73(5):461–4.

129. Tomte O, Draegni T, Mangschau A, Jacobsen D, Auestad B, Sunde K. A comparison of intravascular and surface cooling techniques in comatose cardiac arrest survivors. *Crit Care Med*. 2011;39(3):443–9.

130. Bullock MR, Chesnut R, Ghajar J, Gordon D, Hartl R, Newell DW, et al. Surgical management of traumatic parenchymal lesions. *Neurosurgery*. 2006;58(3 Suppl):S25–46.

131. Mendelow AD, Gregson BA, Fernandes HM, Murray GD, Teasdale GM, Hope DT, et al. Early surgery versus initial conservative treatment in patients with spontaneous supratentorial intracerebral haematomas in the International Surgical Trial in Intracerebral Haemorrhage (STICH): a randomised trial. *Lancet*. 2005;365(9457):387–97.

132. Mendelow AD, Gregson BA, Mitchell PM, Murray GD, Rowan EN, Gholkar AR. Surgical trial in lobar intracerebral haemorrhage (STICH II) protocol. *Trials*. 2011;12:124.

133. Gregson BA, Rowan EN, Mitchell PM, Unterberg A, McColl EM, Chambers IR, et al. Surgical trial in traumatic intracerebral hemorrhage (STITCH(Trauma)): study protocol for a randomized controlled trial. *Trials*. 2012;13:193.

134. Mendelow AD, Gregson BA, Rowan EN, Francis R, McColl E, McNamee P, et al. Early Surgery versus Initial Conservative Treatment in Patients with Traumatic Intracerebral Hemorrhage (STITCH[Trauma]): the first randomized trial. *J Neurotrauma*. May 21 2015. [Epub ahead of print]

135. Li LM, Timofeev I, Czosnyka M, Hutchinson PJ. Review article: the surgical approach to the management of increased intracranial pressure after traumatic brain injury. *Anesth Analg*. 2010;111(3):736–48.

136. Hutchinson P, Timofeev I, Kirkpatrick P. Surgery for brain edema. *Neurosurg Focus*. 2007;22(5):E14.

137. Taylor A, Butt W, Rosenfeld J, Shann F, Ditchfield M, Lewis E, et al. A randomized trial of very early decompressive craniectomy in children with traumatic brain injury and sustained intracranial hypertension. *Childs Nerv Syst*. 2001;17(3):154–62.

138. Cooper DJ, Rosenfeld JV, Murray L, Arabi YM, Davies AR, D'Urso P, et al. Decompressive craniectomy in diffuse traumatic brain injury. *N Engl J Med*. 2011;364(16):1493–502.

139. Kolias AG, Hutchinson PJ, Menon DK, Manley GT, Gallagher CN, Servadei F. Letter to the Editor: Decompressive craniectomy for acute subdural hematomas. *J Neurosurg*. 2014;120(5):1247–9.

140. Hutchinson PJ, Corteen E, Czosnyka M, Mendelow AD, Menon DK, Mitchell P, et al. Decompressive craniectomy in traumatic brain injury: the randomized multicenter RESCUEicp study (www.RESCUEicp.com). *Acta Neurochir Suppl*. 2006;96:17–20.

141. Wijdicks EF, Sheth KN, Carter BS, Greer DM, Kasner SE, Kimberly WT, et al. Recommendations for the management of cerebral and cerebellar infarction with swelling: a statement for healthcare professionals from the American Heart Association/American Stroke Association. *Stroke*. 2014;45(4):1222–38.

142. Vahedi K, Hofmeijer J, Juettler E, Vicaut E, George B, Algra A, et al. Early decompressive surgery in malignant infarction of the middle cerebral artery: a pooled analysis of three randomised controlled trials. *Lancet Neurol*. 2007;6(3):215–22.

143. Kirkman MA, Citerio G, Smith M. The intensive care management of acute ischemic stroke: an overview. *Intensive Care Med*. 2014.

144. Juttler E, Schweickert S, Ringleb PA, Huttner HB, Kohrmann M, Aschoff A. Long-term outcome after surgical treatment for space-occupying cerebellar infarction: experience in 56 patients. *Stroke*. 2009;40(9):3060–6.

145. Adamo MA, Deshaies EM. Emergency decompressive craniectomy for fulminating infectious encephalitis. *J Neurosurg*. 2008;108(1):174–6.

146. Perez-Bovet J, Garcia-Armengol R, Buxo-Pujolras M, Lorite-Diaz N, Narvaez-Martinez Y, Caro-Cardera JL, et al. Decompressive craniectomy for encephalitis with brain herniation: case report and review of the literature. *Acta Neurochir (Wien)*. 2012;154(9):1717–24.

CHAPTER 8

Ethical and legal issues in neurocritical care

Leslie M. Whetstine, David W. Crippen, and W. Andrew Kofke

The place of bioethics in medicine generally, and neurocritical care in particular, has evolved over the past several decades, spurred at least in part by the extraordinary advances in life-supporting and life-sustaining technology. Nonetheless, bioethics as a discipline has maintained a consistent adherence to a core set of principles that include beneficence, nonmaleficence, autonomy, and justice (1).

1. *Beneficence* is the active obligation to remove harm when possible, promote welfare, and act in the best interest of the patient and of society at all times.

2. *Nonmaleficence* is the passive obligation to do no harm to a patient.

3. *Autonomy* is an individual's right to hold views and make choices according to their own values, so long as those actions don't impinge on the rights of others.

4. *Justice* is the provision of fair, equitable treatment in light of what is due or owed to persons.

The spectrum of bioethics is huge so this chapter will overview ethical and legal issues relevant to neurocritical care.

Ethical decision-making

The American College of Physicians' *Ethics Manual* provides an excellent overview of the major ethical issues in medicine (summarized in Table 8.1) and a structured approach to dealing with ethical dilemmas (2). Important elements of this approach are discussed in detail in the following sections.

The primary wishes of the patient

Ethical considerations always presuppose that the wishes of the patient are paramount and the primary driver in medical treatment decision-making (2). In coming to a treatment decision, the problem should first be framed within the relevant context, and then the physiological facts, medical uncertainties, benefits, and harms of various treatment options elucidated. In the course of this process a decision maker must be identified. For a competent patient this can only be the person themselves but for an incompetent patient the decision maker may be the primary caring clinician or a surrogate, depending on the jurisdiction. Clear and understandable information about treatment options and their likely outcome should be provided to the patient or their decision maker. In forming the treatment decision, it is crucial that the wishes and values of the patient are established, either from the patient themselves or their appointed surrogate. A health professional's values should never override those of a patient.

The concept of patient autonomy in decision-making based on provision of comprehensive information about the benefits and risks of treatment is illustrated by the 1914 Schloendorff case in the United States (Box 8.1) in which the judge found that a patient has a right to refuse medical intervention despite a physician's judgement that it is medically indicated (3). This ruling was fundamental in establishing the principle of informed consent. The right of competent patients to refuse any and all treatment, based on the right to self-determination and informed consent, is supported internationally. In the *Sidaway* v. *Bethlem Royal Hospital and Maudesley Hospital Health Authority* case in the United Kingdom, Lord Scarman ruled in 1985 (4):

> A doctor who operates without the consent of his patient is, save in cases of emergency or mental disability, guilty of the civil wrong of trespass to the person: he is also guilty of the criminal offence of assault. The existence of the patient's right to make his own decision, which may be seen as a basic human right protected by the common law, is the reason why a doctrine embodying a right of the patient to be informed of the risks of surgical treatment has been developed …

Doctor–patient relationship

Clinicians' obligations are to hold the welfare and best interests of their patients as the primary goal, even if there are conflicting personal, societal, or institutional pressures to make non-patient-centred decisions. Thus what is medically most appropriate for the patient always takes precedence over issues such as cost containment or bed triage. In countries where medical care is based on a fee for service, decisions regarding patient care should never include considerations of a patient's financial or social status, or clinician or institution compensation. Such principles are simply an extension of the notions of professionalism in which clinician self-interest is irrelevant.

The role of legal processes in clinical decision-making

Although case law can be useful in guiding difficult clinical decisions, law and ethics are not synonymous. Laws tend to be

Table 8.1 Major areas in bioethics

Major ethical category	Subtopics	
Professionalism		
Physician–patient relationship	Initiation and discontinuation	Obligations in healthcare system catastrophes
	Evaluations for a third party	Disability certification
	Confidentiality	Complementary/alternative care
	The medical record	Medical care to self, family, friends, VIPs
	Disclosure	Physician–patient sexual contact
	Reproduction decisions	Boundaries and privacy
	Genetic testing	Gifts from patients
	Medical risk to physician and patient	
Care of patients near the end of life	Making decisions	Futile treatments
	Advance care planning	Determination of death
	Withdrawing or withholding treatment	Physician-assisted suicide and euthanasia
	Artificial nutrition and hydration	Disorders of consciousness
	'Do-Not-Resuscitate' orders	Solid organ transplantation
Ethics of practice	Dealing with the changing practice environment	Financial conflicts of interest
	Financial arrangements with patients	Advertising
The physician and society	Obligations of the physician to society	Ethics committees
	Resource allocation	Medicine and the law
	Relation of physician to government	Expert witnesses
	Cross-cultural issues	Strikes and other joint actions by physicians
	Volunteerism	Futile care conflicts
Physician's relationship to other clinicians	Attending physicians and physicians in training	Peer review
	Consultation and shared care	Conflicts within a healthcare team
	The impaired physician	
Research	Protection of human subjects	Scientific publication
	Use of human biological materials	Sponsored research
	Placebo controls	Public announcement of research discoveries
	Innovative medical therapies	

Data from Snyder L, 'American College of Physicians Ethics Manual: sixth edition', *Annals of Internal Medicine*, 3, 156 (1 Pt 2), pp. 73–104.

prohibitive and tell us what not to do (e.g. don't kill), whereas ethics inform us about what we should do (e.g. act in the patient's best interests). Furthermore, ethical obligations often demand that we go beyond what the law requires. For example, whilst a young mother can legitimately refuse an appendicectomy because she doesn't want to live with a scar, one could make the ethical claim that exercising that legal right might violate the obligation of beneficence that she owes to her family. In this way the law informs ethics, rather than being the final arbiter of right and wrong.

Confidentiality

It is an ethical as well as a professional obligation to maintain confidentiality when providing medical care to a patient. This may be more difficult in the digital age when clinicians have little control over how clinical data are managed or stored. Moreover,

good medical care typically mandates electronic communications between physicians and other healthcare workers, and thus it is incumbent on institutions to develop infrastructures, such as firewalls and e-mail encryption systems, to facilitate communication whilst safeguarding privacy.

There are also work habits that can diminish the possibility of breaches of confidentiality such as not discussing patient information in public areas, using institutional rather than public communication tools, and not discussing the condition of any patient (including 'VIP' or celebrity patients) with individuals who are not approved by the patient.

Clinicians should also not assume that all family members and visitors are familiar with a patient's past medical history, and must never discuss this or new diagnoses with anyone not approved by the patient or their surrogate. Notably, physicians have no

Box 8.1 Schloendorff—issues in rights to self determination

Ms Schloendorff suffered from stomach problems and consented to exploratory surgery under ether to determine the nature of a lump that had been found on palpation. She clearly stated that she did not wish any surgery other than the exploration at that time. During the ether examination the doctor located and removed a large tumour despite the patient's previous instructions to the contrary.

In the court opinion, Justice Cardozo famously penned 'Every human being of adult years and sound mind has a right to determine what shall be done with his own body; and a surgeon who performs an operation without his patient's consent, commits an assault, for which he is liable in damages. This is true except in cases of emergency where the patient is unconscious and where it is necessary to operate before consent can be obtained'.

Data from Poland SC, 'Landmark Legal Cases in Bioethics'. Bioethical Issues: Scope Notes Archive; 1997' [cited 2014. Accessed January 16, 2014]; Available from: https://repository.library.georgetown.edu/bitstream/handle/10822/556889/sn33.pdf?sequence=1

obligation to keep secret from the sentient patient relevant information provided by family or friends, but must not provide a private, social context of a disease presentation to others without patient consent. For example, if a patient develops a stroke whilst in a sexual relationship with someone other than their spouse or partner, the clinician's duty of confidentiality remains to the patient and, assuming that they would wish this information to be kept private, informing the family of the circumstances of the disease onset is inappropriate.

Assessing capacity to provide informed consent

The notion of informed consent presupposes that consent be obtained and that it be informed, that is, that it is based on due consideration of the risks and benefits of a given choice or choices. This principle applies to both clinical activities and research involving human subjects. The process of procuring informed consent and the information provided to achieve that consent is extremely important and a physician must always provide information that is understandable to allow a reasoned decision to be made by the patient. Concurrently the physician must make an assessment of the patient's competence to understand and synthesize the issues into a cogent decision. Notably the consent needs to be freely given and not be coerced.

The capacity to make an informed decision is a judgement usually made by the physician, and is defined as *the ability to receive and express information and to make a choice consonant with that information and one's values* (2). Whilst seemingly straightforward, this assessment may not necessarily be so in critically ill neurological patients where the ability to receive, understand, and express information can be complicated by the underlying disease process. For example, a patient with a frontal lobe tumour might have impaired executive functioning, or an acutely quadriplegic patient might not consent to life-saving treatment because of clinical depression. In such difficult cases psychiatric assessment can be useful, and advice from local ethics committees, court, or other legal authorities may be required depending on local statutes.

Once a condition of incompetence has been determined a surrogate decision-maker must be identified. The process for this

Box 8.2 Howe—cannot legally remove a proxy in the United States

Ms Barbara Howe was a patient with a debilitating brain condition (amyotrophic lateral sclerosis) that left her 'locked in' and therefore unable to move or communicate. During her 4 years in this condition as an inpatient at Massachusetts General Hospital, there was disagreement between the attending physicians and her family regarding prognosis and patient comfort (81). The patient's daughter believed that her mother exhibited some recognition of her environment justifying continued aggressive intensive care, including mechanical ventilation. The physicians believed that there was no potential for improvement and that the patient was in perpetual distress. Complicating the situation, the patient's health insurance company served notice that it would cut off funding for her hospital services, on the basis that the patient was now receiving custodial care.

In March 2005, the hospital filed suit in Massachusetts family court to revoke Ms Howe's daughter as the patient's healthcare proxy. Probate and Family Court Judge John M. Smoot ruled that the daughter's authority as her mother's healthcare proxy should stand and that the hospital could not discontinue life support.

Data from Kowalczyk L, 'Woman dies at MGH after battle over care: daughter fought for life support', Boston Globe, 8 June 2005.

varies between jurisdictions. One widely accepted approach is to prioritize the identification of a surrogate decision maker in the following rank order—pre-designated proxy, spouse, adult children, parent, and other relative/friend. For an incompetent patient with no legally appointed surrogate, a decision maker may be appointed by the hospital or local legal authority depending on local laws and customs. In many jurisdictions, such as the United Kingdom, the clinician acts on the incompetent patient's behalf, informing relatives or friends of clinical decisions whilst seeking their agreement, rather than asking them to make them. In any event, it is important that surrogates understand that they are deciding what is in the patient's best interests, not what they would want for themselves. For example, a Jehovah's Witness surrogate cannot refuse blood transfusion in a non-Jehovah's Witness incompetent adult based on their own values. Concurrently the physician should be evaluating the capacity of the surrogate and also any potential conflicts, such as the surrogate receiving money that is contingent on the patient being alive or dead. In some jurisdictions it can be difficult to remove a legal proxy, as illustrated in the Howe case in the United States (Box 8.2), although this is not true everywhere.

In some jurisdictions, including the United States, a duly appointed surrogate retains the right to make treatment decisions on behalf of a patient in the long term. Further, even if the decisions of a proxy who has the patient's best interests in mind seem ill-considered to the healthcare team, such decisions may be supported by a court. This principle was exemplified by the Wanglie case (Box 8.3) in which a proxy's reliance on a miracle was legally supported. There is a contrasting approach in other jurisdictions. For example, the Canadian government Consent and Capacity boards can be asked to consider whether a designated decision-maker is making decisions in a patient's best interest and can order the proxy to make different decisions or even replace him or her (5). This board tends to rely heavily on the input of the local

Box 8.3 Wanglie—waiting for a miracle legally supported

In 1989, Helga Wanglie, aged 86, fractured her hip and was treated at Hennepin County Medical Center (HCMC) in Minneapolis, Minnesota (82). She was ultimately discharged to a nursing home. Subsequently, she developed respiratory failure and became ventilator dependent for several months but experienced cardiopulmonary arrest, with severe and irreversible anoxic brain injury. Her husband resisted an ethics committee recommendation to limit life support, and requested that Mrs Wanglie be transferred back to HCMC for continued life support. This was done.

Over the next several months, repeated evaluations confirmed that Mrs Wanglie was in a persistent vegetative state (PVS) and ventilator dependent. The medical staff considered her to be moribund. However, the immediate family insisted that all forms of treatment be continued, though they did agree to a do-not-resuscitate order. Some of the family's desires were based on the patient's strong religious background ('only God can decide'). There was no living will or specific discussion of end-of-life desires.

On 8 February 1991, the hospital filed papers with the Fourth Judicial District Court, Hennepin County, asking the court to find Mr Wanglie incompetent to speak for his wife and to appoint an independent guardian, who presumably would permit unilateral withdrawal of the ventilator against the family's wishes.

The court ruled that Mr Wanglie was 'the most suitable and best qualified person', from among the available potential guardians, to serve as guardian for his wife. The court decided the case strictly as a guardianship matter and did not address the appropriateness of treatment (83). In essence this judgment determined that an individual who knows the patient and his or her value system can better approximate the patient's wishes regarding end-of-life decisions than can healthcare providers.

Data from Jecker NS and Schneiderman LJ, 'When families request that "everything possible" be done', *Journal of Medicine and Philosophy*, 1995, 20, 2, pp. 145–163; and Cantor NL, 'Can healthcare providers obtain judicial intervention against surrogates who demand "medically inappropriate" life support for incompetent patients?', *Critical Care Medicine*, 1996, 24, 5, pp. 883–887.

clinical team. An overview of international norms confirms that the arrangements in the United States are not universal and that the surrogate's decision in the Wanglie case would have been overturned or the surrogate replaced in other jurisdictions (6).

Care of patients near the end of their lives

Consumer demand for healthcare resources has been and will continue to be a political as well as a social issue. Wellness has always been a high priority, and populations have gone to great lengths to achieve it. In antiquity, little was known about the physiological processes of the human body that led to or away from wellness so the demand for wellness produced many questionable manipulations. Ancient Egyptian medicine was mentioned in Homer's *Odyssey* around 700 BC (7), bloodletting, the oldest known medical procedure, was a treatment for virtually any ill until the early nineteenth century (8), and trephining, the oldest form of surgery involving

drilling a hole in the skull to allow egress of bad 'humours', was widely practised (9). Demand for these and many other counterintuitive medical treatments demonstrate the public's willingness and determination to seek wellness through any means, including those with no convincing evidence of efficacy. Modern medicine offers new technologies that appear to promise (falsely) near immortality.

The introduction of life-sustaining technologies and the growth of bioethics

The advent of life-support technology and intensive care units (ICUs) in the 1950s radically altered the course of medicine and introduced a new and complex set of ethical issues (10). Prior to these advancements there were relatively few bedside ethical dilemmas with respect to end-of-life care, resource allocation, medical futility, or surrogate decision-making but, after their introduction, accurately prognosticating which patients would actually benefit from complex life-supporting interventions became important although difficult. This lead to carte blanch treatment with little consideration or discussion about what would happen to patients who might survive but not recover a reasonable quality of life. The yield of such a strategy ultimately becomes apparent in an individual but, by that point, patients have often been treated with various life-supporting measures, including mechanical ventilation, dialysis, enteral feeding tubes, and even recurrent rounds of cardiopulmonary resuscitation (CPR). Death is too often perceived as the enemy of modern medicine and doctors sometimes see it as their ultimate failure. Technology has become regarded as an imperative despite the 'life-in-death' prospect it often creates (11).

As a result of technological advances, the following questions have become increasingly pervasive in the ICU:

1. Should patients be able to refuse, or be refused, artificial life support even if death will result?

2. If patients are not competent to decide whether or not to refuse life-supporting treatments, who should be enabled to decide for them?

3. What is the role of medical professionals in this process?

4. What should be done if the patient is not terminally ill but unlikely to regain functional independence to a degree that it is acceptable to them?

As advances in technology and medical care forced such questions, the nascent field of bioethics grew in earnest (12).

In the early days after the introduction of life-sustaining technologies, there was significant concern in some jurisdictions that removal of life support could be regarded as murder such that it could not be forgone no matter how little benefit or how much suffering it might cause. Indeed, for a time in the United States, hotline phone numbers were posted in neonatal ICUs inviting notification to authorities that life support was about to be withdrawn from a patient (13). However, as societal and medical attitudes evolved, a consensus on the legitimacy of forgoing (withholding or withdrawing) life-supporting treatment gradually emerged. This shift was advanced by case law, and evaluated through philosophical and theological enquiry.

The criminality and civil liability of withdrawing life support was tested in the Barber case in the United States (Box 8.4) (14) and the Bland case in the United Kingdom (Box 8.5) (15). Both legal decisions determined that withdrawal of life-supporting treatment (WLST) must be viewed in terms of benefits and burdens. If there

Box 8.4 Barber—non-criminality of terminating life support

The Quinlan decision (Box 8.11) authorized a surrogate to speak on behalf of the patient, but it was unclear whether physicians would be free legally to abide by wishes regarding termination of life support. In 1983, *Barber* v. *Superior Court* clarified the potential for criminality following removal of life support. Two California physicians performed surgery on a patient, who experienced cardiopulmonary arrest postoperatively and was rendered persistently vegetative. The patient was placed on a mechanical ventilator and enterally fed, and physicians determined that the vegetative state would most likely be permanent. Upon request of the patient's family, the physicians removed the artificial life-support systems, and the patient died several days later.

The surgeons were charged with murder by the state of California and went to trial. The court held that the actions of the defendants did not volitionally cause harm and that withdrawal of life support constituted further appropriate medical care. The court held that the physicians were not liable in their actions stating that 'Further treatment would be considered disproportionate to any positive outcome' (14).

Data from Compton J. Barber v. Superior Court (People) (1983) 147 Cal. App. 3d 1006 [195 Cal. Rptr. 484]. 1983 [cited 2012 November 27, 2012]; Available from: http://law.justia.com/cases/california/calapp3d/147/1006.html

is a reasonable chance of recovery, the benefits of therapy will outweigh the burdens but when there is no such chance of recovery, life support can be defined as extraordinary. The Barber and Bland decisions held that doctors could honour requests to discontinue

Box 8.5 Bland—stopping nutrition for an incompetent patient

Anthony Bland sustained an anoxic injury at age 17 years and had survived for 3 years in a PVS with life supported entirely through artificial enteral nutrition (15). He had no advance directive and had not expressed his wishes for such a circumstance. Both his physicians and his parents believed that stopping support was in the patient's best interests but there were uncertain regarding the criminality of such an act. They thus petitioned the UK courts for an opinion on the matter, and the court agreed that removing such support was legal finding that the physicians:

1. 'may lawfully discontinue all life-sustaining treatment and medical supportive measures designed to keep the defendant alive in his existing persistent vegetative state including the termination of ventilation nutrition and hydration by artificial means'; and

2. 'may lawfully discontinue and thereafter need not furnish medical treatment to the defendant except for the sole purpose of enabling him to end his life and die peacefully with the greatest dignity and the least of pain suffering and distress'.

Data from United_Kingdom_House_of_Lords. Airedale NHS Trust (Respondents) v. Bland (acting by his Guardian ad Litem) (Appellant). 1993 [cited 2013 November 15, 2013]; Available from: http://www.bailii.org/uk/cases/UKHL/1992/5.html

extraordinary life support without being guilty of homicide or subject to civil liability.

Ethics is of course not a by-product of modernity but has permeated medicine since its inception. The Hippocratic oath has long served as the enchiridion for practitioners instructed by the primary precept *primum non nocere*—first do no harm. However, the medical culture of Hippocrates and subsequent physicians was one dominated by paternalism even well into the twentieth century. Patients were expected to abide by doctors' orders under the pretence that 'doctor knows best'. Bioethicist Robert Veatch refers to this tendency for doctors to want to make decisions for patients as the generalization of expertise (16). Because doctors are experts in medicine they may also regard themselves as authorities in all spheres of medical decision-making for all patients, despite the unique differences that individuals have with respect to their expectations of treatment goals and interpretation of quality of life. Such philosophical conundrums spawned an international dialogue on the rights of patients (17). The differences of opinion that emerged between healthcare consumers and providers eventually led to involvement of legal systems for the purpose of primary guidance and finally to legal mandates with respect to forgoing treatment (18).

Withholding and withdrawing treatment

To forgo treatment means either to withhold a treatment before it is started or to withdraw a treatment after it has been started. While ethics and the law traditionally regard withholding and withdrawing as equivalent actions, withdrawing therapy tends to be more difficult for families and sometimes even for clinicians (19). When treatment is withdrawn the patient typically dies, leaving the uneasy feeling that those who withdrew the treatment caused the death or were somehow complicit in it. On the other hand, if a treatment could never be withdrawn, patients might reasonably decline potentially beneficial treatment for fear of being reliant on long-term life-support. Time trials are often necessary to determine whether a treatment will be effective in a given individual, meaning that judgements cannot always be made in advance but often only sometime after life-supporting therapy has been implemented when prognosis becomes clearer. Thus, by regarding withholding and withdrawing as ethically equivalent options, patients or surrogates are able to reassess care goals and plans as time progresses.

Neurocritical care encompasses a significant element of care to patients who are near the end of life, mandating therapies directed to control of distressing symptoms and concurrent empathic physical, psychological, and spiritual support. Such treatment can only be decided after review of the patient's condition in the light of the likelihood and quality of survival and in association with consideration of the suffering that may be incurred in achieving such outcomes. Decisions are typically made in the context of the patient's values and previous known wishes (written or verbal), perceptions of the nature of the terminal illness, and understanding of the logical equivalence of not starting versus withdrawing support at a later time.

Principle of double effect

Though not without debate, there has long been a distinction between killing a patient versus allowing a patient to die (20). The law, as well as the dominant Judeo-Christian ethical framework in the Western world, does not regard forgoing burdensome medical treatment as an act of suicide or killing, a distinction rooted in Catholic tradition and buttressed by the principle of double effect (PDE). This construct, attributed to Thomas Aquinas, asks whether it is morally legitimate to perform an act that has two or more consequences, one of which is good and rightly intended and another that is bad but unintended (21). Although the PDE has its origins in a faith tradition, it is also used in secular philosophical analysis most clearly illustrated in palliative care where it is considered an ethical obligation to alleviate pain and discomfort during the dying process (22). In this context, the PDE justifies the actions of a clinician who administers increasing doses of morphine knowing that this may hasten death, provided the intent is only to relieve pain. Although there are many critics of the PDE (23), its application is pervasive in both medicine and law.

The PDE was referenced by the US Supreme Court in its 1997 ruling on physician-assisted suicide in the case of *Vacco* v. *Quill* (24). The court held that there is a fundamental difference between directly causing death and removing life support that allows a patient to die of a natural disease process. The opinion concludes:

> The distinction comports with fundamental legal principles of causation and intent. First, when a patient refuses life sustaining medical treatment, he dies from an underlying fatal disease or pathology; but if a patient ingests lethal medication prescribed by a physician, he is killed by that medication. (25)

When a competent patient refuses treatment or determines that the treatment creates burdens disproportionate to benefits, forgoing interventions is therefore regarded as allowing the patient to die rather than an act of killing. Accordingly it is licit for technology that is prolonging the natural dying process to be removed so that a patient can die from their underlying disease, whereas killing a patient is wrong because the patient dies as a result of an intentional act. The latter is often categorized as euthanasia and is currently deemed a violation of ethics and the law in nearly all countries except Belgium, Luxembourg, the Netherlands, Albania, and Colombia (26). Some argue that the end result of these two processes is identical despite verbal gymnastics to obscure that fact (27). That is, the patient will ultimately die whether he or she dies because of their underlying disease or by an overdose of medication, or whether the physician intends death or not. These arguments raise particularly thorny problems, but the distinction remains despite such disagreement.

Futile care

The usual definition of futile treatment is that which is not effective in bringing about a desired therapeutic goal (28). For example, if a patient demands craniotomy to allow evil humours to escape from their brain, physicians are not mandated to perform the procedure because it is not effective at any level and may in fact be deleterious. Medically futile treatments need not, and ought not, to be given because they violate overarching standards of care. This position is supported by UK and New Zealand legal opinions (4). Moreover, several international professional societies have argued that medically futile treatment is unethical as well as inappropriate. These include the Italian Society of Anaesthesia, Analgesia, Resuscitation and Intensive Care (29), the American Medical Association (30,31), the American Society of Critical Care Medicine (32), and the UK General Medical Council (33).

The situation is unsettled in the United States where the patient or proxy can often successfully demand futile or unreasonable treatments. Under current US definitions, any treatment that sustains vital signs is not necessarily considered futile because a therapeutic goal, that is, maintenance of life, can be achieved (34). Thus, if a surrogate demands dialysis for acute kidney injury in a

100-year-old terminally ill patient with dementia who can never improve under any circumstances, a physician cannot claim medical futility and unilaterally refuse treatment. However, the situation in the United States is slowly shifting. Since 1999, Texas law allows physicians to discontinue extraordinary life-sustaining treatment against the objections of the family if such treatment is determined to be medically futile, this is agreed by an ethics committee and the family is given ten days to seek another hospital that will treat the patient. Virginia law is similar but the law in California law is vague, invoking 'generally accepted health care standards'. Ethicists in many other states have not lobbied for a Texas-style law because of the philosophical difficulties associated with defining futile care and the expected opposition from right-to-life advocates. This is despite the American Medical Association's code of ethics supporting the notion that futile treatment should not be provided, even if demanded by a patient or surrogate (30,31). At the time of writing, case law in the United States continues to be piecemeal and there is no overriding legal precedent one way or the other.

Requests by surrogates to provide or continue support in the context of futile care creates myriad conflicts within families, and with caregivers, institutions, and legal authorities. The complexity of the interplay between medical, social, religious, and family factors may lead to requests to 'do everything possible' or advice that 'we are waiting for a miracle', rather than to a decision to withdraw life support congruent with medical advice. The desire to continue inappropriate or futile care based on an expected miracle has been upheld in the United States (Box 8.3), but in similar circumstances in Canada it is likely that the surrogate would have been overruled or replaced (5). In the United Kingdom, as illustrated in the Bland case (Box 8.5), the courts have determined that there is no requirement to provide futile care.

The expectations of the public for the delivery of futile and inappropriate care are international. In one study, 73% of Israeli and European ICUs frequently admitted patients with no realistic hope of survival despite only 33% of treating physicians believing that such patients should have been admitted (35). The dominant causes of moral distress reported by ICU nurses in this study were the requirement to deliver futile care, unsuccessful patient advocacy and difficulties with communication of unrealistic prospects to patients and families. More recently, 87% of 114 Canadian ICU physician directors reported that futile care was provided in their ICU, and 48% of ICU patients supported the provision of open-ended care regardless of the chances for good recovery (36). As discussed later in the chapter, diminishing resources mean that this is not just an issue of ethics, but also of economics and distributive justice.

Advance directives and surrogate decision makers

A recurring theme in the neurocritical care unit (NCCU) is the difficulty in determining the wishes and desires of patients who do not have capacity to make decisions. As discussed earlier, a surrogate decision maker (sometimes called a proxy) is charged with making decisions on behalf of a patient who cannot speak on their own behalf. Ideally the surrogate should make the same decision the patient would make but, since most people do not explicitly state their medical preferences in advance, the surrogate is typically placed in the position of having to interpret general statements that may not directly pertain to the current medical condition or status. People have an understandable tendency to avoid topics that force consideration of personal debility and, when they do, often use terms like 'I don't want to live like a vegetable' rather than providing clear guidance on which surrogates and clinicians could act. Nonetheless, advanced planning is becoming more common and allows an individual to indicate care preferences and identify a surrogate decision maker ahead of time. Although advance directives, or living wills, are legal documents they should ideally be created with advice from medical professionals. Failure to do so can result in medically naive documents that, for example, forbid intubation under any circumstance including during elective surgery. Physicians should routinely discuss care issues and expectations when patients are competent and institutions should routinely enquire about the availability of advance directives and offer assistance in creating one on admission to hospital. Lack of availability of an a priori designated surrogate should prompt a search (including via social media) for a proxy and failing that it may be necessary to appoint a guardian, according to local regulations. In some jurisdictions the physician becomes the surrogate by default.

Common law has long protected a competent patient's right to refuse medical treatment, but what should be done regarding end-of-life care in an incompetent person if he or she has not previously indicated their wishes is less clear. Whilst a surrogate must make some kind of choice, the criteria by which they should do so is seldom apparent. In the Cruzan case (Box 8.6), the court held that requiring clear and convincing evidence of the incompetent patient's wishes is constitutional and that if such evidence is presented, withdrawal of life support is lawful (37). This position is supported in the Bland case in the United Kingdom and by case law in New Zealand and South Africa (15).

The Cruzan case proved to be pivotal in the battleground between right-to-life and right-to-die advocates, all of whom

developed progressive interest in using the legal system to bolster their causes (38–40). A spokesperson for the Society for the Right to Die publicly noted:

> While it's been a horrible agony for the Cruzans, having intimate private details on the public stage, and having to defend themselves, we owe them a debt for educating us and giving so much impetus to living wills and legislation that helps people plan ahead. (41)

The leader of a Georgia antiabortion group disagreed noting:

> I sympathize with the hardship of caring for a helpless woman, but I have no sympathy for a family who solves their problems by starving their daughter to death when there were hundreds of bona fide offers to care for her regardless of her condition. Even a dog in Missouri cannot be legally starved to death. (41)

The Cruzan action also reinforced the value of advance directives in avoiding intra-family differences of opinion and even court battles (42). If it can be proved that an incompetent patient has given an authoritative opinion as to the direction of his or her medical care, this is clear and convincing evidence that trumps differing opinions of surrogates or even a court. However, in the absence of an advance directive providing clarity regarding a patient's values and preferences, decisions should be made in the patient's best interests, informed by a family member or surrogate best acquainted with the patient.

Even with advance directives and prior statements as to wishes, disagreements and concerns over their interpretation continue to lead to legal proceedings. The 2001 California case of Robert Wendland (Box 8.7) (43) illustrates the problems that arise when surrogates are forced to rely on general statements made by the patient, and when family members disagree as to what such statements actually mean.

Another example of family disagreement and court involvement is the case of Terri Schiavo (Box 8.8), a patient in a persistent vegetative state (PVS) whose family disagreed about her wishes in the absence of an advance directive. This case confirmed that surrogates are able to speak on behalf of a patient but confirmed that their judgement is less authoritative than that of a competent patient. Clearly this brings particular difficulty when there is family disagreement. While a competent patient can refuse treatment, even beneficial treatment, a surrogate must never act contrary to a patient's best interest. Notably in the United Kingdom, physicians have no duty to provide futile care despite family or patient wishes to the contrary (15), and this is now a common position in many other countries.

Advance directives are not a panacea and do not always dictate a clear course of action. This is illustrated by the 1987 *Evans* v. *Bellevue* case (Box 8.9) which found that while a competent patient's refusal of treatment is protected, a surrogate will likely be held to a higher standard such that ambiguity usually results in a decision to support life (44).

Surrogate decision-making on behalf of patients who are not legally competent because of their age (e.g. children), or due to certain medical conditions (e.g. learning difficulties, developmental disabilities, or dementia) pose particular problems. Surrogates should still use the best interest standard of decision-making, assessing the burdens and benefits of treatment from a hypothetical 'reasonable person standard' to the extent that this is possible (45). The supposition is that reasonable people would, on balance, refuse treatments that carry greater risks or burdens than potential benefits, but would accept those that offer benefit without obviously

---

Box 8.6 Cruzan—requirement to know patient's wishes prior to withdrawing care, the case for advance directives

The 1990 Nancy Cruzan case was the first of many similar cases to reach the US Supreme Court, where it would finally cohere sporadic case law regarding incompetent patients and the right to refuse treatment (41). Ms Cruzan was a young woman who was involved in a motor vehicle accident that resulted in a PVS. Physicians inserted a long-term feeding tube. After an extended delay, the patient's parents requested that the feeding tube be removed so that she could die naturally. The hospital refused to do so without approval from the state court.

The US Supreme Court ultimately held that, whereas autonomous individuals may invoke the right to refuse medical treatment under the 'due process of law' clause, surrogates for incompetent persons are not enabled to exercise such rights until they satisfy the burden of proof required by the state. Missouri (where Ms Cruzan's injury occurred) required 'clear and convincing' evidence of the patient's wishes before life support could be removed. The US Supreme Court held that states had the right to select and enforce their evidentiary standard (84).

Data from Lewin T, 'Nancy Cruzan dies, outlived by a debate over the right to die', *New York Times*, December 27, 1990 [cited 2012 November 27, 2012]; Available from: http://www.nytimes.com/1990/12/27/us/nancy-cruzan-dies-outlived-by-a-debate-over-the-right-to-die.html; and Arnold RM and Kellum J, 'Moral justifications for surrogate decision making in the intensive care unit: Implications and limitations', *Critical Care Medicine*, 2003, 31, Suppl 5, pp. S347–S353.

Box 8.7 Wendland—family disagreement as to patient's wishes with minimal consciousness

Robert Wendland suffered a traumatic brain injury during a motor vehicle accident in 1993. Ultimately he was diagnosed in a minimally conscious state where he could follow some simple commands (he could grab a block, for example) but was profoundly cognitively and physically disabled, unable to communicate, and could not perform any activities of daily living. He was sustained by artificial nutrition and hydration (ANH). Over a period of 2 years Wendland repeatedly pulled the feeding tube out until his wife requested it not be reinserted. His wife and children contended that Wendland was unable to recognize himself or others and that he would find this quality of life objectionable based on previous declarations he had made. Wendland's wife argued that he was clear in his previous wishes, declaring that if he couldn't be 'a father, husband, or a provider', or if he was 'ever in a diaper', he would refuse treatment. Wendland did not have advance directives granting his wife authority to make medical decisions for him, and problems arose when Wendland's mother disagreed with his wife's decision.

After 6 years of court proceedings, the California Supreme Court ultimately ruled that Wendland's wife could forgo ANH if she presented clear and convincing evidence of his wishes, or if she could establish that forgoing ANH was in his best interests. The court held that Wendland's general declarations were too vague and that his wife would have to provide 'an exact on all fours account of his wishes' before the ANH could be removed. In other words, Mr Wendland would have to have predicted his current situation and specifically proscribed it. Phrases like 'not wanting to live like a vegetable' were found to be too general and unpersuasive.

This ruling only applied to conscious, non-terminally ill patients. It can be assumed that if Wendland had been in a PVS the court may well have decided differently. Since he was not permanently unconscious, and because it was determined that he should be afforded greater protection as an incompetent person, the court ruled that his wife could not forgo ANH. Wendland died from pneumonia during the legal battle (43).

Data from Nelson LJ and Cranford RE, 'Michael Martin and Robert Wendland: beyond the vegetative state', *The Journal of Contemporary Health Law and Policy*, 1999, 15, 2, pp. 427–453.

Box 8.8 Schiavo—family disagreement as to a patient's wishes with persistent vegetative state

In 1990, Terry Schiavo experienced a cardiac arrest of unknown aetiology and entered a PVS (40,41). During the subsequent months, computed tomography brain scans showed severe atrophy of the cerebral hemispheres, and electroencephalograms were flat, indicating no functional activity of the cerebral cortex.

Her husband and her paternal family vehemently disagreed about what types of medical treatment Ms Schiavo would want in her current situation (42). The patient's husband was considered her legal guardian under Florida law, which designates the spouse as the decision maker if the patient has not previously specified another decision maker. The paternal family however did not accept the diagnosis of PVS, insisting that Ms Schiavo could improve with continued rehabilitation. They also objected to the 'starvation' that would result from withdrawal of feeding. Advised by physicians that there would be no improvement, the husband requested that ANH be stopped.

Ms Schiavo had no advance directive, though her husband maintained that she had spoken about not wanting to be sustained artificially if there was no hope of recovery. Her parents disagreed with the husband, and the situation escalated to intense public and media support of one side or the other by multiple special interest groups. The issue quickly spilled into court. Ultimately, after years of political manipulation and court investigation, the patient's husband wishes prevailed and Ms Schiavo's feeding tube was removed. She died shortly thereafter. Autopsy revealed that her brain anatomy was incompatible with cortical activity consistent with awareness of her environment (43).

Data from various sources (see References).

(Box 8.10) (3). The Saikewicz case represents a scenario in which the guardian of an institutionalized individual with severe learning difficulties and an inability to communicate refused treatment on his behalf based on what would traditionally be deemed to be 'best interests'. The guardian considered the burdens of chemotherapy

causing pain and suffering. However, jurisdictions vary in the authority of a proxy to agree to WLSTs because any surrogate, be it a family member or appointed guardian, may have some conflicts in their ability to make end-of-life decisions no matter how well intended their motives. The issue with an appointed guardian not permitted to give permission for WLST in the United States was illustrated in the Tschumy case in 2012 (46).

Surrogate decision-making involves making judgements about quality of life for others. This is inherently suspect because quality of life is fundamentally a subjective concept and discussions about medical interventions cannot be considered without evaluating their effect on quality of life. The goal is to assess quality of life by objectively examining benefits and burdens of treatment without making social worth judgements about individuals. The case of Joseph Saikewicz illustrates how this concept is used clinically

---

Box 8.9 Wirth—ambiguous advance directive with a potentially reversible condition

Tom Wirth was a 47-year-old patient diagnosed with aids-related complex (ARC) and suffering from probable toxoplasmosis which was causing lesions in his brain. Wirth was unable to communicate his wishes but had executed a living will stating: 'I direct that life sustaining procedures should be withheld or withdrawn if I have illness, disease, or injury or experience extreme mental deterioration, such that there is no reasonable expectation of recovering or regaining a meaningful quality of life.'

Wirth also had a durable power of attorney (DPA) authorized to make treatment decisions on his behalf. The court ruled that there was sufficient ambiguity in the living will, however, to prevent the DPA from forgoing treatment because, although the patient was terminally ill, he was only temporarily incapacitated since toxoplasmosis was reversible.

Box 8.10 Saikewicz—best interests of a mentally disabled patient in refusing chemotherapy for new-onset malignancy

In 1976, Joseph Saikewicz was a 67-year-old man who had been institutionalized for more than 50 years. He was profoundly cognitively and physically disabled and interacted only by grunts and gestures. Saikewicz developed leukaemia that, if treated aggressively with chemotherapy, could result in a temporary 2–13 months of remission, although this was less likely in a patient older than 60. The question was whether Saikewicz would have to undergo treatment or if a guardian could refuse on his behalf despite his never having been competent.

The court ruled that Saikewicz had the right to refuse treatment grounded in his fundamental right to privacy and informed consent. This ruling was curious because the notion that Saikewicz could have refused or consented was a fiction because he never had decisional capacity. However, the standards of surrogate decision-making had yet to be clearly defined, so the court was navigating in uncharted territory (3).

Data from Poland SC, 'Landmark Legal Cases in Bioethics Bioethical Issues: Scope Notes Archive 1997' [cited 2014 Accessed January 16, 2014]; Available from: https://repository.library.georgetown.edu/bitstream/handle/10822/556889/sn33.pdf?sequence=1

Box 8.11 Quinlan—stopping ventilator support for an incompetent patient

The 1976 case of Karen Ann Quinlan was the first major dispute to centre on an incompetent patient's right to refuse treatment (85). Ms Quinlan was diagnosed as being in a PVS after mixing drugs and alcohol. She was mechanically ventilated and fed enterally. Eventually, her family requested that the mechanical ventilator be removed and she be allowed to die naturally. The physicians refused to comply, expecting death would follow and that this death would be attributed to those who removed the support modalities. The family sued to force the issue.

A New Jersey appellate court held that the government had an interest in maintaining the 'sanctity of life' and that removing life support (however artificial) was tantamount to criminal homicide. The New Jersey Supreme Court eventually heard the case, and held that Ms Quinlan's father, as a surrogate, was the authoritative decision maker with the incompetent patient's best interests in mind (86). Accordingly, Ms Quinlan was removed from the ventilator, but she did not die until 9 years later because she unexpectedly breathed and continued to receive artificial nutrition.

Data from Hughes CJ, 'In the matter of Karen Quinlan, an alleged incompetent', 70 N.J. 10; 355 A.2d 647; 1976 N.J. LEXIS 181; 79 A.L.R.3d. 1976 March 31, 1976 [cited 2014 February 5, 2014]; Available from: http://euthanasia.procon.org/sourcefiles/In_Re_Quinlan.pdf; and Kennedy IM, 'Focus: current issues in medical ethics. The Karen Quinlan case: problems and proposals', *Journal of Medical Ethics*, 1976, 2, 1, pp. 3–7.

(many) with the benefits (few) and advised that the treatment be forgone. Importantly, this recommendation was not made because the patient was disabled but because the means to attaining (an unlikely) temporary remission would have been cruel and inhumane. This case determined that it is possible to use the best interest standard to make decisions for individuals who have never expressed a preference regarding treatment, and for those who have never had such decisional capacity.

Inevitably there are times when physicians disagree with a surrogate's interpretation of burdens and benefits and a stalemate occurs, increasing the pressure for legal resolution. A surrogate's reasoning may be based on unrealistic expectations in any circumstance but may be particularly associated with certain religions. For example, Islam and Judaism do not support withdrawal of care (47), nor do some religious and cultural traditions in India (48). While refusal of the clinical team to follow what they believe to be unrealistic surrogate decisions may be impossible in some countries, it is supported in others such as South Africa (49), Canada (5), and Germany (50). In the United States, three professional critical care societies support a shared-decision model, believing that this can minimize intractable disagreements, but do not support the notion that physicians are the ultimate decision makers (51).

Limitations of care

Although withdrawing and withholding care are equivalent from an ethical perspective, there is legal variation in different jurisdictions. In the United Kingdom, the concept that medical treatment can lawfully be withdrawn was articulated by Lord Browne-Wilkinson in the Bland case (Box 8.5) (15). Such rulings mean that treatment must never be withheld based on the notion that it cannot be withdrawn. One of the early legal precedents supporting the practice of limitation of care in an incompetent patient was the Quinlan case described in Box 8.11.

Full supportive treatment is usually indicated initially after admission to the NCCU because it is often impossible to accurately prognosticate early after an acute neurological event and families often need time to come to terms with an event that has a likely poor prognosis. Thus it is common for discussions and decisions to limit or withdraw care to occur over several days, allowing time for family updates and education about likely outcomes. When decisions to limit treatment are made they generally fall along a continuum:

a. Do everything except CPR.

b. Specific treatment limitations including vasoactive drugs, dialysis, intubation, ventilator support, antibiotics, and dialysis.

c. Withdrawal of all life-supporting therapies and provision of comfort care only.

Each institution must develop its own protocols and nomenclature consistent with local laws, culture, and regulations. Often a 'Do Not Resuscitate' order, or some similar descriptor, is applied to indicate where on the continuum of care limitation the patient resides. Notably, anything that constitutes support is subject to withdrawal, following the principle of allowing a disease process to run its natural course. Such support includes not only ventilator and haemodynamic support, but also antibiotics, fluids, and, in some specific circumstances and in certain jurisdictions, nutrition (see 'Limitation of Artificial Nutrition and Hydration').

Once a decision has been made to move to comfort care, organ donation should be considered prior to withdrawal of life-sustaining therapies (see Chapter 30).

Limitation of artificial nutrition and hydration

As noted earlier, the outcome of critically ill neurological patients is often uncertain in the acute phase and it may be difficult to limit care early in the course of an illness. However, this is the period during which removing ventilation and haemodynamic support is most likely to lead to death. When treatment is continued for a period of time to allow better assessment of prognosis, the patient may become more stable and therefore less dependent on ventilator or haemodynamic support. Thus 'early' withdrawal of support after acute brain injury is likely to result in more rapid death, lower risk of survival with severe disability, and a lower societal burden, although at the risk of greater uncertainty about prognosis and insufficient time for considered decisions by surrogates (52). Conversely, delayed withdrawal is associated with less uncertainty about prognosis and more time for surrogates to come to terms with the prognosis, but at the risk of a prolonged dying process and a higher risk of survival with severe disability. At this stage, nutrition and hydration may be the only remaining life-support measures in place and their cessation is ethical if it is clear that the patient would not wish to survive with the likely level of disability and quality of life. However, removal of hydration and nutrition inevitably results in a longer period before death ensues and there are concerns about discomfort in sentient patients. Together, these considerations have fuelled many disagreements regarding this aspect of end-of-life care, and forgoing enteral and parenteral nutrition is contentious.

Artificial nutrition and hydration are rightly considered life-supporting therapies in patients who are unable to seek and ingest food and water independently. They are therefore logically no different than any other form of intensive care support in that they may both benefit and harm a patient. Very often, and understandably, surrogate decision makers may not grasp or accept this concept and are uncomfortable withholding such therapy. The US Supreme Court established in 1990 that artificial nutrition and hydration are medical treatments and can removed in the same way as any other treatment intervention (see Box 8.6), though this concept has been challenged. Additionally, the Brophy (Box 8.12) and Bland (Box 8.5) cases confirmed the legitimacy of removing artificial nutrition and hydration in vegetative patients (15). There is broad international legal support for this practice including in the United States, United Kingdom, New Zealand, and South Africa (53), although in the United Kingdom the General Medical Council, based on case law, recommends seeking a judicial order when contemplating stopping nutrition (33).

Organ donation

As well as being in a patient's best interests, withdrawal of life support may lead to a positive outcome for others in the form of organ donation. In a brain-dead organ donor the ethical issues are relatively straightforward because the patient is pronounced dead based on neurological criteria prior to consideration of organ donation. Given the critical need for organs and a growing shortage of donors, donation after circulatory death (DCD) is playing an increasingly important role (see Chapter 30) (54). In the NCCU, controlled DCD is possible following a decision to WLST when death is predicted to occur within a relatively short timescale, usually 60 or 120 minutes after treatment withdrawal. In such circumstances, death is declared following cardiac arrest using the usual cardiorespiratory criteria of irreversible cessation of circulatory and respiratory functions.

DCD is now widely practised in a number of countries despite continued controversy in many. The main point of contention is whether the usual cardiorespiratory criteria are adequate to

---

Box 8.12 Brophy—stopping nutrition for an incompetent patient

The Paul Brophy case extended the Quinlan ruling (3). Mr Brophy experienced a ruptured cerebral aneurysm on 22 March 1983, resulting in a PVS. A percutaneous gastrostomy tube was placed, through which he was fed and hydrated. After months of no improvement, the patient's wife requested that the feeding tube be removed and her husband be allowed to die naturally. Mr Brophy's physicians refused to withdraw the tube because they believed that doing so was euthanasia, and the matter went to court.

Ultimately, the Massachusetts Supreme Judicial Court authorized Mr Brophy's wife to transfer him to a facility that would honour her wishes. This ruling was based on evidence that Mr Brophy had previously expressed a wish that he did not want to be maintained on artificial life support should he ever require it. The Brophy case was the first case in the United States in which courts authorized a patient in PVS to die following the withdrawal of artificially supplied nutrition and hydration.

Data from Poland SC, 'Landmark Legal Cases in Bioethics Bioethical Issues: Scope Notes Archive 1997' [cited 2014 Accessed January 16, 2014]; Available from: https://repository.library.georgetown.edu/bitstream/handle/10822/556889/sn33.pdf?sequence=1

---

determine death when the need for speed is paramount but the integrity of the 'dead donor rule' (DDR) must be maintained. Additional issues relate to the use of medications or interventions that preserve organ function but offer no benefit to, and/or may potentially harm, the donor or whether the delays that are inherent in withdrawing treatment to allow identification of potential recipients and mobilization of the retrieval team are reasonable.

The dead donor rule and autoresuscitation

The DDR stipulates that patients cannot be killed for or by the removal of organs for donation (55). Much attention has been given to the minimum period of continuous cardiorespiratory arrest that is sufficient to permit the diagnosis of death and indicate the point at which organ retrieval might begin without breaching the DDR. A review of the continuous observation of asystole, apnoea, and unresponsiveness concluded that a period of no less than 2 minutes and no more than 5 minutes of observation is adequate to allow the confirmation of death (56). Thus a minimum period of 5 minutes of continuous cardiorespiratory arrest prior to the start of organ retrieval has been recommended in the United Kingdom (57), Canada (58), and the United States (59), and 10 minutes or longer in some parts of Europe (60).

Despite such evidence, some critics argue that DCD violates the DDR and that donors may be dying but not yet dead when organs are retrieved (61). This argument is based entirely on the perceived risk of spontaneous resumption of cardiac function sometime after the onset of apparently irreversible asystole, the so-called Lazarus phenomenon or autoresuscitation. The anxiety is that autoresuscitation might result in a (partial) return of neurological function. Critics of DCD point out that autoresuscitation is a poorly understood phenomenon that has not been sufficiently studied and that it cannot be guaranteed that it will not occur within 5 minutes after asystole. They argue that removing organs during a period of time in which a patient could spontaneously resume circulation would be considered homicide. A recent review identified 32 reported cases of autoresuscitation all after failed CPR, with times ranging from a few seconds to 33 minutes (62). The continuity of observation and methods of monitoring were highly inconsistent between reports but, in the eight studies reporting continuous electrocardiogram (ECG) monitoring and exact times, autoresuscitation did not occur beyond 7 minutes after failed CPR. In the absence of CPR, as in the context of controlled DCD after WLST, autoresuscitation has not been reported. Further, it is important to recognize that the time for return of circulation in reports of autoresuscitation is the time after asystole at which the circulation was noticed to have returned spontaneously. This is quite different to the specific recommendations for the confirmation of death by cardiorespiratory criteria cited earlier which require a period of 5 minutes of continuous observation for asystole, apnoea, and unresponsiveness before death can be confirmed (57,58). Any spontaneous return of cardiac or respiratory activity during this period should prompt a further 5-minute observation from the next point of cardiorespiratory arrest. Clinical observation should be supplemented with continuous ECG and intra-arterial blood pressure monitoring during WLST on the NCCU. Given such restrictions, the possibility of a spontaneous recovery of functional cardiac activity appears remote in the extreme, and has not been reported (62).

Determining when someone is 'irreversibly' dead is fundamental to the ethical and legal delivery of controlled DCD. Critics continue to argue that death cannot be declared with certainty because it is not an instant event but a process, and that intervening in the process would mistake a dying patient for a dead one (63). Advocates of controlled DCD argue that because resuscitation is proscribed as part of WLST a patient could not possibly be resuscitated because it would be a violation of their wishes to do so. On the other hand, opponents counter that this confuses respect for an ethical norm with the reality of a clinical situation. Ethically and legally a patient cannot be assaulted with life support if refused or deemed not in their best interests but this does not change the empirical reality that one cannot be dead faster just because resuscitation is refused or organ donation is a possibility. Critics point out that we do not routinely regard people as dead 5 minutes after cessation of spontaneous circulation otherwise we would never attempt CPR.

Interventions to benefit the recipient

The processes of warm and cold ischaemia threaten the viability of potentially transplantable organs. Cold ischaemia is minimized by virological screening and tissue typing of the potential donor prior to death, thereby allowing early identification of potential recipients and the earliest possible transplantation. While this requires additional ante-mortem blood sampling, it is supported in most jurisdictions with the informed agreement of the patient's next of kin. To minimize warm ischaemia it is necessary as a minimum to maintain the potential donor on the current level of cardiorespiratory support until the retrieval team is mobilized and ready in the operating theatre to begin the retrieval process.

Ante-mortem medications such as heparin or phentolamine are sometimes recommended in DCD protocols to optimize potentially transplantable organ function. The US Institute of Medicine recommends that these be considered on a case-by-case basis rather than as a blanket policy (64). In the United Kingdom, the Donation Ethics Committee advises that interventions aimed solely at maintaining or optimizing organ function are ethically acceptable providing they do not cause harm or distress (65). Thus heparin would be contraindicated in a patient with an intracranial haemorrhage.

None of the interventions necessary to facilitate controlled DCD, even the prolongation of current levels of cardiorespiratory support until the retrieval team is mobilized, are easy to accommodate under a narrow interpretation of 'best interests'. It is difficult to see how continued treatment can be in a patient's physical interests if such treatment has already been judged to be futile. However, if the best interest concept is extended to include the broader wishes and aspirations of a patient, an indication that they would wish to donate their organs after death, such as through registration with a national donation registry or discussion with the next of kin, can be interpreted by clinicians as authorization to take reasonable steps to facilitate donation (65). Such an approach is in line with other aspects of healthcare delivery where the best interests concepts is not limited to best 'medical' interests, but incorporates the patient's wishes and beliefs when competent, and their spiritual and religious welfare.

While not relevant to NCCU practice, there is a specific issue relating to uncontrolled DCD that is worthy of mention. This is the use of extracorporeal membrane oxygenation (ECMO) to preserve organ function during confirmation of the suitability for donation (66,67). Some DCD protocols, notably in Spain, restore vital organ perfusion after death is confirmed but avoid brain perfusion by placement of a balloon catheter to occlude blood flow to the brain (66). Despite myriad plausible ethical concerns, the Barcelona protocol receives widespread public support in Spain, one of the countries with the highest rates of organ donation anywhere in the world. However, reproducing this level of success and introducing ECMO as a routine to facilitate uncontrolled DCD are unlikely to be straightforward in other countries. It is also likely to be prohibitively expensive.

Allocation of resources for critical care

All of the ethical issues discussed so far in this chapter converge at the interface between quality of care and resource constraint. Significant international disparities in mores and financial resources have created a variety of approaches to the ethical issues that are raised by limited healthcare resources. The reader is referred elsewhere for a detailed discussion of these issues (6).

Crippen sampled global attitudes about ICU resource allocation by surveying online subscribers to the Critical Care Medicine List, an international multidisciplinary group of nearly 1000 critical care providers from 12 countries in five continents (68). Nearly all countries surveyed sustain a 'closed' economic system in which there is a finite amount of money to spend on healthcare and most or all citizens are indemnified against the cost of illness. In general terms, healthcare costs are capped in such systems so nations must prioritize resources. Invariably, this means not offering some treatments or interventions with a poor benefit/expense ratio to allow general services to be financed for the entire population.

The one country that stands out from the rest of the world is the United States where the healthcare system indemnifies only a portion of its population at great expense and runs on a 'customer satisfaction' maxim. Facing the prospect of unlimited expenses, third-party reimbursers (insurance companies) ration implicitly (i.e. without public debate) by denying payment on technicalities after services have been rendered or through a pre-certification process that can limit care deemed appropriate by treating physicians.

In times of financial constraint, or in the face of high levels of healthcare inflation as is now the norm, healthcare systems are expected to do more with less. Healthcare services around the world are therefore caught between the immovable object of diminishing resources and the seemingly irresistible force of increasing demand. Distributive justice refers to societal and individual duty to individuals in need (69). In the context of constrained resources, including in healthcare systems, it can involve withholding resources with little benefit to society or individuals, or redirecting them to benefit more individuals. Thus decisions may have to be made that limit expensive but futile care for a few in favour of providing care that benefits many. Such political and societal decisions are enormously complex.

Healthcare rationing

Healthcare rationing has become a reality in critical care because of national resource allocation systems that limit the availability of ICU beds or, in reimbursement-driven healthcare systems, because insurers and hospitals limit access to expensive therapies. Kerz reviewed rationing of healthcare and reported that German intensivists conflicted by societal versus patient pressure had occasionally limited therapy that they believed had poor risk–benefit for a patient without disclosing this to the individual (50,70). Similar implicit rationing has been reported in the United Kingdom (71), Canada (5), New Zealand (72), South Africa (49), Switzerland (70), and Norway (70). In Italy, Law 229 established the general principles of healthcare, including equality of access to quality care and assurance of dignity, but also, and perhaps paradoxically, the need for savings in resource utilization (29). Within this context, ICU bed availability in Italy is a form of implicit economic rationing, and limiting treatment is a relatively common occurrence and has even been suggested as a quality metric.

Although decisions to ration healthcare are ultimately politically driven, politicians tend to refrain from pursuing policies on explicit rationing as too controversial and likely to threaten their own political aspirations. Political reticence to grapple publicly with these important issues is an international phenomenon that has been reviewed elsewhere (70). The National Institute for Health and Care Excellence in the United Kingdom, which approves drugs and treatments based on efficacy and cost-effectiveness, is an example of national explicit rationing that appears to receive public and clinical support (71). In the United States, attempts to control end-of-life costs led to opponents creating the spectre of 'death panels', thus stalling any attempt to develop an explicitly discussed rationing policy.

Limiting inappropriate admission to intensive care units

One element of limiting inappropriate or futile care is the development and enforcement of explicit ICU admission and discharge criteria. The Italian Society of Anaesthesia, Analgesia, Resuscitation and Intensive Care developed guidelines outlining the clinical appropriateness of admission to an ICU that include the presence of an acute but reversible pathology, a reasonable likelihood of benefit from intensive care taking likely treatment costs into account, and a reasonable expectation that the acute critical illness will resolve as a result of the provision of intensive care (29). Although other nations have promulgated similar guidance (49,72), there are notably difficulties with uniform implementation of policies to limit ICU admission primarily related to disparate local laws and culture. Further, different recommendations within an individual country add to these difficulties. For example, the Society of Critical Care Medicine in the United States recommends giving admission priority to patients most likely to benefit from ICU care (73), whereas the American Thoracic Society recommends admission on a first come, first served basis (51).

Limiting futile care

Although many patients and surrogates opt for palliative care when it becomes clear that technology cannot cure but will only protract the dying process, an increasing number have an unrealistic understanding and expectation of what ICU interventions can actually accomplish (74). There are several reasons why patients and surrogates may demand care that is deemed inappropriate (if not futile) by physicians. First, although withholding and withdrawing life support are regarded as equivalent in law and medical ethics, patients and surrogates often view them as starkly different. Second, the Internet and popular media have become the new resource for families seeking more optimistic opinions but often promulgate poorly authenticated opinions from pseudo-experts. Third, the ethical principle of autonomy is increasingly cited as justification for interventions based on a belief that any chance for life is better than no chance.

Many of the issues of limitations of healthcare resources have not been addressed because they are either sociopolitically too volatile or arouse the interests of too many special interest groups to permit consensus. For example, although many publications and focus groups extol communication as a way to persuade surrogates to accept limitation of care decisions in the interests of individuals and sometimes society more broadly, virtually all stop short of supporting refusal by physicians of providing inappropriate or futile care (75). Further, physicians do not have an admirable track record of predicting death so there is always the potential for unexpected survival. Reporting of such cases is often widespread and surrogates cite such reports as reasons for continuing care. Saying no to an intervention, such as ICU admission, can be seen by some as synonymous with hastening death and a way to save money. There is also an increasingly held view that healthcare 'consumers' have a right to access as many resources as they need or wish and that in developed nations society must underwrite that care no matter the cost.

Making best use of intensive care resources

Intensive care is the most expensive resource in a hospital and its provision is complicated by limited healthcare resources, particularly after a global financial crisis that is directly affecting the delivery of healthcare worldwide (76). It is undisputed that the daily cost of maintaining a patient in a critical care bed is already high and will continue to rise (77), or that healthcare systems will become untenable if inappropriate care, including inappropriate admission to ICU, is provided on demand (78).

One way to limit waste of healthcare resources (including intensive care) on those who cannot conceivably gain benefit is to establish objective limits on its provision based on accumulating global databases that can accurately predict outcome and therefore define outcome futility on the basis of objective bedside physiological data and premorbid status. Based on these considerations, Crippen explored the creation of a system that would maintain the cost-effectiveness and affordability of healthcare by prioritizing and thus rationing healthcare resources by refusing them (79).

In this model, demonstrated effectiveness of particular treatments would be recorded in a world clinical database and providers would consult this in order to prioritize treatment for an individual. Such databases would be made accessible electronically and, when based on outcome data of many thousands of patients with a similar condition, used to inform a decision to withhold treatment on outcome futility grounds. Such an arrangement would involve saying no to a treatment or intervention, such as admission to an ICU, which would be expensive out of proportion to its benefit. Although such a plan is employed in Rie's Oregonian ICU, those with sufficient personal funds are empowered to authorize and personally pay for whatever futile care they desire (80), a situation that would be unacceptable in many other countries. It seems certain that many of the concepts espoused in a cost-effectiveness assessment, however it is delivered, are likely to become elements of health systems worldwide.

References

1. Beauchamp T, Childress J. *Principles of Biomedical Ethics*. London: Oxford; 1994.
2. Snyder L. American College of Physicians Ethics Manual: sixth edition. *Ann Intern Med*. 2012;156(1 Pt 2):73–104.
3. Poland SC. Landmark legal cases in bioethics. *Bioethical Issues: Scope Notes 33*; 1997. [Online] https://repository.library.georgetown.edu/bitstream/handle/10822/556889/sn33.pdf?sequence=1
4. *United Kingdom House of Lords. Sidaway (A.P.) (Appellant) v. Bethlem Royal Hospital and the Maudesley Hospital Health Authority and Others (Respondents)*. [1985] http://www.bailii.org/uk/cases/UKHL/1985/1html
5. Wax R. Canada: where are we going? In Crippen D (ed) *ICU Resource Allocation in the New Millennium Will We Say No?* New York: Springer; 2013:123–9.
6. Crippen D. *ICU Resource Allocation in the New Millennium. Will We Say No?* New York: Springer; 2013.
7. Fadl A. *Comparison Between Egyptian and Medieval Medicine*. Aldokkancom; 2012. [Online] http://www.aldokkan.com/science/medicine.htm
8. Seigworth GR. Bloodletting over the centuries. *N Y State J Med*. 1980;80(13):2022–8.
9. Phisick. *Ancient Skulls Ancient Skills*. Phisick; 2012 [Online] http://phisick.com/article/an-abc-of-craniotomy/ancient-skulls-ancient-skills/
10. Luce JM, White DB. A history of ethics and law in the intensive care unit. *Crit Care Clin*. 2009;25(1):221–37.
11. Dickinson GE, Pearson AA. Death education in selected medical schools as related to physicians' attitudes and reactions toward dying patients. *Annu Conf Res Med Educ*. 1977;16:31–6.
12. Wanzer SH, Adelstein SJ, Cranford RE, Federman DD, Hook ED, Moertel CG, et al. The physician's responsibility toward hopelessly ill patients. *N Engl J Med*. 1984;310(15):955–9.
13. White M. The end at the beginning. *Ochsner J*. 2011;11(4):309–16.
14. *Compton J. Barber v. Superior Court (People) (1983)* 147 Cal. App. 3d 1006 [195 Cal. Rptr. 484]. [http://law.justia.com/cases/california/calapp3d/147/1006.html]
15. *United Kingdom House of Lords. Airedale NHS Trust (Respondents) v. Bland (acting by his Guardian ad Litem) (Appellant)*. [1993] http://www.bailii.org/uk/cases/UKHL/1992/5.html
16. Institute of Society Ethics and the Life Sciences. *Values, Expertise, and Responsibility in the Life Sciences*. Hastings-on-Hudson, NY: Institute of Society, Ethics and the Life Sciences; 1973.
17. Goold SD, Williams B, Arnold RM. Conflicts regarding decisions to limit treatment: a differential diagnosis. *JAMA*. 2000;283(7):909–14.
18. Luce JM, Alpers A. End-of-life care: what do the American courts say? *Crit Care Med*. 2001;29(2 Suppl.):N40–N5.
19. Slomka J. The negotiation of death: clinical decision making at the end of life. *Soc Sci Med*. 1992;35(3):251–9.
20. Kelly D. *Medical Care at the End of Life: A Catholic Perspective*. Washington, DC: Georgetown University Press; 2006.
21. Boyle JM Jr. Toward understanding the principle of double effect. *Ethics*. 1980;90(4):527–38.
22. Luce JM, Alpers A. Legal aspects of withholding and withdrawing life support from critically ill patients in the United States and providing palliative care to them. *Am J Respir Crit Care Med*. 2000;162(6):2029–32.
23. McIntyre A. Doing away with double effect. *Ethics*. 2001;111(2):219–55.
24. Lyons E. In incognito: the principle of double effect in American constitutional law. *Fla Law Rev*. 2005;57(3):469–563.
25. *Rehnquist CJ. Dennis C. VACCO, Attorney General of New York, et al., Petitioners, v. Timothy E. QUILL et al.* 521 U.S. 793117 S.Ct. 2293138 L.Ed.2d 834 [1997].
26. Sulmasy DP. Killing and allowing to die: another look. *J Law Med Ethics*. 1998;26(1):55–64.
27. Rachels J. Active and passive euthanasia. *N Engl J Med*. 1975;292(2):78–80.
28. Luce JM. Physicians do not have a responsibility to provide futile or unreasonable care if a patient or family insists. *Crit Care Med*. 1995;23(4):760–6.
29. Luchetti M, Marraro GA. Italy: where have we been? In Crippen D (ed) *ICU Resource Allocation in the New Millennium Will We Say No?* New York: Springer; 2013:47–57.
30. Burnett LB. Second critique of Buchman and Chalfin's analysis. In Crippen D (ed) *ICU Resource Allocation in the New Millennium Will We Say No?* New York: Springer; 2013:217–26.
31. American Medical Association. *Opinion 2.035—Futile Care. AMA Policy on End-of-Life Care*. American Medical Association; 1994. [Online] https://www.ama-assn.org/ama/pub/physician-resources/medical-ethics/code-medical-ethics/opinion2035.page
32. Truog RD, Campbell ML, Curtis JR, Haas CE, Luce JM, Rubenfeld GD, et al. Recommendations for end-of-life care in the intensive care unit: a consensus statement by the American College of Critical Care Medicine. *Crit Care Med*. 2008;36(3):953–63.
33. General Medical Council. *Treatment and Care Towards the End of Life: Good Practice in Decision Making*. General Medical Council; 2010. [Online] http://www.gmc-uk.org/static/documents/content/End_of_life_9_May_2013.pdf
34. Crippen D. Medical treatment for the terminally ill: the 'risk of unacceptable badness'. *Crit Care*. 2005;9(4):317–18.
35. Piers RD, Azoulay E, Ricou B, DeKeyser Ganz F, Decruyenaere J, Max A, et al. Perceptions of appropriateness of care among European and Israeli intensive care unit nurses and physicians. *JAMA*. 2011;306(24):2694–703.
36. Palda VA, Bowman KW, McLean RF, Chapman MG. "Futile" care: Do we provide it? Why? A semistructured, Canada-wide survey of intensive care unit doctors and nurses. *J Crit Care*. 2005;20(3):207–13.
37. Colby WH. Cruzan: clear and convincing? Missouri stands alone. *Hastings Cent Rep*. 1990;20(5):5–6.
38. WFRTDS. *World Federation of Right to Die Societies* website. 1980. [Online] http://www.worldrtd.net
39. NLRC. *National Right to Life* website. 1968. [Online] http://www.nrlc.org
40. NDY. *Not Dead Yet. The Resistance*; 2014. [Online] http://www.notdeadyet.org
41. Lewin T. Nancy Cruzan dies, outlived by a debate over the right to die. *N Y Times*. 1990;27 December. http://www.nytimes.com/1990/12/27/us/nancy-cruzan-dies-outlived-by-a-debate-over-the-right-to-die.html
42. Silveira MJ, Kim SYH, Langa KM. Advance directives and outcomes of surrogate decision making before death. *N Engl J Med*. 2010;362(13):1211–18.

43. Nelson LJ, Cranford RE. Michael Martin and Robert Wendland: beyond the vegetative state. *J Contemp Health Law Policy.* 1999;15(2):427–53.

44. Di Somma AV. Evans v. Bellevue Hospital. *Issues Law Med.* 1988;4(2):235–8.

45. Kopelman LM. The best interests standard for incompetent or incapacitated persons of all ages. *J Law Med Ethics.* 2007;35(1):187–96.

46. Simons A. Guardians can't end life support, judge rules. *Minneapolis Star Tribune.* 2012;18 October.

47. Segal E. Israel: where have we been? In Crippen D (ed) *ICU Resource Allocation in the New Millenium.* New York: Springer; 2013:39–45.

48. Kofke WA, Sharma D. Predicting survival in NeuroICU patients. *J Neurosurg Anesthesiol.* 2011;23(3):177–8.

49. Hodgson E, Hardcastle TC. South Africa: where have we been? In Crippen D (ed) *ICU Resource Allocation in the New Millennium Will We Say No?* New York: Springer; 2013:75–87.

50. Kerz T. Germany: where are we going? In Crippen D (ed) *ICU Resource Allocation in the New Millennium Will We Say No?* New York: Springer; 2013:131–8.

51. Sprung CL. Third critique of Buchman and Chalfin's analysis. In Crippen D (ed) *ICU Resource Allocation in the New Millennium Will We Say No?* New York: Springer; 2013:227–34.

52. Smith M. Treatment withdrawal and acute brain injury: an integral part of care. *Anaesthesia.* 2012;67(9):941–5.

53. Norton Rose Fulbright. *Euthanasia and Patient's Right to Refuse Treatment.* Norton Rose Fulbright; 2010. [Online] http://www.nortonrosefulbright.com/knowledge/publications/44188/euthanasia-and-patients-right-to-refuse-treatment

54. Kootstra G, Daemen JHC, Oomen APA. Categories of non-heart-beating donors. *Transplant Proc.* 1995;27(5):2893–4.

55. Truog RD, Miller FG, Halpern SD. The dead-donor rule and the future of organ donation. *N Engl J Med.* 2013;369(14):1287–9.

56. Ethics Committee. Recommendations for nonheartbeating organ donation. A position paper by the Ethics Committee, American College of Critical Care Medicine, Society of Critical Care Medicine. *Crit Care Med.* 2001;29(9):1826–31.

57. Department of Health and Academy of Royal Medical Colleges. *A Code of Practice for the Diagnosis of Death.* London: Department of Health and Academy of Royal Medical Colleges; 2007. http://www.aomrc.org.uk/

58. The Canadian Council for Donation and Transplantation. *Donation after Cardiocirculatory Death: A Canadian Forum.* The Canadian Council for Donation and Transplantation; 2005. [Online] http://www.organsandtissues.ca/s/wp-content/uploads/2011/11/Donation-Cardiocirculatory-Death-English.pdf

59. Committee on Non-Heart-Beating Transplantation II. *Non-Heart-Beating Organ Transplantation: Practice and Protocols.* Washington, DC: The National Academies Press; 2000.

60. Domínguez-Gil B, Haase-Kromwijk B, Van Leiden H, Neuberger J, Coene L, Morel P, et al. Current situation of donation after circulatory death in European countries. *Transplant Int.* 2011;24(7):676–86.

61. Marquis D. Are DCD donors dead? *Hastings Cent Rep.* 2010;40(3):24–31.

62. Hornby K, Hornby L, Shemie SD. A systematic review of autoresuscitation after cardiac arrest. *Crit Care Med.* 2010;38(5):1246–53.

63. Whetstine L, Streat S, Darwin M, Crippen D. Pro/con ethics debate: when is dead really dead? *Crit Care.* 2005;9(6):538–42.

64. Potts JT, Herdman R, Institute of Medicine. *Non-Heart-Beating Organ Transplantation: Medical and Ethical Issues in Procurement.* Washington DC: National Academies Press; 1998.

65. UK Donation Ethics Committee. *An Ethical Framework for Controlled Donation after Circulatory Death.* Academy of Medical Royal Colleges; 2011. [Online] http://www.aomrc.org.uk/doc_download/9322-an-ethical-framework-for-controlled-donation-after-circulatory-death

66. Fondevila C, Hessheimer AJ, Flores E, Ruiz A, Mestres N, Calatayud D, et al. Applicability and results of Maastricht type 2 donation after cardiac death liver transplantation. *Am J Transplant.* 2012;12(1):162–70.

67. Marchan SJG, Meneu-Diaz JC, Elola-Olaso A, Perez-Saborido B, Yiliam F, Calvo A, et al. Liver transplantation using uncontrolled non-heart-beating donors under normothermic extracorporeal membrane oxygenation. *Liver Transplant.* 2009;15(9):1110–8.

68. Crippen D. CCM-L. BMJ 2004;328:1180

69. Lamont J, Favor C. Distributive justice. In Zalta EN (ed) *The Stanford Encyclopedia of Philosophy* (Spring 2013 edn). [Online] http://plato.stanford.edu/archives/spr2013/entries/justice-distributive/

70. Kerz T. Germany: where have we been? In Crippen D (ed) *ICU Resource Allocation in the New Millennium Will We Say No?* New York: Springer; 2013:25–31.

71. Batchelor AM. United Kingdom: where have we been? In Crippen D (ed) *ICU Resource Allocation in the New Millennium Will We Say No?* New York: Springer; 2013:89–96.

72. Streat S. New Zealand: where have we been? In Crippen D (ed) *ICU Resource Allocation in the New Millennium: Will We Say No?* New York: Springer; 2013:65–73.

73. ACCM. Guidelines for ICU admission, discharge, and triage. *Crit Care Med.* 1999;27(3):633–8.

74. Crippen D. *End-of-Life Communication in the ICU.* New York: Springer; 2008.

75. Lynn J, Teno JM, Phillips RS, Wu AW, Desbiens N, Harrold J, et al. Perceptions by family members of the dying experience of older and seriously ill patients. *Ann Internal Med.* 1997;126(2):97–106.

76. Lim C, Sander T. Does misery love company? Civic engagement in economic hard times. *Soc Sci Res.* 2013;42(1):14–30.

77. Luce JM, Rubenfeld GD. Can health care costs be reduced by limiting intensive care at the end of life? *Am J Resp Crit Care Med.* 2002;165(6):750–4.

78. Obama B. Securing the future of American health care. *N Engl J Med.* 2012;367(15):1377–81.

79. Crippen D. The Fair and Equitable Health Care Act. In Crippen D (ed) *ICU Resource Allocation in the New Millennium Will We Say No?* New York: Springer; 2013:247–50.

80. Rie MA. The Oregonian ICU: multitiered monetarized morality in health insurance law. *J Law Med Ethics.* 1995;23(2):149–66.

81. Kowalczyk L. Woman dies at MGH after battle over care: daughter fought for life support. *Boston Globe.* 2005;8 June.

82. Jecker NS, Schneiderman LJ. When families request that 'everything possible' be done. *J Med Philos.* 1995;20(2):145–63.

83. Cantor NL. Can healthcare providers obtain judicial intervention against surrogates who demand "medically inappropriate" life support for incompetent patients? *Crit Care Med.* 1996;24(5):883–7.

84. Arnold RM, Kellum J. Moral justifications for surrogate decision making in the intensive care unit: implications and limitations. *Crit Care Med.* 2003;31(5 Suppl.):S347–S53.

85. Hughes CJ. *In the Matter of Karen Quinlan, an Alleged Incompetent. 70 N.J. 10; 355 A.2d 647; 1976 N.J. Lexis 181; 79 A.L.R.3d.* 1976; 31 March. [Online] http://euthanasia.procon.org/sourcefiles/In_Re_Quinlan.pdf

86. Kennedy IM. Focus: current issues in medical ethics. The Karen Quinlan case: problems and proposals. *J Med Ethics.* 1976;2(1):3–7.

CHAPTER 9

Intracranial pressure monitoring

Federico Villa and Giuseppe Citerio

Intracranial pressure (ICP) is defined as the pressure exerted inside the dura mater onto the brain tissue by external forces, such as those caused by cerebrospinal fluid (CSF) and blood. Historically, ICP is synonymous with CSF pressure and is defined as the pressure exerted against a needle introduced into the CSF space to just prevent escape of fluid (1). In the adult, approximately 87% of the intracranial volume is occupied by the brain, 9% by CSF in the ventricles, cisterns, and subarachnoid space, and 4% by blood. In normal conditions, these volumes, encased within the dura mater, produce a low pressure that is reflected throughout the central nervous system (CNS).

Conventionally, the normal mean ICP in adults is 5–10 mmHg (2). Head and body position, as well as pressure transmitted from other body compartments such as thorax and abdomen can cause important variations in ICP, mainly by reducing venous blood return from the head to the central circulation (3). In particular, the supine position may cause an increase in ICP as can high intrathoracic or elevated abdominal pressure (4). In physiological conditions, baseline ICP and the amplitude of the pulsatile components of the ICP waveform remain constant despite a variety of transient perturbations. The brain parenchyma is nearly incompressible and, because CSF is produced and absorbed at a constant rate, the volume of the blood in the cranial cavity is therefore almost constant. Thus, a continuous outflow of venous blood from the cranial cavity is required to make room for continuous incoming arterial blood. In health, ICP is determined by cerebral blood flow (CBF) and CSF circulation. Davson's equation describes this relationship and states that ICP is the sum of sagittal sinus pressure and the product of CSF formation rate and resistance to CSF outflow (5). Normal values for sagittal sinus pressure, CSF formation rate, and resistance to CSF outflow are 5–8 mmHg, 0.3–0.4 mL/min, and 6–10 mmHg/mL/min, respectively. The production of CSF and equivalent re-adsorption dynamically maintains CSF volume, and therefore ICP, within the normal range, with fluctuations of only around 1 mmHg in normal healthy adult subjects.

The existence of clinically relevant pressure gradients within the CNS is the subject of debate (6,7). Uniformly distributed ICP can be seen when CSF circulates freely between all its natural pools, equilibrating pressure throughout. When little or no CSF volume remains in the intracranial cavity, for example, because of brain swelling, the assumption of one, uniform value of ICP is questionable and there is considerable experimental and clinical evidence that ICP is not then evenly distributed throughout the CNS. Moreover, in patients with focal intracranial lesions, interhemispheric ICP gradients exist (6). These disappear with time and this may indicate an increase in the size of the lesion. The clinical relevance of such ICP gradients must be considered in patients with mass lesions, and the ICP monitoring probe should be located in the damaged hemisphere, as described later in this chapter.

ICP therefore depends on the relative constancy of the constituents within the intracranial cavity, that is, CSF, blood, and brain tissue. The following equation describes this relationship:

$$V_{CSF} + V_{BLOOD} + V_{BRAIN} + V_{OTHER} = V_{INTRACRANIAL\ SPACE} = Constant$$

where 'other' encompass all the pathological volumes, such as haematomas, oedema, and tumours.

The importance of these relationships is that, because the skull cannot easily accommodate any additional volume, ICP is a direct consequence of the volumes of brain tissue, blood, and CSF, and compensation for any added volume within its space. Small increases in the volume of any of the components of the intracranial cavity can be offset by an equal, compensatory decrease in the others. For example, if a new intracranial volume, such as haematoma, tumour, or oedema, is introduced, venous blood and CSF are displaced and initially there is little change in the ICP (Figure 9.1). In this way, small changes in the volume of one of the intracranial constituents are buffered so that there is minimal change in ICP, reflecting the compensatory reserve of the cranial space. However, when the compensatory capacity is exhausted, further increases in a constituent of intracranial volume may lead to a substantial increase in ICP.

At very high levels of ICP the amplitude of the ICP wave decreases as CBF is reduced by a reduction in intracranial compliance and perfusion pressure. Changes induced by the heart rate, systemic blood pressure, fluid status, and intrathoracic pressure invoke transient changes, compensated by CSF displacements into the lumbar space and are considered part of the steady state. For example, coughing often produces ICP exceeding 30–50 mmHg but with rapid return to baseline levels.

The ICP waveform is normally pulsatile, and the mean level is commonly referred to as the ICP. Rhythmic fluctuations superimposed on this are associated with cardiac and respiratory activity, reflecting their cyclical effects on cerebral blood volume (CBV). The respiratory contribution to the ICP waveform is the result of fluctuations in arterial blood pressure and cerebral venous outflow during the respiratory cycle, generated by pressure changes in the thoracic cavity. Changes in these pulsatile fluctuations can be the earliest signs that the ICP is beginning to rise, as a reflection of the increased transmission of pressure waves through a less compliant brain.

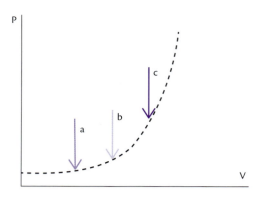

Fig. 9.1 Pressure–volume curve. Note that in the normal range, towards the origin of the x-axis (point a), intracranial pressure remains normal in spite of small additions of volume until a point of decompensation (point b) occurs. After this, each subsequent increment in volume results in an even larger increment in intracranial pressure (point c).

Reproduced with permission from Citerio G. *ICP Monitoring in Encyclopedia of Intensive Care Medicine*, Vincent JL, Hall JB eds. Springer Verlag Ed 2012.

Although ICP levels greater than 15 mmHg are considered abnormal, data from the Traumatic Coma Data Bank (8) show that it is an ICP equal to or greater than 20 mmHg that is associated with poor outcome after severe traumatic brain injury (TBI) (9). Moreover, the time spent over this threshold is important. The proportion of hourly ICP readings greater than 20 mmHg is a highly significant contributor to the poor outcome noted. Episodic ICP measurements are unable to provide information regarding severity and duration of insult. Using continuous, high-resolution capture of elevated ICP over time and computer analysis, a more accurate estimation of the time spent over the threshold, expressed as an area under the curve or 'pressure × time dose' (PTD) of intracranial hypertension, has been evaluated (10,11). Increasing elevated intracranial PTD is associated with mortality. Although this approach is clinically useful, it is quite simplistic and, as early as 1977, Miller stressed the uncertainty of the concept of any threshold for ICP, and the need for adaptability in treating intracranial hypertension (12). This has indeed subsequently proven to be correct (13).

There is strong correlative evidence that high ICP is associated with a greater likelihood of impaired recovery after acute brain injury, and that markedly uncontrolled intracranial hypertension, leading to global ischaemia and cerebral herniation, are predictive of poor outcome. More importantly, ICP is known to be an important cause of secondary brain injury, and high ICP is consistently associated with a worse neurological outcome in patients following TBI and other neurological emergencies. Therefore ICP monitoring in the presence of a suspected disequilibrium of intracranial volumes has a sound physiological as well as clinical rationale.

This chapter will provide an historical overview of the concept of ICP, of its physiological determinants, and of the technology available to monitor ICP.

Historical overview

Although cerebral swelling and the consequences of opening the skull were understood by Galen, Hippocrates, and early Egyptian physicians, the modern understanding of volume regulation within the intracranial cavity began with Kellie and Monro. In their 1783 *Observations on the structure and function of the nervous system* they wrote:

> For, as the substance of the brain, like that of other solids of our body, is nearly incompressible, the quantity of blood within the head must be the same, or very nearly the same at all times, whether in health or disease, in life or after death, those cases only excepted in which water or other matter is effused, or secreted from the blood vessels; for in these a quantity of blood, equal in bulk to the effused matter, will be pressed out of the cranium.

These concepts were formalized physiologically in 1824, and became known as the Monro–Kellie doctrine. This states that, once the fontanelles and sutures are closed, the brain becomes enclosed in a non-expandable case of bone and that changes in ICP can therefore be attributed to a volume change in one or more of the constituents of intracranial contents.

Physiological exploration of human CSF started in the late nineteenth century when Heinrich Quincke published his studies on the diagnostic and therapeutic applications of lumbar puncture at a medical congress in 1891 (Verhandlungen des Congresses für Innere Medizin, Zehnter Congress, Wiesbaden 10. pp. 321–31). He credited Walter Essex Wynter with the use, in 1889, of lumbar cannulation as a treatment of raised ICP in patients with tuberculous meningitis. Quincke subsequently standardized the technique and introduced a method to measure the pressure of the CSF by connecting the lumbar puncture needle to a fine glass pipette in which the fluid was allowed to rise. In the first decades of the last century, lumbar CSF pressure measurement was refined and considered to be a good and reliable indicator of ICP. However, even at that time, reports were published demonstrating that patients showing clinical signs of brain compression can have normal lumbar CSF pressure and that they were at high risk of dying during the lumbar puncture procedure. The reasons for this phenomenon were believed, quite rightly, to be the possibility of inducing brainstem compression through tentorial or tonsillar herniation during the release of CSF from the lumbar region (Figure 9.2).

Partly because of this apparent dissociation between ICP and clinical symptoms, emphasis switched from ICP measurement towards a focus on the relationship between craniospinal volume and pressure, particularly the importance of the elastic properties of the craniospinal system. Ryder was the first to characterize the craniospinal volume–pressure relationship as non-linear, describing it as a hyperbolic function, which implies an increase in elastance as pressure increases (14). Furthermore, it was also partly the work of Ryder that demonstrated a differential between intraventricular and lumbar CSF pressures, thereby restoring confidence in ICP measurement. In 1895, Bayliss reported that it was impossible to obtain valid ICP measurements below the tentorium during the later stages of progressive supratentorial brain compression (15,16). For this reason, and the risk of underestimation of ICP if the two systems do not communicate, measurement of lumbar CSF pressure fell into disuse for the diagnosis of intracranial hypertension. Researchers moved to direct puncture and cannulation of the ventricular system.

The first true ICP measurements were performed by Guillaume and Janny in 1951 using an electromagnetic transducer to measure ventricular fluid pressure signals in patients with various intracranial lesions (17–19). However, it was not until the 1960s, when Lundberg published his now classic monograph (20,21), that interest in clinical ICP measurement was rekindled (22–28). Using ventricular fluid pressure recording in brain

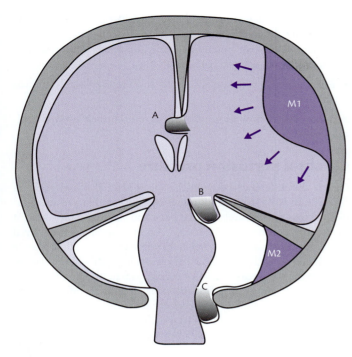

Fig. 9.2 Schematic representation of brain herniation syndromes. According to the Monro–Kellie doctrine, an increased volume and pressure in one compartment of the brain may cause shift of brain tissue to a compartment in which the pressure is lower. M1 is an expanding supratentorial lesion; M2 is an expanding mass in the posterior fossa. A Increased pressure on one side of the brain may cause tissue to push against and slip under the falx cerebri toward the other side of the brain, B Uncal (lateral transtentorial) herniation. Increased ICP from a lateral lesion pushes tissue downward, initially compressing third cranial nerve and, subsequently, ascending reticular activating system, leading to coma, C Infratentorial herniation. Downward displacement of cerebellar tissue through the foramen magnum producing medullar compression and coma.
Reproduced with permission from Citerio G. *ICP Monitoring in Encyclopedia of Intensive Care Medicine*, Vincent JL, Hall JB eds. Springer Verlag Ed 2012.

tumour patients over several weeks, Lundberg was the first to delineate the frequency with which raised ICP occurs clinically, and showed that, at times, ICP could reach pressures as high as 100 mmHg. Lundberg also described three types of spontaneous pressure wave fluctuations:

◆ *A waves* or 'plateau waves' have amplitudes of 50–100 mmHg, and last 5–20 minutes. These are always associated with intracranial pathology and commonly with impending brain herniation. It has been postulated that, as cerebral perfusion pressure (CPP) becomes inadequate to meet metabolic demand, cerebral vasodilatation occurs in an attempt to restore adequate perfusion and, as a consequence, CBV increases. This leads to a vicious cycle where further decreases in CPP cause additional plateau waves and, if adequate flow is not restored, lead to irreversible ischaemic brain injury.

◆ *B waves* are oscillating waves up to 50 mmHg in amplitude with a frequency of 0.5–2/min. They are believed to be related to vasomotor centre instability and occur when CPP is unstable or at the lower limit of pressure autoregulation.

◆ *C waves* are oscillating waves up to 20 mmHg in amplitude with a frequency of 4–8/min. They have been documented in healthy individuals and are believed to occur because of interactions between cardiac and respiratory cycles.

A and B waves are always pathological and require intervention to reduce ICP and maintain CPP (6,29,30).

Lundberg, anticipating modern practice, wrote in 1965:

> The greatest value of recording the ventricular fluid pressure is the information it gives in cases of severe injury of the brain without hematoma. In these cases, intervention to decrease ICP by such means as hypertonic solutions, hyperventilation, hypothermia, drainage of fluid and removal of localized contusions, may be more rationally applied. (9,23,31–43)

It was therefore Lundberg who suggested the absolute need for the continuous monitoring of ICP because, without it, the correct timing and evaluation of the efficacy of the therapy is impossible.

Intracranial pressure waveform and cerebral compliance

The ICP waveform reflects the arterial waveform (Figure 9.3). Brain tissue pressure and ICP increase with each cardiac cycle and the ICP waveform can thus be seen as a modified arterial pressure wave with three distinct components that are related to distinct physiological parameters (1,44):

1. The first peak (P1) is the 'percussive' wave and related to the transmission of arterial pressure from the choroid plexus to the ventricle. It is sharp and fairly constant in amplitude.

2. The second peak (P2), the 'tidal' wave, represents the rebound after initial arterial percussion and is related to brain tissue compliance. It generally increases as compliance decreases. A marked decrease in cerebral compliance is present if the amplitude of the P2 waveform exceeds that of P1.

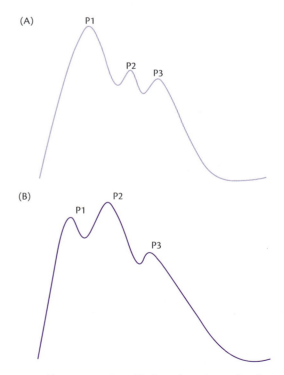

Fig. 9.3 Intracranial pressure waveforms. The figure shows the waveform in a compliant system (A) and a high pressure wave recorded from a noncompliant system (B).
Reproduced with permission from Citerio G. *ICP Monitoring in Encyclopedia of Intensive Care Medicine*, Vincent JL, Hall JB eds. Springer Verlag Ed 2012.

3. The third wave (P3) occurs because if the closure of the aortic valve, and therefore represents the dicrotic notch.

If the craniospinal system is closed, the ICP waveform changes as ICP increases. Initially the amplitudes of both P1 and P2 increase, and then P2 increases to a greater extent than P1 so that P2 becomes predominant. As ICP rises further, all peaks finally become indistinguishable. These modifications are blunted or abolished when the system is not closed, as in the presence of a CSF leak.

A rise in ICP is unfortunately a delayed phenomenon that occurs only when intracranial compensatory mechanisms have become exhausted. Therefore, earlier indicators of an impending imbalance of the system would help the clinician in the timely detection of a potentially dangerous situation. A potential way of improving the detection of intracranial hypertension is to identify the early changes in the ICP waveform that can be extracted from continuous ICP signals. In this way, impending ICP elevation can be recognized prior to its occurrence. In an early study, Contant et al. investigated several ICP metrics to differentiate transient from refractory ICP elevation (45,46), but this seminal work has not yet translated into the clinic or been integrated into clinical monitoring systems. However, investigation of these issues is still ongoing and, in association with the development of improved computation systems and algorithms, it is likely that systems for the prediction of intracranial hypertension will be developed (26,31,47–52).

Marmarou, interested in CSF dynamics, was the first to provide a full mathematical description of the craniospinal volume–pressure relationship. He developed a mathematical model of the CSF system which produced a general solution for CSF pressure (12,53,54). The model parameters have subsequently been verified experimentally in an animal model of hydrocephalus. As a corollary, Marmarou also demonstrated that the non-linear craniospinal volume–pressure relationship could be described as a straight-line segment relating the logarithm of pressure to volume, implying a mono-exponential relationship between volume and pressure. The slope of this relationship is termed the pressure–volume index (PVI), that is the notional volume required to raise ICP tenfold (13,23,55–59). PVI is expressed by the formula:

$$PVI = \Delta V / \left(\log_{10} P_o / P_m \right)$$

where ΔV expresses the volume (in mL) added or withdrawn from the ventricular system, P_o the initial pressure, and P_m the final pressure.

Unlike elastance, that is, the change in pressure per unit change in volume (dP/dV), or its inverse, compliance, that is, change in volume per unit change in pressure (dV/dP), the PVI characterizes the craniospinal volume–pressure relationship over the whole physiological range of ICP. However, the PVI calculated from the pressure change resulting from a rapid injection or withdrawal of fluid from the CSF space has found limited use as a measure of reduced craniospinal compliance both clinically and experimentally. This is likely in part to be related to the disadvantages of the PVI method, which include the following:

◆ Manipulation of the CSF access system (e.g. ventricular drain) to test the PVI increases the risk of infection.

◆ Variability exists between measurements because of the difficulty of manually injecting consistent volumes of fluid at a constant rate of injection—as a result an average of repeated measures is usually required, further increasing the infection risk.

◆ Cerebral autoregulation status can affect PVI estimation despite a normal CPP, and the PVI may overestimate the tolerance of the intracranial system to volume loads in patients with disturbed cerebral autoregulation (14,60,61).

◆ The procedure is time-consuming and requires highly trained personal.

Because of these limitations, the PVI is not routinely used in clinical practice.

Cerebral perfusion pressure

CPP is the difference between the mean arterial blood pressure (MAP) and ICP (16,62,63). It represents the vascular pressure gradient across the cerebral vascular beds and should be measured at the level of these beds (18,59,64–66). A correct setting of the arterial blood pressure transducer level is therefore crucial for the accurate calculation of CPP. At a 30° head elevation, hydrostatic pressure forces mean that measured MAP is approximately 15 mmHg lower if the transducer is 'zeroed' at the external auditory meatus compared to the mid-axillary level, resulting in an underestimation of actual CPP. Conversely, if the arterial blood pressure transducer is placed at mid-axillary level, CPP is overestimated. It is the authors' practice to keep both transducers (ICP and MAP) at the level of the tragus.

Cerebral blood flow is determined by both CPP and cerebrovascular resistance (CVR):

$$CBF = CPP / CVR$$

CVR (and thus CBF) are affected by a number of physiological variables including arterial carbon dioxide gas tension, which has a near linear relationship with CBF within the physiological range (producing a 3% increase of CBF for each mmHg of $PaCO_2$ increase) (21,67–70), and cerebral metabolic rate for oxygen and glucose, which has a direct relationship with CBF (see Chapters 2 and 3). Another example is core body and brain temperatures. An increase in temperature produces a rise in cerebral metabolism and a coupled increase in CBF. The key point is that when intracranial compliance is reduced, even a small increase in CBF and CBV will increase ICP.

Physiologically, cerebral pressure autoregulation has been defined as the ability of the cerebral vasculature to maintain flow over a wide range of CPP (~ 50–150 mmHg) (23,25,27,67,71–74). This process, termed pressure autoregulation, occurs because of reflex variations in arterial calibre and is a fundamental physiological premise governing the CPP/CBF relationship. In subjects with intact autoregulation, a rise in systemic blood pressure within the limits of cerebral autoregulation results in constriction of cerebral vessels and secondary reduction in CBV, and thus in ICP. The opposite occurs during reduction in arterial pressure. On the other hand, in patients with deranged autoregulation the cerebral vasculature is non-reactive and a rise in blood pressure leads to an increase in CBF, CBV, and ICP.

The critical CBF threshold for the development of irreversible tissue damage after TBI is 15–18 mL/100 g/min. Techniques for measuring CBF at the bedside are largely experimental so most clinicians use CPP as a surrogate of CBF. However, Czosnyka has demonstrated that deranged autoregulation after TBI makes it difficult to derive a relationship between CPP and CBF (75–79). Several methods have been developed to assess the state of cerebral autoregulation after brain injury. Among these, the pressure reactivity index (PRx) is derived from calculation of a moving correlation coefficient between mean ICP and MAP over a few minutes (77,79–82). PRx can be measured at the bedside using computer-based analysis of the ICP and MAP signals. Patients with intact autoregulation have a PRx less than 0 (minimum value −1), that is, there is no or negative correlation between ICP and MAP, and an increase in MAP is likely to produce a reduction in ICP. On the other hand, patients with disturbed autoregulation (PRx > 0.2, maximum value 1) have a positive correlation between ICP and MAP and an increase in MAP will result in a rise in ICP. It is important to note that during calculation of PRx no constituent of intracranial volume should be changed by external interventions such as CSF drainage. Abnormal values of PRx, indicating impaired autoregulation and disturbed cerebrospinal pressure reactivity, have been demonstrated to be predictive of a poor outcome following TBI (22).

Indications and prognostic value of intracranial pressure

Clinically, increased ICP may be suggested by the presence of headache, and the Cushing triad of hypertension, bradycardia, and irregular respiratory pattern or apnoea. Increases in ICP can lead to brain herniation syndromes if not reversed or relieved (83–86). Under such circumstances outcome is largely dependent on the primary pathology and the reversal or progression of herniation.

High ICP is correlated with acute neurological deterioration (87,88). Nearly one-third of severely head injured patients develop clinically manifest neurological deterioration during their hospital course, including a spontaneous decrease in Glasgow Coma Scale (GCS) motor score of at least 2 points, a further loss of pupillary reactivity, development of pupillary asymmetry of 1 mm or more, and deterioration in neurological status sufficient to warrant immediate medical or surgical intervention (89,90). The most powerful predictor of neurological worsening is the presence of intracranial hypertension (ICP ≥ 20 mmHg), either initially or during the neurological deterioration. The almost sixfold higher mortality rate in the subgroup of patients who develop such deterioration clearly indicates the need for earlier identification of impending intracranial hypertension, as well as earlier and more effective treatment.

In every condition in which a pathological increase in one of the constituents of intracranial volume is likely, ICP monitoring should be considered, weighing the benefits that the knowledge of ICP will bring to the patient's management against the costs and (small) risks of the procedure.

Traumatic brain injury

Although several researchers have demonstrated the prognostic value of ICP monitoring after TBI (8,91–103), there are no randomized studies that support the use of ICP monitoring to guide management. In a multicentre, randomized controlled trial conducted in Bolivia and Ecuador (BEST-TRIP), 324 patients with severe TBI were randomly assigned to receive either guideline-based management guided by monitored ICP or treatment guided by imaging and clinical examination in the absence of ICP monitoring (102,104–106). This study found that care focused on maintaining monitored ICP at 20 mmHg or less was not superior to care based on imaging and clinical examination in terms of the primary

outcome, that is, a composite of survival time, impaired consciousness, functional status at 3 and 6 months, and neuropsychological status at 6 months. Misinterpretation of these data might lead to the conclusion that ICP monitoring and management after TBI should be abandoned, but this would be inappropriate. Even the Principal Investigator of BEST-TRIP agrees that the use of a safe and accurate quantitative index of ICP that monitors the temporal changes in ICP and response to treatment is much preferable to interventions based on semi-empirical assessment or waiting for pupillary changes to learn that we have been unsuccessful in adequately treating the patient (13,91,102,104,107–111).

Marmarou, reporting on data from the National Institute of Health's Traumatic Coma Data Bank, showed that following the usual clinical predictors of age, admission motor score, and abnormal pupils, the proportion of hourly ICP recordings greater than 20 mmHg was the next most significant predictor of poor outcome after TBI (9,109,112). Other data from large prospective trials carried out in single centres, and from well-controlled multicentre studies, have also provided most convincing evidence for a direct relationship between ICP and outcome (11,92,94,96,98,113–119).

It is the authors' opinion that, given its ease of use, safety, and cost-effectiveness, ICP monitoring should remain a key part of the monitoring strategy after TBI because of the possible catastrophic and often rapid consequences of increased ICP. However, clinical methods for interpreting ICP in the setting of individual patients must be developed, and ICP should be interpreted in association with other physiological variables that assess the adequacy of brain perfusion, such as brain tissue oxygenation (see Chapter 11).

The Brain Trauma Foundation guidelines make the following evidence-based recommendations for ICP monitoring after TBI (53):

◆ *Level I*—there are insufficient data to support a Level I recommendation for this topic.

◆ *Level II*—ICP should be monitored in all salvageable patients with a severe TBI (GCS score of 3–8 after resuscitation) and an abnormal computed tomography (CT) scan, which is defined in this guideline as one that reveals haematomas, contusions, swelling, herniation, or compressed basal cisterns.

◆ *Level III*—ICP monitoring is indicated in patients with severe TBI with a normal CT scan if two or more of the following features are noted at admission: age over 40 years, unilateral or bilateral motor posturing, or systolic blood pressure less than 90 mmHg.

Subarachnoid haemorrhage

Following aneurysmal subarachnoid haemorrhage (SAH), ICP is elevated in more than 50% of cases, usually as an immediate response to aneurysm rupture (120–124). This is particularly evident when a re-bleeding episode occurs. The rise in ICP that accompanies SAH has been attributed to several factors including the volume of the initial haemorrhage, CSF outflow obstruction causing hydrocephalus, diffuse vasoparalysis, and cerebral swelling following massive bleeding. Intracranial hypertension after SAH has been associated with several detrimental effects, including delayed cerebral ischaemic deficits, and changes in cerebral metabolism and blood flow. Intracranial hypertension in patients with SAH has a profound impact on outcome, but unequivocal benefits of ICP monitoring and management have not been demonstrated.

This might in part be related to the complexity of the underlying pathophysiology, including reduced CBF, impaired autoregulation, decreased CO_2 reactivity, systemic abnormalities such as decreased intravascular volume, and biochemical abnormalities such as excitotoxicity, each of which may contribute individually to poor outcome. Despite this it seems reasonable to consider ICP monitoring in patients with poor grade SAH, particularly those who are comatose or sedated and in whom prompt and accurate clinical detection of an ongoing intracranial problem, such as cerebral oedema or hydrocephalus, is not possible. The American Heart Association/American Stroke Association (AHA/ASA) guidelines recommend that SAH-associated acute symptomatic hydrocephalus should be managed by cerebrospinal fluid diversion (125).

It has been suggested that ICP monitoring should be undertaken in patients with more severe SAH (World Federation of Neurosurgeons score ≥ 3), and that a ventricular catheter should be used as the ICP monitoring device because it offers the possibility of therapeutic draining of CSF to treat hydrocephalus (126).

Miscellaneous

There is no strong evidence for ICP monitoring in other neurosurgical emergencies (127), although it can reasonably be used in any acute brain pathology that may be associated with increased ICP and a risk of brain compartmental herniation. These include metabolic disorders, brain ischaemia (128), haemorrhagic stroke (15), and meningitis/encephalitis (129,130). The AHA/ASA guidelines for the management of intracerebral haemorrhage (15) recommend that:

♦ ICP monitoring and treatment should be considered in patients with a GCS score less than 8, those with clinical evidence of transtentorial herniation, or those with significant intraventricular haemorrhage or hydrocephalus, and that it might be reasonable

to maintain CPP between 50 and 70 mmHg, depending on the status of cerebral autoregulation

♦ ventricular drainage as treatment for hydrocephalus is reasonable in patients with a decreased level of consciousness.

In Reye's syndrome, which is characterized by substantial brain swelling, there is evidence that an ICP monitoring and management strategy similar to that used for severe TBI is associated with reduced mortality and morbidity (17,19).

The duration of monitoring will depend on normalization of ICP, and is highly dependent on individual patient characteristics and underlying pathology. It is the authors' policy to stop monitoring 12–48 hours after the cessation of interventions to control ICP, and after normalization of $PaCO_2$.

Intracranial pressure monitoring techniques

A summarized comparison of the different ICP measurement technologies is shown in Table 9.1.

Non-invasive intracranial pressure monitoring

Several techniques for the non-invasive (i.e. without trephining the skull) assessment of ICP have been proposed over the years (20). These are usually episodic rather than continuous estimations and are not really a monitoring system. They include transcranial Doppler ultrasonography (22,24,26,28), tympanic membrane displacement (29), and optic nerve sheath diameter (32–43).

Transcranial Doppler has been used to estimate ICP by calculating the difference between systolic and diastolic flow velocity, divided by the mean flow velocity, that is, the pulsatility index (PI). The PI has been found to correlate with invasively measured ICP, with correlation coefficients varying between 0.439 and 0.938 (31). Apart from being imprecise, the technique requires training and there are large intra- and interoperator differences. Moreover, the

Table 9.1 Comparison of the different systems available for ICP monitoring

Technology	Accuracy	Rate of infection	Rate of haemorrhaging	Cost per patient	Miscellaneous
External ventricular drainage	High	Low to moderate	Low	Relatively low	Can be used for drainage of CSF and infusion of antibiotics
Microtransducer ICP monitoring devices	High	Low	Low	High	Some transducers have problems with high zero drift
Transcranial Doppler ultrasonography	Low	None	None	Low	High percentage of unsuccessful measurements
Tympanic membrane displacement	Low	None	None	Low	High percentage of unsuccessful measurements
Optic nerve sheath diameter	Low	None	None	Low	Can potentially be used as a screening method of detecting raised ICP
MRI/CT	Low	None	None	Low	MRI has potential for being used for non-invasive estimation of ICP
Fundoscopy (papilloedema)	Low	None	None	Low	Can be used as a screening method of detecting raised ICP, but not in cases of sudden raise in ICP, that is, trauma

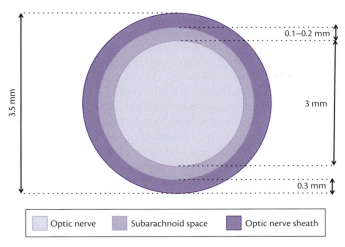

Fig. 9.4 Schematic of the optic nerve image surrounded by its sheath.
Reproduced from Kristiansson H *et al.*, 'Measuring Elevated Intracranial Pressure through Noninvasive Methods: A Review of the Literature', *Journal of Neurosurgical Anesthesiology*, 25, 4, copyright 2013, with permission from Wolters Kluwer.

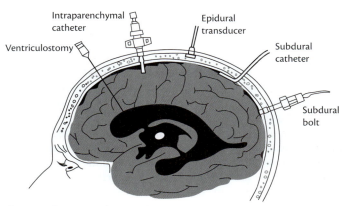

Fig. 9.5 Different sites of ICP monitoring.
Reproduced with permission from Citerio G. *ICP Monitoring in Encyclopedia of Intensive Care Medicine*, Vincent JL, Hall JB eds. Springer Verlag Ed 2012.

technique cannot be used in 15% of patients because of the lack of an acoustic window.

A technique using the measurement of optic nerve sheath diameter (ONSD) has recently been introduced for the non-invasive detection of raised ICP, particularly in patients with severe brain injury, and is physiologically interesting. The optic nerve is part of the CNS and surrounded by a dural sheath. Between the sheath and the white matter is a small subarachnoid space (< 0.2 mm) which communicates with the intracranial subarachnoid space. In cases of increased ICP, the sheath expands (Figure 9.4). Unfortunately the specificity and positive predictive value of ONSD for ICP greater than 20 mmHg are substantially less in patients demonstrating acute fluctuation of ICP between high and normal, the very population in whom knowledge of ICP is important (44). This may be because of delayed reversal of nerve sheath distension. ONSD measurement is of clinical interest because enlargement of the sheath on initial CT scan has been associated with increased mortality after severe TBI. However, the method of measuring ONSD using CT itself needs further confirmation, as does the link between early ONSD enlargement and raised ICP (45). Thus, ONSD measurement is currently not a clinical tool.

The non-invasive techniques for measuring ICP are captivating because they are without the risks of invasive methods. However, they fail to measure ICP sufficiently accurately to be used as routine alternatives to invasive measurement, or to offer continuous monitoring of intracranial dynamics. Currently, invasive techniques are the only options for accurate measurement of ICP (31).

Invasive intracranial pressure monitoring techniques

The optimal ICP monitoring device should be accurate, reliable, cost-effective, and cause minimal patient morbidity (53), concepts first described by Lundberg in 1965 (23). Accuracy and reliability are defined by the Association for the Advancement of Medical Instrumentation (AAMI) standards (http://www.aami.org/standards/index.html). An ICP measuring device should have the following specifications—pressure range 0–100 mmHg, accuracy ± 2 mmHg in the 0–20 mmHg range, and maximum error of 10% in the 20–100 mmHg range. According to the available evidence, ICP

monitoring devices have been ranked according to their accuracy, reliability, and cost as follows (Figure 9.5) (5):

1. Intraventricular devices incorporating a fluid-coupled catheter and an external strain gauge transducer

2. Intraventricular devices incorporating microstrain gauge or fiberoptic technology

3. Parenchymal pressure transducer devices

4. Subdural devices

5. Subarachnoid fluid-coupled devices

6. Epidural devices.

Ventricular catheters

Measurement of ventricular fluid pressure is the established reference standard for measuring ICP (60). A catheter placed into one of the ventricles through a burr hole and connected to an external strain gauge transducer is the most accurate, low-cost, and reliable method of monitoring ICP (62) (Figure 9.5). This method has been proven to be reliable over time, and permits periodic recalibration and therapeutic drainage of CSF.

The major pitfalls of this standard ventricular system are that obstruction of the catheter can occur, and for correct interpretation the external transducer must be maintained at a fixed reference point, usually the external auditory meatus. Changes in position of the transducer may lead to inaccurate assessment of ICP during clinical use. The small holes at the tip of the catheter can become obliterated by blood clots or fibrin deposits and, if this happens, CSF drainage will generate significant pressure gradients between the ventricular catheter lumen and the ventricles resulting in a gross underestimate of ICP. Moreover, a traditional ventricular catheter connected to an external strain gauge transducer system allows only intermittent ICP monitoring when the ventricular drain is closed. Another potential pitfall is the recording of ICP while the ventricular catheter is draining CSF. In this situation the recorded ICP is always equal to or lower than the drainage level because of the hydrostatic laws of communicating vessels. If the actual ICP value is higher it will be underestimated. Some commercially available ventricular catheters have a pressure transducer within their lumen, allowing simultaneous ICP monitoring and CSF drainage.

It is the authors' opinion that, before making a clinical decision based on ICP measured via a ventricular catheter, the correct position of the transducers should be verified and the 'three-way' tap system between catheter and transducer system checked to ensure that CSF is not being drained during ICP measurement. Dependence on such human factors, as well as the need for calibration and choice of reference level, is a major disadvantage to monitoring ICP using a ventricular catheter.

Although surgical placement of the external ventricular catheter is often seen as a minor procedure with few risks, it can be associated with serious haemorrhagic and infectious complications. Based on a meta-analysis, the overall haemorrhagic complication rate from ventriculostomy placement by neurosurgeons is approximately 7%, with a risk of significant haemorrhage of approximately 0.8% (64). An important caveat has to be kept in mind when considering these figures, namely that normal coagulation variables are advocated before inserting external ventricular drains (EVDs) in order to reduce the haemorrhagic risk.

Catheter-related ventriculitis and meningitis are potentially life-threatening complications caused by direct catheter contamination during introduction or by subsequent retrograde bacterial colonization of the catheter (67,68,70). Ventriculostomy-related infection (VRI) is characterized by (67):

◆ one or more positive CSF culture or Gram's stain

◆ progressively declining CSF glucose level

◆ increasing CSF protein profiles

◆ worsening CSF pleocytosis

◆ a paucity of clinical symptoms other than fever.

The use of closed drainage systems, aseptic CSF sampling techniques, and prompt removal of unneeded ventricular catheters minimizes the risk of catheter-related infections. The quoted incidence of VRI is wide, ranging from 0% to greater than 20%, depending on the definition of infection used and the clinical characteristics of the study population. A large meta-analysis evaluating 23 major studies of ventriculostomy use in 5261 patients with 5733 EVD insertions confirmed a cumulative rate of positive CSF culture of 8.80% per patient, or 8.08% per EVD placement. As noted in other reports, studies that defined infection using clinical indicators in addition to a positive CSF culture showed an infection rate of 6.62% per patient or 6.10% per EVD. Risk factors for VRI include those that are known to be associated with CSF infection, such as intraventricular and subarachnoid haemorrhage, operated depressed cranial vault fracture, skull base fracture with CSF leak, intracranial surgery, ventriculostomy irrigation, duration of ventricular catheterization, and systemic infection (67). In addition, factors that are possibly associated with CSF infection, including the site of ventriculostomy insertion, corticosteroid use, CSF pleocytosis, catheter manipulations, and CSF leak around the catheter insertion site, are also likely risk factors for VRI.

The most commonly found pathogens in VRI have traditionally been skin flora, but Gram-negative organisms are increasingly being recognized as causative agents. No recommendations can be made regarding the administration of prophylactic antibiotics for EVDs (80), but it is not the authors' practice to use antibiotic prophylaxis while a ventriculostomy is in place. However, the use of a comprehensive care bundle (83,85), and antibiotic or silver-impregnated catheters (131–135), may decrease the incidence of catheter-related CSF infection. In high-risk populations, antibiotic-impregnated catheters delay the occurrence of infection compared with non-antibiotic coated systems, and a recent meta-analysis supports the general use of antibiotic-coated ventricular catheters to minimize the risk of VRI (87).

Intraparenchymal transducers
The most common alternative location for ICP monitoring is the brain parenchyma, and ICP measurements that correlate well with the 'gold standard' values obtained from intraventricular catheters can be obtained using intraparenchymal microtransducers (89).

Table 9.2 Comparison of the different invasive transducers available for ICP monitoring

	Technology	Rate of infection	Rate of haemorrhaging	Technical errors	Zero drift
Camino ICP Monitor	Fibreoptic	8.5% 4.75%	2.50% (0.66% clinical significant) 1.1%	4.5% 10% 3.14%	Mean 7.3 ± 5.1 mmHg (range −17 to 21 mmHg) Mean −0.67 mmHg (range −13 to 22 mmHg) Mean 3.5 ± 3.1 mmHg (range 0 to 12 mmHg)
Codman MicroSensor	Strain gauge	0% 0%	0% ~ 0.3% (0% clinical significant)	n/a	Mean 0.9 ± 0.2 mmHg (range −5 to 4 mmHg) Mean 0.1 ± 1.6 mmHg/100 hours of monitoring Mean 2.0 mmHg (range −6 to 15 mmHg)
Raumedic Neurovent-P ICP sensor	Strain gauge	0%	2.02% (0% clinical significant)	n/a	Mean 0.8 ± 2.2 mmHg (range −4 to +8 mmHg) 1.7 ± 1.36 mmHg (range −2 to 3 mmHg) In vitro: 0.6 ± 0.96 mmHg (range 0 to 2 mmHg)
Pressio	Strain gauge	n/a	n/a	n/a	Mean −0.7 ± 1.6 mmHg/100 hours of monitoring In vitro: 7-day drift <0.05 mmHg
Spiegelberg	Pneumatic	0%	0%	3.45%	Mean < ± 2 mmHg

Such devices are of two types—solid-state devices based on pressure-sensitive resistors forming a Wheatstone bridge, or those that incorporate a fibreoptic design (FOD).

Fibreoptic devices, such as the Camino ICP Monitor (Integra LifeSciences, Plainsboro Township, New Jersey, USA) (95,100,110) transmit light via a fibreoptic cable towards a displaceable mirror at the tip. Changes in ICP distort the mirror and the differences in intensity of the reflected light are translated into an ICP value. Solid state devices, such as the Codman MicroSensor (Codman & Shurtleff, Raynham, MA, USA) (136,137), the Raumedic Neurovent-P ICP sensor (Raumedic, Helmbrechts, Germany) (102,104,106), and the Pressio sensor (Sophysa, Orsay, France) (138), belong to the group of piezoelectric strain gauge devices. When the transducer is bent because of a change in ICP its resistance changes and this is converted into an ICP value. Intraparenchymal ICP probes are usually placed in the right frontal region at a depth of approximately 2 cm. The Codman and Raumedic sensors are compatible with magnetic resonance imaging (MRI) without any danger to the patient but the Camino and Pressio sensors contain ferromagnetic components and are not.

All microtransducers share a common drawback—it is not possible to recalibrate them after placement. Although both types of system are very accurate at the time of insertion, there is a degree of zero drift over time (91,102,104,107–111), which can result in a measurement error after several days (65). Zero drift expresses the difference between the starting ICP value when the sensor is calibrated (0 mmHg) and the measured value after removal. A large difference between these two values, rarely encountered in clinical practice, indicates that the ICP measured while the device was in use was not the actual ICP at any given moment. It is always advisable to check any catheter for zero drift at removal. Data regarding differences between microtransducer ICP monitoring devices are summarized in Table 9.2.

The overall safety of microtransducer-based ICP monitoring devices is good, with clinically significant complications, such as infection and haematoma, occurring infrequently in centres with sufficient experience in their use. The cost of these microtransducers is higher than conventional ventricular systems.

Subdural (109,112) and epidural (113–116) monitors are less accurate than intraparenchymal devices, and lower ICP values are measured in the subdural than epidural space (65). Such monitors are now rarely used in clinical practice.

References

1. Andrews PJD, Citerio G. Intracranial pressure. Part one: historical overview and basic concepts. *Intensive Care Med.* 2004;30(9):1730–3.
2. Bradley KC. Cerebrospinal fluid pressure. *J Neurol Neurosurg Psychiatr.* 1970;33(3):387–97.
3. Citerio G, Vascotto E, Villa F, Celotti S, Pesenti A. Induced abdominal compartment syndrome increases intracranial pressure in neurotrauma patients: a prospective study. *Crit Care Med.* 2001;29(7):1466–71.
4. Huseby JS, Luce JM, Cary JM, Pavlin EG, Butler J. Effects of positive end-expiratory pressure on intracranial pressure in dogs with intracranial hypertension. *J Neurosurg.* 1981;55(5):704–5.
5. Davson H, Domer FR, Hollingsworth JR. The mechanism of drainage of the cerebrospinal fluid. *Brain.* 1973;96(2):329–36.
6. Sahuquillo J, Poca MA, Arribas M, Garnacho A, Rubio E. Interhemispheric supratentorial intracranial pressure gradients in head-injured patients: are they clinically important? *J Neurosurg.* 1999;90(1):16–26.
7. Mindermann T. Pressure gradients within the central nervous system. *J Clin Neurosci.* 1999;6(6):464–6.
8. Marmarou A, Anderson R, Ward J, Choi S, Young H, Eisenberg H, et al. NINDS Traumatic Coma Data Bank: intracranial pressure monitoring methodology. *J Neurosurg.* 1991;75(1S):21–7.
9. Marmarou A, Anderson R, Ward J, Choi S, Young H, Eisenberg H, et al. Impact of ICP instability and hypotension on outcome in patients with severe head trauma. *J Neurosurg.* 1991;75(1S):59–66.
10. Vik A, Nag T, Fredriksli OA, Skandsen T, Moen KG, Schirmer-Mikalsen K, et al. Relationship of "dose" of intracranial hypertension to outcome in severe traumatic brain injury. *J Neurosurg.* 2008;109(4):678–84.
11. Sheth KN, Stein DM, Aarabi B, Hu P, Kufera JA, Scalea TM, et al. Intracranial pressure dose and outcome in traumatic brain injury. *Neurocrit Care.* 2012;18(1):26–32.
12. Miller JD, Becker DP, Ward JD, Sullivan HG, Adams WE, Rosner MJ. Significance of intracranial hypertension in severe head injury. *J Neurosurg.* 1977;47(4):503–16.
13. Chesnut RM. Intracranial pressure monitoring: headstone or a new head start. The BEST TRIP trial in perspective. *Intensive Care Med.* 2013;39(4):771–4.
14. Ryder HW, Espey FF, Kristoff FV, Evans JP. Observations on the interrelationships of intracranial pressure and cerebral blood flow. *J Neurosurg.* 1951;8(1):46–58.
15. Morgenstern LB, Hemphill JC, Anderson C, Becker K, Broderick JP, Connolly ES, et al. Guidelines for the management of spontaneous intracerebral hemorrhage. *Stroke.* 2010;41(9):2108–29.
16. Bayliss WM, Hill L, Gulland GL. On intra-cranial pressure and the cerebral circulation: Part I. Physiological; Part II. Histological. *J Physiol (Lond).* 1895;18(4):334–62.
17. Chi CS, Law KL, Wong TT, Su GY, Lin N. Continuous monitoring of intracranial pressure in Reye's syndrome—5 years experience. *Acta Paediatr Jpn.* 1990;32(4):426–34.
18. Guillaume J, Janny P. [Continuous intracranial manometry; importance of the method and first results]. *Rev Neurol (Paris).* 1951;84(2):131–42.
19. Haller J. Intracranial pressure monitoring in Reye's syndrome. *Hosp Pract.* 1980;15(2):101–8.
20. Kristiansson H, Nissborg E, Bartek J, Andresen M, Reinstrup P, Romner B. Measuring elevated intracranial pressure through non-invasive methods: a review of the literature. *J Neurosurg Anesthesiol.* 2013;25(4):372–85.
21. Lundberg N. Continuous recording and control of ventricular fluid pressure in neurosurgical practice. *Acta Psychiatr Scand Suppl.* 1960;36(149):1–193.
22. Melo JRT, Di Rocco F, Blanot S, Cuttaree H, Sainte-Rose C, Oliveira-Filho J, et al. Transcranial Doppler can predict intracranial hypertension in children with severe traumatic brain injuries. *Childs Nerv Syst.* 2011;27(6):979–84.
23. Lundberg N, Troupp H, Lorin H. Continuous recording of the ventricular-fluid pressure in patients with severe acute traumatic brain injury. A preliminary report. *J Neurosurg.* 1965;22(6):581–90.
24. Schatlo B, Gläsker S, Zauner A, Thompson BG, Oldfield EH, Pluta RM. Continuous neuromonitoring using transcranial Doppler reflects blood flow during carbon dioxide challenge in primates with global cerebral ischemia. *Neurosurgery.* 2009;64(6):1148–54.
25. Bynke HG, Lundberg NG. Studies on the relationship between variations in ventricular fluid pressure and degree of papilloedema. A preliminary report. *Acta Neurol Scand.* 1961;37:34–40.
26. Hu X, Glenn T, Scalzo F, Bergsneider M, Sarkiss C, Martin N, et al. Intracranial pressure pulse morphological features improved detection of decreased cerebral blood flow. *Physiol Meas.* 2010;31(5):679–95.
27. Lundberg N, Kjallquist A, Bien C. Reduction of increased intracranial pressure by hyperventilation. A therapeutic aid in neurological surgery. *Acta Psychiatr Scand Suppl.* 1959;34(139):1–64.
28. Czosnyka M, Smielewski P, Piechnik S, Schmidt EA, Al-Rawi PG, Kirkpatrick PJ, et al. Hemodynamic characterization of intracranial pressure plateau waves in head-injury patients. *J Neurosurg.* 1999;91(1):11–19.

29. Shimbles S, Dodd C, Banister K, Mendelow AD, Chambers IR. Clinical comparison of tympanic membrane displacement with invasive intracranial pressure measurements. *Physiol Meas.* 2005;26(6):1085–92.

30. Kim D-J, Czosnyka Z, Kasprowicz M, Smielewski P, Baledent O, Guerguerian A-M, *et al.* Continuous monitoring of the Monro-Kellie doctrine: is it possible? *J Neurotrauma.* 2012;29(7):1354–63.

31. Raboel PH, Bartek J, Andresen M, Bellander BM, Romner B. Intracranial pressure monitoring: invasive versus non-invasive methods—a review. *Crit Care Res Pract.* 2012;2012:1–14.

32. Rajajee V, Fletcher JJ, Rochlen LR, Jacobs TL. Comparison of accuracy of optic nerve ultrasound for the detection of intracranial hypertension in the setting of acutely fluctuating vs stable ICP: post-hoc analysis of data from a prospective, blinded single center study. *Crit Care.* 2012;16(3):R79.

33. Soldatos T, Chatzimichail K, Papathanasiou M, Gouliamos A. Optic nerve sonography: a new window for the non-invasive evaluation of intracranial pressure in brain injury. *Emerg Med J.* 2009;26(9):630–4.

34. Killer HE, Laeng HR, Flammer J, Groscurth P. Architecture of arachnoid trabeculae, pillars, and septa in the subarachnoid space of the human optic nerve: anatomy and clinical considerations. *Br J Ophthalmol.* 2003;87(6):777–81.

35. Le A, Hoehn ME, Smith ME, Spentzas T, Schlappy D, Pershad J. Bedside sonographic measurement of optic nerve sheath diameter as a predictor of increased intracranial pressure in children. *Ann Emerg Med.* 2009;53(6):785–91.

36. Beare NAV, Kampondeni S, Glover SJ, Molyneux E, Taylor TE, Harding SP, *et al.* Detection of raised intracranial pressure by ultrasound measurement of optic nerve sheath diameter in African children. *Trop Med Int Health.* 2008;13(11):1400–4.

37. Bäuerle J, Lochner P, Kaps M, Nedelmann M. Intra- and interobserver reliability of sonographic assessment of the optic nerve sheath diameter in healthy adults. *J Neuroimaging.* 2012;22(1):42–5.

38. Masquère P, Bonneville F, Geeraerts T. Optic nerve sheath diameter on initial brain CT, raised intracranial pressure and mortality after severe TBI: an interesting link needing confirmation. *Crit Care.* 2013;17(3):151.

39. Rajajee V, Thyagarajan P, Rajagopalan R. Optic nerve ultrasonography for detection of raised intracranial pressure when invasive monitoring is unavailable. *Neurol India.* 2010;58(5):812.

40. Rajajee V, Vanaman M, Fletcher JJ, Jacobs TL. Optic nerve ultrasound for the detection of raised intracranial pressure. *Neurocrit Care.* 2011;15(3):506–15.

41. Geeraerts T, Launey Y, Martin L, Pottecher J, Vigué B, Duranteau J, *et al.* Ultrasonography of the optic nerve sheath may be useful for detecting raised intracranial pressure after severe brain injury. *Intensive Care Med.* 2007;33(10):1704–11.

42. Geeraerts T, Newcombe VFJ, Coles JP, Abate MG, Perkes IE, Hutchinson PJA, *et al.* Use of T2-weighted magnetic resonance imaging of the optic nerve sheath to detect raised intracranial pressure. *Crit Care.* 2008;12(5):R114.

43. Dubourg J, Javouhey E, Geeraerts T, Messerer M, Kassai B. Ultrasonography of optic nerve sheath diameter for detection of raised intracranial pressure: a systematic review and meta-analysis. *Intensive Care Med.* 2011;37(7):1059–68.

44. Nenekidis I, Geiser M, Riva C, Pournaras C, Tsironi E, Vretzakis G, *et al.* Blood flow measurements within optic nerve head during on-pump cardiovascular operations. A window to the brain? *Interact Cardiovasc Thorac Surg.* 2011;12(5):718–22.

45. Masquère P, Bonneville F, Geeraerts T. Optic nerve sheath diameter on initial brain CT, raised intracranial pressure and mortality after severe TBI: an interesting link needing confirmation. *Crit Care.* 2013;17(3):151.

46. Contant CF, Robertson CS, Crouch J, Gopinath SP, Narayan RK, Grossman RG. Intracranial pressure waveform indices in transient and refractory intracranial hypertension. *J Neurosci Methods.* 1995;57(1):15–25.

47. Hamilton RB, Baldwin K, Fuller J, Vespa P, Hu X, Bergsneider M. Intracranial pressure pulse waveform correlates with aqueductal cerebrospinal fluid stroke volume. *J Appl Physiol.* 2012;113(10):1560–6.

48. Asgari S, Bergsneider M, Hamilton R, Vespa P, Hu X. Consistent changes in intracranial pressure waveform morphology induced by acute hypercapnic cerebral vasodilatation. *Neurocrit Care.* 2011;15(1):55–62.

49. Hu X, Xu P, Asgari S, Vespa P, Bergsneider M. Forecasting ICP elevation based on prescient changes of intracranial pressure waveform morphology. *IEEE Trans Biomed Eng.* 2010;57(5):1070–8.

50. Hamilton R, Xu P, Asgari S, Kasprowicz M, Vespa P, Bergsneider M, *et al.* Forecasting intracranial pressure elevation using pulse waveform morphology. *Conf Proc IEEE Eng Med Biol Soc.* 2009;2009:4331–4.

51. Hu X, Xu P, Scalzo F, Vespa P, Bergsneider M. Morphological clustering and analysis of continuous intracranial pressure. *IEEE Trans Biomed Eng.* 2009;56(3):696–705.

52. Eide PK. A new method for processing of continuous intracranial pressure signals. *Med Eng Phys.* 2006;28(6):579–87.

53. Brain Trauma Foundation, American Association of Neurological Surgeons, Congress of Neurological Surgeons. Guidelines for the management of severe traumatic brain injury. *J Neurotrauma.* 2007;24 Suppl 1:S1–106.

54. Marmarou A, Shulman K, LaMorgese J. Compartmental analysis of compliance and outflow resistance of the cerebrospinal fluid system. *J Neurosurg.* 1975;43(5):523–34.

55. Maset AL, Marmarou A, Ward JD, Choi S, Lutz HA, Brooks D, *et al.* Pressure-volume index in head injury. *J Neurosurg.* 1987;67(6):832–40.

56. Shapiro K, Marmarou A, Shulman K. Characterization of clinical CSF dynamics and neural axis compliance using the pressure-volume index: I. The normal pressure-volume index. *Ann Neurol.* 1980;7(6):508–14.

57. Tain R-W, Bagci AM, Lam BL, Sklar EM, Ertl-Wagner B, Alperin N. Determination of cranio-spinal canal compliance distribution by MRI: Methodology and early application in idiopathic intracranial hypertension. *J Magn Reson Imaging.* 2011;34(6):1397–404.

58. Tans JT, Poortvliet DC. Intracranial volume-pressure relationship in man. Part 2: Clinical significance of the pressure-volume index. *J Neurosurg.* 1983;59(5):810–16.

59. Raabe A, Czosnyka M, Piper I, Seifert V. Monitoring of intracranial compliance: correction for a change in body position. *Acta Neurochir.* 1999;141(1):31–6.

60. Andrews PJD, Citerio G, Longhi L, Polderman K, Sahuquillo J, Vajkoczy P, *et al.* NICEM consensus on neurological monitoring in acute neurological disease. *Intensive Care Med.* 2008;34(8):1362–70.

61. Lavinio A, Rasulo FA, De Peri E, Czosnyka M, Latronico N. The relationship between the intracranial pressure-volume index and cerebral autoregulation. *Intensive Care Med.* 2009;35(3):546–9.

62. Kochanek PM, Adelson PD, Ashwal S, Bell MJ, Bratton S, Carson S, *et al.* Chapter 3. Indications for intracranial pressure monitoring. *Pediatr Crit Care Med.* 2012;13:S11–17.

63. White H, Venkatesh B. Cerebral perfusion pressure in neurotrauma: a review. *Anesth Analg.* 2008;107(3):979–88.

64. Bauer DF, Markert JM. Meta-analysis of hemorrhagic complications from ventriculostomy placement by neurosurgeons. *Neurosurgery.* 2011;69(2):255–60.

65. Jones HA. Arterial transducer placement and cerebral perfusion pressure monitoring: a discussion. *Nurs Crit Care.* 2009;14(6):303–10.

66. Tasker RC. Intracranial pressure: influence of head-of-bed elevation, and beyond. *Pediatr Crit Care Med.* 2012;13(1):116–17.

67. Lozier AP, Sciacca RR, Romagnoli MF, Connolly ES. Ventriculostomy-related infections: a critical review of the literature. *Neurosurgery.* 2002;51(1):170–81.

68. Bota DP, Lefranc F, Vilallobos HR, Brimioulle S, Vincent J-L. Ventriculostomy-related infections in critically ill patients: a 6-year experience. *J Neurosurg.* 2005;103(3):468–72.

69. Murkin JM. Cerebral autoregulation: the role of CO2 in metabolic homeostasis. *Semin Cardiothorac Vasc Anesth*. 2007;11(4):269–73.

70. Mayhall CG, Archer NH, Lamb VA, Spadora AC, Baggett JW, Ward JD, et al. Ventriculostomy-related infections. A prospective epidemiologic study. *N Engl J Med*. 1984;310(9):553–9.

71. Bayliss WM. On the local reactions of the arterial wall to changes of internal pressure. *J Physiol (Lond)*. 1902;28(3):220–31.

72. Aaslid R, Lindegaard K, Sorteberg W. Cerebral autoregulation dynamics in humans. *Stroke*. 1989;20(1):45–52.

73. van Beek AH, Claassen JA, Rikkert MGO, Jansen RW. Cerebral autoregulation: an overview of current concepts and methodology with special focus on the elderly. *J Cereb Blood Flow Metab*. 2008;28(6):1071–85.

74. Panerai RB. Cerebral autoregulation: from models to clinical applications. *Cardiovasc Eng*. 2008;8(1):42–59.

75. Czosnyka M, Smielewski P, Kirkpatrick P, Menon DK, Pickard JD. Monitoring of cerebral autoregulation in head-injured patients. *Stroke*; 1996;27(10):1829–34.

76. Czosnyka M, Smielewski P, Lavinio A, Pickard JD, Panerai R. An assessment of dynamic autoregulation from spontaneous fluctuations of cerebral blood flow velocity: a comparison of two models, index of autoregulation and mean flow index. *Anesth Analg*. 2008;106(1):234–9.

77. Czosnyka M, Brady K, Reinhard M, Smielewski P, Steiner LA. Monitoring of cerebrovascular autoregulation: facts, myths, and missing links. *Neurocrit Care*. 2009;10(3):373–86.

78. Czosnyka M, Czosnyka Z, Momjian S, Pickard JD. Cerebrospinal fluid dynamics. *Physiol Meas*. 2004;25(5):R51–76.

79. Czosnyka M, Smielewski P, Kirkpatrick P, Laing RJ, Menon D, Pickard JD. Continuous assessment of the cerebral vasomotor reactivity in head injury. *Neurosurgery*. 1997;41(1):11–17.

80. Ratilal B, Costa J, Sampaio C. Antibiotic prophylaxis for surgical introduction of intracranial ventricular shunts. *Cochrane Database Syst Rev*. 2006;3:CD005365.

81. Czosnyka M, Smielewski P, Timofeev I, Lavinio A, Guazzo E, Hutchinson P, et al. Intracranial pressure: more than a number. *Neurosurg Focus*. 2007;22(5):E10.

82. Sánchez-Porras R, Santos E, Czosnyka M, Zheng Z, Unterberg AW, Sakowitz OW. "Long" pressure reactivity index (L-PRx) as a measure of autoregulation correlates with outcome in traumatic brain injury patients. *Acta Neurochir*. 2012;154(9):1575–81.

83. Honda H, Jones JC, Craighead MC, Diringer MN, Dacey RG, Warren DK. Reducing the incidence of intraventricular catheter-related ventriculitis in the neurology-neurosurgical intensive care unit at a tertiary care center in St Louis, Missouri: an 8-year follow-up study. *Infect Control Hosp Epidemiol*. 2010;31(10):1078–81.

84. Kalanuria A, Geocadin R, Püttgen H. Brain code and coma recovery: aggressive management of cerebral herniation. *Semin Neurol*. 2013;33(02):133–41.

85. Stenehjem E, Armstrong WS. Central nervous system device infections. *Infect Dis Clin North Am*. 2012;26(1):89–110.

86. Stevens RD, Huff JS, Duckworth J, Papangelou A, Weingart SD, Smith WS. Emergency neurological life support: intracranial hypertension and herniation. *Neurocrit Care*. 2012;17 Suppl 1:S60–5.

87. Sonabend AM, Korenfeld Y, Crisman C, Badjatia N, Mayer SA, Connolly ES. Prevention of ventriculostomy-related infections with prophylactic antibiotics and antibiotic-coated external ventricular drains: a systematic review. *Neurosurgery*. 2011;68(4):996–1005.

88. Juul N, Morris GF, Marshall SB, Marshall LF. Intracranial hypertension and cerebral perfusion pressure: influence on neurological deterioration and outcome in severe head injury. The Executive Committee of the International Selfotel Trial. *J Neurosurg*. 2000;92(1):1–6.

89. Vender J, Waller J, Dhandapani K, McDonnell D. An evaluation and comparison of intraventricular, intraparenchymal, and fluid-coupled techniques for intracranial pressure monitoring in patients with severe traumatic brain injury. *J Clin Monit Comput*. 2011;25(4):231–6.

90. Morris GF, Juul N, Marshall SB, Benedict B, Marshall LF. Neurological deterioration as a potential alternative endpoint in human clinical trials of experimental pharmacological agents for treatment of severe traumatic brain injuries. Executive Committee of the International Selfotel Trial. *Neurosurgery*. 1998;43(6):1369–72.

91. Martínez-Mañas RM, Santamarta D, de Campos JM, Ferrer E. Camino intracranial pressure monitor: prospective study of accuracy and complications. *J Neurol Neurosurg Psychiatr*. 2000;69(1):82–6.

92. Treggiari M, Schutz N, Yanez N, Romand J. Role of intracranial pressure values and patterns in predicting outcome in traumatic brain injury: a systematic review. *Neurocrit Care*. 2007;6(2):104–12.

93. Eide PK. Comparison of simultaneous continuous intracranial pressure (ICP) signals from a Codman and a Camino ICP sensor. *Med Eng Phys*. 2006;28(6):542–9.

94. Badri S, Chen J, Barber J, Temkin NR, Dikmen SS, Chesnut RM, et al. Mortality and long-term functional outcome associated with intracranial pressure after traumatic brain injury. *Intensive Care Med*. 2012;38(11):1800–9.

95. Piper I, Barnes A, Smith D, Dunn L. The Camino intracranial pressure sensor: is it optimal technology? An internal audit with a review of current intracranial pressure monitoring technologies. *Neurosurgery*. 2001;49(5):1158–64.

96. Stocchetti N, Zanaboni C, Colombo A, Citerio G, Beretta L, Ghisoni L, et al. Refractory intracranial hypertension and "second-tier" therapies in traumatic brain injury. *Intensive Care Med*. 2008;34(3):461–7.

97. Eide P. Comparison of simultaneous continuous intracranial pressure (ICP) signals from a Codman and a Camino ICP sensor. *Med Eng Phys*. 2006;28(6):542–9.

98. Stocchetti N, Rossi S, Buzzi F, Mattioli C, Paparella A, Colombo A. Intracranial hypertension in head injury: management and results. *Intensive Care Med*. 1999;25(4):371–6.

99. Gelabert-Gonzalez M, Ginesta-Galan V, Sernamito-Garcia R, Allut A, Bandin-Dieguez J, Rumbo R. The Camino intracranial pressure device in clinical practice. Assessment in a 1000 cases. *Acta Neurochir*. 2006;148(4):435–41.

100. Münch E, Weigel R, Schmiedek P, Schürer L. The Camino intracranial pressure device in clinical practice: reliability, handling characteristics and complications. *Acta Neurochir*. 1998;140(11):1113–20.

101. Stein S, Georgoff P, Meghan S, Mirza K. 150 years of treating severe traumatic brain injury: a systematic review of progress in mortality. *J Neurotrauma*. 2010;27(7):134353.

102. Stendel R, Heidenreich J, Schilling A, Akhavan-Sigari R, Kurth R, Picht T, et al. Clinical evaluation of a new intracranial pressure monitoring device. *Acta Neurochir*. 2003;145(3):185–93.

103. Morton R, Lucas TH, Ko A, Browd SR, Ellenbogen RG, Chesnut RM. Intracerebral abscess associated with the Camino intracranial pressure monitor: case report and review of the literature. *Neurosurgery*. 2012;71(1):E193–8.

104. Citerio G, Piper I, Cormio M, Galli D, Cazzaniga S, Enblad P, et al. Bench test assessment of the new Raumedic Neurovent-P ICP sensor: a technical report by the BrainIT group. *Acta Neurochir*. 2004;146(11):1221–6.

105. Chesnut RM, Temkin N, Carney N, Dikmen S, Rondina C, Videtta W, et al. A Trial of Intracranial-Pressure Monitoring in Traumatic Brain Injury. *N Engl J Med*. 2012;367(26):2471–81.

106. Citerio G, Piper I, Chambers IR, Galli D, Enblad P, Kiening K, et al. Multicenter clinical assessment of the Raumedic Neurovent-P intracranial pressure sensor: a report by the BrainIT group. *Neurosurgery*. 2008;63(6):1152–8.

107. Al-Tamimi YZ, Helmy A, Bavetta S, Price SJ. Assessment of zero drift in the Codman intracranial pressure monitor: a study from 2 neurointensive care units. *Neurosurgery*. 2009;64(1):94–8.

108. Morgalla MH, Dietz K, Deininger M, Grote EH. The problem of long-term ICP drift assessment: improvement by use of the ICP drift index. *Acta Neurochir*. 2002;144(1):57–60.

109. Gray WP, Palmer JD, Gill J, Gardner M, Iannotti F. A clinical study of parenchymal and subdural miniature strain-gauge transducers for monitoring intracranial pressure. *Neurosurgery*. 1996;39(5):927–31.

110. Gopinath SP, Robertson CS, Contant CF, Narayan RK, Grossman RG. Clinical evaluation of a miniature strain-gauge transducer for monitoring intracranial pressure. *Neurosurgery*. 1995;36(6):1137–40.

111. Koskinen L-OD, Olivecrona M. Clinical experience with the intra-parenchymal intracranial pressure monitoring Codman MicroSensor system. *Neurosurgery*. 2005;56(4):693–8.

112. Hong W-C, Tu Y-K, Chen Y-S, Lien L-M, Huang S-J. Subdural intracranial pressure monitoring in severe head injury: clinical experience with the Codman MicroSensor. *Surg Neurol*. 2006;66 Suppl 2:S8–S13.

113. Eide PK. Comparison of simultaneous continuous intracranial pressure (ICP) signals from ICP sensors placed within the brain parenchyma and the epidural space. *Med Eng Phys*. 2008;30(1):34–40.

114. Poca MA, Sahuquillo J, Topczewski T, Peñarrubia MJ, Muns A. Is intracranial pressure monitoring in the epidural space reliable? Fact and fiction. *J Neurosurg*. 2007;106(4):548–56.

115. Poca M, Martínez-Ricarte F, Sahuquillo J, Lastra R, Torné R, Armengol M. Intracranial pressure monitoring with the Neurodur-P epidural sensor: a prospective study in patients with adult hydrocephalus or idiopathic intracranial hypertension. *J Neurosurg*. 2008;108(5):934–42.

116. Eide P. Comparison of simultaneous continuous intracranial pressure (ICP) signals from ICP sensors placed within the brain parenchyma and the epidural space. *Med Eng Phys*. 2008;30(1):34–40.

117. Lu C-W, Czosnyka M, Shieh J-S, Smielewska A, Pickard JD, Smielewski P. Complexity of intracranial pressure correlates with outcome after traumatic brain injury. *Brain*. 2012;135(Pt 8):2399–408.

118. Citerio G, Stocchetti N. Intracranial pressure and outcome in severe traumatic brain injury: the quest for evidence continues. *Intensive Care Med*. 2008;34(7):1173–4.

119. Stocchetti N, Citerio G. Treating intracranial hypertension in traumatic brain injury: be cold! *Intensive Care Med*. 2008;34(9):1737.

120. Mack WJ, King RG, Ducruet AF, Kreiter K, Mocco J, Maghoub A, et al. Intracranial pressure following aneurysmal subarachnoid hemorrhage: monitoring practices and outcome data. *Neurosurg Focus*. 2003;14(4):e3.

121. Voldby B, Enevoldsen EM. Intracranial pressure changes following aneurysm rupture. Part 1: clinical and angiographic correlations. *J Neurosurg*. 1982;56(2):186–96.

122. Voldby B, Enevoldsen EM. Intracranial pressure changes following aneurysm rupture. Part 2: associated cerebrospinal fluid lactacidosis. *J Neurosurg*. 1982;56(2):197–204.

123. Voldby B, Enevoldsen EM. Intracranial pressure changes following aneurysm rupture. Part 3: Recurrent hemorrhage. *J Neurosurg*. 1982;56(6):784–9.

124. Heuer GG, Smith MJ, Elliott JP, Winn HR, Leroux PD. Relationship between intracranial pressure and other clinical variables in patients with aneurysmal subarachnoid hemorrhage. *J Neurosurg*. 2004;101(3):408–16.

125. Connolly ES, Rabinstein AA, Carhuapoma JR, Derdeyn CP, Dion J, Higashida RT, et al. Guidelines for the management of aneurysmal subarachnoid hemorrhage: a guideline for healthcare professionals from the American Heart Association/American Stroke Association. *Stroke*. 2012;43(6):1711–37.

126. Coppadoro A, Citerio G. Subarachnoid hemorrhage: an update for the intensivist. *Minerva Anestesiol*. 2011;77(1):74–84.

127. Forsyth RJ, Wolny S, Rodrigues B. Routine intracranial pressure monitoring in acute coma. *Cochrane Database Syst Rev*. 2010;2:CD002043.

128. Jauch EC, Saver JL, Adams HP, Bruno A, Connors JJB, Demaerschalk BM, et al. Guidelines for the early management of patients with acute ischemic stroke. *Stroke*. 2013;44(3):870–947.

129. Sala F, Abbruzzese C, Galli D, Grimaldi M, Abate MG, Sganzerla EP, et al. Intracranial pressure monitoring in pediatric bacterial meningitis: a fancy or useful tool? A case report. *Minerva Anestesiol*. 2009;75(12):746–9.

130. Odetola FO, Clark SJ, Lamarand KE, Davis MM, Garton HJ. Intracranial pressure monitoring in childhood meningitis with coma: A national survey of neurosurgeons in the United States. *Pediatr Crit Care Med*. 2011;12(6):e350–6.

131. Wong GKC, Ip M, Poon WS, Mak CWK, Ng RYT. Antibiotics-impregnated ventricular catheter versus systemic antibiotics for prevention of nosocomial CSF and non-CSF infections: a prospective randomised clinical trial. *J Neurol Neurosurg Psychiatr*. 2010;81(10):1064–7.

132. Eymann R, Chehab S, Strowitzki M, Steudel WI, Kiefer M. Clinical and economic consequences of antibiotic-impregnated cerebrospinal fluid shunt catheters. *J Neurosurg Pediatr*. 2008;1(6):444–50.

133. Abla AA, Zabramski JM, Jahnke HK, Fusco D, Nakaji P. Comparison of two antibiotic-impregnated ventricular catheters: a prospective sequential series trial. *Neurosurgery*. 2011;68(2):437–42.

134. Stevens EA, Palavecino E, Sherertz RJ, Shihabi Z, Couture DE. Effects of antibiotic-impregnated external ventricular drains on bacterial culture results: an in vitro analysis. *J Neurosurg*. 2010;113(1):86–92.

135. Gutiérrez-González R, Boto GR. Do antibiotic-impregnated catheters prevent infection in CSF diversion procedures? Review of the literature. *J Infect*. 2010;61(1):9–20.

136. Signorini DF, Shad A, Piper IR, Statham PF. A clinical evaluation of the Codman MicroSensor for intracranial pressure monitoring. *Br J Neurosurg*. 1998;12(3):223–7.

137. Piper IR, Miller JD. The evaluation of the wave-form analysis capability of a new strain-gauge intracranial pressure MicroSensor. *Neurosurgery*. 1995;36(6):1142–4.

138. Lescot T, Reina V, Le Manach Y, Boroli F, Chauvet D, Boch A-L, et al. In vivo accuracy of two intraparenchymal intracranial pressure monitors. *Intensive Care Med*. 2011;37(5):875–9.

CHAPTER 10

Monitoring cerebral blood flow

Chandril Chugh and W. Andrew Kofke

Most brain-oriented therapies in neurointensive care are directed towards the maintenance of nutritive cerebral blood flow (CBF). It is thus informative in many circumstances to monitor CBF as part of a multimodal brain monitoring approach to determine the need for, guide, and assess the effectiveness of brain-directed therapy. Technologies for CBF assessment can be conceptually categorized as those providing single CBF determinations, based on imaging or non-imaging methods, and those providing continuous monitoring at the bedside. The monitors can be further categorized as invasive or non-invasive. Despite the fact that many decisions taken during neurointensive care are intended to support or produce adequate CBF, there are only a few approaches that are available for direct titration of therapy to CBF.

Imaging-based assessment of cerebral blood flow

Several imaging modalities are able to quantify CBF. These are discussed in detail in Chapter 15 and only a brief overview will be provided here.

Computed tomography perfusion scanning

The computed tomography (CT) perfusion technique allows rapid qualitative and quantitative evaluation of cerebral perfusion by generating maps of CBF, cerebral blood volume (CBV), and mean transit time (MTT) (1,2). CT perfusion is used to assess CBF in a variety of other circumstances including cerebral vasospasm, assessment of cerebrovascular reserve, and preoperative assessment in patients in whom carotid resection is planned, but primarily to determine viable blood flow in patients with acute stroke (3). The ischaemic penumbra is characterized by decreased CBF, normal to increased CBV, and increased MTT, whereas the infarcted tissue has decreased CBF and CBV with increased MTT (4). MTT maps have been shown to be specific indicators of stroke, whereas CBF and CBV assist in distinguishing between ischaemic and infarcted tissue (5). CT perfusion does not provide a quantitative measure of CBF in mL/100 g/min but demonstrates interregional CBF disparities. Further discussion of the technique with illustrative figures can be found in Chapter 15 (Figures 15.2 and 15.3).

CT perfusion is also used to measure cerebrovascular reserve (see Chapter 3) in conjunction with an acetazolamide challenge (6). It differentiates areas with chronic low CBF due to low metabolic demand from tissue where CBF is inadequate to meet metabolic demands, that is, those at risk of ischaemia. Acetazolamide produces vasodilation by increasing local carbon dioxide concentration, but cerebral vessels in ischaemic tissue do not respond to acetazolamide because they are already maximally dilated (7). In this way, acetazolamide delineates the areas at high risk of insufficient nutritive flow due to an inability to compensate for physiological derangements such as hypoxaemia, decreased systemic blood pressure, or anaemia.

CT perfusion is also increasingly used to assess the perfusion effects of cerebral vasospasm after subarachnoid haemorrhage (SAH); patients with severe vasospasm have low CBF and CBV compared to those with no vasospasm (8). CBF and MMT thresholds of 35 mL/100 g/min and 5.5 seconds respectively have been reported for the detection of delayed cerebral ischaemia (9).

Arterial spin labelling perfusion functional magnetic resonance imaging

Arterial spin labelling (ASL) is a magnetic resonance imaging (MRI) technique that uses protons in arterial blood en route to the brain as an endogenous tracer, negating the need for administration of exogenous tracers. Unlike blood oxygen level-dependent functional magnetic resonance imaging (fMRI), ASL perfusion fMRI creates quantifiable and stable time series data from which absolute CBF can be calculated (10,11). Perfusion fMRI is not as fast as the CT-based techniques and requires transfer of a potentially unstable patient to the MRI scanner. However, no pharmacological contrast is required, there is no radiation exposure, and the flow images can be superimposed over the anatomical images from a structural MRI scan. Serial assessment of response to physiological changes can be made in the scanner (11). Difficulties relate to issues with the management of critically ill patients in the MRI scanner with its unique attendant risks related to magnet precautions. In addition, this does not provide rapid bedside information. Nonetheless, the resolution is probably the best available (Figure 10.1).

Positron emission tomography

Positron emission tomography (PET) provides rapid CBF measurements in three dimensions, but without the regional resolution or quantitation provided by stable xenon (Xe)-CT CBF (see 'Stable Xenon Computed Tomography') or perfusion MRI measurements. It uses $H_2^{15}O$ as a tracer which rapidly distributes throughout the brain in proportion to CBF and is then rapidly washed out, permitting serial flows to be measured (Figure 10.2). Radiation dose limits the number of repetitive studies and data are not available to clinicians in a sufficiently rapid manner to allow therapeutic titration based on measured CBF. PET also entails transporting the patient, who usually also requires CT for structural information, to another imaging suite (12,13). Furthermore, the technology is available in only a few major medical centres, limiting its use predominantly to research purposes.

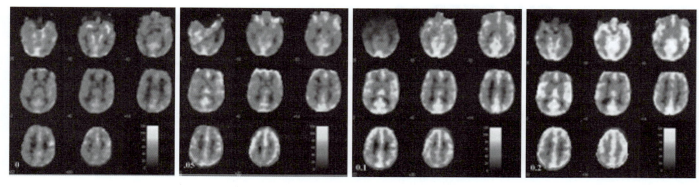

Fig. 10.1 Magnetic resonance imaging continuous arterial spin labelling images of the mean quantitative cerebral blood flow (CBF) images at four remifentanil dosing conditions noted in lower left of each figure as 0.0, 0.05, 0.1, and 0.2 mcg/kg/min. Note the increased CBF with larger doses of remifentanil related to effects of increasing $PaCO_2$. Reproduced with permission from Kofke WA *et al.*, 'Remifentanil-induced cerebral blood flow effects in normal humans: dose and ApoE genotype', *Anesthesia & Analgesia*, 105, 1, pp. 167–175, copyright 2007, with permission from Wolters Kluwer and International Anesthesia Research Society.

Single-photon emission computed tomography

Single-photon emission computed tomography (SPECT) entails the administration of hexamethylpropyleneamineoxime (HMPAO), a radioactive tracer which, like $H_2^{15}O$ in PET, is distributed through the brain in proportion to CBF. However, unlike in PET, the tracers used in SPECT remain in the brain for several hours and can therefore be injected in the intensive care unit prior to transfer of the patient to the imaging suite. In general, SPECT suffers from a lack of quantification without the resolution available with CT perfusion, stable Xe-CT CBF, and perfusion MRI. It also requires transport to an imaging suite distant from the CT scanner and cannot easily be repeated to assess the effects of therapeutic interventions. Reports have described methods that provide better quantification of SPECT data (14,15), which may represent an advance that will make this technology more widely applicable in neurointensive care unit (NICU) patients in the future.

Stable xenon computed tomography

The stable Xe-CT CBF method involves inhalation of 26–33% stable xenon gas which becomes dissolved in the blood and is transported to the brain. Its concentration is then measured simultaneously in

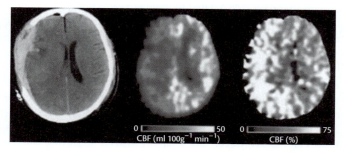

Fig. 10.2 Positron emission tomography images early after head injury. X-ray CT, PET CBF, and PET OEF images are shown 16 hours after injury following evacuation of a subdural haematoma. Note the small amount of residual subdural blood with minimal midline shift and the marked reductions in CBF and increases in OEF in the cerebral hemisphere underlying the evacuated subdural haematoma. CBF, cerebral blood flow; CT, computed tomography; OEF, oxygen extraction fraction; PET, positron emission tomography.
Reprinted by permission from Macmillian Publishers Ltd: *Journal of Cerebral Blood Flow & Metabolism*, Coles JP *et al.*, 'Incidence and mechanisms of cerebral ischemia in early clinical head injury', 24, 2, pp. 202–211, copyright 2004.

the brain and expired gas, the latter being a surrogate for arterial concentration (16). As xenon is radiopaque, its distribution in the brain over time (measured by serial CT scans) can be used to calculate CBF. The method iteratively computes solubility throughout the brain and uses the adjusted solubility for pixel-by-pixel CBF calculations, providing valuable information in disease states in which solubility and therefore CBF are not uniform throughout the brain.

The validity of the Xe-CT technique in clinical practice has been questioned because of the inherent vasodilatory properties of xenon which may increase CBF and confound measured values. However, this effect can be minimized by using multiple early images and weighting calculations to the early portion of the wash-in curve (16–18). Correlation between Xe-CT and an autoradiographic CBF gold standard method in animals is excellent (19) and, moreover, values obtained in normal controls undergoing stable Xe-CT demonstrated a non-hyperaemic CBF. Thus, regardless of concerns about its potential CBF-increasing effects, stable Xe-CT CBF is a versatile and useful tool, especially in the evaluation of low flow conditions.

Stable Xe-CT CBF measurement can be repeated within 15 minutes, so a response to therapy can be observed using repeat studies. The fact that a reactivity challenge can be readily performed whilst a patient is in the CT scanner is a major advantage as these data can be obtained during the course of obtaining a structural CT scan (Figure 10.3) (6,20). Moreover, with the advent of portable CT scanners, this information can be acquired at the bedside (21). This technique is not available in the United States due to Food and Drug Administration regulatory obstacles in approving stable xenon, although xenon use is approved for anaesthesia use in Europe (22) and in Japan for Xe-CT CBF (Howard Yonas, University of New Mexico, personal communication).

Non-imaging-based, non-invasive assessment of cerebral blood flow

There are several non-imaging-based methods of assessing CBF that can be used at the bedside.

Transcranial Doppler ultrasonography

Transcranial Doppler (TCD) ultrasonography uses reflected ultrasound from basal cerebral arteries and the Doppler principle to determine the velocity of blood (in cm/sec) in the insonated

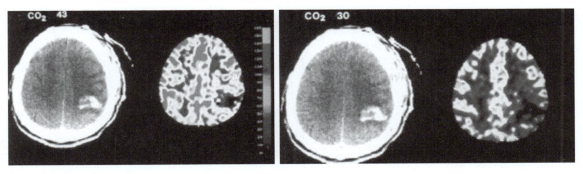

Fig. 10.3 Non-contrast scan (left of each panel) showing a left parietal intraparenchymal haemorrhage with concomitant Xe-CT CBF scan (right of each panel) performed sequentially at $PaCO_2$ levels of 5.7 kPa (43 mmHg) and 4.0 kPa (30 mmHg) demonstrating CBF reactivity to changing $PaCO_2$. Note the higher CBF with higher $PaCO_2$ in the left panel and correspondingly lower CBF in the right panel. The CBF scale is shown in the left panel.
CBF, cerebral flow; Xe-CT, stable xenon computed tomography.

artery. It yields real-time dynamic information regarding blood flow velocity (BFV), providing a continuous waveform similar to the arterial blood pressure (ABP) waveform (Figure 10.4A). Insonated arteries typically include those in the proximal arteries of the circle of Willis. It is important to note that TCD ultrasonography is not a quantitative flow monitor measuring absolute CBF in mL/100 g/min, but a technique that provides non-quantitative information regarding the presence and character of blood flow. There are some situations in which TCD changes may reflect changes in CBF, particularly with abrupt changes in arterial inflow (Figure 10.4A, B) (23).

Although the information provided by TCD is very useful, neurointensivists must be aware of several factors that may artefactually alter the BFV value obtained. These include the following:

♦ *Insonation angle*: the reproducibility of TCD recordings depends on a constant angle of insonation for a given vessel. This is an important operator-dependent factor which becomes less important as the insonation angle becomes more parallel to the vessel being examined.

♦ *Vessel diameter*: decreases in vessel calibre may result in an increase in measured BFV in the face of decreasing CBF.

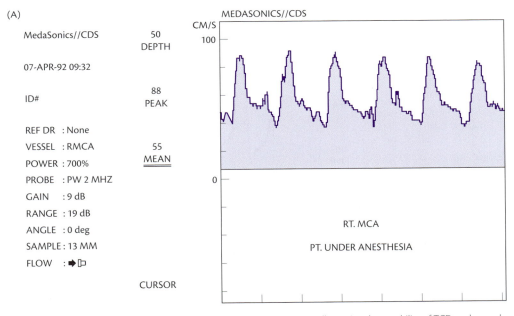

Fig. 10.4 Transcranial Doppler ultrasound monitoring of the MCA during carotid endarterectomy, illustrating the capability of TCD to detect abruptly decreased CBF, emboli, and hyperaemia.
(A) TCD baseline during carotid endarterectomy, before instrumentation of the carotid artery.
(B) Cross-clamping of the carotid artery showing decreased distal BFV.
(C) Unclamping with emboli to the MCA after unclamping the carotid artery.
(D) Reperfusion hyperaemia in the MCA after unclamping the carotid artery.
BFV, blood flow velocity; MCA, middle cerebral artery; TCD, transcranial Doppler ultrasonography.
Reproduced from Hassler W *et al.*, 'Transcranial Doppler ultrasonography in raised intracranial pressure and in intracranial circulatory arrest', *Journal of Neurosurgery*, 68, 5, pp. 745–751, copyright 1988, with permission from *Journal of Neurosurgery*.

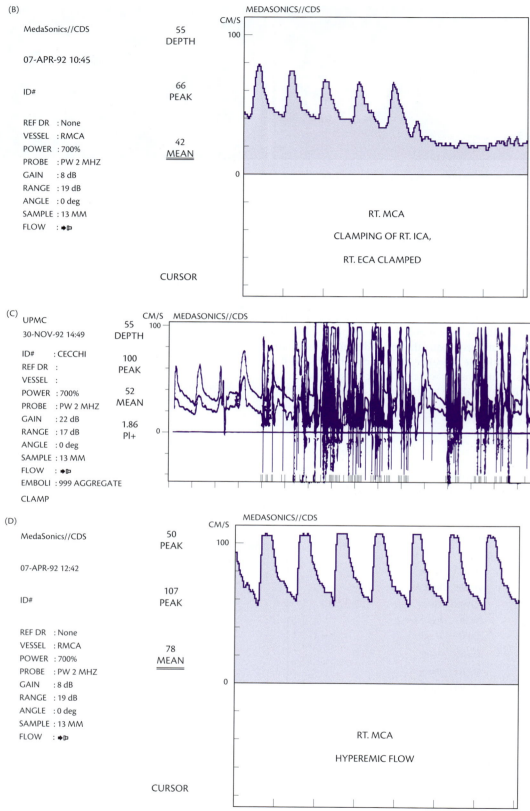

(B)

MedaSonics//CDS

07-APR-92 10:45

ID#

REF DR : None
VESSEL : RMCA
POWER : 700%
PROBE : PW 2 MHZ
GAIN : 8 dB
RANGE : 19 dB
ANGLE : 0 deg
SAMPLE : 13 MM
FLOW : ➡️▷

55
DEPTH

66
PEAK

42
MEAN

CURSOR

MEDASONICS//CDS

CM/S
100

0

RT. MCA

CLAMPING OF RT. ICA,

RT. ECA CLAMPED

(C) UPMC

30-NOV-92 14:49

ID# : CECCHI
REF DR :
VESSEL :
POWER : 700%
PROBE : PW 2 MHZ
GAIN : 22 dB
RANGE : 17 dB
ANGLE : 0 deg
SAMPLE : 13 MM
FLOW : ➡️▷
EMBOLI : 999 AGGREGATE

CLAMP

55
DEPTH

100
PEAK

52
MEAN

1.86
PI+

CM/S
100

MEDASONICS//CDS

0

(D)

MedaSonics//CDS

07-APR-92 12:42

ID#

REF DR : None
VESSEL : RMCA
POWER : 700%
PROBE : PW 2 MHZ
GAIN : 8 dB
RANGE : 19 dB
ANGLE : 0 deg
SAMPLE : 13 MM
FLOW : ➡️▷

50
PEAK

107
PEAK

78
MEAN

CURSOR

CM/S
100

MEDASONICS//CDS

0

RT. MCA

HYPEREMIC FLOW

Fig. 10.4 (continued)

♦ *Physiological factors*: haematocrit, partial pressure of arterial carbon dioxide ($PaCO_2$), systemic blood pressure, and temperature can also influence BFV, although changes may also reflect actual changes in CBF.

TCD has several uses in the NICU including assessment of cerebral vasospasm, vascular reactivity, intracranial pressure (ICP), arterial patency, flow direction, and the detection of emboli (Figure 10.4C) and hyperaemia (Figure 10.4D) (24). Although it can be used at the bedside, it is difficult and labour-intensive. The potential value of TCD ultrasonography as a monitor is illustrated by reports of its use during induction of anaesthesia (25), and of its value in guiding therapy during an aneurysmal rupture (26). Training is required to acquire and identify a signal from a cerebral artery and, once acquired, maintaining acquisition of a good signal for monitoring purposes can be challenging. Minor changes in the angle of insonation related to routine nursing interventions can result in loss or degradation of the TCD signal, or changes in the BFV recorded. Thus, well-trained and motivated staff are needed to use TCD ultrasonography successfully in the NICU. TCD is most optimally used for monitoring purposes when data are acquired hourly or with each clinical neurological examination, thus providing a useful trend indicator over hours or days.

Cerebral vasospasm

With narrowing of a basal cerebral artery, BFV increases even as flow decreases. TCD ultrasonography has thus found a routine place in the NICU as a screening and monitoring tool for cerebral vasospasm (27–29). It may demonstrate early changes indicative of vasospasm prior to the onset of a clinically evident ischaemic deficit. However, some studies have shown that increased BFV in patients with SAH can be associated with hyperaemia more often than vasospasm, possibly related to the use of nimodipine (30). Further, TCD ultrasonography is unable to detect distal spasm, thus possibly giving a false sense of safety if BFV is normal. Although TCD ultrasonography has value as a screening tool for vasospasm, it has insufficient sensitivity and specificity to be the sole criterion on which to base important therapeutic decisions in patients with SAH. TCD criteria for diagnosis of vasospasm are reviewed in Chapter 18.

Cerebrovascular reserve

TCD may also be used to assess the extent of vasodilatory cerebrovascular reserve and, in the context of SAH, provide indirect information regarding capability to increase flow to a vasodilatory stimulus, and thus the likelihood of a vasospastic condition producing clinically evident symptoms (31,32). However, it is unclear whether this approach can differentiate hyperaemia from vasospasm. Analogous to stable Xe-CT, TCD can also be used to determine the extent of vascular reserve in other contexts, thereby providing a semi-quantitative indicator of the severity of injury to a given vascular bed (6,33,34).

Reactivity assessment is performed during manipulation of cerebral perfusion pressure (CPP) or carbon dioxide tension. For a given change in mean arterial pressure (MAP), within the normal autoregulatory range, there should be no change in BFV, and a CPP-induced change in BFV therefore indicates abnormal pressure autoregulation (76). Carbon dioxide reactivity is assessed by increasing inspired CO_2 or by increasing tissue CO_2 via administration of acetazolamide; BFV normally increases by 3–4% per mmHg increase in $PaCO_2$. An absent response implies lack of cerebrovascular reserve

such that the brain may not tolerate minor perturbations in oxygen delivery. CO_2 reactivity index can be defined (35) as:

$$\left(V_2 - V_1\right)/\left(\Delta \text{ end-tidal } CO_2\right)$$

where V_2 is BFV after the change in end-tidal CO_2 and V_1 is the BFV before the CO_2 change. A normal mean (± standard deviation) CO_2 reactivity index is 1.78 (± 0.48). In patients with cerebrovascular disease, the index varies from 0.15 to 2.6. Failure of the brain to respond to rises in CO_2 with a normal increase in BFV implies the presence of maximal vasodilation and impaired vascular reserve.

Intracranial pressure

As ICP increases or CPP decreases, the character of the TCD waveform changes to a more 'spiky' appearance with increased pulsatility (36,37). This is the basis of the pulsatility index (PI) which is defined as follows (38):

$$PI = \left(\text{systolic flow velocity} - \text{end-diastolic velocity}\right)/ \\ \text{mean diastolic velocity}$$

As diastolic perfusion is increasingly compromised, the cerebral circulation takes on more characteristics of the higher-resistance peripheral circulation with a lower diastolic flow velocity. Ultimately the diastolic flow velocity becomes zero, as ICP exceeds diastolic blood pressure. This results in a progressive increase in PI with the increase in ICP.

TCD ultrasonography cannot directly measure ICP or CPP, but may be used to make general inferences about CPP and indicate when ICP exceeds diastolic blood pressure (39,40). TCD-based ICP and CPP assessment is based predominantly on retrospective reports. Notably, use of PI to reliably predict ICP or CPP is not recommended based on a prospective quantitative assessment (41), although there may be some value in following PI trends where direct ICP measurement is not feasible, such as in fulminant hepatic encephalopathy (42).

Increases in ICP into the 20–30 mmHg range, although of epidemiological significance, have not been shown to have substantial physiological significance in terms of a dangerous decrement in CBF. As ICP increases, cerebral vasodilation occurs in a compensatory fashion, and the actual CBF tends not to be in the 'ischaemic' range at lower ICPs. However, with further ICP increases, approaching diastolic arterial pressure and infringing on the critical closing pressure of the cerebral microvasculature (see Chapter 3), flow which ordinarily is continuous throughout the cardiac cycle becomes discontinuous, eventually decreasing to zero during diastole (43,44). This is consistent with the theoretical conclusions of Giulioni and colleagues who suggested, based on considerations of intracranial elastance and vasomotor tone, that systolic increase and diastolic decrease in BFV should occur when ICP reaches the 'breakpoint' value (36). They suggest that the PI should thus be a useful indicator of high ICP, likely at the extremes. In such situations of zero diastolic flow, ICP should theoretically be in the 40–60 mmHg range (44). An ICP of 48 mmHg is the average level at which patients progressing to brain death have been observed initially to sustain a systolic spike pattern on TCD with an oscillating pattern developing at 62.5 mmHg (45).

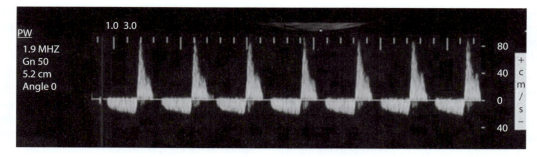

Fig. 10.5 TCD waveform in a patient declared brain dead by clinical tests. Note the reversal of diastolic blood flow in the left middle cerebral artery. CBF, cerebral blood flow; ICP, intracranial pressure; TCD, transcranial Doppler ultrasonography.

Hassler et al. (37) clearly showed the relationship between ICP and phasic blood pressure and how TCD waveform can reflect ICP encroachment on diastolic flow when ICP exceeds diastolic pressure. As CPP progressively decreases to levels associated with no CBF, there is diastolic reversal of flow on TCD presumably due to blood 'bouncing' backwards off an oedematous brain, also shown in a case report of brain death (Figure 10.5—compare with a normal TCD trace in Figure 10.4A) (46). Thus, TCD ultrasonography may be useful as a screening tool for brain death in that the absence of diastolic reversal rules out brain death. This phenomenon has been reported in several reports, and meta-analysis of such reports indicates general support for the notion that TCD can be useful in the assessment for brain death (47). However, it is important to consider the diastolic blood pressure when making such assessments. A strikingly similar TCD waveform can be generated in a totally sentient patient with aortic insufficiency and diastolic pressure low enough to be in the range of normal ICP (24).

Flow patency

Patients may be admitted to the NICU after thrombolysis or procedures to the middle cerebral or internal carotid arteries, and TCD ultrasonography can used to confirm continued patency of the relevant blood vessel(s) (48). As clinical symptoms may not occur until the vessel is completely occluded, or may not occur at all, TCD ultrasonography may be used to indicate when flow in the monitored vessel is decreasing.

Emboli detection

Emboli can be readily detected with TCD ultrasonography, most commonly in the context of cardiac or carotid surgery. This is illustrated in Figure 10.4C, showing embolic released into the cerebral circulation after carotid unclamping during carotid endarterectomy. In the NICU, TCD ultrasonography can help determine the adequacy of anticoagulation to suppress cerebral emboli in patients with artificial cardiac valves or patients and tenuous proximal vascular patency (49,50). However, emboli are very common in some situations without obvious neurological sequelae and thus determination that a given frequency of emboli in a given patient warrants major changes in therapy is presently a matter of clinical judgement.

Hyperaemia detection

Hyperaemia can be a major problem in some clinical conditions, such as after arteriovenous malformation resection and carotid endarterectomy, in hepatic failure, and in systemic hypertension.

TCD ultrasonography can be used to ascertain the presence of cerebral hyperfusion syndrome (51,52).

Near-infrared spectroscopy

Near-infrared spectroscopy (NIRS), which is described in detail in Chapter 11, has been used to assess CBF based on induced changes in SaO_2, using oxyhaemoglobin as a tracer (53,54). Modern NIRS technologies, such as acousto-optic NIRS, yield continuous CBF information (55). Another approach is the use of diffuse correlation spectroscopy (DCS) to provide continuous regional CBF and possibly also continuous regional cerebral metabolic rate of oxygen ($CMRO_2$) and oxygen extraction fraction (OEF) data (21,56–58). The acousto-optic and DCS methods only measure changes in flow from an arbitrary baseline, although quantitatively, but this can be problematic if the baseline value is abnormal. Investigators are actively evaluating possible solutions to this problem. The injection of indocyanine green, combined with NIRS, can provide a quantitative blood flow index, although it is necessarily discontinuous (59–63). A report by Diop and colleagues proposes combining continuous DCS with infrequent indocyanine green injections to yield a continuous NIRS monitor of regional CBF, $CMRO_2$, and OEF (64). This remains an investigational, but attractive, notion.

[133]Xenon

The ^{133}Xe technique depends on the measurement of the concentration of radioactive xenon in the brain tissue using gamma detectors placed over the scalp externally (65). [133]Xe can be inhaled or administered by intravenous or intra-arterial (carotid) injection. Its brain concentration is measured by the gamma detectors, and assessment of regional CBF is possible depending on the number and location of detectors. The advantage of this method is that very low quantities of xenon are needed, removing the potential for side effects of the xenon on CBF. The measurements can be performed at the bedside by appropriately trained staff (66). Its drawback is that it is not very sensitive in low flow states and may miss blood flow in the deep tissues or conversely in the cortex because of persistent flow to the deeper structures. The ^{133}Xe method has generally fallen out of favour in clinical practice but is occasionally still used in research.

Invasive assessment of cerebral blood flow

There are several invasive monitors of CBF that can be used at the bedside.

Arteriovenous oxygen content difference

The arteriovenous oxygen content (AVO_2) difference measurement is based on the Fick equation using arterial and jugular venous blood samples:

$$CMRO_2 = CBF \times (A - VO_2)$$

and

$$(A - VO_2) = CMRO_2 / CBF$$

where $CMRO_2$ is cerebral metabolic rate for oxygen, CBF is cerebral blood flow, and $A - VO_2$ is the difference in oxygen content of arterial and jugular venous blood (see Chapter 11).

Given a stable cerebral metabolic rate, changes in AVO_2 difference across the brain will thus represent changes in global CBF. Obviously, it cannot be used to provide quantitative or regional CBF measurements, but it can be used at the bedside in a serial manner, or continuously if a fibreoptic catheter is used. The AVO_2 difference provides information regarding the adequacy of global CBF relative to cerebral metabolic rate and to infer changes in CBF over time (67–69). The primary problem with this technique arises in situations of heterogeneous CBF or metabolic rate (where hyperaemic regions overshadow focally ischaemic areas of the brain), and in conditions of changing metabolic rate when its information can be misleading.

Thermal Diffusion flowmetry

Tissue cortical CBF (CoCBF) can be continuously measured by thermal diffusion flowmetry (TDF) using a commercially available intraparenchymal probe. This technique is based on the thermal conductivity of cortical tissues using a catheter with two thermistors embedded at the tip of a polyurethane catheter. One thermistor is heated to a few degrees above tissue temperature and the more proximally located thermistor functions as a temperature probe. Temperature differences between the two reflect heat transfer and this can be translated into regional CBF measurements. The monitor produces a real-time simultaneous measure of absolute perfusion and temperature at the cortical measurement site. A microprocessor continuously converts the temperature difference to CBF in mL/100 g/min (70).

TDF CoCBF measurements have been investigated in traumatic brain injury (TBI), SAH, epilepsy, and arteriovenous malformation surgery (71–73). After TBI, continuous monitoring of CoCBF may assist in differentiating oligaemic versus hyperaemic elevations in ICP, and in the assessment of pressure autoregulation and CO_2 reactivity. Theoretically, the use of hyperventilation in the management of intracranial hypertension may be monitored by TDF, reducing the risk of inducing cerebral ischaemia, but there are currently no data to support this hypothesis. This technology has been validated versus Xe-CT CBF in critically ill patients (72,74). Although it provides continuous monitoring of absolute regional CBF, it is unable to assess global brain perfusion.

Laser Doppler flowmetry

Laser Doppler flowmetry (LDF) is based on the principle of Doppler shift. Monochromatic laser light reflected from stationary tissue is unchanged in frequency but when reflected from moving blood cells undergoes a frequency shift and is therefore able to measure the velocity of red blood cells in the cortical circulation (75). LDF requires placement of the probe directly on the cortex or dura. Although it is very positional, LDF provides continuous second-to-second CBF information in the region of interest but is limited by arbitrary units. By its nature, it also provides only regional information (75). LDF is not widely used clinically.

Monitoring cerebral autoregulation

Dynamic time domain analysis of cerebrovascular autoregulation using TCD ultrasonography, ICP, brain tissue oxygen partial pressure ($PtiO_2$), or NIRS is a current topic of investigation with promising reports of potential efficacious and valid bedside use as a continuous monitor of autoregulatory status (76–86). These are often referred to as Mx, Prx, ORx, and COx for TCD-, ICP-, $PtiO_2$-, and NIRS-derived autoregulatory assessments respectively.

It has been suggested that autoregulation monitoring can be used to develop a patient-specific autoregulation curve and allow the determination of an optimal CPP for an individual patient (77,78,80,85,87–90). TCD techniques assess the correlation coefficient between MAP and BFV to determine Mx in real time at the bedside. A strong correlation of BFV with MAP suggests poor autoregulation, whereas a lack of correlation indicates normal autoregulation. Using this technique Czosnyka and colleagues observed a U-shaped curvilinear relationship between BFV and mean arterial blood pressure (MABP), with more impaired autoregulation at MABP readings of lower than 75 mmHg and greater than 125 mmHg (80). This approach to continuous autoregulation monitoring suffers from the previously described drawbacks of using TCD as a bedside monitor.

Pressure reactivity index

In the presence of dysautoregulation, increasing MABP results in increased ICP, and this relationship has been used as another correlation-based marker of autoregulatory reserve. The so-called pressure reactivity index, or PRx, is derived from the moving correlation between slow-wave changes in ICP and ABP and has been used as a continuous monitor of autoregulation (85,91). Steiner et al., in a retrospective study, reported the use of PRx monitoring in TBI patients to determine the optimal CPP, which was defined as the CPP range in which autoregulation was most preserved, that is, the correlation coefficient was closest to zero (87). Patients managed within this optimal CPP range had better outcomes. Moreover, those with dysautoregulation related to higher ABP with corresponding ICP elevation had worse outcomes, suggesting that autoregulation monitoring to ensure adherence to an individual's optimal CPP might be an outcome-altering intervention after TBI. Notably, PRx, as with TCD-based autoregulation studies, has a U-shaped curvilinear relationship with variations in CPP. Moreover, further complementing this information are observations of abnormally high and low OEF at these ABP extremes (92). Such findings are underscored by the reports of a significant ischaemic burden in TBI patients (93), suggesting a delicate balance between hypotension-associated hypoperfusion and hypertension-associated oedema/ICP exacerbation, both of which may worsen regional ischaemia. Taken together, these studies underscore the notion that there is an individualized optimal MAP after TBI which can be ascertained with autoregulation monitoring.

Oxygen reactivity indices

Autoregulation monitoring using a $PtiO_2$-derived pressure reactivity index (ORx) (86) and a NIRS-derived cerebral oximetry index (COx) (77,78,81,84,90,94) have also been described. The latter provides a non-invasive assessment of autoregulation which would be feasible as a bedside monitor not only on the NICU but also in other environments such as acute stroke units.

Overall, autoregulation monitoring remains largely investigational but seems to have some potential to emerge as a useful clinical tool.

References

1. Koenig M, Klotz E, Luka B, Venderink DJ, Spittler JF, Heuser L. Perfusion CT of the brain: diagnostic approach for early detection of ischemic stroke. *Radiology*. 1998;209(1):85–93.
2. Nabavi DG, Cenic A, Craen RA, Gelb AW, Bennett JD, Kozak R, *et al.* CT assessment of cerebral perfusion: experimental validation and initial clinical experience. *Radiology*. 1999;213(1):141–9.
3. Von Kummer R, Allen KL, Holle R, Bozzao L, Bastianello S, Manelfe C, *et al.* Acute stroke: usefulness of early CT findings before thrombolytic therapy. *Radiology*. 1997;205(2):327–33.
4. Wintermark M, Maeder P, Thiran JP, Schnyder P, Meuli R. Quantitative assessment of regional cerebral blood flows by perfusion CT studies at low injection rates: a critical review of the underlying theoretical models. *Eur Radiol*. 2001;11(7):1220–30.
5. Kikuchi K, Murase K, Miki H, Kikuchi T, Sugawara Y, Mochizuki T, *et al.* Measurement of cerebral hemodynamics with perfusion weighted MR imaging: comparison with pre- and post-acetazolamide 133Xe-SPECT in occlusive carotid disease. *AJNR Am J Neuroradiol*. 2001;22(2):248–54.
6. Pindzola RR, Balzer JR, Nemoto EM, Goldstein S, Yonas H, Pindzola RR, *et al.* Cerebrovascular reserve in patients with carotid occlusive disease assessed by stable xenon-enhanced CT cerebral blood flow and transcranial Doppler. *Stroke*. 2001;32(8):1811–17.
7. Lee T, Lev MH, Eastwood JD, Provenzale JM, Azhari T, Herzau MA. Effect of choice of artery in the measurement of cerebral blood flow in stroke by CT perfusion (abstr). *Radiology*. 2001;221(P):481.
8. Nabavi DG, LeBlanc LM, Baxter B, Lee DH, Fox AJ, Lownie SP, *et al.* Monitoring cerebral perfusion after subarachnoid hemorrhage using CT. *Neuroradiology*. 2001;43(1):7–16.
9. Sanelli PC, Ugorec I, Johnson CE, Tan J, Segal AZ, Fink M, *et al.* Using quantitative CT perfusion for evaluation of delayed cerebral ischemia following aneurysmal subarachnoid hemorrhage. *AJNR Am J Neuroradiol*. 2011:2047–53.
10. Detre JA, Zhang W, Roberts DA, Silva AC, Williams DS, Grandis DJ, *et al.* Tissue specific perfusion imaging using arterial spin labeling. *NMR Biomed*. 1994;7:75–82.
11. Kofke WA, Blissitt PA, Rao H, Wang J, Addya K, Detre J. Remifentanil-induced cerebral blood flow effects in normal humans: dose and ApoE genotype. *Anesth Analg*. 2007;105(1):167–75.
12. Kanno I, Iida H, Miura S, Murakami M. Optimal scan time of oxygen-15-labeled water injection method for measurement of cerebral blood flow. *J Nucl Med*. 1991;32(10):1931–4.
13. Iida H, Kanno I, Miura S. Rapid measurement of cerebral blood flow with positron emission tomography. *Ciba Found Symp*. 1991;163:23–37.
14. Pupi A, De Cristofaro MTR, Bacciottini L, Antoniucci D, Formiconi AR, Mascalchi M, *et al.* An analysis of the arterial input curve for technetium-99m-HMPAO: quantification of rCBF using single-photon emission computed tomography. *J Nucl Med*. 1991;32(8):1501–6.
15. Murase K, Tanada S, Fujita H, Sakaki S, Hamamoto K. Kinetic behavior of technetium-99m-HMPAO in the human brain and quantification of cerebral blood flow using dynamic SPECT. *J Nucl Med*. 1992;33(1):135–43.
16. Yonas H. Use of xenon and ultrafast CT to measure cerebral blood flow. *AJNR Am J Neuroradiol*. 1994;15(4):794–5.
17. Good WF, Gur D. Xenon-enhanced CT of the brain: effect of flow activation on derived cerebral blood flow measurements. *AJNR Am J Neuroradiol*. 1991;12(1):83–5.
18. Kashiwagi S, Yamashita T, Nakano S, Kalender W, Polacin A, Takasago T, *et al.* The wash-in/washout protocol in stable xenon CT cerebral blood flow studies. *AJNR Am J Neuroradiol*. 1992;13(1):49–53.
19. Gur D, Yonas H, Jackson DL, Wolfson SK, Jr., Rockette H, Good WF, *et al.* Simultaneous measurements of cerebral blood flow by the xenon/CT method and the microsphere method. A comparison. *Invest Radiol*. 1985;20(7):672–7.
20. Darby J, Yonas H, Marks E, Durham S, Snyder R, Nemoto E. Acute CBF response to dopamine-induced hypertension after subarachnoid hemorrhage. *J Neurosurg*. 1994;80:857–64.
21. Kim MN, Durduran T, Frangos S, Edlow BL, Buckley EM, Moss HE, *et al.* Noninvasive measurement of cerebral blood flow and blood oxygenation using near-infrared and diffuse correlation spectroscopies in critically brain-injured adults. *Neurocrit Care*. 2010;12(2):173–80.
22. Derwall M, Coburn M, Rex S, Hein M, Rossaint R, Fries M. Xenon: recent developments and future perspectives. *Minerva Anestesiol*. 2009;75(1-2):37–45.
23. Kofke W, Brauer P, Policare R, Penthany S, Barker D, Horton J. Middle cerebral artery blood flow velocity and stable xenon-enhanced computed tomographic blood flow during balloon test occlusion of the internal carotid artery. *Stroke*. 1995;26:1603–6.
24. Kofke W. Transcranial Doppler ultrasonography in anesthesia. In: Babikian V, Wechsler L (eds) *Transcranial Doppler Ultrasonography*. St. Louis: Mosby; 1993:190–215.
25. Kofke W, Dong M, Bloom M, Policare R, Janosky J, Sekhar L. Transcranial Doppler ultrasonography with induction of anesthesia for neurosurgery. *J Neurosurg Anesthesiol*. 1994;6:89–97.
26. Eng C, Lam A, Byrd S, Newel lD. The diagnosis and management of a perianesthetic cerebral aneurysmal rupture aided with transcranial Doppler ultrasonography. *Anesthesiology*. 1993;78(1):191–4.
27. Sloan M. Detection of vasospasm following subarachnoid hemorrhage. In: Babikian V, Wechsler L (eds) *Transcranial Doppler Ultrasonography*. St. Louis: Mosby; 1993:105–27.
28. Harders A, Gilsbach J. Time course of blood velocity changes related to vasospasm in the circle of Willis measured by transcranial Doppler ultrasound. *J Neurosurg*. 1987;66:718.
29. Seiler RW, Grolimund P, Aaslid R, Huber P, Nornes H. Cerebral vasospasm evaluated by transcranial ultrasound correlated with clinical grade and CT-visualized subarachnoid hemorrhage. *J Neurosurg*. 1986;64:594.
30. Clyde BL, Resnick DK, Yonas H, Smith HA, Kaufmann AM, Muizelaar JP, *et al.* The relationship of blood velocity as measured by transcranial Doppler ultrasonography to cerebral blood flow as determined by stable xenon computed tomographic studies after aneurysmal subarachnoid hemorrhage. *Neurosurgery*. 1996;38(5):896–905.
31. Hassler W, Chioffi F. CO2 reactivity of cerebral vasospasm after aneurismal subarachnoid haemorrhage. *Acta Neurochir (Wien)*. 1989;98:167–75.
32. Shinoda J, Kimura T, Funakoshi T, Araki Y, Imao Y. Acetazolamide reactivity on cerebral blood flow in patients with subarachnoic haemorrhage. *Acta Neurochir (Wien)*. 1991;109(3–4):102–8.
33. Pindzola RR, Sashin D, Nemoto EM, Kuwabara H, Wilson JW, Yonas H, *et al.* Identifying regions of compromised hemodynamics in symptomatic carotid occlusion by cerebrovascular reactivity and oxygen extraction fraction. *Neurol Res*. 2006;28(2):149–54.
34. Rogg J, Rutigliano M, Yonas H, Johnson DW, Pentheny S, Latchaw RE. The acetazolamide challenge: imaging techniques designed to evaluate cerebral blood flow reserve. *AJR Am J Roentgenol*. 1989;153(3):605–12.

35. Miller J, Smith R, Holaday H. Carbon dioxide reactivity in the evaluation of cerebral ischemia. *Neurosurgery*. 1992;30:518.

36. Giulioni M, Ursino M, Alvisi C. Correlations among intracranial pulsatility, intracranial hemodynamics, and transcranial Doppler wave form: literature review and hypothesis for future studies. *Neurosurgery*. 1988;22:807.

37. Hassler W, Steinmetz H, Gawlowski J. Transcranial Doppler ultrasonography in raised intracranial pressure and in intracranial circulatory arrest. *J Neurosurg*. 1988;68:745.

38. DeWitt L, Rosengart A, Teal P. Transcranial Doppler ultrasonography: normal values. In Babikian V, Wechsler L (eds) *Transcranial Doppler Ultrasonography*. St. Louis, MO: Mosby; 1993:29–38.

39. Homburg A, Jobsen M, Enevoldsen E. Transcranial Doppler recordings in raised intracranial pressure. *Acta Neurol Scand*. 1993;87:488.

40. Goraj B, Rifkinson-Mann S, Leslie D, Lansen T, Kasoff S, Tenner MS. Correlation of intracranial pressure and transcranial Doppler resistive index after head trauma. *AJNR Am J Neuroadiol*. 1994;15:1333.

41. Zweifel C, Czosnyka M, Carrera E, De Riva N, Pickard JD, Smielewski P. Reliability of the blood flow velocity pulsatility index for assessment of intracranial and cerebral perfusion pressures in head-injured patients. *Neurosurgery*. 2012;71(4):853–61.

42. Bindi ML, Biancofiore G, Esposito M, Meacci L, Bisa M, Mozzo R, et al. Transcranial Doppler sonography is useful for the decision-making at the point of care in patients with acute hepatic failure: a single centre's experience. *J Clin Monit Comput*. 2008;22(6):449–52.

43. Early CB, Dewey RC, Pieper HP, Hunt WE. Dynamic pressure flow relationships of brain blood flow in the monkey. *J Neurosurg*. 1974;41(5):590–6.

44. Dewey R, Pieper H, Hunt W. Experimental cerebral hemodynamics. Vasomotor tone, critical closing pressure, and vascular bed resistance. *J Neurosurg*. 1974;41:597.

45. Thomas K, Doberstein C, Martin NA, Zane C, Becker D. Physiological correlation of transcranial Doppler waveform patterns in brain dead patients. In *Proceedings of the 5th International Symposium and Tutorials on Intracranial Hemodynamics: Transcranial Doppler CBF and Other Modalities*. Seattle, WA: The Institute of Applied Physiology and Medicine; 1991.

46. Karakitsos D, Samonis G, Georgountzos V, Karabinis A. Fulminant listerial infection of the central nervous system in an otherwise healthy patient: a case report. *J Med Case Rep*. 3:7838.

47. Monteiro L, Bollen C, Huffelen A, Ackerstaff RA, Jansen NG, Vught A. Transcranial Doppler ultrasonography to confirm brain death: a meta-analysis. *Intensive Care Med*. 2006;32(12):1937–44.

48. Giller C, Mathews D, Purdy P, Kopitnik T, Batjer H, Samson D. The transcranial Doppler appearance of acute carotid artery occlusion. *Ann Neurol*. 1992;31:101.

49. Telman G, Kouperberg E, Schlesinger I, Yarnitsky D. Cessation of microemboli in the middle cerebral artery after a single dose of aspirin in a young patient with embologenic lacunar syndrome of carotid origin. *Isr Med Assoc J*. 2006;8(10):724–5.

50. Poppert H, Sadikovic S, Sander K, Wolf O, Sander D. Embolic signals in unselected stroke patients: prevalence and diagnostic benefit. *Stroke*. 2006;37(8):2039–43.

51. Steiger HJ, Schaffler L, Boll J, Liechti S. Results of microsurgical carotid endarterectomy. A prospective study with transcranial Doppler and EEG monitoring, and elective shunting. *Acta Neurochir (Wien)*. 1989;100(1–2):31–8.

52. Lindegaard K, Lundar T, Wiberg J, Sjoberg D, Aaslid R, Nornes H. Variations in middle cerebral artery blood flow investigated with noninvasive transcranial blood velocity measurments. *Stroke*. 1987;18:1025.

53. Edwards AD, Wyatt JS, Richardson C, Delpy DT, Cope M, Reynolds EO. Cotside measurement of cerebral blood flow in ill newborn infants by near infrared spectroscopy. *Lancet*. 1988;2(8614):770–1.

54. Elwell CE, Cope M, Edwards AD, Wyatt JS, Delpy DT, Reynolds EO. Quantification of adult cerebral hemodynamics by near-infrared spectroscopy. *J Appl Physiol*. 1994;77(6):2753–60.

55. Schytz HW, Guo S, Jensen LT, Kamar M, Nini A, Gress DR, et al. A new technology for detecting cerebral blood flow: a comparative study of ultrasound tagged NIRS and 133Xe-SPECT. *Neurocrit Care*. 2012;17(1):139–45.

56. Culver JP, Durduran T, Cheung C, Furuya D, Greenberg JH, Yodh AG. Diffuse optical measurement of hemoglobin and cerebral blood flow in rat brain during hypercapnia, hypoxia and cardiac arrest. *Adv Exp Med Biol*. 2003;510:293–7.

57. Durduran T, Yu G, Burnett MG, Detre JA, Greenberg JH, Wang J, et al. Diffuse optical measurement of blood flow, blood oxygenation, and metabolism in a human brain during sensorimotor cortex activation. *Opt Lett*. 2004;29(15):1766–8.

58. Yodh AG. Diffuse optics for monitoring brain hemodynamics. *Conf Proc IEEE Eng Med Biol Soc*. 2009;2009:1991–3.

59. De Visscher G, Leunens V, Borgers M, Reneman RS, Flameng W, van Rossem K. NIRS mediated CBF assessment: validating the indocyanine green bolus transit detection by comparison with coloured microsphere flowmetry. *Adv Exp Med Biol*. 2003;540:37–45.

60. De Visscher G, van Rossem K, Van Reempts J, Borgers M, Flameng W, Reneman RS. Cerebral blood flow assessment with indocyanine green bolus transit detection by near-infrared spectroscopy in the rat. *Comp Biochem Physiol A Mol Integr Physiol*. 2002;132(1):87–95.

61. Gora F, Shinde S, Elwell CE, Goldstone JC, Cope M, Delpy DT, et al. Noninvasive measurement of cerebral blood flow in adults using near-infrared spectroscopy and indocyanine green: a pilot study. *J Neurosurg Anesthesiol*. 2002;14(3):218–22.

62. Kuebler WM, Sckell A, Habler O, Kleen M, Kuhnle GE, Welte M, et al. Noninvasive measurement of regional cerebral blood flow by near-infrared spectroscopy and indocyanine green. *J Cereb Blood Flow Metab*. 1998;18(4):445–56.

63. Roberts I, Fallon P, Kirkham FJ, Lloyd-Thomas A, Cooper C, Maynard R, et al. Estimation of cerebral blood flow with near infrared spectroscopy and indocyanine green. *Lancet*. 1993;342(8884):1425.

64. Diop M, Verdecchia K, Lee TY, St Lawrence K. Calibration of diffuse correlation spectroscopy with a time-resolved near-infrared technique to yield absolute cerebral blood flow measurements. *Biomedical Optics Express*. 2011;2(7):2068–82.

65. Obrist W, Thompson HK Jr, King C, Wang H. Determination of regional CBF by inhalation of 133-Xenon. *Circ Res*. 1967;20(1):124–35.

66. Obrist W, Langfitt TW, Jaggi JL, Cruz J, Gennarelli TA. CBF and metabolism in comatose patients with acute head injury. Relationship to intracranial hypertension. *J Neurosurg*. 1984;61:241–53.

67. Bushnell D, Gupta S, Barnes W, Litocy F, Niemiro M, Steffen G. Evaluation of cerebral perfusion reserve using 5% CO2 and SPECT neuroperfusion imaging. *Clin Nucl Med*. 1991;16 (4):263.

68. Schmidt JF. Changes in human cerebral blood flow estimated by the (A-V)O2 difference method. *Dan Med Bull*. 1992;39(4):335–42.

69. Cruz J, Gennarelli TA, Alves WM. Continuous monitoring of cerebral hemodynamic reserve in acute brain injury: relationship to changes in brain swelling. *J Trauma*. 1992;32(5):629–38.

70. Carter LP, Erspamer R, White WL, Yamagata S. Cortical blood flow during craniotomy for aneurysm. *Surg Neurol*. 1982;17(3):204–8.

71. Jaeger M, Soehle M, Schuhmann MU, Winkler D, Meixensberger J, Jaeger M, et al. Correlation of continuously monitored regional cerebral blood flow and brain tissue oxygen. *Acta Neurochir (Wien)*. 2005;147(1):51–6.

72. Vajkoczy P, Horn P, Thome C, Munch E, Schmiedek P. Regional cerebral blood flow monitoring in the diagnosis of delayed ischemia following aneurysmal subarachnoid hemorrhage. *J Neurosurg*. 2003;98(6):1227–34.

73. Dickman CA, Carter LP, Baldwin HZ, Harrington T, Tallman D. Continuous regional cerebral blood flow monitoring in acute craniocerebral trauma. *Neurosurgery*. 1991;28(3):467–72.

74. Vajkoczy P, Roth H, Horn P, Lucke T, Thome C, Hubner U, et al. Continuous monitoring of regional cerebral blood flow: experimental and clinical validation of a novel thermal diffusion microprobe. *J Neurosurg*. 2000;93(2):265–74.

75. Frerichs K, Feurestein G. Laser-Doppler flowmetry. A review of its application for measuring cerebral and spinal cord blood flow. *Mol Chem Neuropathol.* 1990;12 (1):55.

76. Czosnyka M, Brady K, Reinhard M, Smielewski P, Steiner LA. Monitoring of cerebrovascular autoregulation: facts, myths, and missing links. *Neurocrit Care.* 2009;10(3):373–86.

77. Brady KM, Lee JK, Kibler KK, Smielewski P, Czosnyka M, Easley RB, et al. Continuous time-domain analysis of cerebrovascular autoregulation using near-infrared spectroscopy. *Stroke.* 2007;38(10):2818–25.

78. Brady KM, Mytar JO, Kibler KK, Hogue CW, Jr., Lee JK, Czosnyka M, et al. Noninvasive autoregulation monitoring with and without intracranial pressure in the naive piglet brain. *Anesth Analg.* 2010;111(1):191–5.

79. Czosnyka M, Smielewski P, Kirkpatrick P, Laing RJ, Menon D, Pickard JD. Continuous assessment of the cerebral vasomotor reactivity in head injury. *Neurosurgery.* 1997;41(1):11–17.

80. Czosnyka M, Smielewski P, Piechnik S, Steiner LA, Pickard JD. Cerebral autoregulation following head injury. *J Neurosurg.* 2001;95(5):756–63.

81. Joshi B, Brady K, Lee J, Easley B, Panigrahi R, Smielewski P, et al. Impaired autoregulation of cerebral blood flow during rewarming from hypothermic cardiopulmonary bypass and its potential association with stroke. *Anesth Analg.* 2010;110(2):321–8.

82. Lang EW, Mehdorn HM, Dorsch NWC, Czosnyka M. Continuous monitoring of cerebrovascular autoregulation: a validation study. *J Neurol Neurosurg Psychiatry.* 2002;72(5):583–6.

83. Soehle M, Czosnyka M, Pickard JD, Kirkpatrick PJ. Continuous assessment of cerebral autoregulation in subarachnoid hemorrhage. *Anesth Analg.* 2004;98(4):1133–9.

84. Zweifel C, Castellani G, Czosnyka M, Carrera E, Brady KM, Kirkpatrick PJ, et al. Continuous assessment of cerebral autoregulation with near-infrared spectroscopy in adults after subarachnoid hemorrhage. *Stroke.* 2010;41(9):1963–8.

85. Zweifel C, Lavinio A, Steiner LA, Radolovich D, Smielewski P, Timofeev I, et al. Continuous monitoring of cerebrovascular pressure reactivity in patients with head injury. *Neurosurg Focus.* 2008;25(4):E2.

86. Jaeger M, Schuhmann MU, Soehle M, Meixensberger J. Continuous assessment of cerebrovascular autoregulation after traumatic brain injury using brain tissue oxygen pressure reactivity. *Crit Care Med.* 2006;34(6):1783–8.

87. Steiner LA, Czosnyka M, Piechnik SK, Smielewski P, Chatfield D, Menon DK, et al. Continuous monitoring of cerebrovascular pressure reactivity allows determination of optimal cerebral perfusion pressure in patients with traumatic brain injury. *Crit Care Med.* 2002;30(4):733–8.

88. Brady K, Joshi B, Zweifel C, Smielewski P, Czosnyka M, Easley RB, et al. Real-time continuous monitoring of cerebral blood flow autoregulation using near-infrared spectroscopy in patients undergoing cardiopulmonary bypass. *Stroke.* 2010;41(9):1951–6.

89. Brady KM, Lee JK, Kibler KK, Easley RB, Koehler RC, Czosnyka M, et al. The lower limit of cerebral blood flow autoregulation is increased with elevated intracranial pressure. *Anesth Analg.* 2009;108(4):1278–83.

90. Brady KM, Mytar JO, Lee JK, Cameron DE, Vricella LA, Thompson WR, et al. Monitoring cerebral blood flow pressure autoregulation in pediatric patients during cardiac surgery. *Stroke.* 2010;41(9):1957–62.

91. Steiner LA, Czosnyka M, Piechnik SK, Smielewski P, Chatfield D, Menon DK, et al. Continuous monitoring of cerebrovascular pressure reactivity allows determination of optimal cerebral perfusion pressure in patients with traumatic brain injury. *Crit Care Med.* 2002;30(4):733–8.

92. Menon DK, Coles JP, Gupta AK, Fryer TD, Smielewski P, Chatfield DA, et al. Diffusion limited oxygen delivery following head injury. *Crit Care Med.* 2004;32(6):1384–90.

93. Coles J, Minhas P, Fryer T, Smielewski P, Aigbirihio F, Donovan T, et al. Effect of hyperventilation on cerebral blood flow in traumatic head injury: clinical relevance and monitoring correlates. *Crit Care Clin.* 2002;30 (9):1950–9.

94. Zweifel C, Castellani G, Czosnyka M, Helmy A, Manktelow A, Carrera E, et al. Noninvasive monitoring of cerebrovascular reactivity with near infrared spectroscopy in head-injured patients. *J Neurotrauma.* 2010;27(11):1951–8.

95. Coles JP, Fryer TD, Smielewski P, Chatfield DA, Steiner LA, Johnston AJ, et al. Incidence and mechanisms of cerebral ischemia in early clinical head injury. *J Cereb Blood Flow Metab.* 2004;24(2):202–11.

CHAPTER 11

Cerebral oxygenation monitoring

Matthew A. Kirkman and Martin Smith

Cerebral oxygenation monitoring assesses the balance between cerebral oxygen delivery and utilization, and therefore the adequacy of cerebral perfusion and oxygen delivery. A mismatch between cerebral oxygen supply and demand results in cerebral hypoxia/ischaemia and is associated with worsened outcome after acute brain injury (ABI). Hypoxia represents an interruption to oxygen supply from whatever cause, whereas ischaemia occurs when there is an interruption to oxygen supply as well as impairment of blood flow (1).

Time-critical windows to prevent or minimize permanent ischaemic neurological injury exist, but often pass silently because detection of compromised cerebral oxygenation is not straightforward and clinical manifestations of cerebral hypoxia may be masked by sedation (2). Global and regional monitors of cerebral oxygenation have been developed in an attempt to address this issue. This chapter briefly outlines the physiology and pathophysiology of cerebral oxygenation, and reviews bedside methods of cerebral oxygenation monitoring, namely jugular venous oxygen saturation ($SjvO_2$), brain tissue oxygen tension ($PtiO_2$), and near-infrared spectroscopy (NIRS)-based cerebral oximetry. Evidence for the utility of cerebral oxygenation-guided therapy is discussed, and the chapter ends with a brief overview of the technological advancements that are likely to shape the future of cerebral oxygenation monitoring in the neurocritical care unit (NCCU).

Physiology of cerebral oxygenation

Oxygen and glucose are both essential substrates for brain function. Cerebral energy is predominantly generated through the oxidation of glucose, although lactate produced by astrocytes may also be used by neurons in an activity-dependent manner (see Chapter 2). The brain has a high metabolic demand and, as a consequence, receives 20% of the cardiac output despite constituting a mere 2% of total adult body weight. The brain has very limited energy stores and is therefore highly susceptible to injurious processes that impair blood flow and oxygen delivery.

Oxygen, once inhaled, is transported from the lungs to the brain via the bloodstream, mostly bound to haemoglobin. At atmospheric pressure, the remainder, a small amount, circulates as dissolved oxygen. Haemoglobin has a high affinity for oxygen in the lungs and this facilitates the binding of oxygen to haemoglobin. Upon reaching the brain, oxygen is readily dissolved into tissue parenchyma where the presence of oxygen pressure gradients facilitates its movement into cells. Once in the cells, oxygen is used in the aerobic metabolism of glucose through the process of oxidative phosphorylation, utilizing adenosine triphosphate (ATP) as substrate. The enzymatic reactions involved in oxidative phosphorylation are localized in the mitochondria, and the cerebral metabolic rate for oxygen ($CMRO_2$) reflects this function of mitochondrial activity. Under normal conditions, $CMRO_2$ in adult humans is approximately 3.3 mL/100 mL/min (3). If there is a significant reduction in cerebral blood flow (CBF) or arterial partial pressure of oxygen (PaO_2), $CMRO_2$ is reduced accordingly but, at a critical point, there is a shift from aerobic to anaerobic metabolism. In an attempt to maintain adequate oxygen delivery to tissue, a decrease in CBF is usually accompanied by an increase in the amount of oxygen extracted from the blood. This is quantified as the oxygen extraction fraction (OEF), the ratio of cerebral oxygen consumption to cerebral oxygen delivery, which is 0.4 (40%) in healthy individuals (4). Autoregulatory mechanisms are also important in ensuring adequate cerebral oxygenation and, under normal conditions, serve to keep global CBF constant over a range of systolic blood pressure (approximately 50–150 mmHg). Regional mechanisms also permit increases in oxygen delivery to those tissue areas most in need, that is, those that are metabolically most active. However, the severe autoregulatory dysfunction that can accompany ABI may result in pathophysiological derangements in cerebral oxygen delivery and metabolism, and lead to cerebral hypoxia/ischaemia.

In addition to systemic oxygenation and CBF, which is in part affected by arterial partial pressure of CO_2 ($PaCO_2$) and the presence of cerebral vasospasm, there are several other important factors that influence cerebral oxygenation. These include cerebral perfusion pressure (CPP), haemoglobin concentration (and its oxygen binding and release capacity), temperature, cardiac output, and seizures (5–10). Manipulation of CPP and $PaCO_2$ therefore affects $PtiO_2$ (7,11). Magnetic resonance imaging (MRI) studies show that systemic hypoxia increases $CMRO_2$ and CBF, and hyperoxia decreases $CMRO_2$ (in a dose-dependent manner) (12). The role of hyperoxia on CBF is unclear, with one MRI study demonstrating a decrease (independently of $PaCO_2$) (13) and another no change in CBF (12).

Hypoxia/ischaemia is a key determinant of outcome after ABI of all types, and early identification (through monitoring) and subsequent treatment might minimize the risk of irreversible tissue damage and improve patient outcome (14).

Monitoring cerebral oxygenation

Several imaging and bedside methods of monitoring global and regional cerebral oxygenation are available. Some monitors assess global ($SjvO_2$) and others regional ($PtiO_2$, NIRS) oxygenation. In addition, different monitors describe different physiological variables and for this reason are not interchangeable. The principles, relative merits, and drawbacks of the three bedside techniques of cerebral oxygenation monitoring are summarized in Table 11.1 and discussed in detail below.

Table 11.1 Bedside monitors of cerebral oxygenation

	Advantages	Disadvantages	Comments
$SjvO_2$	Real-time Represents the balance between cerebral blood flow and metabolism Global trend monitor	Insensitive to regional changes Invasive procedure—risk of vein thrombosis, haematoma, carotid puncture Assumes stable $CMRO_2$ to infer CBF changes	First bedside measure of cerebral oxygenation Largely superseded by $PtiO_2$ monitoring
$PtiO_2$	Real-time Represents the balance between cerebral blood flow and metabolism Focal monitor	Monitors small region of interest—position of probe is crucial Invasive Small degree of zero and sensitivity drift 1-hour 'run-in' period required	Bedside gold standard for cerebral oxygenation monitoring $PtiO_2$-guided therapy may improve outcome when combined with ICP/CPP-guided therapy May identify CPP targets for optimal brain oxygenation
NIRS	Real-time Non-invasive Assessment of several regions of interest simultaneously	Lack of standardization between commercial devices Extracerebral circulation may 'contaminate' cerebral oxygenation measurements 'Thresholds' for cerebral hypoxia/ischaemia undetermined Current devices only monitor relative changes in oxygenation	Research devices offer the potential for monitoring metabolic variables, blood flow, absolute chromophore concentration, and mitochondrial cytochrome redox state

ABI, acute brain injury; CBF, cerebral blood flow; $CMRO_2$, cerebral metabolic rate for oxygen; CPP, cerebral perfusion pressure; ICP, intracranial pressure; NIRS, near infrared spectroscopy; $PtiO_2$, brain tissue oxygen tension; $SjvO_2$, jugular venous oxygen saturation.

Imaging

Modern cerebral imaging techniques provide sophisticated haemodynamic and metabolic information over multiple regions of interest, which assists clinicians in assessing the adequacy of CBF and cerebral oxygenation after ABI (see Chapter 15). Examples include positron emission tomography (PET), perfusion computed tomography (CT), stable-xenon-enhanced CT (XeCT), single-photon emission CT (SPECT), and perfusion MRI. Some of these modalities also permit the quantification of parameters such as cerebral blood volume (CBV), $CMRO_2$, and OEF.

PET is considered the gold standard for detecting cerebral ischaemia (15) and provides a quantitative measurement of cerebral perfusion and metabolism with high spatial resolution (16). The administration of the ^{15}O-radioisotope permits the quantification of CBF, CBV, OEF, and $CMRO_2$ using PET and this has allowed the elucidation of the pathophysiology of traumatic brain injury (TBI) (17) (Figure 11.1) and been used to assess the effects of hyperoxia on brain tissue oxygenation (18,19). Perfusion CT is a relatively inexpensive and readily accessible imaging modality for the quantification of CBF and CBV, but relies on the administration of contrast agents and identification of regions of interest prior to scanning. XeCT utilizes inhaled (non-radioactive) xenon

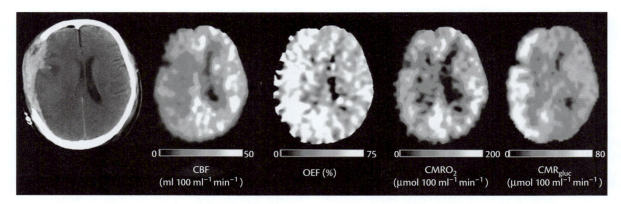

CBF
(ml 100 ml^{-1} min^{-1})　　OEF (%)　　$CMRO_2$
(µmol 100 ml^{-1} min^{-1})　　CMR_{gluc}
(µmol 100 ml^{-1} min^{-1})

Fig. 11.1 Imaging of cerebral ischaemia. The figure shows a non-contrast CT scan and PET-derived CBF, OEF, oxygen metabolism ($CMRO_2$), and glucose metabolism (CMR_{gluc}) images obtained after evacuation of a subdural haematoma. Note the marked reduction in CBF, slight decrease in $CMRO_2$, and large increase in OEF suggestive of cerebral ischaemia in cerebral hemisphere underlying the evacuated subdural haematoma. The substantial increase in CMR_{gluc} implies a switch to non-oxidative metabolism of glucose in order to meet underlying metabolic demand.

CBF, cerebral blood flow; CMR_{gluc}, cerebral metabolic rate for glucose; $CMRO_2$, cerebral metabolic rate for oxygen; CT, computed tomography; OEF, oxygen extraction fraction; PET, positron emission tomography.

Reproduced from Cole JP, 'Imaging after brain injury', *British Journal of Anaesthesia*, 2007, 99, pp. 49–60, by permission of Oxford University Press and the Board of Management and Trustees of the *British Journal of Anaesthesia*.

to quantify both global and regional CBF, but has limited value in the presence of pulmonary disease. SPECT involves the use of the radioisotope ^{99m}Tc and is only semi-quantitative, relying on comparisons of the regions of interest with 'normal' contralateral cerebrum or cerebellum. Perfusion MRI permits the quantification of CBV, has the advantage of avoiding exposure to ionizing radiation, and, when combined with diffusion-weighted MRI, can be used to identify an ischaemic 'penumbra' after ABI. Blood oxygenation level-dependent (BOLD) MRI is able to quantify $CMRO_2$ and OEF, but improvements in sensitivity are required prior to its routine clinical application (20). MRI is more expensive than CT imaging and the scanning time is longer, limiting its use in unstable patients (21).

All imaging modalities have common pitfalls. They require the transfer of patients to imaging facilities, which can itself adversely affect cerebral oxygenation, particularly in those with borderline $PtiO_2$ (22). In addition, imaging provides only a 'snapshot' of cerebral physiology at a particular moment in time and, because pathological changes after ABI are dynamic, might miss important episodes of cerebral hypoxia/ischaemia. Finally, access to some imaging modalities (e.g. PET) is limited outside specialist centres.

Jugular venous saturation monitoring

Jugular venous oxygen saturation monitoring was the first bedside measure of cerebral oxygenation. Blood can be sampled intermittently from a catheter whose tip lies in the jugular venous bulb, or oxygen saturation measured continuously using a fibreoptic catheter. As well as having considerable historical relevance, $SvjO_2$ monitoring formed the basis of our understanding of cerebral oxygenation changes after ABI.

$SjvO_2$ represents a global measure of cerebral oxygenation and provides a non-quantitative estimate of the adequacy of cerebral perfusion (23). Simplistically, when cerebral oxygen supply is insufficient to meet demand the brain extracts more oxygen from haemoglobin resulting in a decreased oxygen saturation of the blood in the jugular bulb. The normal range of $SjvO_2$ is 55–75%, and interpretation of changes is relatively straightforward (Table 11.2).

The arterial to jugular venous oxygen content concentration difference and other derived variables have been studied extensively as an assessment of CBF (24). $SjvO_2$ monitoring has some intraoperative applications (25) although its primary role is in the NCCU where it has been used to detect impaired cerebral perfusion after TBI and subarachnoid haemorrhage (SAH), and to optimize CPP and therapeutic hyperventilation (26–28). The ischaemic 'threshold' following TBI is generally considered to be represented by $SjvO_2$ values less than 50% for 10 minutes or longer (28). Multiple or prolonged episodes of jugular venous desaturations (28), as well as $SjvO_2$ values over 75% (29), are poor prognostic indicators. The Brain Trauma Foundation cites level 3 evidence to support the maintenance of $SjvO_2$ greater than 50% after TBI (30), but no interventional trials have demonstrated outcome benefit from $SjvO_2$-directed therapy.

There are several limitations of $SjvO_2$ monitoring. It is an invasive technique with risks of haematoma and carotid puncture during catheter insertion, and jugular vein or sinus thrombosis during prolonged monitoring. The catheter must be correctly sited to avoid contamination from the extracranial circulation which is minimal when the catheter tip lies at the level of the lower border of the first cervical vertebra on a lateral cervical spine radiograph. The facial vein is the first large extracranial vein draining into the internal jugular vein and rapid aspiration of blood samples (> 2 mL/min) will result in contamination of samples from this source. Further, since $SjvO_2$ is a global measure it is unable to detect regional ischaemia (31). Notably, areas of critically low perfusion can be missed by $SjvO_2$ monitoring as their effluent blood might have only a small impact on the flow-weighted $SjvO_2$ value which will then be predominantly determined by venous return from well-perfused areas, and therefore normal. Evidence from a combined PET and $SjvO_2$ monitoring study demonstrated that more than 13% of the brain must become ischaemic before the $SjvO_2$ falls below 50% (32). $SjvO_2$ values accurately reflect global cerebral oxygenation only if the dominant jugular bulb is cannulated but, despite this, the right side is almost exclusively chosen in clinical practice (33). Although widely used for decades, $SjvO_2$ monitoring is being superseded by $PtiO_2$ monitoring.

Brain tissue oxygen tension monitoring

Intraparenchymal $PtiO_2$ monitoring is increasingly being utilized whenever intracranial pressure (ICP) monitoring is indicated, and has become the 'gold standard' bedside monitor of cerebral oxygenation (34,35). Whilst $PtiO_2$ values can be influenced by CBF, $PtiO_2$ is not a direct measure of blood flow but a complex and dynamic variable representing the interaction between cerebral oxygen delivery and demand (oxygen metabolism) (35), as well as tissue oxygen diffusion gradients (36). PET studies have identified correlations between $PtiO_2$, regional CBF (37), and regional venous oxygen saturation (38) and, as such, $PtiO_2$ is likely to represent a balance between CBF, OEF, and PaO_2.

$PtiO_2$ is influenced by several physiological variables in addition to PaO_2, including mean arterial pressure (MAP) and CPP (7,39). Whilst reductions in $PtiO_2$ may occur because of reduced CBF, $PtiO_2$ can also be decreased in the presence of normal CBF reflecting the key influence of PaO_2 (18), and also because of increased brain tissue gradients for oxygen diffusion following ABI (40). $PtiO_2$ should therefore be considered as a biomarker of cellular function rather than a simple monitor of hypoxia/ischaemia, making it an appropriate therapeutic target after ABI.

Table 11.2 Interpretation of changes in jugular venous oxygen saturation

$SjvO_2$	Relative cerebral blood flow and metabolic changes	Causes
Normal (55–75%)	CBF and $CMRO_2$ balanced	
Low (< 50%)	↓ CBF or ↑ $CMRO_2$	↓ ABP
		↓ PaO_2
		↓ $PaCO_2$
		↑ ICP or ↓ CPP
		Seizures
High (> 80%)	↑ CBF or ↓ $CMRO_2$	Failure of oxygen utilization (cellular metabolic failure)
		Cerebral hyperaemia
		Arteriovenous shunting
		Brain death

ABP, arterial blood pressure; CBF, cerebral blood flow; $CMRO_2$, cerebral metabolic rate for oxygen; CPP, cerebral perfusion pressure; ICP, intracranial pressure; $PaCO_2$, arterial partial pressure of carbon dioxide; PaO_2, arterial partial pressure of oxygen; $SjvO_2$, jugular venous oxygen saturation.

Technological and practical aspects

PtiO$_2$ monitoring devices used in clinical practice incorporate closed polarographic Clark-type cells with reversible electrochemical electrodes. The catheters are approximately 0.5 mm in diameter and can be inserted into the brain parenchyma using single or multiple lumen bolts, through a burr-hole or at craniotomy. The PtiO$_2$ probe is usually placed in subcortical white matter and measures local PtiO$_2$ within a radius of approximately 17 mm^2 (41).

The correct placement of the probe should be confirmed with a non-enhanced cranial CT scan as knowledge of location is important for correct interpretation of readings. A 'run-in' period is required because PtiO$_2$ readings are unreliable in the first hour after insertion. It is important to perform an 'oxygen challenge' when first commencing PtiO$_2$ monitoring, and then on a daily basis, to ensure both the function and responsiveness of the probe. FiO$_2$ is increased to 1.0 for approximately 20 minutes and a normal response is indicated by an increase in baseline PtiO$_2$ of 200% or more at the 20-minute point compared to baseline, although responsiveness will obviously be influenced by pulmonary function (42).

As highlighted earlier, knowledge of the location of the probe is crucial when interpreting PtiO$_2$ values. Some recommend that PtiO$_2$ monitoring should be conducted in 'at risk' perilesional tissue, such as the region immediately surrounding intracerebral haemorrhages or contusions (Figure 11.2D and 11.2E), and in appropriate vascular territories in cases of aneurysmal SAH. PtiO$_2$ values in these 'at-risk' regions are lower than in normal appearing brain tissue (43). For the neurosurgeon, attempting such precise placement can be technically challenging, occasionally producing an undesired intralesional location (Figure 11.2F). Conversely, it is sometimes technically impossible to place a PtiO$_2$ probe near a lesion (Figure 11.2B) and some argue for routine placement in 'normal appearing' areas of brain (Figure 11.2A, C). Thus, in many instances, and especially after diffuse cerebral injury, PtiO$_2$ is measured in normal appearing frontal subcortical white matter, preferably in the non-dominant (right) side. Notably, heterogeneity of brain oxygenation even in 'undamaged' areas of brain is well recognized (44). Placement directly into an area with no expected blood flow, for example, in an infarction or haemorrhage (Figure 11.2F), does not yield useful information.

The measured PtiO$_2$ value is influenced by the composition of the microvasculature and the relative dominance of arterial or venous vessels in the region of interest around the probe. PtiO$_2$ is assumed to largely reflect venous PO$_2$ because venous vessels constitute more than 70% of the cortical microvasculature (37). Since normal arterial PO$_2$ is approximately 12 kPa (90 mmHg) and cerebral venous PO$_2$ is 4.66 kPa (35 mmHg), a wide range of values for PtiO$_2$ is observed (45).

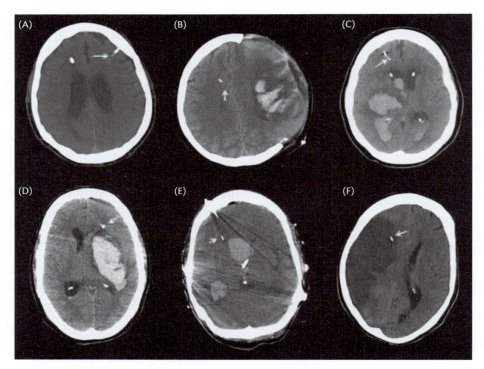

Fig. 11.2 Brain tissue PO$_2$ probe locations relative to injury on post-placement computerized tomography scan.
(A) Diffuse injury and global cerebral oedema with a left frontal probe—note the right frontal EVD.
(B) Focal injury with contralateral probe placement.
(C) Focal injury (right basal ganglia ICH) with ipsilateral probe placement—note the bilateral external ventricular drains.
(D) Perilesional probe placement (large left basal ganglia ICH).
(E) Perilesional probe placement (right basal ganglia ICH)—note the effacement of the lateral ventricle and left frontal EVD.
(F) Probe placement within right MCA infarction.
EVD, external ventricular drain; ICH, intracerebral haemorrhage; MCA, middle cerebral artery.

Adapted with kind permission from Springer Science + Business Media: *Neurocritical Care*, 'Intracranial multimodal monitoring for acute brain injury: a single institution review of current practices', 2010, 12, pp. 188–198, Stuart RM *et al.*, Neurocritical Care Society.

Indications

PtiO$_2$ monitoring is primarily used in the management of TBI and poor-grade aneurysmal SAH, but in some centres also during cerebral angiography (46) and surgery for intracranial aneurysms (47) and arteriovenous malformations (48). Low PtiO$_2$ is associated with poor outcome after severe TBI (44,49–53), with evidence for a dose–response relationship (44). The Brain Trauma Foundation recommends incorporating the monitoring and management of PtiO$_2$ as a complement to ICP/CPP-guided management in patients with severe TBI (30). After SAH an association between low PtiO$_2$ and outcome has been reported in some (54,55) but not all (56,57) studies. Nevertheless, guidelines from the Neurocritical Care Society recommend PtiO$_2$ monitoring in comatose SAH patients (58) as it can identify patients at high risk of delayed cerebral ischaemia (DCI) (57,59). PtiO$_2$ is a valid complement to transcranial Doppler and radiological monitoring after SAH, but its focal nature means that it will miss vasospasm arising in remote brain regions. PtiO$_2$ monitoring has raised questions about the efficacy of triple H therapy (hypertension, haemodilution, and hypervolaemia) in the treatment of DCI after SAH. Induced hypertension improves CBF and PtiO$_2$, whereas hypervolaemia and haemodilution have negligible or even negative effects (60). As a result, induced hypertension alone is now the preferred treatment of DCI (58).

PtiO$_2$ monitoring has been used to identify CPP targets for optimal brain tissue oxygenation in comatose patients with intracerebral haemorrhage (ICH), and reduction in perihaematomal PtiO$_2$ is correlated with poor outcome (61). Further, brain tissue hypoxia improves as ICP reduces and CPP increases following decompressive craniectomy, suggesting that PtiO$_2$ monitoring might assist in the selection of those who might benefit from surgical decompression (62).

Despite a current lack of evidence from randomized controlled trials confirming the utility of PtiO$_2$-directed therapy on outcome following ABI, PtiO$_2$ monitoring and management is widely considered to be a useful complement to ICP/CPP standard care.

Thresholds for therapy

Normal brain PtiO$_2$ values are considered to be in the region of 4.66–6.65 kPa (35–50 mmHg) (63), and a PtiO$_2$ value less than 2.66 kPa (<20 mmHg) is often used as the threshold for commencing brain resuscitative measures (43,50,52,53,64–67). Although PtiO$_2$ thresholds for intervention have been determined from patient outcomes as opposed to a biologically confirmed level at which ischaemic damage occurs (44,68), PET studies suggest that the ischaemic threshold lies below 1.86 kPa (14 mmHg) (7). The Brain Trauma Foundation recommends that a threshold for critical brain hypoxia of less than 2 kPa (< 15 mmHg) should be used to start oxygenation-directed management after TBI (30), and PtiO$_2$ less than 1.33 kPa (< 10 mmHg) is generally accepted to indicate severe brain hypoxia (44).

From a clinical perspective however, it is the severity, duration, and chronological trend of cerebral hypoxia rather than isolated absolute PtiO$_2$ values that are the key determinants of outcome (44,52,53). Critical values should therefore be considered within a range rather than as a precise threshold, and ischaemia best defined as the burden of tissue hypoxia, that is, its duration as well as depth (44). Further, it is unclear whether a PtiO$_2$ value above a certain threshold ensures adequate cerebral oxygenation, or whether (or how) to treat a mildly elevated ICP in the face of normal PtiO$_2$.

Brain tissue oxygen tension-guided management

There is currently no consensus for the treatment of low PtiO$_2$, although a stepwise approach has been recommended in a manner akin to treatment of intracranial hypertension (Figure 11.3) (69). Understanding the factors that affect PtiO$_2$ is crucial in determining treatment of brain hypoxia/ischaemia. The most widely studied influences on cerebral oxygenation are ICP/CPP (6) and CBF, with regional CBF correlating well with PtiO$_2$ (70). Pathological and sustained increases in ICP can result in reduced CPP and secondary cerebral hypoxia/ischaemia, but interestingly outcome after severe TBI appears also to be influenced by low PtiO$_2$ values independently of ICP and CPP (53). Secondary hypoxic brain insults may go unnoticed when therapy is guided by ICP/CPP monitoring in isolation (52,53), highlighting the importance of multimodal neuromonitoring. Since CPP and MAP augmentation may significantly increase cerebral oxygenation (7), PtiO$_2$ monitoring has been used to define individual CPP thresholds to prevent brain tissue hypoxia (71). However, the CPP threshold to avoid secondary brain ischaemia after TBI varies (72), confirming the importance of an individualized approach to therapy.

PtiO$_2$ monitoring may also assist in the management of elevated ICP. Mannitol and hypertonic saline are both widely used to treat intracranial hypertension, but hypertonic saline appears to be better at improving PtiO$_2$ whilst simultaneously reducing ICP (73,74). PtiO$_2$ monitoring may also have a role in targeting optimal PaCO$_2$ during moderate hyperventilation to treat intracranial hypertension because of the risk of cerebral ischaemia even with modest reductions in PaCO$_2$ (75). Concomitant intracranial hypertension and low PtiO$_2$ may suggest the need for more aggressive interventions such as decompressive craniectomy (76).

Optimization of systemic physiological variables after ABI may also be guided by PtiO$_2$ monitoring. In one study, manipulation of ventilation, CPP, and sedation levels was successful in improving PtiO$_2$ in over two-thirds of cases (69). However, which intervention or combination of interventions is/are most effective remains unclear. In fact it appears that it is the responsiveness of the hypoxic brain to a given intervention that is the prognostic factor, with reversal of hypoxia being associated with reduced mortality (69). Although increasing FiO$_2$ effectively improves PtiO$_2$, the outcome effect of normobaric hyperoxia is still debated (77). Further, one study using XeCT-measured CBF found that increasing FiO$_2$ did not improve PtiO$_2$ in hypoperfused brain regions which are the tissue areas most in need of oxygen (78). The PaO$_2$/FiO$_2$ ratio is strongly associated with cerebral hypoxia (79) and suggests that PtiO$_2$-guided lung-protective strategies might minimize the risk of treatment-related secondary cerebral hypoxia/ischaemia. Anaemia-associated cerebral hypoxia can be corrected by red cell transfusion, so PtiO$_2$ monitoring might also guide transfusion therapy after ABI (80,81).

Outcome of brain tissue oxygen tension-guided therapy

There is a large body of evidence corroborating the relationship between low PtiO$_2$ and deleterious outcome after ABI, although studies that have investigated the outcome effects of PtiO$_2$-directed therapy and compared this to standard ICP/CPP-guided management have reached conflicting results (Table 11.3) (50,64,65,67,82,128,129). These varied outcome effects may in part be due to the heterogeneity of the study populations, and differences in study design and PtiO$_2$ thresholds for intervention. Of particular note, a standardized approach to PtiO$_2$-directed therapy is rarely described and many

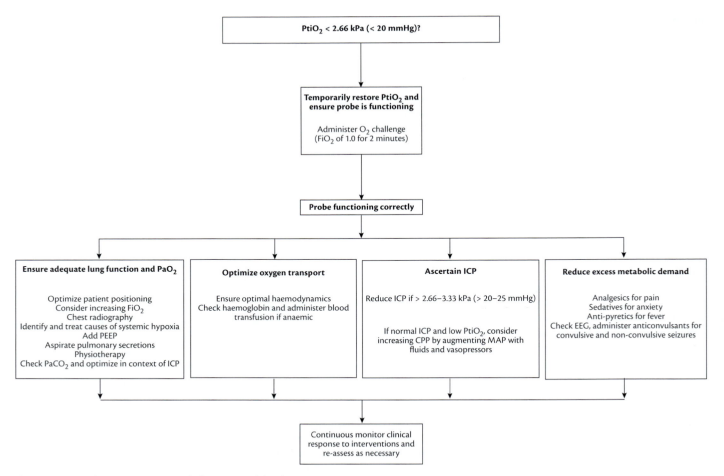

Fig. 11.3 Proposed management protocol of a patient with low brain tissue oxygen tension.
CPP, cerebral perfusion pressure; EEG, electroencephalography; ICP, intracranial pressure; MAP, mean arterial pressure; PaCO$_2$, arterial partial pressure of carbon dioxide; PEEP, positive end-expiratory pressure; PtiO$_2$, brain tissue oxygen tension.

studies report data from a single centre. Only two studies are truly prospective, and both are hampered by small sample size (64,82). However, a systematic review found overall outcome benefits from PtiO$_2$-directed therapy compared to ICP/CPP-guided therapy alone (odds ratio of favourable outcome of 2.1) (66).

Thus, it seems likely that integrating PtiO$_2$ monitoring as an additional physiological therapeutic target might improve outcome after TBI, particularly if used in conjunction with more established targets such as ICP and CPP. This hypothesis is being tested in a prospective, randomized controlled trial evaluating the impact of PtiO$_2$-directed therapy in patients with TBI (Brain Tissue Oxygen Monitoring in Traumatic Brain Injury—BOOST 2: http://clinical-trials.gov/ct2/show/NCT00974259).

Advantages and disadvantages of PtiO$_2$ monitoring

PtiO$_2$ monitoring provides real-time data and allows rapid detection of cerebral ischaemia at the bedside (47). It offers the potential for selective monitoring of critically perfused tissue if the probe is correctly sited. However, the focal nature of the technique can also be disadvantageous because it may miss important pathology remote from the monitored region. Under certain circumstances, such as diffuse injury, PtiO$_2$ may reflect global brain oxygenation (31).

Readings from PtiO$_2$ monitoring are unreliable in the first hour, perhaps due to microscopic injury at the probe interface at the time

of insertion (83). The early hours after ABI may be a critical time for the development of cerebral hypoxia/ischaemia, and any changes will be missed during this 'run-in' period. PtiO$_2$ monitoring is an invasive procedure but is nonetheless relatively safe. A small (usually clinically insignificant) iatrogenic haematoma is identified in fewer than 2% of cases. This compares favourably to intraparenchymal ICP monitoring and is much lower than that associated with ventricular catheters (84). No probe-related infections have been reported (44), although technical complication rates (dislocation or defect) may reach 13.6% (84). The probes are subject to a small amount of drift over time, with clinical data suggesting a low mean zero and sensitivity drift of 0.15 kPa (1.1 mmHg) and 0.19 kPa (1.4 mmHg) respectively (85).

Cerebral-near infrared spectroscopy

NIRS is a non-invasive technique that allows the real-time monitoring of cerebral oxygenation over multiple regions of interest. NIRS-based cerebral oximetry has been utilized in the perioperative setting, particularly during carotid (86) and cardiac surgery (87,88). However, despite interest in the clinical application of NIRS for over three decades, widespread translation into routine clinical practice has not occurred and its application in brain injury, where it might be expected to have a key monitoring role, is undefined.

Table 11.3 Summary of studies comparing outcome following brain tissue oxygen tension-directed therapy versus intracranial pressure/cerebral perfusion pressure-directed therapy in patients with severe traumatic brain injury

Reference	Study type	Country	PtiO$_2$-guided therapy (n)	ICP/ CPP-guided therapy (n)	PtiO$_2$ probe location	PtiO$_2$ threshold for intervention	Endpoint(s)	Principal findings
Adamides et al., 1998 (82)	Prospective	Australia	20	10	Mass lesion: CL Diffuse injury: NDH	2.66 kPa (20 mmHg)	GOS at 6 months	No significant difference in mean GOS score between the two groups (PtiO$_2$ group = 3.55, ICP/CPP group = 4.40; P = 0.19)
Meixensberger et al., 2003 (50)	Retrospective (historical controls)	Germany	53	40	MIH, FL	1.33 kPa (10 mmHg)	GOS at 6 months	A non-significant trend towards improved outcomes in the PtiO$_2$ group (GOS 4 or 5 in PtiO$_2$ group = 65%, in ICP/CPP group = 54%) (P = 0.27)
Stiefel et al., 2005 (128)	Retrospective (historical controls)	USA	28	25	MIH, NAB, FL	3.33 kPa (25 mmHg)	In-hospital mortality	Mortality rate in PtiO$_2$ group (25%) significantly lower than ICP/CPP group (44%) (P < 0.05).
Martini et al. 2009 (129)	Retrospective cohort study	USA	123	506	MIH, NAB, FL	2.66 kPa (20 mmHg)	In-hospital mortality, FIM at hospital discharge.	Slightly worse adjusted mortality in PtiO$_2$ group compared to ICP/CPP group (adjusted mortality difference 4.4%, 95% CI −3.9% to 13%). Worse functional outcomes at discharge in the PtiO$_2$ group (adjusted FIM score difference −0.75, 95% CI −1.41 to −0.09)
McCarthy et al., 2009 (64)	Prospective	USA	81	64	NDH	2.66 kPa (20 mmHg)	In-hospital mortality, GOS every 3 months post-discharge.	No significant difference in mortality rates between PtiO$_2$ group (31%) and ICP/CPP group (36%) (P = 0.52). A non-significant trend towards better outcome (GOS 4 or 5) in PtiO$_2$ group (79%) compared to ICP/CPP group (61%) (P = 0.09)
Narotam et al., 2009 (65)	Retrospective (historical controls)	USA	139	41	NAB	2.66 kPa (20 mmHg)	GOS at 6 months	Higher mean GOS score in PtiO$_2$ group (3.55 ± 1.75) compared to ICP/CPP group (2.71 ± 1.65) (P < 0.01). OR for good outcome in PtiO$_2$ group = 2.09 (95% CI = 1.03–4.24). A reduced mortality rate was observed in the PtiO$_2$ group (26% vs 41.5%; RR reduction 37%) despite higher ISS scores in PtiO$_2$ group
Spiotta et al., 2010 (67)	Retrospective (historical controls)	USA	70	53	MIH, FL	2.66 kPa (20 mmHg)	In-hospital mortality, GOS at 3 months	Mortality rates significantly lower in PtiO$_2$ group (26%) than ICP/CPP group (45%) (P < 0.05). A favourable outcome (GOS score of 4 or 5) was also observed more commonly in the PtiO$_2$ group (64% vs 40%; P = 0.01)

CI, confidence interval; CL, contralateral to mass lesion; CPP, cerebral perfusion pressure; FIM, functional independence measure; FL, frontal lobe; GOS, Glasgow Outcome Score; ICP, intracranial pressure; ISS, injury severity score; LOS, length of stay; MAP, mean arterial pressure; MIH, most injured hemisphere; NAB, normal appearing brain; NDH, non-dominant hemisphere; OR, odds ratio; PtiO$_2$, brain tissue oxygen tension; RR, relative risk.
Data from various studies (see References).

Technological aspects

The technical details of NIRS have been reviewed in detail elsewhere (89) and only a brief summary will be provided here. NIRS systems are based on the transmission and absorption of near infrared (NIR) light (wavelength range 700–950 nm) as it passes through tissue. Several biological molecules, termed chromophores, have distinct absorption spectra in the NIR and their concentrations can be determined by their relative absorption of light in the NIR range. From a clinical perspective, oxyhaemoglobin (O_2Hb) and deoxyhaemoglobin (HHb) are the most commonly measured chromophores, but cytochrome c oxidase (CCO) may ultimately prove clinically more important and was in fact the subject of early clinical NIRS studies (90,91). In adults, NIR light cannot pass across the whole head so the light source and detecting devices (the optodes) are placed a few centimetres apart on the same side of the head. This is called reflectance spectroscopy and allows examination of the superficial cortex.

In a non-scattering medium, where light travels in a straight line between source and detector, there is a linear relationship between the attenuation of light and the absolute concentration of the absorber (chromophore) of interest, as described by the Beer–Lambert law (Figure 11.4A). However in a highly scattering medium, such as biological tissue, light attenuation is determined by both light absorption and scattering (Figure 11.4B). Differential spectroscopy, utilizing a modification of the Beer–Lambert law, assumes that light scattering remains constant during the measurement period and that measured changes in attenuation are due only to changes in absorption. This technique can be applied *in vivo* but allows only changes in chromophore concentration from an arbitrary baseline point to be measured. Multiple scattering events also increase the optical pathlength of the light through the tissue. This further complicates the estimation of chromophore concentration using differential spectroscopy which is dependent on the application of an a priori defined differential pathlength factor to take account of the additional distance travelled by the scattered light. To overcome these issues most commercial cerebral oximeters use multidistance, or spatially resolved, spectroscopy in which multiple closely-spaced detectors measure light attenuation as a function of source-detector separation (Figure 11.4C) (89). By combining these measures with an estimation of the wavelength dependency of light scattering, it is possible to derive a scaled absolute haemoglobin concentration, that is, the relative proportions of O_2Hb and HHb, from which regional cerebral oxygen saturation ($rScO_2$) can be calculated (92):

$$rScO_2 = \left[O_2Hb / O_2Hb + HHb \right] \times 100\%$$

NIRS interrogates arterial, venous, and capillary blood within the field of view. The derived saturation represents a tissue oxygen saturation measured from these three compartments and reflects the balance between cerebral oxygen delivery and utilization. Many systems incorporate two or more channels allowing monitoring of multiple regions of interest simultaneously. Although most commercial cerebral oximeters provide an absolute measure of $rScO_2$ and display this as a simple percentage value, the lack of standardization makes comparisons between studies and devices difficult (93,94). $rScO_2$ is thus best used as a trend monitor.

Cerebral oximeters generally use two wavelengths of NIR light limiting them to measurement of two chromophores, namely O_2Hb and HHb. Advanced NIRS systems, such as those used by research laboratories,

incorporate additional wavelengths and this brings improved accuracy as well as the possibility of monitoring additional chromophores such as CCO (89,93). Some devices, including frequency (or domain)- resolved spectroscopy and time-resolved spectroscopy (TRS) systems, are also able to measure light scattering and absorption in tissue directly, and allow measurement of absolute chromophore concentration, CBF, and cerebral metabolic variables (95,96).

In the research setting, NIRS has been used to measure OEF (7), and regional CBF and CBV using dye-dilution techniques with indocyanine green as the intravascular tracer (98). Good correlation between NIRS- and CT perfusion-derived CBF measurements has been reported in animals (99). Through derivation of cerebral oximetry indices, NIRS has also been used to assess cerebral autoregulation non-invasively (100).

Thresholds for therapy

The 'normal' range of $rScO_2$ is usually stated to be 60–75% but there is substantial intra- and interindividual baseline variability (101), supporting the use of cerebral oximetry values only as a trend monitor (94). Claims for absolute $rScO_2$ thresholds for the determination of cerebral hypoxia/ischaemia are unfounded and, in any case, likely to be patient- and disease-specific (102). Like other measures of cerebral oxygenation, $rScO_2$ is influenced by multiple physiological variables including arterial oxygen saturation, $PaCO_2$, systemic blood pressure, haematocrit, CBV and the cerebral arterial:venous ratio (94).

Near infrared spectroscopy-guided management

In the last decade, there has been a rapid expansion in the clinical experience of cerebral oximetry in the perioperative setting and there is some evidence from retrospective studies that NIRS-guided brain protection protocols might lead to a reduction in neurological complications after cardiac surgery (87,88).

A logical application of NIRS is following ABI where secondary ischaemic injury is common and adversely affects outcome. However, there has been limited research in this area and no outcome studies (89,103). Although low $rScO_2$ values have been associated with poor outcome after ABI (104), the application of NIRS in brain injury is hampered by the inability to define NIRS-derived thresholds for hypoxia/ischaemia, and lack of a gold standard against which to compare NIRS-derived variables (91). Further, the difficulties in describing and interpreting NIRS variables in the normal brain are exacerbated by the optical complexity of the injured brain. Factors such as intracranial haematoma, cerebral oedema, and subarachnoid blood present significant challenges since they may invalidate some of the assumptions upon which NIRS algorithms are based. Indeed, this has been utilized to advantage in studies aiming to identify intracranial haematomas (105,106) and cerebral oedema (107) using NIRS.

A small observational study of 18 TBI patients identified an association between increasing length of time at which $rScO_2$ values were below 60% and intracranial hypertension, low CPP, and mortality (104). In another study comparing changes in $rScO_2$ and $PtiO_2$ after severe TBI, $rScO_2$ less than 60% was found to be moderately accurate for the prediction of 'severe' brain hypoxia ($PtiO_2 < 1.6$ kPa (< 12 mmHg)) but poor at detecting 'moderate' hypoxia ($PtiO_2$ 1.6–2 kPa (12–15 mmHg)), highlighting the different physiological variables and brain regions monitored by the two techniques (108).

NIRS has also been used to monitor cortical oxygenation during cerebral vasospasm after SAH. In one study, the rate of decline of $rScO_2$ was 3.5%/min greater in patients who developed

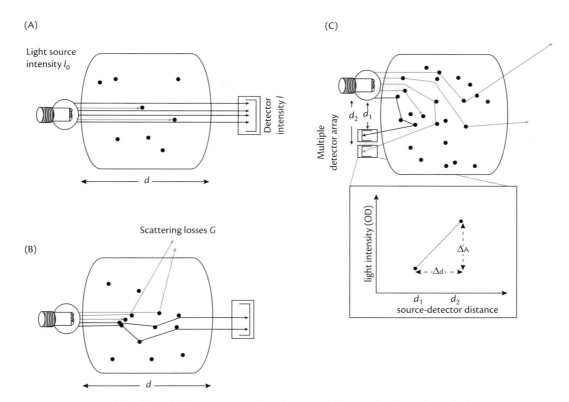

Fig. 11.4 Diagrammatic representation of the effects of light scattering in biological tissue and the principles of spatially resolved spectroscopy.
(A) The idealized situation, not applicable *in vivo*, where light attenuation between a source and detector is dependent only on its absorption by chromophores. In this case the attenuation of light at a given wavelength is described by the Beer–Lambert law. Chromophore concentration can be accurately calculated using the measured degree of light attenuation by the chromophore in association with knowledge of the source-detector separation and relevant absorption coefficient.

$$A = \frac{I}{I_o} = \varepsilon.c.d$$

(B) Differential spectroscopy, utilizing a modification of the Beer Lambert law, can be applied *in vivo*. This technique assumes that light scattering remains constant during the measurement period and that measured changes in attenuation are due only to changes in absorption. Therefore only *changes* in chromophore concentration from an arbitrary baseline point can be measured. The scale of the measured changes in chromophore concentration is dependent on the application of a differential pathlength factor which accounts for the additional path taken by the scattered light and must be defined a priori.

$$A = \frac{I}{I_o} = \varepsilon.c.d.DPF + G$$

A, light attenuation; c, chromophore concentration; d, source-detector distance; DPF, differential pathlength factor; ε, absorption coefficient; G, scattering losses; I, incident light intensity; I_o, detected light intensity.
(C) Multidistance (spatially resolved) spectroscopy incorporates an array of closely spaced detectors and measures light attenuation as a function of source–detector separation (lower panel). By combining these measures with an estimation of the wavelength dependency of light scattering, a scaled absolute haemoglobin concentration, that is, the relative proportions of oxyhaemoglobin and deoxyhaemoglobin, can be derived, and cerebral tissue oxygen saturation calculated:

$$rScO_2 = \left[O_2Hb / O_2Hb + HHb \right] \times 100$$

where O_2Hb = oxyhaemoglobin and HHb = deoxyhaemoglobin.
Reproduced from Ghosh A *et al.*, 'Cerebral near-infrared spectroscopy in adults: a work in progress', *Anesthesia & Analgesia*, 115, pp. 1373–1383, copyright 2012, with permission from Wolters Kluwer Health and International Anesthesia Research Society.

vasospasm during coil embolization than in those who did not (109). In another, angiographic-proven vasospasm was predicted with 100% sensitivity and 85.7% specificity using TRS, which was able to confirm vasospasm in patients in whom transcranial Doppler was not diagnostic (110). In this study, the reliability of repeated NIRS measurements over time was improved by the use of CT image-guidance to position the NIRS optodes, allowing consistent measurement of the same cortical area on consecutive days.

CCO is the terminal complex of the electron transfer chain and catalyses over 95% of oxygen metabolism. NIRS-derived measurement of CCO has been validated in animal studies as a measure of cellular energy status (111), and changes in the concentration of cerebral CCO have been measured in human adults using an optimized multiwavelength NIRS system (112). Monitoring of CCO concentration, in addition to oxygenation variables, may aid in the determination of ischaemic thresholds following ABI by providing additional information about cellular metabolic failure

(91). A customised broadband spectroscopy (BBS) system has been used to demonstrate correlation between changes in CCO concentration and cerebral oxygen delivery in healthy volunteers (112), and increases in CCO concentration during normobaric hyperoxia following TBI (113). Although the lack of a gold standard against which to compare CCO concentration remains an obstacle to its interpretation, the development of mathematical models of brain haemodynamics and metabolism allows *in silico* derivation of physiological variables which can be compared with measured signals to facilitate their interpretation (114).

Advantages and disadvantages

NIRS has potential advantages over other neuromonitoring techniques. It is non-invasive, has high temporal and spatial resolution, and offers simultaneous measurement over multiple regions of interest. During carotid surgery, NIRS-based cerebral oximetry has similar accuracy and reproducibility in the detection of cerebral ischaemia compared to other monitoring modalities, and some advantages in terms of simplicity and temporal resolution (115).

There are several concerns over the clinical application of NIRS, particularly 'contamination' of the signal by extracranial tissue. Some commercial cerebral oximeters use two detectors and a subtraction-based algorithm to deal with this problem. It is assumed that the detecting optode closest to the emitter receives light that has passed mainly through the scalp and that arriving at the farthest detector has passed mainly through brain tissue. Although there is weighting in favour of intracerebral tissue with an interoptode spacing (between emitter and detector) greater than 4 cm (116), the proprietary algorithms on which these assumptions are based are often not published. In any case, even though NIRS has high sensitivity and specificity for intracranial changes when appropriate $rScO_2$ thresholds are chosen (117), it is still prone to some degree of extracerebral contamination (118). This may be particularly problematic during low CBF states. The NIRS-derived CCO signal is highly specific for intracerebral changes potentially making it a superior biomarker to haemoglobin-based NIRS variables (119).

Future technology

A number of technological developments are likely to influence the way in which cerebral oxygenation is monitored in the future. To support the development of routine invasive multimodality neuromonitoring, a multiparameter probe incorporating ICP, $PtiO_2$, and temperature measurements is already available and quantification of CBF is likely to become incorporated into such a device. Advances in $PtiO_2$ technology should allow for improved insertion techniques and more durable devices that are less likely to malfunction (120). The stereotactic placement of invasive probes may help target regions of interest with improved accuracy and might find a place in selected patients. Cerebral arterial oxygen saturation has been estimated using fibreoptic pulse oximetry (121), and a prototype invasive probe that combines NIRS and indocyanine green dye dilution has been used in the simultaneous monitoring of ICP, CBF, and CBV, avoiding the NIRS signal contamination by extracerebral tissues inherent to transcranial systems (122). Optoacoustic technology may also provide an opportunity for the non-invasive monitoring of cerebral venous oxygenation status (123).

In the future, a single NIRS-based device may be able to provide non-invasive monitoring of cerebral oxygenation, haemodynamics, and cellular metabolic status over multiple regions of interest.

Supercontinuum light sources allow the combination of TRS and BBS to yield absolute measurements of optical absorption and scattering across a range of wavelengths, and thus of absolute concentrations of multiple chromophores. A prototype device combining diffuse correlation spectroscopy and NIRS for the bedside measurement of CBF and cerebral oxygenation respectively has also been described (124). Finally, NIRS systems that characterize the cerebral haemodynamic and metabolic responses associated with neuronal function and dysfunction, in addition to identifying cerebral hypoxia/ischaemia, are being developed. Combining NIRS and electroencephalography (EEG) provides a unique opportunity to acquire, non-invasively and simultaneously, regional cerebral electrophysiological and haemodynamic data and thereby inform on neurovascular coupling mechanisms. A combined NIRS/EEG system using a co-located 'opto-electrode' which can house both an EEG electrode and optical probe from an NIRS system has been described for research use (125). However, substantial technological advances are necessary before any of these techniques can be introduced into clinical practice (91).

Multimodal cerebral monitoring, particularly NIRS, generates large and complex datasets, and systems that analyse and present information in a user-friendly format at the bedside are essential to maximize its clinical relevance (see Chapter 13) (126,127). Incorporation of mathematical models of cerebral physiology will facilitate the interpretation of complex datasets and also allow derivation and display of unmeasured but clinically relevant variables such as $CMRO_2$ (127).

References

1. Zauner A, Daugherty WP, Bullock MR, Warner DS. Brain oxygenation and energy metabolism: part I – biological function and pathophysiology. *Neurosurgery*. 2002;51(2):289–301.
2. Tisdall MM, Smith M. Multimodal monitoring in traumatic brain injury: current status and future directions. *Br J Anaesth*. 2007;99:61–7.
3. Ito H, Kanno I, Fukuda H. Human cerebral circulation: positron emission tomography studies. *Ann Nucl Med*. 2005;19:65–74.
4. Derdeyn CP, Videen TO, Yundt KD, Fritsch SM, Carpenter DA, Grubb RL, *et al*. Variability of cerebral blood volume and oxygen extraction: stages of cerebral haemodynamic impairment revisited. *Brain*. 2002;125:595–607.
5. van Santbrink H, Maas AI, Avezaat CJ. Continuous monitoring of partial pressure of brain tissue oxygen in patients with severe head injury. *Neurosurgery*. 1996;38:21–31.
6. Doppenberg EM, Zauner A, Bullock R, Ward JD, Fatouros PP, Young HF. Correlations between brain tissue oxygen tension, carbon dioxide tension, pH, and cerebral blood flow—a better way of monitoring the severely injured brain? *Surg Neurol*. 1998;49:650–4.
7. Johnston AJ, Steiner LA, Coles JP, Chatfield DA, Fryer TD, Smielewski P, *et al*. Effect of cerebral perfusion pressure augmentation on regional oxygenation and metabolism after head injury. *Crit Care Med*. 2005;33:189–95.
8. Rao GS, Durga P. Changing trends in monitoring brain ischemia: from intracranial pressure to cerebral oximetry. *Curr Opin Anaesthesiol*. 2011;24: 48794.
9. Hemphill JC, 3rd, Knudson MM, Derugin N, Morabito D, Manley GT. Carbon dioxide reactivity and pressure autoregulation of brain tissue oxygen. *Neurosurgery*. 2001;48:377–83.
10. Hadolt I, Litscher G. Noninvasive assessment of cerebral oxygenation during high altitude trekking in the Nepal Himalayas (2850-5600 m). *Neurol Res*. 2003;25:183–8.
11. Stocchetti N, Chieregato A, De Marchi M, Croci M, Benti R, Grimoldi N. High cerebral perfusion pressure improves low values of local

brain tissue O2 tension (PtiO2) in focal lesions. *Acta Neurochir Suppl.* 1998;71:162–5.

12. Xu F, Liu P, Pascual JM, Xiao G, Lu H. Effect of hypoxia and hyperoxia on cerebral blood flow, blood oxygenation, and oxidative metabolism. *J Cereb Blood Flow Metab.* 2012;32:1909–18.

13. Floyd TF, Clark JM, Gelfand R, Detre JA, Ratcliffe S, Guvakov D, et al. Independent cerebral vasoconstrictive effects of hyperoxia and accompanying arterial hypocapnia at 1 ATA. *J Appl Physiol.* 2003;95:2453–61.

14. Kirkman MA. Debate—does a reversible penumbra exist in intracerebral haemorrhage? *Br J Neurosurg.* 2011;25:523–5.

15. Rohlwink UK, Figaji AA. Methods of monitoring brain oxygenation. *Childs Nerv Syst.* 2010;26:453–64.

16. Dagal A, Lam AM. Cerebral blood flow and the injured brain: how should we monitor and manipulate it? *Curr Opin Anaesthesiol.* 2011;24:131–7.

17. Menon DK. Brain ischaemia after traumatic brain injury: lessons from 15O2 positron emission tomography. *Curr Opin Crit Care.* 2006;12:85–9.

18. Nortje J, Coles JP, Timofeev I, Fryer TD, Aigbirhio FI, Smielewski P, et al. Effect of hyperoxia on regional oxygenation and metabolism after severe traumatic brain injury: preliminary findings. *Crit Care Med.* 2008;36:273–81.

19. Diringer MN, Aiyagari V, Zazulia AR, Videen TO, Powers WJ. Effect of hyperoxia on cerebral metabolic rate for oxygen measured using positron emission tomography in patients with acute severe head injury. *J Neurosurg.* 2007;106:526–9.

20. Shiino A, Yamauchi H, Morikawa S, Inubushi T. Mapping of cerebral metabolic rate of oxygen using DSC and BOLD MR imaging: a preliminary study. *Magn Reson Med Sci.* 2012;11:109–15.

21. Singer OC, Sitzer M, du Mesnil de Rochemont R, Neumann-Haefelin T. Practical limitations of acute stroke MRI due to patient-related problems. *Neurology.* 2004;62:1848–9.

22. Swanson EW, Mascitelli J, Stiefel M, MacMurtrie E, Levine J, Kofke WA, et al. Patient transport and brain oxygen in comatose patients. *Neurosurgery.* 2010;66:925–31.

23. Schell RM, Cole DJ. Cerebral monitoring: jugular venous oximetry. *Anesth Analg.* 2000;90:559–66.

24. Macmillan CS, Andrews PJ. Cerebrovenous oxygen saturation monitoring: practical considerations and clinical relevance. *Intensive Care Med.* 2000;26:1028–36.

25. Matta BF, Lam AM, Mayberg TS, Shapira Y, Winn HR. A critique of the intraoperative use of jugular venous bulb catheters during neurosurgical procedures. *Anesth Analg.* 1994;79:745–50.

26. Murr R, Schurer L. Correlation of jugular venous oxygen saturation to spontaneous fluctuations of cerebral perfusion pressure in patients with severe head injury. *Neurol Res.* 1995;17:329–33.

27. Chan KH, Dearden NM, Miller JD, Andrews PJ, Midgley S. Multimodality monitoring as a guide to treatment of intracranial hypertension after severe brain injury. *Neurosurgery.* 1993;32:547–52.

28. Robertson CS, Gopinath SP, Goodman JC, Contant CF, Valadka AB, Narayan RK. SjvO2 monitoring in head-injured patients. *J Neurotrauma.* 1995;12:891–6.

29. Macmillan CS, Andrews PJ, Easton VJ. Increased jugular bulb saturation is associated with poor outcome in traumatic brain injury. *J Neurol Neurosurg Psychiatry.* 2001;70:101–4.

30. Brain Trauma Foundation, American Association of Neurological Surgeons, Congress of Neurological Surgeons. Guidelines for the management of severe traumatic brain injury. *J Neurotrauma.* 2007;24(Suppl):S1–106.

31. Gupta AK, Hutchinson PJ, Al-Rawi P, Gupta S, Swart M, Kirkpatrick PJ, et al. Measuring brain tissue oxygenation compared with jugular venous oxygen saturation for monitoring cerebral oxygenation after traumatic brain injury. *Anesth Analg.* 1999;88:549–53.

32. Coles JP, Fryer TD, Smielewski P, Chatfield DA, Steiner LA, Johnston AJ, et al. Incidence and mechanisms of cerebral ischemia in early clinical head injury. *J Cereb Blood Flow Metab.* 2004;24:202–11.

33. Lam JM, Chan MS, Poon WS. Cerebral venous oxygen saturation monitoring: is dominant jugular bulb cannulation good enough? *Br J Neurosurg.* 1996;10:357–64.

34. Nortje J, Gupta AK. The role of tissue oxygen monitoring in patients with acute brain injury. *Br J Anaesth.* 2006;97:95–106.

35. Rose JC, Neill TA, Hemphill JC, 3rd. Continuous monitoring of the microcirculation in neurocritical care: an update on brain tissue oxygenation. *Curr Opin Crit Care.* 2006;12:97–102.

36. Rosenthal G, Hemphill JC, 3rd, Sorani M, Martin C, Morabito D, Obrist WD, et al. Brain tissue oxygen tension is more indicative of oxygen diffusion than oxygen delivery and metabolism in patients with traumatic brain injury. *Crit Care Med.* 2008;36:1917–24.

37. Scheufler KM, Rohrborn HJ, Zentner J. Does tissue oxygen-tension reliably reflect cerebral oxygen delivery and consumption? *Anesth Analg.* 2002;95:1042–8.

38. Gupta AK, Hutchinson PJ, Fryer T, Al-Rawi PG, Parry DA, Minhas PS, et al. Measurement of brain tissue oxygenation performed using positron emission tomography scanning to validate a novel monitoring method. *J Neurosurg.* 2002;96:263–8.

39. McLeod AD, Igielman F, Elwell C, Cope M, Smith M. Measuring cerebral oxygenation during normobaric hyperoxia: a comparison of tissue microprobes, near-infrared spectroscopy, and jugular venous oximetry in head injury. *Anesth Analg.* 2003;97:851–6.

40. Menon DK, Coles JP, Gupta AK, Fryer TD, Smielewski P, Chatfield DA, et al. Diffusion limited oxygen delivery following head injury. *Crit Care Med.* 2004;32:1384–90.

41. Kleinig TJ, Helps SC, Ghabriel MN, Manavis J, Leigh C, Blumbergs PC, et al. Hemoglobin crystals: A pro-inflammatory potential confounder of rat experimental intracerebral hemorrhage. *Brain Res.* 2009;1287:164–72.

42. Rosenthal G, Hemphill JC, Sorani M, Martin C, Morabito D, Meeker M, et al. The role of lung function in brain tissue oxygenation following traumatic brain injury. *J Neurosurg.* 2008;108:59–65.

43. Longhi L, Pagan F, Valeriani V, Magnoni S, Zanier ER, Conte V, et al. Monitoring brain tissue oxygen tension in brain-injured patients reveals hypoxic episodes in normal-appearing and in peri-focal tissue. *Intensive Care Med.* 2007;33:2136–42.

44. van den Brink WA, van Santbrink H, Steyerberg EW, Avezaat CJ, Suazo JA, Hogesteeger C, et al. Brain oxygen tension in severe head injury. *Neurosurgery.* 2000;46:868–76.

45. Alves OL, Daugherty WP, Rios M. Arterial hyperoxia in severe head injury: a useful or harmful option? *Curr Pharm Des.* 2004;10:2163–76.

46. Carvi y Nievas M, Toktamis S, Hollerhage HG, Haas E. Hyperacute measurement of brain-tissue oxygen, carbon dioxide, pH, and intracranial pressure before, during, and after cerebral angiography in patients with aneurysmatic subarachnoid hemorrhage in poor condition. *Surg Neurol.* 2005;64:362–7.

47. Jodicke A, Hubner F, Boker DK. Monitoring of brain tissue oxygenation during aneurysm surgery: prediction of procedure-related ischemic events. *J Neurosurg.* 2003;98:515–23.

48. Ibanez J, Vilalta A, Mena MP, Topczewski T, Noguer M, et al. Intraoperative detection of ischemic brain hypoxia using oxygen tissue pressure microprobes. [In Spanish]. *Neurocirugia (Astur).* 2003;14:483–9.

49. Wintermark M, Chiolero R, van Melle G, Revelly JP, Porchet F, Regli L, et al. Relationship between brain perfusion computed tomography variables and cerebral perfusion pressure in severe head trauma patients. *Crit Care Med.* 2004;32:1579–87.

50. Meixensberger J, Jaeger M, Vath A, Dings J, Kunze E, Roosen K. Brain tissue oxygen guided treatment supplementing ICP/CPP therapy after traumatic brain injury. *J Neurol Neurosurg Psychiatry.* 2003;74:760–4.

51. van Santbrink H, vd Brink WA, Steyerberg EW, Carmona Suazo JA, Avezaat CJ, Maas AI. Brain tissue oxygen response in severe traumatic brain injury. *Acta Neurochir (Wien).* 2003;145:429–38.

52. Chang JJ, Youn TS, Benson D, Mattick H, Andrade N, Harper CR, et al. Physiologic and functional outcome correlates of brain tissue hypoxia in traumatic brain injury. *Crit Care Med.* 2009;37:283–90.

53. Oddo M, Levine JM, Mackenzie L, Frangos S, Feihl F, Kasner SE, et al. Brain hypoxia is associated with short-term outcome after severe

traumatic brain injury independently of intracranial hypertension and low cerebral perfusion pressure. *Neurosurgery.* 2011;69:1037–45.

54. Ramakrishna R, Stiefel M, Udoetuk J, Spiotta A, Levine JM, Kofke WA, et al. Brain oxygen tension and outcome in patients with aneurysmal subarachnoid hemorrhage. *J Neurosurg.* 2008;109:1075–82.

55. Vath A, Kunze E, Roosen K, Meixensberger J. Therapeutic aspects of brain tissue pO2 monitoring after subarachnoid hemorrhage. *Acta Neurochir Suppl.* 2002;81:307–9.

56. Meixensberger J, Vath A, Jaeger M, Kunze E, Dings J, Roosen K. Monitoring of brain tissue oxygenation following severe subarachnoid hemorrhage. *Neurol Res.* 2003;25:445–50.

57. Kett-White R, Hutchinson PJ, Al-Rawi PG, Gupta AK, Pickard JD, Kirkpatrick PJ. Adverse cerebral events detected after subarachnoid hemorrhage using brain oxygen and microdialysis probes. *Neurosurgery.* 2002;50:1213–21.

58. Diringer MN, Bleck TP, Claude Hemphill J, 3rd, Menon D, Shutter L, Vespa P, et al. Critical care management of patients following aneurysmal subarachnoid hemorrhage: recommendations from the Neurocritical Care Society's Multidisciplinary Consensus Conference. *Neurocrit Care.* 2011;15:211–40.

59. Jaeger M, Schuhmann MU, Soehle M, Nagel C, Meixensberger J. Continuous monitoring of cerebrovascular autoregulation after subarachnoid hemorrhage by brain tissue oxygen pressure reactivity and its relation to delayed cerebral infarction. *Stroke.* 2007;38:981–6.

60. Muench E, Horn P, Bauhuf C, Roth H, Philipps M, Hermann P, et al. Effects of hypervolemia and hypertension on regional cerebral blood flow, intracranial pressure, and brain tissue oxygenation after subarachnoid hemorrhage. *Crit Care Med.* 2007;35:1844–51.

61. Ko SB, Choi HA, Parikh G, Helbok R, Schmidt JM, Lee K, et al. Multimodality monitoring for cerebral perfusion pressure optimization in comatose patients with intracerebral hemorrhage. *Stroke.* 2011;42:3087–92.

62. Stiefel MF, Heuer GG, Smith MJ, Bloom S, Maloney-Wilensky E, Gracias VH, et al. Cerebral oxygenation following decompressive hemicraniectomy for the treatment of refractory intracranial hypertension. *J Neurosurg.* 2004;101:241–7.

63. Hoffman WE, Charbel FT, Edelman G. Brain tissue oxygen, carbon dioxide, and pH in neurosurgical patients at risk for ischemia. *Anesth Analg.* 1996;82:582–6.

64. McCarthy MC, Moncrief H, Sands JM, Markert RJ, Hall LC, Wenker IC, et al. Neurologic outcomes with cerebral oxygen monitoring in traumatic brain injury. *Surgery.* 2009;146:585–90.

65. Narotam PK, Morrison JF, Nathoo N. Brain tissue oxygen monitoring in traumatic brain injury and major trauma: outcome analysis of a brain tissue oxygen-directed therapy. *J Neurosurg.* 2009;111:672–82.

66. Nangunoori R, Maloney-Wilensky E, Stiefel M, Park S, Andrew Kofke W, Levine JM, et al. Brain tissue oxygen-based therapy and outcome after severe traumatic brain injury: a systematic literature review. *Neurocrit Care.* 2012;17:131–8.

67. Spiotta AM, Stiefel MF, Gracias VH, Garuffe AM, Kofke WA, Maloney-Wilensky E, et al. Brain tissue oxygen-directed management and outcome in patients with severe traumatic brain injury. *J Neurosurg.* 2010;113:571–80.

68. Valadka AB, Gopinath SP, Contant CF, Uzura M, Robertson CS. Relationship of brain tissue PO2 to outcome after severe head injury. *Crit Care Med.* 1998;26:1576–81.

69. Bohman LE, Heuer GG, Macyszyn L, Maloney-Wilensky E, Frangos S, Le Roux PD, et al. Medical management of compromised brain oxygen in patients with severe traumatic brain injury. *Neurocrit Care.* 2011;14:361–9.

70. Hemphill JC, 3rd, Morabito D, Farrant M, Manley GT. Brain tissue oxygen monitoring in intracerebral hemorrhage. *Neurocrit Care.* 2005;3:260–70.

71. Jaeger M, Schuhmann MU, Soehle M, Meixensberger J. Continuous assessment of cerebrovascular autoregulation after traumatic brain injury using brain tissue oxygen pressure reactivity. *Crit Care Med.* 2006;34:1783–8.

72. Jaeger M, Dengl M, Meixensberger J, Schuhmann MU. Effects of cerebrovascular pressure reactivity-guided optimization of cerebral perfusion pressure on brain tissue oxygenation after traumatic brain injury. *Crit Care Med.* 2010;38:1343–7.

73. Oddo M, Levine JM, Frangos S, Carrera E, Maloney-Wilensky E, Pascual JL, et al. Effect of mannitol and hypertonic saline on cerebral oxygenation in patients with severe traumatic brain injury and refractory intracranial hypertension. *J Neurol Neurosurg Psychiatry.* 2009;80:916–20.

74. Al-Rawi PG, Tseng MY, Richards HK, Nortje J, Timofeev I, Matta BF, et al. Hypertonic saline in patients with poor-grade subarachnoid hemorrhage improves cerebral blood flow, brain tissue oxygen, and pH. *Stroke.* 2010;41:122–8.

75. Rangel-Castilla L, Lara LR, Gopinath S, Swank PR, Valadka A, Robertson C. Cerebral hemodynamic effects of acute hyperoxia and hyperventilation after severe traumatic brain injury. *J Neurotrauma.* 2010;27:1853–63.

76. Strege RJ, Lang EW, Stark AM, Scheffner H, Fritsch MJ, Barth H, et al. Cerebral edema leading to decompressive craniectomy: an assessment of the preceding clinical and neuromonitoring trends. *Neurol Res.* 2003;25:510–15.

77. Beynon C, Kiening KL, Orakcioglu B, Unterberg AW, Sakowitz OW. Brain tissue oxygen monitoring and hyperoxic treatment in patients with traumatic brain injury. *J Neurotrauma.* 2012;29:2109–23.

78. Hlatky R, Valadka AB, Gopinath SP, Robertson CS. Brain tissue oxygen tension response to induced hyperoxia reduced in hypoperfused brain. *J Neurosurg.* 2008;108:53–8.

79. Oddo M, Nduom E, Frangos S, MacKenzie L, Chen I, Maloney-Wilensky E, et al. Acute lung injury is an independent risk factor for brain hypoxia after severe traumatic brain injury. *Neurosurgery.* 2010;67:338–44.

80. Leal-Noval SR, Rincon-Ferrari MD, Marin-Niebla A, Cayuela A, Arellano-Orden V, Marín-Caballos A, et al. Transfusion of erythrocyte concentrates produces a variable increment on cerebral oxygenation in patients with severe traumatic brain injury: a preliminary study. *Intensive Care Med.* 2006;32:1733–40.

81. Smith MJ, Stiefel MF, Magge S, Frangos S, Bloom S, Gracias V, et al. Packed red blood cell transfusion increases local cerebral oxygenation. *Crit Care Med.* 2005;33:1104–8.

82. Adamides AA, Cooper DJ, Rosenfeldt FL, Bailey MJ, Pratt N, Tippett N, et al. Focal cerebral oxygenation and neurological outcome with or without brain tissue oxygen-guided therapy in patients with traumatic brain injury. *Acta Neurochir (Wien).* 2009;151:1399–409.

83. van den Brink WA, Haitsma IK, Avezaat CJ, Houtsmuller AB, Kros JM, Maas AI. Brain parenchyma/pO2 catheter interface: a histopathological study in the rat. *J Neurotrauma.* 1998;15:813–24.

84. Dings J, Meixensberger J, Jager A, Roosen K. Clinical experience with 118 brain tissue oxygen partial pressure catheter probes. *Neurosurgery.* 1998;43:1082–95.

85. Meixensberger J, Dings J, Jager A, Roosen K. Die Gewebesauerstoffmessung im Gehirn—Was ist bewiesen? *Intensivmed Notfmed.* 1998;35:s072–079.

86. Pennekamp CW, Moll FL, de Borst GJ. The potential benefits and the role of cerebral monitoring in carotid endarterectomy. *Curr Opin Anaesthesiol.* 2011;24:693–7.

87. Fedorow C, Grocott HP. Cerebral monitoring to optimize outcomes after cardiac surgery. *Curr Opin Anaesthesiol.* 2010;23:89–94.

88. Vohra HA, Modi A, Ohri SK. Does use of intra-operative cerebral regional oxygen saturation monitoring during cardiac surgery lead to improved clinical outcomes? *Interact Cardiovasc Thorac Surg.* 2009;9:318–22.

89. Ghosh A, Elwell C, Smith M. Cerebral near-infrared spectroscopy in adults: a work in progress. *Anesth Analg.* 2012;115:1373–83.

90. Kakihana Y, Matsunaga A, Yasuda T, Imabayashi T, Kanmura Y, Tamura M. Brain oximetry in the operating room: current status and future directions with particular regard to cytochrome oxidase. *J Biomed Opt.* 2008;13:033001.

91. Smith M, Elwell C. Near-infrared spectroscopy: shedding light on the injured brain. *Anesth Analg.* 2009;108:1055–7.

92. Suzuki S, Takasaki S, Ozaki T, Kobayashi, Y. A tissue oxygenation monitor using NIR spatially resolved spectroscopy. *SPIE Proc.* 1999;3597:582–92.

93. Ferrari M, Quaresima V. Near infrared brain and muscle oximetry: from discovery to current applications. *J Near Infrared Spectrosc.* 2012;20:1–14.

94. Highton D, Elwell C, Smith M. Noninvasive cerebral oximetry: is there light at the end of the tunnel? *Curr Opin Anaesthesiol.* 2010;23:576–81.

95. Diop M, Verdecchia K, Lee TY, St Lawrence K. Calibration of diffuse correlation spectroscopy with a time-resolved near-infrared technique to yield absolute cerebral blood flow measurements. *Biomed Opt Express.* 2011;2:2068–81.

96. Verdecchia K, Diop M, Lee TY, St Lawrence K. Quantifying the cerebral metabolic rate of oxygen by combining diffuse correlation spectroscopy and time-resolved near-infrared spectroscopy. *J Biomed Opt.* 2013;18:27007.

97. Brown DW, Hadway J, Lee TY. Near-infrared spectroscopy measurement of oxygen extraction fraction and cerebral metabolic rate of oxygen in newborn piglets. *Pediatr Res.* 2003;54:861–7.

98. Ferrari M, Mottola L, Quaresima V. Principles, techniques, and limitations of near infrared spectroscopy. *Can J Appl Physiol.* 2004;29:463–87.

99. Diop M, Elliott JT, Tichauer KM, Lee TY, St Lawrence K. A broadband continuous-wave multichannel near-infrared system for measuring regional cerebral blood flow and oxygen consumption in newborn piglets. *Rev Sci Instrum.* 2009;80:054302.

100. Ono M, Joshi B, Brady K, Easley RB, Zheng Y, Brown C, *et al.* Risks for impaired cerebral autoregulation during cardiopulmonary bypass and postoperative stroke. *Br J Anaesth.* 2012;109:391–8.

101. Thavasothy M, Broadhead M, Elwell C, Peters M, Smith M. A comparison of cerebral oxygenation as measured by the NIRO 300 and the INVOS 5100 Near-Infrared Spectrophotometers. *Anaesthesia.* 2002;57:999–1006.

102. Hunt K, Tachtsidis I, Bleasdale-Barr K, Elwell C, Mathias C, Smith M. Changes in cerebral oxygenation and haemodynamics during postural blood pressure changes in patients with autonomic failure. *Physiol Meas.* 2006;27:777–85.

103. Smith M. Shedding light on the adult brain: a review of the clinical applications of near-infrared spectroscopy. *Phil Trans R Soc.* 2011;369:4452–69.

104. Dunham CM, Ransom KJ, Flowers LL, Siegal JD, Kohli CM. Cerebral hypoxia in severely brain-injured patients is associated with admission Glasgow Coma Scale score, computed tomographic severity, cerebral perfusion pressure, and survival. *J Trauma.* 2004;56:482–9.

105. Robertson CS, Gopinath SP, Chance B. A new application for near-infrared spectroscopy: detection of delayed intracranial hematomas after head injury. *J Neurotrauma.* 1995;12:591–600.

106. Salonia R, Bell MJ, Kochanek PM, Berger RP. The utility of near infrared spectroscopy in detecting intracranial hemorrhage in children. *J Neurotrauma.* 2011;29:1047–53.

107. Gill AS, Rajneesh KF, Owen CM, Yeh J, Hsu M, Binder DK. Early optical detection of cerebral edema in vivo. *J Neurosurg.* 2011;114:470–7.

108. Leal-Noval SR, Cayuela A, Arellano-Orden V, Marín-Caballos A, Padilla V, Ferrándiz-Millón C, *et al.* Invasive and noninvasive assessment of cerebral oxygenation in patients with severe traumatic brain injury. *Intensive Care Med.* 2010;36:1309–17.

109. Bhatia R, Hampton T, Malde S, Kandala NB, Muammar M, Deasy N, *et al.* The application of near-infrared oximetry to cerebral monitoring during aneurysm embolization: a comparison with intraprocedural angiography. *J Neurosurg Anesthesiol* 2007;19:97–104.

110. Yokose N, Sakatani K, Murata Y, Awano T, Igarashi T, Nakamura S, *et al.* Bedside monitoring of cerebral blood oxygenation and hemodynamics after aneurysmal subarachnoid hemorrhage by quantitative time-resolved near-infrared spectroscopy. *World Neurosurg.* 2010;73:508–13.

111. Springett R, Wylezinska M, Cady EB, Cope M, Delpy DT. Oxygen dependency of cerebral oxidative phosphorylation in newborn piglets. *J Cereb Blood Flow Metab.* 2000;20:280–9.

112. Tisdall MM, Tachtsidis I, Leung TS, Elwell CE, Smith M. Near-infrared spectroscopic quantification of changes in the concentration of oxidized cytochrome c oxidase in the healthy human brain during hypoxemia. *J Biomed Opt.* 2007;12:024002.

113. Tisdall MM, Tachtsidis I, Leung TS, Elwell CE, Smith M. Increase in cerebral aerobic metabolism by normobaric hyperoxia after traumatic brain injury. *J Neurosurg.* 2008;109:424–32.

114. Banaji M, Mallet A, Elwell CE, Nicholls P, Cooper CE. A model of brain circulation and metabolism: NIRS signal changes during physiological challenges. *PLoS Comput Biol.* 2008;4:e1000212.

115. Moritz S, Kasprzak P, Arlt M, Taeger K, Metz C. Accuracy of cerebral monitoring in detecting cerebral ischemia during carotid endarterectomy: a comparison of transcranial Doppler sonography, near-infrared spectroscopy, stump pressure, and somatosensory evoked potentials. *Anesthesiology.* 2007;107:563–9.

116. Germon TJ, Evans PD, Barnett NJ, Wall P, Manara AR, Nelson RJ. Cerebral near infrared spectroscopy: emitter-detector separation must be increased. *Br J Anaesth.* 1999;82:831–7.

117. Al-Rawi PG, Smielewski P, Kirkpatrick PJ. Evaluation of a near-infrared spectrometer (NIRO 300) for the detection of intracranial oxygenation changes in the adult head. *Stroke.* 2001;32:2492–500.

118. Davie SN, Grocott HP. Impact of extracranial contamination on regional cerebral oxygen saturation: a comparison of three cerebral oximetry technologies. *Anesthesiology.* 2012;116:834–40.

119. Kolyva C, Ghosh A, Tachtsidis I, Highton D, Cooper CE, Smith M, *et al.* Cytochrome c oxidase response to changes in cerebral oxygen delivery in the adult brain shows higher brain-specificity than haemoglobin. *Neuroimage.* 2013;85 Pt 1:234–44.

120. Stuart RM, Schmidt M, Kurtz P, Waziri A, Helbok R, Mayer SA, *et al.* Intracranial multimodal monitoring for acute brain injury: a single institution review of current practices. *Neurocrit Care.* 2010;12:188–98.

121. Phillips JP, Langford RM, Chang SH, Maney K, Kyriacou PA, Jones DP. Cerebral arterial oxygen saturation measurements using a fiber-optic pulse oximeter. *Neurocrit Care.* 2010;13:278–85.

122. Keller E, Froehlich J, Muroi C, Sikorski C, Muser M. Neuromonitoring in intensive care: a new brain tissue probe for combined monitoring of intracranial pressure (ICP) cerebral blood flow (CBF) and oxygenation. *Acta Neurochir Suppl.* 2011;110:217–20.

123. Petrov IY, Petrov Y, Prough DS, Deyo DJ, Cicenaite I, Esenaliev RO. Optoacoustic monitoring of cerebral venous blood oxygenation through extracerebral blood. *Biomed Opt Express.* 2012;3:125–36.

124. Kim MN, Durduran T, Frangos S, Frangos S, Mesquita RC, Levine JM, *et al.* Continuous optical monitoring of cerebral hemodynamics during head-of-bed manipulation in brain-injured adults. *Neurocrit Care.* 2010;12:173–80

125. Cooper RJ, Hebden JC, O'Reilly H, Mitra S, Michell AW, Everdell NL, *et al.* Transient haemodynamic events in neurologically compromised infants: a simultaneous EEG and diffuse optical imaging study. *Neuroimage.* 2011;55:1610–16.

126. Oddo M, Villa F, Citerio G. Brain multimodality monitoring: an update. *Curr Opin Crit Care.* 2012;18:111–18.

127. Hemphill JC, Andrews P, De Georgia M. Multimodal monitoring and neurocritical care bioinformatics. *Nat Rev Neurol.* 2011;7:451–60.

128. Stiefel MF, Spiotta A, Gracias VH, Garuffe AM, Guillamondegui O, Maloney-Wilensky E, *et al.* Reduced mortality rate in patients with severe traumatic brain injury treated with brain tissue oxygen monitoring. *J Neurosurg.* 2005;103:805–11.

129. Martini RP, Deem S, Yanez ND, Chesnut RM, Weiss NS, Daniel S, *et al.* Management guided by brain tissue oxygen monitoring and outcome following severe traumatic brain injury. *J Neurosurg.* 2009;111:644–9.

CHAPTER 12

Brain tissue biochemistry

Imoigele Aisiku and Claudia Robertson

Cerebral microdialysis (MD) was introduced as an *in vivo* biochemical monitoring tool for basic science studies almost 40 years ago. It was evaluated in the human brain in 1990 (1) and its clinical use first reported in 1992 by Persson and colleagues who demonstrated 25-fold increases in brain extracellular fluid (ECF) glutamate, aspartate, and taurine, and increases in the lactate:pyruvate ratio (LPR) under conditions of stress or increased energy utilization in brain-injured patients (2). In 1995, commercially available MD instrumentation was introduced for clinical use, facilitating the translation of a laboratory-based technique into clinical practice (3).

Brain tissue oxygen tension (PtiO$_2$) monitoring provides the earliest signs of cerebral hypoxia/ischaemia after acute brain injury (see Chapter 11), but MD provides additional information. Not only is cerebral MD a monitor for the detection of ischaemic events, it also monitors the supply of substrate and its cellular metabolism, including the consequences of reduced tissue oxygenation on brain metabolism. Cerebral MD is the only neuromonitoring tool that can provide information on the brain's biochemical/metabolic status which can be used to guide the management of critically ill brain-injured patients in real time at the bedside (4).

The principal substances measured during routine cerebral MD monitoring are markers of cerebral hypoxia/ischaemia, excitotoxic states, tissue damage, and inflammation (5–7). These can generally be categorized as:

- energy-related metabolites: glucose, lactate, pyruvate, LPR, adenosine, and xanthine
- neurotransmitters: glutamate, aspartate, and gamma-aminobutyric acid (GABA)
- markers of tissue damage and inflammation: glycerol, potassium, and cytokines
- exogenous substances: including drugs.

Principles of cerebral microdialysis

MD is a technique that can be used *in vitro* and *in vivo* to measure endogenous and exogenous molecules of various sizes without the need for tissue sampling. It provides large amounts of information about tissue biochemistry in the research and clinical setting with the advantage of semicontinuous sampling. Cerebral MD provides a facsimile of brain tissue biochemistry which has significantly improved our understanding of cerebral physiology and pathophysiology (8).

A semipermeable dialysis membrane is introduced into brain parenchyma in a region of interest and a commercially available, semi-automated analyser is available for the bedside monitoring of glucose, lactate, pyruvate, glycerol, and glutamate on the collected samples, usually at hourly intervals (7). MD samples can also be assayed 'off-line' in the laboratory for a multitude of other substances making MD a 'universal' biosensor capable of monitoring essentially every small and medium-sized molecule in the interstitial fluid that is able to traverse the dialysis membrane (9).

Although the following methodology relates to monitoring the brain, it can easily be adapted to other organ systems.

Microdialysis catheter

The cerebral MD catheter is a thin tubing composed of inner and outer concentric tubes with a semipermeable polyamide dialysis membrane (0.6 mm) at its tip (Figure 12.1) (10). The dialysis membrane functions like a blood capillary, with diffusion driving the movement of chemical substances from the brain ECF into an isotonic perfusion fluid that is continuously flushed along the inner side of the membrane to maintain the concentration gradient across it. The perfusion fluid is infused at a constant rate, using a precision micropump, through the outer (inlet) tube to the dialysis membrane where bi-directional exchange of molecules between interstitial and perfusion fluid takes place (Figure 12.2). Now termed the microdialysate, the perfusion fluid then flows via the inner (outlet) tube to the distal end of the catheter where it is collected into a small microvial for analysis at the bedside or subsequently in the laboratory. The microdialysate contains any molecule that has diffused across the dialysis member from the brain ECF. Notably concentrations of molecules in the dialysate do not equal their tissue concentrations but reflect a constant fraction of the tissue concentration (see later). This is termed the relative recovery fraction.

The choice of perfusion fluid is important as it can influence the concentration of molecules recovered or even enzymatic function in the surrounding tissue. Commercially available perfusion fluid for clinical monitoring is an un-buffered solution with an ionic composition similar to that of the brain ECF. This ensures that there is no significant transfer of major cations (sodium, potassium, and calcium) or anions (chloride) across the MD membrane.

Recovery of measured substances

Unless there is total equilibration between the brain ECF and perfusion fluid the concentration of a given substance in the microdialysate will be lower than its actual concentration in the ECF. The relationship between dialysate and ECF concentrations is termed the relative recovery and is defined as the concentration in the dialysate expressed as a percentage of the concentration in the interstitial fluid. The final concentration of substances in the dialysate depends on the balance between substrate delivery to,

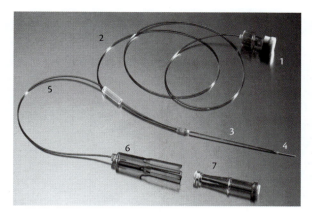

Fig. 12.1 Components of clinical microdialysis catheter.
1. Pump connector
2. Inlet tube
3. Microdialysis catheter
4. Microdialysis membrane
5. Outlet tube
6. Microvial holder
7. Microvial for collection of microdiasylate

Reproduced with permission from Tisdall MM and Smith M, 'Cerebral microdialysis: research technique or clinical tool', *British Journal of Anaesthesia*, 2006, 97, pp. 18–25, by permission of Oxford University Press and the Board of Management and Trustees of the *British Journal of Anaesthesia*.

and uptake from, the brain ECF and also on several factors related to the MD technique itself (8). Low perfusate flow rate and long dialysis membrane allows a higher recovery rate, although longer membranes decrease anatomical specificity. If the membrane is sufficiently long and the perfusate flow sufficiently slow, the concentration of a substance in the dialysate will approach that in the interstitial fluid, that is, recovery will be close to 100%. Another factor affecting recovery is the dialysis membrane pore size, also known as the molecular weight cut-off (8). The size of the molecules of interest therefore plays a crucial role in the selection of the dialysis membrane type. The markers of cerebral metabolism studied measured at the bedside, including glucose, pyruvate, lactate,

glycerol, and glutamate, are typically small and a 20 kDa molecular weight cut-off catheter can be used, whereas monitoring of larger molecules such as cytokines requires 100 kDa molecular weight cut-off membranes. In general, as the molecular weight of a substance increases, the probe efficiency and accuracy of the sample decreases (11). In clinical practice a perfusate flow rate of 0.3 μL/min, a membrane length of 10 mm, and a 20 kDa molecular weight cut-off catheter are commonly used and this combination results in recovery of commonly measured analytes of around 65%–70% (12). At higher flow rates, which allow greater sampling temporal resolution, recovery declines. At a flow rate of 1.0 μL/min recovery is between 21% and 34% for the same molecules. Figure 12.3 shows a typical setup of the bedside equipment required for cerebral MD monitoring.

Markers of ischaemia and cell damage

Each sampled substance acts as a marker of a particular cellular process associated with hypoxia, ischaemia, and cellular energy failure, allowing cerebral MD to be used to monitor pathophysiological changes in brain tissue as well as the response to treatment. Lactate, pyruvate, glucose, glycerol, and glutamate are the most useful biochemical variables in the clinical setting (3,5,7,13).

Cerebral energy metabolism

Glucose is the essential energy substrate for the brain where it is almost entirely oxidized to carbon dioxide and water. Although the brain represents only 2% of body weight, it receives 15% of the cardiac output and is responsible for 20% of total body oxygen consumption and 25% of glucose utilization (see Chapter 3) (14). With a global blood flow of 50–55 mL/100 g/min and a metabolic rate for oxygen of around 3.3 mL/100 g/min, the brain extracts approximately 40–50% of delivered oxygen and 10% of glucose from the arterial blood (15). Although there can be significant regional and temporal differences, these values provide a critical baseline and reference point for the understanding and interpretation of measured MD variables.

Glucose is initially transported from the ECF into the cellular cytoplasm where it is metabolized to pyruvate in a process that yields two molecules of adenosine triphosphate (ATP) for each molecule of glucose. Under aerobic conditions, the majority of pyruvate enters the tricarboxylic acid cycle within the mitochondria where subsequent metabolism, through electron complex mediated reduction of oxygen, yields another 36 molecules of ATP (Figure 12.4) (15). This highly efficient aerobic conversion of glucose to water and carbon dioxide is responsible for over 95% of cerebral energy requirements under normal circumstances. In hypoxic conditions, pyruvate is anaerobically converted to lactate in a process which yields only two molecules of ATP.

Lactate can also be formed under aerobic conditions in the central nervous system (CNS). *In vivo* and *in vitro* studies confirm that the physiological stimulation of a given brain region triggers a rapid activation of glycogenolysis and glycolysis, which in turn results in synthesis and release of lactate (16). Mitochondrial failure, which is common after brain injury, also results in higher lactate concentrations because of the inability of cells to utilize delivered oxygen and glucose. There is considerable evidence that synaptic activity *in vitro* can be maintained when lactate is the only metabolic substrate (17). Changes in brain ECF lactate and pyruvate levels can be

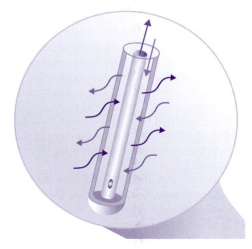

Fig. 12.2 Schematic showing the bi-directional diffusion of molecules across a microdialysis membrane.
With courtesy from M Dialysis AB, Stockholm, Sweden.

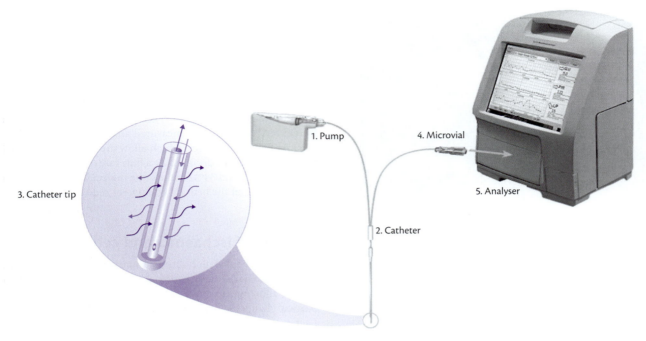

Fig. 12.3 Components of a clinical microdialysis system.
1. Microdialysis pump
2. Microdialysis catheter
3. Microdialysis catheter tip showing exchange of molecules across the dialysis membrane
4. Microvial for collection of the microdialysate
5. Bedside analyser.
With courtesy from M Dialysis AB, Stockholm, Sweden.

measured *in vivo* by MD which, in combination with glucose concentration, forms the basis by which the metabolic analysis using MD is accomplished.

Glucose and the LPR are the most clinically useful MD markers.

Glucose

Although glucose is the main energy source for the brain, there are no significant cerebral glucose stores so a continued supply is essential in order to sustain normal metabolic activity. MD provides a means by which the balance between cerebral glucose delivery and utilization can be determined. A low brain ECF glucose concentration can be a reflection of decreased cerebral glucose delivery because of hypoperfusion or systemic hypoglycaemia, or cerebral hyperglycolysis secondary to hypoxia/ischaemia and anaerobic metabolism (14). It is therefore important to interpret cerebral MD glucose concentration within the context of systemic blood glucose levels and other monitored intracranial variables including $PtiO_2$.

Lactate:pyruvate ratio

Although lactate was previously believed to be a metabolically inactive waste product of anaerobic metabolism, there is increasing evidence that it is a key intermediary in normal metabolic pathways. Lactate fuels energy-requiring processes and, in the context of cerebral metabolic function whereby astrocytes are a major source of lactate production in response to glutamate released by neurons, lactate may become a preferred fuel for neurons, especially in traumatic or hypoxic brain injury (18). It seems likely that brain tissue can also utilize lactate produced elsewhere in the body and this pathway may be preferentially selected in

instances where there is an increased systemic lactate source (19). Increased arterial lactate levels have been shown to be associated with increased cerebral lactate uptake and elevated brain lactate concentration in the presence of reductions in brain glucose uptake and brain tissue glucose concentrations (20,21). However, it remains unclear whether arterial lactate is the driving force for such increased cerebral lactate levels or whether it is reduced uptake of glucose that drives the increased cerebral lactate levels.

For the reasons just described, the LPR rather than lactate level alone is usually utilized clinically. Based on the near equilibrium between the ratios of lactate:pyruvate and cytosolic free $NADH:NAD^+$, cytosolic free NADH is an important trigger or sensor of regional cerebral blood flow. The re-oxidation of NADH to NAD^+ is a step of vital importance for brain cells, especially in the activated state, because, without continuing replenishment of NAD^+, glycolysis cannot proceed and ATP cannot be generated (22). The increase in blood flow triggered by NADH, and indicated by the LPR, whilst indicative of the presence of glycolysis and anaerobic metabolism, is not always indicative of increased cerebral metabolism (23).

Two distinct types of elevated LPR, related to the mechanism of the physiological perturbations, are described (24). Type 1 changes are associated with reduced ECF pyruvate and elevated lactate concentrations secondary to classic ischaemia, whereas type 2 is characterized by diminished pyruvate concentration in the absence of tissue hypoxia (25). This 'non-ischaemic' type 2 elevation in LPR may reflect impairment of the glycolytic pathway in the presence of adequate (or reduced) glucose supply because of mitochondrial

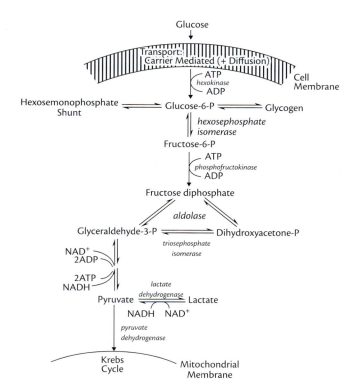

Fig. 12.4 Overview of glucose metabolism. Glucose that enters the cell is converted into pyruvate through glycolysis. Pyruvate is converted either to acetyl-CoA through pyruvate dehydrogenase and enters the citric acid cycle, or to lactate through lactate dehydrogenase. The latter is favoured when pyruvate cannot be converted to acetyl-CoA for entry into the citric acid cycle, as is the case during hypoxic/ischaemic conditions.

ADP, adenosine diphosphate; ATP, adenosine triphosphate; glucose-6-P, glucose-6-phosphate; fructose-6-P, fructose-6-phosphate; glyceraldehyde-3-P, glyceraldehyde-3-phosphate; dihydroxyacetone-P, dihydroxyacetone phosphate; NADH/NAD+, nicotinamide adenine dinucleotide.

Reproduced from Springer, *Neurocritical Care*, 2011, 15, pp. 609–622, 'Potential non-hypoxic/ischemic causes of increased cerebral interstitial fluid lactate/pyruvate ratio: a review of available literature', Larach DB *et al.*, Neurocritical Care Society. With kind permission from Springer Science and Business Media.

dysfunction (4,26), or inadequate availability or entry of glucose into this pathway possibly because of shunting of glucose to competing metabolic pathways such as the pentose phosphate pathway (27). Decreased metabolic flux through the glycolytic pathway poses a bioenergetic threat to the brain and, regardless of the mechanism, decreased brain ECF glucose concentration is a poor prognostic indicator after traumatic brain injury (TBI) (3). Because lactate and pyruvate have very similar molecular weights, the LPR is independent of relative recovery *in vivo* (28).

The normal LPR is around 20 and levels higher than 25 are often considered to be an early sign of metabolic abnormalities (7). However, a tissue hypoxic threshold for an abnormal LPR has not been clearly established (29), and different thresholds for abnormality, ranging from 20 to 40, are applied in clinical studies by different research groups.

It should be noted that elevated lactate levels are seen in the context of ischaemia only if there is sufficient glucose substrate (26) and, for this reason, the lactate/glucose ratio is occasionally assessed. However, because of the potential role of lactate in normal cerebral metabolism, elevation of the lactate:glucose ratio might

also occur because of functional adaptation processes after brain injury. This underscores the importance of interpreting the LPR in a clinical context and, as feasible, in association with other brain monitoring variables such as brain tissue PO$_2$.

Cellular tissue damage

Failure of cellular metabolism allows intracellular influx of calcium, induction of phospholipases, and subsequent enzymatic degradation of cell membrane triglycerides. This results in release of free fatty acids and glycerol into the brain ECF making glycerol a reliable marker of cell death and possibly also a marker of tissue hypoxia and cellular energy failure (30). However, glycerol levels increase relatively slowly after cellular energy failure and remain elevated after metabolism is restored, making it a somewhat unresponsive biomarker to guide acute dynamic management of brain injury (31,32).

Alterations in systemic glycerol concentration can impact on MD glycerol concentration, for example, as a result of peripheral catecholamine-induced lipolysis or because of systemic administration of glycerol containing substances commonly found in medication preparations (5). Simultaneous measurement of systemic glycerol levels from a reference MD catheter allows improved interpretation of brain ECF glycerol levels but this is rarely performed in the clinical setting.

Neurotransmitters

L-glutamate is a non-essential amino acid with multiple roles in the CNS, including involvement in a variety of cellular metabolic pathways and mediation of normal synaptic activity. Glutamate is the primary excitatory neurotransmitter with more than 90% of excitatory synapses utilizing glutamate. Brain ischaemia may lead to cellular depolarization and release of glutamate, aspartate, and other excitatory amino acids (EAAs), and also to reduced glutamate reuptake leading to increased ECF glutamate concentration (33). Release of EAAs is a proposed mechanism of secondary brain injury and animal studies have demonstrated that brain ECF glutamate concentration is significantly elevated in global cerebral ischaemia (34). MD monitoring of glutamate and other EAA levels may have clinical utility as a marker of brain injury and cerebral energy failure.

Novel analytes

Novel analytes, including *N*-acetylaspartate (NAA), nitric oxide (NO) metabolites, and cytokines have recently received increased attention. NAA is a neuronal marker present in high concentration in the CNS and its depletion is a marker of neuronal damage and death. Belli and colleagues used cerebral MD to investigate 19 patients with TBI and demonstrated that NAA concentrations were 34% lower in non-survivors compared to survivors (35). A non-recoverable fall in NAA was observed in non-survivors beyond day 4, with a concomitant rise in LPR and glycerol suggesting that bioenergetic failure contributed to the poor outcome.

Nitrate and nitrite (NOx) are the oxidative metabolites of NO, a key modulator of vascular tone, neuronal communication, and inflammation. NO may be beneficial in acute brain injury via its role in the maintenance of cerebrovascular reactivity but, at higher concentrations such as those seen in inflammation, it can be detrimental. Low NOx concentrations have been correlated with decreased cerebral blood flow, diminished cerebrovascular reactivity, and poor outcome after TBI and subarachnoid haemorrhage

(SAH) (36–38). Although instrumentation for NOx measurement is available it is not widely used in neurocritical care.

There is increasing interest in the role of inflammatory mediators such as cytokines in brain injury pathophysiology. The temporal profile of 42 cytokines has been analysed following TBI with varying responses identified for individual cytokines (39). Tumour necrosis factor, interleukin (IL) 7, and IL-8 peaked during the first day after injury, IL-1 receptor antagonist (IL-1ra), and IL-6 peaked on day two, and many other mediators later. There was a large variation in cytokine response between different patients with similar severity and patterns of brain injury and also marked heterogeneity between brain and systemic cytokine concentrations, arguing for measurement of brain levels with MD. A relatively large dialysate volume is needed for cytokine analysis so the temporal resolution is limited with current clinical MD equipment. Moreover, substantial inter- and intraindividual variability between cytokine values has been reported (40).

Clinical applications of microdialysis

The MD technique is performed clinically using a commercially available catheter inserted into brain parenchyma with the catheter tip positioned approximately 2 cm deep in the region of interest. The catheter can be implanted through a cranial access device or at the time of surgery. The volume of tissue interrogated by a MD catheter is limited to a few cubic millimetres around its tip which means that only local tissue biochemistry is monitored. It is therefore crucial that the catheter tip is accurately placed in the tissue of interest (41), and commercially available catheters have an incorporated gold tip visible on computed tomography so that the correct location can be verified by a post-insertion scan.

There remains debate about whether the catheter should be located in areas of normal-appearing brain or in tissue regarded as being 'at risk,' but there is agreement that it should not be placed in contusional tissue (13). Engstrom and colleagues investigated placement of MD catheters in 'at-risk' and normal appearing brain and found a difference in glucose, lactate, LPR, glutamate, and glycerol levels between the two catheter locations (41). It has been suggested that locating the probe in normal brain evaluates global cerebral metabolic status whereas probes in pericontusional tissue provide information on the microenvironment of potentially salvageable tissue (42). A consensus statement published by a group of clinical MD experts in 2015 recommends strongly that catheters should be placed in 'at-risk' tissue (13). In TBI this is the area of tissue adjacent to a focal lesion (pericontusional area) and in SAH the parent vascular territory, that is, the area most at risk from vasospasm. After diffuse axonal injury, placement in the right frontal lobe is recommended.

Insertion of the MD catheter causes some disruption of local tissue, including mild astrogliosis, macrophage infiltration, and microhaemorrhages along the catheter tract (43). Whilst these have no clinical effect impact, they can result in unreliable MD values early after catheter placement, and a 'run-in' period of around 1 hour should be allowed. Since MD is an invasive technique there is the possibility of complications such as haemorrhage and infection. No major procedure-related complications have been reported despite the widespread use of MD in many centres worldwide over two decades, but the risk of their development should always be borne in mind (5).

Table 12.1 Normal values of cerebral microdialysis analytes

Microdialysate concentration	Normal value	Normal value
Glucose (mmol/L)	1.7 (0.9)	2.1 (0.2)
Lactose (mmol/L)	2.9 (0.9)	3.1 (0.3)
Pyruvate (µmol/L)	166 (47)	151 (12)
Lactate:pyruvate ratio	23 (4)	19 (2)
Glyceral (µmol/L)	82 (44)	82 (12)
Glutamate (µmol/L)	16 (16)	14.0 (3.3)

Baseline values of commonly measured variables have been estimated during wakefulness using MD catheters inserted into normal posterior frontal cerebral cortex in nine patients undergoing neurosurgery (44), and in patients with SAH (45). These have been used to define 'normal' values against which pathophysiological states can be evaluated (Table 12.1), although it is important to interpret MD data in terms of trends as opposed to absolute values. The pathophysiological changes identified by commonly measured variables are shown in Table 12.2.

Cerebral MD is potentially useful in identifying cerebral ischaemia and metabolic distress in many different clinical scenarios including TBI, SAH, ischaemic stroke, brain tumours, epilepsy, and during neurosurgery (5), but is usually reserved for patients with significant or severe brain injury. However, evidence of improved outcomes of cerebral MD-guided therapy in any clinical entity is lacking.

Traumatic brain injury

The vast majority of clinical data to date have been obtained from studies in patients with severe TBI. This is a devastating condition characterized by primary brain damage related to the initial impact and subsequent, secondary, injury mediated by complex

Table 12.2 Microdialysis biomarkers and injury patterns

MD variable	Secondary injury process	Comments
Low glucose	Hypoxia/ischaemia Reduce cerebral glucose supply Cerebral hyperglycolysis	Should be interpreted in association with serum glucose concentration
Increased lactate: pyruvate ratio	Hypoxia/ischaemia Reduction in cellular redox state Reduced cerebral glucose supply Mitochondrial dysfunction	Most reliable biomarker of ischaemia Independent of catheter recovery Tissue hypoxic threshold for raised LPR not established
Increased glycerol	Hypoxia/ischaemia Cell membrane degradation	Increased glycerol may also occur because of spill over from systemic glycerol or from the formation of glycerol from glucose
Increased glytamate	Hypoxia/ischaemia Excitotoxicity	Wide variability in glutamate levels within and between patients

biochemical and inflammatory cascades that results in brain ischaemia and a non-ischaemic metabolic crisis (see Chapter 17) (26). Although the pathophysiology of severe TBI is complex, two factors are of crucial importance—reduction of substrate delivery below critical thresholds and the inability of brain cells to utilize delivered oxygen and glucose because of failing cellular metabolism. Metabolic monitoring of the injured brain reveals the frequency, duration, and adverse effects of the widespread metabolic dysfunction that occurs after TBI, and also those brain regions at risk of secondary injury and neuronal loss (5,46,47).

Typical changes in biomarkers

Reductions in brain ECF glucose and elevation of the LPR have been associated with intracranial hypertension, severe tissue hypoxia/ischaemia, and poor outcome after severe TBI. In one study using PtiO$_2$ and cerebral MD monitoring, cerebral glucose decreased whereas lactate, LPR, and glutamate increased when PtiO$_2$ fell below 1.3 kPa (10 mmHg) (4).

Regional hyperglycolysis as well as critical supply of glucose and oxygen can lead to cerebral hypoglycaemia after TBI (26). Whatever the underlying cause, brain ECF glucose concentration consistently less than 0.66 mmol/L in the first 50 hours post injury is associated with poor outcome (48). There are no data confirming whether interventions targeted to increase brain glucose influence outcome, although there are data suggesting that abnormally elevated glucose can be deleterious.

Correlation between elevated LPR and clinical markers of severe brain injury were identified in early clinical studies (49,50), and more recently with outcome (47). Elevations in LPR may precede a rise in ICP, thereby providing early warning of brain energy crisis and potentially extending the window for therapeutic intervention before irreversible tissue damage has occurred (51). A persistently elevated LPR may be predictive of subsequent tissue atrophy (52) and, given that the LPR often remains elevated for a considerable period of time after TBI, the window of opportunity for neuroprotection might be longer than previously thought.

Brain ECF glycerol concentration is typically elevated in the first 24 hours after TBI and declines during the ensuing 72 hours (30). Secondary rises in glycerol are associated with ongoing ischaemic events including intracranial hypertension, low cerebral perfusion pressure (CPP), low PtiO$_2$, and seizures. However, most studies identify no correlation between glycerol levels and outcome after TBI so the clinical role of monitoring brain ECF glycerol concentration remains uncertain.

Wide variations in the concentration of the EAAs have been detected after TBI, with extremely high levels being associated with secondary ischaemia (53).

Intracranial and cerebral perfusion pressure

Timofeev and colleagues prospectively collected observational multimodal neuromonitoring data in 97 patients with severe TBI and identified a significant and independent relationship between perilesional tissue biochemistry and abnormalities in other monitored variables (47). LPR increased in response to a decrease in PtiO$_2$ and CPP, and increase in ICP. The relationship between CPP and tissue biochemistry was also dependent on the state of autoregulation as assessed by the pressure reactivity index (PRx). In agreement with previous studies (54), significantly higher levels of cerebral lactate, glycerol, LPR, and lactate:glucose ratio were identified in perilesional tissue compared to normal brain and

these differences remained significant after adjustment for the influences of other important physiological parameters, namely ICP, CPP, PtiO$_2$, and PRx, suggesting that they may reflect inherent tissue properties related to the initial injury. However, deranged tissue chemistry within individuals, especially in perilesional tissue, occurred even when pre-defined physiological targets were met. Whereas the baseline differences between perilesional and normal brain tissue can reflect the injury type and severity, variability in response to physiological challenges provides more important feedback to guide treatment, supporting the use of cerebral MD as a part of a multimodal monitoring approach to guide individualized therapy after TBI.

In a study in which more than 7350 hourly samples of commonly measured MD variables were obtained in 90 patients with severe TBI, Nelson and colleagues performed extensive statistical analysis and computer-based linear and non-linear pattern recognition methods to explore the relationship between ICP, CPP, and MD biomarkers (6). The highly perturbed metabolism, likely to predominately represent long-term metabolic patterns, was only weakly correlated with ICP and CPP suggesting that disturbances other than pressure and/or flow have a dominant influence on tissue biochemistry after TBI. This is a consistent finding across studies (54,55), many of which have identified little correlation between elevated LPR and ICP and CPP, again suggesting non-ischaemic causes for monitored increases in LPR (56). Using an ICP pulse morphological analysis algorithm (57) one group found no correlation between MD-derived LPR and either vasoconstriction or vasodilation identified by monophasic morphologic ICP pulse changes (58).

Taken together these data strongly suggest non-vascular mediated metabolic derangements in some patients after TBI, changes which can only be identified at the bedside by cerebral MD monitoring. Despite this, a relationship between improved clinical outcome and treatment guided by biochemical monitoring data has not yet been demonstrated.

Metabolic crisis

Metabolic crisis after TBI is characterized by a reduction in oxidative metabolism, increased glucose consumption, and a resultant imbalance in the tissue redox state. Positron emission tomography (PET) is able to provide detailed information about cerebral metabolism after brain injury but such data are difficult to acquire in critically ill patients. Moreover, PET is only able to provide a metabolic 'snapshot' at a particular moment in time and therefore unable to quantify the duration and trends of metabolic derangements or their response to treatment (see Chapter 15). Cerebral MD on the other hand is able to capture this metabolic crisis, defined as a low glucose concentration and/or elevation in the LPR in biochemical terms, in real time (52,59). As noted earlier, a tissue metabolic crisis can occur in the presence or absence of cerebral ischaemia, although a prolonged crisis from whatever cause is associated with poor neurological outcome (26,59). Adequate haemodynamic resuscitation and control of ICP does not prevent a metabolic crisis in some patients, and this is a strong independent predictor of poor neurological outcome if it persists beyond 72 hours after the initial injury (60).

Inflammatory cytokines

Inflammatory mediators have extensive physiological and pathophysiological effects after TBI and are one of the numerous novel biomarkers that can be analysed using cerebral MD. Although individual cytokines have multiple effects, in general terms they are either pro- or anti-inflammatory with the eventual inflammatory state of the tissue depending on the complex interplay of multiple cytokines. Initial studies investigating cytokine responses after brain injury were performed in serum and cerebrospinal fluid but more recently direct monitoring of the cytokine response has been undertaken in animals and humans using cerebral MD (61–64). In a study by Hillman and colleagues, paired MD catheters with high cut-off (100 kDa) membranes were inserted into 14 comatose patients with SAH or TBI (62). Macroscopic tissue injury was strongly linked to IL-6 but not IL-1β activation, and IL-6 release was stimulated by local ischaemia. Hutchinson and colleagues studied 15 patients with severe TBI and found no significant relationship between IL-1α and -β, IL-1ra, and energy-related molecules, but a significant correlation between reductions in ICP and increases in IL-1β and IL-1α (40). Temporal changes in cytokines have also been demonstrated after brain injury. In one study, the highest concentrations in IL-1β, IL-6, and IL-8 occurred during the first 24 hours after injury following which there was a gradual decline, although, in contrast, the average concentration of IL-10 did not vary over time (65). In this study there was also substantial variation in the correlation between cytokine concentration and ICP and $PtiO_2$, and no difference in cytokine concentrations in patients with and without radiographic evidence of cerebral oedema.

Age has been found to play an important role in tissue biochemical and inflammatory responses to brain injury. Mellagard and colleagues evaluated standard MD variables and eight cytokines (IL-1β, IL-6, IL-10, IL-8, MIP-1β, RANTES, FGF2, and VEGF), and found that patients of 65 years of age or older had significantly higher glycerol and glutamate concentrations and a higher LPR compared to younger patients (66). However, age dependency of the cytokine responses varied markedly. There were no age differences in the response of IL-1b, IL-10, and IL-8, whereas there were age differences for MIP-1b, RANTES, VEGF, and IL-6 responses but no clear correlation with increasing age. There are many unresolved methodological issues with the use of MD to study the cytokine response after TBI, but this study demonstrates that it is feasible to recover cytokines over a prolonged period using MD.

Outcome

A large observational study of 223 patients suggested that brain ECF biochemical markers are independently associated with 6-month outcome after severe TBI (47). During the initial 72 hours of monitoring, median glycerol levels were higher in patients who died and LPR and lactate levels lower in those with a favourable outcome. Brain ECF glucose and LPR were significant independent positive predictors of mortality, whereas pyruvate was an independent negative predictor. Averaged over the total monitoring period, glutamate and LPR were significantly higher in patients who died.

Patterns of change in MD-derived biochemical variables may also offer prognostic information. Chamoun and colleagues identified two patterns of glutamate response in 165 patients with severe TBI (67). Those in whom glutamate normalized over time (i.e. started low and remained low or started high and decreased over time) had lower mortality and better outcome compared to those in whom glutamate increased over time or started high and remained high. Several studies have also attempted to identify critical MD substrate levels that predict poor outcome. In a small study of 34 patients, all those with a favourable outcome after severe TBI had a LPR lower than 37 and glycerol concentration less than 72 mmol/L (68).

Subarachnoid haemorrhage

Abnormalities in brain tissue biochemistry are common early after SAH, with the degree of disturbance reflecting the severity of the initial haemorrhage (69). Significantly elevated levels of lactate and pyruvate reflect the hypermetabolic state of the injured brain and are associated with global oedema on the initial CT scan (70). High ICP is associated with a severely deranged cerebral metabolism and poor outcome after SAH (71). Moreover, intracranial hypertension is associated with intense activation of cerebral and systemic inflammation and is likely underestimated as a pro-inflammatory trigger in the pathogenesis of complications after SAH (72). Future therapies targeting anti-inflammatory responses in plasma may help to reduce the inflammatory cascade responsible for development of intracranial hypertension. Cerebral oedema after SAH is possibly related to glutamate-mediated excitotoxicity, and large increases in glutamate, aspartate, and GABA concentration have been identified early after ictus and associated with cerebral ischaemia (73). The increases in glutamate may lead to worsened neuronal injury and poor outcome (69). Some authors have reported a decrease in glutamate levels during targeted temperature management after SAH and suggested that this represents the mechanism of the potential neuroprotective effects of hypothermia (74).

Cerebral ECF lactate levels are also elevated in the early phase (1–5 days) after SAH, but this may be indicative of hyperglycolysis rather than brain hypoxia (75). Low brain ECF glucose and high LPR are associated with a poor outcome after SAH (76,77).

The initial biochemical disturbances after SAH often settle and secondary elevations in the LPR, lactate, and glutamate concentrations, and reductions in glucose, between days 5 and 10 after the ictus are likely related to vasospasm-induced cerebral ischaemia (78). In one study, patients who developed a delayed ischaemic neurological deficit had significantly higher lactate, glutamate and LPR compared with those who remained asymptomatic (45). A recent international multi-disciplinary consensus conference on the critical care management of SAH identified a positive tendency for cerebral MD to predict delayed cerebral ischaemia (DCI) and outcome after SAH (79).

The metabolic changes associated with cerebral ischaemia can be detected by cerebral MD before the onset of symptomatic vasospasm in up to 83% of patients (80,81). In one study, an ischaemic pattern of biochemical changes preceded the onset of clinical symptoms in all 17 patients who developed DCI (82). The mean delay from the peak in the LPR to the occurrence of symptoms was 23 hours (range 4–50 hours), and 11 hours from the identification of the ischaemic metabolic pattern to presentation of a clinical deficit. Ischaemia-related biochemical abnormalities can be reversed following the institution of standard treatments for vasospasm suggesting that brain tissue biochemistry might be a target for treatment after SAH, although this has not been tested in clinical outcome studies.

On the other hand, several studies have failed to show a relationship between some MD biomarkers and ischaemia after SAH. Sakowitz and colleagues found that cerebral energy metabolism and extracellular NOx concentrations were not correlated with DCI (83). Moreover, MD measured endothelin-1, a substance which is implicated in the development of cerebral vasospasm, does not correlate with the development of clinical symptoms of vasospasm (80).

Metabolic monitoring after SAH may identify patients who might benefit from interventions such as endovascular treatment of vasospasm or decompressive craniectomy for intracranial hypertension by the early detection of those at risk (42). Importantly, LPR and PtiO₂ may be abnormal in many instances when ICP is normal, and biochemical disturbances may precede increases in ICP after SAH, suggesting that they may be more sensitive at detecting cerebral compromise than ICP alone (84).

Although numerous MD biomarkers have been reported to have variable correlations with DCI and mortality after SAH, most studies are observational with small sample sizes and varying methodology (79). Thus, although cerebral MD can identify cerebral ischaemia in the setting of SAH its clinical utility has still not been clearly elucidated.

Other clinical conditions

Cerebral MD has also been utilized, but to a lesser extent than after TBI and SAH, in a variety of other neurological disorders in which cerebral ischaemia is key part of the pathophysiological processes. These include ischaemic stroke, brain tumours, and during vascular neurosurgery. Changes in the concentration of glucose, lactate, pyruvate, and glutamate have been associated with CSF drainage, brain retraction, and temporary vessel clipping during craniotomy for aneurysm surgery (85). Cerebral MD has also been used in conjunction with electroencephalography (EEG) monitoring to identify the biochemical changes associated with seizure activity, but only in small studies or case series. Large increases in ECF glutamate concentration were associated with seizure activity in a study of four patients undergoing hippocampal EEG and microdialysis monitoring during temporal lobe epilepsy surgery (86).

Application of proteomics to cerebral MD is an exciting field of research that has potential to provide new insights into the pathophysiology of brain injury. Metabolic distress after TBI has been associated with a differential proteome suggestive of cellular destruction (59), and, in a study investigating a proteome-wide screening after SAH, several isoforms of glyceraldehyde-3-phosphate dehydrogenase were almost twofold higher in patients who developed symptomatic vasospasm whereas heat-shock cognate 71 kDa proteins isoforms were decreased by 50% (81). These changes were identified on average 3.8 days before the onset of clinical symptoms.

Many investigators are exploring the clinical use of cerebral MD beyond its neuromonitoring capabilities. MD offers the potential for quantifiable assays of multiple drugs including anticonvulsants and neuroprotectants, and holds promise for more accurate and effective CNS drug dose determination (87). It allows evaluation of the effects of new drugs at clinically relevant target sites in the brain and measures the pharmacologically active free level of a drug, thereby providing an excellent platform for drug delivery studies.

Conclusion

An understanding of brain tissue biochemistry is a complex but important area of experimental and clinical neuroscience. Cerebral MD provides substantial and novel information about the biochemistry of the acutely injured brain at the bedside. The 'routine' clinical application of MD is already a standard part of multimodal monitoring in many technically advanced neurocritical care units, but remains a research tool in others.

Mechanistic insights derived from MD studies have already translated into clinical applications and it is likely that future studies will provide further mechanistic information as well as identify therapeutic targets. Although there are many exciting possibilities for the application of cerebral MD, there are currently insufficient data to recommend a clinical role beyond monitoring in TBI and SAH. The interpretation and application of data from other clinical scenarios represents the next wave of the clinical and basic science investigation of the MD technique. There is still much to be learned about the biochemistry of different types of neurological injury, the impact of therapeutics and neuroprotectants, and ultimately about the functional outcome of patients. Well-organized multicentre studies are required to identify new MD biomarkers and determine thresholds values that should prompt clinical intervention.

References

1. Hillered L, Persson L, Ponten U, Ungerstedt U. Neurometabolic monitoring of the ischaemic human brain using microdialysis. *Acta Neurochir (Wien)*. 1990;102:91–7.
2. Persson L, Hillered L. Chemical monitoring of neurosurgical intensive care patients using intracerebral microdialysis. *J Neurosurg*. 1992;76:72–80.
3. Goodman JC, Robertson CS. Microdialysis: is it ready for prime time? *Curr Opin Crit Care*. 2009;15:110–17.
4. Hlatky R, Valadka AB, Goodman JC, Contant CF, Robertson CS. Patterns of energy substrates during ischemia measured in the brain by microdialysis. *J Neurotrauma*. 2004;21:894–906.
5. Hillered L, Vespa PM, Hovda DA. Translational neurochemical research in acute human brain injury: the current status and potential future for cerebral microdialysis. *J Neurotrauma*. 2005;22:3–41.
6. Nelson DW, Thornquist B, MacCallum RM, Nystrom H, Holst A, Rudehill A, *et al.* Analyses of cerebral microdialysis in patients with traumatic brain injury: relations to intracranial pressure, cerebral perfusion pressure and catheter placement. *BMC Med*. 2011;9:21.
7. Tisdall MM, Smith M. Cerebral microdialysis: research technique or clinical tool. *Br J Anaesth*. 2006;97:18–25.
8. Chefer VI, Thompson AC, Zapata A, Shippenberg TS. Overview of brain microdialysis. *Curr Protoc Neurosci*. 2009;Chapter 7:Unit7.
9. Ungerstedt U, Rostami E. Microdialysis in neurointensive care. *Curr Pharm Des*. 2004;10:2145–52.
10. Peerdeman SM, Girbes AR, Vandertop WP. Cerebral microdialysis as a new tool for neurometabolic monitoring. *Intensive Care Med*. 2000;26:662–9.
11. Bungay PM, Morrison PF, Dedrick RL. Steady-state theory for quantitative microdialysis of solutes and water in vivo and in vitro. *Life Sci*. 1990;46:105–19.
12. Hutchinson PJ, O'Connell MT, Al-Rawi PG, Maskell LB, Kett-White R, Gupta AK, *et al.* Clinical cerebral microdialysis: a methodological study. *J Neurosurg*. 2000;93:37–43.
13. Hutchinson PJ, Jalloh I, Helmy A, Carpenter KL, Rostami E, Bellander BM, *et al.* Consensus statement from the 2014 international microdialysis forum. *Intensive Care Med*. 2015;41:1517–28.
14. Ghosh A, Smith M. Brain tissue biochemistry. In Matta B, Menon D, Smith M (eds) *Core Topics in Neuroanaesthesia and Neurocritical Care*. Cambridge: Cambridge University Press; 2010:85–100.
15. Magistretti PJ. Neuroscience. Low-cost travel in neurons. *Science* 2009;325:1349–51.
16. Okada Y, Lipton P. *Glucose, Oxidative Energy Metabolism and Neural Function in Brain Slices—Glycolysis plays a key role*. New York: Springer Science; 2014.
17. Roberts E. *Handbook of the Support of Energy Metabolism in the Central Nervous System with Substrates other than Glucose*. New York: Springer Science; 2007.

18. Berthet C, Lei H, Thevenet J, Gruetter R, Magistretti PJ, Hirt L. Neuroprotective role of lactate after cerebral ischemia. *J Cereb Blood Flow Metab.* 2009;29:1780–9.

19. Bouzat P, Oddo M. Lactate and the injured brain: friend or foe? *Curr Opin Crit Care.* 2014;20:133–40.

20. Meierhans R, Brandi G, Fasshauer M, Sommerfeld J, Schupbach R, Bechir M, et al. Arterial lactate above 2 mM is associated with increased brain lactate and decreased brain glucose in patients with severe traumatic brain injury. *Minerva Anestesiol.* 2012;78:185–93.

21. Nemoto EM, Hoff JT, Severinghaus JW. Lactate uptake and metabolism by brain during hyperlactatemia and hypoglycemia. *Stroke.* 1974;5:48–53.

22. Vlassenko AG, Rundle MM, Raichle ME, Mintun MA. Regulation of blood flow in activated human brain by cytosolic NADH/NAD+ ratio. *Proc Natl Acad Sci U S A.* 2006;103:1964–9.

23. Mintun MA, Vlassenko AG, Rundle MM, Raichle ME. Increased lactate/pyruvate ratio augments blood flow in physiologically activated human brain. *Proc Natl Acad Sci U S A.* 2004;101:659–64.

24. Vespa PM. The implications of cerebral ischemia and metabolic dysfunction for treatment strategies in neurointensive care. *Curr Opin Crit Care.* 2006;12:119–23.

25. Hillered L, Persson L, Nilsson P, Ronne-Engstrom E, Enblad P. Continuous monitoring of cerebral metabolism in traumatic brain injury: a focus on cerebral microdialysis. *Curr Opin Crit Care.* 2006;12:112–18.

26. Vespa P, Bergsneider M, Hattori N, Wu HM, Huang SC, Martin NA, et al. Metabolic crisis without brain ischemia is common after traumatic brain injury: a combined microdialysis and positron emission tomography study. *J Cereb Blood Flow Metab.* 2005;25:763–74.

27. Dusick JR, Glenn TC, Lee WN, Vespa PM, Kelly DF, Lee SM, et al. Increased pentose phosphate pathway flux after clinical traumatic brain injury: a [1,2-13C2]glucose labeling study in humans. *J Cereb Blood Flow Metab.* 2007;27:1593–602.

28. Persson L, Valtysson J, Enblad P, Warme PE, Cesarini K, Lewen A, et al. Neurochemical monitoring using intracerebral microdialysis in patients with subarachnoid hemorrhage. *J Neurosurg.* 1996;84:606–16.

29. Johnston AJ, Steiner LA, Coles JP, Chatfield DA, Fryer TD, Smielewski P, et al. Effect of cerebral perfusion pressure augmentation on regional oxygenation and metabolism after head injury. *Crit Care Med.* 2005;33:189–95.

30. Clausen T, Alves OL, Reinert M, Doppenberg E, Zauner A, Bullock R. Association between elevated brain tissue glycerol levels and poor outcome following severe traumatic brain injury. *J Neurosurg.* 2005;103:233–8.

31. Li AL, Zhi DS, Wang Q, Huang HL. Extracellular glycerol in patients with severe traumatic brain injury. *Chin J Traumatol.* 2008;11:84–8.

32. Merenda A, Gugliotta M, Holloway R, Levasseur JE, Alessandri B, Sun D, et al. Validation of brain extracellular glycerol as an indicator of cellular membrane damage due to free radical activity after traumatic brain injury. *J Neurotrauma;* 2008;25:527–37.

33. Magistretti PJ. Role of glutamate in neuron-glia metabolic coupling. *Am J Clin Nutr.* 2009;90:875S–880S.

34. Azarias G, Perreten H, Lengacher S, Poburko D, Demaurex N, Magistretti PJ, et al. Glutamate transport decreases mitochondrial pH and modulates oxidative metabolism in astrocytes. *J Neurosci.* 2011;31:3550–9.

35. Belli A, Sen J, Petzold A, Russo S, Kitchen N, Smith M, et al. Extracellular N-acetylaspartate depletion in traumatic brain injury. *J Neurochem.* 2006;96:861–9.

36. Goodman JC, Feng YQ, Valadka AB, Bryan RJ, Robertson CS. Measurement of the nitric oxide metabolites nitrate and nitrite in the human brain by microdialysis. *Acta Neurochir Suppl.* 2002;81:343–5.

37. Hlatky R, Goodman JC, Valadka AB, Robertson CS. Role of nitric oxide in cerebral blood flow abnormalities after traumatic brain injury. *J Cereb Blood Flow Metab.* 2003;23:582–8.

38. Reinert M, Zauner A, Khaldi A, Seiler R, Bullock R. Microdialysis nitric oxide levels and brain tissue oxygen tension in patients with subarachnoid hemorrhage. *Acta Neurochir Suppl.* 2001;77:155–7.

39. Helmy A, Carpenter KL, Menon DK, Pickard JD, Hutchinson PJ. The cytokine response to human traumatic brain injury: temporal profiles and evidence for cerebral parenchymal production. *J Cereb Blood Flow Metab.* 2011;31:658–70.

40. Hutchinson PJ, O'Connell MT, Rothwell NJ, Hopkins SJ, Nortje J, Carpenter KL, et al. Inflammation in human brain injury: intracerebral concentrations of IL-1alpha, IL-1beta, and their endogenous inhibitor IL-1ra. *J Neurotrauma.* 2007;24:1545–57.

41. Engstrom M, Polito A, Reinstrup P, Romner B, Ryding E, Ungerstedt U, et al. Intracerebral microdialysis in severe brain trauma: the importance of catheter location. *J Neurosurg.* 2005;102:460–9.

42. Kitagawa R, Yokobori S, Mazzeo AT, Bullock R. Microdialysis in the neurocritical care unit. *Neurosurg Clin N Am.* 2013;24:417–26.

43. Benveniste H, Diemer NH. Cellular reactions to implantation of a microdialysis tube in the rat hippocampus. *Acta Neuropathol.* 1987;74:234–8.

44. Reinstrup P, Stahl N, Mellergard P, Uski T, Ungerstedt U, Nordstrom CH. Intracerebral microdialysis in clinical practice: baseline values for chemical markers during wakefulness, anesthesia, and neurosurgery. *Neurosurgery.* 2000;47:701–9.

45. Schulz MK, Wang LP, Tange M, Bjerre P. Cerebral microdialysis monitoring: determination of normal and ischemic cerebral metabolisms in patients with aneurysmal subarachnoid hemorrhage. *J Neurosurg.* 2000;93:808–14.

46. Petzold A, Tisdall MM, Girbes AR, Martinian L, Thom M, Kitchen N, et al. In vivo monitoring of neuronal loss in traumatic brain injury: a microdialysis study. *Brain.* 2011;134:464–83.

47. Timofeev I, Carpenter KL, Nortje J, Al-Rawi PG, O'Connell MT, Czosnyka M, et al. Cerebral extracellular chemistry and outcome following traumatic brain injury: a microdialysis study of 223 patients. *Brain.* 2011;134:484–94.

48. Vespa PM, McArthur D, O'Phelan K, Glenn T, Etchepare M, Kelly D, et al. Persistently low extracellular glucose correlates with poor outcome 6 months after human traumatic brain injury despite a lack of increased lactate: a microdialysis study. *J Cereb Blood Flow Metab.* 2003;23:865–77.

49. Hutchinson PJ, Al-Rawi PG, O'Connell MT, Gupta AK, Maskell LB, Hutchinson DB, et al. On-line monitoring of substrate delivery and brain metabolism in head injury. *Acta Neurochir Suppl.* 2000;76:431–5.

50. Zauner A, Doppenberg EM, Woodward JJ, Choi SC, Young HF, Bullock R. Continuous monitoring of cerebral substrate delivery and clearance: initial experience in 24 patients with severe acute brain injuries. *Neurosurgery.* 1997;41:1082–91.

51. Belli A, Sen J, Petzold A, Russo S, Kitchen N, Smith M. Metabolic failure precedes intracranial pressure rises in traumatic brain injury: a microdialysis study. *Acta Neurochir (Wien).* 2008;150:461–9.

52. Marcoux J, McArthur DA, Miller C, Glenn TC, Villablanca P, Martin NA, et al. Persistent metabolic crisis as measured by elevated cerebral microdialysis lactate-pyruvate ratio predicts chronic frontal lobe brain atrophy after traumatic brain injury. *Crit Care Med.* 2008;36:2871–7.

53. Hutchinson PJ, Gupta AK, Fryer TF, Al-Rawi PG, Chatfield DA, Coles JP, et al. Correlation between cerebral blood flow, substrate delivery, and metabolism in head injury: a combined microdialysis and triple oxygen positron emission tomography study. *J Cereb Blood Flow Metab.* 2002;22:735–45.

54. Vespa PM, O'Phelan K, McArthur D, Miller C, Eliseo M, Hirt D, et al. Pericontusional brain tissue exhibits persistent elevation of lactate/pyruvate ratio independent of cerebral perfusion pressure. *Crit Care Med.* 2007;35:1153–60.

55. Nelson DW, Bellander BM, MacCallum RM, Axelsson J, Alm M, Wallin M, et al. Cerebral microdialysis of patients with severe traumatic brain injury exhibits highly individualistic patterns as visualized by cluster analysis with self-organizing maps. *Crit Care Med.* 2004;32:2428–36.

56. Larach DB, Kofke WA, Le RP. Potential non-hypoxic/ischemic causes of increased cerebral interstitial fluid lactate/pyruvate ratio: a review of available literature. *Neurocrit Care.* 2011;15:609–22.

57. Hu X, Xu P, Scalzo F, Vespa P, Bergsneider M. Morphological clustering and analysis of continuous intracranial pressure. *IEEE Trans Biomed Eng.* 2009;56:696–705.

58. Asgari S, Vespa P, Bergsneider M, Hu X. Lack of consistent intracranial pressure pulse morphological changes during episodes of microdialysis lactate/pyruvate ratio increase. *Physiol Meas.* 2011;32:1639–51.

59. Lakshmanan R, Loo JA, Drake T, Leblanc J, Ytterberg AJ, McArthur DL, et al. Metabolic crisis after traumatic brain injury is associated with a novel microdialysis proteome. *Neurocrit Care.* 2010;12:324–36.

60. Stein NR, McArthur DL, Etchepare M, Vespa PM. Early cerebral metabolic crisis after TBI influences outcome despite adequate hemodynamic resuscitation. *Neurocrit Care.* 2012;17:49–57.

61. Folkersma H, Breve JJ, Tilders FJ, Cherian L, Robertson CS, Vandertop WP. Cerebral microdialysis of interleukin (IL)-1beta and IL-6: extraction efficiency and production in the acute phase after severe traumatic brain injury in rats. *Acta Neurochir (Wien).* 2008;150:1277–84.

62. Hillman J, Aneman O, Persson M, Andersson C, Dabrosin C, Mellergard P. Variations in the response of interleukins in neurosurgical intensive care patients monitored using intracerebral microdialysis. *J Neurosurg.* 2007;106:820–5.

63. Hutchinson PJ, O'Connell MT, Rothwell NJ, Hopkins SJ, Nortje J, Carpenter KL, et al. Inflammation in human brain injury: intracerebral concentrations of IL-1alpha, IL-1beta, and their endogenous inhibitor IL-1ra. *J Neurotrauma.* 2007;24:1545–57.

64. Mellergard P, Aneman O, Sjogren F, Pettersson P, Hillman J. Changes in extracellular concentrations of some cytokines, chemokines, and neurotrophic factors after insertion of intracerebral microdialysis catheters in neurosurgical patients. *Neurosurgery.* 2008;62:151–7.

65. Perez-Barcena J, Ibanez J, Brell M, Crespi C, Frontera G, Llompart-Pou JA, et al. Lack of correlation among intracerebral cytokines, intracranial pressure, and brain tissue oxygenation in patients with traumatic brain injury and diffuse lesions. *Crit Care Med.* 2011;39:533–40.

66. Mellergard P, Sjogren F, Hillman J. The cerebral extracellular release of glycerol, glutamate, and FGF2 is increased in older patients following severe traumatic brain injury. *J Neurotrauma.* 2012;29:112–18.

67. Chamoun R, Suki D, Gopinath SP, Goodman JC, Robertson C. Role of extracellular glutamate measured by cerebral microdialysis in severe traumatic brain injury. *J Neurosurg.* 2010;113:564–70.

68. Paraforou T, Paterakis K, Fountas K, Paraforos G, Chovas A, Tasiou A, et al. Cerebral perfusion pressure, microdialysis biochemistry and clinical outcome in patients with traumatic brain injury. *BMC Res Notes.* 2011;4:540.

69. Staub F, Graf R, Gabel P, Kochling M, Klug N, Heiss WD. Multiple interstitial substances measured by microdialysis in patients with subarachnoid hemorrhage. *Neurosurgery.* 2000;47:1106–15.

70. Zetterling M, Hallberg L, Hillered L, Karlsson T, Enblad P, Ronne EE. Brain energy metabolism in patients with spontaneous subarachnoid hemorrhage and global cerebral edema. *Neurosurgery.* 2010;66:1102–10.

71. Nagel A, Graetz D, Schink T, Frieler K, Sakowitz O, Vajkoczy P, et al. Relevance of intracranial hypertension for cerebral metabolism in aneurysmal subarachnoid hemorrhage. *J Neurosurg.* 2009;111:94–101.

72. Graetz D, Nagel A, Schlenk F, Sakowitz O, Vajkoczy P, Sarrafzadeh A. High ICP as trigger of proinflammatory IL-6 cytokine activation in aneurysmal subarachnoid hemorrhage. *Neurol Res.* 2010;32:728–35.

73. Hutchinson PJ, O'Connell MT, Al-Rawi PG, Kett-White CR, Gupta AK, Maskell LB, et al. Increases in GABA concentrations during cerebral ischaemia: a microdialysis study of extracellular amino acids. *J Neurol Neurosurg Psychiatry.* 2002;72:99–105.

74. Maloney-Wilensky E, Le RP. The physiology behind direct brain oxygen monitors and practical aspects of their use. *Childs Nerv Syst.* 2010;26:419–30.

75. Oddo M, Levine JM, Frangos S, Maloney-Wilensky E, Carrera E, Daniel RT, et al. Brain lactate metabolism in humans with subarachnoid hemorrhage. *Stroke.* 2012;43:1418–21.

76. Cesarini KG, Enblad P, Ronne-Engstrom E, Marklund N, Salci K, Nilsson P, et al. Early cerebral hyperglycolysis after subarachnoid haemorrhage correlates with favourable outcome. *Acta Neurochir (Wien).* 2002;144:1121–31.

77. Kett-White R, Hutchinson PJ, Al-Rawi PG, Gupta AK, Pickard JD, Kirkpatrick PJ. Adverse cerebral events detected after subarachnoid hemorrhage using brain oxygen and microdialysis probes. *Neurosurgery.* 2002;50:1213–21.

78. Sarrafzadeh AS, Haux D, Ludemann L, Amthauer H, Plotkin M, Kuchler I, et al. Cerebral ischemia in aneurysmal subarachnoid hemorrhage: a correlative microdialysis-PET study. *Stroke.* 2004;35:638–43.

79. Hanggi D. Monitoring and detection of vasospasm II: EEG and invasive monitoring. *Neurocrit Care.* 2011;15:318–23.

80. Kastner S, Oertel MF, Scharbrodt W, Krause M, Boker DK, Deinsberger W. Endothelin-1 in plasma, cisternal CSF and microdialysate following aneurysmal SAH. *Acta Neurochir (Wien).* 2005;147:1271–9.

81. Maurer MH, Haux D, Sakowitz OW, Unterberg AW, Kuschinsky W. Identification of early markers for symptomatic vasospasm in human cerebral microdialysate after subarachnoid hemorrhage: preliminary results of a proteome-wide screening. *J Cereb Blood Flow Metab.* 2007;27:1675–83.

82. Skjoth-Rasmussen J, Schulz M, Kristensen SR, Bjerre P. Delayed neurological deficits detected by an ischemic pattern in the extracellular cerebral metabolites in patients with aneurysmal subarachnoid hemorrhage. *J Neurosurg.* 2004;100:8–15.

83. Sakowitz OW, Wolfrum S, Sarrafzadeh AS, Stover JF, Dreier JP, Dendorfer A, et al. Relation of cerebral energy metabolism and extracellular nitrite and nitrate concentrations in patients after aneurysmal subarachnoid hemorrhage. *J Cereb Blood Flow Metab.* 2001;21:1067–76.

84. Nagel A, Graetz D, Vajkoczy P, Sarrafzadeh AS. Decompressive craniectomy in aneurysmal subarachnoid hemorrhage: relation to cerebral perfusion pressure and metabolism. *Neurocrit Care.* 2009;11:384–94.

85. Xu W, Mellergard P, Ungerstedt U, Nordstrom CH. Local changes in cerebral energy metabolism due to brain retraction during routine neurosurgical procedures. *Acta Neurochir (Wien).* 2002;144:679–83.

86. Thomas PM, Phillips JP, Delanty N, O'Connor WT. Elevated extracellular levels of glutamate, aspartate and gamma-aminobutyric acid within the intraoperative, spontaneously epileptiform human hippocampus. *Epilepsy Res.* 2003;54:73–9.

87. Helmy A, Carpenter KL, Hutchinson PJ. Microdialysis in the human brain and its potential role in the development and clinical assessment of drugs. *Curr Med Chem.* 2007;14:1525–37.

CHAPTER 13

Multimodal brain monitoring and neuroinformatics

Hooman Kamel and J. Claude Hemphill III

Multimodal brain monitoring is the concurrent use of two or more monitoring modalities to assess aspects of brain physiology and function. In the neurocritical care unit (NCCU), multimodal monitoring has come to mean the use of multiple advanced neuromonitoring tools to evaluate cerebral haemodynamic and metabolic function in patients in whom clinical neurological assessment is limited because of sedation or depressed consciousness [1,2].

Interest in multimodal monitoring has evolved because of the recognition that reliance on a single parameter usually provides an incomplete picture of the injured brain. For example, knowledge of cerebral perfusion pressure (CPP), a key variable in the management of critically ill brain-injured patients, provides no information about the adequacy of brain perfusion in an individual patient. Initial attempts at multimodal monitoring have shown that this paradigm raises a host of questions including which set of monitors provides the optimal monitoring set-up, how clinically incongruent data from different monitors should be reconciled, and how the large volume of data generated in the context of multimodal brain monitoring is best acquired and analysed.

The central purpose of neurocritical care for patients with acute central nervous system catastrophes such as stroke and trauma is the prevention, identification, and treatment of secondary brain and spinal cord injury [3]. Mechanisms of secondary spinal cord injury are less well understood than those of the brain, and spinal monitoring methods are similarly more limited. Thus, the focus of this chapter is the monitoring of secondary brain injury which occurs when cells or brain tissue made vulnerable by a primary brain injury, such as ischaemic stroke, aneurysmal subarachnoid haemorrhage (SAH), or traumatic brain injury (TBI), progress to irreversible cell damage or death. While much of the primary brain injury, such as a diffuse axonal injury after TBI or hypoxic/ischaemic injury at the time of aneurysm rupture, may be irreversible, secondary brain injury represents a cascade of cellular injury that is potentially reversible or modifiable. Furthermore, secondary brain insults, such as hypotension, hypoglycaemia, hypoxaemia, fever, and seizures, may potentially further injure vulnerable brain cells and regions [4–6]. The term penumbra, although initially used to describe a zone of ischaemic tissue surrounding an area of infarction after acute ischaemic stroke, is now used more broadly to describe an area of vulnerable but potentially salvageable brain tissue after any brain injury type.

Neuromonitoring is the fundamental way in which secondary brain injury and insults are identified, with the purpose of guiding interventions to treat or reverse these abnormalities. An optimal neuromonitoring strategy should consider several different

factors, including the utilization of complementary methods to identify and confirm evolving tissue injury, use of continuous or high-frequency data, safety and ease of implementation, and ability to use the neuromonitoring information for therapeutic, not just prognostic, information. Many of the initial forays into multimodal brain monitoring have taken the relatively simplistic approach of understanding how new tools, such as brain tissue oxygen tension ($PtiO_2$) or cerebral microdialysis monitoring, relate to the more traditional measures of intracranial pressure (ICP) and CPP [7–10]. However, emphasis is now also being placed on the development of new indices that describe physiological phenomena of interest, such as cerebral autoregulation [11], and new methods of data analysis, such as dynamic Bayesian networks, that treat overall conditions as 'states' rather than examining single physiological variables at a time [12].

Individual neuromonitoring tools are described in detail in other chapters in this book. The aim of this chapter is to consider how neuromonitoring methods should be considered together in a unified monitoring strategy and how current and future informatics methods can, and should, be used to improve the process and potential of multimodal brain monitoring.

Modes of brain monitoring: getting to multimodal

Multimodal monitoring is already integral to the way in which neurocritical care is delivered. If a patient undergoes intermittent neurological examination and concurrent and frequent checks of systemic arterial blood pressure, then multimodal monitoring using a clinical and physiological monitor is being performed. In this way, an assumption of the intrinsic value of using multiple different monitoring methods has been present throughout modern critical care. There is indirect evidence that coordinated care with an emphasis on close neuromonitoring serves to improve outcomes in neurocritical care [13]. Whilst the fundamental value of multimodal monitoring is generally accepted, there are several unanswered questions:

1. What are the strengths and shortcomings of current monitors, individually or in combination?

2. What information is provided from new advanced neuromonitoring tools that augments or supplants traditional tools?

3. How can the voluminous data now accessible from neuromonitoring be more effectively understood and utilized by clinicians

to guide interventions targeted to prevent or minimize secondary brain injury?

Current neuromonitoring tools can be divided into three broad categories—clinical, physiological, and metabolic.

Clinical monitoring

While often not expressed as such, the clinical neurological examination is probably the most commonly used, and certainly the most familiar, neuromonitor. The clinical neurological examination forms the basis of the assessment of the severity of injury, and typically directs the initial diagnostic workup and treatment. Grading scales, such as the Glasgow Coma Scale (GCS) and the NIH Stroke Scale, are used to provide structure and inter-rater consistency to the clinical assessment (14,15). Thus, when nursing assessment of the GCS is undertaken at regular intervals at the bedside, an intermittent (clinical) neuromonitoring strategy is implemented to detect clinical deterioration that may be related to secondary brain injury. However, the application of the neurological examination as a neuromonitor for secondary brain injury has significant shortcomings. Reversible ischaemia cannot be clinically distinguished from infarction, patients in deep coma may have severe ongoing secondary injury mechanisms but limited ability to manifest clinical changes, and sedatives and metabolic disturbances may confound the reliability of clinical assessment (16). Despite these shortcomings, clinical examination is the standard neuromonitoring tool used in virtually all patients on the NCCU.

Physiological monitoring

Physiological monitoring of multiple different parameters, such as systemic blood pressure, oxygen saturation, body temperature, and numerous other cardiovascular variables, is the mainstay of monitoring in all intensive care units (ICUs), including neurocritical care (17). While cardiovascular monitoring may primarily be implemented to detect arrhythmias and blood pressure changes that affect cardiac function, when conducted in the context of monitoring for secondary brain injury a common goal would be to avoid hypotension that decreases cerebral blood flow (CBF), hypoxaemia that decreases arterial oxygen delivery, and hypertension that might predispose to worsening cerebral haemorrhage or oedema.

ICP monitoring provides a direct measure of the impact of intracranial processes on cerebral compliance and pressure and, with knowledge of mean arterial pressure (MAP), allows the calculation of CPP (CPP = MAP – ICP). The most common use of cardiovascular monitors in the context of brain injury is therefore in targeting a minimum threshold of systemic blood pressure, ICP, and/or CPP. The use of monitoring in this way assumes that, if the measured parameter is not below a predefined threshold, blood flow and oxygen delivery to the injured brain is sufficient. This has led to 'one-size-fits-all' recommendations of thresholds of ICP less than 20 mmHg and CPP greater than 60 mmHg (18), using values derived from cohort studies that identify them as reasonable cut-off points. Whilst such thresholds are useful estimates for a population, they may not (and often do not) identify the critical threshold in an individual patient because of substantial interpatient variability. On the other hand, neurophysiological monitoring techniques such as electroencephalography (EEG) or evoked potentials (EPs) have the advantage of directly monitoring the electrical activity of the injured brain; studies have shown that EEG changes may

detect early ischaemia and EP brainstem functional integrity (19). However, metabolic disturbances and sedative medications may confound the use of direct brain monitors, especially EEG, as secondary brain injury detection tools. Thus, the most prevalent use of EEG in the NCCU is currently as a monitor for clinical and subclinical status epilepticus (20).

Advanced neuromonitoring

Advanced neuromonitoring techniques, such as those that measure cerebral oxygenation, CBF, and cerebral interstitial metabolites, have emerged as tools that might address some of the shortcomings of clinical and physiological neuromonitors. The ability to directly measure $PtiO_2$ (21,22), the arteriovenous oxygen difference ($AVDO_2$), quantitative regional CBF, markers of anaerobic metabolism such as the lactate/pyruvate ratio and extracellular glutamate concentration (23–25), and brain temperature represents exciting advances that bring the concepts of secondary brain injury monitoring of multiple pathophysiological pathways to the forefront of clinical care. However, each of these new parameters comes from the institution of at least one new monitoring device or method, and a fundamental question is whether these monitors provide information which is more relevant than prior accepted measures such as ICP, CPP, or P_aO_2.

There are studies suggesting that cerebral metabolism, as detected by one or more of these advanced monitoring tools, is compromised even though other conventionally monitored parameters, such as ICP and CPP, are within an acceptable range (26). However, much of the work to date has focused on understanding the relationship between the newer parameters and existing measures. For example, $PtiO_2$ has been shown to represent an interaction between CBF and oxygen diffusion (27) and, at a steady state of dissolved arterial oxygen, acute changes in $PtiO_2$ track closely with changes in CBF. CPP thresholds for cerebral 'metabolic crisis', usually defined as a microdialysis-monitored lactate/pyruvate ratio higher than 40, have been investigated after TBI and SAH (28,29). However, in the light of a recent clinical trial which did not demonstrate the superiority of ICP monitoring-guided management with a target treatment threshold of less than 20 mmHg in patients with severe TBI (30), it may be time to consider whether newer metabolic monitors in the context of multimodal monitoring should take a more primary role in neurocritical care monitoring.

Imaging

Imaging is ubiquitous in the management of critically ill neurological patients but serves principally as an anatomical snapshot at a particular moment in time, and is thus distinguished from a neuromonitoring tool. However, integration of anatomical imaging information with physiological data from computed tomography (CT) or magnetic resonance imaging (MRI) perfusion (and perhaps in the future with MRI or positron emission tomography functional imaging) with clinical, physiological, and metabolic neuromonitoring data is an important goal. Initial studies have identified relationships between physiological parameters such as lactate/pyruvate ratio and regional brain atrophy after TBI (29).

Data analysis as a neuromonitor

It is a basic axiom that monitoring is only as useful as the interpretation of the data generated by a monitor; monitors don't determine treatment, physicians, nurses, and other clinical providers do. Although bedside clinicians have been using some form of monitoring data since the origins of critical care, cautionary tales are often brought to bear regarding the lack of utility of certain monitoring paradigms, most notably the pulmonary artery catheter in sepsis and general critical care (31).

The overall care of critically ill neurological patients continues to improve, with secular trends in improved outcome and evidence of benefit of neurocritical care as a general concept to patient outcome (32). What this suggests is that bedside clinicians already perform data analysis as part of their decision-making approach to clinical care, and that there is substantial value in this. However, in almost all current clinical situations this analysis involves bedside review of raw data presented by either a paper or electronic medical record, with clinical decisions based on experience, intuition, and art, rather than on advanced data presentation and analysis. Importantly, the advent of new neuromonitoring tools, the regulatory-mandated move to electronic medical records in many countries (33), and the increasing recognition of the complexity of secondary brain injury mechanisms have converged to create a sense that further advances will be strongly dependent on the ability to acquire, store, analyse, and utilize neuromonitoring data in better ways. In a sense, it is data analysis that is the neuromonitor, not the device that generates the data.

Data acquisition, integration, and storage

In order for neuromonitoring data to be used efficiently, it must be able to be viewed, stored, and reviewed. Currently there are often more than 30 parameters generating data continuously and/or at a high frequency, and most of this information is viewed only if a bedside clinician happens to be looking at the monitor interface, or if a pre-programmed alarm alerts the clinician to pay attention to a specific parameter. Paper charts remain the most common way of recording monitoring data in critical care units, although they are being replaced in large numbers of centres and countries by electronic medical records which acquire data 'automatically' and continuously, and populate a database often after clinician review for accuracy of the information acquired. Unfortunately, most electronic critical care records merely recapitulate the format of the paper chart, with many parameters entered hourly regardless of the temporal resolution of the source monitor. Additionally, commercially available critical care charting systems have major disadvantages related to their ability to acquire, store, and retrieve disparate datasets. In order to perform any meaningful advanced analysis of bedside neuromonitoring data beyond simple review of intermittent (usually hourly) raw data, a robust data acquisition, integration, and storage system is required.

Ideally an ICU monitoring system would facilitate a comprehensive and integrated view of all available clinical, radiographic, laboratory, and physiological data, but current systems fall substantially short of this ideal (34). Several barriers stand in the way of meaningful integration of neuromonitoring data. First, most monitoring devices are not designed to be interoperable, in contrast to the way that modern consumer computers work seamlessly together. Most ICU medical devices are stand-alone proprietary systems and this prevents easy integration of their data output. To address this, the American Society for Testing and Materials recently adopted the concept of the 'integrated clinical environment' to ensure improved

compatibility of future medical device designs (35). Second, meaningful integration of monitoring data requires highly precise time synchronization of different data streams, so that clinicians can be confident that the apparent correlations between different monitoring modalities reflect true *in vivo* processes rather than an artefact of misaligned data. Third, like any other form of data collection in the busy environment of the ICU, data collected by neuromonitors are subject to false inputs, such as apparent ICP elevations that occur when a patient is repositioned. While bedside nurses can use clinical judgement to remove artefactual values when recording data in bedside paper flowcharts, automated neuromonitoring devices require sophisticated algorithms to detect and exclude such artefacts (36). Ironically, confidence that clinically recorded data are accurate is an advantage of the paper chart on which all values are hand-recorded (and checked) by a bedside nurse.

Several data acquisition systems designed for multimodal neuromonitoring have been developed and implemented. While some are commercially available as software or hardware solutions (37), most systems to date have been 'one-off' solutions built within an institution to serve the needs of researchers with a specific interest in physiological informatics (34,38,39). These systems are generally in two basic forms—*kiosk* systems in which a computerized data acquisition unit is brought to the patient bedside and connected to the output ports of various monitors, and *distributed* systems in which data from bedside monitors are sent continuously to a remote server (Figure 13.1). A kiosk system is usually less expensive but only allows data acquisition from one patient at a time, and only when connected and turned on. An example of a kiosk system is the CNS data acquisition monitor (Moberg Research Inc., Ambler, PA), which has specific software written to allow direct data input from many critical care devices and physiological monitors (3). Distributed systems are costlier because they require set-up in multiple ICU beds and a remote server for storage. However, a distributed system is always in place and collects data without requiring a data acquisition device to be attached and turned on. A major disadvantage to all current systems is that adding data from new devices usually requires specific software patches, unlike the 'plug-and-play' approach now expected in consumer electronic devices and computers.

Barriers related to data security and systems architecture also make implementation of data transmission and storage challenging. Much of the problem in this regard derives from the fact that different hospitals, governmental agencies, and regulatory oversight groups have different rules for the protection of data. This creates individual data silos that make it difficult to share data from multiple sites for the purposes of clinical practice, research, or quality assurance. Certain groups, such as the Brain-IT consortium, have overcome such obstacles in the short term by allowing investigators from various sites to add data to a group database voluntarily rather than having data automatically populate an external (to a single institution) database (40,41).

Data storage was previously considered a barrier because of the volume of frequently collected data. However, rapid and continual advances in database storage solutions and cloud computing have lessened the impact of this on the advancement of neurocritical care bioinformatics. Consequently, the principal issue regarding data storage relates to rapidity of data retrieval from large databases, rather than the ability to store the data in the first place. Methods that allow tiered storage based on likelihood of need, such as most

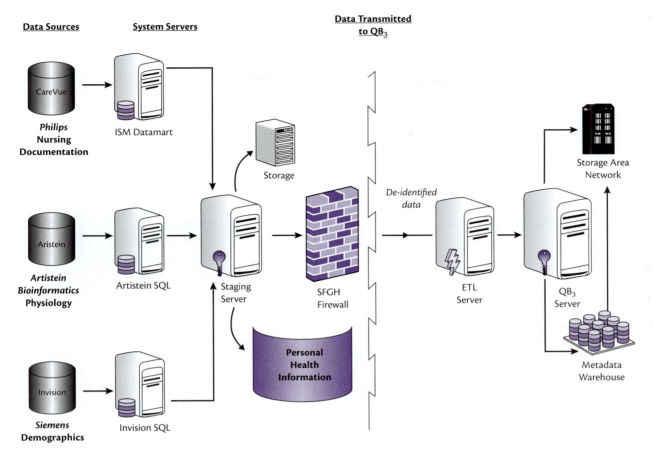

Fig. 13.1 Schematic of data integration across multiple sources. Primary data is derived from three different sources (intensive care charting software (Philips), a locally developed physiology data acquisition system (Aristein), the electronic health record (Siemens)) and integrated into a single staging server. Personal health information is redacted and data is transmitted to an external server where it is then available for research analysis.

ETL, extract/transform/load; QB3, California Institute for Quantitative Biosciences; SFGH, San Francisco General Hospital; SQL, structured query language.

Image courtesy of Drs Norm Aleks, Stuart Russell, and Geoff Manley.

recent data or data of acutely hospitalized patients, are important to provide timely data access so that clinicians can utilize advanced data analyses at the bedside.

Data analysis: simple to advanced

The promise of multimodal monitoring derives from the hypothesis that more advanced integrated analysis of data from multiple different monitors, or new analytical techniques applied to traditional parameters, will provide insights into disease pathophysiology and treatment that are not apparent from current methods of data analysis (Table 13.1). Certainly this has been the case in other areas, such as the Human Genome Project, where development of new statistical and analytic methods was a necessary accompaniment to improved methods of gene sequencing (42). Initial attempts at more advanced data analysis of multimodal neurocritical care data have yielded interesting insights and helped to focus the challenge of developing clinically relevant analytical tools for this complex data-stream.

One effort has focused on developing more informative indices from raw data of single parameters. An example would include assessment of 'fever burden' as the area under the curve between body temperature and a specific threshold cut-off point

(e.g. 37.5°C), with the hypothesis that this new *index* describes the impact of fever more fully than simply identifying a single fever spike (43). Another example is the use of the pressure reactivity index (PRx), which is a measure of intracranial compliance derived as a running correlation coefficient between ICP and MAP (44). These methods create new individual parameters derived from raw data that may prove to be more informative than the original data streams. Other methods attempt to integrate and analyse across multiple data parameters with the goal of interpreting multimodality monitoring for the purpose of predicting events and outcomes. These can be divided into two main methodologies—*data-driven methods* and *model-based methods*.

Data-driven methods

Data-driven methods can generally be thought of as using existing known data to predict an outcome of interest. Supervised learning involves training on an existing dataset where outcomes are known, whereas unsupervised learning, sometime referred to as 'data mining', has the identification of unforeseen associations between parameters as its goal.

A commonly used and familiar data-driven method is multivariable regression analyses, in which all data points are assumed of value and used to create a linear mathematical equation to

Table 13.1 Methods of data analysis used or proposed in multimodal neuromonitoring

Method	Example
Arithmetic	Cerebral perfusion pressure (CPP = MAP – ICP)
Index	Fever burden (area under the curve)
	PRx (correlation coefficient)
Data-driven methods	Regression analysis
	Decision trees
	Neural network
	Data mining
Model-based methods	Dynamic Bayesian networks (DBN)
	Dynamical systems models

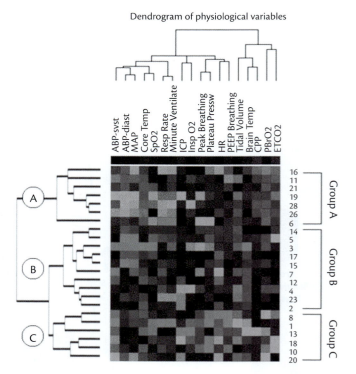

Fig. 13.2 Self-organizing heat map of physiological variables. Heat maps have been commonly used in genetics when genes are displayed across the top row and related genes cluster. In this physiology heat map, genes are replaced by physiological variables that hierarchically cluster on the basis of association within and across three groups of patients. As would be expected, MAP and ABP cluster together. In this specific case, ICP and inspiratory oxygen (or fraction of inspired oxygen) unexpectedly clustered, leading to the identification of previously unrecognized ICP elevations during bedside suctioning in this set of mechanically ventilated traumatic brain injury patients.

ABP, arterial blood pressure; ETCO$_2$, end tidal carbon dioxide; HR, heart rate; ICP, intracranial pressure; O$_2$, oxygen; PbtO$_2$, brain tissue oxygen tension; PEEP, positive end-expiratory pressure; SpO$_2$, systemic oxygen saturation.

Data from Sorani MD *et al.*, 'New approaches to physiological informatics in neurocritical care', *Neurocritical Care*, 2007, 7, 1, pp. 45–52.

associate with an outcome of interest. For example, Hemphill used multivariate linear regression with a time lag to demonstrate that changes in the inspired fraction of oxygen and MAP predicted a subsequent change in PtiO$_2$ several minutes later (45). However, there are shortcomings to regression analysis, such as challenges with time-series data, assumption of linear relationships between predictors, and difficulty handling missing data. These all limit its ultimate utility for multimodal monitoring analytics.

Without making assumptions about linearity, relationships between multiple prognostic factors and treatment decisions can be analysed using decision trees. After being grouped together at the top of a decision tree, a cohort of patients can then be subdivided in a series of steps corresponding to prognostic factors (e.g. a dichotomized age cut-off) and treatment decisions (e.g. receipt of a drug). Such decision trees have been used to identify groups of patients with a poor prognosis for neurological recovery after TBI (46). Artificial neural networks represent even more powerful tools for performing non-linear multivariable analysis, and this is especially useful for modelling complex data to detect previously unknown patterns. This technique has been used to delineate complex patient-specific metabolic states on the basis of microdialysis data (47). Similarly, discrete clusters of physiological data that portend the risk of future infection, organ failure, and death have been identified in trauma patients (48). Other quantitative methods based on measures of variability, such as time-series analysis, have been used to demonstrate that decreased variability in ICP more strongly predicts outcomes than mean ICP (49).

In a more general approach, the overall degree of randomness within a series of data can be quantified using a measure termed approximate entropy. Among critically ill patients, decreased approximate entropy in heart rate measurements has been shown to correlate with a higher risk of mortality (50). Such studies demonstrate that advanced bioinformatics using data-driven methods can uncover previously unrecognized relationships in existing data (Figure 13.2) that may ultimately allow better clinical prognostication and identify novel therapeutic targets (51).

Model-based methods

Other advanced bioinformatics approaches seek to use model-based analytical methods to identify previously unrecognized physiological states with the goal of shifting patients from an undesirable physiological state to a more desirable one (52,53). At a basic level, dynamical systems models can be used to describe the evolution of systems over time on the basis of classic mechanics, such as theories of pressure–volume–flow relationships. This approach has been fruitfully used to model the interaction between cerebrovascular reserve, cerebral haemodynamics during blood pressure changes, and the relationship between CPP and autoregulatory status (54). However, dynamical system models assume linear relationships between model parameters, and this limits their use in the non-linear and complex biological environment encountered during neurocritical care (55,56). Such complexity may be better captured and understood with dynamic Bayesian networks, a method which is powerfully suited to describe environments with a high degree of uncertainty. In this approach, patients are assigned a priori a distribution of probabilities of being in different physiological states, and these probabilities are then updated with new empirical data that are weighted based on the prior likelihood. The Avert-IT project, sponsored by the Brain-IT European neurocritical care informatics consortium, seeks to use dynamic Bayesian modelling of demographic, clinical, and physiological data from patients with TBI to identify those at risk of transitioning from a stable status (free of hypotension) to another, more unstable status (hypotensive) and thus at risk of secondary brain injury (57). The advantage of an explicitly Bayesian approach to real-time data analysis at the bedside is that it takes away from clinicians some of the work of considering pre-test probabilities, and automatically incorporates it into the analysis and display of incoming data.

As neuromonitoring expands, and the amount of available continuous clinical data expands with it, this type of clinical decision support will become increasingly important if clinicians are to be able to make best use of available data. Without such advanced model-based methods, it may be difficult to continuously incorporate already-obtained physiological data into the clinical assessment. For example, in two previously-healthy patients who both present similarly with a Hunt–Hess grade 4 SAH, there may be a tendency to interpret incoming physiological information in the same background context. On the other hand, application of machine-based dynamic Bayesian modelling may be better able to build different background contexts for these two patients over the course of their hospitalization, incorporating subtle differences, such as minor degrees of acute kidney injury. Such a model-based method may then make better use of new data collected later during hospitalization than would a clinician who had not been able to fully incorporate the wealth of complex physiological data that had accrued during this time.

Data visualization

Clinicians often underestimate the importance of interfaces and tools used to visualize monitoring data in the NCCU. This likely comes from the fact that data visualization is itself the process of how information is viewed in order to integrate and develop a 'picture' of the patient's condition. An example of how data visualization is taken for granted by the end user is CT imaging. CT scans generate quantitative raw numerical data in Hounsfield units, but this is converted to greyscale which is then translated to an image based on the 'anatomical' location of the pixel and its greyscale value from Hounsfield units (58). This translation of raw data for the purposes of ease and interpretability is rarely if ever considered by clinicians viewing CT scans, and this is precisely the point. Good data visualization tools operate in the background and make it easier for clinicians to care for patients and improve workflow. The current state of data visualization in neurointensive care is analogous to viewing CT scans using absolute Hounsfield unit numbers, with no image generation except that in the mind of the clinician reviewing the raw data.

Ironically, the advent of electronic critical care charting tools and medical records has brought to light the value, through familiarity, of prior data visualization tools. Most notably, the paper chart that has historically been used as a bedside tool in many NCCUs served as a data visualization tool in which clinicians became familiar with the location on the chart of different variables such as medications, vital signs, fluid balance, and ventilation parameters. Anecdotally, the switch to electronic records has led many senior clinicians to lament the challenge of finding the data that they want from the interface offered as part of the electronic chart. These examples of long-standing adaptation to a prior paradigm (paper bedside chart) and translation of numeric data into intuitively meaningful information (CT scan) serve as useful constructs to improve the ways in which multimodal data visualization are developed.

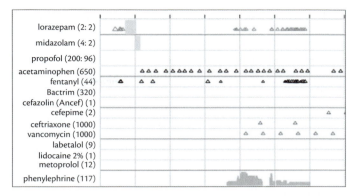

Fig. 13.3 Data visualization tool for medications. Different symbols are used to provide organizational information about medication administration. Medications are grouped according to category (sedatives; antipyretics and opiates; antibiotics; vasoactive drugs). Individual triangles denote single dosing while continuous blocks indicate dose of infusions. In this example, an increase in benzodiazepine sedatives precedes antipyretic fever treatment. Subsequent pressor use (phenylephrine) is then followed by antibiotic administration. This is a pattern in a patient with sepsis and early pattern recognition could potentially lead to earlier intervention.
Image courtesy of Drs Norm Aleks, Stuart Russell, and Geoff Manley.

In designing data visualization tools and interfaces to enhance the usability of multimodal neuromonitoring data it seems most prudent to concentrate initially on those applications which might be used consistently across providers, rather than emphasizing a different data visualization environment in which each provider selects the data that they want. Several different approaches have already been tested including the use of a separate monitoring screen to display time-synchronized physiological data across several parameters, with the ability to change the time-scale (e.g. seconds, minutes, or hours) and identify trends and relationships based on visual inspection. Also, 'dashboards' in which different colours are used to alert providers to uncompleted tasks, such as venous thromboprophylaxis or sedation holds, have been described (59). Novel ways of viewing medication administration based on dose and timing could also help providers identify emerging clinical events (Figure 13.3). Finally, in order to enhance usability, new ways of interpreting data and improved data visualization methods, such as graphical representation of area under the curve as an indicator of secondary brain insults such as fever or ICP 'burden', are required. It is fair to say that without intuitive data visualization tools that improve the ability to integrate new multimodal neuromonitoring data into routine bedside workflow, advances in multimodal monitoring are unlikely to be widely adopted by clinicians outside focused clinical research settings.

Workflow

Workflow is the sequence of steps required to complete a specific task. In the neurointensive care environment, in which the task is to provide comprehensive 24/7 care to a critically ill neurological patient, workflow is complex and involves interrelationships between numerous care providers (nurses, neurointensivist, consulting physicians, resident doctors, pharmacists, therapists, etc.) all of whom have their own specific tasks and associated workflow. Just as advanced data visualization in neurocritical care has received relatively little attention, the way in which workflow influences the use of multimodal neuromonitoring is also underappreciated. Suffice it to say that, if the introduction of multimodal neuromonitoring makes it slower and more challenging to care for a patient, it is unlikely to be integrated into routine clinical practice. Conversely, if multimodal neuromonitoring streamlines and focuses care, it is likely to be embraced even by those who are not cognizant with its specific biological or informatics underpinnings.

Workflow in hospitals is a major interest of patient safety advocates. The use of checklists, pre-procedure 'time-out', and double-checks for blood transfusions are all examples of modifications to workflow introduced with the goal of error reduction (60). The introduction of new technology into routine medical workflow has also been studied in other contexts. For example, the impact of workflow changes after the introduction of a radiology picture archiving and communication system (PACS) to replace printed films was studied in a single institution (61). The average time searching for individual images dropped from 16 to 2 minutes, saving 21.5 physician years and over $1 million annually. Further, removing the need for film printing reduced file clerk needs by half and freed up over 2000 square feet of prior storage space, saving over $3 million annually (61).

Patel and colleagues have developed a cognitive workflow model which focuses on the process of information transfer between providers in critical care, and identified seven 'critical zones' in which interactions with the opportunity for streamlining or breakdown in care delivery occur (Figure 13.4) (62). These include re-orientation and preliminary planning, goal formulation, goal execution, transfers, admissions, reassessment, and handover. Each of these critical zones has specific activities, such as nursing change of shift, ward rounds, post-round order execution, and discharge to another

ward, associated with it. By understanding the process of knowledge acquisition and transfer between providers at these various critical zones, it may be possible to develop improved (and possibly safer) ways of delivering bedside critical care. Furthermore, this process may also depend on the usefulness of information transferred, and the expertise of the practitioner.

Any new multimodal neuromonitoring approach must be introduced into an existing paradigm of clinical care, and it is important to consider its impact on overall workflow. As the final point where information is translated into bedside action, neurocritical care workflow represents the execution of the process of monitoring, data acquisition and integration, advanced analysis, and visualization. Advances in multimodal neuromonitoring must therefore be coupled with ways to improve workflow by providing more streamlined patient assessment, simplifying the complex critical care environment, and improving communication and consistency across providers from different backgrounds and with different levels of expertise. The idea of simulating critical care workflow is now being considered, just as simulation is routine in anaesthesia, emergency medicine, and resuscitation (63).

Future directions

Multimodal monitoring and accompanying developments in neuroinformatics are very much in their infancy. While the concept of multimodality monitoring is inherent to the practice of neurocritical care, its optimal application in the research, and particularly clinical, environment remains far from clarified. The idea of identifying clinically important and treatable parameters not immediately obvious from raw bedside data is compelling, and

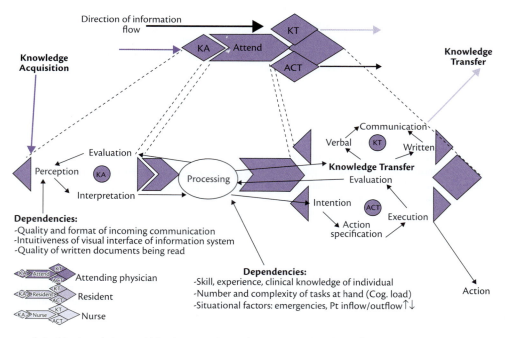

Fig. 13.4 Workflow diagram of physician knowledge acquisition, interpretation, and action. Internal workings of an attending physician that take place in order to accept, interpret, process, and act upon information arriving from a source. Dependent factors for perception of arriving information as well as the processing of the information are also depicted. Similar depiction would apply for any other member (resident/nurse) in the clinical workflow, although the dependencies for the concerned individual may differ.

ACT, actions; KA, knowledge acquisition; KT, knowledge transfer.

Data from Malhotra S et al., 'Workflow modeling in critical care: piecing together your own puzzle', *Journal of Biomedical Informatics*, 2007, 40, 2, pp. 81–92, with permission from Elsevier .

potentially of great significance to patients (13). Certainly this concept has precedent in history, most notably in the development of CT imaging, which was initially shunned by many as too complex and impractical. However, it should also be acknowledged by those focused in this field that widespread translation to the clinic will also be dependent on the development of user-friendly interfaces that improve the workflow of bedside clinicians who are not even aware of the advanced analytics going on 'behind the scene'.

Therefore, it is probably most reasonable to consider multimodal monitoring as a concept that includes many different steps, such as:

1. data generation from devices that are monitoring the organ of interest (e.g. brain)

2. data storage for immediate and longer-term use

3. real-time advanced analysis that feeds back parameters into the medical record for treating clinicians to use

4. intuitive, user-friendly interfaces that encourage clinician use

5. improvements to workflow efficiency among bedside providers that are facilitated by multimodal monitoring.

Taken as such, the implementation of multimodal monitoring is a substantive task that will require (and deserves) collaboration between neurointensivists, bedside nurses, engineers, computer scientists, physiological researchers, computer interface design experts, and experts in workflow. At its core though, multimodal monitoring is about bringing order to chaos, and improving the 'art of managing extreme complexity' (64).

References

1. Anderson NE, Mason DF, Fink JN, Bergin PS, Charleston AJ, Gamble GD. Detection of focal cerebral hemisphere lesions using the neurological examination. *J Neurol Neurosurg Psychiatry*. 2005;76(4):545–9.

2. Josephson SA, Hills NK, Johnston SC. NIH Stroke Scale reliability in ratings from a large sample of clinicians. *Cerebrovasc Dis (Basel)*. 2006;22(5–6):389–95.

3. Hemphill JC, Andrews P, De Georgia M. Multimodal monitoring and neurocritical care bioinformatics. *Nat Rev Neurol*. 2011;7(8):451–60.

4. Chesnut RM, Marshall LF, Klauber MR, Blunt BA, Baldwin N, Eisenberg HM, et al. The role of secondary brain injury in determining outcome from severe head injury. *J Trauma*. 1993;34(2):216–22.

5. Graham DI, Lawrence AE, Adams JH, Doyle D, McLellan DR. Brain damage in fatal non-missile head injury without high intracranial pressure. *J Clin Pathol*. 1988;41(1):34–7.

6. Graham DI, Ford I, Adams JH, Doyle D, Teasdale GM, Lawrence AE, et al. Ischaemic brain damage is still common in fatal non-missile head injury. *J Neurol Neurosurg Psychiatry*. 1989;52(3):346–50.

7. Gopinath SP, Valadka AB, Uzura M, Robertson CS. Comparison of jugular venous oxygen saturation and brain tissue PO2 as monitors of cerebral ischemia after head injury. *Crit Care Med*. 1999;27(11):2337–45.

8. Spiotta AM, Stiefel MF, Gracias VH, Garuffe AM, Kofke WA, Maloney-Wilensky E, et al. Brain tissue oxygen-directed management and outcome in patients with severe traumatic brain injury. *J Neurosurg*. 2010;113(3):571–80.

9. Narotam PK, Morrison JF, Nathoo N. Brain tissue oxygen monitoring in traumatic brain injury and major trauma: outcome analysis of a brain tissue oxygen-directed therapy. *J Neurosurg*. 2009;111(4):672–82.

10. Stiefel MF, Spiotta A, Gracias VH, Garuffe AM, Guillamondegui O, Maloney-Wilensky E, et al. Reduced mortality rate in patients with severe traumatic brain injury treated with brain tissue oxygen monitoring. *J Neurosurg*. 2005;103(5):805–11.

11. Budohoski KP, Czosnyka M, de Riva N, Smielewski P, Pickard JD, Menon DK, et al. The relationship between cerebral blood flow autoregulation and cerebrovascular pressure reactivity after traumatic brain injury. *Neurosurgery*. 2012;71(3):652–60.

12. Crump C, Saxena S, Wilson B, Farrell P, Rafiq A, Silvers CT. Using Bayesian networks and rule-based trending to predict patient status in the intensive care unit. *AMIA Annu Symp Proc*. 2009;2009:124–8.

13. Pineda JA, Leonard JR, Mazotas IG, Noetzel M, Limbrick DD, Keller MS, et al. Effect of implementation of a paediatric neurocritical care programme on outcomes after severe traumatic brain injury: a retrospective cohort study. *Lancet Neurol*. 2013;12(1):45–52.

14. Lyden P, Brott T, Tilley B, Welch KM, Mascha EJ, Levine S, et al. Improved reliability of the NIH Stroke Scale using video training. NINDS TPA Stroke Study Group. *Stroke*. 1994;25(11):2220–6.

15. Teasdale G, Jennett B, Murray L, Murray G. Glasgow coma scale: to sum or not to sum. *Lancet*. 1983;2(8351):678.

16. Vespa PM, Nuwer MR, Nenov V, Ronne-Engstrom E, Hovda DA, Bergsneider M, et al. Increased incidence and impact of nonconvulsive and convulsive seizures after traumatic brain injury as detected by continuous electroencephalographic monitoring. *J Neurosurg*. 1999;91(5):750–60.

17. Dellinger RP, Levy MM, Rhodes A, Annane D, Gerlach H, Opal SM, et al. Surviving Sepsis Campaign: International Guidelines for Management of Severe Sepsis and Septic Shock: 2012. *Crit Care Med*. 2013;41(2):580–637.

18. Bratton SL, Chestnut RM, Ghajar J, McConnell Hammond FF, Harris OA, Hartl R, et al. Guidelines for the management of severe traumatic brain injury. IX. Cerebral perfusion thresholds. *J Neurotrauma*. 2007;24 Suppl 1:S59–64.

19. Claassen J, Hirsch LJ, Kreiter KT, Du EY, Connolly ES, Emerson RG, et al. Quantitative continuous EEG for detecting delayed cerebral ischemia in patients with poor-grade subarachnoid hemorrhage. *Clin Neurophysiol*. 2004;115(12):2699–710.

20. Friedman D, Claassen J, Hirsch LJ. Continuous electroencephalogram monitoring in the intensive care unit. *Anesth Analg*. 2009;109(2):506–23.

21. van Santbrink H, Maas AI, Avezaat CJ. Continuous monitoring of partial pressure of brain tissue oxygen in patients with severe head injury. *Neurosurgery*. 1996;38(1):21–31.

22. Gupta AK, Hutchinson PJ, Fryer T, Al-Rawi PG, Parry DA, Minhas PS, et al. Measurement of brain tissue oxygenation performed using positron emission tomography scanning to validate a novel monitoring method. *J Neurosurg*. 2002;96(2):263–8.

23. Hillered L, Persson L, Ponten U, Ungerstedt U. Neurometabolic monitoring of the ischaemic human brain using microdialysis. *Acta Neurochir (Wien)*. 1990;102(3–4):91–7.

24. Vespa PM, McArthur D, O'Phelan K, Glenn T, Etchepare M, Kelly D, et al. Persistently low extracellular glucose correlates with poor outcome 6 months after human traumatic brain injury despite a lack of increased lactate: a microdialysis study. *J Cereb Blood Flow Metab*. 2003;23(7):865–77.

25. Goodman JC, Valadka AB, Gopinath SP, Uzura M, Robertson CS. Extracellular lactate and glucose alterations in the brain after head injury measured by microdialysis. *Crit Care Med*. 1999;27(9):1965–73.

26. Rose JC, Neill TA, Hemphill JC, 3rd. Continuous monitoring of the microcirculation in neurocritical care: an update on brain tissue oxygenation. *Curr Opin Crit Care*. 2006;12(2):97–102.

27. Rosenthal G, Hemphill JC, 3rd, Sorani M, Martin C, Morabito D, Obrist WD, et al. Brain tissue oxygen tension is more indicative of oxygen diffusion than oxygen delivery and metabolism in patients with traumatic brain injury. *Crit Care Med*. 2008;36(6):1917–24.

28. Schmidt JM, Ko SB, Helbok R, Kurtz P, Stuart RM, Presciutti M, et al. Cerebral perfusion pressure thresholds for brain tissue hypoxia and metabolic crisis after poor-grade subarachnoid hemorrhage. *Stroke*. 2011;42(5):1351–6.

29. Marcoux J, McArthur DA, Miller C, Glenn TC, Villablanca P, Martin NA, et al. Persistent metabolic crisis as measured by elevated cerebral microdialysis lactate-pyruvate ratio predicts chronic frontal lobe brain atrophy after traumatic brain injury. *Crit Care Med*. 2008;36(10):2871–7.

30. Chesnut RM, Temkin N, Carney N, Dikmen S, Rondina C, Videtta W, *et al*. A trial of intracranial-pressure monitoring in traumatic brain injury. *N Engl J Med*. 2012;367(26):2471–81.

31. Hadian M, Pinsky MR. Evidence-based review of the use of the pulmonary artery catheter: impact data and complications. *Crit Care*. 2006;10 Suppl 3:S8.

32. Kramer AH, Zygun DA. Do neurocritical care units save lives? Measuring the impact of specialized ICUs. *Neurocrit Care*. 2011;14(3):329–33.

33. Sittig DF, Singh H. Electronic health records and national patient-safety goals. *N Engl J Med*. 2012;367(19):1854–60.

34. Goldstein B, McNames J, McDonald BA, Ellenby M, Lai S, Sun Z, *et al*. Physiologic data acquisition system and database for the study of disease dynamics in the intensive care unit. *Crit Care Med*. 2003;31(2):433–41.

35. Ropper A, Gress D, Diringer M, Green D, Mayer S, Bleck T. *Neurological and Neurosurgical Intensive Care* (4th edn). Philadelphia, PA: Lippincott Williams & Wilkins; 2004.

36. Otero A, Felix P, Barro S, Palacios F. Addressing the flaws of current critical alarms: a fuzzy constraint satisfaction approach. *Artif Intell Med*. 2009;47(3):219–38.

37. Smielewski P, Czosnyka M, Steiner L, Belestri M, Piechnik S, Pickard JD. ICM+: software for on-line analysis of bedside monitoring data after severe head trauma. *Acta Neurochir Suppl*. 2005;95:43–9.

38. Sorani MD, Hemphill JC, 3rd, Morabito D, Rosenthal G, Manley GT. New approaches to physiological informatics in neurocritical care. *Neurocrit Care*. 2007;7(1):45–52.

39. Gomez H, Camacho J, Yelicich B, Moraes L, Biestro A, Puppo C. Development of a multimodal monitoring platform for medical research. *Conf Proc IEEE Eng Med Biol Soc*. 2010;1:2358–61.

40. Chambers I, Gregson B, Citerio G, Enblad P, Howells T, Kiening K, *et al*. BrainIT collaborative network: analyses from a high time-resolution dataset of head injured patients. *Acta Neurochir Suppl*. 2008;102:223–7.

41. Piper I, Chambers I, Citerio G, Enblad P, Gregson B, Howells T, *et al*. The brain monitoring with Information Technology (BrainIT) collaborative network: EC feasibility study results and future direction. *Acta Neurochir (Wien)*. 2010;152(11):1859–71.

42. Hanauer DA, Rhodes DR, Sinha-Kumar C, Chinnaiyan AM. Bioinformatics approaches in the study of cancer. *Curr Mol Med*. 2007;7(1):133–41.

43. Badjatia N, Fernandez L, Schmidt JM, Lee K, Claassen J, Connolly ES, *et al*. Impact of induced normothermia on outcome after subarachnoid hemorrhage: a case-control study. *Neurosurgery*. 2010;66(4):696–700.

44. Czosnyka M, Brady K, Reinhard M, Smielewski P, Steiner LA. Monitoring of cerebrovascular autoregulation: facts, myths, and missing links. *Neurocrit Care*. 2009;10(3):373–86.

45. Hemphill JC, 3rd, Morabito D, Farrant M, Manley GT. Brain tissue oxygen monitoring in intracerebral hemorrhage. *Neurocrit Care*. 2005;3(3):260–70.

46. Andrews PJ, Sleeman DH, Statham PF, McQuatt A, Corruble V, Jones PA, *et al*. Predicting recovery in patients suffering from traumatic brain injury by using admission variables and physiological data: a comparison between decision tree analysis and logistic regression. *J Neurosurg*. 2002;97(2):326–36.

47. Nelson DW, Bellander BM, Maccallum RM, Axelsson J, Alm M, Wallin M, *et al*. Cerebral microdialysis of patients with severe traumatic brain injury exhibits highly individualistic patterns as visualized by cluster analysis with self-organizing maps. *Crit Care Med*. 2004;32(12):2428–36.

48. Cohen MJ, Grossman AD, Morabito D, Knudson MM, Butte AJ, Manley GT. Identification of complex metabolic states in critically injured patients using bioinformatic cluster analysis. *Crit Care*.14(1):R10.

49. Kirkness CJ, Burr RL, Mitchell PH. Intracranial pressure variability and long-term outcome following traumatic brain injury. *Acta Neurochir Suppl*. 2008;102:105–8.

50. Papaioannou VE, Maglaveras N, Houvarda I, Antoniadou E, Vretzakis G. Investigation of altered heart rate variability, nonlinear properties of heart rate signals, and organ dysfunction longitudinally over time in intensive care unit patients. *J Crit Care*. 2006;21(1):95–103.

51. Buchman TG. Novel representation of physiologic states during critical illness and recovery. *Crit Care*. 2010;14(2):127.

52. Buchman TG. Physiologic stability and physiologic state. *J Trauma*. 1996;41(4):599–605.

53. Buchman TG. Nonlinear dynamics, complex systems, and the pathobiology of critical illness. *Curr Opin Crit Care*. 2004;10(5):378–82.

54. Ursino M, Lodi CA, Rossi S, Stocchetti N. Estimation of the main factors affecting ICP dynamics by mathematical analysis of PVI tests. *Acta Neurochir Suppl*. 1998;71:306–9.

55. Coveney PV, Fowler PW. Modelling biological complexity: a physical scientist's perspective. *J R Soc Interface*. 2005;2(4):267–80.

56. Godin PJ, Buchman TG. Uncoupling of biological oscillators: a complementary hypothesis concerning the pathogenesis of multiple organ dysfunction syndrome. *Crit Care Med*. 1996;24(7):1107–16.

57. Lozier AP, Sciacca RR, Romagnoli MF, Connolly ES, Jr. Ventriculostomy-related infections: a critical review of the literature. *Neurosurgery*. 2008;62 Suppl 2:688–700.

58. Brooks RA. A quantitative theory of the Hounsfield unit and its application to dual energy scanning. *J Comput Assist Tomogr*. 1977;1(4):487–93.

59. Salazar A, Tyroch AH, Smead DG. Electronic trauma patient outcomes assessment tool: performance improvement in the trauma intensive care unit. *J Trauma Nurs*. 2011;18(4):197–201.

60. Pronovost P, Needham D, Berenholtz S, Sinopoli D, Chu H, Cosgrove S, *et al*. An intervention to decrease catheter-related bloodstream infections in the ICU. *N Engl J Med*. 2006;355(26):2725–32.

61. Srinivasan M, Liederman E, Baluyot N, Jacoby R. Saving time, improving satisfaction: the impact of a digital radiology system on physician workflow and system efficiency. *J Healthc Inf Manag*. 2006;20(2):123–31.

62. Malhotra S, Jordan D, Shortliffe E, Patel VL. Workflow modeling in critical care: piecing together your own puzzle. *J Biomed Inform*. 2007;40(2):81–92.

63. Razzouk E, Cohen T, Almoosa K, Patel V. Approaching the limits of knowledge: the influence of priming on error detection in simulated clinical rounds. *AMIA Annu Symp Proc*. 2011;2011:1155–64.

64. Gawande A. The checklist. *New Yorker*. 2007;10 December.

CHAPTER 14

Electrophysiology in the intensive care unit

Neha S. Dangayach and Jan Claassen

The management of all critically ill patients relies heavily on continuous cardiac and respiratory monitoring but continuous neurological monitoring is not a standard of care for most intensive care unit (ICU) patients, although commonplace in the neurocritical care unit (NCCU). Clinical neurological examination by nurses and physicians is the cornerstone of neurological monitoring but may miss changes in neurological status in sedated patients and those with an impaired level of consciousness. Imaging studies, such as computed tomography (CT), magnetic resonance imaging (MRI), and Doppler ultrasound, like serial clinical examination, provide only a snapshot in time. Additional limitations, particularly for imaging studies, include contraindications to MRI such as pacemakers, supine positioning during the scan which may precipitate intracranial pressure (ICP) crises, in-hospital transportation of unstable critically ill patients, and the difficulty of monitoring some physiologic parameters, such as ICP, during the scan. Neurophysiological techniques such as electroencephalography allow continuous monitoring of the brain at the bedside, while electromyography and evoked potential studies can be conducted once or repeatedly as required. Medication effects, diurnal variations in level of consciousness or state changes, and structural lesions may add to the variability of neurophysiological monitoring data and necessitate contextual interpretation. Issues of practicality, including maintenance of high-quality recordings, artefacts inherent to the ICU, non-specificity of findings, controversial observations, and time-consuming interpretation must also be considered. However, neurophysiology offers diagnostic and monitoring information that is not available from other multimodal monitoring techniques. Each neurophysiological modality has been studied in different populations of critically ill patients, albeit some more extensively than others. Each has specific uses and limitations in critically ill neurological patients.

Electroencephalography

The electroencephalogram (EEG) reflects voltages generated by excitatory postsynaptic potentials from apical dendrites of synchronized neocortical pyramidal cells. Electrodes placed on the surface of the scalp are able to capture this electrical activity and identify different physiological states such as wakefulness and sleep, and to diagnose pathological electrical activity such as seizures and encephalopathic states. The EEG is described based on amplitude, frequency, symmetry, and patterns. Although amplitude is measured quantitatively in microvolts it is generally reported as low or high compared to normal or to a previously measured baseline. Frequency is measured in Hertz (Hz; cycles per second) and is generally characterized as slow or fast activity. There are four classical frequency bands—delta (< 4 Hz), theta (4–8 Hz), alpha (8–13 Hz), and beta (13–30 Hz)—that identify various physiological and behavioural states (Figure 14.1). Symmetry of the EEG from hemisphere to hemisphere can be assessed visually or by computer processing and is used to detect unilateral problems which often have a cerebrovascular origin. Specific EEG patterns such as those associated with seizures or herpes encephalitis can provide diagnostic information.

EEG montage

An EEG montage refers to the arrangement of the different electrodes that are placed to record electrical activity from different areas of the brain. EEG voltages are potential differences between two recording points and by convention electrically negative potentials are recorded as upward deflections on an EEG recording and positive potentials as downward deflections. The 10–20 system refers to a standardized agreement of electrode location on the scalp surface which provides a reproducible method for placing a relatively small number of EEG electrodes (typically 21) between different studies (Figure 14.2) (1). The American Clinical Neurophysiological Society has produced guideline statements on EEG and the clinical nomenclature used in various clinical situations including in the ICU (2). An adequate number of electrodes is essential to ensure that EEG activity from a small region of interest is recorded, and to analyse accurately the distribution of more diffuse activity. A smaller number of electrodes may be appropriate for special circumstances, but is not considered comprehensive. Occasionally, additional electrodes placed between or below those representing the standard placements are needed in order to record localized activity.

A grounding electrode should always be used except in situations (e.g. ICU and operating theatres) where other electrical equipment is attached to the patient and double grounding must be avoided. The patient ground electrode must be connected only to the appropriate jack of the input jack box and never to the equipment chassis or other earth ground. Interelectrode impedances should routinely be checked before recording and electrode impedance should normally not exceed 5000 Ohms (5 kΩ.) Electrode impedances should be re-checked during the recording if patterns that might be artefactual appear.

EEG can also be monitored using intracranial electrodes, either with subdural electrode arrays, also referred to as grids, or via intraparenchymal electrodes. Such invasive EEG electrode

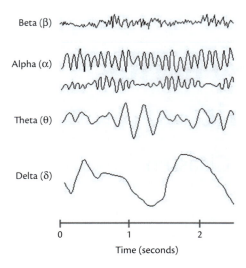

Fig. 14.1 Electroencephalogram waveforms. The electroencephalogram has been somewhat arbitrarily divided into four frequency ranges. From the highest to the lowest frequency these waves are:
- *Beta waves*—frequency range 15–30 Hertz and amplitude of about 30 μV
- *Alpha waves*—frequency range 8–14 Hz and amplitude of 30–50 μV
- *Theta waves*—frequency range 3–8 Hz and amplitude of 50–100 μV
- *Delta waves*—frequency range 0.5–4 Hz and amplitude of 100–200 μV.
A flat-line trace indicates no EEG activity.
Adapted from *The Brain From Top to Bottom*, http://thebrain.mcgill.ca, with permission. ⊚

configurations can yield additional information regarding specific origin of EEG signals which might otherwise be missed with standard scalp electrodes.

Types of EEG recordings

Based on the clinical scenario and available resources, different types of EEG monitoring can be chosen for recording in the ICU. These include spot or single EEG typically lasting no longer than 30 minutes, serial spot EEGs, continuous surface EEG monitoring

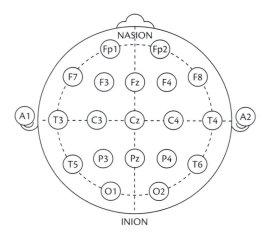

Fig. 14.2 The standard electroencephalogram montage. The 10–20 system is an internationally recognized technique to describe the position of scalp electrodes for EEG measurement, description, and interpretation. The 10 and 20 refer to the fact that the actual distances between adjacent electrodes are either 10% or 20% of the total front-to-back or right-to-left distance of the skull.
Figure from Wikimedia commons based on guidelines of the International Federation of Clinical Neurophysiology.

with or without quantitative EEG, and EEG with cortical or depth electrodes with or without other (multimodality) neuromonitoring. With advances in computer technology enabling digital recording and storage of large volumes of EEG data, neurophysiological monitoring has become more integrated with other neuromonitoring techniques.

Using only a single EEG recording in the ICU is similar to making a clinical assessment once only in a patient with a fluctuating neurological course. Serial or continuous EEG (cEEG) allows the identification of evolving EEG patterns and provides a better correlation with clinical course than a single recording. Logistic challenges for cEEG monitoring include cost and availability of technicians, equipment, and analytical software, maintenance of electrodes to allow high-quality recordings long term, and the availability of electrophysiologists to review and interpret the large volume of data produced (3). Despite these problems, cEEG monitoring provides a unique opportunity for the diagnosis and management of various disease states in the NCCU.

Some of the important applications of electrophysiological monitoring in the ICU setting are listed in Box 14.1.

Quantitative EEG

cEEG generates large amounts of data that are time-consuming to interpret, so quantitative EEG (qEEG) tools that allow rapid screening of long-term recordings have been developed (4). Many qEEG parameters are based on fast Fourier transformation (FFT) of the digital EEG signal and the creation of power spectra. FFT decomposes the EEG signal into power by frequency ranges, thereby generating a set of discrete data values that can be tracked over time. A Fourier transform converts time (or space) to frequency and vice versa, and a FFT allows rapid computation of such transformations. qEEG can be displayed either as numbers, or graphically as compressed spectral arrays (CSAs), histograms, or staggered arrays (Figure 14.3). qEEG graphs may reveal subtle changes over time that may not be evident when reviewing raw EEG data. Additionally, FFT-based power spectra can also be plotted as power in a specific frequency spectrum over total or different specific frequency spectra

---

Box 14.1 Applications of electrophysiological monitoring in the intensive care unit

- Diagnosis and management of status epilepticus
- Titration of antiepileptic and sedative medications
- Detection of non-convulsive seizures in patients with an unexplained decrease in level of consciousness
- Detection of periodic electrographic patterns diagnostic of certain disease states like herpes encephalitis or hepatic encephalopathy
- Detection of cerebral ischaemia, particularly due to vasospasm after subarachnoid haemorrhage
- Prognostication in comatose patients, for example, after traumatic brain injury or cardiac arrest
- Integration with multimodality monitoring in comatose patients, using both surface and depth electrode monitoring, after acute brain injury including high-grade subarachnoid haemorrhage or severe traumatic brain injury.

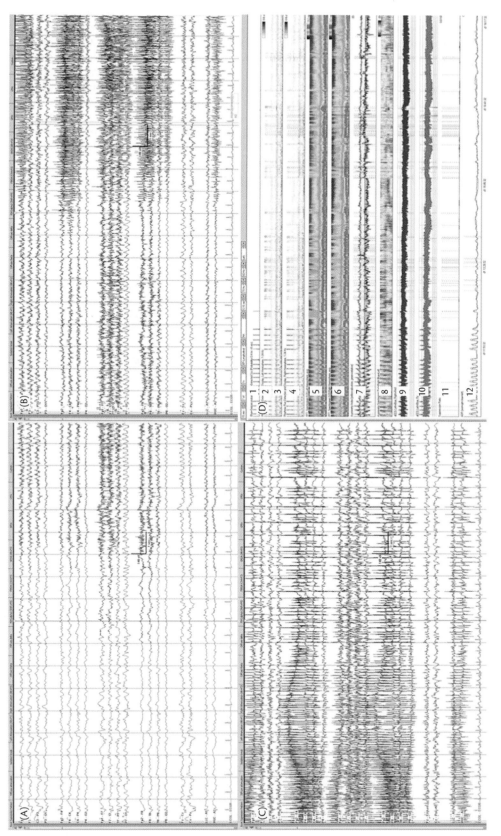

Fig. 14.3 A 47-year-old woman with a history of cerebral palsy, epilepsy controlled on carbamazepine was admitted with increasing seizures frequency associated with hyponatraemia and sub-therapeutic antiepileptic drug levels. Secondary generalized tonic–clonic seizures were controlled with carbamazepine, phenobarbital, levetiracetam, and phenytoin.

(A–C) Contiguous surface EEG recording displaying secondary generalized seizures.

(D) Quantitative EEG instruments:

Top row—seizure probability index.

Rows 2 and 3—rhythmic run detection and display (the darker colours indicate increasing rhythmicity).

Rows 4 and 5—compressed spectral array (darker > lighter indicates increased intensity, y-axis low to high frequencies).

Rows 6 and 7—asymmetry index.

Row 8—asymmetry relative spectrogram.

Rows 9 and 10—amplitude integrated interval.

Row 11—suppression ratio (duration of suppressed EEG; i.e. < 5 mv for > 0.5 s).

Row 12—alpha delta ratio (power of alpha frequency divided by delta frequency).

(e.g. alpha over delta ratio) or as spectral edge frequencies (e.g. the frequency below which 75% of the EEG record resides) (5,6).

Other EEG data reduction display formats include the cerebral function analysing monitor (CFAM), EEG density modulation, automated analysis of segmented EEG, and the bispectral index monitor (7,8). Rhythmicity indices, such as the rhythmic run detector (see Figure 14.3), indicate increasing periodic activity or rhythmicity (9). Spectral measures are well suited for signals with easily identifiable signatures in the frequency domain, while temporal recurrences in the time domain are useful for the detection of patterns which may have a much more complicated frequency domain representation because of compound morphologies or non-periodic repetitions. For complex signals, recurrence analysis provides a convenient and complementary measure to spectral characteristics that can be used either as a sole analysis method or to augment existing seizure detection or prediction algorithms. Applying more sophisticated analytical algorithms, such as empirical orthogonal functional analysis, to the spectral analysis data may further aid the detection of seizures and brain ischaemia (10). In practice, a combination of measures may yield the highest success rate for the analysis of the wide range of patterns of interest in acutely brain-injured patients. Detailed descriptions of the various qEEG methods have been published elsewhere (11–14).

With the advent of powerful microprocessors, data processing of this type can now be performed in real time at the bedside. qEEG analysis equipment is readily available and most manufacturers have integrated it to some extent into their software packages. Importantly, qEEG should never be interpreted in isolation but always in the context of the underlying raw EEG and always by those with proper training in electroencephalography. It is unrealistic to expect 24-hour coverage by a trained electroencephalographer in all NCCUs but it is now possible for well-trained NCCU staff to obtain qEEG recordings and seek interpretation through a web-based link from a remotely stationed specialist with access to at least one excerpt of the correlating raw EEG (15,16).

Automated seizure detection

Early seizure detection software was primarily based on machine learning algorithms and analyses of seizures in patients in epilepsy monitoring units (EMUs) with ictal activity that has a clear onset and offset, and easy to recognize changes in maximum EEG frequency. Unfortunately, artefacts and non-seizure related EEG changes result in low sensitivity and specificity for detecting seizures outside an EMU and particularly in the ICU. Further, seizures in the ICU are rarely classic in nature. Borderline-type seizure activity is frequently encountered leading to a high false-negative rate with automated seizure detection algorithms.(17) Additionally many EEG patterns encountered in the ICU do not fulfil classic seizure definitions and are often described by the term 'ictal-interictal continuum'(18). Compared to classic seizures these EEG patterns are less organized and lack clear on- and offset (3). Substantial research effort has been spent on defining such patterns unequivocally (10,19). Automated seizure detection software has been used on ICU EEG datasets to train algorithms and, anecdotally, appears to have increased specificity and sensitivity for seizure detection on the ICU. Again, none of the algorithms are sufficiently accurate to replace trained interpretation of the raw EEG and, given the variability of qEEG findings encountered following acute brain injury, there is some doubt that this will ever be accomplished.

Seizure detection programs make use of specialized EEG processing software that can be used to screen large amounts of cEEG data and mark sections containing activity that are suggestive of seizures. Based on an FFT analysis of the EEG, CSA graphs can be generated to determine the occurrence of subclinical seizures. Once the CSA 'signature' of a seizure in an individual patient has been determined it can quickly be used to screen a 24-hour recording and quantify the seizure frequency (20). Paroxysmal events may at times be identified using the CFAM, though the sensitivity of this system for detecting partial seizures is limited. Gotman and Vespa et al. have developed automated seizure detection algorithms with limited success (21,22).

Depth and surface EEG recording as part of multimodality monitoring

Invasive multimodality brain monitoring is increasingly used in comatose patients with severe brain injury and has many promising applications including early detection of evolving brain injury, prevention of secondary injury such as vasospasm, and individualizing treatment in the aftermath of acute brain injury. A number of different devices are available to measure and track either upstream effectors or downstream indicators of neuronal health, including neuronal activity, and brain tissue metabolism, oxygenation, and perfusion (23). These modalities are described in detail elsewhere in this book. Surface and depth EEG monitoring may become an integral part of multimodality monitoring, although few studies have investigated this to date (24–28).

Following acute brain injury, electrographic seizures have been associated with tachycardia, tachypnoea, elevated ICP, increased cerebral perfusion pressure (CPP), elevated lactate:pyruvate ratio monitored by microdialysis, reduction in jugular bulb oxygen saturation followed by decreasing partial brain tissue oxygenation, and a delayed increase in regional cerebral blood flow (CBF) (24–26,28,29). There may be differences between focal depth seizures (Figure 14.4) and more widespread seizures detected on surface EEG, with the latter requiring higher levels of cerebral glucose to be sustained (27). Depth seizures may be associated with a worse functional outcome than surface seizures and are clearly associated with a poorer prognosis than no seizures in the setting of a relatively preserved EEG background (27).

EEG applications

There are multiple applications for EEG monitoring in critically ill neurological patients.

Subclinical seizures and status epilepticus

Acute seizures and status epilepticus (SE) are common in all acute brain injury types and not restricted to patients with pre-existing epilepsy or those admitted with seizures or SE (Figure 14.5). A substantial proportion of seizures seen in the NCCU setting are non-convulsive in nature and therefore detectable only if EEG monitoring is employed. Although some patients with non-convulsive seizures (NCSz) may have very subtle clinical signs such as face and limb myoclonus, nystagmus, eye deviation, pupillary abnormalities, and autonomic instability (30–33), many have purely electrographic seizures (34,35). None of these clinical manifestations, even if present, are specific for NCSz and cEEG is necessary to confirm or refute the diagnosis of NCSz. The underlying aetiologies for convulsive SE and non-convulsive SE (NCSE) are similar and include structural brain lesions, infections, metabolic derangements,

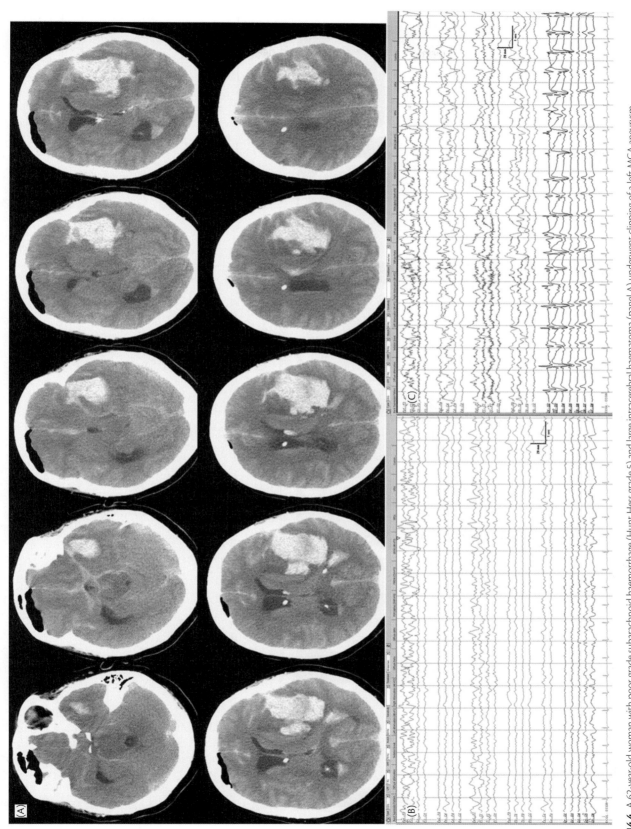

Fig. 14.4 A 62-year-old woman with poor grade subarachnoid haemorrhage (Hunt Hess grade 5) and large intracerebral haematoma (panel A) underwent clipping of a left MCA aneurysm.

(A) Cranial CT scan demonstrating large intracerebral haemorrhage.

(B) and (C) Surface EEGs are artefact contaminated but depth recordings at the bottom of the panels show intermittent runs of ictal discharges.

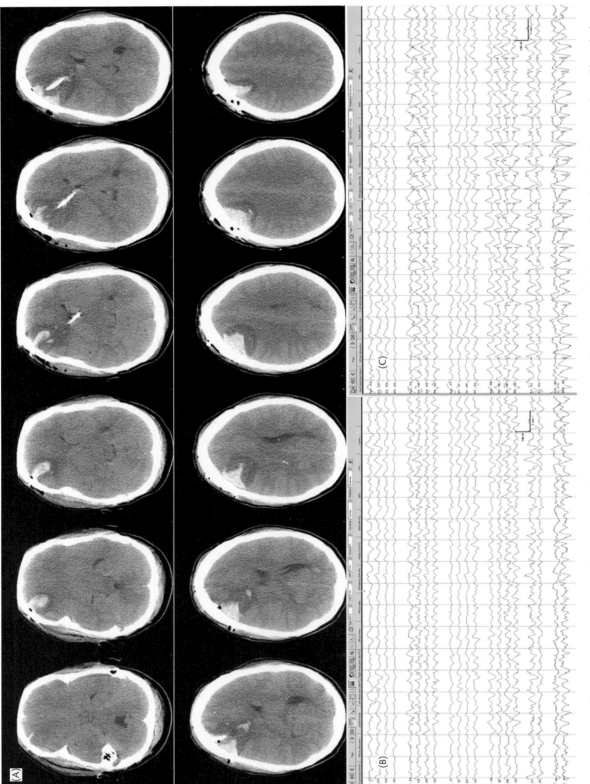

Fig. 14.5 A 30-year-old woman presented post-partum day 6 with decreased mental status. Her poor mental status persisted after clot evacuation and angiography suggested reversible cerebral vasoconstriction syndrome (Call–Flemming syndrome).

(A) Cranial CT shows a right frontal intracerebral haemorrhage.

(B) and (C) Surface EEG revealed ongoing electrographic seizures arising from the right hemisphere which were controlled by levetiracetam and phenytoin.

toxins, alcohol withdrawal and epilepsy, all of which are common diagnoses in the critically ill (36).

NCSz occur in 48% and NCSE in 14% of patients with generalized convulsive SE (GCSE) following control of convulsions (37). In ICUs, patients without any clinical signs of seizure activity, and after excluding those with a history of neurological disease, 8% have been reported to have NCSE (35,38). However, in the NCCU, up to 34% patients may have NCSz and up to 76% NCSE (39). Patients receiving continuous intravenous antiepileptic drugs (AEDs) for the treatment of refractory SE should always be monitored with cEEG since subclinical seizures may occur in more than half during treatment. Further, the majority of such patients have subclinical seizures after discontinuation of therapy and cEEG should therefore be monitored to detect or exclude ongoing seizure activity in any patient who does not quickly regain consciousness after a convulsive seizure. This includes those who are sedated and/or paralysed during the treatment of SE in whom level of consciousness cannot be assessed adequately.

NCSE is associated with high morbidity and mortality in critically ill patients (40–43). Experimental models and pathological studies confirming neuronal damage from SE pertain primarily to GCSE and, as no randomized controlled study has conclusively proven that treating NCSz or NCSE alters outcome, it is not entirely clear if treating these EEG phenomena is beneficial. However, overwhelming evidence has emerged that NCSz and NCSE have potential to further damage the injured brain. Studies have demonstrated elevations of neuron-specific enolase (NSE) (44,45), brain interstitial glutamate (25), lactate:pyruvate ratio (46,47), and ICP (47), brain tissue hypoxia (29,46), increasing mass effect (47–49), and hippocampal atrophy on follow-up MRI (50) after NCSz and NCSE.

Duration of monitoring

There are no prospective studies that have evaluated different durations of cEEG monitoring in patients with SE. One compared routine EEG to continuous video EEG and found that routine EEG monitoring detected fewer than half of electrographic seizures identified by cEEG (11% versus 27%) (51). In a retrospective analysis of electrographic data obtained from patients with depressed conscious level from an undetermined cause, 20% did not have a first seizure until after 24 hours of monitoring and 13% until more than 48 hours after monitoring was begun (52). However, the yield from further cEEG monitoring is low in a patient not in coma if no clinical or electrographic ictal activity is detected within the first 24 hours of monitoring (34). Recently published guidelines recommend that delays in initiating cEEG monitoring should be minimized as the cumulative duration of SE affects neurological outcomes and mortality (53). These guidelines further recommend at least 48 hours of monitoring for comatose patients with acute brain injury and at least 24 hours for those not in coma.

EEG findings

Efforts are underway to standardize, at least for research purposes, definitions of ictal and ictal-interictal EEG patterns (19). A wide range of epileptiform discharges has been described following SE (54,55), and controversy exists regarding the interpretation and therapeutic implications of periodic epileptiform discharges (PEDs) that do not meet formal seizure criteria (18,56). Periodic lateralized epileptiform discharges (PLEDs) may be both ictal and interictal (57,58) and additional information regarding their nature can be

Table 14.1 Common electroencephalographic patterns

EEG pattern	Clinical association
PLEDS	Acute ischaemic stroke
	Herpes encephalitis
FIRDA	ICP dysregulation
	Hydrocephalus after SAH
Alpha or beta coma	Treatment with barbiturates or benzodiazepines
Generalized slowing	Metabolic encephalopathies
Triphasic waves	Metabolic encephalopathies
Burst suppression	Induced by propofol, barbiturates, or benzodiazepines in the treatment of SE
	Post-cardiac arrest
Arrhythmic theta/delta activity	Various medications

FIRDA, frontal intermittent rhythmic delta; PLEDs, periodic lateralized epileptiform discharges; SAH, subarachnoid haemorrhage.

determined by using serial EEG data (55,59), focal hyperperfusion on single-photon-emission CT (60), and increased metabolism on fluorodeoxyglucose positron emission tomography (61). PEDs may represent ictal activity in the comatose patient if they are associated with some type of evolution in frequency, amplitude, and location. Supplementary testing, including a trial of benzodiazepines, imaging, measurement of serum markers, and invasive brain monitoring, may guide the physician in managing patients with these EEG findings (62).

The importance of focal findings and EEG pattern recognition in critical care lies in generating appropriate differential diagnoses and prognosis, and some common EEG patterns are shown in Table 14.1. Another frequent EEG pattern in encephalopathic ICU patients is ictal or interictal appearing activity that is triggered by stimulation or arousal. This evoked activity is typically on the ictal-interictal continuum and has been termed stimulus-induced rhythmic, periodic, or ictal discharges (SIRPIDs) (63). As with most ICU seizures there is usually no clinical correlate, although a small portion of patients do exhibit focal motor seizures that are consistently elicited by alerting stimuli (64).

Metabolic and infectious encephalopathy

Critically ill patients are susceptible to many toxic, metabolic, and electrolyte imbalances that may cause both mental status changes and seizures. The incidence of non-convulsive seizures in conditions such as hypo- and hyperglycaemia, hyponatraemia, hypocalcaemia, drug intoxication or withdrawal, uraemia, liver dysfunction, hypertensive encephalopathy, and sepsis has been variably reported to lie between 55% and 22% (41). Sepsis and acute kidney injury may also be associated with electrographic seizures (36,40). While certain periodic discharges are more closely related to systemic metabolic abnormalities, such as triphasic waves in hepatic encephalopathy, the significance of others such as PLEDs, recently renamed as lateralized periodic discharges (LPDs), is controversial.

A benzodiazepine trial may be useful to differentiate ictal from non-ictal EEG patterns in selected critically ill patients. However, almost all periodic discharges including periodic triphasic waves seen in metabolic encephalopathy are attenuated by benzodiazepines (65) and, unless there is clinical improvement accompanying the EEG change, the test remains non-diagnostic. Unfortunately, clinical improvement can take a substantial amount of time even if the EEG activity of NCSE is aborted with benzodiazepines and it is important to recognize that lack of immediate clinical improvement does not exclude NCSE and that the use of benzodiazepines simply helps determine its presence or absence.

Traumatic brain injury

Between 15% and 22% of patients with moderate or severe traumatic brain injury (TBI) develop convulsive seizures and although the incidence of NCSz is less well-studied rates between 18% and 28% have been reported (66–68). As well as being used to diagnose seizures, EEG monitoring after TBI may be used to monitor clinical course, to guide titration of sedative medications (particularly during the management of raised ICP) and to diagnose post-traumatic complications. The goal is to individualize therapeutic approaches in order to detect and treat secondary brain injury as early as possible and prevent further ischaemic damage (69). Craniotomy defects create breach artefact (i.e. higher amplitude of EEG activity due to the skull defect) and scalp oedema and subgaleal haemorrhages may lead to attenuation of the EEG, and must be taken into account when interpreting the EEG after TBI.

High-dose benzodiazepines, propofol, or barbiturate infusions may be needed to manage intracranial hypertension after TBI and EEG may be used as an endpoint of such therapy. Burst suppression has been proposed as a titration goal during such treatment. A simple two-channel left and right hemisphere recording is sufficient to titrate the therapeutic dose needed to induce burst suppression, monitor steady-state conditions, and avoid unnecessarily high doses which may result in significant cardiovascular side effects.

A number of EEG findings are associated with outcome following TBI including seizures, periodic discharges, lack of sleep architecture, and EEG reactivity. A qEEG monitoring approach using changes in the EEG variability has been used to predict outcome after TBI (70,71). In this study, data reduction was achieved by focusing on the percentage of alpha-frequencies (PA) at multiple electrodes and determination of PA variability (PAV) over time. A low PAV, and particularly a decrease in PAV over time, strongly correlated with fatal outcome especially in patients presenting with low Glasgow Coma Scale (GCS) score. In particular, PAV during the initial 3 days after injury was significantly associated with outcome independent of clinical and radiological variables. Another interesting approach to outcome prediction after TBI utilizes EEG background attenuation and low-amplitude EEEG events (72). In a study of 32 TBI patients, periods of EEG suppression were quantification to derive the EEG silence ratio (ESR), and outcome at 6 month was closely related to the ESR during the first 4 days after injury (73). Limitations of this method include artificial increases of the ESR by some sedative agents, and ESR monitoring is most useful in comatose TBI patients undergoing sedation with benzodiazepines and opioids. In the Co-operative Study for Brain Depolarisation (COSBID), patients with TBI underwent electrocorticographic recordings with subdural electrodes and prolonged depolarizations were associated with isoelectricity or PEDs, prolonged depression of spontaneous activity, and occurrence in temporal clusters, all of which were associated with poor prognosis (74).

Subarachnoid haemorrhage

In patients with SAH, seizures may occur at the time of the ictus, at any point during the hospital stay, and long after discharge.

While the underlying mechanisms differ, all seizures are associated with worse outcome after SAH. Studies have reported convulsive seizures rates of 4–9% at the time of the initial bleed often in the setting of a focal clot or rebleeding episode (75). However, several more recent cEEG studies suggest that the incidence of electrographic seizures following SAH, especially in comatose patients, is actually much higher. In the Columbia series of 570 patients who underwent cEEG for altered mental status or suspicion of seizures, 19% of 108 SAH patients had seizures, primarily NCSz, and 70% of the patients with seizures went on to develop NCSE (76).

Quantitative analysis of cEEG has been used to detect delayed cerebral ischaemia (DCI) after SAH (Figure 14.6) (70,76,77). The qEEG parameter that best correlates with clinically significant ischaemia is controversial but most authors agree that using a ratio of fast over slow activity (e.g. alpha over delta activity, or relative alpha variability) is the most practical approach (12,13,70) A number of qEEG parameters including trend analysis of total power (1–30 Hz) (77), variability of relative alpha (6–14 Hz/1–20 Hz) (70), and post-stimulation alpha:delta ratio (PSADR, 8–13 Hz/1–4 Hz) (76) have been shown to correlate with DCI or angiographic vasospasm. In a retrospective study of 34 poor-grade SAH patients monitored from postoperative day 2–14, a reduction in the post-stimulation ratio of alpha and delta frequency with a power of greater than 10% relative to baseline in six consecutive epochs of cEEG was 100% sensitive and 76% specific for DCI, whilst a reduction of more than 50% in a single epoch was 89% sensitive and 84% specific (76). All studies have found that focal ischaemia sometimes results in global or bilateral changes in the EEG, and importantly that EEG changes may precede clinical deterioration by several days (70). Rathakrishnan and colleagues measured relative alpha power and variability in the anterior brain quadrants and termed this the composite alpha index (CAI) (78). In 12 patients with DCI, the sensitivity of predicting clinical deterioration with cEEG improved from 40% to 67%, and clinical improvement from 8% to 50%, using this modification of more usual methods. In three patients in this study, cEEG was predictive of deterioration more than 24 hours prior to clinical changes. Tracking the daily mean alpha power accurately has also been used to identify DCI recurrence and poor responders to first-line therapy at pre-clinical stages (79). A small feasibility study reported that intracortical mini-depth electrodes may have a role in detecting ischaemia from vasospasm in poor-grade SAH patients, and that it may be superior to scalp EEG and allow automated detection, particularly using the alpha:delta ratio (80). cEEG monitoring provides independent prognostic information in patients with poor-grade SAH, even after controlling for clinical and radiological findings, and unfavourable findings include PEDS, electrographic SE, and the absence of sleep architecture (81).

The combined use of somatosensory evoked potentials (SSEPs) and cEEG monitoring is a unique example of dynamic brain monitoring (82). The temporal variation of these two parameters evaluated by continuous monitoring can establish whether treatments are properly tailored to the neurological changes induced by the lesions responsible for secondary brain damage. Using a logistic regression model, progressive deterioration on the basis of EEG was associated with a 24% increased risk of dying compared to no worsening of the EEG (82). SSEP changes were also significantly associated with outcome; for patients with worsening SSEPs, the odds of dying increased to approximately 32%.

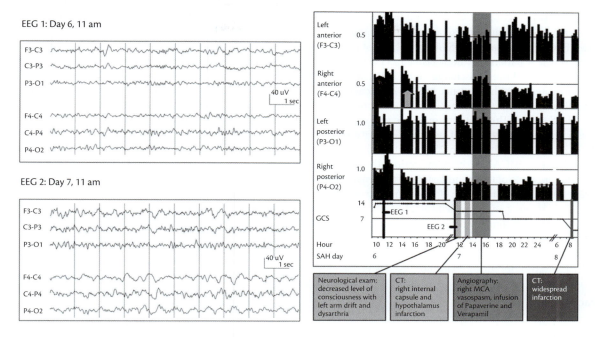

Fig. 14.6 Detection of delayed cerebral ischaemia from vasospasm after subarachnoid haemorrhage. A 57-year-old woman was admitted with acute subarachnoid haemorrhage (admission Hunt–Hess grade 4) from a right posterior communicating aneurysm that was clipped. cEEG was performed from SAH days 3 to 8 (right panel). The alpha:delta ratio (ADR) progressively decreased after day 6, particularly in the right anterior region (thick vertical grey arrow), to settle into a steady trough level later that night, reflecting loss of fast frequencies and increased slowing over the right hemisphere in the raw cEEG. On day 7, the GCS dropped from 14 to 12 and a CT scan showed a right internal capsule and hypothalamic infarction. Angiography demonstrated severe distal right MCA and left vertebral artery spasm intra-arterial verapamil and papaverine were infused. This resulted in a marked but transient increase of the right anterior and posterior alpha/delta ratios (right panel).

Reprinted from *Clinical Neurophysiology*, 115, 12, Claassen J *et al.*, 'Quantitative continuous EEG for detecting delayed cerebral ischemia in patients with poor-grade subarachnoid hemorrhage', pp. 2699–2710, Copyright 2004, with permission from Elsevier.

Intracerebral haemorrhage

ICH is associated with a 3–19% rate of in-hospital convulsive seizures (49,83–86), and 18–21% of patients have cEEG-confirmed NCSz (48,49). Vespa et al. demonstrated that NCSz were associated with increased midline shift and a trend toward worse outcome even after controlling for haemorrhage volume (48). In another study, Claassen et al. found that NCSz were associated with haematoma expansion and mass effect and a trend towards poorer outcome (49). In addition, PEDs were an independent predictor of poor outcome after ICH but it remains unclear whether their presence should change management.

Ischaemic stroke

It has long been known that cerebral infarction may result in polymorphic delta activity, loss of fast activity and sleep spindles and focal EEG attenuation. These EEG findings reflect abnormal CBF and cerebral metabolic rate of oxygen as demonstrated by positron emission tomography and xenon-CT-CBF imaging (87,88). EEG is very sensitive for ischaemia and usually demonstrates changes at the time of reversible neuronal dysfunction when CBF is in the 25–30 mL/100 g/min range (89). It is also very sensitive at detecting restoration of blood flow and may demonstrate recovery of brain function from reperfusion earlier than the clinical examination (90).

A population-based cEEG study in 177 patients with acute ischaemic stroke (AIS) reported a 7% incidence of seizures (> 70% of them NCSz) in the acute (within 24 hours) phase (86), and hospital-based studies have reported rates of acute clinical seizures following ischaemic stroke ranging from 2% to 9% (83,84). Acute clinical seizures are associated with increased mortality after AIS (83,84,91,92). In a prospective study of 232 stroke patients (177 ischaemic and 55 haemorrhagic strokes), EEG recording was performed within 24 hours of admission to hospital and follow-up lasted 1 week (93). Fifteen patients (6.5%) had early (within 24 hours) seizures and ten of these had focal SE with or without secondary generalization. There were sporadic epileptiform focal abnormalities in 10% and PLEDs in 6%. SE was identified in more than 70% of the patients with PLEDs and multivariate analysis confirmed that early epileptic manifestations were independently associated with PLEDs (93).

EEG may be of additional value by confirming or excluding definite stroke after resolution of symptoms in lacunar and posterior circulation syndromes of presumed ischaemic origin, and for prognostication of short-term functional status in lacunar and anterior circulation syndromes (94,95) In the subacute setting of ischaemic stroke, EEG may be of prognostic value for disability, dependency, and death at 6 months. In a study of 110 ischaemic stroke patients, the pairwise-derived Brain Symmetry Index (pdBSI) and (delta + theta)/(alpha + beta) ratio (DTABR) were significantly correlated with the modified Rankin Scale (mRS) score at 6 months (96). Dependency was independently predicted by the National Institute for Health Stroke Scale (NIHSS) and DTABR with odds ratios (ORs) of 1.22 and 2.25 respectively. Six-month mortality was independently associated with age at stroke onset (OR 1.18), NIHSS (OR 1.11), and DTABR (OR 2.04).

In a study of EEG power spectra analysis, six of ten patients displayed a peak in the EEG power spectrum at 5–10 Hz and all six had a Glasgow outcome score (GOS) of 3 and level of consciousness (LOC) score of 7 or higher at discharge, whereas the patients without faster EEG activity had a GOS of 2 and LOC of 6 or lower (97). In contrast, the 4 patients without faster EEG activity had a GOS of 2 and LOC 6 or lower. Discharge GOS, LOC, and NIHSS significantly correlated with the presence of 5- to 10-Hz activity but not with age, time to hemicraniectomy, duration of hospital stay, or baseline NIHSS scores. Three-month outcome was significantly correlated with age and the presence of faster EEG activity. In a prospective study of cEEG monitoring in 25 patients with malignant middle cerebral artery (MCA) territory infarction, the absence of delta activity and presence of theta and fast beta frequencies within the focus were found to be predictive of a benign course, whereas diffuse generalized slowing and slow delta activity in the ischaemic hemisphere predicted a malignant course (98). Decrease in CPP is associated with a reduction in faster EEG activity (99) and rapid improvements in background EEG activity have been observed when CPP/CBF increase following mannitol therapy or haemodilution (100,101).

Post-cardiac arrest

In patients with post-cardiac arrest hypoxic-ischaemic encephalopathy, the presence of seizures has important prognostic value and may also be a contributor to decreased conscious level (102). In addition, as therapeutic hypothermia is more widely implemented after cardiac arrest (see Chapter 25), cEEG may become an important tool for identifying NCSz especially during re-warming (103). Convulsive and non-convulsive SE is common in comatose post-cardiac arrest patients undergoing therapeutic hypothermia and most seizures occur within 12 hours. About 20–35% of cardiac arrest patients develop NCSz and NCS (34,104,105) and outcomes are poor in those who go on to NCSE and convulsive SE (102,106,107).

In patients treated with hypothermia after cardiac arrest, EEG monitoring during the first 24 hours after resuscitation can contribute to the prediction of both good and poor neurological outcome. Low-voltage EEG after 24 hours predicts poor outcome with a sensitivity almost twice that of the bilateral absence of SSEP responses (108). EEG reactivity has a particularly high predictive accuracy for outcome after cardiac arrest in those treated with hypothermia (109). In a study of 111 patients with prolonged coma, continuous amplitude-integrated EEG and SSEP monitoring, repeated sampling of NSE and brain MRI were undertaken (110). In patients with NSE blood concentration greater than 33 ng/mL, all ten who underwent MRI had extensive brain injury, 12 of 16 had absent cortical responses on SSEP monitoring, and all six who underwent autopsy had extensive severe histological damage. NSE levels also correlated with EEG pattern but less uniformly because only 11 of 17 patients with NSE blood concentration less than 33 ng/mL had electrographic SE, although only one recovered. A reactive cEEG pattern correlated with NSE blood concentration less than 33 ng/mL. In summary, hypothermia-treated cardiac arrest patients with good neurological outcome have different early qEEG suppression and epileptiform activity compared to those with poor outcome (110).

A scoring system based on a combination of clinical and EEG findings has been used to predict the absence of early cortical SSEP response and, in settings without access to SSEPs, may aid decision-making in a subset of comatose cardiac arrest survivors (111). In 192 post-cardiac arrest patients of whom 103 were hypothermic and 89 normothermic, myoclonic SE was invariably associated with death as were malignant EEG patterns and global cerebral oedema on cranial CT scan (112). qEEG and auditory P300 event-related potentials were studied in 42 conscious survivors of cardiac arrest 3 months after the incident and no difference was found in any assessment of cognitive function between those treated with hypothermia and normothermia (113). Sixty-seven per cent of patients in the hypothermia group and 44% in the normothermia group were cognitively intact or had only very mild impairment, whereas severe cognitive deficits were present in 15% and 28% of patients in the hypothermia and normothermia groups respectively. All qEEG parameters were more normal in the hypothermia-treated group, but these differences did not reach statistical significance.

Postoperative patients

Seizures can occur in any postoperative setting in which there is an acute neurological injury, a high risk of metabolic derangement, or neurotoxicity. Postoperative cEEG monitoring may be indicated in selected patients undergoing surgery for supratentorial lesions or those with pre-existing epilepsy (114,115). Other high-risk groups for seizure development include patients undergoing cardiac surgery (116) and solid organ transplantation (117,118), although the incidence of NCSz and NCSE in these patient groups has not been studied systematically.

Evoked potentials

Evoked potentials (EPs) are used for diagnosis and monitoring in the ICU and operating theatre. EPs are electrical potentials recorded from the nervous system following presentation of a stimulus and evaluate conduction along neural pathways. EPs can be auditory, visual, or electrical and are essentially an event (stimulus)-gated averaged EEG recording. The amplitude of EPs is orders of magnitude smaller than EEG signals and requires signal averaging and precise localization of the recording electrode to measure a response (119). For example, when measuring a SSEP multiple stimuli are applied rapidly and the cortical responses from a fixed time segment (e.g. 0–120 milliseconds) following the stimuli are averaged. The EEG signal averages out at each time point following the stimulus, whereas the peaks and troughs of the evoked response increase in amplitude. At the end of the repetitive simulations the average of all the time segments produces the displayed EP. Diagnostic EPs are evaluated on the basis of their latency and amplitudes of the waveform peaks and troughs compared to laboratory-established norms in healthy individuals, or to contralateral recordings in an individual patient. In the operating theatre, EPs are compared to initial baselines.

SSEPs allow assessment of the integrity of different sensory pathways from the periphery to the central integrator. The latency is the time taken for a stimulus to travel between two measurement points, such as between the stimulating electrode and the cortical recording electrode, and is expressed in milliseconds. The amplitude is typically reported in microvolts (μV) and, by convention, negative signals are displayed as upward deflections and positive as downward. SSEPs are the second most frequently used electrophysiological investigation after EEG in the NCCU and are less affected by sedation and hypothermia than EEG (120). EPs have many other advantages over EEG and other techniques and these are summarized in Box 14.2 (121).

<table>
<tr><td>Box 14.2</td><td>Advantages of evoked potential monitoring</td></tr>
</table>

Box 14.2 Advantages of evoked potential monitoring

- Non-invasive
- May be used serially
- Provides objective quantitative values that can be tracked over time and compared between patients
- Relatively stable in the presence of mild hypothermia
- Relatively resistant to many commonly used sedatives
- Provides information about subcortical structures
- Inexpensive.

On the downside, significant technical expertise is required to record and interpret EPs, strict grounding and electrical safety procedures have to be followed, and in awake patients EPs may be perceived as painful.

Types of evoked potentials

Evoked potentials can be sensory or motor and there are several types of sensory EPs.

Somatosensory evoked potentials

SSEPs test the integrity of the dorsal column-lemniscal system (121). This pathway is responsible for carrying light touch, vibration, and deep proprioception via the sensory component of spinal nerves to the dorsal root ganglion and then via the dorsal column of the spinal cord to the cuneate (upper extremities) and gracilis nuclei (lower extremities), both located in the lower brainstem. The tracts cross over at the level of the medulla and project via the medial lemniscus to the ventroposterior lateral thalamus and then to the primary somatosensory cortex Brodmann area 3,2,1 and finally to a wide network of cortical areas involved in somatosensory processing. Although different peripheral spinal nerves can be used for assessing the integrity of the dorsal column-medial leminscal system, the median and tibial nerves are most often stimulated during SSEP monitoring (Table 14.2).

The SSEP stimulus is a brief electric pulse delivered by a pair of electrodes placed on the skin above the relevant nerve, with a ground electrode placed between the stimulation and the recording sites. The recording electrodes can be standard disc or plate electrodes. For upper limb median nerve SSEP recording, stimulating electrodes are placed over the anterolateral wrist area. Recording electrodes are located at the clavicle between the heads of the sternocleidomastoid muscles (Erb's point) to confirm transmission of the impulse from the peripheral nerve, on the skin overlying cervical bodies 6–7 to confirm entry into the central nervous system and over the cortex to identify the cortical potential. Cortical recording electrodes are placed according to the international 10–20 system depending on the stimulated nerve. For example, CP3 and CP4 are used for median nerve SSEPs. For tibial nerve SSEPs, stimulating electrodes are placed at the ankle between the Achilles tendon and medial malleolus and recording electrodes in the popliteal fossa, over the lumbar vertebra and over the cortex. This electrode configuration produces a standard pattern of EP waveforms from each recording electrode (Figure 14.7). For clinical purposes the early responses, known as 'short latency' SSEP signals, are used. These are usually the waveforms recorded at about 20 milliseconds after

Table 14.2 Normal values for evoked potentials from healthy volunteers

	Recording site	Latency, mean (ms)	Latency, upper limit (ms)
Median SSEP			
N9	Erb's point (brachial plexus)	9.8	11.5
N13	Cervical spine (C7)	13.3	14.5
N20	Contralateral cortex (CP3 or CP4)	19.8	23.0
Intervals median			
CCT (P14–N20)	—	5.6	6.6
Tibial SSEP			
N8	Popliteal fossa	8.5	10.5
N22	Lumbar spine (L1)	21.8	25.2
P30	Fz–Cv7	29.2	34.7
P39	Cz–Fz	38.0	43.9
Intervals tibial			
N22–P30	—	7.4	10.2
P30–P39	—	8.7	13.4

CCT, central conduction time; SSEP, somatosensory evoked potential.

This table was published in *Monitoring in Neurocritical Care*, Le Roux P *et al.* (eds), 'Brainstem Auditory Evoked Potentials and Somatosensory Evoked Potentials', Carrera E *et al.*, pp. 175, Copyright Elsevier 2010.

stimulation and designated N20. The later signal components are more susceptible to the effects of medications and level of consciousness. Although they are currently neglected during clinical monitoring, they carry significant information that may be utilized in the future (121).

At least two bipolar channels (e.g. CPz–FPz and CP3–CP4) should be used to record the cortical component of the SSEP whose waveform is obtained by averaging between 500 and 2000 stimuli. It is necessary to repeat at least two independent averages to demonstrate reproducibility. SSEPs are recorded using a broad pass-band filter with high-pass and low-pass filters typically set to 30 and 2000 Hz respectively. Notch filters are used to eliminate electrical noise (60 Hz) but can sometimes produce an oscillatory 'ringing' artefact.

Brainstem auditory evoked potentials

Brainstem auditory evoked potentials (BAEPs) are produced by an auditory stimulus which activates the cochlea, auditory nerve, and the brainstem auditory pathways (122). The first 10 milliseconds of the recorded signal represent conduction of the stimulus through the brainstem and this is the BAEP (122). Recording electrodes are placed between Cz (according to the international 10–20 system) and the ipsilateral ear. The normal BAEP typically shows five to six waves which are attributed to different generators and labelled with corresponding Roman numerals (Figure 14.8):

- Wave I—auditory nerve
- Wave II—auditory nerve as it exits the porus acoustics or the cochlear nerve

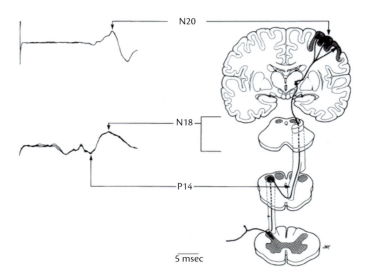

Fig. 14.7 Median nerve somatosensory evoked potential (SSEP) recording. From the bottom of the figure upwards, the four anatomical sections are:
- cervical spinal cord axial section
- brainstem axial section
- midbrain axial section
- brain coronal section including basal ganglia and cortex.

The waveforms reflect recording made from cortical and cervical electrodes.

This figure was published in *Monitoring in Neurocritical Care*, Le Roux P *et al.* (eds), 'Brainstem Auditory Evoked Potentials and Somatosensory Evoked Potentials', Carrera E *et al.*, pp. 175, Copyright Elsevier 2010.

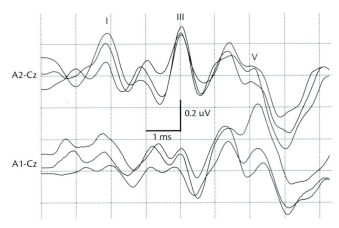

Fig. 14.8 Brainstem auditory evoked potentials (BAEPs). The figure shows a BAEP in response to a 90 db click in a 49-year-old woman with a right frontal brain tumour. Although the exact identity of short-latency BAEP waveforms remains somewhat uncertain, commonly recognized generators include:
- the distal auditory nerve (wave I)
- the auditory nerve as it exits the porus acousticus or the cochlear nucleus (wave II)
- the cochlear nucleus or ipsilateral superior olivary nucleus (wave III)
- the superior olivary nucleus or axons of the lateral lemniscus (wave IV)
- the inferior colliculus and ventral lateral lemniscus (wave V).

Because waves II and IV are less reliably recorded across individuals, clinical interpretation is based primarily on assessment of waves I, III, and V.

This figure was published in Carrera E *et al.*, 'Evoked Potentials', in LeRoux PD *et al.* (eds), *Monitoring in Neurocritical Care*, Copyright Elsevier 2013.

- ◆ Wave III—cochlear nucleus or ipsilateral superior olivary nucleus
- ◆ Wave IV—superior olivary nucleus or axons of lateral lemniscus
- ◆ Wave V—inferior colliculus and ventral lateral lemniscus.

The stimulus used to generate a BAEP consists of a brief 'click', typically delivered at approximately 10 Hz. The stimuli are presented to one ear at a time using headphones or ear inserts whilst the non-stimulated ear is 'masked' with white hissing noise to prevent sound stimulation being conducted through the cranium. Standard surface or needle electrodes may be used to record BAEPs which are typically recorded using a two-channel montage from the ipsilateral ear to vertex (channel 1) and contralateral ear to vertex (channel 2). Averaging of 2000–4000 stimuli is typically required and, as with SSEPs, at least two independent averages must be recorded to prove reproducibility of waveforms. BAEPs are recorded using a broad pass-band filter with the high-pass filter typically set to 100 Hz or 150 Hz and the low-pass filter to 3000 Hz.

If the auditory nerve is damaged, wave I will be absent. The absence of waves II–V with a recordable wave I indicates structural or functional disruption of the auditory pathway between the site of the absent wave and the auditory cortex.

Visual evoked potentials

Visual evoked responses (VEPs) are monitored from a recording electrode over or near to the visual cortex following the application of a visual stimuli such as a flashing light or a flickering checkerboard (123). Measured from the primary recording electrodes over the primary visual cortex, these stimuli typically produced a negative deflection at approximately 75 milliseconds (N75) and a positive deflection at approximately 100 milliseconds (P100). VEPs are rarely used in the ICU.

Motor evoked potentials

Motor evoked potential (MEPs) interrogate the integrity of the motor pathway and are primarily used in the operating theatre. They are generated using magnetic stimulation at or close to the primary motor cortex and recorded from electrodes placed in relevant muscles. MEPs are rarely used in the ICU.

Evoked potential monitoring in the intensive care unit

In the ICU, EPs are primarily used for prognostication, particularly after cardiac arrest and TBI. Diagnostically, they have largely been replaced by imaging studies, invasive neuromonitoring (e.g. brain tissue oxygen monitoring and cerebral microdialysis) and cEEG. However, serial and even continuous EP monitoring is possible (120,124) and may be considered where continuous invasive or other non-invasive neuromonitoring modalities are of limited value or contraindicated such as in evolving spinal cord or brainstem injury. The reader is referred to recently published consensus recommendations for the use of EPs in the ICU for further information (125).

Technical considerations

There are many issues that must be taken into account during EP monitoring on the ICU.

Effect of sedative medications

The subcortical components of EPs are relatively unaffected by level of consciousness and sedative medications but the cortical components are more easily depressed in a dose-dependent manner (126,127). However, interpeak changes are more stable and comparing left- and right-sided recordings may be useful, particularly during SSEP monitoring. Neuromuscular blockade does not affect SSEPs, VEPs, or BAEPs but is contraindicated during MEP monitoring (119).

Electrical artefact

Electrical artefact or 'noise' may interfere with recordings in the ICU and this will influence the accuracy and interpretation of the recordings (128). Notch filters may eliminate electrical artefact but can introduce a 'ringing' oscillatory artefact.

Hypothermia

Therapeutic temperature modulation or mild therapeutic hypothermia is increasingly being used in the ICU. The prognostic accuracy of EP variables that have been associated with outcome, such as the N20 SSEP after cardiac arrest, is not significantly affected by mild hypothermia (33°C) (129).

Risks

EP studies are non-invasive and considered safe. However, several ICU-specific considerations regarding electrical safety must be kept in mind (130). ICU patients are at a high risk for electrical injury and induction of cardiac arrhythmias and, to reduce these risks, all electrical equipment must be appropriately grounded (122).

Indications

There are several indications for EP monitoring in the ICU.

Post-cardiac arrest

EPs can be used for prognostication after cardiac arrest and absence of short latency (N20) SSEPs is the most reliable predictor of poor outcome in anoxic-ischaemic encephalopathy. Neurological examination does not reliably predict the presence or absence of specific SSEP patterns, particularly the N20 responses (131). In a meta-analysis of 4500 patients with post-cardiac arrest cerebral anoxia, bilaterally absent N20s within the first week had 100% specificity for the prediction of poor outcome (132). A prospective study of 407 cardiac arrest patients demonstrated bilaterally absent N20s in 45% of patients who were comatose at 72 hours and all of these had poor outcome (133).

Combining SSEPs with other predictors of outcome after cardiac arrest, such as EEG or serum markers of neuronal injury, improves prognostic accuracy (134,135). However, whilst some predictions can be made for poor recovery it is much more difficult to predict good outcome. In a prospective study of 111 cardiac arrest patients who underwent therapeutic hypothermia, none with absent SSEPs 24 hours after discontinuation of sedation had a favourable neurological outcome (109). In a retrospective study of 185 post-cardiac arrest patients treated with therapeutic hypothermia, 36 had bilaterally absent SSEPs and only one made a good recovery (136). In a smaller control study of 60 cardiac arrest patients, 30 of whom underwent therapeutic hypothermia, no patient (in either hypothermia or normothermia groups) with absent SSEPs at 24 hours post arrest regained consciousness (129). In contrast, a recent study reported recovery of consciousness and normal cognitive function in two post-cardiac arrest patients treated with hypothermia with absent or minimally detectable cortical N20 responses on day 3 after arrest (136). In summary, SSEPs have a high specificity for poor outcome in comatose post-cardiac arrest patients and are easy to use, low cost, and minimally affected by drugs and metabolic derangements. A major limitation is their relative low sensitivity for poor outcome (137).

The large majority of studies supporting the robust prognostic accuracy of SSEPs were conducted before the use of hypothermia and further investigation of their prognostic accuracy in patients treated with hypothermia, with investigators blinded to the test result to avoid a self-fulfilling prophecy, is crucial. However, a recent meta-analysis of the use of SSEPs to predict neurological outcome in patients treated with therapeutic hypothermia after cardiopulmonary resuscitation demonstrated that the false positive rate assessed the false positive of a bilaterally absent SSEP N20 response was low and comparable with that reported in patients treated with normothermia (138).

Several other SSEP variables are associated with outcome after cardiac arrest but they are less robust than absent cortical SSEP responses. These include central conduction time (CCT), the time from cervicomedullary (N20) to cortical (P14) peaks, the N20-to-P25 amplitude ratio (139), and the N70 latency (140). False positives are common (between 4% and 15%) and make it impractical to base treatment decisions on these parameters. Late SSEP components may be better associated with long-term cognitive outcome than short-latency components but are not routinely used (141).

The role of BAEPs after cardiac arrest has not been systematically studied. In one study they were not found to be useful for prognostication (129), although in a small cohort study of 13 patients, middle latency auditory evoked responses (MLAEPs) were absent in all patients who died or remained in a persistent vegetative state (142). A recent study combined EEG and BAEPs in patients with post-anoxic coma and used two sets of recordings, the first performed within 24 hours post cardiac arrest and under mild hypothermia and the second after 1 day under normothermic conditions (143). A deterioration of auditory discrimination between the two sets of recordings had a 100% positive predictive value for non-survival. Tracking auditory discrimination in comatose patients over time could provide new insight into the chances of awakening in a quantitative and automatic fashion during early stages of coma.

Traumatic brain injury

Following TBI, bilaterally absent cortical SSEP responses in the presence of intact peripheral and spinal potentials is associated with poor outcome (144). In a review of studies (n = 44) addressing the prediction of outcome after severe brain injury using SSEPs, the positive likelihood ratio, positive predictive value and sensitivity for normal SEPs predicting favourable outcome were 4.04, 71.2%, and 59.0% respectively, and 11.41, 98.5%, and 46.2% respectively for bilaterally absent SEPs predicting unfavourable outcome (144). The false-positive rate of bilaterally absent SEPs for the prediction of poor outcome was less than 0.5%.

Serial EPs may allow early detection of the onset of recovery after TBI. For example, reduction of latency or normalization of amplitude may occur earlier than clinical signs of recovery (Figure 14.9) (124,145). Moreover, serial EPs can provide early warning of the development of secondary brain injury including haematoma enlargement, increased ICP, brainstem herniation, and cerebral ischaemia (146,147). Poor long-term functional outcome (death or vegetative state at 2 years) has been reported in comatose patients with traumatic brainstem lesions and absent N20s who did not recover consciousness within 48 hours of the injury (148), although it must be remembered that recovery of the N20 does not necessarily equate to recovery of brain function. Prolongation or absent CCT is associated with poor 1-year cognitive and behavioural function after TBI (149). Although rare, reappearance of previously absent bilateral SSEPs may occur after TBI and has been described

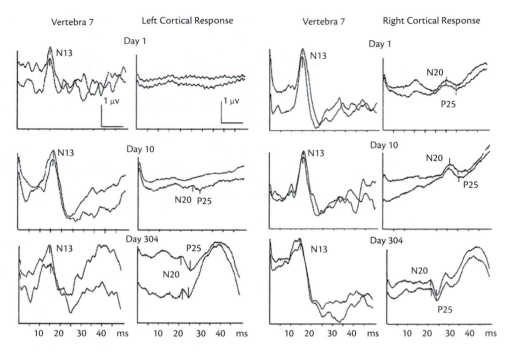

Fig. 14.9 Recovery of somatosensory evoked potential (SSEP) after TBI. This 14-year-old boy was admitted in a deep coma (GCS score 3) with severe diffuse axonal injury associated with elevated intracranial pressure. GCS score improved on day 13 post TBI but he did not move his left side purposefully until day 26. The initial median nerve SSEP was severely abnormal. Left cortical recordings were absent, and right hemispheric responses were prolonged with severely decreased amplitude. For the left cortical projections, the first indication of recovery was documented with somatosensory evoked potentials on day 10. Over the next few days, these somatosensory evoked potential findings improved. Twenty-three days after injury, latencies of the right cortical projection were within normal limits, whereas amplitudes remained reduced. One year after the accident, he suffered from minimal residual speech impairment and has returned fully to his former activities.

in some patients with good outcome after infratentorial haemorrhage or following hemicraniectomy (150).

Ischaemic and haemorrhagic stroke

The role of EPs in outcome prediction after AIS and intracerebral haemorrhage (ICH) is limited and less well studied than after TBI or coma from toxic or metabolic causes. Although several EP observations can be associated with the anatomical location of a stroke, EP is rarely used clinically to guide clinical management. BAEPs obtained within 24 hours of malignant MCA territory stroke may identify patients at risk of malignant oedema (151). Recovery of motor function after putaminal or thalamic ICH generally parallels normalization of SSEP components (152) but SSEPs do not provide the same predictive accuracy of poor outcome in coma from other neurological injuries. BAEP and SSEP abnormalities are observed in SAH patients with poor functional outcome (147,153) and as in other pathologies bilaterally absent cortical potentials carry a dismal prognosis (147).

Brain death

In a review of different international practice parameters and guidelines for determining brain death, it was reported that there is a lack of consensus on the exact criteria for defining brain death due to differences in cultural perceptions and beliefs, but about 40% recommended some confirmatory testing (154). Many practice parameters and guidelines accept EPs as one option for a confirmatory test (154) but the American Academy of Neurology's recently updated guidelines on the determination of brain death do not include SSEPs as a recommended ancillary test (155).

On serial examination, patients evolving to brain death lose subcortical SSEPs and all BAEP responses, and loss of median nerve

SSEP non-cephalic P14, and its cephalic referenced reflection N14 as well as the N18, is seen in brain death (156,157). However, the disadvantages of relying on SSEPs or BAEPs for the confirmation of brain death are multiple, including the fact that they cannot be interpreted by all clinicians and, most importantly, that there is a likelihood of false-positive and false-negative results.

Spinal cord injury

After spinal cord injury (SCI) SSEPs can assist in localizing the level of injury and in determining prognosis for functional outcome. Latencies and amplitudes of tibial SSEPs change over time after SCI and the early presence of a tibial SSEP is associated with a favourable functional and neurological outcome (158). Median and ulnar SSEP are valuable to indicate the level of injury, degree of sensory impairment, and to predict the outcome of hand function even in unconscious patients (159).

SSEPs and MEPs have similar significance in predicting functional outcome of ambulatory capacity, hand and bladder function, as clinical examination (160). The electromyogram (EMG), neurographic, and reflex recordings of acute SCI patients with spinal shock are more sensitive than clinical examination in assessing associated damage of peripheral motor pathways and allow the possibility of predicting the development of muscle tone or muscle atrophy (161).

Event-related potentials

Event-related potentials (ERPs) are long-latency potentials visualized by applying signal-averaging techniques to the EEG and are thought to reflect more complex cognitive processing of stimuli. Examples of ERPs include P300, N100, and mismatch negativity (MMN). The N100 is thought to represent attention (162), the P300 is elicited by a rare task-related stimulus, and the MMN by an 'odd-ball' sound in a sequence of sounds (163). A meta-analysis compared the predictive ability of late-stage EPs for awakening from coma due to ischaemia, haemorrhage, trauma, anoxic injury, and metabolic aetiologies, and the presence of an N100 had a sensitivity of 71% and specificity of 57% for good outcome across several studies (164). The MMN had a sensitivity of 38% and specificity of 91% for good outcome and P300 a sensitivity of 62% and specificity of 77%. MMN has a relatively high specificity for recovery of wakefulness, particularly after anoxic injury. Fischer and colleagues found it to be the most powerful prognostic indicator for awakening from coma and used it as the initial criterion to develop a decision tree for prognostication after cardiac arrest (165).

Electromyography and nerve conduction studies

In addition to a focused clinical history and neurological examination, electrodiagnostic test, such as EMG and nerve conduction velocity studies (NCSs), may assist in the diagnosis and prognosis of patients with neuromuscular disease (see Chapter 22). Some basic terminologies for understanding EMG and NCS are important. These are discussed briefly in the following sections but for a detailed description the reader is referred elsewhere (166).

Nerve conduction studies

NCSs can be motor, sensory, or mixed. Motor conduction responses are recorded in millivolts and sensory or mixed studies in microvolts. The active recording electrode, also known as G1, is placed on the centre of a muscle belly over the motor endplate and the reference electrode (G2) distally over the tendon. The stimulating electrode is placed over the nerve that supplies the muscle with the cathode closest to the recording electrode. The latency is recorded as the time from the stimulus to the initial compound muscle action potential (CMAP) deflection from baseline, and the amplitude from the baseline to the negative peak of the CMAP. Motor conduction velocity can be calculated after two sites, one distal and one proximal, have been stimulated. The CMAP is a biphasic potential with an initial negativity.

Ring recording electrodes are used for sensory nerve conduction studies. A sensory nerve action potential (SNAP), a compound potential representing a summation of all sensory fibre action potentials, is recorded. Similar to motor studies, latency, amplitude, duration, and conduction velocity is recorded for each SNAP. In patients with neuropathic lesions and axonal loss, the primary abnormalities are a reduction in the amplitude of the SNAP, CMAP, or both. Conduction velocities and latencies may be normal as long as the largest and fastest conducting axons remain intact.

Myelin is essential for salutatory conduction so in patients with demyelinating lesions there will be marked slowing in conduction velocities and prolongation of distal latencies. Essentially any motor, sensory or mixed nerve conduction velocity slower than 35 m/s in the arms or 30 m/s in the legs signifies unequivocal demyelination. Conduction blocks are also seen in acquired demyelination where there is also a reduction in the CMAP amplitude depending on the site of stimulation and the conduction block. In myopathies, SNAPs and CMAPs will usually be normal. There are additional reflexes and potentials that can be recorded during NCSs including the late responses of the F-wave and H-reflex. The F wave is the second of two voltage changes observed after electrical stimulation is applied above the distal region of a nerve and the H-reflex (Hoffmann's reflex) a reaction of muscles after electrical stimulation of innervating sensory fibres. Temporal dispersion occurs as individual nerve fibres fire at slightly different times and is normally more prominent at proximal stimulation sites because slower fibres progressively lag behind faster fibres.

Electromyogram

The motor unit comprises a motor nerve and all the muscles fibres that it innervates. It acts as a single functional unit with all the fibres contracting synchronously. Each muscle fibre produces an action potential and the summation of the individual potentials within the motor unit is the motor unit action potential (MUAP). EMG evaluates the electrophysiological activity from multiple motor units.

A concentric needle electrode is used to measure the EMG. The shaft of the needle serves as the reference electrode and the active electrode runs as a very small wire through the centre of the needle. Once the appropriate muscle is identified using anatomical landmarks, the first part of the examination assesses insertional and spontaneous activity at rest. Increased insertional muscle activity is defined as any electrical activity other than endplate potentials that lasts longer than 300 milliseconds after brief needle movement. Spontaneous activity is any activity at rest that lasts longer than 3 seconds. Next, MUAPs are recorded during minimal activation or contraction of the muscle and assessed for duration, amplitude, and number of phases. Recruitment and activation refers to the change in the frequency and number of firing MUAPs as the patient slowly increases force and tries to maximally contract the muscle under examination. Activation is the ability to fire the available MUAPs faster and recruitment refers to the ability to 'recruit' more MUAPs as the strength of muscle contraction increases. MUAPs are abnormal in different types of myopathy (see Chapter 22).

Electrodiagnostics in the intensive care unit

There are several indications for EMG and NCS are useful in the ICU. These include the following:

◆ Rapidly progressive ascending or descending weakness, with or without sensory signs/symptoms, and impending respiratory failure.

◆ The diagnosis of critical illness polymyoneuropathy.

◆ Difficulty in weaning mechanical ventilator despite improvement of underlying systemic illness.

◆ Patients with known diagnoses of myasthenia gravis or other neuromuscular disease presenting with an acute exacerbation

◆ A 'train of 4' technique, using a peripheral nerve stimulator, can be used to monitor the depth of neuromuscular blockade in patients receiving neuromuscular blocking agents to facilitate ventilation in severe ARDS or to prevent shivering during therapeutic hypothermia (167). The minimal current intensity (MCI) for recording a train of four responses is documented and then the responses are recorded at different current strengths, for example, 20, 40, 60, and 80 mA. Depending on the underlying indication for neuromuscular blockade, a target train of 4 is chosen. 0 out of 4 represents the most profound degree of neuromuscular block, 3 out of 4 the weakest, and 4 out of 4 indicates no blockade although some receptors may still be blocked.

Limitations

There are several limitations to performing EMGs and NCSs in critically ill patients including frequent occurrences of electrical interference, electrode contact problems associated with peripheral oedema and cool extremities due to the use of vasopressors, limited patient cooperation, reduced access to sites for electric stimulation and recording because of catheters and dressings, and the use of therapeutic anticoagulation. Patients with neuromuscular emergencies are often intubated and sedated which makes EMG limited to the study of insertional activity. These difficulties can be overcome to some extent. For example, hot packs can be used for warming cool limbs and electrical interference can be minimized by using an isolated electrical outlet although this is often insufficient on its own. Increasing the low-frequency filter during needle examination may allow identification of fibrillation potentials. Sound can also be used to identify fibrillation potentials and small, polyphasic motor unit potentials even if they are hidden within an electrical artefact. A 50 Hz artefact may particularly interfere with F-wave recordings and sensory responses, although signal averaging may help overcome these problems. Fortunately, motor nerve conduction studies are usually less affected.

Attention to electrical safety is also crucially important in the ICU. Proper grounding is essential and stimulation in a region of fluid spills should be avoided to prevent current leak. Patients with external pacemakers cannot undergo NCSs and although those with implanted pacemakers can be studied it is prudent to avoid repetitive stimulation.

A better yield is obtained if EMG recording is performed in patients who are minimally sedated and able to cooperate, so timing the study when a patient can tolerate minimal or no sedation safely may facilitate a diagnostic recording.

Indications

There are several conditions in which EMG and NCSs offer a high diagnostic yield (see also Chapter 22) (166).

Acute axonal and demyelinating polyneuropathies

Patients with clinical features suggestive of an acute polyneuropathy cannot be diagnosed solely on the basis of clinical features. Electrodiagnostic tests are required to classify these disorders into axonal and demyelinating variants which is important both for management and prognosis. The incidence of acute polyneuropathy variants is variably reported depending on many factors including clinical definitions, underlying triggering factors, and also on the electrophysiological criteria used to confirm the diagnosis and whether this was based on single or serial studies (168). In Ho's criteria for diagnosing Guillain–Barré syndrome, evidence of 'unequivocal temporal dispersion' was included among the parameters to assess demyelination (169), but Hadden and colleagues replaced this with conduction block defined as a proximal CMAP:distal CMAP amplitude ratio less than 0.5 (170). Acute motor and sensory axonal neuropathy is diagnosed by the absence of demyelinating features, as in Ho's criteria, and reduction of SNAP amplitude to lower than 50% of the lower limit of normal in at least two nerves (168).

Myasthenic syndromes

Acute neuromuscular weakness from a variety of causes can lead to respiratory failure. In patients presenting for the first time, electrodiagnostic studies with repetitive nerve stimulation and single-fibre EMG are important for diagnosis and management (171).

Critical illness myopathy and neuropathy

EMGs and NCSs are the gold standard for diagnosing critical illness polyneuropathy (CIP) and critical illness myopathy (CIM), although some authors suggest that the diagnosis can also be made clinically (172,173). CIM is more difficult to diagnose than CIP because diagnostic EMG findings require patient cooperation (173). CIP is usually an acute axonal polyneuropathy which can be sensory, motor, or both (174).

References

1. Jasper HH. The ten-twenty electrode system of the International Federation of Electroencephalography. *Clin Neurophysiol.* 1958;10:367–80.
2. Berger S, Schürer L, Härtl R, Messmer K, Baethmann A. Reduction of post-traumatic intracranial hypertension by hypertonic/hyperoncotic saline/dextran and hypertonic mannitol. *Neurosurgery.* 1995;37:98–108.
3. Hirsch J, Claassen J. The current state of treatment of status epilepticus. *Curr Neurol Neurosci Rep.* 2002;2:345–56.
4. Treatment of convulsive status epilepticus. Recommendations of the Epilepsy foundation of America's Working Group on Status Epilepticus. *JAMA.* 1993;270:854–9.
5. Suzuki A, Mori N, Hadeishi H, Yoshioka K, Yasui N. Computerized monitoring system in neurosurgical intensive care. *J Neurosci Methods.* 1988;26:133–9.
6. Agarwal R, Gotman J, Flanagan D, Rosenblatt B. Automatic EEG analysis during long-term monitoring in the ICU. *Electroencephalogr Clin Neurophysiol.* 1998;107:44–58.
7. Newton DE. Electrophysiological monitoring of general intensive care patients. *Intensive Care Med.* 1999;25:350–2.
8. Maynard DE, Jenkinson JL. The cerebral function analysing monitor. Initial clinical experience, application and further development. *Anaesthesia.* 1984;39:678–90.
9. Hirsh L, Brenner R (eds). *Atlas of EEG in Critical Care.* Chichester: Wiley-Blackwell; 2010.
10. Albers DJ, Claassen J, Schmidt JM, Hripcsak G. A methodology for detecting and exploring non-convulsive seizures in patients with SAH. Presented at *2013 International Symposium on Nonlinear Theory and its Applications* (NOLTA2013); 8–12 September; Santa Fe, CA; 2013.
11. Tong S, Thankor NV (eds). *Quantitative EEG Analysis Methods and Clinical Applications.* Norwood, MA: Artech House; 2009.
12. Foreman B, Claassen J. Quantitative EEG for the detection of brain ischemia. *Crit Care.* 2012;16:216.
13. Friedman D, Claassen J, Hirsch LJ. Continuous electroencephalogram monitoring in the intensive care unit. *Anesth Analg.* 2009;109:506–23.
14. Hirsch LB, Brenner R (eds). *Atlas of EEG in Critical Care.* Hoboken, NJ: Wiley-Blackwell, 2010.
15. Scheuer ML, Wilson SB. Data analysis for continuous EEG monitoring in the ICU: seeing the forest and the trees. *J Clin Neurophysiol.* 2004;21:353–78.
16. Chamberlin N, Dingledine R. GABAergic inhibition and the induction of spontaneous epileptiform activity by low chloride and high potassium in the hippocampal slice. *Brain Res.* 1988;445:12.
17. Tasker RC, Boyd SG, Harden A, Matthew DJ. The cerebral function analysing monitor in paediatric medical intensive care: applications and limitations. *Intensive Care Med.* 1990;16:60–8.
18. Pohlmann-Eden B, Hoch DB, Cochius JI, Chiappa KH. Periodic lateralized epileptiform discharges—a critical review. *J Clin Neurophysiol.* 1996;13:519–30.
19. Hirsch LJ, LaRoche SM, Gaspard N, Gerard E, Svoronos A, Herman ST, et al. American Clinical Neurophysiology Society's Standardized Critical Care EEG Terminology: 2012 version. *J Clin Neurophysiol.* 2013;30:1–27.
20. Claassen J, Baeumer T, Hansen HC. [Continuous EEG for monitoring on the neurological intensive care unit. New applications and uses for therapeutic decision making]. *Nervenarzt.* 2000;71:813–21.

21. Gotman J. Automatic detection of seizures and spikes. *J Clin Neurophysiol.* 1999;16:130–40.

22. Vespa PM, Nenov V, Nuwer MR. Continuous EEG monitoring in the intensive care unit: early findings and clinical efficacy. *J Clin Neurophysiol.* 1999;16:1–13.

23. Wartenberg KE, Schmidt JM, Mayer SA. Multimodality monitoring in neurocritical care. *Crit Care Clin.* 2007;23:507–38.

24. Miller CM, Vespa PM, McArthur DL, Hirt D, Etchepare M. Frameless stereotactic aspiration and thrombolysis of deep intracerebral hemorrhage is associated with reduced levels of extracellular cerebral glutamate and unchanged lactate pyruvate ratios. *Neurocrit Care.* 2007;6:22–9.

25. Vespa P, Prins M, Ronne-Engstrom E, Caron M, Shalmon E, Hovda DA, et al. Increase in extracellular glutamate caused by reduced cerebral perfusion pressure and seizures after human traumatic brain injury: a microdialysis study. *J Neurosurg.* 1998;89:971–82.

26. Waziri A, Claassen J, Stuart RM, Arif H, Schmidt JM, Mayer SA, et al. Intracortical electroencephalography in acute brain injury. *Ann Neurol.* 2009;66:366–77.

27. Claassen J, Perotte A, Albers D, Kleinberg S, Schmidt JM, Tu B, et al. Nonconvulsive seizures after subarachnoid hemorrhage: multimodality detection and outcomes. Ann Neurol. 2013;74(1):53–64.

28. Nangunoori R, Maloney-Wilensky E, Stiefel M, Park S, Andrew Kofke W, Levine JM, et al. Brain tissue oxygen-based therapy and outcome after severe traumatic brain injury: a systematic literature review. *Neurocrit Care.* 2012;17:131–8.

29. Ko SB, Ortega-Gutierrez S, Choi HA, Claassen J, Presciutti M, Schmidt JM, et al. Status epilepticus-induced hyperemia and brain tissue hypoxia after cardiac arrest. *Arch Neurol* 2011;68:1323–6.

30. Jirsch J, Hirsch LJ. Nonconvulsive seizures: developing a rational approach to the diagnosis and management in the critically ill population. *Clin Neurophysiol.* 2007;118:1660–70.

31. Husain AM, Horn GJ, Jacobson MP. Non-convulsive status epilepticus: usefulness of clinical features in selecting patients for urgent EEG. *J Neurol Neurosurg Psychiatry.* 2003;74:189–91.

32. Kaplan PW. Behavioral manifestations of nonconvulsive status epilepticus. *Epilepsy Behav.* 2002;3:122–39.

33. Lowenstein DH, Aminoff MJ. Clinical and EEG features of status epilepticus in comatose patients. *Neurology.* 1992;42:100–4.

34. Claassen J, Mayer SA, Kowalski RG, Emerson RG, Hirsch LJ. Detection of electrographic seizures with continuous EEG monitoring in critically ill patients. *Neurology.* 2004;62:1743–8.

35. Oddo M, Carrera E, Claassen J, Mayer SA, Hirsch LJ. Continuous electroencephalography in the medical intensive care unit. *Crit Care Med.* 2009;37:2051–6.

36. Abou Khaled KJ, Hirsch LJ. Advances in the management of seizures and status epilepticus in critically ill patients. *Crit Care Clin.* 2006;22:637–59.

37. DeLorenzo RJ, Waterhouse EJ, Towne AR, Boggs JG, Ko D, DeLorenzo GA, et al. Persistent nonconvulsive status epilepticus after the control of convulsive status epilepticus. *Epilepsia.* 1998;39:833–40.

38. Towne AR, Waterhouse EJ, Boggs JG, Garnett LK, Brown AJ, Smith JR, Jr, et al. Prevalence of nonconvulsive status epilepticus in comatose patients. *Neurology.* 2000;54:340–5.

39. Jordan KG. Neurophysiologic monitoring in the neuroscience intensive care unit. *Neurol Clin.* 1995;13:579–626.

40. Oddo M, Carrera E, Claassen J, Mayer SA, Hirsch LJ. Continuous electroencephalography in the medical intensive care unit. *Crit Care Med.* 2009;37:2051–6.

41. Young GB, Jordan KG, Doig GS. An assessment of nonconvulsive seizures in the intensive care unit using continuous EEG monitoring: an investigation of variables associated with mortality. *Neurology.* 1996;47:83–9.

42. Krumholz A, Sung GY, Fisher RS, Barry E, Bergey GK, Grattan LM. Complex partial status epilepticus accompanied by serious morbidity and mortality. *Neurology.* 1995;45:1499–504.

43. Litt B, Wityk RJ, Hertz SH, Mullen PD, Weiss H, Ryan DD, et al. Nonconvulsive status epilepticus in the critically ill elderly. *Epilepsia.* 1998;39:1194–202.

44. DeGiorgio CM, Correale JD, Gott PS, Ginsburg DL, Bracht KA, Smith T, et al. Serum neuron-specific enolase in human status epilepticus. *Neurology.* 1995;45:1134–7.

45. Rabinowicz AL, Correale JD, Bracht KA, Smith TD, DeGiorgio CM. Neuron-specific enolase is increased after nonconvulsive status epilepticus. *Epilepsia.* 1995;36:475–9.

46. Claassen J, Perotte A, Albers D, Kleinberg S, Schmidt JM, Tu B, et al. Nonconvulsive seizures after subarachnoid hemorrhage: multimodal detection and outcomes. *Ann Neurol.* 2013;74(1):53–64.

47. Vespa PM, Miller C, McArthur D, Eliseo M, Etchepare M, Hirt D, et al. Nonconvulsive electrographic seizures after traumatic brain injury result in a delayed, prolonged increase in intracranial pressure and metabolic crisis. *Crit Care Med.* 2007;35:2830–6.

48. Vespa PM, O'Phelan K, Shah M, Mirabelli J, Starkman S, Kidwell C, et al. Acute seizures after intracerebral hemorrhage: a factor in progressive midline shift and outcome. *Neurology.* 2003;60:1441–6.

49. Claassen J, Jette N, Chum F, Green R, Schmidt M, Choi H, et al. Electrographic seizures and periodic discharges after intracerebral hemorrhage. *Neurology.* 2007;69:1356–65.

50. Vespa PM, McArthur DL, Xu Y, Eliseo M, Etchepare M, Dinov I, et al. Nonconvulsive seizures after traumatic brain injury are associated with hippocampal atrophy. *Neurology.* 2010;75:792–8.

51. Pandian JD, Cascino GD, So EL, Manno E, Fulgham JR. Digital video-electroencephalographic monitoring in the neurological-neurosurgical intensive care unit: clinical features and outcome. *Arch Neurol.* 2004;61:1090–4.

52. Claassen J, Mayer SA. Continuous electroencephalographic monitoring in neurocritical care. *Curr Neurol Neurosci Rep.* 2002;2:534–40.

53. Brophy GM, Bell R, Claassen J, Alldredge B, Bleck TP, Glauser T, et al. Guidelines for the evaluation and management of status epilepticus. *Neurocrit Care.* 2012;17:3–23.

54. Treiman DM. Electroclinical features of status epilepticus. *J Clin Neurophysiol.* 1995;12:343–62.

55. Garzon E, Fernandes RM, Sakamoto AC. Serial EEG during human status epilepticus: evidence for PLED as an ictal pattern. *Neurology.* 2001;57:1175–83.

56. Husain AM, Mebust KA, Radtke RA. Generalized periodic epileptiform discharges: etiologies, relationship to status epilepticus, and prognosis. *J Clin Neurophysiol.* 1999;16:51–8.

57. Kaplan PW. Assessing the outcomes in patients with nonconvulsive status epilepticus: nonconvulsive status epilepticus is underdiagnosed, potentially overtreated, and confounded by comorbidity. *J Clin Neurophysiol.* 1999;16:341–52.

58. Niedermeyer E, Ribeiro M. Considerations of nonconvulsive status epilepticus. *Clin Electroencephalogr.* 2000;31:192–5.

59. Treiman DM, Walton NY, Kendrick C. A progressive sequence of electroencephalographic changes during generalized convulsive status epilepticus. *Epilepsy Res.* 1990;5:49–60.

60. Assal F, Papazyan JP, Slosman DO, Jallon P, Goerres GW. SPECT in periodic lateralized epileptiform discharges (PLEDs): a form of partial status epilepticus? *Seizure.* 2001;10:260–5.

61. Handforth A, Cheng JT, Mandelkern MA, Treiman DM. Markedly increased mesiotemporal lobe metabolism in a case with PLEDs: further evidence that PLEDs are a manifestation of partial status epilepticus. *Epilepsia.* 1994;35:876–81.

62. Claassen J. How I treat patients with EEG patterns on the ictal-interictal continuum in the neuro ICU. *Neurocrit Care.* 2009;11:437–44.

63. Hirsch LJ, Claassen J, Mayer SA, Emerson RG. Stimulus-induced rhythmic, periodic, or ictal discharges (SIRPIDs): a common EEG phenomenon in the critically ill. *Epilepsia.* 2004;45:109–23.

64. Hirsch LJ, Pang T, Claassen J, Chang C, Khaled KA, Wittman J, et al. Focal motor seizures induced by alerting stimuli in critically ill patients. *Epilepsia.* 2008;49:968–73.

65. Fountain NB, Waldman WA. Effects of benzodiazepines on triphasic waves: implications for nonconvulsive status epilepticus. *J Clin Neurophysiol.* 2001;18:345–52.

66. Annegers JF, Grabow JD, Groover RV, Laws ER, Jr., Elveback LR, Kurland LT. Seizures after head trauma: a population study. *Neurology.* 1980;30:683–9.

67. Temkin NR, Dikmen SS, Wilensky AJ, Keihm J, Chabal S, Winn HR. A randomized, double-blind study of phenytoin for the prevention of post-traumatic seizures. *N Engl J Med.* 1990;323:497–502.

68. Vespa P. Continuous EEG monitoring for the detection of seizures in traumatic brain injury, infarction, and intracerebral hemorrhage: "to detect and protect". *J Clin Neurophysiol.* 2005;22:99–106.

69. Jones PA, Andrews PJ, Midgley S, Anderson SI, Piper IR, Tocher JL, *et al.* Measuring the burden of secondary insults in head-injured patients during intensive care. *J Neurosurg. Anesthesiol.* 1994;6:4–14.

70. Vespa PM, Nuwer MR, Juhasz C, Alexander M, Nenov V, Martin N, *et al.* Early detection of vasospasm after acute subarachnoid hemorrhage using continuous EEG ICU monitoring. *Electroencephalogr Clin Neurophysiol.* 1997;103:607–15.

71. Vespa PM, Boscardin WJ, Hovda DA, McArthur DL, Nuwer MR, Martin NA, *et al.* Early and persistent impaired percent alpha variability on continuous electroencephalography monitoring as predictive of poor outcome after traumatic brain injury. *J Neurosurg.* 2002;97:84–92.

72. Rae-Grant AD, Barbour PJ, Reed J. Development of a novel EEG rating scale for head injury using dichotomous variables. *Electroencephalogr Clin Neurophysiol.* 1991;79:349–57.

73. Theilen HJ, Ragaller M, Tscho U, May SA, Schackert G, Albrecht MD. Electroencephalogram silence ratio for early outcome prognosis in severe head trauma. *Crit Care Med.* 2000;28:3522–9.

74. Hartings JA, Watanabe T, Bullock MR, Okonkwo DO, Fabricius M, Woitzik J, *et al.* Spreading depolarizations have prolonged direct current shifts and are associated with poor outcome in brain trauma. *Brain.* 2011;134:1529–40.

75. Hasan D, Schonck RS, Avezaat CJ, Tanghe HL, van Gijn J, van der Lugt PJ. Epileptic seizures after subarachnoid hemorrhage. *Ann Neurol.* 1993;33:286–91.

76. Claassen J, Hirsch LJ, Kreiter KT, Du EY, Connolly ES, Emerson RG, *et al.* Quantitative continuous EEG for detecting delayed cerebral ischemia in patients with poor-grade subarachnoid hemorrhage. *Clin Neurophysiol.* 2004;115:2699–710.

77. Labar DR, Fisch BJ, Pedley TA, Fink ME, Solomon RA. Quantitative EEG monitoring for patients with subarachnoid hemorrhage. *Electroencephalogr Clin Neurophysiol.* 1991;78:325–32.

78. Rathakrishnan R, Gotman J, Dubeau F, Angle M. Using continuous electroencephalography in the management of delayed cerebral ischemia following subarachnoid hemorrhage. *Neurocrit Care.* 2011;14:152–61.

79. Claassen J, Hansen HC. Early recovery after closed traumatic head injury: somatosensory evoked potentials and clinical findings. *Crit Care Med.* 2001;29:494–502.

80. Stuart RM, Waziri A, Weintraub D, Schmidt MJ, Fernandez L, Helbok R, *et al.* Intracortical EEG for the detection of vasospasm in patients with poor-grade subarachnoid hemorrhage. *Neurocrit Care.* 2010;13:355–8.

81. Claassen J, Hirsch LJ, Frontera JA, Fernandez A, Schmidt M, Kapinos G, *et al.* Prognostic significance of continuous EEG monitoring in patients with poor-grade subarachnoid hemorrhage. *Neurocrit Care.* 2006;4:103–12.

82. Bosco E, Marton E, Feletti A, Scarpa B, Longatti P, Zanatta P, *et al.* Dynamic monitors of brain function: a new target in neurointensive care unit. *Crit Care.* 2011;15:R170.

83. Bladin CF, Alexandrov AV, Bellavance A, Bornstein N, Chambers B, Coté R, *et al.* Seizures after stroke: a prospective multicenter study. *Arch Neurol.* 2000;57:1617–22.

84. Arboix A. [Epileptic crisis and cerebral vascular disease]. *Rev Clin Esp.* 1997;197:346–50.

85. Faught E, Peters D, Bartolucci A, Moore L, Miller PC. Seizures after primary intracerebral hemorrhage. *Neurology.* 1989;39:1089–93.

86. Szaflarski JP, Rackley AY, Kleindorfer DO, Khoury J, Woo D, Miller R, *et al.* Incidence of seizures in the acute phase of stroke: a population-based study. *Epilepsia.* 2008;49:974–81.

87. Nagata K, Tagawa K, Hiroi S, Shishido F, Uemura K. Electroencephalographic correlates of blood flow and oxygen metabolism provided by positron emission tomography in patients with cerebral infarction. *Electroencephalogr Clin Neurophysiol.* 1989;72:16–30.

88. Tolonen U, Sulg IA. Comparison of quantitative EEG parameters from four different analysis techniques in evaluation of relationships between EEG and CBF in brain infarction. *Electroencephalogr Clin Neurophysiol.* 1981;51:177–85.

89. Astrup J, Siesjo BK, Symon L. Thresholds in cerebral ischemia—the ischemic penumbra. *Stroke.* 1981;12:723–5.

90. Jordan KG. Nonconvulsive status epilepticus in acute brain injury. *J Clin Neurophysiol.* 1999;16:332–40.

91. Arboix A, Comes E, Massons J, Garcia L, Oliveres M. Relevance of early seizures for in-hospital mortality in acute cerebrovascular disease. *Neurology.* 1996;47:1429–35.

92. Vernino S, Brown RD, Jr., Sejvar JJ, Sicks JD, Petty GW, O'Fallon WM. Cause-specific mortality after first cerebral infarction: a population-based study. *Stroke.* 2003;34:1828–32.

93. Mecarelli O, Pro S, Randi F, Dispenza S, Correnti A, Pulitano P, *et al.* EEG patterns and epileptic seizures in acute phase stroke. *Cerebrovasc Dis.* 2011;31:191–8.

94. Sheorajpanday RV, Nagels G, Weeren AJ, De Deyn PP. Quantitative EEG in ischemic stroke: correlation with infarct volume and functional status in posterior circulation and lacunar syndromes. *Clin Neurophysiol.* 2011;122:884–90.

95. Sheorajpanday RV, Nagels G, Weeren AJ, De Surgeloose D, De Deyn PP. Additional value of quantitative EEG in acute anterior circulation syndrome of presumed ischemic origin. *Clin Neurophysiol.* 2010;121:1719–25.

96. Sheorajpanday RV, Nagels G, Weeren AJ, van Putten MJ, De Deyn PP. Quantitative EEG in ischemic stroke: correlation with functional status after 6 months. *Clin Neurophysiol.* 2011;122:874–83.

97. Diedler J, Sykora M, Juttler E, Veltkamp R, Steiner T, Rupp A. EEG power spectrum to predict prognosis after hemicraniectomy for space-occupying middle cerebral artery infarction. *Cerebrovasc Dis.* 2010;29:162–9.

98. Burghaus L, Hilker R, Dohmen C, Bosche B, Winhuisen L, Galldiks N, *et al.* Early electroencephalography in acute ischemic stroke: prediction of a malignant course? *Clin Neurol Neurosurg.* 2007;109:45–9.

99. Diedler J, Sykora M, Bast T, Poli S, Veltkamp R, Mellado P, *et al.* Quantitative EEG correlates of low cerebral perfusion in severe stroke. *Neurocrit Care.* 2009;11:210–6.

100. Huang Z, Dong W, Yan Y, Xiao Q, Man Y. Effects of intravenous mannitol on EEG recordings in stroke patients. *Clin Neurophysiol.* 2002;113:446–53.

101. Wood JH, Polyzoidis KS, Epstein CM, Gibby GL, Tindall GT. Quantitative EEG alterations after isovolemic-hemodilutional augmentation of cerebral perfusion in stroke patients. *Neurology.* 1984;34:764–8.

102. Rossetti AO, Logroscino G, Liaudet L, Ruffieux C, Ribordy V, Schaller MD, *et al.* Status epilepticus: an independent outcome predictor after cerebral anoxia. *Neurology.* 2007;69:255–60.

103. Hovland A, Nielsen EW, Kluver J, Salvesen R. EEG should be performed during induced hypothermia. *Resuscitation.* 2006;68:143–6.

104. Krumholz A, Stern BJ, Weiss HD. Outcome from coma after cardiopulmonary resuscitation: relation to seizures and myoclonus. *Neurology.* 1988;38:401–5.

105. Wright WL, Geocadin RG. Postresuscitative intensive care: neuroprotective strategies after cardiac arrest. *Semin Neurol.* 2006;26:396–402.

106. Legriel S, Bruneel F, Sediri H, Hilly J, Abbosh N, Lagarrigue MH, *et al.* Early EEG monitoring for detecting postanoxic status epilepticus during therapeutic hypothermia: a pilot study. *Neurocrit Care.* 2009;11:338–44.

107. Rittenberger JC, Popescu A, Brenner RP, Guyette FX, Callaway CW. Frequency and timing of nonconvulsive status epilepticus in comatose post-cardiac arrest subjects treated with hypothermia. *Neurocrit Care.* 2012;16:114–22.

108. Cloostermans MC, van Meulen FB, Eertman CJ, Hom HW, van Putten MJ. Continuous electroencephalography monitoring for early prediction of neurological outcome in postanoxic patients after cardiac arrest: a prospective cohort study. *Crit Care Med.* 2012;40:2867–75.

109. Rossetti AO, Oddo M, Logroscino G, Kaplan PW. Prognostication after cardiac arrest and hypothermia: a prospective study. *Ann Neurol.* 2010;67:301–7.

110. Wennervirta JE, Ermes MJ, Tiainen SM, Salmi TK, Hynninen MS, Särkelä MO, et al. Hypothermia-treated cardiac arrest patients with good neurological outcome differ early in quantitative variables of EEG suppression and epileptiform activity. *Crit Care Med.* 2009;37:2427–35.

111. Daubin C, Guillotin D, Etard O, Gaillard C, du Cheyron D, Ramakers M, et al. A clinical and EEG scoring system that predicts early cortical response (N20) to somatosensory evoked potentials and outcome after cardiac arrest. *BMC Cardiovasc Disord.* 2008;8:35.

112. Fugate JE, Wijdicks EF, Mandrekar J, Claassen DO, Manno EM, White RD, et al. Predictors of neurologic outcome in hypothermia after cardiac arrest. *Ann Neurol.* 2010;68:907–14.

113. Tiainen M, Poutiainen E, Kovala T, Takkunen O, Happola O, Roine RO. Cognitive and neurophysiological outcome of cardiac arrest survivors treated with therapeutic hypothermia. *Stroke.* 2007;38:2303–8.

114. Matthew E, Sherwin AL, Welner SA, Odusote K, Stratford JG. Seizures following intracranial surgery: incidence in the first post-operative week. *Can J Neurol Sci.* 1980;7:285–90.

115. Foy PM, Copeland GP, Shaw MD. The incidence of postoperative seizures. *Acta Neurochir (Wien).* 1981;55:253–64.

116. Llinas R, Barbut D, Caplan LR. Neurologic complications of cardiac surgery. *Prog Cardiovasc Dis.* 2000;43:101–12.

117. Wijdicks EF, Plevak DJ, Wiesner RH, Steers JL. Causes and outcome of seizures in liver transplant recipients. *Neurology.* 1996;47:1523–5.

118. Vaughn BV, Ali, II, Olivier KN, Lackner RP, Robertson KR, Messenheimer JA, et al. Seizures in lung transplant recipients. *Epilepsia.* 1996;37:1175–9.

119. Freye E. Cerebral monitoring in the operating room and the intensive care unit—an introductory for the clinician and a guide for the novice wanting to open a window to the brain. Part II: Sensory-evoked potentials (SSEP, AEP, VEP). *J Clin Monit Comput.* 2005;19:77–168.

120. Moulton RJ, Brown JI, Konasiewicz SJ. Monitoring severe head injury: a comparison of EEG and somatosensory evoked potentials. *Can J Neurol Sci.* 1998;25:S7–11.

121. Cruccu G, Aminoff MJ, Curio G, Guerit JM, Kakigi R, Mauguiere F, et al. Recommendations for the clinical use of somatosensory-evoked potentials. *Clin Neurophysiol.* 2008;119:1705–19.

122. Carrera E, Emerson RG, Claassen J. Brainstem auditory evoked potentials and somatosensory evoked potentials. In Le Roux P, Levine JM, Kofke WA (eds) *Monitoring in Neurocritical Care.* Philadelphia, PA: Elsevier; 2013:236–245.

123. Moller AR. *Intraoperative Neurophysiological Monitoring* (2nd edn). Totowa, NJ: Humana Press; 2006.

124. Fossi S, Amantini A, Grippo A, Innocenti P, Amadori A, Bucciardini L, et al. Continuous EEG-SEP monitoring of severely brain injured patients in NICU: methods and feasibility. *Neurophysiol Clin.* 2006;36:195–205.

125. Guerit JM, Amantini A, Amodio P, Andersen KV, Butler S, de Weerd A, et al. Consensus on the use of neurophysiological tests in the intensive care unit (ICU): electroencephalogram (EEG), evoked potentials (EP), and electroneuromyography (ENMG). *Neurophysiol Clin.* 2009;39:71–83.

126. Drummond JC, Todd MM, Schubert A, Sang H. Effect of the acute administration of high dose pentobarbital on human brain stem auditory and median nerve somatosensory evoked responses. *Neurosurgery.* 1987;20:830–5.

127. Liu EH, Wong HK, Chia CP, Lim HJ, Chen ZY, Lee TL. Effects of isoflurane and propofol on cortical somatosensory evoked potentials during comparable depth of anaesthesia as guided by bispectral index. *Br J Anaesth.* 2005;94:193–7.

128. Zandbergen EG, Hijdra A, de Haan RJ, van Dijk JG, Ongerboer de Visser BW, Spaans F, et al. Interobserver variation in the interpretation of SSEPs in anoxic-ischaemic coma. *Clin Neurophysiol.* 2006;117:1529–35.

129. Tiainen M, Kovala TT, Takkunen IS, Roine RO. Somatosensory and brainstem auditory evoked potentials in cardiac arrest patients treated with hypothermia. *Crit Care Med.* 2005;33:1736–40.

130. Seaba P. Electrical safety. *Am J EEG Technol.* 1980;20:1–13.

131. Bouwes A, Binnekade JM, Verbaan BW, Zandbergen EG, Koelman JH, Weinstein HC, et al. Predictive value of neurological examination for early cortical responses to somatosensory evoked potentials in patients with postanoxic coma. *J Neurol.* 2012;259:537–41.

132. Zandbergen EG, de Haan RJ, Stoutenbeek CP, Koelman JH, Hijdra A. Systematic review of early prediction of poor outcome in anoxic-ischaemic coma. *Lancet.* 1998;352:1808–12.

133. Zandbergen EG, Hijdra A, Koelman JH, Hart AA, Vos PE, Verbeek MM, et al. Prediction of poor outcome within the first 3 days of postanoxic coma. *Neurology.* 2006;66:62–8.

134. Meynaar IA, Oudemans-van Straaten HM, van der Wetering J, et al. Serum neuron-specific enolase predicts outcome in post-anoxic coma: a prospective cohort study. *Intensive Care Med.* 2003;29:189–95.

135. Young GB, Doig G, Ragazzoni A. Anoxic-ischemic encephalopathy: clinical and electrophysiological associations with outcome. *Neurocrit Care.* 2005;2:159–64.

136. Leithner C, Ploner CJ, Hasper D, Storm C. Does hypothermia influence the predictive value of bilateral absent N20 after cardiac arrest? *Neurology.* 2010;74:965–9.

137. Samaniego EA, Persoon S, Wijman CA. Prognosis after cardiac arrest and hypothermia: a new paradigm. *Curr Neurol Neurosci Rep.* 2011;11:111–19.

138. Kamps MJA, Horn J, Oddo M, Fugate JE, Storm C, Cronberg T, et al. Prognostication of neurologic outcome in cardiac arrest patients after mild therapeutic hypothermia: a meta-analysis of the current literature. *Intensive Care Med.* 2013; 39: 1671–82.

139. Walser H, Mattle H, Keller HM, Janzer R. Early cortical median nerve somatosensory evoked potentials. Prognostic value in anoxic coma. *Arch Neurol.* 1985;42:32–8.

140. Zandbergen EG, Koelman JH, de Haan RJ, Hijdra A, Group PR-S. SSEPs and prognosis in postanoxic coma: only short or also long latency responses? *Neurology.* 2006;67:583–6.

141. Prohl J, Rother J, Kluge S, de Heer G, Liepert J, Bodenburg S, et al. Prediction of short-term and long-term outcomes after cardiac arrest: a prospective multivariate approach combining biochemical, clinical, electrophysiological, and neuropsychological investigations. *Crit Care Med.* 2007;35:1230–7.

142. Yvert B, Crouzeix A, Bertrand O, Seither-Preisler A, Pantev C. Multiple supratemporal sources of magnetic and electric auditory evoked middle latency components in humans. *Cereb Cortex.* 2001;11:411–23.

143. Tzovara A, Rossetti AO, Spierer L, Grivel J, Murray MM, Oddo M, et al. Progression of auditory discrimination based on neural decoding predicts awakening from coma. *Brain.* 2013;136:81–9.

144. Carter BG, Butt W. Review of the use of somatosensory evoked potentials in the prediction of outcome after severe brain injury. *Crit Care Med.* 2001;29:178–86.

145. Claassen J, Hansen HC. Early recovery after closed traumatic head injury: Somatosensory evoked potentials and clinical findings. *Crit Care Med.* 2001;29:494–502.

146. Sleigh JW, Havill JH, Frith R, Kersel D, Marsh N, Ulyatt D. Somatosensory evoked potentials in severe traumatic brain injury: a blinded study. *J Neurosurg.* 1999;91:577–80.

147. Ritz R, Schwerdtfeger K, Strowitzki M, Donauer E, Koenig J, Steudel WI. Prognostic value of SSEP in early aneurysm surgery after SAH in poor-grade patients. *Neurol Res.* 2002;24:756–64.

148. Christophis P. The prognostic value of somatosensory evoked potentials in traumatic primary and secondary brain stem lesions. *Zentralbl Neurochir.* 2004;65:25–31.

149. Furlonger AJ, Sleigh JW, Havill JH, Marsh NV, Kersel DA. Cognitive and psychosocial outcome in survivors of severe traumatic brain injury: correlations with cerebral perfusion pressure, frontal lobe damage and somatosensory evoked potentials. *Crit Care Resusc.* 2000;2:246–52.

150. Rumpl E, Prugger M, Gerstenbrand F, Hackl JM, Pallua A. Central somatosensory conduction time and short latency somatosensory evoked potentials in post-traumatic coma. *Electroencephalogr Clin Neurophysiol.* 1983;56:583–96.

151. Burghaus L, Liu WC, Dohmen C, Bosche B, Haupt WF. Evoked potentials in acute ischemic stroke within the first 24 h: possible predictor of a malignant course. *Neurocrit Care.* 2008;9:13–16.

152. Kato H, Sugawara Y, Ito H, Onodera K, Sato C, Kogure K. Somatosensory evoked potentials following stimulation of median and tibial nerves in patients with localized intracerebral hemorrhage: correlations with clinical and CT findings. *J Neurol Sci.* 1991;103:172–8.

153. Schick U, Dohnert J, Meyer JJ, Vitzthum HE. Prognostic significance of SSEP, BAEP and serum S-100B monitoring after aneurysm surgery. *Acta Neurol Scand.* 2003;108:161–9.

154. Wijdicks EF. Brain death worldwide: accepted fact but no global consensus in diagnostic criteria. *Neurology.* 2002;58:20–5.

155. Wijdicks EF, Varelas PN, Gronseth GS, Greer DM, American Academy of Neurology. Evidence-based guideline update: determining brain death in adults: report of the Quality Standards Subcommittee of the American Academy of Neurology. *Neurology.* 2010;74:1911–18.

156. Buchner H, Ferbert A, Hacke W. Serial recording of median nerve stimulated subcortical somatosensory evoked potentials (SEPs) in developing brain death. *Electroencephalogr Clin Neurophysiol.* 1988;69:14–23.

157. Sonoo M, Tsai-Shozawa Y, Aoki M, Nakatani T, Hatanaka Y, Mochizuki A, et al. N18 in median somatosensory evoked potentials: a new indicator of medullary function useful for the diagnosis of brain death. *J Neurol Neurosurg Psychiatry.* 1999;67:374–8.

158. Spiess M, Schubert M, Kliesch U, EM-SCI Study group, Halder P. Evolution of tibial SSEP after traumatic spinal cord injury: baseline for clinical trials. *Clin Neurophysiol.* 2008;119:1051–61.

159. Curt A, Dietz V. Traumatic cervical spinal cord injury: relation between somatosensory evoked potentials, neurological deficit, and hand function. *Arch Phys Med Rehabil.* 1996;77:48–53.

160. Curt A, Dietz V. Electrophysiological recordings in patients with spinal cord injury: significance for predicting outcome. *Spinal Cord.* 1999;37:157–65.

161. Curt A, Dietz V. Neurologic recovery in SCI. *Arch Phys Med Rehabil.* 1999;80:607–8.

162. Papageorgiou C, Giannakakis GA, Nikita KS, Anagnostopoulos D, Papadimitriou GN, Rabavilas A. Abnormal auditory ERP N100 in children with dyslexia: comparison with their control siblings. *Behav Brain Funct.* 2009;5:26.

163. Duncan CC, Barry RJ, Connolly JF, Fischer C, Michie PT, Näätänen R, et al. Event-related potentials in clinical research: guidelines for eliciting, recording, and quantifying mismatch negativity, P300, and N400. *Clin Neurophysiol.* 2009;120:1883–908.

164. Daltrozzo J, Wioland N, Mutschler V, Kotchoubey B. Predicting coma and other low responsive patients outcome using event-related brain potentials: a meta-analysis. *Clin Neurophysiol.* 2007;118:606–14.

165. Fischer C, Dailler F, Morlet D. Novelty P3 elicited by the subject's own name in comatose patients. *Clin Neurophysiol.* 2008;119:2224–30.

166. Preston DC, Shapiro B. *Electromyography and Neuromuscular Disorders* (2nd edn). Philadelphia, PA: Elsevier Butterworth Heinemann; 2005.

167. Lagneau F, Benayoun L, Plaud B, Bonnet F, Favier J, Marty J. The interpretation of train-of-four monitoring in intensive care: what about the muscle site and the current intensity? *Intensive Care Med.* 2001;27:1058–63.

168. Uncini A, Manzoli C, Notturno F, Capasso M. Pitfalls in electrodiagnosis of Guillain-Barre syndrome subtypes. *J Neurol Neurosurg Psychiatry.* 2010;81:1157–63.

169. Ho TW, Mishu B, Li CY, Gao CY, Cornblath DR, Griffin JW, et al. Guillain-Barre syndrome in northern China. Relationship to Campylobacter jejuni infection and anti-glycolipid antibodies. *Brain.* 1995;118 (Pt 3):597–605.

170. Hadden RD, Cornblath DR, Hughes RA, Zielasek J, Hartung HP, Toyka KV, et al. Electrophysiological classification of Guillain-Barre syndrome: clinical associations and outcome. Plasma Exchange/Sandoglobulin Guillain-Barre Syndrome Trial Group. *Ann Neurol.* 1998;44:780–8.

171. Chaudhuri A, Behan PO. Myasthenic crisis. *QJM.* 2009;102:97–107.

172. Morris C, Trinder JT. Electrophysiology adds little to clinical signs in critical illness polyneuropathy and myopathy. *Crit Care Med.* 2002;30:2612.

173. Latronico N. Neuromuscular alterations in the critically ill patient: critical illness myopathy, critical illness neuropathy, or both? *Intensive Care Med.* 2003;29:1411–13.

174. Bolton CF, Gilbert JJ, Hahn AF, Sibbald WJ. Polyneuropathy in critically ill patients. *J Neurol Neurosurg Psychiatry.* 1984;47:1223–31.

CHAPTER 15

Neuroimaging

Yanrong Zhang, Peter Komlosi,
Mingxing Xie, and Max Wintermark

Neuroimaging is a critical tool in the management of patients in the neurocritical care unit (NCCU). It is used to diagnose, monitor, and guide treatment for a variety of conditions, and may assist in prognosis. This chapter will review the imaging modalities available during the management of critically ill neurological patients, and discuss the typical imaging features of the most common pathological conditions encountered during neurocritical care.

Structural imaging modalities

Computed tomography (CT) and magnetic resonance imaging (MRI) are routine imaging tools used to identify structural lesions in neurological patients.

Non-contrast computed tomography

Owing to its non-invasiveness, speed of data acquisition, and ease of access, non-contrast computed tomography (NCCT) is the preferred imaging modality for the initial evaluation of many intracranial lesions, especially in the acute setting of traumatic brain injury (TBI), acute ischaemic stroke (AIS), and subarachnoid haemorrhage (SAH), and also for patients on the NCCU who require prompt identification of potential surgically remedial lesions, such as acute haemorrhage or herniation, in whom timely surgical intervention is associated with improved outcome (1). Many patients may be unstable or agitated, so the rapid imaging times of NCCT are crucial.

Modern CT scanners are able to acquire volumetric data, improving the evaluation of intracranial and spinal structures in reconstructed three-dimensional (3D) images. The principal disadvantage of NCCT is the use of ionizing radiation, although technological CT advancements such as dose modulation have effectively reduced the amount of radiation exposure. It is also limited in the assessment of lesions in the middle and posterior cranial fossas where 'beam-hardening' artefacts from thick surrounding bone structures obscure the brain tissue images.

Magnetic resonance imaging

Clinical MRI is based on the relaxation properties of the hydrogen nuclei of water molecules following excitement by radiofrequency waves. The hydrogen nuclei (protons) of body tissue water become aligned with the direction of the magnetic field inside a magnetic resonance (MR) scanner. A radio frequency is briefly turned on, and this is absorbed and flips the spin of the protons in the magnetic field. After the electromagnetic field is turned off, the spin of the protons relaxes back to the original states and they become realigned with the static magnetic field. As protons relax back to their original states, they re-emit energy at the same radiofrequency and this is detected by a receiving coil in the scanner. MRI produces particularly good images of soft tissue, and greater contrast between different tissue types than NCCT.

By varying the manner in which images are obtained, the soft tissue contrast of the visualized anatomical structures can be altered (Table 15.1). On T1-weighted images, water and fluid-containing tissues are dark and fat-containing tissues bright, whereas on T2-weighted images water and fluid-containing tissues are bright. T1-weighted images are therefore best suited to imaging anatomy and T2 tissue oedema. MRI thus has the potential to provide much more information on tissue status than CT, but there are many factors that limit its use in critically ill patients including long scan duration and MR-related safety issues (see later) (2,3).

There are several distinct MRI sequences that can be used to enhance image acquisition.

Fluid-attenuated inversion recovery

Fluid-attenuated inversion recovery (FLAIR) is an MRI sequence used to null the signal from fluids so that cerebrospinal fluid (CSF) is suppressed during brain imaging, making periventricular and subcortical T2 bright lesions more conspicuous. On FLAIR images, focal bright grey matter (e.g. contusions) and white matter abnormalities (e.g. diffuse axonal injury involving the fornix and corpus callosum) are more easily appreciated against the adjacent 'nulled' (dark) CSF-filled ventricles and subarachnoid spaces (4,5). FLAIR also has increased sensitivity for the presence of acute or subacute SAH, which appears as bright signals within the sulci and cisterns (6,7).

Gradient-echo

Gradient-echo (GRE) T2*-weighted images, and their most modern counterpart, susceptibility-weighted images (SWI), are very sensitive for the detection of intracranial blood (8–10).

Diffusion-weighted imaging

Diffusion-weighted imaging (DWI) explores the random motion of water molecules in the body, and the rate of water diffusion of tissue at specific locations is reflected by the intensity of each image voxel. On clinical MR scanners, the diffusion sensitivity is easily varied by changing the parameter known as the b value; generally the larger the b value the greater the degree of signal attenuation from water molecules. To enable meaningful interpretation, DWI is typically performed using at least two b values.

Because the movement of water molecules is the reflection of the surrounding cellular environment, DWI reveals early pathological abnormalities. For example, in the acute phase after AIS, cytotoxic oedema results in 'restricted' diffusion of water which appears 'bright' on DWI. This 'restricted' diffusion must not be

Table 15.1 Signal changes displayed in computed tomography and magnetic resonance imaging sequences in different pathological conditions

Conditions	CT density	DWI intensity	T1 intensity	T2 intensity	GRE/SWI intensity
Acute ischaemic stroke	≅	↑	≅	≅	≅
Subacute ischaemic stroke	↓	↑	↓	↑	≅
Chronic ischaemic stroke	↓↓	↑ or ↓	↓	↑	≅
Hyperacute haemorrhage	≅	≅	≅	↑	↓
Acute haemorrhage	↑	↓	↑	↓	↓
Subacute haemorrhage	≅	↓	↑	↑	↓
Chronic haemorrhage	↓	↓	↑	↓	↓
Traumatic axonal injury	≅	↑	≅	≅	↓ in haemorrhagic cases
Epilepsy	≅	↑	≅	≅	≅

DWI, diffusion weighted; GRE, gradient-echo; SWI, susceptibility weighted images.

confused with 'T2 shine through', which occurs when a bright, usually chronic, lesion on T2 imaging also appears bright on DWI. Confusion between these can be avoided by obtaining apparent diffusion coefficient (ADC) maps, which are based on quantitative differences of tissue diffusion independent of T2 effects. An area of infarction after AIS is thus typically 'bright' on DWI and 'dark' on ADC. DWI becomes positive in stroke patients within 5–10 minutes of symptom onset, whereas CT often does not detect changes of acute ischaemia/infarction for up to 4–6 hours.

DWI can also be used to assess the connectivity of white matter axons in the central nervous system. In an isotropic medium such as water inside a glass, water molecules move randomly in all directions because of turbulence and Brownian motion, but in biological tissues diffusion is anisotropic. For example, water molecules inside a neuronal axon move principally along the axis of the neural fibre, but have a low probability of crossing the myelin membrane. This property is exploited in a variant of DWI called diffusion tensor imaging (DTI) which can be used to examine the connectivity of different regions in the brain (tractography) (11,12), or areas of neural degeneration and demyelination in diseases like multiple sclerosis (13–15).

Safety issues

There are many factors that interfere with the routine use of MRI in critically ill patients. These include the relatively long image acquisition times, interference from metallic implants (pacemakers, defibrillators, cochlear implants), and the requirement for specialized, MRI-compatible, monitoring equipment (2,3).

The MRI environment is hazardous because of the static magnetic field and risk of radiofrequency heating. Ferromagnetic objects are pulled towards the centre of the magnet, risking injury to patients. Pacemakers or hearing implants may also be dislodged or inactivated. Therefore, a safety check for metallic foreign bodies, implantable devices, equipment, and other contraindications should always be undertaken prior to MRI. The reader is directed elsewhere for detailed discussion of MRI safety issues (16).

Angiography

Digital subtraction angiography (DSA) is the established diagnostic tool for imaging intracranial and cervical vessels, but the non-invasive modalities of CT angiography (CTA) and MR angiography (MRA) are increasingly used alternatives.

Digital subtraction angiography

DSA utilizes computerized X-ray imaging equipment for image acquisition, and subtraction of the images acquired prior to injection of iodinated contrast agent injection from the subsequent images after contrast. In this way, the bony or dense soft tissue images are removed. Although DSA is considered the gold standard for the evaluation of cerebrovascular diseases, it is an invasive procedure with an associated procedural risk. The rate of neurological complications ranges from 0.3% to 1.3%, of which 0.07–0.5% are permanent (17–20). The vast majority are minor and transient (e.g. groin haematomas, femoral artery injury, and minor allergic reactions), although more severe complications, such as cerebral infarction, seizure, and death can occur.

Spinal angiography imposes the same risks as cerebral angiography, and increases the risk of cord infarction due to spinal artery embolus. Therefore, it should only be performed when a vascular malformation is displayed by another imaging technology or in a patient with SAH and normal pan-cerebral angiographic findings in whom a spinal source is strongly suspected (20).

With the rapid progress of CTA and MRA, DSA is now rarely used for initial diagnostic purposes and reserved for endovascular interventions to treat cerebral aneurysms and other cerebrovascular malformations, or to recannulate a stenosed or occluded artery.

Computed tomography angiography

Using multidetector-row computed tomography (MDCT) technology, CTA can assess the entire vasculature from the aortic arch to the circle of Willis quickly in a single data acquisition with excellent 3D spatial resolution. The acquisition time is typically less than 10 seconds, that is, within a single breath-hold during injection of intravenous contrast. Multiplanar reformatted images, maximum intensity projection images (MIP), and 3D reconstructions of axial CTA source images provide images comparable, or even superior, to those obtained with conventional DSA (Figures 15.1 and 15.2) (21,22).

The advantages of CTA lie in the short imaging time, wide availability, logistical ease of imaging critically ill patients, fewer artefacts relative to MRA, availability of extra-luminal information not available with DSA, and excellent sensitivity for intracranial aneurysms. On the other hand, CTA does not provide the dynamic, real-time information of DSA. The increased usage of MDCT technology has led to a significantly increased radiation dose to patients, and

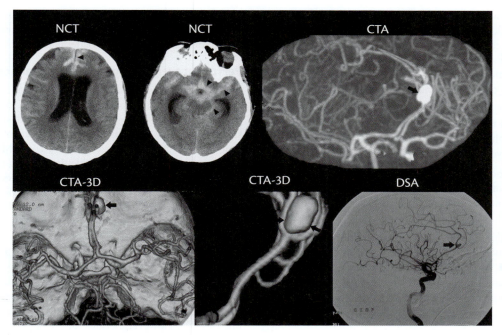

Fig. 15.1 A 45-year-old patient was admitted with thunderclap headache, nausea, and vomiting. Non-contrast computed tomography (NCT) brain scan demonstrated diffuse subarachnoid haemorrhage (arrowheads), and bilateral enlargement of the ventricles. Computed tomographic angiography (CTA) and digital subtraction angiography (DSA) identified a ruptured saccular aneurysm at the right pericallosal-calloso-marginal bifurcation (arrows).

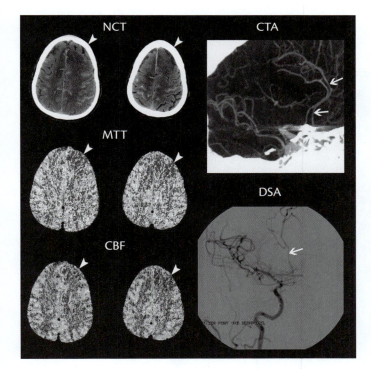

Fig. 15.2 A 40-year-old patient underwent coiling for a ruptured anterior communicating artery aneurysm and 5 days later experienced new symptoms of apathy and altered mental state. Non-contrast computed tomography (NCT) scan of the brain demonstrated extensive residual subarachnoid haemorrhage, as well as an area of loss of the grey–white matter differentiation (white arrowheads) in the left frontal lobe. Perfusion-CT demonstrated increased mean transit time (MTT) and decreased cerebral blood flow (CBF) (arrowheads), suggestive of vasospasm in this area and also in the right frontal lobe. CT angiography (CTA) and digital subtraction angiography (DSA) confirmed the suspicion of moderate vasospasm in both A2 and A3 segments of the anterior cerebral arteries (white arrows).

neuroradiologists now apply techniques to reduce the dose associated with neuro-CT imaging protocols (23). In addition, the use of X-ray contrast agent is associated with a risk of allergic reaction and acute kidney injury. As a result, CTA should be used with caution in patients with renal disease or diabetes.

Magnetic resonance angiography

MRA can be performed using one of three techniques—time-of-flight (TOF), phase-contrast, and contrast-enhanced. Contrast-enhanced MRA uses a contrast agent which changes the relaxation time of blood whereas TOF and phase-contrast techniques exploit two MRI in-flow effects, saturation and phase effects, which differentiate flowing blood from static tissue. TOF MRA is the most widely used technique, and two-dimensional TOF MRA is sensitive to slow velocity blood flow and therefore recommended for venous evaluation. On the other hand, 3D TOF works well for high arterial flow areas such as the circle of Willis. There are several advantages of MRA over DSA and CTA including no exposure to ionizing radiation and, in the case of TOF MRA, no contrast material. Disadvantages of MRA include the relatively long scanning time compared to CTA, its somewhat limited spatial resolution for small aneurysms, and overestimation of the degree of stenosis because of signal loss immediately distal to a stenosis on TOF MRA (24).

Functional imaging modalities

As technology advances, functional CT and MRI techniques are becoming more widely used in clinical practice.

Perfusion computed tomography

Perfusion CT (PCT) consists of continuous scanning of a region of interest in the brain during the injection of a bolus of contrast medium as it washes in and washes out through the cerebral vasculature. There is a linear relationship between contrast agent concentration and X-ray attenuation, with the contrast agent causing a transient increase in attenuation proportional to the amount of contrast agent in the region of interest. PCT data are analysed utilizing mathematical models and custom software to calculate quantitative values of several variables describing cerebral perfusion (25–28):

- The mean transit time (MTT) is the time taken for a theoretical instantaneous bolus of iodinated contrast to cross the capillary network in each voxel of the brain.

- The cerebral blood volume (CBV) indicates the volume of blood per unit of brain mass (normal range in grey matter: 4–6 mL/100 g), and the CBV map is calculated from the area under the time–density curves.

- Cerebral blood flow (CBF) indicates the volume of blood flow flowing per unit of brain mass per minute (normal range in grey matter: 60–80 mL/100 g/min), and the relationship between CBF and CBV is expressed by the equation:

$$CBF = \frac{CBV}{MTT}$$

The main advantages of PCT are its wide availability and quantitative accuracy (25,28). It has multiple applications in the NCCU. PCT is able to differentiate the reversible ischaemic penumbra and irreversible infarct core after AIS (Figure 15.3) (25,29) and, after SAH, can diagnose and quantify the severity of cerebral vasospasm

(30). In patients with TBI, PCT can be used for the early diagnosis of contusions and also to assess cerebral vascular autoregulation and guide treatment of brain oedema (31,32).

Perfusion-weighted magnetic resonance imaging

MRI can also be used to assess brain perfusion. Perfusion-weighted imaging (PWI) monitors the passage of a contrast agent bolus through brain capillaries as a transient loss of signal because of the susceptibility (T2*) effects of the contrast agent. A haemodynamic time–signal intensity curve is produced, and MTT, CBF, and CBV perfusion maps subsequently calculated using the same principles as for PCT. The T1-weighted signal of the contrast material can also be used to assess the permeability of the blood–brain barrier (33).

Arterial spin labelling (ASL) is an MRI technique that uses the blood signal as an endogenous tracer and can therefore be used to assess cerebral perfusion without the need for exogenous tracers. Because of its non-invasiveness, ASL can be repeated over time and therefore used to track changes in CBF during disease progression or treatment interventions. Importantly, ASL yields an absolute measure of CBF and change in flow is expressed in physiologically meaningful units rather than as a percentage change from baseline (34–37). However, because of the large amount of processing involved, this method largely remains a research tool.

PWI is often used in combination with DWI in stroke patients to assess the infarct core and ischaemic penumbra. The DWI abnormality represents the infarct core, and the DWI–PWI mismatch, that is, the area that is abnormal on PWI but not yet abnormal on DWI, the ischaemic penumbra (Figure 15.4) (38).

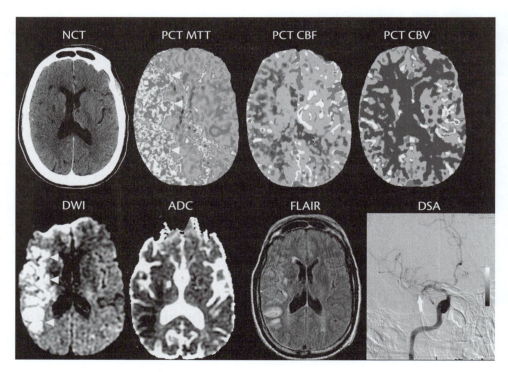

Fig. 15.3 A 67-year-old patient was admitted to the emergency department with a left hemiparesis. The non-contrast head CT scan (NCT) showed patchy areas of hypodensity and blurry grey–white matter junctions in the right middle cerebral artery territory. The perfusion CT scan (PCT) demonstrated delayed mean transit time (MTT) (arrowheads), decreased cerebral blood flow (CBF), and decreased cerebral blood volume (CBV). The lesion was 'bright' on diffusion-weighted imaging (DWI) and fluid-attenuated inversion recovery (FLAIR) MR sequences, and 'dark' on apparent diffusion coefficient (ADC) maps, consistent with an acute infarction. Digital subtraction angiography (DSA) identified an occlusion at the right M1 bifurcation (arrow) as the cause of the infarction.

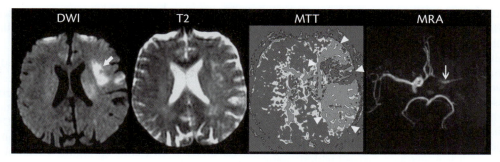

Fig. 15.4 Diffusion-weighted imaging (DWI) of a 70-year-old patient with aphasia and right hemiplegia showed reduced diffusion in the left frontal lobe (arrow), reflecting irreversibly damaged infarct core. The T2-weighted images show a faint increased corresponding signal indicating that the infarct is acute. Mean transit time (MTT) maps calculated from the perfusion-weighted imaging (PWI) show an area of hypoperfusion (arrowheads) that is larger than the infarct core on DWI. This PWI/ DWI 'mismatch' represents the ischaemic penumbra. Magnetic resonance angiography (MRA) displays an occlusion of the left middle cerebral artery (arrow).

Single-positron emission computed tomography imaging

In single-positron emission computed tomography (SPECT) perfusion studies, the radioisotope technetium-99m is attached to a delivery compound, either hexamethylpropyleneamine oxime (HMPAO) or ethyl cysteinate dimer (ECD). After intravenous injection it crosses the blood–brain barrier and is taken up by the neuronal and glial cells where it remains trapped for several hours. Imaging can thus be performed anytime within a few hours after injection (39). SPECT imaging of brain perfusion can be used at the bedside and is feasible in children.

One specific indication for SPECT is in the investigation of seizures. Because SPECT uses a retention tracer for measurement of cerebral perfusion, the radiopharmaceutical can be administered at the moment of the seizure and imaging performed later, after stabilization of the patient, to identify the active epileptic focus (40).

Ictal SPECT studies, complemented by interictal investigations (Figure 15.5) and co-registered with CT or MRI anatomical images are indicated in focal epilepsy for the localization of the epileptic focus before epilepsy surgery. SPECT perfusion can also be used in patients with acute and chronic cerebrovascular diseases (41).

Application of neuroimaging techniques in neurocritical care

Neuroimaging plays a key role in the management of critically ill neurological patients. This section will outline the typical imaging features of the most common conditions encountered on the NCCU.

Cerebral oedema

Cerebral oedema results from a pathological increase in the total amount of brain water content, and consequent increase in brain

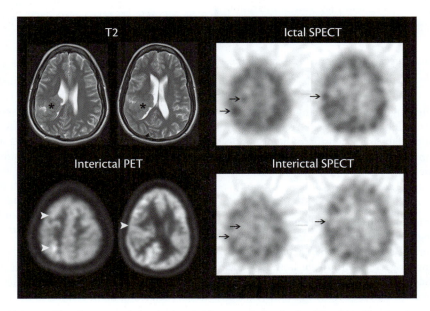

Fig. 15.5 A 28-year-old female with intractable epilepsy was admitted to hospital for presurgical evaluation. T2-weighted imaging showed an abnormal area of deeply infolded cortex extending from the posterior aspect of the insular cortex deep into the right parietal lobe and lined by abnormally lobulated grey matter. It extends to the body of the right lateral ventricle and protruding into it (star). The interictal positron emission tomography (PET) scan shows increased metabolic activity (brighter signal) in the right frontal lobe and posterior right parietal lobe (arrowheads). The interictal single-positron emission computed tomography (SPECT) scan shows three areas of decreased radioisotope uptake (lighter grey)—two in the right parietal lobe and one in right temporal lobe (arrows). These same areas showed increased uptake (darker grey) on the ictal SPECT, indicating that these are the likely sites of the seizure focus.

volume. There are three types of brain oedema—cytotoxic, vaso-genic, and interstitial. Cytotoxic oedema is characterized by an increase in intracellular water content and caused by an energy depletion that results in an imbalance of neurotransmitters and failure of active ion-pumps that normally maintain cellular home-ostasis. Ischaemia and profound metabolic derangements are the most common causes of cytotoxic oedema which involves both grey matter and white matter. Vasogenic oedema on the other hand results from disruption of the blood–brain barrier, leading to extravasation of fluid from the intravascular into the extravascular and extracellular spaces. It is primarily associated with tumours, inflammatory lesions, traumatic tissue damage, and haemorrhage, and predominantly involves the white matter. Interstitial oedema results from obstructive hydrocephalus in which there is an increase in trans-ependymal flow of CSF from the intraventricular compart-ment to the brain parenchyma, leading to CSF infiltration of the extracellular space of the periventricular white matter.

CT is poor at differentiating different types of brain oedema because it displays any water content increase as an abnormal dark area. MRI however shows oedema as dark on T1-weighted sequences and bright on T2-weighted and FLAIR sequences. On DWI, cyto-toxic oedema is bright because of the diffusion restriction, whereas vasogenic oedema appears grey or dark. Contrast-enhanced CT/MRI is helpful to delineate the oedema and reveal BBB leakage in vasogenic oedema (42).

Intracranial mass effect

Intracranial mass effect results from a large tumour, haemorrhage, or severe oedema sufficient to cause displacement and distortion of normal brain structures. This is manifest as sulcal effacement, mid-line shift, obstructive hydrocephalus, and herniation (Figure 15.6). The displacement of brain tissue can compress blood vessels, cra-nial nerves, and vital structures of the brainstem (medullary res-piratory and cardiac rhythm centres), and may lead to infarction and death.

Brain herniation

Different types of brain herniation can be encountered—subfalcine, transtentorial, and tonsillar.

Subfalcine herniation

In subfalcine herniation the cingulate or supracingulate gyri are pushed beneath the falx. These changes are easily recognized on CT or MRI as deviation of the falx and extension of hemispheric structures across the midline. Midline shift is easily measured by imaging software, and its degree is a useful guide to clinical man-agement and prognostication (43).

Transtentorial herniation

Transtentorial herniation is usually caused by a supratentorial mass or severe oedema displacing the medial temporal lobe downward through the tentorial incisura. It may involve the uncus anteriorly, the parahippocampal or lingual gyri posteriorly, or both. CT and MRI may demonstrate widening of the ipsilateral ambient cis-tern and effacement of the contralateral ambient cistern (44,45). An ascending transtentorial herniation can also occur when an infratentorial mass pushes the pons, vermis, and adjacent portions of the cerebellar hemispheres upward through the incisura. CT and MRI display symmetrical effacement of the ambient cisterns and acute hydrocephalus from compression of the Sylvian aqueduct. An

occipital lobe infarction may occur if the posterior cerebral artery is compressed between the temporal lobe and the crus cerebri (46).

Tonsillar herniation

Tonsillar herniation occurs when the cerebral tonsils are forced through the foramen magnum into the cervical spinal canal, usu-ally as a result of uncontrolled intracranial hypertension. Eventually the medulla is compressed leading to dysfunction and then failure of the vital respiratory and cardiac centres. Displacement of the cerebellar tonsils below the level of the foramen magnum is clearly seen on CT or MRI, although sagittal MR images display the tonsil-lar herniation most clearly (47).

Hydrocephalus

Hydrocephalus is defined as the abnormal enlargement of the ven-tricles and is of two types—communicating and obstructive.

Communicating hydrocephalus

In communicating hydrocephalus there is no obstruction between the ventricles and subarachnoid spaces. It results either from an overproduction of CSF (e.g. choroid plexus papilloma) or defec-tive CSF absorption in conditions such as SAH, meningitis, and leptomeningeal carcinomatosis. The typical appearance of commu-nicating hydrocephalus on CT and MRI is symmetrical expansion of all the ventricles with effacement of cerebral sulci. Because of the high pressure, CSF may leak from the ventricles into the brain leading to interstitial oedema that can be easily recognized on MRI.

Obstructive hydrocephalus

In obstructive hydrocephalus, CSF flow is obstructed within the ventricular system or at the level of its outlets into the subarachnoid space. Therefore only the ventricles proximal to the obstruction are seen to be dilated on CT or MRI. Both modalities are useful in iden-tifying the site of obstruction as well as its aetiology (Figure 15.6). With relatively new MRI sequences, such as 3D constructive inter-ference in the steady state (3D CISS), MRI can now scrutinize CSF flow at various sites (48).

Traumatic brain injury

Imaging is critical both for the initial diagnosis and subsequent management of TBI (see Chapter 17). Primary injuries, such as skull fractures, cortical contusions, haematomas, and traumatic axonal injury (TAI), result directly from the initial mechanical damage and are readily imaged using a variety of CT and MRI techniques (Figure 15.7). For the diagnosis of TBI in the acute set-ting, NCCT is the modality of choice as it quickly and accurately identifies intracranial haematomas that require urgent neurosurgi-cal evacuation. CT with thin slices and 3D reconstructions is the preferred imaging modality to assess skull fractures. MRI has better diagnostic sensitivity for lesions such as TAI.

Extradural haematoma

An extradural haematoma (EDH) is an abnormal blood accumula-tion between the dura mater and inner table of the skull, and is usually related to blunt trauma to the head, often to the temporal region. It may be associated with an overlying calvarial skull frac-ture. The source of haemorrhage is arterial in 85% of cases, but venous EDHs are occasionally seen in an occipital location sec-ondary to traumatic laceration of venous sinuses (49). On NCCT, an EDH appears as a biconvex, extra-axial, bright fluid collection

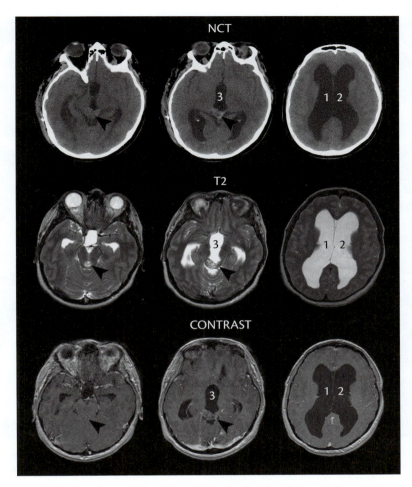

Fig. 15.6 A 30-year-old patient was admitted with nausea and vomiting. A non-contrast head CT (NCT) showed a heterogeneous mass lesion cantered in the tectum of the midbrain (black arrowheads) and causing obstructive hydrocephalus with enlargement of the lateral (numbers 1 and 2) and third (number 3) ventricles. Corresponding findings were observed on the T2-weighted magnetic resonance images. The post-gadolinium T1-weighted images (contrast) demonstrated the mass to be enhancing in a multiseptated pattern (black arrowhead).

(Figure 15.8). EDHs do not typically cross cranial suture lines because the dura is tightly adherent to the inner table at these sites. However, they can extend from the right to the left or from the supratentorial to infratentorial space, in contrast to subdural haematomas (SDHs) which are limited by the falx and the tentorium. The presence of alternating crescent-shaped dark regions within an otherwise bright EDH (the 'swirl' sign) may represent areas of active (ongoing) bleeding (50).

Subdural haematoma

SDHs may also be caused by brain trauma and usually have a venous origin. They often evolve rapidly and compress brain tissue, resulting in progressive neurological deterioration and death. On NCCT, an acute SDH appears as a crescent-shaped, bright, extra-axial fluid collection, which can extend along the falx and/or the tentorium. After a few days, SDHs become increasingly isodense to grey matter on CT, and this can make their detection difficult. A SDH can result from very minor head trauma and, under such circumstances, may progress unnoticed into a 'chronic' subdural haematoma (CSDH) which typically appears homogeneously dark relative to grey matter. The MRI appearance of an SDH is analogous to that on CT, with the age of the haematoma influencing the signal characteristics on

T1- and T2-weighted images. MRI is more sensitive than CT in the detection of a small SDH, especially in the tentorial and interhemispheric locations (50).

Traumatic axonal injury

TAI, also commonly referred to as diffuse axonal injury or shear injury, is characterized by widespread damage to the axons of the brainstem, parasagittal white matter of the cerebral cortex, corpus callosum, and at the grey–white matter junction of the cerebral cortex. The changes associated with TAI are thought to be responsible for the majority of global cognitive defects seen after TBI, particularly with regard to difficulties with memory and information processing (51).

TAI is difficult to diagnose on CT because more than 80% are non-haemorrhagic (52). However, advanced MRI sequences (as opposed to conventional MRI) can detect haemorrhagic and non-haemorrhagic TAI lesions more sensitively. Haemorrhagic lesions demonstrate focal susceptibility and signal loss because of the paramagnetic effects of deoxyhaemoglobin on GRE and SWI (53). DWI and FLAIR can identify non-haemorrhagic lesions in the corpus callosum, at the grey–white matter interface and in the dorsolateral aspect of the brain stem (Figure 15.7) (54,55).

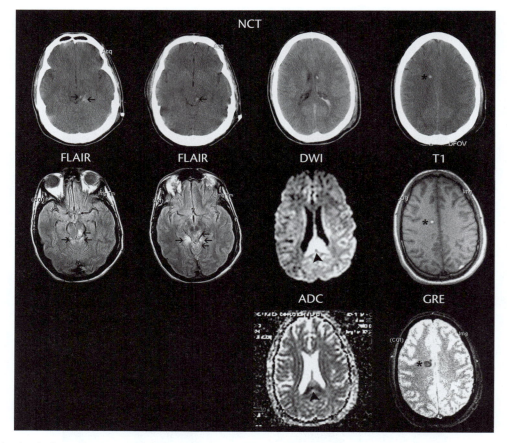

Fig. 15.7 A 45-year-old patient had a transient cognitive disorder after traumatic brain injury. Non-contrast cranial CT (NCT) demonstrated a small haemorrhagic focus in the left dorsolateral midbrain and in the adjacent left upper vermis (arrows). This was confirmed on fluid-attenuated inversion recovery (FLAIR) magnetic resonance images, which also demonstrated several additional injuries in the brainstem and upper vermis (arrows). The NCT also shows a small amount of intraventricular blood and a punctate focus of haemorrhage at the right frontal grey–white matter junction (star) which is also visualized on gradient-echo (GRE) magnetic resonance images (star). Diffusion-weighted imaging (DWI) demonstrated restricted diffusion in the splenium of the corpus callosum (arrowhead), which appears dark on apparent diffusion coefficient (ADC) maps. All these features are typically encountered after haemorrhagic and non-haemorrhagic traumatic axonal injury.

As previously discussed, DTI can provide information about brain microstructure by quantifying isotropic and anisotropic water diffusion. Water diffusion has a directional asymmetry (anisotropy) in organized tissues such as brain white matter (56). Where axons are aligned in white matter fibre tracts, diffusion along the axons is greater than that perpendicular to the axons but, when axonal injury occurs, diffusion anisotropy decreases (57). In this way disrupted axonal tracts can be imaged.

Subarachnoid haemorrhage

SAH is the accumulation of blood in the space between the arachnoid membrane and pia mater surrounding the brain. Intracranial aneurysms are the cause of SAH in 85% of cases (see Chapter 18) (58), but SAH can also occur secondary to trauma or intraparenchymal haemorrhage. Non-contrast cranial CT is the primary screening tool for patients in whom SAH is suspected (59). The sensitivity of CT for SAH is more than 95% in the first 12 hours after the ictus. Beyond 12 hours, normal CT findings do not rule out the diagnosis of acute SAH, and a lumbar puncture is indicated if there is a high index of clinical suspicion (60).

Acute SAH appears as a bright filling of the subarachnoid spaces around the brain (sulci, ventricles, and cisterns) on NCCT

(Figures 15.1 and 15.2). After several days, the initial high-attenuation of blood and clot tends to decrease, and changes to an intermediate grey relative to normal brain parenchyma. The distribution of the subarachnoid blood load can help localize the ruptured aneurysm. For example, blood in the anterior interhemispheric fissure or the adjacent frontal lobe is highly suggestive of rupture of an anterior communicating artery aneurysm. CT also allows for some degree of prognostication because the blood load, and presence of localized clots in the subarachnoid space, are correlated with a higher incidence of delayed symptomatic arterial vasospasm (61).

In the first few days after the ictus, MRI with proton density and especially FLAIR images is as sensitive as NCCT in detecting SAH. However, later, when the subarachnoid brightness on CT scans decreases, MRI becomes better at detecting SAH, with FLAIR and T2* images being the most sensitive techniques (62,63).

Vascular imaging in SAH

DSA is considered the gold standard for the identification of intracranial aneurysms and of aneurysm-related complications. It also represents a treatment modality as it permits coiling of ruptured and unruptured aneurysms, and endovascular treatment of vasospasm, including angioplasty and/or intra-arterial injection of vasodilators (64).

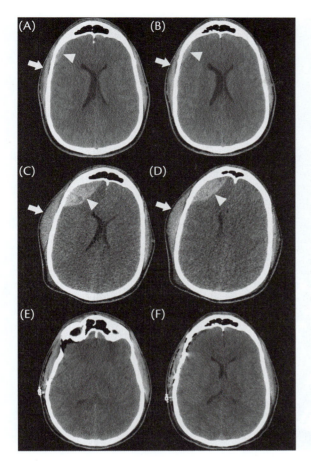

Fig. 15.8 Images of a 19-year-old patient involved in a high-speed motor vehicle accident. The admission non-contrast brain CT (NCT) demonstrated a small right frontal epidural haematoma (A and B arrowheads), which increased in size over a few hours (C and D arrowheads), before being surgically evacuated (E and F). A right parietal subgaleal haematoma was also present (A–D arrows).

CTA and MRA are now feasible alternatives to conventional angiography. CTA has 83–96% sensitivity and 97–100% specificity for aneurysm detection overall, although the sensitivity for smaller aneurysms is lower (40–91% for those < 3 mm diameter) (Figure 15.1) (65–67). Similarly, MRA is highly sensitive and specific for the detection of intracranial aneurysms but, like CTA, has lower sensitivity for smaller (< 3 mm diameter) aneurysms (66,67).

Cerebral vasospasm is a major cause of delayed neurologic morbidity after SAH. Vasospasm-related cerebral ischaemia occurs in 20–30% of patients (68), and is associated with a 1.5- to 3-fold increase in mortality in the first 2 weeks after SAH (69). Transcranial Doppler ultrasonography is a widely used technique for the detection of vasospasm, but has clear limitations (see Chapter 10) (70). The standard for the anatomical demonstration of cerebral vasospasm is DSA, but CTA has emerged as a reliable and accurate alternative that offers the potential for rapid diagnosis and monitoring (71). The very rapid acquisition of CTA images is a major advantage in unstable patients. CTA can be supplemented with PCT to provide an accurate and non-invasive assessment of the haemodynamic effects of vasospasm (Figure 15.2) (30,72,73), including quantification of CBF in the regions of interest (74).

Intraventricular haemorrhage

Intraventricular haemorrhage is usually associated with other lesions such as intraparenchymal haematoma, SAH, or TAI and has a poor prognosis (75). Blood enters the ventricles from contiguous extension from a parenchymal haematoma, shearing of subependymal veins that line the ventricular cavities, or retrograde reflux of a SAH through the foramina of the fourth ventricle.

Intracerebral haemorrhage

Intraparenchymal haematomas display five characteristic stages on CT and MRI—hyperacute (< 12 hours), acute (12 hours to 2 days), early subacute (2–7 days), late subacute (8 days to 1 month), and chronic (> 1 month to years) (76,77).

A hyperacute intracerebral haematoma consists of a matrix of red blood cells (RBC), white blood cells, and platelet thrombi intermixed with protein-rich serum. Because RBCs retain intracellular oxygenated haemoglobin, which has a density equal to that of the adjacent normal brain parenchyma, the haemorrhage can be difficult to delineate on NCCT in the early stages. However, a hyperacute haematoma has T1-grey or dark and T2-bright appearance on MRI. CTA is often performed in the acute phase after intracerebral haemorrhage (ICH) to identify extravasation of intravenous contrast in the centre or edge of the haematoma, the so-called spot sign (see Chapter 19). A positive spot sign suggests active bleeding and is predictive of early haematoma expansion and poor outcome compared to spot sign-negative patients.

After a few hours, the density of the haematoma increases with the extrusion of the serum, and vasogenic oedema develops in the adjacent brain tissue. This leads to developing brightness of the clot on NCCT, and a surrounding dark rim due to the serum and vasogenic oedema in the adjacent brain tissue. As the acute stage progresses, RBCs in the clot dehydrate and shrink, and the intracellular haemoglobin becomes progressively deoxygenated, so that the haematoma appears T1-grey or dark and T2-dark on MRI.

During the subsequent early subacute phase of ICH, the intracellular deoxyhaemoglobin is gradually converted to methaemoglobin and released into the extracellular space in the late subacute stage. On CT, the haematoma therefore becomes isodense to adjacent brain parenchyma. Injection of contrast media can delineate the haematoma because its periphery may show enhancement due to the disruption of the BBB because of local inflammation. On MRI, the haematoma is T1-bright and T2-dark in the early subacute stage, and T1- and T2-bright in the late subacute stage.

In the final, chronic, stage of haematoma evolution, macrophages and astroglial cells surround the haematoma and slowly phagocytize it. Extracellular methaemoglobin is converted by, and stored within, macrophages as haemosiderin and ferritin. On NCCT, a small dark brain defect typically remains and sometimes residual bright calcifications. Occasionally, focal atrophy leads to enlargement of neighbouring sulci. On MRI, chronic haematomas appear as T1-dark and T2-centrally bright surrounded by a rim of darkness (Figure 15.9). The high sensitivity of T2*-GRE MR sequences for the susceptibility effects of paramagnetic and superparamagnetic substances increases the number of haemorrhagic lesions that can be identified (78). A major limitation of this modality is that it cannot estimate the age of the haematomas.

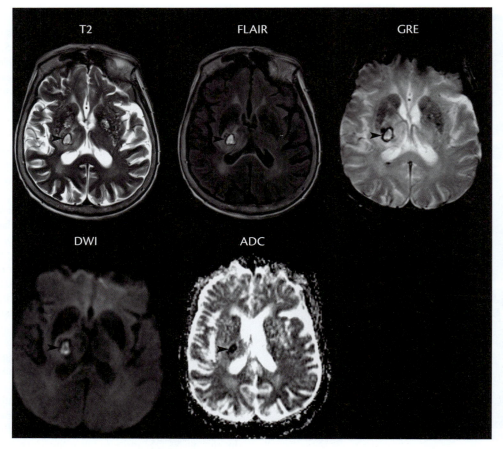

Fig. 15.9 An 89-year-old patient was admitted with a left motor deficit and numbness. Within the right thalamus, T2-weighted, fluid-attenuated inversion recovery (FLAIR), and gradient-echo (GRE) images showed a focus with increased T2 signal and a peripheral rim of low signal (black arrowhead). Diffusion-weighted imaging (DWI) also demonstrated a bright signal at the centre, corresponding to a dark signal on the apparent diffusion coefficient (ADC) map (black arrowhead). These findings are consistent with a chronic lacunar infarct with a haemorrhagic component.

Ischaemic stroke

Neuroimaging plays a critical role in the diagnosis and acute management of AIS. Early imaging is used to differentiate between ischaemic and haemorrhagic strokes, exclude stroke mimics, confirm and localize the area of ischaemia and clot if present, differentiate infarct core and penumbra, and assess the risk of haemorrhagic transformation.

NCCT is commonly used to rapidly exclude intracranial haemorrhage after stroke onset but, in the absence of haemorrhage, it may appear completely normal in the hyperacute phase. Early signs of brain infarction on NCCT include hyperdense arteries (see 'Vascular imaging'), sulcal effacement, effacement of grey structures including the insular ribbon sign and disappearing basal ganglia sign, and, later in the evolution of the infarct, hypodensity. Compared with DWI, NCCT is insensitive (25%) for the detection of ischaemia in the first 3 hours after stroke onset, but its sensitivity increases in the first 6 hours to 40–60%. Despite this, NCCT remains the acute imaging modality most commonly used to rule out ICH and some stroke mimics that would obviate the need for recanalization therapy.

Using GRE and other T2* sequences, MRI is equally sensitive to NCCT at excluding haemorrhage, but far more sensitive for the detection of non-haemorrhagic stroke mimics. Conventional T2-weighted and FLAIR images, in association with post-contrast T1-weighted images, identify non-haemorrhagic lesions such as tumours, metabolic disorders (e.g. hypoglycaemi), and seizure foci (79). DWI is the most sensitive method for the delineation of hyperacute ischaemia. The infarct core has restricted diffusion and this appears bright on DWI and dark on ADC maps. DWI is able to detect changes within minutes after the onset of ischaemia (80,81). Direct visualization of the infarct core and assessment of brain tissue viability is the main advantage of MR over CT in the assessment of AIS. Although signs of cerebral ischaemia on T2-weighted and FLAIR images are not visible until several hours post stroke, a 'mismatch' between positive DWI and negative FLAIR allows for the identification of patients within 3 hours of symptom onset with high specificity and positive predictive value (82,83).

Vascular imaging

Vascular imaging in stroke is used to detect arterial thrombus and characterize collateral flow. The presence of a bright thrombus or embolus in the middle cerebral artery creates a linear brightness on NCCT, often called the 'hyperdense artery sign'. It is seen in approximately one-third of AIS patients, and associated with poor radiological and clinical outcome. Similarly, because of the high concentration of deoxyhaemoglobin in the acute thrombus, T2*-weighted images delineate intraluminal clots as areas of linear or dot-shaped dark signal. CTA demonstrates arterial abnormalities in up to 95% of patients with acute ischaemic infarcts, and evaluates the intra- and extracranial vasculature with a single injection of contrast, revealing the location of the clot as well as the extent of atherosclerotic disease (84).

In the setting of AIS, CBF is compromised to the affected brain territory. The central core of tissue that dies immediately is often called the infarct core, and this is surrounded by an area of brain that is hypoperfused but still viable. It is this latter region of brain, often called the ischaemic penumbra, which is potentially salvageable by acute reperfusion therapy (see Chapter 20). Intravenous tissue plasminogen activator (rt-PA) is approved for thrombolysis after AIS within a short time (0–4.5 hours) from symptom onset (85), but this narrow time window significantly limits its usage and fewer than 10% of AIS patients are applicable for such treatment (86). It has been suggested that intravenous rt-PA, or other reperfusion therapies, could be safely administered in an extended time window in selected patients with a sufficient volume of salvageable penumbra (87,88). MRI could be used to identify those suitable for later intervention and allow a much larger percentage of stroke patients to be safely treated. DWI reflects irreversibly damaged tissue whereas PWI demonstrates an overall area of hypoperfusion. The volumetric difference between these abnormal regions, called the PWI/DWI 'mismatch', represents the MR correlate of the ischaemic penumbra (Figure 15.4). On the other hand, there is no difference in the PWI and DWI volumes (i.e. there is a PWI/DWI 'match') in patients with no penumbral (i.e. 'salvageable') tissue. The Diffusion and Perfusion Imaging Evaluation for Understanding Stroke Evolution (DEFUSE) study showed that early reperfusion is associated with a more favourable clinical response in patients with a PWI/DWI mismatch profile, and that those without a mismatch do not benefit from reperfusion (38). The optimal definition of mismatch remains uncertain but, in many studies, is defined as a PWI lesion of at least 10 cm^3 or at least 120% of the DWI lesion volume (89,90). A subgroup analysis of the DEFUSE study demonstrated that a mismatch ratio of 2.6 provided the highest sensitivity (90%) and specificity (83%) for identifying patients in whom reperfusion is likely to be associated with a favourable clinical response (91).

To differentiate the infarct core from the penumbra, PCT imaging relies on the difference in cerebral autoregulation between these two regions. In the penumbra, where autoregulation is intact or only mildly impaired, MTT is prolonged because of arterial occlusion but CBV is maintained or increased because of compensatory vasodilatation and recruitment of collaterals. In the infarct core, where autoregulation is severely impaired, MTT is prolonged in association with a reduction in CBV (Figure 15.3). By combining MTT and CBV, PCT has the ability to reliably identify reversible ischaemic penumbra and irreversible infarct core after AIS.

Haemorrhagic transformation

Haemorrhagic transformation is a serious complication of AIS that is associated with an 11-fold increase in mortality (92). Combined data from six major stroke trials confirm that severe haemorrhage with significant mass effect occurs in around 5% of patients treated with rt-PA within 3 hours after symptom onset, and in up to 6% of those treated between 3 and 6 hours (93). However, haemorrhagic transformation is a multifactorial phenomenon, with damage to the blood–brain barrier and subsequent vascular leakage one of the contributing mechanisms (94). Although often triggered

by reperfusion, it can occur spontaneously (95,96). Imaging can potentially be used to detect early blood–brain barrier damage and thereby identify patients who are more likely to develop haemorrhagic transformation after reperfusion. CT and MR both allow assessment of the integrity of the blood–brain barrier (97–99), and patients with abnormal barrier permeability are at increased risk of haemorrhagic transformation (98,99). Other imaging biomarkers associated with an increased risk of haemorrhagic transformation include CT hypodensity involving more than one-third of the middle cerebral artery territory, and a large volume of infarct on DWI (100).

Epilepsy

Imaging plays an important role in the pre-surgical assessment of patients with refractory epilepsy. SPECT and positron emission tomography (PET) techniques can define seizure onset zone and outline resection margins in those in whom surgery is planned. In general, cerebral metabolism and CBF are markedly increased during an epileptic seizure and decreased in the interictal period (101). Ictal SPECT has substantially higher specificity and positive predictive value than interictal studies (102), with ictal hyperperfusion restricted to the ictal-onset zones unless the seizure propagates (Figure 15.5). The accuracy of ictal SPECT analysis is enhanced when comparing ictal and interictal perfusion imaging data.18F-FDG-PET is routinely restricted to interictal studies, where it can provide useful localizing information with regards to the epileptogenic focus. The brain region with marked hypometabolism is considered to contain the epileptogenic zone, although this area tends to be larger than the actual seizure onset zone (103,104). The advantages of PET over SPECT include superior spatial resolution, and the potential for metabolic rather than blood-flow imaging (Figure 15.5) (105).

Epileptogenic lesions may also be visualized on structural imaging such as MRI, particularly using T1-weighted spoiled gradient recalled pulse sequences, T2, and FLAIR images. Contrast can be used to further delineate a lesion detected on non-contrast images, for example, in patients with a suspected brain tumour. MRI, SPECT, and PET image fusion allows direct correlation of the anatomical abnormalities identified on MRI with the metabolic and perfusion abnormalities detected on FDG-PET and SPECT respectively.

References

1. Wilberger JE, Jr., Harris M, Diamond DL. Acute subdural hematoma: morbidity and mortality related to timing of operative intervention. *J Trauma*. 1990;30(6):733–6.
2. Weintraub MI, Khoury A, Cole SP. Biologic effects of 3 Tesla (T) MR imaging comparing traditional 1.5 T and 0.6 T in 1023 consecutive outpatients. *J Neuroimaging*. 2007;17(3):241–5.
3. Shellock FG, Crues JV. MR procedures: biologic effects, safety, and patient care. *Radiology*. 2004;232(3):635–52.
4. Topal NB, Hakyemez B, Erdogan C, Bulut M, Koksal O, Akkose S, et al. MR imaging in the detection of diffuse axonal injury with mild traumatic brain injury. *Neurol Res*. 2008;30(9):974–8.
5. Hammoud DA, Wasserman BA. Diffuse axonal injuries: pathophysiology and imaging. *Neuroimaging Clin N Am*. 2002;12(2):205–16.
6. Mohamed M, Heasly DC, Yagmurlu B, Yousem DM. Fluid-attenuated inversion recovery MR imaging and subarachnoid hemorrhage: not a panacea. *AJNR Am J Neuroradiol*. 2004;25(4):545–50.
7. Lummel N, Schoepf V, Burke M, Brueckmann H, Linn J. 3D fluid-attenuated inversion recovery imaging: reduced CSF artifacts

and enhanced sensitivity and specificity for subarachnoid hemorrhage. *AJNR Am J Neuroradiol.* 2011;32(11):2054–60.

8. Copenhaver BR, Shin J, Warach S, Butman JA, Saver JL, Kidwell CS. Gradient echo MRI: implementation of a training tutorial for intracranial hemorrhage diagnosis. *Neurology.* 2009;72(18):1576–81.

9. Lobel U, Sedlacik J, Sabin ND, Kocak M, Broniscer A, Hillenbrand CM, *et al.* Three-dimensional susceptibility-weighted imaging and two-dimensional T2*-weighted gradient-echo imaging of intratumoral hemorrhages in pediatric diffuse intrinsic pontine glioma. *Neuroradiology.* 2010;52(12):1167–77.

10. Bradley WG, Jr. MR appearance of hemorrhage in the brain. *Radiology.* 1993;189(1):15–26.

11. Kasahara K, Hashimoto K, Abo M, Senoo A. Voxel- and atlas-based analysis of diffusion tensor imaging may reveal focal axonal injuries in mild traumatic brain injury—comparison with diffuse axonal injury. *Magn Reson Imaging.* 2012;30(4):496–505.

12. Palacios EM, Sala-Llonch R, Junque C, Roig T, Tormos JM, Bargallo N, *et al.* White matter integrity related to functional working memory networks in traumatic brain injury. *Neurology.* 2012;78(12):852–60.

13. Senda J, Watanabe H, Tsuboi T, Hara K, Watanabe H, Nakamura R, *et al.* MRI mean diffusivity detects widespread brain degeneration in multiple sclerosis. *J Neurol Sci.* 2012;319(1–2):105–10.

14. Harrison DM, Shiee N, Bazin PL, Newsome SD, Ratchford JN, Pham D, *et al.* Tract-specific quantitative MRI better correlates with disability than conventional MRI in multiple sclerosis. *J Neurol.* 2013;260(2):397–406.

15. Filippi M, Riccitelli G, Mattioli F, Capra R, Stampatori C, Pagani E, *et al.* Multiple sclerosis: effects of cognitive rehabilitation on structural and functional MR imaging measures—an explorative study. *Radiology.* 2012;262(3):932–40.

16. Reddy U, White MJ, Wilson SR. Anaesthesia for magnetic resonance imaging. *Contin Educ Anaesth Crit Care Pain.* 2012;12(3):140–4.

17. Burger IM, Murphy KJ, Jordan LC, Tamargo RJ, Gailloud P. Safety of cerebral digital subtraction angiography in children: complication rate analysis in 241 consecutive diagnostic angiograms. *Stroke.* 2006;37(10):2535–9.

18. Leffers AM, Wagner A. Neurologic complications of cerebral angiography. A retrospective study of complication rate and patient risk factors. *Acta Radiol.* 2000;41(3):204–10.

19. Willinsky RA, Taylor SM, TerBrugge K, Farb RI, Tomlinson G, Montanera W. Neurologic complications of cerebral angiography: prospective analysis of 2,899 procedures and review of the literature. *Radiology.* 2003;227(2):522–8.

20. Cloft HJ, Joseph GJ, Dion JE. Risk of cerebral angiography in patients with subarachnoid hemorrhage, cerebral aneurysm, and arteriovenous malformation: a meta-analysis. *Stroke.* 1999;30(2):317–20.

21. Ledezma CJ, Wintermark M. Multimodal CT in stroke imaging: new concepts. *Radiol Clin North Am.* 2009;47(1):109–16.

22. Tan JC, Dillon WP, Liu S, Adler F, Smith WS, Wintermark M. Systematic comparison of perfusion-CT and CT-angiography in acute stroke patients. *Ann Neurol.* 2007;61(6):533–43.

23. Smith AB, Dillon WP, Gould R, Wintermark M. Radiation dose-reduction strategies for neuroradiology CT protocols. *AJNR Am J Neuroradiol.* 2007;28(9):1628–32.

24. Wikstrom J, Bjornerud A, McGill S, Johansson L. Venous saturation slab causes overestimation of stenosis length in two-dimensional time-of-flight magnetic resonance angiography. *Acta Radiol.* 2009;50(1):55–60.

25. Wintermark M, Flanders AE, Velthuis B, Meuli R, van Leeuwen M, Goldsher D, *et al.* Perfusion-CT assessment of infarct core and penumbra: receiver operating characteristic curve analysis in 130 patients suspected of acute hemispheric stroke. *Stroke.* 2006;37(4):979–85.

26. Wintermark M. Brain perfusion-CT in acute stroke patients. *Eur Radiol.* 2005;15 Suppl 4:D28–31.

27. Wintermark M, Sesay M, Barbier E, Borbély K, Dillon WP, Eastwood JD, *et al.* Comparative overview of brain perfusion imaging techniques. *J Neuroradiol.* 2005;32(5):294–314.

28. Wintermark M, Fischbein NJ, Smith WS, Ko NU, Quist M, Dillon WP. Accuracy of dynamic perfusion CT with deconvolution in detecting acute hemispheric stroke. *AJNR Am J Neuroradiol.* 2005;26(1):104–12.

29. Wintermark M, Sincic R, Sridhar D, Chien JD. Cerebral perfusion CT: technique and clinical applications. *J Neuroradiol.* 2008;35(5):253–60.

30. Wintermark M, Ko NU, Smith WS, Liu S, Higashida RT, Dillon WP. Vasospasm after subarachnoid hemorrhage: utility of perfusion CT and CT angiography on diagnosis and management. *AJNR Am J Neuroradiol.* 2006;27(1):26–34.

31. Wintermark M, Chiolero R, Van Melle G, Revelly JP, Porchet F, Regli L, *et al.* Cerebral vascular autoregulation assessed by perfusion-CT in severe head trauma patients. *J Neuroradiol.* 2006;33(1):27–37.

32. Wintermark M, van Melle G, Schnyder P, Revelly JP, Porchet F, Regli L, *et al.* Admission perfusion CT: prognostic value in patients with severe head trauma. *Radiology.* 2004;232(1):211–20.

33. Kassner A, Mandell DM, Mikulis DJ. Measuring permeability in acute ischemic stroke. *Neuroimaging Clin N Am.* 2011;21(2):315–25.

34. Kim J, Whyte J, Wang J, Rao H, Tang KZ, Detre JA. Continuous ASL perfusion fMRI investigation of higher cognition: quantification of tonic CBF changes during sustained attention and working memory tasks. *Neuroimage.* 2006;31(1):376–85.

35. Chng SM, Petersen ET, Zimine I, Sitoh YY, Lim CC, Golay X. Territorial arterial spin labeling in the assessment of collateral circulation: comparison with digital subtraction angiography. *Stroke.* 2008;39(12):3248–54.

36. Yan L, Li C, Kilroy E, Wehrli FW, Wang DJ. Quantification of arterial cerebral blood volume using multiphase-balanced SSFP-based ASL. *Magn Reson Med.* 2012;68(1):130–9.

37. Fujiwara Y, Kimura H, Miyati T, Kabasawa H, Matsuda T, Ishimori Y, *et al.* MR perfusion imaging by alternate slab width inversion recovery arterial spin labeling (AIRASL): a technique with higher signal-to-noise ratio at 3.0 T. *Magma.* 2012;25(2):103–11.

38. Albers GW, Thijs VN, Wechsler L, Kemp S, Schlaug G, Skalabrin E, *et al.* Magnetic resonance imaging profiles predict clinical response to early reperfusion: the diffusion and perfusion imaging evaluation for understanding stroke evolution (DEFUSE) study. *Ann Neurol.* 2006;60(5):508–17.

39. Catafau AM. Brain SPECT in clinical practice. Part I: perfusion. *J Nucl Med.* 2001;42(2):259–71.

40. Wintermark M, Sesay M, Barbier E, Borbély K, Dillon WP, Eastwood JD, *et al.* Comparative overview of brain perfusion imaging techniques. *Stroke.* 2005;36(9):e83–99.

41. Ueda T, Yuh WT. Single-photon emission CT imaging in acute stroke. *Neuroimaging Clin N Am.* 2005;15(3):543–51, x.

42. Unterberg AW, Stover J, Kress B, Kiening KL. Edema and brain trauma. *Neuroscience.* 2004;129(4):1021–9.

43. Yuh EL, Cooper SR, Ferguson AR, Manley GT. Quantitative CT improves outcome prediction in acute traumatic brain injury. *J Neurotrauma.* 2012;29(5):735–46.

44. Laine FJ, Shedden AI, Dunn MM, Ghatak NR. Acquired intracranial herniations: MR imaging findings. *AJR Am J Roentgenol.* 1995;165(4):967–73.

45. Wijdicks EF, Miller GM. MR imaging of progressive downward herniation of the diencephalon. *Neurology.* 1997;48(5):1456–9.

46. Jauss M, Muffelmann B, Krieger D, Zeumer H, Busse O. A computed tomography score for assessment of mass effect in space-occupying cerebellar infarction. *J Neuroimaging.* 2001;11(3):268–71.

47. Endo M, Ichikawa F, Miyasaka Y, Yada K, Ohwada T. Capsular and thalamic infarction caused by tentorial herniation subsequent to head trauma. *Neuroradiology.* 1991;33(4):296–9.

48. Dincer A, Ozek MM. Radiologic evaluation of pediatric hydrocephalus. *Childs Nerv Syst.* 2011;27(10):1543–62.

49. Scheibl A, Calderon EM, Borau MJ, Prieto RM, González PF, Galiana GG. Epidural hematoma. *J Pediatr Surg.* 2012;47(2):e19–21.

50. Provenzale J. CT and MR imaging of acute cranial trauma. *Emerg Radiol.* 2007;14(1):1–12.

51. King JT, Jr., Carlier PM, Marion DW. Early Glasgow Outcome Scale scores predict long-term functional outcome in patients with severe traumatic brain injury. *J Neurotrauma.* 2005;22(9):947–54.

52. Meythaler JM, Peduzzi JD, Eleftheriou E, Novack TA. Current concepts: diffuse axonal injury-associated traumatic brain injury. *Arch Phys Med Rehabil.* 2001;82(10):1461–71.

53. Tong KA, Ashwal S, Holshouser BA, Shutter LA, Herigault G, Haacke EM, et al. Hemorrhagic shearing lesions in children and adolescents with posttraumatic diffuse axonal injury: improved detection and initial results. *Radiology.* 2003;227(2):332–9.

54. Marquez de la Plata C, Ardelean A, Koovakkattu D, Srinivasan P, Miller A, Phuong V, et al. Magnetic resonance imaging of diffuse axonal injury: quantitative assessment of white matter lesion volume. *J Neurotrauma.* 2007;24(4):591–8.

55. Ezaki Y, Tsutsumi K, Morikawa M, Nagata I. Role of diffusion-weighted magnetic resonance imaging in diffuse axonal injury. *Acta Radiol.* 2006;47(7):733–40.

56. Basser PJ, Jones DK. Diffusion-tensor MRI: theory, experimental design and data analysis—a technical review. *NMR Biomed.* 2002;15(7-8):456–67.

57. Qin W, Zhang M, Piao Y, Guo D, Zhu Z, Tian X, et al. Wallerian degeneration in central nervous system: dynamic associations between diffusion indices and their underlying pathology. *PLoS One.* 2012;7(7):e41441.

58. van Gijn J, Kerr RS, Rinkel GJ. Subarachnoid haemorrhage. *Lancet.* 2007;369(9558):306–18.

59. Perry JJ, Spacek A, Forbes M, Wells GA, Mortensen M, Symington C, et al. Is the combination of negative computed tomography result and negative lumbar puncture result sufficient to rule out subarachnoid hemorrhage? *Ann Emerg Med.* 2008;51(6):707–13.

60. McCormack RF, Hutson A. Can computed tomography angiography of the brain replace lumbar puncture in the evaluation of acute-onset headache after a negative noncontrast cranial computed tomography scan? *Acad Emerg Med.* 2010;17(4):444–51.

61. Fisher CM, Kistler JP, Davis JM. Relation of cerebral vasospasm to subarachnoid hemorrhage visualized by computerized tomographic scanning. *Neurosurgery.* 1980;6(1):1–9.

62. Noguchi K, Seto H, Kamisaki Y, Tomizawa G, Toyoshima S, Watanabe N, Comparison of fluid-attenuated inversion-recovery MR imaging with CT in a simulated model of acute subarachnoid hemorrhage. *AJNR Am J Neuroradiol.* 2000;21(5):923–7.

63. Fiebach JB, Schellinger PD, Geletneky K, Wilde P, Meyer M, Hacke W, et al. MRI in acute subarachnoid haemorrhage; findings with a standardised stroke protocol. *Neuroradiology.* 2004;46(1):44–8.

64. Chappell ET, Moure FC, Good MC. Comparison of computed tomographic angiography with digital subtraction angiography in the diagnosis of cerebral aneurysms: a meta-analysis. *Neurosurgery.* 2003;52(3):624–31.

65. Karamessini MT, Kagadis GC, Petsas T, Karnabatidis D, Konstantinou D, Sakellaropoulos GC, et al. CT angiography with three-dimensional techniques for the early diagnosis of intracranial aneurysms. Comparison with intra-arterial DSA and the surgical findings. *Eur J Radiol.* 2004;49(3):212–23.

66. Tipper G, JM UK-I, Price SJ, Trivedi RA, Cross JJ, Higgins NJ, et al. Detection and evaluation of intracranial aneurysms with 16-row multi-slice CT angiography. *Clin Radiol.* 2005;60(5):565–72.

67. White PM, Wardlaw JM, Easton V. Can noninvasive imaging accurately depict intracranial aneurysms? A systematic review. *Radiology.* 2000;217(2):361–70.

68. Kassell NF, Sasaki T, Colohan AR, Nazar G. Cerebral vasospasm following aneurysmal subarachnoid hemorrhage. *Stroke.* 1985;16(4):562–72.

69. Treggiari-Venzi MM, Suter PM, Romand JA. Review of medical prevention of vasospasm after aneurysmal subarachnoid hemorrhage: a problem of neurointensive care. *Neurosurgery.* 2001;48(2):249–61.

70. Suarez JI, Qureshi AI, Yahia AB, Parekh PD, Tamargo RJ, Williams MA, et al. Symptomatic vasospasm diagnosis after subarachnoid hemorrhage: evaluation of transcranial Doppler ultrasound and cerebral angiography as related to compromised vascular distribution. *Crit Care Med.* 2002;30(6):1348–55.

71. Yoon DY, Choi CS, Kim KH, Cho BM. Multidetector-row CT angiography of cerebral vasospasm after aneurysmal subarachnoid hemorrhage: comparison of volume-rendered images and digital subtraction angiography. *AJNR Am J Neuroradiol.* 2006;27(2):370–7.

72. Chaudhary SR, Ko N, Dillon WP, Yu MB, Liu S, Criqui GI, et al. Prospective evaluation of multidetector-row CT angiography for the diagnosis of vasospasm following subarachnoid hemorrhage: a comparison with digital subtraction angiography. *Cerebrovasc Dis.* 2008;25(1–2):144–50.

73. Binaghi S, Colleoni ML, Maeder P, Uské A, Regli L, Dehdashti AR, et al. CT angiography and perfusion CT in cerebral vasospasm after subarachnoid hemorrhage. *AJNR Am J Neuroradiol.* 2007;28(4):750–8.

74. Klimo P, Jr., Schmidt RH. Computed tomography grading schemes used to predict cerebral vasospasm after aneurysmal subarachnoid hemorrhage: a historical review. *Neurosurg Focus.* 2006;21(3):E5.

75. Atzema C, Mower WR, Hoffman JR, Holmes JF, Killian AJ, Wolfson AB, et al. Prevalence and prognosis of traumatic intraventricular hemorrhage in patients with blunt head trauma. *J Trauma.* 2006;60(5):1010–7; discussion 7.

76. Alemany Ripoll M, Stenborg A, Sonninen P, Terent A, Raininko R. Detection and appearance of intraparenchymal haematomas of the brain at 1.5 T with spin-echo, FLAIR and GE sequences: poor relationship to the age of the haematoma. *Neuroradiology.* 2004;46(6):435–43.

77. Aygun N, Masaryk TJ. Diagnostic imaging for intracerebral hemorrhage. *Neurosurg Clin N Am.* 2002;13(3):313–34.

78. Lin DD, Filippi CG, Steever AB, Zimmerman RD. Detection of intracranial hemorrhage: comparison between gradient-echo images and b(0) images obtained from diffusion-weighted echo-planar sequences. *AJNR Am J Neuroradiol.* 2001;22(7):1275–81.

79. Vroomen PC, Buddingh MK, Luijckx GJ, De Keyser J. The incidence of stroke mimics among stroke department admissions in relation to age group. *J Stroke Cerebrovasc Dis.* 2008;17(6):418–22.

80. Provenzale JM, Sorensen AG. Diffusion-weighted MR imaging in acute stroke: theoretic considerations and clinical applications. *AJR Am J Roentgenol.* 1999;173(6):1459–67.

81. Gonzalez RG, Schaefer PW, Buonanno FS, Schwamm LH, Budzik RF, Rordorf G, et al. Diffusion-weighted MR imaging: diagnostic accuracy in patients imaged within 6 hours of stroke symptom onset. *Radiology.* 1999;210(1):155–62.

82. Thomalla G, Rossbach P, Rosenkranz M, Siemonsen S, Krützelmann A, Fiehler J, et al. Negative fluid-attenuated inversion recovery imaging identifies acute ischemic stroke at 3 hours or less. *Ann Neurol.* 2009;65(6):724–32.

83. Thomalla G, Cheng B, Ebinger M, Hao Q, Tourdias T, Wu O, et al. DWI-FLAIR mismatch for the identification of patients with acute ischaemic stroke within 4.5 h of symptom onset (PRE-FLAIR): a multicentre observational study. *Lancet Neurol.* 2011;10(11):978–86.

84. Verro P, Tanenbaum LN, Borden NM, Sen S, Eshkar N. CT angiography in acute ischemic stroke: preliminary results. *Stroke.* 2002;33(1):276–8.

85. Schellinger PD, Warach S. Therapeutic time window of thrombolytic therapy following stroke. *Curr Atheroscler Rep.* 2004;6(4):288–94.

86. Bambauer KZ, Johnston SC, Bambauer DE, Zivin JA. Reasons why few patients with acute stroke receive tissue plasminogen activator. *Arch Neurol.* 2006;63(5):661–4.

87. Hacke W, Albers G, Al-Rawi Y, Bogousslavsky J, Davalos A, Eliasziw M, et al. The Desmoteplase in Acute Ischemic Stroke Trial (DIAS): a phase II MRI-based 9-hour window acute stroke thrombolysis trial with intravenous desmoteplase. *Stroke.* 2005;36(1):66–73.

88. Furlan AJ, Eyding D, Albers GW, Al-Rawi Y, Lees KR, Rowley HA, et al. Dose Escalation of Desmoteplase for Acute Ischemic Stroke (DEDAS): evidence of safety and efficacy 3 to 9 hours after stroke onset. *Stroke.* 2006;37(5):1227–31.

89. Schaefer PW. Imaging acute stroke is rapidly evolving. *Neuroimaging Clin N Am.* 2011;21(2):xv.

90. Olivot JM, Mlynash M, Thijs VN, Kemp S, Lansberg MG, Wechsler L, *et al.* Optimal Tmax threshold for predicting penumbral tissue in acute stroke. *Stroke.* 2009;40(2):469–75.

91. Kakuda W, Lansberg MG, Thijs VN, Kemp SM, Bammer R, Wechsler LR, *et al.* Optimal definition for PWI/DWI mismatch in acute ischemic stroke patients. *J Cereb Blood Flow Metab.* 2008;28(5):887–91.

92. Berger C, Fiorelli M, Steiner T, Schäbitz WR, Bozzao L, Bluhmki E, *et al.* Hemorrhagic transformation of ischemic brain tissue: asymptomatic or symptomatic? *Stroke.* 2001;32(6):1330–5.

93. Hacke W, Donnan G, Fieschi C, Kaste M, von Kummer R, Broderick JP, *et al.* Association of outcome with early stroke treatment: pooled analysis of ATLANTIS, ECASS, and NINDS rt-PA stroke trials. *Lancet.* 2004;363(9411):768–74.

94. Wang X, Lo EH. Triggers and mediators of hemorrhagic transformation in cerebral ischemia. *Mol Neurobiol.* 2003;28(3):229–44.

95. Lyden PD, Zivin JA. Hemorrhagic transformation after cerebral ischemia: mechanisms and incidence. *Cerebrovasc Brain Metab Rev.* 1993;5(1):1–16.

96. Lapchak PA. Hemorrhagic transformation following ischemic stroke: significance, causes, and relationship to therapy and treatment. *Curr Neurol Neurosci Rep.* 2002;2(1):38–43.

97. Hjort N, Wu O, Ashkanian M, Sølling C, Mouridsen K, Christensen S, *et al.* MRI detection of early blood-brain barrier disruption: parenchymal enhancement predicts focal hemorrhagic transformation after thrombolysis. *Stroke.* 2008;39(3):1025–8.

98. Aviv RI, d'Esterre CD, Murphy BD, Hopyan JJ, Buck B, Mallia G, *et al.* Hemorrhagic transformation of ischemic stroke: prediction with CT perfusion. *Radiology.* 2009;250(3):867–77.

99. Hom J, Dankbaar JW, Soares BP, Schneider T, Cheng SC, Bredno J, *et al.* Blood-brain barrier permeability assessed by perfusion CT predicts symptomatic hemorrhagic transformation and malignant edema in acute ischemic stroke. *AJNR Am J Neuroradiol.* 2011;32(1):41–8.

100. Selim M, Fink JN, Kumar S, Caplan LR, Horkan C, Chen Y, *et al.* Predictors of hemorrhagic transformation after intravenous recombinant tissue plasminogen activator: prognostic value of the initial apparent diffusion coefficient and diffusion-weighted lesion volume. *Stroke.* 2002;33(8):2047–52.

101. Duncan JS. Imaging and epilepsy. *Brain.* 1997;120 (Pt 2):339–77.

102. Zaknun JJ, Bal C, Maes A, Tepmongkol S, Vazquez S, Dupont P, *et al.* Comparative analysis of MR imaging, ictal SPECT and EEG in temporal lobe epilepsy: a prospective IAEA multi-center study. *Eur J Nucl Med Mol Imaging.* 2008;35(1):107–15.

103. Park CK, Kim SK, Wang KC, Hwang YS, Kim KJ, Chae JH, *et al.* Surgical outcome and prognostic factors of pediatric epilepsy caused by cortical dysplasia. *Childs Nerv Syst.* 2006;22(6):586–92.

104. Ollenberger GP, Byrne AJ, Berlangieri SU, Rowe CC, Pathmaraj K, Reutens DC, *et al.* Assessment of the role of FDG PET in the diagnosis and management of children with refractory epilepsy. *Eur J Nucl Med Mol Imaging.* 2005;32(11):1311–16.

105. Meltzer CC, Adelson PD, Brenner RP, Crumrine PK, Van Cott A, Schiff DP, *et al.* Planned ictal FDG PET imaging for localization of extratemporal epileptic foci. *Epilepsia.* 2000;41(2):193–200.

PART 3

Specific conditions

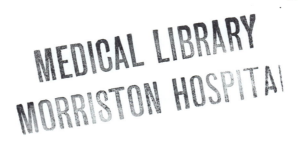

CHAPTER 16

Postoperative care

Nicolas Bruder and Lionel Velly

Postoperative complications are common after intracranial procedures. In a prospective study of 486 patients, 54.5% of the 431 who were extubated during the 4 hours following surgery suffered at least one complication (1). Nausea or vomiting occurred in 38% of patients, and respiratory, cardiovascular, and neurological complications in 2.8%, 6.7%, and 5.7% respectively. In retrospective studies, the overall major complication rates are variably reported between 13% and 27.5% (2).

The 30-day mortality rate after intracranial tumour surgery is around 2.2% (3,4). Although the overall risk of perioperative death has decreased over the last decades, mortality is probably not the best outcome measure for quality of care after neurosurgery (4). In our institution during the years 2000–2001, in-hospital mortality was 2% but the frequency of postoperative complications in the first 48 hours after elective surgery was 14.4%, and major neurological events represented 45% of these complications (intracranial haemorrhage in 20% and seizures in 15%). Risk factors for mortality after intracranial tumour surgery include tumour type, age older than 60 years, and biopsy compared to craniotomy (3). The most frequent cause of early postoperative death relate to the tumour itself, but intracranial bleeding accounts for about one-third of perioperative mortality. The risks associated with other intracranial procedures are roughly similar to those for tumour surgery. For example, symptomatic haemorrhage occurs in 2.1% of patients after functional neurosurgery and results in permanent deficit or death in 1.1% (5).

Indications for postoperative admission to neurointensive care

The need for neurointensive care after neurosurgery is dependent on many factors, and varies for elective and emergency procedures.

Elective craniotomy

The rationale for admitting patients to a neurocritical care unit (NCCU) after uncomplicated elective craniotomy is the relatively high rate of postoperative complications compared to other surgery types, and the need to recognize and treat intracranial complications as early as possible. The outcome after urgent reoperation for haemorrhage is independently associated with the Glasgow Coma Scale (GCS) score before reoperation and the time interval between primary surgery and reoperation (6). However, the identification of intracranial haemorrhage may be difficult in the first hours after craniotomy. Drowsiness or mild confusion may be the only early clinical signs and these may be interpreted as delayed anaesthetic recovery. Headaches and mild hemiparesis may also occur and,

when temporary, can also be associated with anaesthesia recovery (7). Close clinical monitoring is mandatory and there should be a low index of suspicion, prompting an urgent computed tomography (CT) scan to confirm an intracranial complication before intracranial hypertension and cerebral herniation ensue.

However, most elective patients do not need active intervention after the first 4 hours following craniotomy and only 15% need to stay in the NCCU for more than 24 hours (8,9). This is a problem for a busy NCCU where bed resources are often scarce, and other care locations are often chosen (see below) if the predicted risk of complications is low (Table 16.1). Risk factors for the development of postoperative complications include failure to extubate the trachea in the operating theatre, duration of surgery more than 4 hours, lateral positioning of the patient during surgery, Karnofsky performance scale score below 80, and intraoperative blood loss greater than 350 mL (10,11). Such factors should be considered when deciding which patients require admission to the NCCU after elective neurosurgery.

In the absence of risk factors and with meticulous neurological monitoring in the recovery room for 4–6 hours, some centres admit postoperative craniotomy patients to a regular neurosurgical ward with good results (12). However, this practice has been validated only in a small number of patients and the financial and personal cost of one undetected major complication is likely to far outweigh the resource benefits of bypassing the NCCU. Most postoperative intracranial haemorrhages occur in the first 6 hours following surgery (13,14), so if intracranial procedures are planned for the morning, prolonged monitoring in the recovery room (or NCCU) prior to return to the ward is feasible. Another solution is the development of intermediate care units, appropriately staffed to perform frequent clinical checks but without the extended monitoring and life support capabilities available in the NCCU.

It is only possible to avoid admission to the NCCU if rapid emergence and tracheal extubation are possible at the end of surgery. Although this practice is widely recommended, a survey of German neuroanaesthetists revealed that only 61% of patients with brain tumours were managed without postoperative ventilation in the 1990s (15). However, there was a trend towards earlier extubation from 1991 to 1997 and, with the developments in neuroanaesthesia, this trend is likely to have continued since then.

In summary, the indication for postoperative intensive care after elective intracranial surgery varies between neurosurgical centres and depends on NCCU capacity, nurse staffing, and competency levels in other clinical areas, as well as intraoperative anaesthesia and surgical management.

Table 16.1 Indications for postoperative admission to different care locations

NCCU	Intermediate care unit	Ward
Major preoperative co-morbidity	Posterior fossa surgery	Small supratentorial tumour without complication
Slow emergence after surgery	Preoperative midline shift > 5 mm (CT scan)	Grade 0 aneurysm
Unexpected neurological deficit after surgery	Duration of surgery > 4 h	Intracranial biopsy without complication
Massive intraoperative blood losses	Age > 70 years	Surgery not involving the brain
Posterior fossa surgery involving cranial nerves IX–XII	Severe postoperative pain	CSF shunt placement
Postoperative seizures	Recurrent postoperative nausea and vomiting	Uncomplicated trans-sphenoidal surgery
Karnofsky index < 80	Hypothermia < 35.5°C at extubation	
	Severe postoperative arterial hypertension	
	Postoperative hypoxaemia	
	Blood loss > 350 mL	

Emergency procedures

There is little doubt that the majority of emergency neurosurgical procedures require postoperative management in the NCCU. Emergency neurosurgery is indicated most frequently for trauma patients or to treat intracranial hypertension and impending brain herniation and, less frequently, to clip an intracranial aneurysm, excise an arteriovenous malformation, treat pituitary apoplexy, or remove a brain abscess or subdural empyema.

After serious head trauma, the benefit of direct transportation to an institution with a neurosurgical unit compared to the nearest hospital is strongly recommended (16), but this can be a challenge for busy neurosurgical centres with limited NCCU beds. Our policy is to admit patients and perform surgery whenever it is indicated, sometimes by admitting the patient directly into the operating theatre (after the CT scan) if the NCCU is full. This ensures timely surgical intervention and allows time to identify a bed, or in extreme circumstances to transfer the patient to another facility after post-surgery stabilization.

General care after craniotomy

Frequent neurological observations undertaken by a trained nurse are mandatory after intracranial neurosurgery irrespective of the care location. In addition, several treatments are needed to prevent postoperative complications or treat side effects of surgery and anaesthesia (Table 16.2).

Postoperative pain, nausea, and vomiting

Although craniotomy is less painful than other major surgical procedures such as thoracic, abdominal, and orthopaedic surgery (17), post-craniotomy pain is often moderate or severe, and frequently underestimated and inadequately treated (18). Pain scores decrease from the first to the second postoperative day and pain is more severe after infratentorial than supratentorial surgery. The increasing use of remifentanil during anaesthesia for craniotomy means that postoperative analgesia requirements must be anticipated before awakening. Scalp nerve blocks or wound infiltrations

Table 16.2 Corticosteroids comparison table (potency of anti-inflammatory and mineralocorticoid effect is relative to hydrocortisone)

Drug	Equivalent glucocorticoid dose (mg)	Route of administration	Potency relative to hydrocortisone		Duration of action (hours)
			Anti-inflammatory	Mineralocorticoid	
Short acting					
Hydrocortisone	20	IM, IV, PO	1	1	8–12
Intermediate acting					
Prednisolone	5	PO	4	0.8	12–36
Prednisolone	5	PO	4	0.8	12–36
Methylprednisolone	4	IM, IV, PO	5	0.5	12–36
Long acting					
Dexamethasone	0.75	IM, IV, PO	30	0	36–54
Betamethasone	0.6	IM, PO	30	0	36–54
Mineralocorticoid					
Fludrocortisone	0	PO	15	150	24–36
Aldosterone	0	PO	0	400	–

Modified from Adrenal cortical steroids. In *Drug Facts and Comparisons*, 2015 edition. Clinical Drug Information, 2014.

with local anaesthesia provide effective early postoperative analgesia, but pain reappears a few hours after the end of surgery (19–21). Importantly, the duration of the analgesic effect of scalp infiltration placed before surgery may be too short to provide long-lasting postoperative analgesia. Paracetamol (acetaminophen) alone does not provide adequate pain relief and should be used in combination with other analgesics including opioids in the early postoperative period (22). Tramadol is effective after craniotomy, does not affect intracranial pressure (ICP) or cerebral perfusion pressure (CPP) (23), but may increase the frequency of nausea and vomiting and induce somnolence (24). Nefopam has anti-shivering and analgesic properties but has been associated with convulsions (25) despite having strong anticonvulsant properties in experimental studies (26). Patient-controlled opioid analgesia is effective and safe after craniotomy, although the adverse effects of opioids in neurosurgical patients, including somnolence, retention of CO_2, and increased ICP, may limit its use (27). Non-steroidal anti-inflammatory drugs (NSAIDs) are rarely used early after craniotomy because they inhibit platelet aggregation and might thereby increase the risk of postoperative bleeding. There are also concerns about the well-known upper gastrointestinal side effects, particularly in patients concurrently receiving corticosteroids. However, there are no data demonstrating adverse consequences of NSAIDs after craniotomy and they can probably be used safely in selected patients.

Nausea occurs in 50% of patients after craniotomy and vomiting in approximately 40% (1,28,29). Emesis is more frequent after infratentorial surgery and in women. Prophylaxis for postoperative nausea and vomiting is often indicated. Ondansetron is safe and has few side effects, but is only partially effective (28–30). Droperidol is more effective than ondansetron and does not induce sedation at doses of 1 mg or less (28). Repeated doses of droperidol may be sedative so the combination of droperidol (< 1 mg) and ondansetron is often used. Corticosteroids are also effective in the prevention of postoperative nausea and vomiting (31).

Corticosteroids

The oedema surrounding brain tumours is mainly vasogenic, and corticosteroids dramatically reduce oedema associated with malignant glioma or brain metastasis. This effect has been known since 1961 (32) and, more recently, diffusion tensor magnetic resonance imaging studies confirm localized decreased water content in the white matter surrounding brain tumours a few days after corticosteroid use (33). A plateau effect is observed after 4–6 days of treatment. Corticosteroids have no effect on cytotoxic or interstitial oedema and should not be used in cerebral ischaemia or after brain trauma (34). Side effects of corticosteroids are frequent, and toxicity has been related to cumulative dose as well as duration of treatment. Hyperglycaemia is the most common complication of steroid use but psychoses can be problematic and are often overlooked or mistakenly presumed to be related to the primary neurological pathology. The administration of corticosteroids should be reviewed regularly in the postoperative period, and high doses tapered rapidly over a few days.

Dexamethasone is the most commonly prescribed corticosteroid for the management of cerebral oedema and has low mineralocorticoid activity. The initial dexamethasone regimen is a bolus dose of 10 mg followed by 4 mg every 6 hours (35), although daily doses of 4–8 mg are usually appropriate (36). Other corticosteroids, for example, methylprednisolone, may also be used but each has specific potencies and anti-inflammatory and mineralocorticoid actions (Table 16.3). Dexamethasone is approximately six times more potent than methylprednisolone.

Prophylactic anticonvulsants

The prophylactic use of antiepileptic drugs after intracerebral surgery is controversial. Their effects on the prevalence of seizures are unclear (37), and they have important and potentially serious side effects (38,39). In 2000, a consensus statement from the Quality Standards Subcommittee of the American Academy of Neurology recommended that prophylactic antiepileptic drugs should not be used routinely in patients with brain tumours and that, if they are, the drug should be stopped in the first week after surgery if the patient remains seizure free (40). However, there is considerable disparity between guidelines and management strategies pursued by neurologists, neurosurgeons, and neuroanaesthetists. In 2005, a clinical practice survey showed that 70% of neurosurgeons routinely used prophylactic antiepileptic drugs in patients undergoing brain tumour resection (41).

Two meta-analyses concluded that prophylactic anticonvulsants are not superior to placebo (no prophylaxis) in the prevention of a post-craniotomy seizure in patients with brain tumours, but are associated with a higher risk of other adverse effects (42,43). Milligan and colleagues compared the efficacy and tolerability of prophylactic levetiracetam with phenytoin after supratentorial surgery (44) and found no difference in efficacy but fewer adverse effects with levetiracetam. The duration of prophylactic therapy in patients without preoperative seizures should be restricted to the first postoperative week (45). Seizures have been reported after posterior fossa surgery but a preventive treatment is seldom required (46).

Table 16.3 Treatments after intracranial tumour surgery

Analgesics	Corticosteroids	Antiepileptics	Thromboprophylaxis	Other
Paracetamol 1 g/6 h + tramadol 100 mg/6–8 h ± nefopam or NSAID Persistent pain: opioid PCA	Dexamethasone Day 1: 12 mg/6 h Day 2: 6 mg/6 h + PPI	Levetiracetam 500 mg/8h or phenytoin 100 mg/8 h or continue other preoperative drug	Consider IPC in all patients LMWH the morning after surgery (after CT scan)	Antibiotic prophylaxis Hormonal treatment after pituitary surgery or craniopharyngioma

IPC, intermittent pneumatic calf compression; LMWH, low molecular weight heparin; NSAID, non-steroidal anti-inflammatory drugs; PCA, patient-controlled analgesia; PPI, proton pump inhibitor.

Chronic antiepileptic treatments in known epileptics should be administered as early as possible in the postoperative period.

Thromboprophylaxis

The risk of venous thromboembolism (VTE) is high after intracranial surgery. Without prophylaxis, the frequency of ultrasonography- or venography-confirmed deep vein thrombosis (DVT) is 20–35% and 2.3–6% for symptomatic events (47). Malignant tumour, prolonged surgery, hemiparesis, and advanced age are risk factors for VTE. The value of both mechanical methods of prophylaxis against DVT, such as intermittent pneumatic compression (IPC) of the calves, and low-molecular-weight heparin (LMWH) or low dose unfractionated heparin (UFH) have been demonstrated. Compression stockings are probably not effective alone (48), but are usually used in combination with IPC. LMWH or IPC decrease the risk of DVT by at least 50%, and at least one method should be employed routinely after intracranial surgery (49). The combination of LMWH and IPC is highly effective (50) but, in large trials, low-dose heparin or LMWH increased the rate of symptomatic haemorrhage (49,51). The potential benefits of heparin must therefore be weighed against the risk of intracranial haemorrhage. For this reason, IPC alone is usually recommended in the early period after craniotomy.

In patients at high risk of developing VTE (see above), heparin is indicated when adequate haemostasis has been established. Otherwise, the optimal delay between surgery and anticoagulation has not been determined. Mechanical prophylaxis (IPC) should be started at the time of surgery and, in our practice, LMWH or UFH treatment is started on the morning after surgery following a cranial CT scan to rule out intracranial bleeding. In some centres, UFH is preferred to LMWH because heparin can be reversed by protamine, but this benefit is unclear and many centres use LMWH without adverse effects.

Antibiotics

Antibiotic prophylaxis is recommended during intracranial surgery as it halves the rate of postoperative infection (52,53). The optimal duration of treatment is unknown but should be less than 24 hours to avoid the development and selection of antibiotic-resistant microorganisms. It is common practice to continue antibiotic prophylaxis in the first few hours after surgery. A first-generation cephalosporin (cefazolin) is usually recommended.

Hormone replacement

Hormone support may be necessary after pituitary or craniopharyngioma surgery. Postoperative thyroid replacement therapy is never an emergency because the half-life of thyroid hormone is several days. Cortisol replacement may be needed after the surgical treatment of Cushing's disease, and is mandatory in patients with preoperative adrenal insufficiency. Hydrocortisone 50 mg 6-hourly is sufficient to prevent relative adrenal insufficiency in the first 24 hours after surgery.

Cranial diabetes insipidus (CDI) is characterized by polyuria and polydipsia, but the signs of polydipsia are absent in sedated postoperative patients (see Chapter 28). CDI may rapidly induce dehydration and hypernatraemia if not diagnosed and treated early. Monitoring urine output and specific gravity or osmolarity is mandatory when there is a risk of CDI. Increased diuresis from intraoperative fluids or residual effects of mannitol can occur, but is usually limited to the early postoperative period, does not induce hypernatraemia and should not be mistaken for CDI. In the context of pituitary surgery, urine output above 250 mL/hour for more than 2 hours and a specific gravity less than 1.005 (urine osmolality < 300 mOsm/kg) is an indication to administer desmopressin (DDAVP) by the oral, nasal, intravenous, or subcutaneous route. In postoperative patients, intravenous administration, in doses of 1–4 mcg as required, is preferred. Oral water intake guided by thirst is an effective and safe way of managing fluid replacement in the majority of awake patients, but intravenous hypotonic fluid replacement may be necessary to limit hypernatraemia in those unable to take oral fluids. Rapid reduction of plasma osmolality may promote cerebral oedema and should be avoided.

Monitoring strategies

Although clinical neurological examination is the mainstay of monitoring postoperative neurosurgical patients, careful attention to systemic and cerebral physiological homeostasis mandates additional monitoring.

Clinical monitoring

The best neurological monitor is repeated clinical examination by a trained observer. Neurological worsening may cause either a focal neurological deficit (motor, speech, or visual deficits) or a decrease in conscious level. Several scores have been described to assess neurological status (54). The Glasgow Coma Scale (GCS), although not validated for postoperative patients, is simple to use and well known by nurses and physicians, explaining its widespread use. The GCS score relies on the best global response and therefore cannot detect focal deficits, so focal neurological status (limb power and pupil responses) must also be documented. As well as monitoring for general neurological changes, attention should also be given to monitoring for procedure-specific deficits. For example, speech deficits after surgery of the left temporal lobe or swallowing disorders after surgery of the cerebropontine angle are deficits of concern after these specific procedures, and clinical monitoring must focus on these in addition to the GCS.

A decrease in consciousness is the most common clinical sign of postoperative intracranial haemorrhage (see 'Intracranial haemorrhage'). However, even small doses of narcotics or hypnotics may exacerbate or unmask focal neurological deficits and decrease consciousness, and may lead to unnecessary brain imaging (7,55).

Haemodynamic monitoring

Hypoxaemia and hypotension are associated with a significant increase in morbidity and mortality after traumatic brain injury (TBI) (56), and this probably also holds true for other brain injury types including the postoperative brain. It is also likely that severe postoperative hypertension may increase the risk of brain haemorrhage, especially shortly after a procedure when the process of fragile surgical haemostasis is ongoing (13). Therefore, continuous arterial blood pressure monitoring is common practice in the postoperative period after neurosurgery, and should be available until blood pressure is stable or intervention to control it is no longer required.

Continuous electrocardiography is mandatory to detect arrhythmias, especially after epilepsy surgery or subarachnoid haemorrhage (SAH) (57,58). Cardiac output monitoring may be necessary in specific situations including pre-existing cardiac failure, SAH-induced cardiomyopathy, and when complex haemodynamic management is required after massive blood losses and sepsis. Echocardiography should also be available to quantify ventricular systolic function if required.

Respiratory monitoring

Oxygen saturation measurement using pulse oximetry is indicated for all postoperative patients. The arterial partial pressure of CO_2 ($PaCO_2$) is a major determinant of cerebral blood flow (CBF) and patients with low intracranial compliance have a significant risk of developing raised ICP during hypercapnia. Blood gas analysis should be performed on admission of neurosurgical patients to the NCCU or recovery room. Administration of opioids or sedatives may lead to an increase in $PaCO_2$ and explain some temporally related neurological changes. Similarly, it seems reasonable to monitor end-tidal CO_2 ($ETCO_2$) in all ventilated neurosurgical patients. Although the gradient between $PaCO_2$ and $ETCO_2$ may vary over time (59), large variations in $ETCO_2$ always indicate a change in $PaCO_2$, and this may go undetected without $ETCO_2$ monitoring.

Intracranial monitoring

Except after SAH and TBI, ICP is rarely routinely monitored in elective postoperative craniotomy patients. In a retrospective study of 514 patients with ICP monitoring after elective supratentorial and infratentorial surgery, 17% had an increase in ICP and this was associated with clinical deterioration in 53% (60). Risk factors for postoperative ICP elevation included resection of glioblastoma, repeat surgery, and surgery lasting more than 6 hours. In a 2012 randomized study after TBI, care based on ICP monitoring was not superior to care based on imaging and clinical examination (61), confirming the results of a previous non-randomized study (62). Such findings do not mean that ICP is not useful in selected patients, but rather that the routine use of ICP monitoring, especially in the postoperative period, is probably not indicated. Conversely, ICP monitoring should be undertaken when clinical examination is unreliable because of sedation or coma, or when there are signs of intracranial hypertension or oedema on brain CT scan or intraoperatively. In this case, ICP monitoring is the only way to measure CPP continuously in order to identify and treat cerebral hypoperfusion.

Transcranial Doppler sonography (TCD) of the middle cerebral artery allows real-time estimation of cerebral perfusion and CO_2 reactivity (see Chapter 10). A low diastolic CBF velocity or a high pulsatility index on TCD suggests a low CPP (Figure 16.1). In this situation, physiological factors that alter CBF, such as hypocapnia, hypotension, and high ICP, should be checked and corrected. The effect of treatments on the cerebral circulation can be followed on successive TCD recordings or with continuous TCD monitoring over a few hours using a specially designed TCD probe fixation. In situations of zero diastolic flow, ICP is approximately equal to or is greater than the diastolic arterial pressure. Conversely, high blood flow velocity may indicate cerebral vasospasm, although it has rarely been reported after elective neurosurgery (Table 16.4). Case reports suggest that vasospasm be more frequent after amygdalo-hippocampectomy for epilepsy surgery (63) or pituitary surgery (64), but it has rarely been reported after uncomplicated tumour surgery (65). Blood flow velocity can also be increased in the postoperative period because of haemodilution, and should not be mistaken for vasospasm (66). Neurological symptoms due to

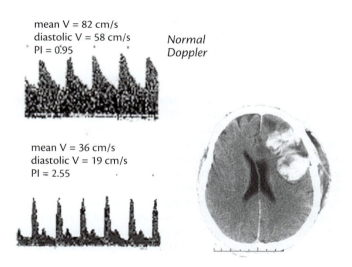

Fig. 16.1 Transcranial Doppler (TCD) sonography to assess cerebral haemodynamics. CT scan (right of panel) showing postoperative frontal haemorrhage and TCD recording showing low velocities (V) and high pulsatility index (PI) suggesting elevated intracranial pressure and low cerebral perfusion pressure (low trace). A normal TCD trace is shown upper left panel. (See Chapter 10 for further discussion of TCD.)

vasospasm may appear as early as 2 days after surgery, and the time course of TCD flow velocity acceleration parallels the development of angiographic vasospasm. If the patient develops symptoms compatible with cerebral vasospasm, immediate cerebral angiography should be performed in order to diagnose and treat this complication appropriately.

Jugular venous bulb oxygen saturation (SjO_2), or the arteriojugular difference in oxygen content ($AJDO_2$), provides information about the balance between brain oxygen demand and supply, and may be useful in distinguishing between cerebral hyperaemia and vasospasm (see Chapter 11). During periods of constant cerebral metabolic rate, changes in CBF parallel changes in SjO_2. SjO_2 below 50% indicates relative hypoperfusion and, in the absence of anaemia, SjO_2 above 75% suggests relative or absolute hyperaemia

Table 16.4 Assessment of cerebral blood flow at the bedside using TCD and SjO_2 and suspected intracranial haemodynamic situation

	SjO_2	CBF	PI	Suspected situation: recommendation
CBFV low	< 55%	Low	> 1.2	Low CPP, high ICP: monitor ICP
	55–75%	Adequate	< 1.2	Low CPP, low CO_2: therapeutic trial
	> 75%	Brain ischaemia		Normal
				Ischaemic lesion: CT scan
CBFV high	< 55%	Low		Cerebral vasospasm: CT angiography
	55–75%	Adequate		Normal or impending vasospasm: repeat TCD
	> 75%	High		Hyperaemia: check blood pressure, CO_2

CBFV, cerebral blood flow velocity; CO_2, arterial carbon dioxide partial pressure; PI, pulsatility index; TCD, transcranial Doppler.

(Table 16.4). Thus, the combination of high blood flow velocity and low SjO_2 strongly suggests diffuse cerebral vasospasm, although a normal SjO_2 value does not rule out focal cerebral ischaemia.

Blood glucose monitoring

Hyperglycaemia has been consistently associated with poor outcome in neurosurgical patients (67–69). Routine glucose monitoring and glycaemic control are indicated in the postoperative period but the targets for glycaemic control remain a matter of debate. One randomized study in elective and emergency neurosurgical patients demonstrated shorter NCCU stay and reduced infection rates with tight glycaemic control, but more frequent episodes of hypoglycaemia (70). Studies in brain trauma patients have demonstrated reduced brain glucose availability and increased brain energy crisis with tight glycaemic control (71,72) and, after acute ischaemic stroke, intensive insulin therapy has been associated with larger infarct size (73). Therefore, both hyperglycaemia and low blood glucose should be avoided in neurosurgical patients justifying systematic blood glucose monitoring and maintenance of blood sugar between 5.0 and 10 mmol/L (90 and 180 mg/dL).

Electroencephalography

Epilepsy is a frequent complication of neurosurgery. Seizures may be clinically evident in some patients and an electroencephalogram (EEG) is needed only to monitor the effectiveness of antiepileptic treatment. However, drowsiness or coma may be due to non-convulsive epilepsy or non-convulsive status epilepticus (NCSE) and these conditions can only be detected with EEG monitoring. In a study of 236 patients with coma and no overt clinical seizure activity, EEG monitoring demonstrated NCSE in 8% (74). In the postoperative period, NCSE is a well-identified cause of coma after various surgical procedures (75–77). Standard single EEG examination may miss the typical features of epilepsy due to intermittent epileptic discharges or difficulties in recognizing a specific pattern such as rhythmic delta waves, for example. When imaging does not identify a cause for a decrease in consciousness in the postoperative period, continuous EEG monitoring (i.e. over several hours or more) should be obtained to rule out NCSE.

Haemodynamic management

Because of the link between the brain and cardiovascular system, hypertension, hypotension, arrhythmias, myocardial failure, and neurogenic pulmonary oedema are common in neurosurgical patients (see Chapter 27) (78–80). Myocardial damage is especially frequent after SAH, and neurogenic pulmonary oedema may occur after TBI, stroke, and intracranial hypertension (81–84). Haemodynamic management may be difficult after neurosurgical emergencies and complex neurosurgical procedures, particularly in the presence of intracranial hypertension, and invasive haemodynamic monitoring is mandatory. Echocardiography may also be of assistance because treatment may be different depending on the presence or absence of neurogenic myocardial dysfunction. Two studies in SAH patients have suggested improved outcome with cardiac output monitoring and goal-directed therapy (85,86).

Hypertension

Hypertension is common after craniotomy (87) and likely to be related to sympathetic stimulation and release of epinephrine (adrenaline) and norepinephrine (noradrenaline). Continuing sedation into the postoperative period does not attenuate this response (88). Hypertension after craniotomy may lead to cerebral oedema and haemorrhage (89,90). A strong association between postoperative hypertension (> 160 mmHg) and intracranial bleeding has been reported (13) and, despite absence of evidence of causality, it seems wise to maintain postoperative blood pressure below 160 mmHg to reduce the risk of intracranial haemorrhage. In addition, it has been demonstrated that intensive blood pressure reduction after acute intracerebral haemorrhage (systolic blood pressure between 130 and 140 mmHg) can attenuate haematoma growth (91).

The early administration of an antihypertensive agent is sometimes required to prevent or limit the rise in blood pressure associated with awakening and tracheal extubation, and labetalol (0.15 mg/kg, as needed), esmolol (1 mg/kg bolus followed with an infusion of 0.2 mg/kg/min), urapidil (0.15 mg/kg, as needed) or nicardipine (0.5 to 1 mg bolus) may be used. After extubation, blood pressure returns toward normal values in 30–60 minutes in most patients. In normotensive patients, a secondary rise in blood pressure may be the first sign of an intracerebral complication.

Early intracranial hypertension has been reported in 18% of patients after elective supratentorial surgery (60), and is significantly associated with clinical deterioration possibly because cerebral hyperaemia combined with systemic hypertension may explain or aggravate cerebral oedema (92). Esmolol, a short-acting beta blocker, has the advantage of limiting the postoperative rise in blood pressure and the cerebral hyperaemic response (93). Intracranial hypertension is more common after craniotomy for ruptured intracranial aneurysms than for other indications. In one study, it was observed in 54% of 433 SAH patients overall (94) and, although more common in poor-grade patients (64%), high ICP occurred postoperatively in 48% of patients with a good clinical grade. The ICP response to treatment was strongly related to patient outcome.

Hypotension

Arterial hypotension is an uncommon complication after intracranial surgery but it is important to recognize and treat it rapidly to avoid cerebral hypoperfusion and ischaemia. Hypotension is most often related to hypovolaemia as a result of urinary losses due to the infusion of mannitol or underestimation of intraoperative blood loss. If hypovolaemia is suspected it is reasonable to test the response to a small fluid challenge with 250 mL of isotonic crystalloid over 10–20 minutes (see Chapter 5). CDI may lead to profound volume loss after pituitary surgery if not diagnosed and treated early. Adrenal insufficiency may also occur after pituitary surgery or in patients on chronic corticosteroid treatment.

Less frequently, myocardial ischaemia may progress to heart failure in patients with coronary artery disease and, if suspected, an electrocardiogram and plasma troponin-I should be obtained. Early postoperative pulmonary embolism should always be considered in cases of refractory hypotension, and the diagnosis may be suspected based on electrocardiographic, arterial blood gases, and chest X-ray findings. Echocardiography is easy to obtain at the bedside and is always positive after massive pulmonary embolism, but may be negative in small embolism. Helical pulmonary CT scanning has the highest sensitivity and specificity to confirm the diagnosis of pulmonary embolism.

Management of common complications

There are many complications that can arise in the postoperative period and some, such as intracranial haemorrhage, require immediate intervention. Early post-procedural neurological evaluation and timely investigations (see earlier sections) when indicated allow early identification of intracranial complications. An algorithm summarizing the approach to a new postoperative neurological deficit is shown in Figure 16.2.

Intracranial haemorrhage

The most feared complication after neurosurgery is intracranial haemorrhage (Figure 16.3). Its reported incidence varies greatly depending on the definition (95). In large retrospective studies, the incidence of intracranial haemorrhage causing clinical deterioration or requiring surgery varies between 0.8% and 2.2% (Table 16.5) (3,13,14,96–98). Approximately 40–60% of such bleeding episodes are intracerebral haematomas (97,98), and the outcome is frequently poor. Most intracranial bleeding occurs within the first 6 hours after surgery (13,14), and risk factors for postoperative bleeding include cerebral amyloid angiopathy, platelet count below 10^9/L, factor XIII and other clotting factor deficiencies, and preoperative treatment with antiplatelet agents or anticoagulants (95).

The risk of postoperative haemorrhage also depends on the surgical procedure (Table 16.6). As discussed earlier, postoperative hypertension is probably the most important and modifiable risk factor for intracerebral haemorrhage, and may in some cases be related to the hyperaemic response during awakening and extubation (92). Although prospective studies proving efficacy are lacking, retrospective studies (13) indicate that postoperative blood pressure control may reduce the risk of postoperative haemorrhage (93). Cerebral bleeding remote from the surgical area is a rare but well-described complication, and is most frequently located in the cerebellum. Remote cerebellar haemorrhage is thought to be related to cerebrospinal fluid (CSF) loss during surgery, intracranial hypotension, cerebellar sag and stretching, or transient occlusion of cerebellar veins leading to venous infarction (99,100). It may also occur after spinal surgery. Cerebellar haemorrhage is frequently asymptomatic but may lead to clinical deterioration requiring surgical evacuation.

Regular neurological monitoring is the best way to detect intracranial bleeding early, and this is the reason why short-acting anaesthetic agents should be used and patients extubated as early as possible after surgery. As already noted, even small doses of hypnotics and narcotics may worsen mild neurological deficits and impair neurological assessment (7,55). Conversely, inadequately

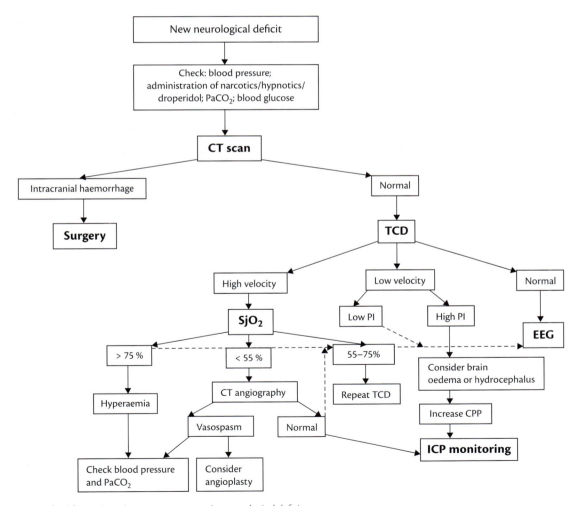

Fig. 16.2 Management algorithm to investigate new postoperative neurological deficits.
EEG, electroencephalography; SjO$_2$, jugular venous bulb oxygen saturation; TCD, transcranial Doppler.

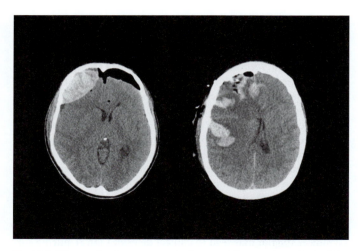

Fig. 16.3 CT scans showing postoperative intracranial haemorrhage. On the left panel, the patient suffered an extradural haematoma after removal of a frontal tumour. The patient was asymptomatic and the haematoma was revealed by a systematic postoperative CT scan the morning after surgery. On the right panel, an intracerebral haemorrhage occurred due to venous infarction after meningioma surgery.

treated pain may predispose to systemic hypertension and the above-noted risk of intracranial haemorrhage.

Not all patients can be awakened and extubated at the end of surgery. Reasons for delayed extubation include preoperative decreased consciousness, prolonged surgery, intraoperative complications (including bleeding and cerebral swelling) and end of surgery hypothermia (temperature < 35.5°C). In some patients, particularly if sedation will be continued for some time, postoperative ICP monitoring is indicated. Transcranial Doppler monitoring of middle cerebral artery blood flow velocity may be used to assess intracranial hypertension and impaired cerebral perfusion non-invasively by the demonstration of low diastolic velocity and high pulsatility index (Figure 16.1). Other non-invasive methods of assessing intracranial pressure, such as optic nerve sheath diameter, are discussed in Chapter 9.

Table 16.5 Rates of intracranial haemorrhage after craniotomy in large (>1000 patients) retrospective studies

Study	Criteria	Complication/ total (%)	Outcome
Fukamachi et al., 1985 (96)		42/1074 (3.9%)	
Kalfas and Little, 1988 (97)	CD	40/4992 (0.8%)	Death 11; poor 7
Palmer et al., 1994 (98)	Surgical evacuation	71/6668 (1.1%)	Death 22
Taylor et al., 1995 (14)	CD	50/2305 (2.2%)	Death 9
Basali et al., 2000 (13)	CD	86/11214 (0.77%)	?
Lassen et al., 2011 (3)	Surgical evacuation	54/2630 (2.1%)	Death 21

CD, clinical deterioration; poor, poor neurologic outcome.

Data from various studies (see References).

Table 16.6 Risk factors for postoperative intracranial haemorrhage

Procedure	Patient risk factor
Large intracerebral tumour (> 30 mL)	Uncontrolled arterial hypertension
Hypervascular tumour	Coagulation disorders
Large arterial-venous malformation resection	Disorders of haemostasis (low platelet count)
Carotid or intracranial artery angioplasty	Cerebral amyloid angiopathy
Thrombolysis for stroke	Treatment with antiplatelet agents

In all cases of unexpected neurological deficit, an urgent brain CT scan is mandatory to allow rapid diagnosis of intracranial complications and immediate treatment to avoid long-term sequelae. Symptomatic haemorrhage should to be evacuated as soon as possible after checking and correcting coagulation status, platelet count, and haemoglobin. After posterior fossa surgery, even small volume haemorrhage may cause significant neurological worsening and the decision to proceed to surgical evacuation can be difficult, although somnolence associated with even a small haemorrhage should prompt reoperation. Progression from coma to irreversible brainstem compression can be very rapid, particularly with posterior fossa haemorrhage. Some features such as duret haemorrhage (brainstem haemorrhage associated with herniation) may occur before obvious signs of clinical deterioration and should prompt urgent consideration of surgery.

Infection

Neurosurgical site infections occur in approximately 4% of craniotomy cases (101), although the rate is variably reported in the literature (102–105). Reoperation to treat central nervous system infections is required in only 0.5% of patients (106). The frequency of meningitis is also low at 1.5–2%. The most important risk factors for postoperative infection and meningitis are postoperative CSF leak (103,104), surgical duration greater than 4 hours, emergency surgery, early reoperation, and Altemeier class (clean, clean-contaminated, contaminated, and dirty type of surgery) (107). *Staphylococcus aureus* and various Gram-negative bacteria are the most common pathogens associated with postoperative infections, although coagulase negative staphylococci, *Propionibacterium acnes*, and streptococci infections may also occur.

The diagnosis of postoperative meningitis is often difficult because the usual clinical signs of fever, nuchal rigidity, headache, and decreased consciousness may be unreliable or appear late. Further, no CSF leucocyte count threshold is sensitive or specific enough for the diagnosis of postoperative meningitis and, although Gram staining is almost 100% specific, it has a very low sensitivity (108). A CSF serum to glucose ratio lower than 0.4 has a high sensitivity and specificity for the diagnosis of bacterial meningitis, but even extreme low glucose is not always confirmatory (109). CSF lactate greater than 4 mmol/L is highly sensitive and specific for the differentiation between bacterial and viral meningitis (110). CSF lactate may also differentiate bacterial from aseptic meningitis, although studies have reported mixed sensitivities and specificities (111). Among cytokines, CSF interleukin 1 beta seems to be the best biochemical marker of infection (112) but is not routinely performed in clinical practice. When bacteriological cultures are negative, a combination of clinical and biochemical markers is the best indicator for antibiotic treatment.

Epilepsy

Supratentorial craniotomy is associated with a relatively high risk of postoperative seizure. Depending on the indications for surgery (Table 16.7), about 15–20% of patients have at least one seizure in the postoperative period (113,114). The majority are partial seizures, either simple partial (focal motor or sensory phenomena without alteration of consciousness), complex partial (with alteration of consciousness), or partial with secondary generalization. Early seizures are likely to be related to surgical injury such as cerebral oedema, local inflammation, excitotoxic damage, oxidative stress, and impairment of neuronal metabolism (115). In addition to the direct risks that they bring to the recently operated brain, seizures may precipitate other serious complications, including intracranial haemorrhage, hypoxaemia, and pulmonary aspiration.

Late postoperative seizures represent actual epilepsy and may require long-term treatment (116). Several risk factors for late seizures have been described and include the nature of the primary intracranial disease (Table 16.7), severity of surgical insult, and pre-operative heraldic seizures (117). Both early and late seizures negatively affect neurological outcome and patients' quality of life.

Tension pneumocephalus

Pneumocephalus, or asymptomatic intracranial air, is a common occurrence after craniotomy (118,119). Significant amounts of intracranial air may persist for up to 14 days after surgery. Transformation of pneumocephalus into tension pneumocephalus (symptomatic intracranial air) is a rare complication (0.5–3%) after sitting craniotomy, and an exceptional complication after non-sitting craniotomy. It has been attributed to a diminution of brain volume, and several contributing factors have been implicated including the use of intraoperative mannitol or hyperventilation, gravitational effects of the sitting position, nitrous oxide anaesthesia, and the presence of a ventriculoperitoneal shunt. Tension pneumocephalus presents with deterioration of consciousness, focal neurological deficit, severe restlessness, and generalized convulsions, and may be a serious and life-threatening emergency. It is easily recognized on a CT scan (Figure 16.4). Two signs suggest

Table 16.7 Risk of seizures after common neurosurgical interventions

Incidence of postoperative seizure	(%)
Intracranial abscess	92%
Arteriovenous malformation	50%
Intracerebral haematoma	10–20%
Cerebral aneurysm	7–40%
Meningioma	36%
Metastasis resection	20%
Suprasellar tumour	5%
Shunt	22%

Reproduced with permission from Shaw MDM and Foy PM, 'Epilepsy after Craniotomy and the Place of Prophylactic Anticonvulsant Drugs: Discussion Paper', *Journal of the Royal Society of Medicine*, 84, 4, p. 3, Copyright © 1991 SAGE publications.

increased tension of the subdural air (120)—a widened interhemispheric space between the tips of the frontal lobes (because subdural air under tension separates and compresses the frontal lobes) that mimics the silhouette of Mount Fuji (121), and the presence of multiple small air bubbles scattered through several cisterns (the 'air bubble sign') (122). Putatively, these air bubbles enter the subarachnoid space through a tear in the arachnoid membrane caused by increased tension of air in the subdural space.

Tension pneumocephalus must be rapidly treated with 100% oxygen. A frontal burr hole to release trapped air under local or general anaesthesia is rarely indicated.

Electrolyte disorders

Hyponatraemia is a frequent complication of neurosurgery and it is important to distinguish between the syndrome of inappropriate secretion of antidiuretic hormone (SIADH) and cerebral salt wasting (CSW) (Table 16.8). SIADH is associated with fluid volume expansion, whereas CSW is a fluid volume-contracted state involving renal loss of sodium. Hence, the treatment of patients with SIADH is fluid restriction whereas the treatment for patients with CSW is salt and water replacement (123). The reader is referred to Chapter 28 for a detailed discussion of the mechanisms and treatment of these conditions.

In severe hyponatraemia (serum sodium < 120 mmol/L) from whatever cause, sodium replacement with 3% NaCl (513 mmol/L) may be required. Symptomatic patients with severe confusion or coma may require a 1 mL/kg 3% (hypertonic) saline load over 3–4 hours. This can be given more rapidly (over 30 minutes) if the patient is actively seizing, bearing in mind the risks of over-rapid sodium correction (see Chapter 28). One mL/kg of 3% NaCl elevates serum sodium by approximately 1 mmol/L.

CDI is a common complication of pituitary surgery and can be transient or permanent. The inability to concentrate urine leaves the patient dehydrated and leads to metabolic abnormalities that can be life-threatening if not recognized and treated with an exogenous arginine vasopressin analogue in a timely manner. The reported incidence of postsurgical CDI varies from 1% to 67% (124), and factors affecting the likelihood of CDI include pituitary tumour size, adherence to surrounding structures, surgical approach, and pathology of pituitary lesion. Postoperative CDI is characterized by urine output greater than 4 mL/kg/h, low urine, and high serum osmolality in the absence of other causes of polyuria (Table 16.9). Once the diagnosis is established, a DDAVP infusion is commenced at 1–4 mcg every 8–24 hours aimed at decreasing the urine output to less than 2 mL/kg/h. Total maintenance fluids (intravenous and oral) should not exceed the insensible losses plus the obligatory urinary losses.

Conclusion

The postoperative period after intracranial neurosurgery is critical. Patients should be carefully monitored and managed in an appropriate environment to identify and treat complications early. It is necessary to control blood pressure, minimize the risk of brain oedema, maintain water and electrolytes homeostasis, and prevent and treat pain. Early post-procedural neurological evaluation is the key to the detection of early intracranial complications. A brain CT scan should be obtained urgently in cases of unexpected neurological deterioration, but a normal CT scan does not rule out

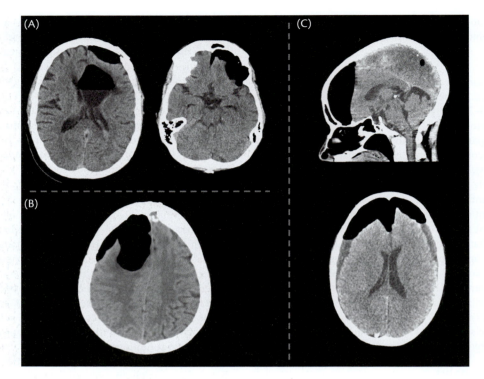

Fig. 16.4 CT scans showing postoperative pneumocephalus.
(A) Postoperative axial brain CT scans from a patient after brain tumour resection with a postoperative focal deficit showing pneumocephalus in the resection cavity and left frontal horn. There is *ex vacuo* dilatation with a stable 7 mm rightward midline shift and effacement of the lateral ventricles.
(B) Postoperative axial brain CT scans from a patient after surgical clipping of a pericallosal right anterior cerebral aneurysm, re-admitted to the ICU with acute left hemiparesis. Axial brain shows a tension pneumocephalus in the right frontal horn resulting in mass effect and effacement of the right frontal lobe sulci. Noted to have eschar on right craniotomy site with likely dehiscence and tracking of air from atmosphere into cranium.
(C) Postoperative sagittal and axial CT scan from a 59-year-old patient's bilateral chronic subdural haematomas demonstrating the 'Mount Fuji sign' with an accumulation of air in the bi-frontal subdural space.

Table 16.8 Clinical features of cerebral salt wasting (CSW) and syndrome of inappropriate antidiuretic hormone secretion (SIADH)

Clinical features	CSW	SIADH
Serum osmolality	Decreased	Decreased
Urine osmolality	Inappropriately high	Inappropriately high
Extracellular fluid volume	Decreased	Increased
Haematocrit	Increased	Normal
Plasma albumin concentration	Increased	Normal
Plasma blood urea nitrogen/creatinine	Increased	Decreased
Plasma potassium	Normal or increased	Normal
Plasma uric acid	Normal or decreased	Decreased
Treatment	Normal saline	Fluid restriction

Determination of extracellular fluid volume is the main method to differentiate CSW from SIADH.

Reprinted from *Trends in Endocrinology & Metabolism*, 14, 4, Palmer BF, 'Hyponatremia in patients with central nervous system disease: SIADH versus CSW', pp. 182–187, Copyright 2003, with permission from Elsevier.

Table 16.9 Clinical features of cranial diabetes insipidus

Urine output of	> 4 mL/kg/h
Serum Na	> 145 mEq/L
Serum osmolality	> 300 mOsm/kg
Urine osmolality	< 300 mOsm/kg
Polyuria persisting	> 30 min

Other causes of polyuria must be ruled out (e.g. administration of mannitol, furosemide, osmotic contrast agents, hyperglycaemia, or excessive fluid administration).

complications such as epilepsy, infection, brainstem compression, or increased ICP. The cause of neurological worsening is sometimes difficult to determine, and cooperation between neurosurgeons, neuroanaesthesiologists, and neurointensivists is critical for the optimal management of postoperative patients.

References

1. Manninen PH, Raman SK, Boyle K, el-Beheiry H. Early postoperative complications following neurosurgical procedures. *Can J Anaesthes*. 1999;46:7–14.
2. Bruder NJ. Awakening management after neurosurgery for intracranial tumours. *Curr Opin Anaesthesiol*. 2002;15:477–82.

3. Lassen B, Helseth E, Ronning P, Scheie D, Johannesen TB, Maehlen J, et al. Surgical mortality at 30 days and complications leading to re-craniotomy in 2630 consecutive craniotomies for intracranial tumors. *Neurosurgery*. 2011;68:1259–68.

4. Solheim O, Jakola AS, Gulati S, Johannesen TB. Incidence and causes of perioperative mortality after primary surgery for intracranial tumors: a national, population-based study. *J Neurosurg*. 2012;116:825–34.

5. Zrinzo L, Foltynie T, Limousin P, Hariz MI. Reducing hemorrhagic complications in functional neurosurgery: a large case series and systematic literature review. *J Neurosurg*. 2012;116:84–94.

6. Chernov MF, Ivanov PI. Urgent reoperation for major regional complications after removal of intracranial tumors: outcome and prognostic factors in 100 consecutive cases. *Neurol Med Chir (Tokyo)*. 2007;47:243–8.

7. Thal GD, Szabo MD, Lopez-Bresnahan M, Crosby G. Exacerbation or unmasking of focal neurologic deficits by sedatives. *Anesthesiology*. 1996;85:21–5.

8. Ziai WC, Varelas PN, Zeger SL, Mirski MA, Ulatowski JA. Neurologic intensive care resource use after brain tumor surgery: an analysis of indications and alternative strategies. *Crit Care Med*. 2003;31:2782–7.

9. Zimmerman JE, Junker CD, Becker RB, Draper EA, Wagner DP, Knaus WA. Neurological intensive care admissions: identifying candidates for intermediate care and the services they receive. *Neurosurgery*. 1998;42:91–101.

10. Rhondali O, Genty C, Halle C, Gardellin M, Ollinet C, Oddoux M, et al. Do patients still require admission to an intensive care unit after elective craniotomy for brain surgery? *J Neurosurg Anesthesiol*. 2011;23:118–23.

11. Asano K, Nakano T, Takeda T, Ohkuma H. Risk factors for postoperative systemic complications in elderly patients with brain tumors. *J Neurosurg*. 2009;111:258–64.

12. Bui JQ, Mendis RL, van Gelder JM, Sheridan MM, Wright KM, Jaeger M. Is postoperative intensive care unit admission a prerequisite for elective craniotomy? *J Neurosurg*. 2011;115:1236–41.

13. Basali A, Mascha EJ, Kalfas I, Schubert A. Relation between perioperative hypertension and intracranial hemorrhage after craniotomy. *Anesthesiology*. 2000;93:48–54.

14. Taylor WA, Thomas NW, Wellings JA, Bell BA. Timing of postoperative intracranial hematoma development and implications for the best use of neurosurgical intensive care. *J Neurosurg*. 1995;82:48–50.

15. Himmelseher S, Pfenninger E. Anaesthetic management of neurosurgical patients. *Curr Opin Anaesthesiol*. 2001;14:483–90.

16. Stevenson MD, Oakley PA, Beard SM, Brennan A, Cook AL. Triaging patients with serious head injury: results of a simulation evaluating strategies to bypass hospitals without neurosurgical facilities. *Injury*. 2001;32:267–74.

17. Dunbar PJ, Visco E, Lam AM. Craniotomy procedures are associated with less analgesic requirements than other surgical procedures. *Anesth Analg*. 1999;88:335–40.

18. Gottschalk A, Berkow LC, Stevens RD, Mirski M, Thompson RE, White ED, et al. Prospective evaluation of pain and analgesic use following major elective intracranial surgery. *J Neurosurg*. 2007;106:210–16.

19. Ayoub C, Girard F, Boudreault D, Chouinard P, Ruel M, Moumdjian R. A comparison between scalp nerve block and morphine for transitional analgesia after remifentanil-based anesthesia in neurosurgery. *Anesth Analg*. 2006;103:1237–40.

20. Biswas BK, Bithal PK. Preincision 0.25% bupivacaine scalp infiltration and postcraniotomy pain: a randomized double-blind, placebo-controlled study. *J Neurosurg Anesthesiol*. 2003;15:234–9.

21. Nguyen A, Girard F, Boudreault D, Fugere F, Ruel M, Moumdjian R, et al. Scalp nerve blocks decrease the severity of pain after craniotomy. *Anesth Analg*. 2001;93:1272–6.

22. Verchere E, Grenier B, Mesli A, Siao D, Sesay M, Maurette P. Postoperative pain management after supratentorial craniotomy. *J Neurosurg Anesthesiol*. 2002;14:96–101.

23. Ferber J, Juniewicz H, Glogowska E, Wronski J, Abraszko R, Mierzwa J. Tramadol for postoperative analgesia in intracranial surgery. Its effect on ICP and CPP. *Neurol Neurochir Pol*. 2000;34:70–9.

24. Jeffrey HM, Charlton P, Mellor DJ, Moss E, Vucevic M. Analgesia after intracranial surgery: a double-blind, prospective comparison of codeine and tramadol. *Br J Anaesth*. 1999;83:245–9.

25. Durrieu G, Olivier P, Bagheri H, Montastruc JL. Overview of adverse reactions to nefopam: an analysis of the French Pharmacovigilance database. *Fundam Clin Pharmacol*. 2007;21:555–8.

26. Czuczwar M, Czuczwar K, Cieszczyk J, Kis J, Saran T, Luszczki JJ, et al. Nefopam enhances the protective activity of antiepileptics against maximal electroshock-induced convulsions in mice. *Pharmacol Rep*. 2011;63:690–6.

27. Morad AH, Winters BD, Yaster M, Stevens RD, White ED, Thompson RE, et al. Efficacy of intravenous patient-controlled analgesia after supratentorial intracranial surgery: a prospective randomized controlled trial. *J Neurosurg*. 2009;111:343–50.

28. Fabling JM, Gan TJ, El-Moalem HE, Warner DS, Borel CO. A randomized, double-blinded comparison of ondansetron, droperidol, and placebo for prevention of postoperative nausea and vomiting after supratentorial craniotomy. *Anesth Analg*. 2000;91:358–61.

29. Kathirvel S, Dash HH, Bhatia A, Subramaniam B, Prakash A, Shenoy S. Effect of prophylactic ondansetron on postoperative nausea and vomiting after elective craniotomy. *J Neurosurg Anesthesiol*. 2001;13:207–12.

30. Fabling JM, Gan TJ, El-Moalem HE, Warner DS, Borel CO. A randomized, double-blind comparison of ondansetron versus placebo for prevention of nausea and vomiting after infratentorial craniotomy. *J Neurosurg Anesthesiol*. 2002;14:102–7.

31. De Oliveira GS, Jr, Castro-Alves LJ, Ahmad S, Kendall MC, McCarthy RJ. Dexamethasone to prevent postoperative nausea and vomiting: an updated meta-analysis of randomized controlled trials. *Anesth Analg*. 2013;116:58–74.

32. Galicich JH, French LA, Melby JC. Use of dexamethasone in treatment of cerebral edema associated with brain tumors. *Lancet*. 1961;81:46–53.

33. Sinha S, Bastin ME, Wardlaw JM, Armitage PA, Whittle IR. Effects of dexamethasone on peritumoural oedematous brain: a DT-MRI study. *J Neurol Neurosurg Psychiatry*. 2004;75:1632–5.

34. Gomes JA, Stevens RD, Lewin JJ, 3rd, Mirski MA, Bhardwaj A. Glucocorticoid therapy in neurologic critical care. *Crit Care Med*. 2005;33:1214–24.

35. Hockey B, Leslie K, Williams D. Dexamethasone for intracranial neurosurgery and anaesthesia. *J Clin Neurosci*. 2009;16:1389–93.

36. Ryan R, Booth S, Price S. Corticosteroid-use in primary and secondary brain tumour patients: a review. *J Neurooncol*. 2012;106:449–59.

37. Komotar RJ, Raper DM, Starke RM, Iorgulescu JB, Gutin PH. Prophylactic antiepileptic drug therapy in patients undergoing supratentorial meningioma resection: a systematic analysis of efficacy. *J Neurosurg*. 2011;115:483–90.

38. Fuller KL, Wang YY, Cook MJ, Murphy MA, D'Souza WJ. Tolerability, safety, and side effects of levetiracetam versus phenytoin in intravenous and total prophylactic regimen among craniotomy patients: a prospective randomized study. *Epilepsia*. 2013;54:45–57.

39. Pulman J, Greenhalgh J, Marson AG. Antiepileptic drugs as prophylaxis for post-craniotomy seizures. *Cochrane Database Syst Rev*. 2013;2:CD007286.

40. Glantz MJ, Cole BF, Forsyth PA, Recht LD, Wen PY, Chamberlain MC, et al. Practice parameter: anticonvulsant prophylaxis in patients with newly diagnosed brain tumors. Report of the Quality Standards Subcommittee of the American Academy of Neurology. *Neurology*. 2000;54:1886–93.

41. Tremont-Lukats IW, Ratilal BO, Armstrong T, Gilbert MR. Antiepileptic drugs for preventing seizures in people with brain tumors. *Cochrane Database Syst Rev*. 2008;2:CD004424.

42. Siomin V, Angelov L, Li L, Vogelbaum MA. Results of a survey of neurosurgical practice patterns regarding the prophylactic use of anti-epilepsy drugs in patients with brain tumors. *J Neurooncol*. 2005;74:211–15.

43. Temkin NR. Antiepileptogenesis and seizure prevention trials with antiepileptic drugs: meta-analysis of controlled trials. *Epilepsia*. 2001;42:515–24.

44. Milligan TA, Hurwitz S, Bromfield EB. Efficacy and tolerability of levetiracetam versus phenytoin after supratentorial neurosurgery. *Neurology.* 2008;71:665–9.

45. Klimek M, Dammers R. Antiepileptic drug therapy in the perioperative course of neurosurgical patients. *Curr Opin Anaesthesiol.* 2010;23:564–7.

46. Suri A, Mahapatra AK, Bithal P. Seizures following posterior fossa surgery. *Br J Neurosurg.* 1998;12:41–4.

47. Samama CM, Albaladejo P, Benhamou D, Bertin-Maghit M, Bruder N, Doublet JD, et al. Venous thromboembolism prevention in surgery and obstetrics: clinical practice guidelines. *Eur J Anaesthesiol.* 2006;23:95–116.

48. Dennis M, Sandercock PA, Reid J, Graham C, Murray G, Venables G, et al. Effectiveness of thigh-length graduated compression stockings to reduce the risk of deep vein thrombosis after stroke (CLOTS trial 1): a multicentre, randomised controlled trial. *Lancet.* 2009;373:1958–65.

49. Gould MK, Garcia DA, Wren SM, Karanicolas PJ, Arcelus JI, Heit JA, et al. Prevention of VTE in nonorthopedic surgical patients: Antithrombotic Therapy and Prevention of Thrombosis, 9th ed: American College of Chest Physicians Evidence-Based Clinical Practice Guidelines. *Chest.* 2012;141:e227S–277S.

50. Goldhaber SZ, Dunn K, Gerhard-Herman M, Park JK, Black PM. Low rate of venous thromboembolism after craniotomy for brain tumor using multimodality prophylaxis. *Chest.* 2002;122:1933–7.

51. Iorio A, Agnelli G. Low-molecular-weight and unfractionated heparin for prevention of venous thromboembolism in neurosurgery: a meta-analysis. *Arch Intern Med.* 2000;160:2327–32.

52. Korinek AM, Baugnon T, Golmard JL, van Effenterre R, Coriat P, Puybasset L. Risk factors for adult nosocomial meningitis after craniotomy: role of antibiotic prophylaxis. *Neurosurgery.* 2006;59:126–33.

53. Barker FG, 2nd. Efficacy of prophylactic antibiotics against meningitis after craniotomy: a meta-analysis. *Neurosurgery.* 2007;60:887–94.

54. Fabregas N, Bruder N. Recovery and neurological evaluation. *Best Pract Res Clin Anaesthesiol.* 2007;21:431–47.

55. Lazar RM, Fitzsimmons BF, Marshall RS, Berman MF, Bustillo MA, Young WL, et al. Reemergence of stroke deficits with midazolam challenge. *Stroke.* 2002;33:283–5.

56. Chesnut RM, Marshall LF, Klauber MR, Blunt BA, Baldwin N, Eisenberg HM, et al. The role of secondary brain injury in determining outcome from severe head injury. *J Trauma.* 1993;34:216–22.

57. Bealer SL, Little JG, Metcalf CS, Brewster AL, Anderson AE. Autonomic and cellular mechanisms mediating detrimental cardiac effects of status epilepticus. *Epilepsy Res.* 2010;91:66–73.

58. Frontera JA, Parra A, Shimbo D, Fernandez A, Schmidt JM, Peter P, et al. Cardiac arrhythmias after subarachnoid hemorrhage: risk factors and impact on outcome. *Cerebrovasc Dis.* 2008;26:71–8.

59. Grenier B, Verchere E, Mesli A, Dubreuil M, Siao D, Vandendriessche M, et al. Capnography monitoring during neurosurgery: reliability in relation to various intraoperative positions. *Anesth Analg.* 1999;88:43–8.

60. Constantini S, Cotev S, Rappaport Z, Pomeranz S, Shalit M. Intracranial pressure monitoring after elective intracranial surgery. A retrospective study of 514 consecutive patients. *J Neurosurg.* 1988;69:540–4.

61. Chesnut RM, Temkin N, Carney N, Dikmen S, Rondina C, Videtta W, et al. A trial of intracranial-pressure monitoring in traumatic brain injury. *N Engl J Med.* 2012;367:2471–81.

62. Cremer OL, van Dijk GW, van Wensen E, Brekelmans GJ, Moons KG, Leenen LP, et al. Effect of intracranial pressure monitoring and targeted intensive care on functional outcome after severe head injury. *Crit Care Med.* 2005;33:2207–13.

63. Lackner P, Koppelstaetter F, Ploner P, Sojer M, Dobesberger J, Walser G, et al. Cerebral vasospasm following temporal lobe epilepsy surgery. *Neurology.* 2012;78:1215–20.

64. Puri AS, Zada G, Zarzour H, Laws E, Frerichs K. Cerebral vasospasm after transsphenoidal resection of pituitary macroadenomas: report of 3 cases and review of the literature. *Neurosurgery.* 2012;71:173–80.

65. Bejjani GK, Sekhar LN, Yost AM, Bank WO, Wright DC. Vasospasm after cranial base tumor resection: pathogenesis, diagnosis, and therapy. *Surg Neurol.* 1999;52:577–83.

66. Bruder N, Cohen B, Pellissier D, Francois G. The effect of hemodilution on cerebral blood flow velocity in anesthetized patients. *Anesth Analg.* 1998;86:320–4.

67. Rovlias A, Kotsou S. The influence of hyperglycemia on neurological outcome in patients with severe head injury. *Neurosurgery.* 2000;46:335–42.

68. McGirt MJ, Woodworth GF, Ali M, Than KD, Tamargo RJ, Clatterbuck RE. Persistent perioperative hyperglycemia as an independent predictor of poor outcome after aneurysmal subarachnoid hemorrhage. *J Neurosurg.* 2007;107:1080–5.

69. Ahmed N, Davalos A, Eriksson N, Ford GA, Glahn J, Hennerici M, et al. Association of admission blood glucose and outcome in patients treated with intravenous thrombolysis: results from the Safe Implementation of Treatments in Stroke International Stroke Thrombolysis Register (SITS-ISTR). *Arch Neurol.* 2010;67:1123–30.

70. Bilotta F, Caramia R, Paoloni FP, Delfini R, Rosa G. Safety and efficacy of intensive insulin therapy in critical neurosurgical patients. *Anesthesiology.* 2009;110:611–19.

71. Oddo M, Schmidt JM, Carrera E, Badjatia N, Connolly ES, Presciutti M, et al. Impact of tight glycemic control on cerebral glucose metabolism after severe brain injury: a microdialysis study. *Crit Care Med.* 2008;36:3233–8.

72. Vespa P, McArthur DL, Stein N, Huang SC, Shao W, Filippou M, et al. Tight glycemic control increases metabolic distress in traumatic brain injury: a randomized controlled within-subjects trial. *Crit Care Med.* 2012;40:1923–9.

73. Rosso C, Corvol JC, Pires C, Crozier S, Attal Y, Jacqueminet S, et al. Intensive versus subcutaneous insulin in patients with hyperacute stroke: results from the randomized INSULINFARCT trial. *Stroke.* 2012;43:2343–9.

74. Towne AR, Waterhouse EJ, Boggs JG, Garnett LK, Brown AJ, Smith JR, Jr, et al. Prevalence of nonconvulsive status epilepticus in comatose patients. *Neurology.* 2000;54:340–5.

75. Burneo JG, Steven D, McLachlan RS. Nonconvulsive status epilepticus after temporal lobectomy. *Epilepsia.* 2005;46:1325–7.

76. Al-Mefty O, Wrubel D, Haddad N. Postoperative nonconvulsive encephalopathic status: identification of a syndrome responsible for delayed progressive deterioration of neurological status after skull base surgery. *J Neurosurg.* 2009;111:1062–8.

77. Devarajan J, Siyam AM, Alexopoulos AV, Weil R, Farag E. Non-convulsive status epilepticus in the postanesthesia care unit following meningioma excision. *Can J Anaesth.* 2011;58:68–73.

78. Laowattana S, Zeger SL, Lima JA, Goodman SN, Wittstein IS, Oppenheimer SM. Left insular stroke is associated with adverse cardiac outcome. *Neurology.* 2006;66:477–83.

79. Oppenheimer S. The anatomy and physiology of cortical mechanisms of cardiac control. *Stroke.* 1993;24:I3–5.

80. Soros P, Hachinski V. Cardiovascular and neurological causes of sudden death after ischaemic stroke. *Lancet Neurol.* 2012;11:179–88.

81. Bruder N, Rabinstein A. Cardiovascular and pulmonary complications of aneurysmal subarachnoid hemorrhage. *Neurocrit Care.* 2011;15(2):257–69.

82. Davidyuk G, Soriano SG, Goumnerova L, Mizrahi-Arnaud A. Acute intraoperative neurogenic pulmonary edema during endoscopic ventriculoperitoneal shunt revision. *Anesth Analg.* 2010;110:594–5.

83. Stollberger C, Wegner C, Finsterer J. Seizure-associated Takotsubo cardiomyopathy. *Epilepsia.* 2011;52:e160–7.

84. Yoshimura S, Toyoda K, Ohara T, Nagasawa H, Ohtani N, Kuwashiro T, et al. Takotsubo cardiomyopathy in acute ischemic stroke. *Ann Neurol.* 2008;64:547–54.

85. Kim DH, Haney CL, Van Ginhoven G. Reduction of pulmonary edema after SAH with a pulmonary artery catheter-guided hemodynamic management protocol. *Neurocrit Care.* 2005;3:11–15.

86. Mutoh T, Kazumata K, Ajiki M, Ushikoshi S, Terasaka S. Goal-directed fluid management by bedside transpulmonary hemodynamic monitoring after subarachnoid hemorrhage. *Stroke.* 2007;38:3218–24.

87. Wong AY, O'Regan AM, Irwin MG. Total intravenous anaesthesia with propofol and remifentanil for elective neurosurgical procedures: an audit of early postoperative complications. *Eur J Anaesthesiol.* 2006;23:586–90.

88. Bruder N, Stordeur JM, Ravussin P, Valli M, Dufour H, Bruguerolle B, *et al.* Metabolic and hemodynamic changes during recovery and tracheal extubation in neurosurgical patients: immediate versus delayed recovery. *Anesth Analg.* 1999;89:674–8.

89. Giraldo EA, Fugate JE, Rabinstein AA, Lanzino G, Wijdicks EF. Posterior reversible encephalopathy syndrome associated with hemodynamic augmentation in aneurysmal subarachnoid hemorrhage. *Neurocrit Care.* 2011;14:427–32.

90. Grande PO. The Lund concept for the treatment of patients with severe traumatic brain injury. *J Neurosurg Anesthesiol.* 2011;23:358–62.

91. Arima H, Anderson CS, Wang JG, Huang Y, Heeley E, Neal B, *et al.* Lower treatment blood pressure is associated with greatest reduction in hematoma growth after acute intracerebral hemorrhage. *Hypertension.* 2010;56:852–8.

92. Bruder N, Pellissier D, Grillot P, Gouin F. Cerebral hyperemia during recovery from general anesthesia in neurosurgical patients. *Anesth Analg.* 2002;94:650–4.

93. Grillo P, Bruder N, Auquier P, Pellissier D, Gouin F. Esmolol blunts the cerebral blood flow velocity increase during emergence from anesthesia in neurosurgical patients. *Anesth Analg.* 2003;96:1145–9.

94. Heuer GG, Smith MJ, Elliott JP, Winn HR, LeRoux PD. Relationship between intracranial pressure and other clinical variables in patients with aneurysmal subarachnoid hemorrhage. *J Neurosurg.* 2004;101:408–16.

95. Seifman MA, Lewis PM, Rosenfeld JV, Hwang PY. Postoperative intracranial haemorrhage: a review. *Neurosurg Rev.* 2011;34:393–407.

96. Fukamachi A, Koizumi H, Nukui H. Postoperative intracerebral hemorrhages: a survey of computed tomographic findings after 1074 intracranial operations. *Surg Neurol.* 1985;23:575–80.

97. Kalfas IH, Little JR. Postoperative hemorrhage: a survey of 4992 intracranial procedures. *Neurosurgery.* 1988;23:343–7.

98. Palmer JD, Sparrow OC, Iannotti F. Postoperative hematoma: a 5-year survey and identification of avoidable risk factors. *Neurosurgery.* 1994;35:1061–4.

99. Friedman JA, Piepgras DG, Duke DA, McClelland RL, Bechtle PS, Maher CO, *et al.* Remote cerebellar hemorrhage after supratentorial surgery. *Neurosurgery.* 2001;49:1327–40.

100. Marquardt G, Setzer M, Schick U, Seifert V. Cerebellar hemorrhage after supratentorial craniotomy. *Surg Neurol* 2002;57:241–51.

101. Korinek AM. Risk factors for neurosurgical site infections after craniotomy: a prospective multicenter study of 2944 patients. The French Study Group of Neurosurgical Infections, the SEHP, and the C-CLIN Paris-Nord. Service Epidemiologie Hygiene et Prevention. *Neurosurgery.* 1997;41:1073–9.

102. Whitby M, Johnson BC, Atkinson RL, Stuart G. The comparative efficacy of intravenous cefotaxime and trimethoprim/sulfamethoxazole in preventing infection after neurosurgery: a prospective, randomized study. Brisbane Neurosurgical Infection Group. *Br J Neurosurg.* 2000;14:13–18.

103. Korinek AM, Golmard JL, Elcheick A, Bismuth R, van Effenterre R, Coriat P, *et al.* Risk factors for neurosurgical site infections after craniotomy: a critical reappraisal of antibiotic prophylaxis on 4,578 patients. *Br J Neurosurg.* 2005;19:155–62.

104. Lietard C, Thebaud V, Besson G, Lejeune B. Risk factors for neurosurgical site infections: an 18-month prospective survey. *J Neurosurg.* 2008;109:729–34.

105. O'Keeffe AB, Lawrence T, Bojanic S. Oxford craniotomy infections database: a cost analysis of craniotomy infection. *Br J Neurosurg.* 2012;26:265–9.

106. Dashti SR, Baharvahdat H, Spetzler RF, Sauvageau E, Chang SW, Stiefel MF, *et al.* Operative intracranial infection following craniotomy. *Neurosurg Focus.* 2008;24:E10.

107. Altemeier W. Review of postoperative wound infections. In *Informal Papers of a Workshop on Control of Operating Room Airborne Bacteria, November 8–10, 1974.* Washington, DC: The National Research Council; 1976:11–27.

108. Schade RP, Schinkel J, Roelandse FW, Geskus RB, Visser LG, van Dijk JM, *et al.* Lack of value of routine analysis of cerebrospinal fluid for prediction and diagnosis of external drainage-related bacterial meningitis. *J Neurosurg.* 2006;104:101–8.

109. Viola GM. Extreme hypoglycorrhachia: not always bacterial meningitis. *Nat Rev Neurol.* 2010;6:637–41.

110. Viallon A, Desseigne N, Marjollet O, Birynczyk A, Belin M, Guyomarch S, *et al.* Meningitis in adult patients with a negative direct cerebrospinal fluid examination: value of cytochemical markers for differential diagnosis. *Crit Care.* 2011;15:R136.

111. Sakushima K, Hayashino Y, Kawaguchi T, Jackson JL, Fukuhara S. Diagnostic accuracy of cerebrospinal fluid lactate for differentiating bacterial meningitis from aseptic meningitis: a meta-analysis. *J Infect.* 2011;62:255–62.

112. Lopez-Cortes LF, Marquez-Arbizu R, Jimenez-Jimenez LM, Jimenez-Mejias E, Caballero-Granado FJ, Rey-Romero C, *et al.* Cerebrospinal fluid tumor necrosis factor-alpha, interleukin-1beta, interleukin-6, and interleukin-8 as diagnostic markers of cerebrospinal fluid infection in neurosurgical patients. *Crit Care Med.* 2000;28:215–19.

113. North JB, Penhall RK, Hanieh A, Hann CS, Challen RG, Frewin DB. Postoperative epilepsy: a double-blind trial of phenytoin after craniotomy. *Lancet.* 1980;1:384–6.

114. Shaw MD, Foy PM. Epilepsy after craniotomy and the place of prophylactic anticonvulsant drugs: discussion paper. *J R Soc Med.* 1991;84:221–3.

115. van Breemen MS, Wilms EB, Vecht CJ. Epilepsy in patients with brain tumours: epidemiology, mechanisms, and management. *Lancet Neurol.* 2007;6:421–30.

116. Manaka S, Ishijima B, Mayanagi Y. Postoperative seizures: epidemiology, pathology, and prophylaxis. *Neurol Med Chir (Tokyo).* 2003;43:589–600.

117. Tellez-Zenteno JF, Dhar R, Hernandez-Ronquillo L, Wiebe S. Long-term outcomes in epilepsy surgery: antiepileptic drugs, mortality, cognitive and psychosocial aspects. *Brain.* 2007;130:334–45.

118. Toung TJ, McPherson RW, Ahn H, Donham RT, Alano J, Long D. Pneumocephalus: effects of patient position on the incidence and location of aerocele after posterior fossa and upper cervical cord surgery. *Anesth Analg.* 1986;65:65–70.

119. Di Lorenzo N, Caruso R, Floris R, Guerrisi V, Bozzao L, Fortuna A. Pneumocephalus and tension pneumocephalus after posterior fossa surgery in the sitting position: a prospective study. *Acta neurochirurgica.* 1986;83:112–15.

120. Schirmer CM, Heilman CB, Bhardwaj A. Pneumocephalus: case illustrations and review. *Neurocrit Care.* 2010;13:152–8.

121. Sadeghian H. Mount Fuji sign in tension pneumocephalus. *Arch Neurol.* 2000;57:1366.

122. Ishiwata Y, Fujitsu K, Sekino T, Fujino H, Kubokura T, Tsubone K, *et al.* Subdural tension pneumocephalus following surgery for chronic subdural hematoma. *J Neurosurg.* 1988;68:58–61.

123. Palmer BF. Hyponatremia in patients with central nervous system disease: SIADH versus CSW. *Trends Endocrinol Metab.* 2003;14:182–7.

124. Schreckinger M, Szerlip N, Mittal S. Diabetes insipidus following resection of pituitary tumors. *Clin Neurol Neurosurg.* 2013;115(2):121–6.

CHAPTER 17

Traumatic brain injury

Hayden White and Bala Venkatesh

Traumatic brain injury (TBI) is defined as an alteration in brain function, or other evidence of brain pathology, caused by an external mechanical force from direct impact, acceleration or deceleration forces, blast waves, or penetrating trauma. The term head injury, although used interchangeably with TBI, may also refer to trauma to other parts of the head such as the scalp and the skull. TBI remains the most common cause of trauma-related death and disability, disproportionately affecting young individuals (1) with the majority being male. Globally, the incidence of TBI is rising, largely from increasing motor vehicle use in low-income countries. Importantly, the cost to all societies in emotional, social, and financial terms is substantial as the disabling effects of the original injury may persist for many years. A further disturbing trend is the increasing age of patients suffering TBI, most likely related to increasing falls in the elderly (see Table 17.1) (2,3).

Over the last 40 years, a number of epidemiological studies have described the causes and outcomes of TBI in developed countries (4–6). All-cause mortality from severe TBI has remained consistent at approximately 30–35% over the last 20 years (4,7,8). Of patients who survive the initial injury and reach a healthcare system but subsequently die, the mortality attributable directly to the TBI is approximately 90%. Despite advances in critical care, resuscitation, and imaging techniques, the management of severe TBI continues to pose a challenge to intensivists. TBI remains a major global health problem with 12-month mortality of about 35% and poor neurological outcome in 55–60% of survivors (4,7).

Classification

Several systems have been used to classify TBI and are based on either the severity of injury, mechanism of injury, pathophysiology, or pathoanatomical location (9). The classification based on injury severity is the most commonly used in clinical practice for triage, direction of targeted therapies, and for research purposes. This is based on the Glasgow Coma Scale (GCS) score at the scene. A GCS score of 3–8 defines severe TBI, 9–13 moderate TBI, and 14–15 mild TBI. Classifications based on clinical scoring systems such as the GCS have limitations. They do not take account of the impact of sedation, hypoxaemia, and circulatory instability on the score, nor other potentially confounding factors such as the age, presence of other injuries, and general physiological status.

TBI has also been classified according to its pathophysiological basis and the evolution of the injury over time which has given rise to the concepts of primary and secondary injury. Primary injury refers to the brain damage sustained at the time of the injury and can be in the form of a contusion, haematoma, diffuse axonal injury, and neuronal damage from mediator release and altered blood–brain barrier (BBB) permeability. Secondary injury refers to pathophysiological processes which occur from the moment of the primary injury and continue into the post injury phase, and can exacerbate brain damage. Secondary injury can occur at any time after the initial injury including during resuscitation, transport, and in the intensive care unit (ICU). A number of secondary physiological insults that can cause secondary brain injury have been described but the most common are hypoxia and hypotension.

Classification of TBI based on the physical mechanism of injury relies on knowledge of the forces applied and their directions. They have utility in modelling injuries and their prevention, but do not have a significant impact on clinical management.

A pathoanatomical approach has been used to classify head injury according to the location and type of the injury (Figure 17.1), and the advent of computed tomography (CT) scanning facilitated more precise classification. The six-category Marshall scoring system is an example (10). This is a descriptive system of CT classification which focuses on the presence or absence of a mass lesion, and differentiates diffuse injuries by signs of increased intracranial pressure (ICP) including compression of basal cisterns and midline shift (Table 17.2). CT classification methods are useful for diagnosis, targeted patient management, outcome prognostication, and standardized enrolment into research trials.

Resuscitation and transfer

It is essential that there is coordinated teamwork and an organized approach to ensure prompt attention to clinical assessment and management after TBI. Retrieval systems, including road and air ambulances, play a major role in this process. Airway protection together with stabilization of the neck and cardiopulmonary systems are integral initial steps to minimize further neurological damage by preventing secondary insults.

Monitoring

Prior to transfer to the ICU, optimizing perfusion and oxygenation at the scene of the injury and in the emergency department are critical. Monitoring haemoglobin oxygen saturation with a pulse oximeter (SpO_2) and blood pressure using a reliable non-invasive or preferably an invasive method to facilitate continuous recordings are essential.

Prevention of hypoxia and hypotension

The impetus for cerebral haemodynamic monitoring in neurotrauma first arose from the original 'talk and die' studies which described a group of head-injured patients who talked and then subsequently died (11–13). At necropsy, hypoxic or ischaemic brain

Table 17.1 Increasing age of patients in TBI studies

	Year of study	n	Median age (years)	Proportion aged > 50 years
Traumatic Coma Data Bank	1984–1987	746	25	15%
UK four-centre study	1986–1988	988	29	27%
European Brain Injury Consortium Core Data Survey	1995	847	38	33%
Rotterdam cohort study	1999–2003	774	42	39%
Austrian Severe TBI study	1999–2004	415	48	45%
TBI outcomes in Australia and NZ	2000–2001	635	42	45%

Reprinted from *The Lancet Neurology*, 7, 8, Maas AI *et al.*, 'Moderate and severe traumatic brain injury in adults', pp. 728–741, copyright 2008, with permission from Elsevier.

damage was observed in a variable proportion of these patients, raising the possibility that post-trauma systemic or cerebral hypoxia might have contributed to their death. The concepts of primary and secondary brain injury were thus developed as outlined earlier. However, the differentiation between primary and secondary injury is somewhat artificial and it is now appreciated that there is temporal overlap between the two (Figure 17.2).

The principal secondary insults causing secondary brain injury are hypoxia and hypotension. Data from the studies of Bouma et al. and Jaggi et al. demonstrated an inverse correlation between cerebral blood flow and neurological outcome after neurotrauma (14,15), and those from the Traumatic Coma Data Bank the importance of hypoxia and hypotension in determining outcome (16). Improved understanding of the pathophysiology of TBI influenced clinical practice in two ways. First, a plethora of monitoring modalities was developed for evaluating cerebral haemodynamics and oxygenation. Second, the concept of 'driving' oxygenated blood through a swollen brain to minimize the risk of cerebral hypoxia/ischaemia became the cornerstone of therapy in patients with severe TBI. The critical circulatory and oxygenation thresholds to prevent secondary injury to the brain are unknown but data from the Traumatic Coma Data Bank point to the importance of maintaining a systolic blood pressure (SBP) greater than 90 mmHg and SpO_2 greater than 90%. In a cohort of 717 patients with severe TBI, Chesnut et al. demonstrated that hypotension (defined as SBP < 90 mmHg) was an independent predictor of outcome and that a single episode of hypotension was associated with a marked increase in morbidity and mortality (16). Similarly, episodes of arterial desaturation (SpO_2 < 90%) were also associated with significant increases in morbidity and mortality, and the presence of

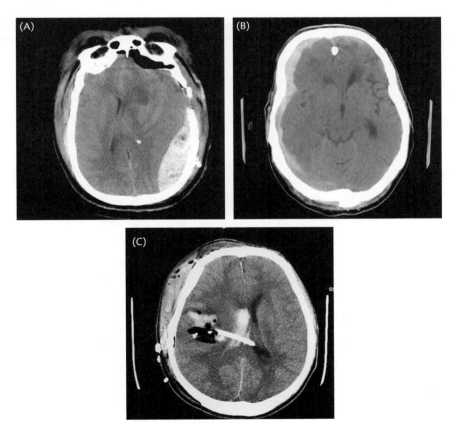

Fig. 17.1 Cranial computed tomography scans showing some consequences of brain trauma.
(A) Large left-sided occipitoparietal extradural haematoma. Note the classic convex nature of the haematoma. There is also a fracture in the temporoparietal region, marked cerebral oedema, midline shift with subfalcine herniation, and intracranial air.
(B) Right-sided acute subdural haematoma. The high density suggests a recent bleed. There is midline shift with ipsilateral loss of Sylvian fissure and sulci.
(C) Severe TBI complicated by intracranial haematoma requiring craniotomy. Note the intraventricular catheter.

Table 17.2 Marshall CT classification of TBI

Structural damage	Definition
Diffuse injury I	No visible pathology
Diffuse injury II	Cisterns present, midline shift 0–5 mm and/or lesion densities present or no mass lesion > 25 mL
Diffuse injury III (swelling)	Cisterns compressed or absent with midline shift 0–5 mm or no mass lesion > 25 mL
Diffuse injury IV (shift)	Midline shift > 5 mm, no mass lesion > 25 mL
Evacuated mass lesion	Any lesion surgically evacuated
Non-evacuated mass lesion	High or mixed-density lesion > 25 mL, not surgically evacuated

hypotension and hypoxaemia simultaneously had an additive effect on poor outcome. Other published studies also support the crucial significance of avoiding hypotension and hypoxaemia, and these are summarized in Table 17.3 (16,17,136–143).

Because hypoxia (PaO$_2$ < 8.0 kPa, < 60 mmHg) is generally considered deleterious, it has been suggested that early intubation and ventilation may be beneficial after severe TBI (16,17). However, data from studies investigating the benefits of pre-hospital intubation are conflicting. One randomized controlled trial reported improved functional outcome with pre-hospital intubation and mechanical ventilation, whereas others have demonstrated adverse outcomes that have been attributed to longer field times, misplaced

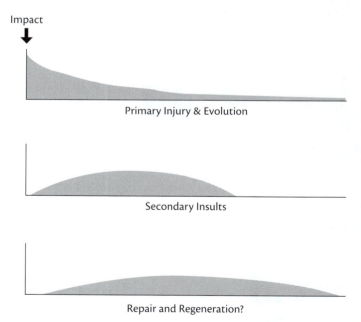

Fig. 17.2 Evolution of the injury and repair processes after brain trauma. A current model of the effects of impact on the brain showing three overlapping and inter-related processes.
Reprinted from *The Lancet*, 306, 7931, Reilly PL *et al.*, 'Patients with head injury who talk and die', pp. 375–377, Copyright 1975, with permission from Elsevier.

tracheal tubes and overly aggressive hyperventilation (18). Concern that hypercapnia may lead to cerebral oedema prompted the use of hyperventilation in earlier guidelines, but it is now accepted that aggressive hyperventilation (PaCO$_2$ < 4.0 kPa (< 30 mmHg)) can lead to severe cerebral ischaemia because of PaCO$_2$-related reductions in cerebral blood flow (CBF) in the early post-injury period (19). Hyperventilation should therefore only be used in the setting of impending cerebral herniation (20–22).

Resuscitation

The resuscitation of patients with severe TBI should follow standard Advanced Trauma Life Support (ATLS) guidelines, including airway protection, stabilization of the neck, and maintenance of cardiopulmonary stability. Primary and secondary surveys should also be carried out according to ATLS guidelines. A few key principles are particularly important:

◆ There is a 5% incidence of associated cervical spine injury in patients with moderate and severe TBI, and a thorough radiological assessment must be undertaken to exclude bony injury to the cervical spine (23). Until the spine is cleared, all patients must be assumed to have an unstable cervical spine and appropriate precautions undertaken (see Chapter 21).

◆ The Brain Trauma Foundation (BTF) recommends avoidance of hypoxia defined as SpO$_2$ less than 90% (level III recommendation) and hypotension defined as SBP lower than 90mm Hg (level II recommendation) (24).

◆ In intubated patients, hypocapnia (PCO$_2$ < 4.0 kPa (<30 mmHg)) should be avoided as prophylactic hyperventilation is associated with poor neurological outcome (19).

◆ Post-resuscitation GCS score is most useful for prognostication because level of consciousness may be impacted by the presence of other injuries, hypoxia, hypotension, and drugs.

Neurological assessment

Overall neurological status is assessed by the GCS, which takes into account a patient's response to command and physical stimuli (see Chapter 26) (25). The GCS was originally developed to grade the severity of TBI and prognosticate outcome but is now used to assess all causes of impaired consciousness and coma. Whilst it is a simple clinical score easily performed by both medical and nursing staff, there are a number of caveats when assessing GCS:

◆ The best response in each of the components of the GCS should be determined following cardiopulmonary stabilization.

◆ GCS score should be defined with regard to patient's vital signs, namely blood pressure, heart rate, and temperature.

◆ GCS score must be interpreted in light of previous or concomitant drug therapy.

◆ The presence of alcohol on the breath or in the serum should always be documented.

◆ It is important to define the responses in descriptive terms rather than only emphasizing the numerical score associated with each response because of considerable interobserver variation in scoring.

◆ Measurement of awareness by the GCS is limited, and subtle changes in brainstem reflexes are not adequately assessed by the GCS.

Table 17.3 Summary of studies outlining the relationship between hypoxia and hypotension and poor neurological outcome

Authors	Year of publication	Sample size	Main findings
Jeffreys and Jones (136)	1981	190	Respiratory failure was a common avoidable factor contributing to death
Gentleman (137)	1992	600	Hypoxia and hypotension have independent and additive adverse effects on outcome
Chestnut et al. (16)	1993	717	Early hypotension was associated with a doubling of mortality (55% vs 27%). If shock was present on admission, the mortality was 65%
Robertson et al. (138)	1995	177	Jugular venous desaturation ($SjvO_2 < 50\%$) was associated with poor neurological outcome
Manley et al. (139)	2001	107	Increases in number of hypotensive episodes increased the odds ratio for death. Hypotension, but not hypoxia, occurring in the initial phase of resuscitation is significantly ($P = 0.009$) associated with increased mortality following brain injury
Jeremitsky et al. (17)	2003	81	Hypoxia was significantly associated with longer intensive care unit length of stay. Hypotension was independently related to mortality
Chi et al. (140)	2006	150	Prehospital hypoxia increased the odds ratio for mortality after TBI
McHugh et al. (141)	2007	6629	Prehospital hypoxia and hypotension were strongly associated with a poorer outcome (odds ratios of 2.1 95% CI (1.7–2.6) and 2.7 95% CI (2.1–3.4) respectively)
Franschmann et al. (142)	2011	339	Hypotension was associated with an increased odds ratio (3.5) for poor neurological outcome.
Oddo et al. (143)	2011	103	Brain tissue hypoxia was associated with poor CNS outcome

Data from various studies (see References).

In an attempt to overcome the limitations of the GCS when assessing overall consciousness, Wijdicks and colleagues proposed the FOUR (Full Outline of UnResponsiveness) score (26,27). The components of the FOUR score include eye movements, motor score, brainstem reflexes, and respiration—each subcomponent is scored out of a maximum of 4 and therefore the maximum score is 16 (see Chapter 26). The FOUR score may be more suitable in the intubated patient than GCS because it does not include verbal responses, although it is seldom used clinically.

Factors predicting lesion progression

Clinical assessment and imaging provide a basis for triage, admission to ICU, monitoring, and initial medical and surgical management pathways. Data from a number of studies have identified clinical and radiological features which predict a high risk of intracranial lesion progression. In a review of 113 patients with TBI exhibiting 229 intraparenchymal haemorrhages (IPHs) initially managed medically, Chang et al. demonstrated that an IPH larger than 5 cm and effacement of basal cisterns on initial CT scan were associated with a later requirement for surgical evacuation (28). Similar observations were reported by Chieregato et al. in the setting of traumatic subarachnoid haemorrhage (tSAH) (29). Furthermore, analyses of the CT scan findings from more than 5000 cases in the IMPACT database are in accord with these observations (30). Outcome was worse in patients with diffuse injuries in CT class III or IV and in those with mass lesions prognosis was better for epidural compared to acute subdural haematoma. Partial obliteration of the basal cisterns, tSAH, and midline shift of 5 mm or more were strongly related to poorer outcome.

Transfer to a neurosurgical unit

Patients with severe TBI should be transported to a specialized neurotrauma centre where there is immediate access to CT scanning, neurosurgery, neurocritical care, and neuromonitoring facilities.

Support for management of severe TBI in specialized neurosurgical centres comes from the data of Patel et al. (31). In this study, patients with severe TBI treated in a non-neurosurgical unit had a 26% increase in mortality and a 2.15-fold increase in odds of death compared with those treated in a neurosurgical unit with comprehensive facilities.

Rapid transport is essential to minimize pre-hospital time. Although the impact of transfer delays on outcome is unknown, early retrieval and transport to a specialized facility are critical (32). Early drainage of acute subdural haematomas (< 4 hours) is associated with improved survival. The mode of transport is crucial in regions where there are long retrieval distances and times, with evidence of improved outcomes with helicopter transfer compared to ground ambulance transport (33). Both inter-hospital and intra-hospital transport is associated with cardiovascular and respiratory deterioration and it is therefore essential that transfer is undertaken by appropriately skilled personnel.

Intensive care management

The intensive care management of severe TBI is complex and involves meticulous general intensive care support and interventions targeted to the injured brain. Treatment focuses on the prevention or treatment of secondary brain injury by optimization of systemic and intracranial physiological variables to minimize secondary insults and improve outcome.

Monitoring

All patients with severe TBI require continuous cardiorespiratory monitoring with ECG, arterial and central venous pressures, ventilatory variables, pulse oximetry, and capnography.

Standard indications exist for monitoring ICP as outlined in the latest (2007) BTF guidelines which recommend that ICP should be monitored in all salvageable patients with a severe TBI (GCS score of 3–8 after resuscitation) and an abnormal cranial CT scan (34).

Level III evidence suggests that ICP monitoring is also indicated in patients with severe TBI with a normal CT scan if two or more of the following features are noted at admission: age over 40 years, unilateral or bilateral motor posturing, or systolic blood pressure lower than 90 mmHg. Other neuromonitoring modalities include brain tissue oxygen tension, cerebral microdialysis, transcranial Doppler (TCD) sonography, and electroencephalography (EEG). TCD is useful in the assessment of cerebral autoregulation and detection of cerebral vasospasm (35). EEG and evoked potentials are used to diagnose non-convulsive status, for titration of barbiturate and assessment of brainstem activity (36,37). These monitoring techniques are discussed in more detail elsewhere in this book (see Chapters 9–14).

Fluid therapy

Euvolaemia is the primary cardiovascular goal. Rapid restoration of circulating blood volume is essential for the maintenance of normotension and prevention of cerebral hypoperfusion.

There is debate about the optimal choice of fluids (crystalloids versus colloids) and their tonicity (hyper- versus isotonic) and in the use of albumin as opposed to synthetic colloids. Fluids are used for two primary indications in neurotrauma—volume restoration and maintenance and hyperosmolar therapy.

Volume restoration

There are no randomized controlled trials to guide the optimal choice or volume of replacement fluid. A post hoc analysis of the Saline versus Albumin Fluid Evaluation (SAFE) study, the SAFE-TBI study, demonstrated that albumin (a hypo-osmolar solution) was associated with greater mortality compared to normal saline (an iso-osmolar solution) after TBI (38). Although the study was not designed to address the precise mechanism behind the increased mortality, the hypo-osmolality of albumin resulting in increased cerebral oedema was proposed as a possibility. As an extrapolation of this argument, it might be prudent to avoid other hypo-osomolar solutions such as gelofusine (osmolality 274 mOsm/kg) and Hartmann's solution (276 mOsm/kg) in the context of severe TBI. A randomized controlled trial examining the utility of a single bolus of 250 mL of hypertonic saline and dextran versus saline for resuscitation in the field did not demonstrate any differences in neurological outcome between the two groups (39).

Hyperosmolar therapy

Hypertonic saline (3%, 7.5%, and 20%) or mannitol are hyperosmolar agents commonly used for the control of intracranial hypertension. Hypertonic saline is administered through a central venous line as intermittent boluses or as a continuous infusion. Regular serum sodium monitoring is required to maintain the target sodium concentration between 145 and 150 mmol/L. Hypertonic saline therapy may be associated with hypernatraemia, hyperchloraemia, a non-anion gap acidosis, and polyuria which can be mistaken for diabetes insipidus.

Mannitol is another osmotic agent that increases plasma osmolality, with two potentially beneficial actions. It increases circulating blood volume and reduces haematocrit, both of which improve cerebral perfusion pressure (CPP) and CBF. This is likely responsible for the immediate actions of mannitol on ICP. Mannitol also induces hyperosmolality resulting in a net efflux of fluid from the swollen brain, thereby reducing cerebral swelling and ICP. This effect presages an intact BBB and, in the presence of a damaged BBB, mannitol may potentially worsen cerebral oedema. Unlike hypertonic saline, mannitol can be administered through a peripheral cannula usually as a 0.25–1 g/kg bolus. Some experts recommend administration only in response to an increase in ICP as a bridge to definitive treatment, whereas others suggest 6-hourly boluses titrated to ICP to achieve a serum osmolality between 290 and 320 mOsm/kg. Higher osmolality levels do not confer additional therapeutic benefit and may be associated with dehydration, hypokalaemia, and renal failure. Mannitol administration is also associated with a raised serum osmolar gap and calculated serum osmolalities are unreliable in the presence of mannitol therapy. Frequent serum osmolality measurements are therefore essential to ensure that the target osmolality is within the specified range.

The BTF makes no level I recommendations with regards to hyperosmolar therapy. There are level II recommendations for the use of mannitol for controlling raised ICP, and level III recommendations for restricting mannitol use, prior to ICP monitoring, in patients with signs of transtentorial herniation or progressive neurological deterioration not attributable to extracranial causes (40).

Indications for surgery

For the most part, the literature regarding the surgical management of severe TBI is lacking in terms of data from randomized controlled trials. Prompt evacuation of mass lesions causing intracranial hypertension is essential, and guidelines have been developed for the traditional based classifications of TBI—extradural, subdural, and intracerebral haematoma (41–43). Haematoma volume greater than 30 cm^3, midline shift greater than 5 mm, or clot thickness less than 15 mm are considered indications for immediate evacuation of an extradural haematomas (43). Patients not meeting these criteria should have serial CT scans to monitor haematoma progression. Indications for surgery for acute subdural haematomas are midline shift greater than 5 mm or clot thickness less than 10 mm (42). Specific criteria for the surgical management of intraparenchymal lesions have not been developed, but those associated with progressive neurological deterioration and increasing ICP should be considered for evacuation (41). An external ventricular drain can be beneficial even in the absence of significant hydrocephalus because drainage of a few millilitres of cerebrospinal fluid (CSF) lowers ICP in patients with reduced intracranial compliance (see Chapter 7).

Although bilateral frontoparietal craniectomy is effective in reducing ICP refractory to maximal medical treatment, a recent large randomized controlled trial of decompressive craniectomy in patients with diffuse TBI and refractory intracranial hypertension (DECRA) was associated with an increase in unfavourable outcome in survivors (44). DECRA has increased rather than resolved the controversy about the indications, technique, timing, and selection of patients for decompressive craniectomy, and it is hoped that the recently completed RESCUE-ICP trial will resolve some of these issues. Given the dismal outcome of patients with high ICP refractory to other therapies, decompressive craniectomy is regarded by many as a potential management strategy in those with a chance of a reasonable functional outcome when all other measures to control ICP have failed.

Coagulopathy

The reported incidence of coagulopathy after TBI varies considerably between studies (10–90%) because of differences in definitions and timing of assessment (45). It is generally estimated that one in three TBI patients will develop some form of coagulopathy, although the incidence is substantially lower in those with mild TBI. Both hypo and hypercoagulable states have been described. Factors predisposing to coagulopathy include release of tissue factor, disseminated intravascular coagulation, fibrinolysis, platelet dysfunction, and activation of protein C. The presence of hypothermia and acidosis may further amplify coagulation disturbances. Conventional clotting screens may not reveal the full extent of the derangement in all patients and thromboelastography is recommended.

Intracranial and cerebral perfusion pressures

In many ways the management of severe TBI has polarized around CPP versus ICP management strategies for control of intracranial hypertension. Despite the fact that these two entities are related (CPP = MAP – ICP), approaches based on the two strategies are very different (46). The goal of both is to maintain cerebral oxygenation, and the main factors determining this are CBF, arterial oxygen content, and the cerebral metabolic rate of oxygen consumption ($CMRO_2$) (47,48). By manipulating ICP and CPP, clinicians aim to improve CBF and therefore cerebral oxygenation. Although raised ICP and low CPP are associated with worse outcome, the optimal targets and absolute effects of both on clinical outcome are less clear (49,50). A number of studies have attempted to answer this question and will be reviewed later in the chapter.

The basics of cerebral perfusion and intracranial pressures

The underlying physiology of cerebral perfusion and intracranial pressures is discussed in detail in Chapters 2 and 9, and only a brief summary will be presented here.

Cerebral perfusion pressure

CPP represents the vascular pressure gradient across the cerebrovascular beds and is a function of CBF and cerebrovascular resistance (CVR). CVR and therefore CBF are influenced by a number of physiological variables and control mechanisms (see Chapter 3) (51–53).

- Metabolic control ('metabolic autoregulation'): CBF is regulated by the balance between cerebral metabolism and oxygen delivery via various vasoactive substances.

- Pressure autoregulation: pressure changes detected by smooth muscle in the arterioles of the brain lead to a change in vessel calibre to maintain CBF over a wide range of systemic and cerebral perfusion pressures; this is fundamental to maintaining cerebral oxygenation (Figure 17.3).

- Chemical control: $PaCO_2$ has a near linear relationship with CBF within the physiological range because of a direct effect of extracellular hydrogen ion concentration on vascular smooth muscle.

- Neural control: smooth muscle actuators in the arterioles affect vessel calibre via sympathetic innervation from inputs in the brainstem; neuronal nitric oxide may play a role in modulating CBF via this mechanism.

Under normal circumstances, CBF is maintained at a relatively constant rate of 50 mL/100 g/min over a wide range of CPP. This is termed autoregulation (Figure 17.3) (54) and is defined as the inherent ability of arteries to vasodilate or vasoconstrict in response to changing perfusion pressure. This process is adaptive and varies from brain region to region. Autoregulation may be impaired to varying degrees following brain injury, leading to a situation where CBF becomes pressure dependent in some brain regions (55). Artificially increasing MAP with vasoconstrictors leads to an increase in cerebral hydrostatic pressure and worsening cerebral oedema in these regions. Alternatively, if autoregulation is intact, increasing MAP and CPP leads to a decrease in ICP via compensatory vasoconstriction (56,57). Several studies have suggested that assessment of cerebral autoregulatory status may be used to guide individualized therapy (58–60).

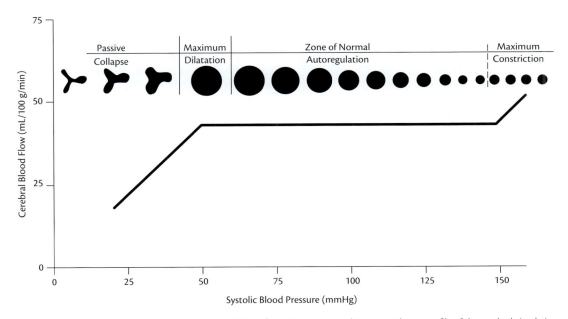

Fig. 17.3 The relationship between systolic blood pressure and cerebral blood flow demonstrating the autoregulatory profile of the cerebral circulation.
Reproduced from White H and Venkatesh B, 'Cerebral perfusion pressure in neurotrauma: a review', *Anesthesia & Analgesia*, 107, 3, pp. 979–988, copyright 2008 with permission from Wolters Kluwer Health and International Anesthesia Research Society. Data from various studies (see References).

The critical threshold of CBF for the development of irreversible brain damage is 15 mL/100 g/min (61). Given the difficulty of measuring CBF at the bedside, other metabolic or oxygenation endpoints have been utilized to assess the impact of CPP manipulation on cerebral metabolism. However, this approach is limited by the lack of consensus on the ideal brain region to sample and the global applicability of regional data. Nevertheless, it does provide some indication of the impact that changes in CPP can have on brain function. Several techniques can be used to monitor cerebral oxygenation including brain tissue oxygen tension probes, near infra-red spectroscopy, and jugular bulb venous oxygen saturation (62–66). Each technique has advantages and limitations as noted in earlier chapters, and the correlation between CPP and cerebral oxygen levels as determined by these techniques is marginal at best. Further, the effects of vasopressors on $CMRO_2$ are variable (67). It is worth noting that the BTF now recommends brain tissue oxygen monitoring as an adjunct to the management of severe TBI (68). In general, once CPP is below the autoregulatory range (for that patient), cerebral oxygenation worsens.

Cerebral microdialysis measures multiple aspects of brain metabolism. Glucose delivery and utilization, lactate:pyruvate ratio (intercellular redox state), glycerol (index of cell membrane breakdown), and glutamate (a measure of cerebral excitotoxicity) can be measured at the bedside (69–72). As with brain oxygenation, the effect that changes in CPP have on metabolic endpoints is also not clear. Microdialysis variables are adversely affected by both high (> 70 mmHg) and low (< 50 mmHg) CPP and more research is necessary to clarify the utility of cerebral microdialysis in directing CPP-guided management.

Intracranial pressure

Being encased in a fixed structure the brain is subject to the principles espoused by Munro (1783) and Kellie (1824) who noted that brain tissue is nearly incompressible and that any change in the volume of individual intracranial contents (brain, blood, and CSF) must occur at the expense of the volume of another element and will ultimately lead to an increase in ICP (73). The relationship between ICP and intracranial volume is described by a non-linear pressure volume curve and, once the compensatory mechanisms (reduction in cerebral blood volume (CBV) or CSF) are exhausted, ICP rises rapidly until cessation of CBF ensues (see Chapter 7).

A number of techniques exist for monitoring ICP but the two most common are an intraventricular catheter and intraparenchymal probe. Each has benefits and limitations (see Chapter 9). An intraventricular catheter is able to drain CSF for ICP control but has a high incidence of catheter-associated ventriculitis (6–11%) (74). Intraparenchymal catheters have a very low infection rate but are subject to drift of the zero reference point. ICP is not necessarily uniformly distributed and significant pressure gradients exist across the tentorial compartments in patients with intracranial hypertension. Furthermore, although raised ICP is associated with worse outcome, the use of ICP monitoring and management has not been shown to improve outcome (75). In a Dutch study, mortality rates were similar when ICP-guided therapy was compared with empirical management of TBI (76). Several other studies have come to similar conclusions although most are retrospective (77,78). A recent study by Chestnut and colleagues compared outcomes in two groups of patients with severe TBI admitted to ICUs in Bolivia and Ecuador (75). Patients were managed using a protocol for monitoring intraparenchymal ICP or a protocol in which treatment was based on imaging and clinical examination. The trial included 324 patients and no difference in outcome including functional status and 6-month mortality could be demonstrated.

The ICP threshold for intervention is controversial and depends on age and clinical diagnosis. For TBI in adults, the BTF recommends the institution of therapy when ICP rises above 20–25 mmHg (79) although there are reports of patients suffering cerebral herniation at lower ICP. ICP monitoring may also be utilized as an indicator for repeat imaging or further intervention as sudden changes in ICP may represent a new or worsening intracranial event. Analysis of ICP waveforms provide information about brain compliance and Lundberg historically classified waves based on a time domain (see Chapter 9) (80). More recently, advanced computer modelling has demonstrated that ICP waveform analysis monitoring can be used to provide an indicator of global cerebral perfusion (81,82).

Cerebral perfusion- and intracranial pressure-based therapy

It is difficult to separate the influence of CPP- and ICP-based treatment of intracranial hypertension as the two are inter-related. There are those who advocate a predetermined CPP target irrespective of ICP and others who allow CPP to decrease as long as ICP is maintained. The BTF has lowered the recommended CPP target (from > 70 mmHg to 50–70 mmHg) over the past few years, and recent research suggests that there is a place for both approaches with treatment being individualized based on the autoregulatory state of the brain.

CPP-based therapy

Rosner and colleagues were among the first to study the effects of aggressive CPP management on outcome after TBI (56,57). They assumed that autoregulation was not absent but shifted to the right, and that a higher CPP was therefore necessary to maintain adequate CBF. Reflex cerebral vasoconstriction would then result in a reduction in ICP because of secondary reductions in intracranial blood volume and cerebral oedema. In this way they described a vasodilatory and vasoconstriction cascade in which a decrease in CPP stimulates cerebral autoregulatory vasodilatation and an increase in CBV and ICP (Figure 17.4). It was assumed that the effects of ICP therapies were transient, potentially toxic and should be used sparingly, and that treatment directed towards maintaining CPP as high as possible, and certainly greater than 70 mmHg, was preferable.

Rosner undertook a non-randomized study of 158 TBI patients in whom CPP was maintained above 70 mmHg (CPP as high as 90 mmHg was allowed in certain circumstances) by the combination of vasoconstrictors, mannitol, and CSF drainage (83). The mortality rate was 29% and there was a favourable recovery at 10.5 months in 59% of patients. ICP averaged 25 ± 12 mmHg and the mean CPP was 83 mmHg. These results compared favourably with those from the Traumatic Coma Data Bank, and the authors concluded that CPP should be maintained above 70 mm Hg at all costs. These findings were subsequently confirmed in a case series published by Young et al. who questioned whether an upper limit of intracranial pressure existed in patients with severe head injury if CPP is maintained (84). They reported four patients with ICP ranging from 36 to 50 mmHg who were managed with CPP at 60 mmHg or greater. On discharge, all were able to perform activities of daily living with minimal disability and the authors concluded that aggressive CPP therapy should be instituted and maintained even though apparently lethal ICP levels may be present.

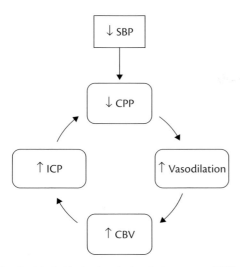

Fig. 17.4 The physiological basis of cerebral perfusion pressure (CPP)-guided management. The CPP management strategy is based on the vasodilatory cascade described by Rosner et al. (83). Increasing blood pressure breaks the vasodilatory stimulus for intracranial hypertension.

CBF, cerebral blood flow; CBV, cerebral blood volume; SBP, systolic blood pressure.

Robertson CS, 'Management of cerebral perfusion pressure after traumatic brain injury', *Anesthesiology* 2001, 95, pp. 1513–1517; and Rosner S, Johnson A, 'Cerebral perfusion pressure: management protocol and clinical results', *Journal of Neurosurgery* 1995, 83, pp. 949–962.

Subsequent studies have, however, questioned this approach. Robertson and colleagues undertook a study in 189 TBI patients and compared CPP-targeted therapy with a standard ICP-targeted management protocol (85). In the CPP-targeted group, CPP was maintained at greater than 70 mmHg and $PaCO_2$ around 4.7 kPa (35 mmHg), whereas in the ICP-targeted group ICP was controlled by hyperventilation to a target $PaCO_2$ of 3.3–4.0 kPa (25–30 mmHg) and CPP was allowed to fall to 50 mmHg. The frequency of reduced cerebral oxygenation (as assessed by jugular desaturation) was 2.5 times higher in the ICP-targeted group, suggesting that CPP-targeted therapy is more effective at maintaining adequate cerebral oxygen delivery, but there was no difference in neurological outcome between the groups. The CPP group had a significantly higher frequency of acute lung injury suggesting that the potential benefits of CPP-based therapy were offset by its complications (86). It was these findings that led the BTF to decrease their recommended CPP level from 70 to 60 mmHg.

Several other studies have also questioned the use of aggressive CPP targets. Lang et al. noted a plateau in brain tissue oxygen tension at CPP between 70 and 90 mmHg (87), and Juul et al., examining patients enrolled in the Selfotel trial, failed to find an independent effect on neurological outcome of CPP higher than 60 mmHg (88). Balestreri et al. subsequently confirmed the dangers of excessively high or low CPP in a retrospective review of 429 patients with TBI (89). In summary it is evident that artificially increasing blood pressure to generate arbitrarily high CPP is not associated with improved outcomes and has potential to produce significant complications.

ICP-based therapy

As previously noted, an ICP threshold in the region of 20–25 mmHg has been adopted by the BTF because higher levels correlate with worse outcome (79). However, it is worth noting that no prospective study has been undertaken (or is likely to be undertaken) to prove that this is the correct threshold. With continuous ICP

monitoring, waveforms can be analysed in the time domain according to the Lundberg classification (80) and these provide prognostic information (see Chapter 9). 'A' waves comprise a steep increase in ICP from baseline to above 40 mmHg and persist for up to 20 minutes, and are always pathological. 'B' waves probably reflect changes in vascular tone and consist of oscillations occurring at 0.5–2 waves/min increasing to approximately 20 mmHg above baseline. 'C' waves which were originally described as oscillations that occur with a frequency of 4–8/min, are of little pathological significance.

Although intraventricular catheters allow drainage of CSF to control ICP, this effect can be limited in the presence of severe brain swelling because the CSF compartment collapses under pressure from oedematous brain. Traditional techniques to reduce ICP have revolved around the use of hyperosmolar therapy to shrink the brain. The ideal osmotic agent would establish a strong transendothelial osmotic gradient across the BBB. Mannitol has been the predominant osmotherapeutic agent for decades but has several limitations including osmotic diuresis leading to hypotension, adverse effects on the kidney and central nervous system including a rebound phenomenon leading to raised ICP (90). Other solutions, particularly hypertonic saline, have been investigated as substitutes.

Animal and human studies have demonstrated that hypertonic saline has clinically desirable physiological effects on CBF, ICP, and inflammatory responses after neurotrauma. Potential benefits include increases in CBF, MAP, and CPP, reduction in ICP, modulation of inflammation, and maintenance of BBB integrity. Studies have demonstrated consistent effectiveness in reducing and maintaining ICP during periods of intracranial hypertension (91,92), findings that have been confirmed by a recent meta-analysis (93). These benefits and the limited side effects have led many units to adopt hypertonic saline in preference to mannitol. However, despite good basic research, no large randomized controlled trials demonstrating improved outcome from hypertonic saline have been performed. Three randomized controlled trials examining pre-hospital boluses of hypertonic saline in TBI failed to demonstrate a benefit (39,94,95).

Lund therapy

Possibly the biggest advocates of ICP-based therapy are the Lund group in Sweden who utilize a unique approach to the management of TBI. The so-called Lund therapy is a theoretical approach to controlling ICP based on physiological and pathophysiological haemodynamic principles of brain volume and perfusion regulation (96). Lund therapy is based on the observation that BBB permeability increases after TBI thereby reducing the effectiveness of the brain's normal volume-regulating mechanisms (96–98). Consequently, brain volume is controlled by forces other than the crystalloid transcapillary force control, such as capillary hydrostatic and plasma oncotic pressure. Enthusiasts of the Lund approach advocate prevention of cerebral oedema and intracranial hypertension while maintaining intravascular volume using colloid volume expanders. Some even recommend the use of antihypertensive treatment such as beta blockers, alpha-2 agonists, and angiotensin II antagonists to counteract the development of brain oedema. Crystalloids are largely avoided in the Lund approach in which 20% albumin is the main volume expander with haemoglobin level maintained above 12 g/dL to maintain cerebral oxygen delivery. Vasoconstrictors are avoided and CPP is allowed to fall to 50 mmHg in adults. Osmotherapy is generally avoided although mannitol and hypertonic saline can be used in the setting of impending brain herniation. Patients remain heavily sedated to reduce stress, and hypothermia is avoided until ICP is under control. CSF may be drained via a ventricular catheter as necessary.

A recent small randomized controlled trial in 60 postoperative patients with brain trauma and SAH demonstrated lower mortality in the patients treated with ICP-targeted (modified Lund) therapy guided by cerebral microdialysis monitoring compared to those treated with CPP-based therapy (99). However, this study has a number of limitations including the inclusion of SAH and TBI patients in the same groups and exclusion from the analysis of TBI patients who did not require surgery. Furthermore, the target haemoglobin concentration of 12.5–14.0 g/dL is contrary to current recommendations. Interpretation of these data is therefore difficult and further research is necessary before a definitive assessment can be made. In a pros/cons debate, Sharma and Vavilala took issue with a number of the treatment measures advocated by proponents of the Lund concept (100–102). Despite various reports of improved neurological outcomes in patients with TBI subsequent to the adoption of a volume-targeted protocol, they noted that the Lund concept has not found significant support elsewhere in the world. Further, some individual components have proved detrimental to TBI outcomes and the Lund concept deemphasizes the treatment goal of CBF optimization via maintenance of adequate brain perfusion. The assumption that the BBB is disrupted and explains the onset of cerebral oedema has also been questioned because oedema may occur in areas of brain not subject to direct injury. Furthermore, oncotic pressure is less likely to influence cerebral oedema than serum sodium levels, and haemoglobin concentration greater than 10 g/dL has not been shown to benefit TBI patients. Moreover the SAFE-TBI study reported a worse neurological outcome in patients receiving colloids as opposed to crystalloids. Although autoregulation can be altered by TBI, these changes are patient specific and may vary regionally within the same patient. Thus there is concern that the antihypertensive therapy advocated by the Lund approach

risks causing cerebral hypoperfusion and focal cerebral ischaemia. Finally, Lund therapy has tended to evolve over time with changes in individual components of the protocol making interpretation of previous studies difficult.

Summary

Current protocols based on CPP and ICP targeted therapy have not been adequately scrutinized and are based on physiological principles and prejudice rather than strong scientific evidence. Further, TBI is a heterogeneous disease with pathophysiological processes that vary regionally and temporally and, as such, there is an increasingly strong argument for individualization of therapy (103,104). Thus it is likely that certain individuals may benefit from CPP-based management while others from ICP-based therapy. Howells et al. compared an ICP based protocol in Uppsala, Sweden with a CPP based protocol in Edinburgh, Scotland evaluating pressure reactivity as a guide to treatment of CPP (59). They concluded that ICP-orientated therapy led to better outcomes in pressure-passive patients, whereas hypertensive CPP therapy was superior in patients with intact autoregulation. It is therefore likely that neuromonitoring technologies will allow further refinement of treatment protocols, but whether this translates into improved outcomes remains to be seen. See Table 17.4.

Multiple trauma

About 50% of patients with severe TBI have associated severe extracranial injuries (105). In a 2012 meta-analysis of three observational TBI studies, International Mission on Prognosis and Clinical Trial Design in TBI (IMPACT), the randomized controlled trial Corticosteroid Randomization After Significant Head Injury (CRASH), and the Trauma Audit and Research Network (TARN) trauma registry study, van Leeuwen et al. investigated the prognostic value of extracranial injuries on mortality after TBI (106). These authors concluded that, while extracranial injuries have an impact on outcome after TBI, this relationship depends on the severity of

Table 17.4 Comparison of CPP management protocols

Therapy	Theoretical concept	Goals	Supporting evidence
Management of cerebral volume and perfusion (97,98)	Disruption of BBB leads to leakage of fluid into cerebral tissue worsening ICH. CPP based therapy leads to increased hydrostatic pressure in the setting of deranged autoregulation and increased ICP.	Reduction in capillary hydrostatic cerebral pressure with antihypertensive therapy. Maintenance of COP with 20% albumin. CPP 60–70 mmHg but as low as 50 mmHg as long as ICP normal	11-patient non-randomized study comparing outcome with that predicted by injury, and 53-patient study comparing with historical controls. Both suggested a good outcome with Lund therapy but the lack of a randomized prospective study has limited the universal acceptance of this therapy
CPP based (56)	Autoregulation after TBI is shifted to the right and therefore a much higher CPP is required to maintain cerebral perfusion	Maintenance of CPP > 70 mmHg with a combination of volume replacement (albumin in the original study), vasopressors and mannitol. CPP could be raised to 80–90 mmHg if necessary	Non-randomized study of 158 patients comparing outcome to the Traumatic Coma Data Bank. Subsequent studies have suggested that there may be significant adverse effects associated with CPP > 70 mmHg
CBF/oxygen extraction coupling (144)	TBI leads to reduced cerebral oxygen extraction with consequent relative cerebral hyperperfusion. Optimizing hyperventilation improves oxygen extraction coupling with better ICP control	Ventilation is manipulated to optimize $SjVO_2$ and ICP	Prospective randomized study with 178 patients and 175 controls. Groups matched by CT rather than randomization. Mortality rate in treatment group was 9% and 30% in control. There are no data comparing ICP and CPP during the study period. Previous studies suggest hyperventilation leads to worse outcome (although these were not guided by $SjVO_2$)

Data from various studies (see References).

TBI (where the relationship is not as strong) and the time of inclusion in the study.

The principles of management of TBI associated with multi-trauma are similar to those of an isolated brain trauma but there are a few important additional considerations:

◆ Hypotension secondary to haemorrhage from extracranial injuries is associated with worse outcome after TBI and therefore the basic principles of resuscitation must be vigorously applied.

◆ There is a higher incidence of associated cervical spine injury (about 5%) in patients with moderate and severe TBI and other trauma, and therefore a thorough radiological assessment must be undertaken to exclude injury to the cervical spine (23). Until the spine is cleared, all patients must be assumed to have an unstable cervical spine and appropriate precautions undertaken.

◆ In situations where a patient with severe TBI needs life-saving non-neurological surgery prior to neuroimaging, there are few data to guide the utility of prophylactic ICP during anaesthesia and surgery. The use of ICP monitoring in these circumstances is variable amongst neurosurgeons.

◆ Intra-abdominal hypertension resulting from bleeding and ileus can result in secondary increases in ICP (107).

◆ The presence of extracranial trauma such as unstable spinal, pelvic, or limb injuries has implications on the positioning of the patient during intensive care and this may impact management of the injured brain. For example, head-up positioning to control ICP may be impossible.

Current guidelines for the management of severe traumatic brain injury

As TBI is the most common cause of death in young adults in First World countries (108,109) a number of organizations have created guidelines for the management of severe TBI. This has been challenging because there is little evidence to support many treatment strategies, and expert opinion varies widely. Even the need for ICP monitoring is questioned because of the lack of conclusive evidence for its benefits. The use of other invasive monitoring techniques, such as brain tissue oxygen tension and microdialysis, has led some institutions to modify basic therapies to respond to changes in these monitored variable rather than the traditional measures of ICP and CPP. This variability in treatment approaches makes standardization difficult and creates problems in the design of large multicentre interventional studies.

Despite these limitations, a number of organizations have attempted to standardize treatment and influential guidelines have been published by the European Brain Injury Consortium (EBIC) and the BTF (24,34,40,49,68,79,110–119). The original BTF guidance was published in 1995 and updated in 2000 and 2007, whereas the 1997 EBIC guidance has yet to be updated. The two guidelines differ in a number of key areas and this can be partly explained by the different approaches taken by their authors. The EBIC guidelines were written in an effort to create some uniformity in the management of TBI between institutions, primarily to facilitate research. As such, they are largely based on expert opinion and tend to be fairly pragmatic. The BTF guidelines on the other hand are largely evidence based (although in many instances the evidence is not strong), and their main message has been to highlight the lack

of rigorous evidence upon which clinical management is based. Despite the differences, the two sets of guidance represent complementary rather than opposing views (120). Much of the emphasis is on preventing or minimizing secondary brain injury and thereby limiting the ultimate burden of brain injury (14,121). Their focus is therefore on the prevention or early treatment of secondary insults, particularly hypoxia and hypotension, which are causes of worsening cerebral ischaemia and secondary brain injury.

The EBIC consortium took a pragmatic approach and did not insist on sophisticated levels of invasive monitoring, known not to be in general use. They describe minimal monitoring requirements during ICU management and recommend maintaining MAP at greater than 90 mmHg and SpO_2 higher than 95%. MAP should be managed with fluid resuscitation to euvolaemia and inotropes/vasopressors as necessary. In ventilated patients, the PaO_2 should be greater than 13.3 kPa (> 100 mmHg) and $PaCO_2$ 4.0–4.7 kPa (30–35 mmHg). Early enteral feeding is advocated as is maintenance of normoglycaemia and normothermia. If ICP monitoring is available and evidence of intracranial hypertension present, treatment should be aimed at maintaining ICP below 20–25 mmHg and CPP between 60 and 70 mmHg. The EBIC guidance for achieving these targets includes the following:

◆ Sedation and analgesia.

◆ Ventilation to maintain $PaCO_2$ 4.0–4.7 kPa (30–35 mmHg).

◆ Vasopressors—although there is no evidence supporting a specific agent.

◆ Osmotherapy—using boluses of mannitol or hypertonic saline.

◆ Consideration of moderate hyperventilation ($PaCO_2$ < 4 kPa (< 30 mmHg)) with monitoring of cerebral oxygenation to minimize the risk of cerebral ischaemia, and possibly barbiturates, if the above therapies fail to control ICP and CPP.

◆ Decompressive craniotomy may be considered in exceptional circumstances.

◆ Steroids should be avoided and nimodipine is not advocated.

Despite dating from 1997, the EBIC guidance is still considered a standard of care in many units. The American Brain Injury Consortium, in their 2010 guidelines, largely replicated the EBIC statement with a few minor modifications (122).

The third (2007) and most recent edition of the BTF guidance was produced following a systematic review of the literature to assess the influence of the use of the earlier (2000) guidelines on mortality and morbidity after TBI. The BTF guidelines are generally more structured than those from the EBIC, and levels of evidence are provided for each recommendation. Rather than providing an overarching approach to TBI, the BTF guidelines are divided into topics such as blood pressure, oxygenation, or hyperosmolar therapy (24,34,40,68,79,110–119). Most of the BTF guidance is supported by only level II or III evidence. In summary (as it appears in the document):

◆ Systolic blood pressure lower than 90 mmHg and PaO_2 less than 8.0 kPa (< 60 mmHg) should be avoided (level II).

◆ Oxygenation should be monitored and hypoxia (PaO_2 ≤ 60 mm Hg or SpO_2 ≤ 90%) avoided (level III)

◆ Mannitol is the osmotic agent of choice for the management of intracranial hypertension (level II), but the current evidence base was insufficiently strong to make recommendations on the use, concentration and method of administration of hypertonic saline.

- Induced hypothermia does not improve mortality but may improve neurological outcome in survivors, although the evidence is weak (level III).

- Treatment for raised ICP should be initiated if the pressure exceeds 20 mmHg (level II).

- CPP should be maintained between 50 and 70 mmHg, although patients with intact autoregulation may tolerate higher CPP. Ancillary monitoring of cerebral oxygenation, blood flow and metabolism may be indicated to guide CPP management (level III).

- If brain oxygen monitoring is employed, jugular venous saturation lower than 50% and brain tissue oxygen tension of less than 2 kPa (< 15 mmHg) should be avoided. There is insufficient evidence to generate a target level for these measurements (level III).

- While barbiturates should not be used routinely, there is a role for the control of refractory intracranial hypertension (level II).

- Nutritional goals should be attained by day 7 (level II).

- Hyperventilation to $PaCO_2$ less than 4.0 kPa (< 30 mmHg) should be avoided unless as a temporizing measure for acute reduction in ICP (level III).

- Steroids should be avoided (level I).

Many countries also produce their own guidelines. In the United Kingdom, the National Institute for Health and Care Excellence (NICE) produces guidelines for a number of clinical conditions including TBI (123). These have recently (2014) been updated but only address issues related to transportation of injured patients, indications for CT scanning and information that should be provided for family members.

Despite an overall improvement in outcome from TBI, the IMPACT study demonstrated a significant difference between centres (124). This reflects a number of factors but the lack of an internationally agreed evidence-based approach to TBI management is believed to be important. As such, more research is necessary to further define and tailor treatments to match the pathophysiology of an individual patient. Units that advocate 'non-standard' therapies, such as the Lund approach, must demonstrate improved outcomes in large trials before they can be considered more widely.

A number of organizations have been established to coordinate research, including the International Initiative for Traumatic Brain Injury Research (InTBIR) under the auspices of the European Commission and the US National Institute for Health (125). Given the difficulties associated with conducting randomized controlled trials in patients with TBI, calls are being made to use comparative effectiveness research in which data from observational studies, case series, systematic reviews, and meta-analyses can be used to augment those generated from randomized controlled trials (2). Guidelines continue to evolve as more evidence comes to light and will hopefully lead to a more uniform approach to TBI management.

Pharmacological agents in neurotrauma

Several agents have been tested in clinical trials with a view to modulating the inflammatory process and subsequent neuronal

death after TBI, and for conferring 'neuroprotection' (1). These include dexanabinol (a cannabinoid antagonist) (126), tirilazad (an amino-steroid), glucocorticoids, magnesium, and NMDA antagonists, although none has been shown to improve morbidity or mortality (127). Drugs currently undergoing clinical trials based on their potential neuroprotective properties include progesterone, erythropoietin hyperoxia, and tranexamic acid (128,129). Ketones are also being investigated for their neuroprotective properties (130).

Other pharmacological measures include the use of levodopa and amantadine for improving patients' level of consciousness (131). Initial trials have reported some recovery response in terms of reduction in spasticity and improved cognitive behaviour and communication. Zolpidem has also been studied in patients with traumatic and anoxic aetiologies of reduced consciousness but results have been variable. Whilst some investigators report enhanced verbal, motor and cognitive functions, these have not been reproduced in other small trials. Moreover the duration of effects of zolpidem is short. Bromocriptine and intrathecal baclofen have also been tried but no large-scale studies have been reported (132,133).

References

1. Rosenfeld JV, Maas AI, Bragge P, Morganti-Kossmann MC, Manley GT, Gruen RL. Early management of severe traumatic brain injury. *Lancet*. 2012;380:1088–98.
2. Maas AI, Menon DK, Lingsma HF, Pineda JA, Sandel ME, Manley GT. Re-orientation of clinical research in traumatic brain injury: report of an international workshop on comparative effectiveness research. *J Neurotrauma*. 2012;29:32–46.
3. Stocchetti N, Paterno R, Citerio G, Beretta L, Colombo A. Traumatic brain injury in an aging population. *J Neurotrauma*. 2012;29:1119–25.
4. Myburgh JA, Cooper DJ, Finfer SR, Venkatesh B, Jones D, Higgins A, et al. Epidemiology and 12-month outcomes from traumatic brain injury in Australia and New Zealand. *J Trauma*. 2008;64:854–62.
5. Fearnside MR, Cook RJ, McDougall P, McNeil RJ. The Westmead Head Injury Project outcome in severe head injury. A comparative analysis of pre-hospital, clinical and CT variables. *Br J Neurosurg*. 1993;7:267–79.
6. Jennett B, Teasdale G, Galbraith S, Pickard J, Grant H, Braakman R, et al. Severe head injuries in three countries. *J Neurol Neurosurg Psychiatry*. 1977;40:291–8.
7. Murray GD, Teasdale GM, Braakman R, Cohadon F, Dearden M, Iannotti F, et al. The European Brain Injury Consortium survey of head injuries. *Acta Neurochir (Wien)*. 1999;141:223–36.
8. Eisenberg HM, Gary HE, Jr., Aldrich EF, Saydjari C, Turner B, Foulkes MA, et al. Initial CT findings in 753 patients with severe head injury. A report from the NIH Traumatic Coma Data Bank. *J Neurosurg*. 1990;73:688–98.
9. Saatman KE, Duhaime AC, Bullock R, Maas AI, Valadka A, Manley GT, et al. Classification of traumatic brain injury for targeted therapies. *J Neurotrauma*. 2008;25:719–38.
10. Marshall LF, Marshall SB, Klauber MR, Van Berkum Clark M, Eisenberg H, et al. The diagnosis of head injury requires a classification based on computed axial tomography. *J Neurotrauma*. 1992;9 Suppl 1:S287–92.
11. Reilly PL, Graham DI, Adams JH, Jennett B. Patients with head injury who talk and die. *Lancet*. 1975;2:375–7.
12. Reilly PL. Brain injury: the pathophysiology of the first hours.'Talk and Die revisited'. *J Clin Neurosci*. 2001;8:398–403.
13. Ramadan A, Berney J, Reverdin A, Rilliet B, Bongioanni F. [Study of the deterioration factors in adult patients with cranio-cerebral injuries who "talk and die"]. *Neurochirurgie*. 1986;32:423–32.
14. Bouma GJ, Muizelaar JP, Choi SC, Newlon PG, Young HF. Cerebral circulation and metabolism after severe traumatic brain injury: the elusive role of ischemia. *J Neurosurg*. 1991;75:685–93.

15. Jaggi JL, Obrist WD, Gennarelli TA, Langfitt TW. Relationship of early cerebral blood flow and metabolism to outcome in acute head injury. *J Neurosurg.* 1990;72:176–82.

16. Chesnut RM, Marshall LF, Klauber MR, Blunt BA, Baldwin N, Eisenberg HM, *et al.* The role of secondary brain injury in determining outcome from severe head injury. *J Trauma.* 1993;34:216–22.

17. Jeremitsky E, Omert L, Dunham CM, Protetch J, Rodriguez A. Harbingers of poor outcome the day after severe brain injury: hypothermia, hypoxia, and hypoperfusion. *J Trauma.* 2003;54:312–9.

18. von Elm E, Schoettker P, Henzi I, Osterwalder J, Walder B. Pre-hospital tracheal intubation in patients with traumatic brain injury: systematic review of current evidence. *Br J Anaesth.* 2009;103:371–86.

19. Muizelaar JP, Marmarou A, Ward JD, Kontos HA, Choi SC, Becker DP, *et al.* Adverse effects of prolonged hyperventilation in patients with severe head injury: a randomized clinical trial. *J Neurosurg.* 1991;75:731–9.

20. Bernard SA, Nguyen V, Cameron P, Masci K, Fitzgerald M, Cooper DJ, *et al.* Prehospital rapid sequence intubation improves functional outcome for patients with severe traumatic brain injury: a randomized controlled trial. *Ann Surg.* 2010;252:959–65.

21. Laird AM, Miller PR, Kilgo PD, Meredith JW, Chang MC. Relationship of early hyperglycemia to mortality in trauma patients. *J Trauma.* 2004;56:1058–62.

22. Seyed Saadat SM, Bidabadi E, Seyed Saadat SN, Mashouf M, Salamat F, Yousefzadeh S. Association of persistent hyperglycemia with outcome of severe traumatic brain injury in pediatric population. *Childs Nerv Syst.* 2012;28:1773–7.

23. Holly LT, Kelly DF, Counelis GJ, Blinman T, McArthur DL, Cryer HG. Cervical spine trauma associated with moderate and severe head injury: incidence, risk factors, and injury characteristics. *J Neurosurg.* 2002;96:285–91.

24. Brain Trauma Foundation; American Association of Neurological Surgeons; Congress of Neurological Surgeons; Joint Section on Neurotrauma and Critical Care, AANS/CNS, Bratton SL, Chestnut RM, *et al.* Guidelines for the management of severe traumatic brain injury. I. Blood pressure and oxygenation. *J Neurotrauma.* 2007;24 Suppl 1:S7–13.

25. Teasdale G, Jennett B. Assessment of coma and impaired consciousness. A practical scale. *Lancet.* 1974;2:81–4.

26. Wijdicks EF, Bamlet WR, Maramattom BV, Manno EM, McClelland RL. Validation of a new coma scale: The FOUR score. *Ann Neurol.* 2005;58:585–93.

27. Wijdicks EF, Rabinstein AA, Bamlet WR, Mandrekar JN. FOUR score and Glasgow Coma Scale in predicting outcome of comatose patients: a pooled analysis. *Neurology.* 2011;77:84–5.

28. Chang EF, Meeker M, Holland MC. Acute traumatic intraparenchymal hemorrhage: risk factors for progression in the early post-injury period. *Neurosurgery.* 2007;61:222–30.

29. Chieregato A, Fainardi E, Morselli-Labate AM, Antonelli V, Compagnone C, Targa L, *et al.* Factors associated with neurological outcome and lesion progression in traumatic subarachnoid hemorrhage patients. *Neurosurgery.* 2005;56:671–80.

30. Maas AI, Marmarou A, Murray GD, Teasdale SG, Steyerberg EW. Prognosis and clinical trial design in traumatic brain injury: the IMPACT study. *J Neurotrauma.* 2007;24:232–8.

31. Patel HC, Bouamra O, Woodford M, King AT, Yates DW, Lecky FE, *et al.* Trends in head injury outcome from 1989 to 2003 and the effect of neurosurgical care: an observational study. *Lancet.* 2005;366:1538–44.

32. Baxt WG, Moody P. The impact of advanced prehospital emergency care on the mortality of severely brain-injured patients. *J Trauma.* 1987;27:365–9.

33. Davis DP, Peay J, Serrano JA, Buono C, Vilke GM, Sise MJ, *et al.* The impact of aeromedical response to patients with moderate to severe traumatic brain injury. *Ann Emerg Med.* 2005;46:115–22.

34. Bratton SL, Chestnut RM, Ghajar J, McConnell Hammond FF, Harris OA, Hartl R, *et al.* Guidelines for the management of severe traumatic brain injury. VI. Indications for intracranial pressure monitoring. *J Neurotrauma.* 2007;24 Suppl 1:S37–44.

35. White H, Venkatesh B. Applications of transcranial Doppler in the ICU: a review. *Intensive Care Med.* 2006;32:981–94.

36. Friedman D, Claassen J, Hirsch LJ. Continuous electroencephalogram monitoring in the intensive care unit. *Anesth Analg.* 2009;109:506–23.

37. Guerit JM, Amantini A, Amodio P, Andersen KV, Butler S, de Weerd A, *et al.* Consensus on the use of neurophysiological tests in the intensive care unit (ICU): electroencephalogram (EEG), evoked potentials (EP), and electroneuromyography (ENMG). *Neurophysiol Clin.* 2009;39:71–83.

38. SAFE Study Investigators; Australian and New Zealand Intensive Care Society Clinical Trials Group; Australian Red Cross Blood Service; George Institute for International Health, Myburgh J, Cooper DJ, *et al.* Saline or albumin for fluid resuscitation in patients with traumatic brain injury. *N Engl J Med.* 2007;357:874–84.

39. Cooper DJ, Myles PS, McDermott FT, Murray LJ, Laidlaw J, Cooper G, *et al.* Prehospital hypertonic saline resuscitation of patients with hypotension and severe traumatic brain injury: a randomized controlled trial. *JAMA.* 2004;291:1350–7.

40. Bratton SL, Chestnut RM, Ghajar J, McConnell Hammond FF, Harris OA, Hartl R, *et al.* Guidelines for the management of severe traumatic brain injury. II. Hyperosmolar therapy. *J Neurotrauma.* 2007;24 Suppl 1:S14–20.

41. Bullock MR, Chesnut R, Ghajar J, Gordon D, Hartl R, Newell DW, *et al.* Surgical management of traumatic parenchymal lesions. *Neurosurgery.* 2006;58:S25–46.

42. Bullock MR, Chesnut R, Ghajar J, Gordon D, Hartl R, Newell DW, *et al.* Surgical management of acute subdural hematomas. *Neurosurgery.* 2006;58:S16–24.

43. Bullock MR, Chesnut R, Ghajar J, Gordon D, Hartl R, Newell DW, *et al.* Surgical management of acute epidural hematomas. *Neurosurgery.* 2006;58:S7–15.

44. Cooper DJ, Rosenfeld JV, Murray L, Arabi YM, Davies AR, D'Urso P, *et al.* Decompressive craniectomy in diffuse traumatic brain injury. *N Engl J Med.* 2011;364:1493–502.

45. Maegele M. Coagulopathy after traumatic brain injury: incidence, pathogenesis, and treatment options. *Transfusion.* 2013;53 Suppl 1:28S–37S.

46. White H, Venkatesh B. Cerebral perfusion pressure in neurotrauma: a review. *Anesth Analg.* 2008;107:979–88.

47. Harper AM. Physiology of cerebral bloodflow. *Br J Anaesth.* 1965;37:225–35.

48. Lassen NA. Control of cerebral circulation in health and disease. *Circ Res.* 1974;34:749–60.

49. Maas AI, Dearden M, Teasdale GM, Braakman R, Cohadon F, Iannotti F, *et al.* EBIC-guidelines for management of severe head injury in adults. European Brain Injury Consortium. *Acta Neurochir (Wien).* 1997;139:286–94.

50. Bullock MR, Povlishock JT. Guidelines for the management of severe traumatic brain injury. Editor's Commentary. *J Neurotrauma.* 2007;24 Suppl 1:vii–viii.

51. Morillo CA, Ellenbogen KA, Fernando Pava L. Pathophysiologic basis for vasodepressor syncope. *Cardiol Clin.* 1997;15:233–49.

52. Jones SC, Radinsky CR, Furlan AJ, Chyatte D, Perez-Trepichio AD. Cortical NOS inhibition raises the lower limit of cerebral blood flow-arterial pressure autoregulation. *Am J Physiol.* 1999;276:H1253–62.

53. McCulloch TJ, Visco E, Lam AM. Graded hypercapnia and cerebral autoregulation during sevoflurane or propofol anesthesia. *Anesthesiology.* 2000;93:1205–9.

54. Steiner LA, Andrews PJ. Monitoring the injured brain: ICP and CBF. *Br J Anaesth.* 2006;97:26–38.

55. Baguley IJ, Nicholls JL, Felmingham KL, Crooks J, Gurka JA, Wade LD. Dysautonomia after traumatic brain injury: a forgotten syndrome? *J Neurol Neurosurg Psychiatry.* 1999;67:39–43.

56. Rosner MJ. Introduction to cerebral perfusion pressure management. *Neurosurg Clin N Am*. 1995;6:761–73.

57. Rosner MJ, Rosner SD, Johnson AH. Cerebral perfusion pressure: management protocol and clinical results. *J Neurosurg*. 1995;83:949–62.

58. Czosnyka M, Smielewski P, Kirkpatrick P, Piechnik S, Laing R, Pickard JD. Continuous monitoring of cerebrovascular pressure-reactivity in head injury. *Acta Neurochir Suppl*. 1998;71:74–7.

59. Howells T, Elf K, Jones PA, Ronne-Engström E, Piper I, Nilsson P, *et al*. Pressure reactivity as a guide in the treatment of cerebral perfusion pressure in patients with brain trauma. *J Neurosurg*. 2005;102:311–17.

60. Steiner LA, Czosnyka M, Piechnik SK, Smielewski P, Chatfield D, Menon DK, *et al*. Continuous monitoring of cerebrovascular pressure reactivity allows determination of optimal cerebral perfusion pressure in patients with traumatic brain injury. *Crit Care Med*. 2002;30:733–8.

61. Cunningham AS, Salvador R, Coles JP, Chatfield DA, Bradley PG, Johnston AJ, *et al*. Physiological thresholds for irreversible tissue damage in contusional regions following traumatic brain injury. *Brain*. 2005;128:1931–42.

62. Gopinath SP, Robertson CS, Contant CF, Hayes C, Feldman Z, Narayan RK, *et al*. Jugular venous desaturation and outcome after head injury. *J Neurol Neurosurg Psychiatry*.1994;57:717–23.

63. Cruz J, Jaggi JL, Hoffstad OJ. Cerebral blood flow and oxygen consumption in acute brain injury with acute anemia: an alternative for the cerebral metabolic rate of oxygen consumption? *Crit Care Med*. 1993;21:1218–24.

64. Stiefel MF, Udoetuk JD, Spiotta AM, Gracias VH, Goldberg A, Maloney-Wilensky E, *et al*. Conventional neurocritical care and cerebral oxygenation after traumatic brain injury. *J Neurosurg*. 2006;105:568–75.

65. Stiefel MF, Udoetuk JD, Storm PB, Sutton LN, Kim H, Dominguez TE, *et al*. Brain tissue oxygen monitoring in pediatric patients with severe traumatic brain injury. *J Neurosurg*. 2006;105:281–6.

66. Kiening KL, Hartl R, Unterberg AW, Schneider GH, Bardt T, Lanksch WR. Brain tissue pO2-monitoring in comatose patients: implications for therapy. *Neurol Res*. 1997;19:233–40.

67. Venkatesh B. Monitoring cerebral perfusion and oxygenation: an elusive goal. *Crit Care Resusc*. 2005;7:195–9.

68. Bratton SL, Chestnut RM, Ghajar J, McConnell Hammond FF, Harris OA, Hartl R, *et al*. Guidelines for the management of severe traumatic brain injury. X. Brain oxygen monitoring and thresholds. *J Neurotrauma*. 2007;24 Suppl 1:S65–70.

69. Nelson DW, Bellander BM, Maccallum RM, Axelsson J, Alm M, Wallin M, *et al*. Cerebral microdialysis of patients with severe traumatic brain injury exhibits highly individualistic patterns as visualized by cluster analysis with self-organizing maps. *Crit Care Med*. 2004;32:2428–36.

70. Bellander BM, Cantais E, Enblad P, Hutchinson P, Nordström CH, Robertson C, *et al*. Consensus meeting on microdialysis in neurointensive care. *Intensive Care Med*. 2004;30:2166–9.

71. Nordstrom CH. Assessment of critical thresholds for cerebral perfusion pressure by performing bedside monitoring of cerebral energy metabolism. *Neurosurg Focus*. 2003;15:E5.

72. Nordstrom CH, Reinstrup P, Xu W, Gardenfors A, Ungerstedt U. Assessment of the lower limit for cerebral perfusion pressure in severe head injuries by bedside monitoring of regional energy metabolism. *Anesthesiology*. 2003;98:809–14.

73. Andrews PJ, Citerio G. Intracranial pressure. Part one: historical overview and basic concepts. *Intensive Care Med*. 2004;30:1730–3.

74. Aucoin PJ, Kotilainen HR, Gantz NM, Davidson R, Kellogg P, Stone B. Intracranial pressure monitors. Epidemiologic study of risk factors and infections. *Am J Med*. 1986;80:369–76.

75. Chesnut RM, Temkin N, Carney N, Dikmen S, Rondina C, Videtta W, *et al*. A trial of intracranial-pressure monitoring in traumatic brain injury. *N Engl J Med*. 2012;367:2471–81.

76. Biersteker HA, Andriessen TM, Horn J, Franschman G, van der Naalt J, Hoedemaekers CW, *et al*. Factors influencing intracranial pressure monitoring guideline compliance and outcome after severe traumatic brain injury. *Crit Care Med*. 2012;40:1914–22.

77. Haddad S, Aldawood AS, Alferayan A, Russell NA, Tamim HM, Arabi YM. Relationship between intracranial pressure monitoring and outcomes in severe traumatic brain injury patients. *Anaesth Intensive Care*. 2011;39:1043–50.

78. Mendelson AA, Gillis C, Henderson WR, Ronco JJ, Dhingra V, Griesdale DE. Intracranial pressure monitors in traumatic brain injury: a systematic review. *Can J Neurol Sci*. 2012;39:571–6.

79. Bratton SL, Chestnut RM, Ghajar J, McConnell Hammond FF, Harris OA, Hartl R, *et al*. Guidelines for the management of severe traumatic brain injury. VIII. Intracranial pressure thresholds. *J Neurotrauma*. 2007;24 Suppl 1:S55–8.

80. Lundberg N. Continuous recording and control of ventricular fluid pressure in neurosurgical practice. *Acta Psychiatr Scand Suppl*. 1960;36:1–193.

81. Lang EW, Lagopoulos J, Griffith J, Yip K, Mudaliar Y, Mehdorn HM, *et al*. Noninvasive cerebrovascular autoregulation assessment in traumatic brain injury: validation and utility. *J Neurotrauma*. 2003;20:69–75.

82. Lang EW, Mehdorn HM, Dorsch NW, Czosnyka M. Continuous monitoring of cerebrovascular autoregulation: a validation study. *J Neurol Neurosurg Psychiatry*. 2002;72:583–6.

83. Rosner MJ, Rosner SD, Johnson AH. Cerebral perfusion pressure: management protocol and clinical results. *J Neurosurg*. 1995;83:949–62.

84. Young JS, Blow O, Turrentine F, Claridge JA, Schulman A. Is there an upper limit of intracranial pressure in patients with severe head injury if cerebral perfusion pressure is maintained? *Neurosurg Focus*. 2003;15:E2.

85. Robertson CS, Valadka AB, Hannay HJ, Contant CF, Gopinath SP, Cormio M, *et al*. Prevention of secondary ischemic insults after severe head injury. *Crit Care Med*. 1999;27:2086–95.

86. Contant CF, Valadka AB, Gopinath SP, Hannay HJ, Robertson CS. Adult respiratory distress syndrome: a complication of induced hypertension after severe head injury. *J Neurosurg*. 2001;95:560–8.

87. Lang EW, Czosnyka M, Mehdorn HM. Tissue oxygen reactivity and cerebral autoregulation after severe traumatic brain injury. *Crit Care Med*. 2003;31:267–71.

88. Juul N, Morris GF, Marshall SB, Marshall LF. Intracranial hypertension and cerebral perfusion pressure: influence on neurological deterioration and outcome in severe head injury. The Executive Committee of the International Selfotel Trial. *J Neurosurg*. 2000;92:1–6.

89. Balestreri M, Czosnyka M, Hutchinson P, Steiner LA, Hiler M, Smielewski P, *et al*. Impact of intracranial pressure and cerebral perfusion pressure on severe disability and mortality after head injury. *Neurocrit Care*. 2006;4:8–13.

90. Wakai A, Roberts I, Schierhout G. Mannitol for acute traumatic brain injury. *Cochrane Database Syst Rev*. 2007;1:CD001049.

91. Vialet R, Albanese J, Thomachot L, Antonini F, Bourgouin A, Alliez B, *et al*. Isovolume hypertonic solutes (sodium chloride or mannitol) in the treatment of refractory posttraumatic intracranial hypertension: 2 mL/kg 7.5% saline is more effective than 2 mL/kg 20% mannitol. *Crit Care Med*. 2003;31:1683–7.

92. Khanna S, Davis D, Peterson B, Fisher B, Tung H, O'Quigley J, *et al*. Use of hypertonic saline in the treatment of severe refractory posttraumatic intracranial hypertension in pediatric traumatic brain injury. *Crit Care Med*. 2000;28:1144–51.

93. Mortazavi MM, Romeo AK, Deep A, Griessenauer CJ, Shoja MM, Tubbs RS, *et al*. Hypertonic saline for treating raised intracranial pressure: literature review with meta-analysis. *J Neurosurg*. 2012;116:210–21.

94. Morrison LJ, Baker AJ, Rhind SG, Rhind SG, Simitciu M, Perreira T, *et al*. The Toronto prehospital hypertonic resuscitation—head injury and multiorgan dysfunction trial: feasibility study of a randomized controlled trial. *J Crit Care*. 2011;26:363–72.

95. Bulger EM, May S, Brasel KJ, Schreiber M, Kerby JD, Tisherman SA, *et al*. Out-of-hospital hypertonic resuscitation following severe traumatic brain injury: a randomized controlled trial. *JAMA*. 2010;304:1455–64.

96. Grande PO. The "Lund Concept" for the treatment of severe head trauma—physiological principles and clinical application. *Intensive Care Med.* 2006;32:1475–84.

97. Asgeirsson B, Grande PO, Nordstrom CH. A new therapy of post-trauma brain oedema based on haemodynamic principles for brain volume regulation. *Intensive Care Med.* 1994;20:260–7.

98. Eker C, Asgeirsson B, Grande PO, Schalen W, Nordstrom CH. Improved outcome after severe head injury with a new therapy based on principles for brain volume regulation and preserved microcirculation. *Crit Care Med.* 1998;26:1881–6.

99. Dizdarevic K, Hamdan A, Omerhodzic I, Kominlija-Smajic E. Modified Lund concept versus cerebral perfusion pressure-targeted therapy: a randomised controlled study in patients with secondary brain ischaemia. *Clin Neurol Neurosurg.* 2012;114:142–8.

100. Grande PO. The Lund concept for the treatment of patients with severe traumatic brain injury. *J Neurosurg Anesthesiol.* 2011;23:358–62.

101. Grande PO. PRO: the "Lund concept" for treatment of patients with severe traumatic brain injury. *J Neurosurg Anesthesiol.* 2011;23:251–5.

102. Sharma D, Vavilala MS. Lund concept for the management of traumatic brain injury: a physiological principle awaiting stronger evidence. *J Neurosurg Anesthesiol.* 2011;23:363–7.

103. Elf K, Nilsson P, Ronne-Engstrom E, Howells T, Enblad P. Cerebral perfusion pressure between 50 and 60 mm Hg may be beneficial in head-injured patients: a computerized secondary insult monitoring study. *Neurosurgery.* 2005;56:962–71.

104. Johnson U, Nilsson P, Ronne-Engstrom E, Howells T, Enblad P. Favorable outcome in traumatic brain injury patients with impaired cerebral pressure autoregulation when treated at low cerebral perfusion pressure levels. *Neurosurgery.* 2011;68:714–21.

105. Sarrafzadeh AS, Peltonen EE, Kaisers U, Kuchler I, Lanksch WR, Unterberg AW. Secondary insults in severe head injury—do multiply injured patients do worse? *Crit Care Med.* 2001;29:1116–23.

106. Van Leeuwen N, Lingsma H, Perel P, Lecky F, Roozenbeek B, Lu J, et al. Prognostic value of major extracranial injury in traumatic brain injury: an individual patient data meta-analysis in 39,274 patients. *Erasmus J Med.* 2011;2:40.

107. Vegar-Brozovic V, Brezak J, Brozovic I. Intra-abdominal hypertension: pulmonary and cerebral complications. *Transplant Proc.* 2008;40:1190–2.

108. Andelic N. The epidemiology of traumatic brain injury. *Lancet Neurol.* 2013;12:28–9.

109. Tennant A. Admission to hospital following head injury in England: incidence and socio-economic associations. *BMC Public Health.* 2005;5:21.

110. Bratton SL, Chestnut RM, Ghajar J, McConnell Hammond FF, Harris OA, Hartl R, et al. Guidelines for the management of severe traumatic brain injury. XV. Steroids. *J Neurotrauma.* 2007;24 Suppl 1:S91–5.

111. Bratton SL, Chestnut RM, Ghajar J, McConnell Hammond FF, Harris OA, Hartl R, et al. Guidelines for the management of severe traumatic brain injury. XIV. Hyperventilation. *J Neurotrauma.* 2007;24 Suppl 1:S87–90.

112. Bratton SL, Chestnut RM, Ghajar J, McConnell Hammond FF, Harris OA, Hartl R, et al. Guidelines for the management of severe traumatic brain injury. XIII. Antiseizure prophylaxis. *J Neurotrauma.* 2007;24 Suppl 1:S83–6.

113. Bratton SL, Chestnut RM, Ghajar J, McConnell Hammond FF, Harris OA, Hartl R, et al. Guidelines for the management of severe traumatic brain injury. XII. Nutrition. *J Neurotrauma.* 2007;24 Suppl 1:S77–82.

114. Bratton SL, Chestnut RM, Ghajar J, McConnell Hammond FF, Harris OA, Hartl R, et al. Guidelines for the management of severe traumatic brain injury. XI. Anesthetics, analgesics, and sedatives. *J Neurotrauma.* 2007;24 Suppl 1:S71–6.

115. Bratton SL, Chestnut RM, Ghajar J, McConnell Hammond FF, Harris OA, Hartl R, et al. Guidelines for the management of severe traumatic brain injury. IX. Cerebral perfusion thresholds. *J Neurotrauma.* 2007;24 Suppl 1:S59–64.

116. Bratton SL, Chestnut RM, Ghajar J, McConnell Hammond FF, Harris OA, Hartl R, et al. Guidelines for the management of severe traumatic brain injury. VII. Intracranial pressure monitoring technology. *J Neurotrauma.* 2007;24 Suppl 1:S45–54.

117. Bratton SL, Chestnut RM, Ghajar J, McConnell Hammond FF, Harris OA, Hartl R, et al. Guidelines for the management of severe traumatic brain injury. V. Deep vein thrombosis prophylaxis. *J Neurotrauma.* 2007;24 Suppl 1:S32–6.

118. Bratton SL, Chestnut RM, Ghajar J, McConnell Hammond FF, Harris OA, Hartl R, et al. Guidelines for the management of severe traumatic brain injury. IV. Infection prophylaxis. *J Neurotrauma.* 2007;24 Suppl 1:S26–31.

119. Bratton SL, Chestnut RM, Ghajar J, McConnell Hammond FF, Harris OA, Hartl R, et al. Guidelines for the management of severe traumatic brain injury. III. Prophylactic hypothermia. *J Neurotrauma.* 2007;24 Suppl 1:S21–5.

120. Moppett IK. Traumatic brain injury: assessment, resuscitation and early management. *Br J Anaesth.* 2007;99:18–31.

121. Xiong Y, Mahmood A, Chopp M. Animal models of traumatic brain injury. *Nat Rev Neurosci.* 2013;14:128–42.

122. American Brain Injury Consortium (ABIC). *Patient Care Guidelines.* Virginia Commonwealth University, 2008. [Online] https://cymbalta.nsc.vcu.edu/ABIC/guidelines/index.cfm

123. Hodgkinson S, Pollit V, Sharpin C, Lecky F. Early management of head injury: summary of updated NICE guidance. *BMJ.* 2014;348:g104.

124. Lingsma HF, Roozenbeek B, Li B, Lu J, Weir J, Butcher I, et al. Large between-center differences in outcome after moderate and severe traumatic brain injury in the international mission on prognosis and clinical trial design in traumatic brain injury (IMPACT) study. *Neurosurgery.* 2011;68:601–7.

125. Tosetti P, Hicks RR, Theriault E, Phillips A, Koroshetz W, Draghia-Akli R, et al. Toward an international initiative for traumatic brain injury research. *J Neurotrauma.* 2013;30:1211–22.

126. Maas AI, Murray G, Henney H, 3rd, Kassem N, Legrand V, Mangelus M, et al. Efficacy and safety of dexanabinol in severe traumatic brain injury: results of a phase III randomised, placebo-controlled, clinical trial. *Lancet Neurol.* 2006;5:38–45.

127. Hatton J. Pharmacological treatment of traumatic brain injury: a review of agents in development. *CNS Drugs.* 2001;15:553–81.

128. Fernandez-Gajardo R, Matamala JM, Carrasco R, Gutierrez R, Melo R, Rodrigo R. Novel therapeutic strategies for traumatic brain injury: acute antioxidant reinforcement. *CNS Drugs.* 2014;28:229–48.

129. Vink R, Nimmo AJ. Novel therapies in development for the treatment of traumatic brain injury. *Expert Opin Investig Drugs.* 2002;11:1375–86.

130. White H, Venkatesh B. Clinical review: ketones and brain injury. *Crit Care.* 2011;15:219.

131. Georgiopoulos M, Katsakiori P, Kefalopoulou Z, Ellul J, Chroni E, Constantoyannis C. Vegetative state and minimally conscious state: a review of the therapeutic interventions. *Stereotact Funct Neurosurg.* 2010;88:199–207.

132. Whyte J, Rajan R, Rosenbaum A, Katz D, Kalmar K, Seel R, et al. Zolpidem and restoration of consciousness. *Am J Phys Med Rehabil.* 2014;93:101–13.

133. Frenette AJ, Kanji S, Rees L, Williamson DR, Perreault MM, Turgeon AF, et al. Efficacy and safety of dopamine agonists in traumatic brain injury: a systematic review of randomized controlled trials. *J Neurotrauma.* 2012;29:1–18.

134. Robertson CS. Management of cerebral perfusion pressure after traumatic brain injury. *Anesthesiology.* 2001;95:1513–17.

135. Maas AI, Stocchetti N, Bullock R. Moderate and severe traumatic brain injury in adults. *Lancet Neurol.* 2008;7:728–41.

136. Jeffreys RV, Jones JJ. Avoidable factors contributing to the death of head injury patients in general hospitals in Mersey Region. *Lancet.* 1981;2:459–61.

137. Gentleman D. Causes and effects of systemic complications among severely head injured patients transferred to a neurosurgical unit. *Int Surg.* 1992;77:297–302.

138. Robertson CS, Gopinath SP, Goodman JC, Contant CF, Valadka AB, Narayan RK. SjvO2 monitoring in head-injured patients. *J Neurotrauma.* 1995;12:891–6.

139. Manley G, Knudson MM, Morabito D, Damron S, Erickson V, Pitts L. Hypotension, hypoxia, and head injury: frequency, duration, and consequences. *Arch Surg.* 2001;136:1118–23.

140. Chi JH, Knudson MM, Vassar MJ, McCarthy MC, Shapiro MB, Mallet S, *et al.* Prehospital hypoxia affects outcome in patients with traumatic brain injury: a prospective multicenter study. *J Trauma.* 2006;61:1134–41.

141. McHugh GS, Engel DC, Butcher I, Steyerberg EW, Lu J, Mushkudiani N, *et al.* Prognostic value of secondary insults in traumatic

brain injury: results from the IMPACT study. *J Neurotrauma.* 2007;24:287–93.

142. Franschman G, Peerdeman SM, Andriessen TM, Greuters S, Toor AE, Vos PE, *et al.* Effect of secondary prehospital risk factors on outcome in severe traumatic brain injury in the context of fast access to trauma care. *J Trauma.* 2011;71:826–32.

143. Oddo M, Levine JM, Mackenzie L, Frangos S, Feihl F, Kasner SE, *et al.* Brain hypoxia is associated with short-term outcome after severe traumatic brain injury independently of intracranial hypertension and low cerebral perfusion pressure. *Neurosurgery.* 2011;69:1037–45.

144. Cruz J, Jaggi JL, Hoffstad OJ. Cerebral blood flow, vascular resistance, and oxygen metabolism in acute brain trauma: redefining the role of cerebral perfusion pressure? *Crit Care Med.* 1995;23:1412–17.

CHAPTER 18

Subarachnoid haemorrhage

Pouya Tahsili-Fahadan and Michael N. Diringer

Subarachnoid haemorrhage (SAH) is a neurological emergency caused by acute extravasation of blood into the subarachnoid space, located between the layers of the meningeal coverings of the brain. The overall mortality is around 33% and a significant number of patients (12–15%) die before reaching hospital (1). More than half of survivors suffer from long-term neurological impairment related to the initial bleed and secondary insults including rebleeding, hydrocephalus, and delayed cerebral ischaemia (DCI). Given the severity and complexity of SAH, the need for multiple procedures, and long length of hospital stays, it is unsurprising that it is associated with significant healthcare costs.

Approximately 85% of cases of non-traumatic SAH are due to rupture of an intracranial saccular aneurysm. Although the overall mortality of aneurysmal SAH (aSAH) has declined over the last few decades, it is still associated with high rates of mortality and morbidity. Other, non-aneurysmal, causes of spontaneous SAH (Table 18.1), such as vascular malformations and perimesencephalic SAH (localized bleeding thought to be of venous origin), are associated with fewer neurological complications and better prognosis than aSAH. This chapter will focus on recent advances in the diagnosis and management of aSAH, with particular reference to its critical care management.

Epidemiology

Intracranial aneurysms are identified in 2–5% of autopsies (2), but rupture occurs in only a small proportion of those harbouring aneurysms. The incidence of aSAH ranges from 2 to 16 cases per 100,000 population per year, varying considerably across different countries with the lowest rates in high-income nations. In the United States, the overall reported incidence of aSAH is 14.5 cases per 100,000 persons per year (3), although the actual rate is likely to be higher because of the high pre-hospital mortality. The incidence of aSAH is 1.24 times higher in women, and the rate of aneurysmal rupture increases with age, peaking between 50 and 60 years. Considering both age and gender together, the highest rates of rupture are seen in males under 45 or over 85 years, and in females between the age of 55 and 85 years (4). aSAH is also more common in African Americans and those of Hispanic origin (5, 6). The overall incidence of SAH has decreased over the past 50 years in most countries (4), but the mean age of initial presentation is rising and this is associated with worsened outcome (1).

Pathophysiology

The anatomy of intracranial arteries is different to their extracranial counterparts. They lack the external elastic lamina that separates the middle (media) and outer (adventitia) layers in the extracranial arterial wall, have a very thin adventitia, and a lower wall-thickness to lumen ratio (7). Saccular aneurysms, also known as berry aneurysms because of their morphology, consist of out-pouchings of the arterial wall and are most commonly located at bifurcations of the large arteries that make up the circle of Willis. The majority of aneurysms arise from the anterior cerebral circulation; 34% from anterior cerebral and anterior communicating arteries, 25% from the posterior communicating artery, 20% the middle cerebral artery, and 7.5% the internal carotid artery (8). In the posterior circulation 7% of aneurysms arise from the basilar artery and 3% from the posterior inferior cerebellar artery. Other locations account for 3.5% of cerebral aneurysms. Multiple aneurysms are present in about 20% of cases (9).

Risk factors for aneurysm development and rupture

The risk factors associated with aneurysm formation are summarized in Table 18.2, and include both environmental and genetic factors. Changes in the structure of intracranial arterial walls, especially thinning of the tunica media and internal elastic lamina, predispose to damage by haemodynamic stress, particularly at branching sites (2). The anatomical distribution of saccular aneurysms and their increased prevalence with age supports this hypothesis.

Although the exact pathophysiology underlying aneurysm formation remains an area of active investigation, histological studies confirm that smooth muscle cells migrate through disruptions of the internal elastic lamina and proliferate. Inflammatory processes are also thought to play a pivotal role in both the formation and enlargement of aneurysms (10), and it has been suggested that 3-hydroxy-3-methylglutaryl-coenzyme A (HMG-CoA) reductase inhibitors (statins) and calcium channel blockers might inhibit aneurysm formation by suppression of nuclear factor kappa B (11). Inflammation affects all three layers of the arterial wall prior to rupture, leading to an irregular and disrupted endothelial surface and loss of smooth muscle cells with invasion of inflammatory cells (7).

Genetic factors also play an important role in the formation of aneurysms. Studies have revealed enhanced expression of genes involved in inflammatory processes and programmed cell death in the walls of unruptured aneurysms compared to normal arteries (12). A neuroimaging study of 8680 individuals found that the incidence of aneurysms increases from 6.8% in the general population to 10.5% in those with a family history of aSAH (13). Although a familial form is recognized, the underlying genes have not been identified.

Table 18.1 Cause of non-traumatic non-aneurysmal subarachnoid haemorrhage

Conditions	Examples
Autoimmune diseases	Primary CNS vasculitis, systemic vasculitis (Behçet's disease, Churg–Strauss syndrome, polyarteritis nodosa, ANCA-associated granulomatosis)
Drugs	Anticoagulant therapy, psychostimulants
Haematological disorders	Bleeding disorders, sickle cell disease
Infections	Borreliosis, mycotic arteritis, Lyme disease, syphilis
Neoplastic disorders	Brain metastases, meningeal carcinomatosis, pituitary apoplexy, primary CNS neoplasms
Vascular diseases	Arterial dissection, arteriovenous malformations, capillary telangiectasis, cavernous malformations, cerebral amyloid angiopathy, cerebral venous thrombosis, dural arteriovenous fistulae, moyamoya disease, spinal artery aneurysm

Non-aneurysmal perimesencephalic SAH (not shown in the table) accounts for 10% of non-traumatic non-aneurysmal SAH.

CNS, central nervous system; SAH, subarachnoid haemorrhage.

The majority of cerebral aneurysms pose a very low risk of bleeding despite the once dominant belief to the contrary (2). The underlying mechanisms of aneurysm rupture remain controversial, but unrecognized genetic predisposition may affect the risk of aneurysm growth and subsequent rupture. On the microscopic level, the severity of endothelial damage, disarrangement of smooth muscle fibres, and inflammatory changes are associated with the risk of rupture (7). Stress induced by haemodynamic changes and the rate of aneurysm growth are also believed to be implicated.

Aneurysmal rupture usually occurs at the dome where the arterial wall is thinnest and most degenerate, and is more likely in recently developed aneurysms that have expanded rapidly over the course of few days or weeks (14). Aneurysm size greater than 7 mm is a risk factor for rupture, as is patient age. The characteristics of the aneurysm are also important, with a higher risk of rupture in symptomatic, large, and posterior circulation aneurysms. In addition, morphological and haemodynamic features should be considered when evaluating the risk of rupture. A history of aSAH or family history of aneurysms (ruptured or not) increases the risk of aSAH, with a threefold risk in patients with three or more affected relatives (15). Recent major social stressors may also increase the risk of aSAH, but there does not appear to be an increased risk during pregnancy, delivery, and the puerperium (16).

Table 18.2 Risk factors for cerebral aneurysms

Modifiable	Non-modifiable
Smoking	Advancing age
Hypertension	Female gender
Heavy alcohol consumption	Black and Hispanic ethnicity
Psychostimulants	Family history in ≥ 2 first-degree relatives
Oral contraceptive use	

Table 18.3 Five-year risk of aneurysm rupture in patients without a history of subarachnoid haemorrhage

| Aneurysm diameter | 5-Year risk of rupture | |
	Anterior circulation[a]	Posterior circulation[b]
Small (2–7 mm)	0%	2.5%
Medium (7–12 mm)	2.6%	14.5%
Large (13–24 mm)	4.5%	18.4%
Giant (> 24 mm)	40%	50%

[a] Non-cavernous internal carotid, anterior and middle cerebral arteries.

[b] Vertebrobasilar and posterior communicating arteries.

Adapted from *The Lancet*, 362, 9378, Wiebers DO *et al.*, 'Unruptured intracranial aneurysms: natural history, clinical outcome, and risks of surgical and endovascular treatment', pp. 103–110, Copyright 2003, with permission from Elsevier.

Preventable measures

The wide availability of advanced neuroimaging techniques has resulted in early recognition of both incidentally identified and symptomatic aneurysms. The International Study of Unruptured Intracranial Aneurysms, a multicentre prospective study, followed the natural course of unruptured cerebral aneurysms in 1692 patients (Table 18.3) (2). Of note, participants in this study were preselected by neurosurgeons as being at low risk of aneurysm rupture, and therefore the higher risks of rupture reported in other studies may be more realistic.

A number of risk factors for aneurysmal rupture are modifiable and thus the target of preventive strategies. In addition to its myriad adverse effects on cerebrovascular, cardiovascular, and renal function, chronic hypertension also increases the risk of aneurysm rupture. In addition, avoidance of smoking and heavy alcohol use is recommended (17). Although a few studies have suggested a role for diet in preventing aSAH, further investigation of this relationship is required. However, it is reasonable to recommend increasing the daily proportion of vegetables.

Screening for aneurysms in high-risk patients may lead to lower mortality and morbidity rates because of pre-emptive treatment before rupture occurs. Non-invasive screening, such as magnetic resonance angiography (MRA), should be considered in individuals with personal history of aSAH or a family history in more than one first-degree relative (18). Screening should also be an option for patients with autosomal dominant polycystic kidney disease because of the high rates of concurrent cerebral aneurysms, but screening frequency should be determined by the presence of cerebral aneurysms in relatives (19).

Clinical presentation

The most common presentation of aSAH, in over 80% of cases, is sudden-onset severe headache. This is classically a 'thunderclap' headache, often described as 'the worst headache of one's life'. Although aneurysm rupture may occur during strenuous exercise, the majority of cases occur during normal daily activities.

A history of a less severe (sentinel) headache in the days or weeks prior to the ictus is present in approximately one-half of patients (20). Sentinel headaches may be related to enlargement of an aneurysm, small leaks, or ruptures, and it is associated with a tenfold increase in the risk of rebleeding (21). However, headache is a common complaint generally and only 1% of headache cases presenting to emergency departments are related to aSAH. A high level of clinical suspicion is required to differentiate sentinel headache from other causes (SAH mimics) including migraine, other intracranial haemorrhage, meningitis, hypertensive encephalopathy, venous sinus thrombosis, pituitary apoplexy, and acute ischaemic stroke. Two other key elements of the presentation of aSAH are nausea and syncope and, together with a thunderclap headache, should markedly raise the suspicion of SAH.

Transient loss of consciousness occurs in about half of patients and is thought to be related to a sudden rise in intracranial pressure (ICP) with intracranial circulatory arrest or oligaemia, or cardiac arrhythmias (22). Other presenting symptoms include confusion, neck pain, blurred vision, diplopia, and photophobia. The common clinical signs of aSAH are meningeal irritation, pre-retinal haemorrhages (Terson's syndrome), sixth cranial nerve palsy due to increased ICP, seizures, and posturing. Focal neurological deficits, including cranial nerve palsies, occur in about 10% of cases of aSAH and their nature depends on the location of the ruptured aneurysm. For example, a third cranial nerve palsy is typically associated with an expanding posterior communicating artery aneurysm. Other focal deficits may be caused by the mass effect of very large aneurysms, thick focal subarachnoid clot, or intraparenchymal haemorrhage.

Respiratory failure and cardiac abnormalities, including elevated troponin levels, arrhythmias, electrocardiogram (ECG) changes, and reversible left ventricular dysfunction may also be present (see below and Chapter 27).

Notably, presenting signs and symptoms of aSAH may be mild and result in missed, delayed, or inaccurate diagnoses in up to 12% of the cases (23). However, the rate of misdiagnosis has significantly decreased because of the wide availability of computed tomography (CT) scanners.

Diagnosis

The diagnosis of SAH is confirmed based imaging findings and, in certain circumstances, lumbar puncture.

Imaging

Non-contrast cranial CT scan remains the preferred diagnostic modality for SAH. The sensitivity of modern scanning techniques for SAH is 100% within 6 hours of headache onset and 85.7% after 6 hours, with an overall sensitivity and specificity of 92.9% and 100% respectively (24). Acute haemorrhage appears as hyperdensity within the basal, perimesencephalic, and interpeduncular cisterns, Sylvian and anterior interhemispheric fissures and sulci, and may extend into the cerebral parenchyma or ventricles (Figure 18.1). CT also assists in the localization of the aneurysm based on the pattern and distribution of the blood load, as well as in identifying early hydrocephalus, mass effect or intra-parenchymal haemorrhage. The modified Fisher scale is a score based on the CT findings after SAH and correlates with the probability of DCI and outcome (Table 18.4).

Magnetic resonance imaging (MRI), including fluid-attenuated inversion recovery (FLAIR), gradient echo (GRE), diffusion- and susceptibility-weighted sequences, has a sensitivity comparable to CT for the diagnosis of SAH and can be used to avoid lumbar

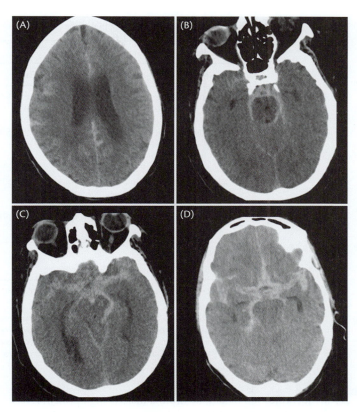

Fig. 18.1 Subarachnoid haemorrhage on non-contrast head CT scan. Non-contrast head CT scans show subarachnoid blood in:
(A) Interhemispheric fissure and frontoparietal sulci.
(B) Prepontine and quadrigeminal cisterns.
(C) Interpeduncular, Sylvian, perimesencephalic, and superior cerebellar cisterns.
(D) Suprasellar and ambient cisterns.
CT, computed tomography.

puncture (see 'Lumbar puncture') in the absence of haemorrhage on CT scan (25). MRI can also detect subacute and chronic haemorrhage and, by providing higher structural resolution than CT, excludes other diagnoses. However, the higher costs of MRI, lack of rapid availability, unfavourable environment for monitoring unstable patients, and a longer duration of scanning precludes its use as the initial imaging choice.

The dilution of red cells by bulk flow of CSF and the presence of anticoagulant factors enhance haemorrhage clearance, and the sensitivity of CT therefore decreases over time. In addition, CT may not confirm SAH if the haemorrhage is small or the haemoglobin very low (< 7 g/dL).

Lumbar puncture

Lumbar puncture is mandatory if there is a high index of clinical suspicion in patients with non-diagnostic imaging findings. It should be performed with care to avoid traumatic puncture since the diagnosis of SAH is dependent on the presence of red blood cells (RBCs) in the CSF. SAH is confirmed by the identification of xanthochromia in a centrifuged CSF sample. As pigment change depends on the breakdown of RBCs and metabolism of haemoglobin it may take up to 12 hours to develop, although it may be detectable as early as 2 hours after the ictus. This may lead to false negative findings in early CSF samples. Other confounding factors

Table 18.4 Grading scales in subarachnoid haemorrhage

	Radiographic grading scales		Clinical grading scales	
Grade	Fisher	Modified Fisher	Hunt and Hess	WFNS
I	No blood on head CT	Minimal or thin SAH without IVH	Asymptomatic or mild headache and neck stiffness	GCS = 15 without motor deficit
II	Diffuse or vertical layers < 1 mm thick, no clots	Minimal or thin SAH with IVH	Moderate to severe headache and neck stiffness ± cranial nerve palsy	GCS = 13–14 without motor deficit
III	Localized subarachnoid clot ± vertical layers > 1 mm thick	Thick SAH without IVH	Mild focal deficit, lethargy or confusion	GCS = 13–14 with motor deficit
IV	IVH or IPH with Diffuse or no SAH	Thick SAH with IVH	Stupor ± hemiparesis	GCS = 7–12 ± motor deficit
V	N/A	N/A	Deep coma ± extensor posturing	GCS = 3–6 ± motor deficit

GCS, Glasgow Coma Scale; IPH, intraparenchymal haemorrhage; IVH, intraventricular haemorrhage; WFNS: World Federation of Neurologic Surgeons.

Fisher: Adapted from Fisher CM et al., 'Relation of cerebral vasospasm to subarachnoid hemorrhage visualized by computerized tomographic scanning', *Neurosurgery*, 6, 1, pp. 1–9, copyright 1980, with permission from Wolters Kluwer and Congress of Neurological Surgeons. Modified Fisher: Adapted from Frontera JA et al., 'Prediction of symptomatic vasospasm after subarachnoid hemorrhage: the modified fisher scale', *Neurosurgery*, 59, 1, pp. 21–27, copyright 2006, with permission from Wolters Kluwer and Congress of Neurological Surgeons.

for the identification of xanthochromia include high protein levels and hyperbilirubinaemia. Spectrophotometry is superior to visual inspection of CSF in such cases but is not routinely available in many centres. Vascular imaging is recommended in patients with clinical features suggestive of SAH in whom CT and CSF analyses are negative.

Vascular imaging

After a diagnosis of SAH is confirmed, vascular imaging should be obtained as soon as possible to evaluate for underlying aneurysm(s) or other vascular pathologies, as well as for treatment planning. Computed tomography angiography (CTA) is replacing conventional (catheter) angiography as the initial diagnostic tool of choice because of its high sensitivity (especially by using a combination of two- and three-dimensional angiography), availability, and ease of use, as well as lower costs, radiation dose, and complication rates. CTA is also preferred over conventional angiography in the first 3–6 hours post ictus if hyperacute endovascular treatment is not being considered as the risk of rebleeding is higher with catheter angiography. A newer technology, multisection CTA combined with matched mask bone elimination (CTA-MMBE), has been developed to improve the quality of CTA in the detection of lesions close to bony structures such as the skull base (26). Of note, small aneurysms (< 3 mm) may be missed on CTA (27). Although controversial, further evaluation by conventional angiography should be considered in the presence of negative CTA studies, especially in cases of diffuse SAH (28). The ability of CTA to determine the best treatment for the aneurysm (i.e. clipping or coiling) is still a matter of debate, and subsequent catheter angiography may be indicated in selected cases.

Magnetic resonance angiography (MRA) is not currently recommended for the evaluation of patients with an established diagnosis of SAH because of its low sensitivity for the detection of small aneurysms.

Catheter angiography is still considered the 'gold standard' for the evaluation of intracranial aneurysms. It not only identifies the aneurysm and allows follow-on endovascular treatment, but also provides valuable information regarding morphology, complications (such as vasospasm), and other vascular aetiologies. Complications of catheter angiography include contrast nephropathy and allergic reactions (both also a risk with CTA), access site injuries including haematoma, arterial dissection and femoral neuropathy, and intracranial complications such as rebleeding, intracranial dissection, and stroke.

The initial angiogram may not identify a source of haemorrhage in as many as 20% of cases of non-traumatic SAH and, in such circumstances, angiography should be repeated in about 1 week (29). However, repeat angiography in CT-proven perimesencephalic SAH with negative angiography is typically unrevealing. Such cases have excellent prognosis and CTA evaluation may suffice (28).

Acute management

Outcome is improved by rapid stabilization, prompt diagnosis and securing of the ruptured aneurysm, and treatment of complications.

Initial stabilization

The initial management of aSAH should focus on assessment of neurological status and careful attention to airway management and respiratory and haemodynamic function. Several clinical grading scales have been developed for the assessment of aSAH severity (Table 18.4), including the Hunt and Hess (30) and World Federation of Neurological Surgeons (WFNS) scales (31). Both are graded based on initial clinical evaluation, have prognostic value (a higher score indicates poorer prognosis), and can be used for treatment planning.

Elective intubation of lethargic or agitated patients facilitates further evaluation and treatment, and prevents hypoventilation or airway obstruction induced by sedation. Assessment of cardiac function should include continuous ECG monitoring and measurement of cardiac enzymes. Baseline echocardiography is recommended in patients with ECG changes, elevated cardiac enzymes, and pre-existing cardiac disease.

Blood pressure control

Both hypertension, particularly prior to repair of the ruptured aneurysm, and hypotension should be avoided. Hypertension is common after SAH and related to a combination of sympathetic activation, pain, anxiety, and elevated ICP. Control of high blood pressure is believed to be important in preventing rebleeding and reduction of environmental stimulation and effective pain control are important in this regard. Although the optimal blood pressure immediately after SAH is not known, it is reasonable to keep systolic blood pressure below 160 mmHg or mean blood pressure below 110 mmHg. Chronic antihypertensive medications should not be resumed initially, especially if they are long acting. Pain management with analgesics may be sufficient to lower blood pressure in some patients, but antihypertensive agents with rapid onset-of-action is required in others. Intermittent doses of the αβ-blocker labetalol or arterial dilator hydralazine are often effective. Alternatively, continuous infusions of calcium channel blockers can be used; nicardipine infusion provides more stable blood pressure control than intermittent boluses (32). Venodilators, such as nitrates or nitroprusside, should be avoided because they may increase ICP (33). In cases of hydrocephalus (see following sections), control of blood pressure should be delayed until CSF drainage is instituted to avoid critical reductions in cerebral perfusion pressure (CPP) (34). Similarly, hypotension induced by sedation, hypovolaemia, or cardiac failure, should be avoided to preserve CPP. Permissive hypertension is usually employed once the aneurysm is secured (see Induced Hypertension).

Early hydrocephalus

Impairment of CSF flow or re-absorption after SAH may lead to development of early hydrocephalus. The incidence of hydrocephalus is higher in patients with poor-grade and large volume aSAH, but not different between patients treated with surgery versus endovascular coiling. Urgent CT should be performed to confirm hydrocephalus and exclude other causes of deterioration in any patient with a decline in level of consciousness.

Early hydrocephalus (from hours to 3 days post-ictus) develops in one-fifth of patients after aSAH (35), and it may occur in the absence of intraventricular haemorrhage. If hydrocephalus is untreated, one-third of patients will deteriorate, one-third will remain unchanged, and one-third will improve. Placement of an external ventricular drain (EVD) typically results in rapid clinical improvement, but whether this increases the risk of rebleeding is controversial (36). Lumbar drainage does not increase the risk of rebleeding and is associated with lower incidence of vasospasm, but it can result in brain herniation in patients with obstructed CSF flow (37).

Rebleeding

Rebleeding may present with sudden neurological deterioration, worsened headache, vomiting, or haemodynamic instability. It occurs in 4–13.6% of patients, with the highest risk in the first 24 hours after ictus. The majority of repeat haemorrhages occur in the first 3–6 hours after the initial bleed (38), although the actual rates may be higher because ultra-early rebleeding may be missed. The rebleeding risk decreases with time after ictus.

Rebleeding is associated with very high mortality and poor neurological outcome in survivors. The risk factors for rebleeding include female gender, serious medical co-morbidities, history of sentinel headache, poor clinical grade on admission, loss of consciousness at the time of initial ictus, systolic blood pressure above 160 mmHg, large aneurysm, early catheter angiography (< 3–6 hours post-ictus), and longer delay in aneurysm treatment (38).

Prior to definitive surgical or endovascular aneurysm repair, measures to minimize the risk of rebleeding focus on prevention of abrupt changes in the transmural pressure across the aneurysm wall. Accordingly, acute hypertension should be treated as discussed previously. Patients should also be maintained in a calm, quiet environment with minimal stimulation and appropriate treatment of pain, anxiety, and agitation. Short-acting opiates are often prescribed, but over-sedation must be avoided as it may interfere with neurological assessment. Valsalva manoeuvers should be minimized by suppression of excessive cough and the administration of stool softeners. In case of lumbar puncture or ventriculostomy, rapid drainage of large volumes of CSF should also be avoided.

Antifibrinolytic agents, such as epsilon aminocaproic acid and tranexamic acid, were previously recommended to reduce the likelihood of rebleeding, but there has been a reduction in their use after the widespread adoption of early treatment of ruptured aneurysms. Treatment courses greater than 72 hours increase the risk of DCI and negate any benefits from reduced rebleeding rates (39). However, recent studies suggest that early short-term use of antifibrinolytics (< 72 hours) reduces rebleeding rates (2.4% versus 10.8%) without an increased risk of vasospasm and DCI (40), and this has renewed interest in their use. Antifibrinolytics should be stopped 2 hours prior to endovascular procedures to minimize the risk of intra-procedural thrombus formation. Regular screening for deep vein thrombosis (DVT) is recommended when using antifibrinolytics which should be avoided in patients predisposed to thromboembolic events.

Treatment of the ruptured aneurysm

A ruptured aneurysm can be repaired by endovascular coiling (Figure 18.2) or surgical clipping (Figure 18.3). Early treatment (within 24–48 hours of ictus) is recommended as this not only prevents rebleeding (17) but also allows safe haemodynamic augmentation to treat DCI.

Prior to the introduction of detachable platinum coils in the early 1990s, aneurysms were primarily treated surgically. The most comprehensive comparison between the two treatment modalities was undertaken in the International Subarachnoid Aneurysm Trial (ISAT), a multicentre prospective randomized clinical trial (41). ISAT included 2143 patients (from 9559 screened) in whom the treating clinical teams agreed that there was clinical equipoise such that each enrolled patient was an equally good candidate for surgical or endovascular treatment. At 1 year, patients treated with

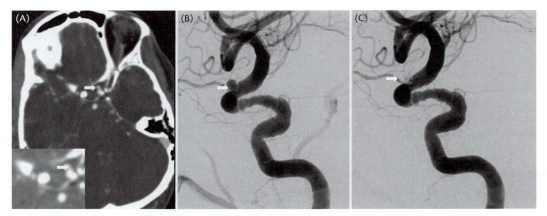

Fig. 18.2 Endovascular coiling of cerebral aneurysm.
(A) CT angiography showed small left ophthalmic artery aneurysm.
(B) Catheter angiography confirming the presence of the aneurysm.
(C) Aneurysm obliterated by endovascular coiling.

endovascular coiling were 24% less likely to have a poor outcome (death or dependency) and had lower complication rates compared to those treated with surgical clipping. Importantly, the incidence of vasospasm was similar for both treatments despite the potential advantage of being able to clear subarachnoid blood during surgery (42). However, long term follow up demonstrated that endovascular treatment was associated with a lower rate of complete aneurysm obliteration (58% versus 81%), and an increased risk of rebleeding and aneurysm recurrence compared to surgery. Over the course of 21 months the need for retreatment was 6.9 times more likely in patients treated with endovascular coiling. Although 5-year survival was lower in coiled patients, the rate of independence in survivors remained equal between the two treatment methods.

Post hoc analyses have confirmed that incomplete obliteration is more common in aneurysms with large neck to dome ratio (43). Insertion of a stent improves the rates of complete obliteration by coiling but at the cost of increased morbidity and mortality that may be related, at least in part, to the need for dual antiplatelet therapy to minimize the risk of stent thrombosis (44). Preliminary data support the use of biologically active coils to achieve complete obliteration, but further studies are warranted in this regard (17).

Various factors in addition to local expertise and patient/advocate preference are used by neurosurgeons and interventional neuroradiologists to select the best treatment modality on an individual basis. Surgical clipping is more appropriate in the presence of mass effect or intraparenchymal haemorrhage greater than 50 mL, and for wide-neck aneurysms. Some aneurysms are only amenable to one approach or the other. For example, basilar aneurysms are almost always treated by endovascular coiling and middle cerebral artery aneurysms often by neurosurgical clipping. In cases suitable for either modality, endovascular treatment is recommended (17). Repeat angiography is recommended when feasible to evaluate for, and treat, remnant or recurrent aneurysms, particularly in the posterior circulation where coiled aneurysms are associated with high rates of incomplete obliteration (45).

Intracranial complications

Once the aneurysm is secured and the risk of rebleeding is minimized, the major intracranial complications after aSAH include seizures, hydrocephalus, and DCI. Meticulous attention to their prevention and early treatment contributes to improved outcome.

Seizures

Although seizure-like activity is seen in about one-quarter of patients, the incidence of true seizures after aSAH is not clear. Differentiating between epileptic and non-epileptic abnormal movements, such as tonic posturing due to increased ICP or herniation, can be difficult. Seizures occurring at the time of haemorrhage are not associated with increased risk of late epilepsy (46). The risk of chronic seizures is higher in patients with history of hypertension (47), prolonged loss of consciousness, poor neurological status on admission, thick subarachnoid clot, rebleeding (48), ruptured middle cerebral artery aneurysm (49), intraparenchymal haematoma or infarct, and hydrocephalus (50).

Seizures occurring prior to treatment of the aneurysm may be related to rebleeding and should prompt an urgent CT scan (41). The risk of seizures after endovascular coiling is about half that after surgical clipping (1.4% versus 3%), especially in patients older than 65 years (41). A small percentage of patients, mostly with the aforementioned risk factors, may develop seizures that persist for more than 1 year, and this is also more likely in those who have undergone surgical clipping (1.3% versus 2.2% for coiling and clipping, respectively) (41).

The implications of seizures on outcome is not clear, with some studies suggesting that clinical seizures per se may not adversely affect functional outcome (48). However, non-convulsive subclinical seizures can be detected on continuous EEG monitoring in 10–20% of cases of poor-grade SAH in whom the prognosis is poor (51). Therefore, continuous EEG is recommended in poor-grade patients with clinical deterioration of unknown aetiology or who fail to improve (52). Other electrographic findings associated with poor outcome include periodic lateralized epileptiform discharges, impaired sleep architecture, and decreased alpha variability.

Due to a lack of randomized clinical trials, the routine prophylactic use of antiepileptic drugs (AEDs), choice of agents, and duration of administration are controversial. Potential side effects and drug interactions must be considered on an individual basis when deciding which AEDs, if any, to administer. Retrospective data suggest that prolonged phenytoin use is associated with worse long-term

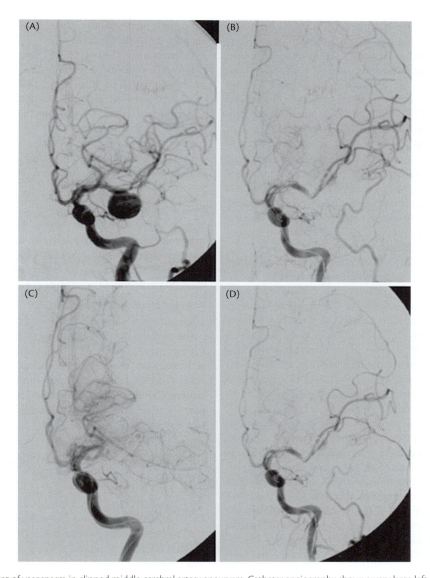

Fig. 18.3 Endovascular treatment of vasospasm in clipped middle cerebral artery aneurysm. Catheter angiography shows a very large left middle cerebral artery aneurysm (A) that was completely obliterated by surgical clipping (B). Severe vasospasm developed later (C), and was reversed by balloon angioplasty and intra-arterial infusion of verapamil (D).

outcome, and its routine use for prophylaxis is not now recommended (53). However, prophylactic administration of AEDs after aSAH is still a common practice in many units even though there are insufficient data to support this practice. If prophylactic AEDs are used in patients with no history of seizures, treatment beyond 3 days post bleed is not indicated (54). Patients who develop seizures, or who have the risk factors described earlier, may benefit from longer treatment courses of between 6 weeks to 6 months (55).

Delayed hydrocephalus

Delayed hydrocephalus affects up to one-quarter of patients and develops from days to weeks after the initial haemorrhage. The exact mechanism is unknown but likely to be multifactorial. Risk factors for the development of delayed hydrocephalus include older age, female gender, poor initial clinical grade, early ventriculomegaly, and the presence of intraventricular haemorrhage (56). Chronic symptomatic hydrocephalus usually requires shunt placement, but

the rate of EVD weaning or fenestration of lamina terminalis has not been shown to affect the need for a shunt (57). Whether rate of shunt dependency differs between those undergoing coiling versus clipping of the aneurysm has not been determined.

Delayed cerebral ischaemia

DCI is a common complication of SAH and is second only to rebleeding in terms of effects on mortality and poor outcome.

Terminology and pathophysiology

Delayed neurological deterioration refers to a clinical deterioration following initial stabilization that may be a result of multiple aetiologies including hydrocephalus, seizures, cerebral oedema, metabolic derangements, fever, infections, and DCI.

Vasospasm is arterial narrowing detected by angiography or transcranial Doppler ultrasonography (TCD). It occurs in 50–70% of patients after aSAH (58) but is not always accompanied by clinical or monitored signs of cerebral ischaemia. Genetic factors and ethnicity influence the risk of vasospasm (59,60). The pathophysiology of vasospasm has been studied extensively. The presence of oxyhaemoglobin in the CSF increases concentrations of endothelin-1, an extremely potent vasoconstrictor, and oxygen free radicals inhibit nitric oxide synthase and lead to structural changes in the intima and media of the arterial wall (61). Systemic and focal inflammatory processes also appear to be implicated in the pathogenesis (62). The best predictor of angiographic vasospasm is the amount and pattern of haemorrhage on the initial CT scan, graded using the modified Fisher scale (Table 18.4) (22). Vasospasm typically affects proximal basal arteries and may lead to a reduction in cerebral blood flow (CBF) and tissue oxygenation. Radiographic vasospasm typically occurs between days 4 and 10 after aneurysmal rupture, with the highest incidence at day 7. It may persist for up to 3 weeks. Only half of those with angiographic vasospasm develop ischaemic symptoms (63).

DCI refers to a state which has the potential to, or actually does, lead to cerebral infarction. It is usually, but not always, associated with clinical symptoms. The absence of obvious symptoms and signs may be related to an inability to assess patients who are sedated or in poor clinical condition, or because of the involvement of less eloquent brain regions. DCI typically occurs in conjunction with angiographic vasospasm, and a causal relationship has long been assumed. However, whether the link between the large vessel narrowing seen on angiography and DCI is in fact causal has recently been challenged. The distribution of regions with low blood flow does not always match the vessels with angiographic narrowing (64), and infarction can occur due to various aetiologies in patients without angiographic vasospasm (65). Further, although large randomized controlled multicentre trials of endothelin antagonists have demonstrated a consistent reduction in angiographic vasospasm this has not been associated with outcome benefits (66). Therefore, it is important to recognize that vasospasm and DCI are different phenomena and that these terminologies should not be applied interchangeably. Other factors that may contribute to the development of DCI include impaired autoregulatory mechanisms in distal vessel branches leading to reduced regional CBF, intravascular volume contraction, and hypercoagulability-related microthrombosis (67).

Prevention

Established strategies to reduce the risk of DCI include the use of nimodipine, prevention of hypovolaemia and hypotension, and removal of subarachnoid blood.

Nimodipine

Nimodipine, a centrally acting calcium channel blocker, has been shown to decrease the incidence of infarction and improve outcome (68), and is the only drug approved for the treatment of aSAH. Oral/enteral nimodipine should be administered to all patients as soon as the diagnosis of aSAH is established, at a dose of 60 mg every 4 hours for 21 days (17). The exact mechanism of action of nimodipine is not clear as it does not appear to decrease the incidence of vasospasm. It may provide benefit via a direct action on neuronal calcium channels. Although hypotension occurs infrequently in well-hydrated patients receiving oral nimodipine, care must be taken to avoid hypotension during intravenous infusion (not available in the United States). Hypotension may be responsive to fluids or, alternatively, administration of smaller and more frequent doses of nimodipine (30 mg every 2 hours orally). In a very small proportion of cases, nimodipine must be discontinued because of hypotension (69).

Other calcium channel blockers may also have a role. Intravenous nicardipine reduces the incidence of vasospasm and DCI, but has no demonstrated outcome benefit (70). Intrathecal administration of nicardipine reduces both radiographic and clinical vasospasm and improves outcome but is associated with side effects including elevated ICP and infection (71). Subarachnoid implantation at the time of surgery of prolonged-release nicardipine has been shown to decrease the rate of vasospasm and DCI (72). Diltiazem has been evaluated only in poorly controlled studies, but no clear benefit on vasospasm has been seen (70).

Prevention of hypovolaemia

Despite general consensus on the importance of the prevention of hypovolaemia, the use of prophylactic hypervolaemia after aSAH is not recommended. In a randomized trial, hypervolaemia failed to show benefit in terms of prevention of vasospasm, improvement of cerebral perfusion, or prognosis (73).

Removal of subarachnoid blood

The amount of subarachnoid blood is the best predictor of vasospasm, and various interventions to enhance blood clearance have been proposed. Intracisternal administration of tissue plasminogen activator (tPA) during and after surgery decreases the rate of vasospasm (74), as does intracisternal urokinase (75). Early reports of lumbar CSF drainage to clear blood have also been promising (76). Further trials are required to establish or refute clinical benefit of all these methods.

Statins

HMG-CoA reductase inhibitors (statins) have neuroprotective properties mediated via activation of endothelial nitric oxide synthase (eNOS) independent of their cholesterol-lowering effects (77). Two early small randomized controlled trials suggested a beneficial effect for statins in the prevention of vasospasm and DCI (78,79). Several more recent studies have evaluated the role of simvastatin 80 mg or pravastatin 40 mg started within 96 hours of ictus and continued for 2–3 weeks in reducing aSAH-associated vasospasm and DCI (80). A meta-analysis of six studies demonstrated a reduced incidence of DCI and a non-significant trend toward lower mortality, but no significant effect on the incidence of vasospasm or functional outcome (81). The reported side effects of treatment were limited to non-significant increase in liver enzymes in 5–10% of cases and myalgia in one.

Pending the results of an ongoing multicentre, placebo-controlled, randomized clinical trial, current guidance recommends continuing treatment in patients already taking a statin prior to admission but not starting the drugs in those who are not (80).

Magnesium

The vasodilatory properties of magnesium result from its action as a non-competitive calcium antagonist, and its neuroprotective actions from inhibition of release of the excitatory neurotransmitter glutamate and reduction of oxidative stress (82). Magnesium is relatively safe, inexpensive and easy to administer, and low serum magnesium levels are observed in about 40% of patients after aSAH. Therefore, one may surmise that magnesium would be of benefit in preventing vasospasm and DCI.

Although multiple studies have investigated the potential beneficial role of magnesium infusion in aSAH, they vary considerably in design, outcome measures, methodologies, and sample size/selection, and thus provide only low to moderate quality evidence (83). Magnesium infusion (64 mmol/day) appears to be safe despite increased rates of hypocalcaemia and hypotension requiring treatment (84). However, a phase III clinical trial, the Intravenous Magnesium sulfate for Aneurysmal Subarachnoid Hemorrhage (IMASH) study, did not show any benefit of magnesium over placebo in either primary (favourable outcome in the extended Glasgow Outcome Scale at 6 months) or secondary outcome measures, or differences in mortality or side effects between the two groups (85). Whilst there is agreement that hypomagnesemia should be avoided after aSAH, routinely inducing hypermagnesaemia is not currently recommended (83).

Other therapies

Several other strategies have been used in an attempt to prevent vasospasm, but further studies are required to establish their clinical benefit (86). Based on animal data, several clinical trials have investigated the ability of the free radical scavenger tirilazad mesylate to prevent vasospasm, but all failed to demonstrate benefit, possibly in part related to uncontrolled pharmacokinetic variables (87). Recent studies have focused on the role of endothelial function in vasospasm and although a dose-dependent reduction in angiographic vasospasm has been demonstrated with the endothelin-1 receptor antagonist clazosentan, this does not translated into improved outcome (66).

Prophylactic transluminal balloon angioplasty is another promising technique that has failed to show a sustained clinical benefit, primarily because of high complication rates and increased mortality (88).

Monitoring

The holy grail of the management of aSAH is the early detection and treatment of DCI before it leads to cerebral infarction. Monitoring for the development of DCI includes clinical, radiographic and physiological methods.

Clinical assessment

Clinical monitoring involves serial neurological examinations at the bedside. Neurological changes associated with DCI often appear gradually, may wax and wane, and are worsened by hypovolaemia and hypotension. Clinical findings include non-specific and non-focal changes in the level of consciousness, focal deficits such as abulia, aphasia, hemiparesis/hemiplegia, and visual field defects. Clinical evidence of vasospasm, however, may be difficult to detect, particularly in sedated or poor-grade patients. One-fifth of cerebral infarcts after poor grade aSAH are clinically asymptomatic, although always associated with worsened outcome (89). Additionally, the clinical findings can be non-specific and DCI must be distinguished from other causes of neurological deterioration such as rebleeding, hydrocephalus, cerebral oedema, seizures, fever, hypoxia, infections, and metabolic abnormalities.

Poor-grade patients are at the highest risk for DCI but are also the most difficult to assess clinically. Therefore, radiological and monitoring tools are frequently employed to evaluate for DCI. These techniques typically assess for physical narrowing of the vessels or decreased regional CBF or oxygenation.

Angiography

Catheter angiography is the gold standard for the diagnosis of large vessel vasospasm, although CTA is an alternative with reasonable sensitivity (80%) and specificity (93%) (90). The positive predictive value of CTA is significantly improved when the endpoint is the absence of vasospasm or presence of severe vasospasm (94% and 100%, respectively), as opposed to mild or moderate vasospasm (54% and 58%, respectively). CTA may overestimate the severity of vasospasm in some cases (91).

Transcranial Doppler ultrasonography

TCD is a non-invasive technique that measures linear blood flow velocity (LBFV) to estimate narrowing of large conducting vessels (see Chapter 10). The thresholds used to confirm the presence of severe vasospasm are LBFV greater than 200 cm/s or velocity ratio between middle cerebral and internal carotid arteries greater than 6 (92). In the posterior circulation, a velocity ratio greater than 2 or 3 between basilar and vertebral arteries has been associated with high sensitivity and specificity for the detection of basilar artery vasospasm (93). The rate of rise in LBFV over days, often defined as greater than 50 cm/s/day, can also be used as a diagnostic criterion of vasospasm. The negative predictive value of TCD is very high, and normal velocities (< 120 cm/s) essentially rule out vasospasm.

TCD has several limitations. Whilst it is a sensitive and specific technique for the detection of middle cerebral artery vasospasm (94), accuracy significantly declines for vasospasm in the anterior and posterior circulation when compared to catheter angiography (Table 18.5) (95). In addition, several factors such as age, blood pressure, ICP, and vascular anatomy may affect the accuracy of TCD measurements. For example, TCD may mistakenly diagnose the increased CBF associated with induced hypertension or fever as worsening vasospasm. The accuracy and reliability of TCD is also dependent on the skills of the operator.

Assessment of cerebral perfusion

As noted earlier, vasospasm does not necessarily lead to DCI. On the other hand, DCI may occur in the absence of vasospasm because of other factors that lead to decreased cerebral perfusion. The assessment of cerebral perfusion for the early diagnosis of DCI may therefore be advantageous. Several techniques are available for the regional measurement of CBF including MR and CT perfusion (CTP), xenon CT, and single photon emission computed tomography (see Chapter 15). CTP techniques have been

Table 18.5 Comparison of transcranial Doppler and digital subtraction angiography for the diagnosis of cerebral vasospasm

Artery	Sensitivity	Specificity	PPV	NPV
ICA	25%	91%	73%	56%
ACA	42%	76%	56%	69%
MCA	67%	99%	97%	78%
BA	77%	79%	63%	88%
VA	44%	88%	54%	82%

ACA, anterior cerebral artery; BA, basilar artery; ICA, internal carotid artery; MCA, middle cerebral artery; NPV, negative predictive value; PPV, positive predictive value; TCD, transcranial Doppler; VA, vertebral artery.

Adapted from Springer and *Neurocritical Care*, 15, 2, 2011, pp. 312–317, 'Detection and monitoring of vasospasm and delayed cerebral ischemia: a review and assessment of the literature', Washington C, Zipfel GJ, Participants in the International Multi-disciplinary Consensus Conference on the Critical Care Management of Subarachnoid Hemorrhage, with kind permission from Springer Science and Business Media.

studied most widely (96), and early CTP assessment, between 0 to 72 hours after ictus, can reliably predict DCI. Early identification of interhemispheric perfusion asymmetry is associated with later development of DCI, especially when combined with other risk factors such as age, clinical presentation, and blood load. When compared to conventional angiography, CTP is able to detect vasospasm with a sensitivity and specificity of 74% and 93%, respectively (90), with mean transit time and CBF variables having the highest sensitivity and specificity for the diagnosis of DCI (97). Data supports the use of CTP for the detection of DCI (98,99), and multimodal assessment with a combination of structural CT, CTA, and CTP warrants further investigation. Important limitations of these techniques include radiation exposure and the side effects of high contrast loads, particularly the risk of acute kidney injury.

Other monitoring techniques

The utility of several other invasive and non-invasive methods for monitoring DCI has been studied and these are discussed in detail in Part 2 of this book. Different substances can be measured directly in brain extracellular fluid using cerebral microdialysis (Chapter 12), and correlation between the levels of glucose, glutamate, lactate, and pyruvate with ischaemia and outcome after SAH has been reported (100). Brain tissue oxygen tension (Chapter 11) has also been used to detect vasospasm-related cerebral ischaemia and predicts outcome after SAH (101), but its validity has been questioned (102). Thermal diffusion CBF monitoring (Chapter 11) has also been used to continuously monitor CBF after SAH (102). Near infrared spectroscopy-derived measures of regional oxygen saturation (Chapter 11) have been used to evaluate the efficacy of treatment after SAH (103,104), but the sensitivity of this technique for the detection of vasospasm has been questioned (105).

Electroencephalography (EEG) has been used for decades to confirm clinical and subclinical seizures, and more recent studies have suggested a role for continuous EEG monitoring in the early identification of DCI in poor-grade patients through the identification of reduced alpha variability (102).

Treatment

Vasospasm and DCI can occur despite prophylactic interventions aimed at their prevention. The threshold to initiate or stop aggressive medical treatment of DCI (haemodynamic augmentation) varies between centres and clinical conditions. In good-grade, low risk patients, neurological deterioration that cannot be explained by another aetiology (e.g. sedation or seizure) should be evaluated urgently with catheter angiography or CTA, and treatment commenced if vasospasm is confirmed. In high-risk, poor-grade patients, such as those with a high Fisher score or documented arterial narrowing at the time of initial angiography, neurological deterioration that cannot be explained by another aetiology should trigger treatment without further evaluation. Patients with poor cardiac function or at high risk of complications from vasopressors may be earlier candidates for alternative, endovascular, treatments and should always undergo diagnostic and therapeutic angiography if DCI is suspected. In general, the decision to start, modify, or stop treatment of DCI should not be based on the findings of any single monitoring method.

The goal of treatment is to improve perfusion and reverse or reduce DCI, and both medical and endovascular approaches are available to treat both vasospasm and DCI (100).

Medical treatment

Haemodynamic augmentation has been the mainstay of the medical treatment of vasospasm and DCI for decades. It refers to a combination of interventions to enhance cerebral perfusion which originally involved a combination of hypervolaemia, hypertension, and haemodilution, known as 'triple-H therapy.' More recent evidence however, emphasizes the combination of hypertension and euvolaemia, with no role for hypervolaemia and resulting haemodilution (106). Since these manipulations (particularly hypertension) may increase the risk of rebleeding, they are usually applied only after repair of the ruptured aneurysm, although haemodynamic augmentation therapy appears to be safe in the presence of other small unruptured and untreated aneurysms (107). The relative contribution of different components of haemodynamic augmentation remains a matter of debate.

Fluid resuscitation

It is believed that, in the setting of cerebral ischaemia, intravascular volume expansion can increase CBF through its effects on preload and cardiac output, and by raising blood pressure. However, hypervolaemia is accompanied by a decline in haematocrit which can theoretically reduce cerebral oxygen delivery. Although hypervolaemia was previously employed in the treatment of DCI, its role has recently been questioned. In any case, the effect of hypervolaemia on cerebral perfusion is modest in comparison to induced hypertension, and it is likely that any benefits of hypervolaemia in the treatment of DCI do not go beyond correction of hypovolaemia (108). It is also associated with more complications than euvolaemia. Nevertheless, in the presence of DCI, a bolus administration of saline has been shown to modestly increase CBF in regions with low baseline flow, and can be used as a first step in its treatment (109). The use of albumin for volume expansion and neuroprotection against DCI has been proposed and a randomized controlled trial of its efficacy is currently underway. In selected poor-grade patients, administration of hypertonic saline may improve cerebral perfusion by decreasing ICP (110). Current guidance recommends maintenance of euvolaemia with avoidance of hypovolaemia after aSAH (111).

Induced hypertension

Induced hypertension is the most effective component of triple-H therapy, and recommended as the primary intervention in patients with DCI without cardiac failure or baseline hypertension (17). Overall, two-thirds of patients with symptomatic DCI improve with induced hypertension. The target blood pressure is usually determined as a percent change from baseline rather than a pre-determined level. Blood pressure should be increased in an incremental, stepwise, fashion with neurological assessment at each new blood pressure level so that a decision can be made whether a higher pressure is required. The agent used to induce hypertension is selected based on its pharmacological properties and the patient's cardiovascular status. Phenylephrine and norepinephrine (noradrenaline) are commonly used, and vasopressin has been recommended in cases unresponsive to other agents (111). Induced hypertension is associated with several important complications including rebleeding, hyponatraemia, cardiac ischaemia, and pulmonary oedema.

Whilst changes in cardiac output do not affect CBF under normal conditions, they may do so in the setting of ischaemia and impaired autoregulation (112). Accordingly, inotropic agents such as dobutamine or milrinone may be useful in patients with ventricular dysfunction who fail to improve with induced hypertension alone (113). Application of intra-aortic balloon pump has also been reported in such circumstances (114).

Haemodilution

The role of haemodilution is not so well understood as the other two components of triple-H therapy, but it is hypothesized that decreased blood viscosity leads to improved CBF. However, haemodilution also results in decreased oxygen carrying capacity and reduced cerebral oxygen delivery (115). The use of haemodilution in the treatment of DCI has been abandoned.

Monitoring

The previous frequent use of pulmonary capillary wedge pressure measured by Swan–Ganz catheters to guide haemodynamic management after SAH is no longer recommended because of the use-associated risks and limited efficacy in this context. Haemodynamic augmentation is now monitored by assessment of clinical status and non-invasive monitors of cardiac output, but usually adjusted based on clinical improvement. Thus, if reaching a previously set blood pressure goal does not lead to neurological improvement, a new goal should be identified. Patients are maintained at the optimal goal for 2–3 days after which haemodynamic augmentation is cautiously weaned over several days during which serial clinical assessments are performed. Any deterioration should prompt return to the previous higher blood pressure target, and the weaning process restarted after 1–2 days. Notably, the clinical consequences of weaning haemodynamic augmentation may not appear for several hours after de-escalation.

Endovascular treatment

In cases where haemodynamic augmentation fails to improve DCI, or is contraindicated, endovascular treatments may be useful (116). Options include balloon angioplasty and intra-arterial infusion of vasodilators for proximal and distal arteries, respectively (Figure 18.3). The optimal timing of initial endovascular treatment or the exact role of medical and endovascular therapies is not clear, although early intervention might be preferable. One retrospective study suggested improved outcome in patients who underwent endovascular intervention within 2 hours of the onset of clinical deterioration (117).

Angioplasty of the proximal segments of constricted vessels leads to dramatic short- and long-lasting changes in their angiographic appearance (118) but major complications, including vessel rupture, dissection, and occlusion as well as bleeding and haemorrhagic infarcts, occur in approximately 5% of procedures and may offset to some degree the potential benefits (88). Since balloon catheters cannot reach more distal branches, vasodilators may be infused in cases of more distal narrowing. Several vasodilating agents have been shown to acutely improve the angiographic appearance of spastic vessels (119), but none have been studied in a randomized clinical trial. Although the intra-arterial infusion of papaverine promptly and significantly reverses vasospasm, and transiently enhances regional blood flow, its clinical benefit is unclear (118). The short duration of action and multiple complications including increased ICP, apnoea, worsening of vasospasm, neurological deterioration, and seizures have led to the replacement of papaverine with other agents (120). Calcium channel blockers, such as nicardipine, nimodipine, and verapamil, have all been shown to reverse vasospasm (118), but further studies are required to determine their

clinical efficacy. Although one study showed superior effects of balloon angioplasty in comparison to intra-arterial papaverine (121), others have failed to demonstrate the superiority of one technique over another (122,123). Repeated endovascular treatment may be required if vasospasm does not resolve with the initial procedure. Continuous intra-arterial infusion of verapamil has been shown to decrease the need for repeated interventions (124).

Systemic complications

Medical complications associated with SAH are common and lead to increased morbidity and mortality. These are covered in detail in Chapters 27 and 28 and only a brief summary of the important issues relating to aSAH will be included here.

Fever

Fever (core body temperature > 38.3°C) develops in up to 75% of aSAH patients overall, and at higher rates in those with poor clinical grade and intraventricular extension of the haemorrhage (125). Fever is associated with disease severity, blood load, intraventricular extension, and occurrence of vasospasm (126). Non-infectious fever typically appears in the first 72 hours and is thought to be due to an inflammatory response or a central process (126). Fever is an independent predictor of poor outcome after aSAH and associated with more cerebral infarcts, elevated ICP, longer hospital stay, and worse cognitive and functional outcome (127). Treatment of fever leads to improvement in microdialysis-defined cerebral metabolic distress (128) and potentially in outcome (129).

Cardiopulmonary complications

Cardiac and pulmonary abnormalities occur frequently after SAH and are associated with DCI, higher mortality, and worse outcome. The most common cardiac problems are mild transient elevation in blood troponin levels and arrhythmias, each in about 35% of cases, and myocardial dysfunction in 25% (130,131). Various electrocardiographic changes are recognized including QT prolongation, ST segment depression, and peaked T-waves ('cerebral T-waves'). These are related to enhanced catecholamine release and do not usually reflect cardiac ischaemia. Dysrhythmias are common in the first 24 hours after ictus and, although usually benign, can be life-threatening in 5% of cases (130). Ventricular dysrhythmias are more common in the presence of elevated troponin levels (132). Correction of electrolyte abnormalities may help prevent arrhythmias.

Neurogenic stress cardiomyopathy, or the 'stunned myocardium,' refers to the transient constellation of chest pain, dyspnoea, hypoxaemia, and cardiogenic shock with pulmonary oedema in association with elevated cardiac enzymes in the context of acute SAH (133). This phenomenon is usually reversible, although mortality may be as high as 12% (134). Management of heart failure is similar to other causes of cardiogenic shock, although attention must also be given to maintenance of cerebral perfusion in the context of aSAH (135).

Cardiogenic and neurogenic pulmonary oedema, acute lung injury (ALI), and acute respiratory distress syndrome frequently occur after aSAH (136). Euvolaemia should be maintained in patients with pulmonary oedema or ALI. Close monitoring and careful management of haemodynamic treatment of vasospasm minimizes the risk of iatrogenic pulmonary oedema (137).

Fluid and electrolyte disturbances

Hypovolaemia develops in about one-third of patients after aSAH, and is associated with higher rates of DCI and worse outcome (138). Central salt wasting, anaemia, and hypoalbuminaemia, in addition to changes in other factors such as vasopressin, atrial natriuretic peptide, renin–angiotensin–aldosterone system, and catecholamines, play a central role in development of aSAH-associated hypovolaemia (139). Intravascular volume monitoring is an important aspect of the medical management of aSAH, but can be very difficult to accurately accomplish (140). Defining and monitoring volume status using central venous pressure measurement has not proved useful and is no longer recommended (139). The use of pulmonary artery catheters is also discouraged because of their high complication rate. Other less-invasive techniques can also be used to monitor volume status with fewer complications, but should not supplant clinical evaluation.

Euvolaemia is the target. It is not clear whether colloids are superior to crystalloids in treatment of volume contraction after aSAH, but isotonic crystalloid fluids are currently recommended for volume replacement. The volume of fluid required to maintain euvolaemia may be decreased by using mineralocorticoid or high-dose glucocorticoid agents (141), and these should be considered in patients with a persistent negative fluid balance whilst being mindful of the risk of steroid-induced hyperglycaemia.

The most common electrolyte disturbance in SAH is hyponatraemia which is seen in 30–50% of patients (142) and associated with higher incidence of vasospasm (143). Hyponatraemia was previously thought to be secondary to the syndrome of inappropriate secretion of antidiuretic hormone (SIADH), but more recent studies have revealed a more complex pathophysiology involving increased secretion of natriuretic peptides and dysregulation of both sodium and water homeostasis leading to hypovolaemic hyponatraemia due to cerebral salt wasting (CSW). Despite this differentiation, it is likely that many patients may suffer from both conditions simultaneously (144). The pathophysiology and treatment of SIADH and CSW are discussed in detail in Chapter 28.

Hyponatraemia in the context of SAH can be treated with restriction of free water, using isotonic intravenous fluids and concentrated enteral feed whilst maintaining euvolaemia, and by minimizing oral intake in awake patients. However, mildly hypertonic (1.25–3.0%) saline or oral sodium chloride supplementation is often used to treat persistent mild hyponatraemia (145). Both mineralocorticoids and glucocorticoids may assist in the prevention and treatment of hyponatraemia if administered early after ictus, but may lead to hyperglycaemia and hypokalaemia (146). ADH antagonists, such as conivaptan, can correct hyponatraemia, but must be used cautiously after SAH to avoid volume contraction secondary to diuresis.

Anaemia

Anaemia occurs in large number of patients within 3–4 days after aSAH. It is more common in females, older and poor-grade patients, and in those undergoing surgical treatment of their aneurysm (147). Anaemia is associated with higher rates of DCI and mortality, and worse neurological outcome in survivors (130,148). Higher haemoglobin concentration (> 11 g/L) is an independent favourable prognostic factor (149). Cerebral hypoxia may develop at higher haemoglobin levels after SAH compared to normal subjects, possibly due to impaired autoregulation (150).

The optimal haemoglobin concentration after SAH has yet to be determined, and there are insufficient data to support either a liberal or restricted transfusion trigger (haemoglobin < 10 g/L and 7 g/L, respectively) (151). Other medical conditions, such as coronary artery disease, must also be considered when choosing the trigger for transfusion. Although transfusion is associated with improved oxygen delivery and brain oxygen tension (152), its effect on outcome is controversial. In addition, blood transfusion is associated with significant complications such as vasospasm, infection, transfusion reactions, transfusion-related lung injury, and multiorgan failure (153). A common practice is to maintain haemoglobin concentration between 8 g/L and 10 g/L with red blood cell transfusion in high-risk patients or those with established vasospasm. Routine measures should be used to minimize blood loss from lab tests and arterial blood gas analysis.

Thromboembolic events

Patients with SAH are at increased risk of deep vein thrombosis (DVT) and pulmonary embolism because of immobility and a hypercoagulable state secondary to systemic inflammatory responses (154). Screening with lower extremity Doppler studies identifies DVTs in about one-fifth of patients (155).

Endocrine complications

Disturbances in endocrine function are common in aSAH and discussed in detail in Chapter 28.

Glycaemic control

Hyperglycaemia, commonly seen in poor-grade patients, is associated with an increased risk of vasospasm and worsened prognosis after aSAH (156). On the other hand, overly aggressive management of systemic glucose concentration has been associated with higher rates of systemic hypoglycaemia, low cerebral glucose concentrations, and higher rates of DCI and poor outcome (157,158). Accordingly, moderate glucose control may be more appropriate after SAH (159), and the current recommendation is to maintain serum glucose below 11 mmol/L and avoid hypoglycaemic events (serum glucose < 4.4 mmol/L).

The hypothalamic–pituitary–adrenal axis

Due to the proximity of many aneurysms to the base of the brain, impairment of the hypothalamic–pituitary–adrenal (HPA) axis is particularly common after aSAH. A wide range of adrenocorticotropic hormone and cortisol level abnormalities have been reported (160). It has been proposed that the diurnal cycle of cortisol release is impaired in the acute phase of aSAH with initially high levels that may be associated with DCI (161) and worse prognosis (162).

HPA axis disruption may last for months to years in up to one-third of the survivors of aSAH, but few studies have systematically investigated the potential benefit of hormonal replacement therapy. Mineralocorticoids appear to be safe when used to prevent hypovolaemia, but the administration of corticosteroids, such as hydrocortisone or methylprednisolone, has been associated with increased mortality and hyperglycaemia without evidence of advantage in reducing DCI, or improving outcome (160).

Acknowledgements

This work was supported in part by NIH (NINDS) grant 5P50NS05597704. We thank Dr Esther Hsiao for helpful suggestions and comments on an initial draft of this chapter and Dr Noushin Yahyavi Firouz Abadi for assistance in selection of radiographic images.

References

1. Nieuwkamp DJ, Setz LE, Algra A, Linn FH, de Rooij NK, Rinkel GJ. Changes in case fatality of aneurysmal subarachnoid haemorrhage over time, according to age, sex, and region: a meta-analysis. *Lancet Neurol.* 2009;8(7):635–42.

2. Wiebers DO, Whisnant JP, Huston J, 3rd, Meissner I, Brown RD, Jr., Piepgras DG, *et al.* Unruptured intracranial aneurysms: natural history, clinical outcome, and risks of surgical and endovascular treatment. *Lancet.* 2003;362(9378):103–10.

3. Shea AM, Reed SD, Curtis LH, Alexander MJ, Villani JJ, Schulman KA. Characteristics of nontraumatic subarachnoid hemorrhage in the United States in 2003. *Neurosurgery.* 2007;61(6):1131–7.

4. de Rooij NK, Linn FH, van der Plas JA, Algra A, Rinkel GJ. Incidence of subarachnoid haemorrhage: a systematic review with emphasis on region, age, gender and time trends. *J Neurol Neurosurg Psychiatry.* 2007;78(12):1365–72.

5. Eden SV, Meurer WJ, Sanchez BN, Lisabeth LD, Smith MA, Brown DL, *et al.* Gender and ethnic differences in subarachnoid hemorrhage. *Neurology.* 2008;71(10):731–5.

6. Labovitz DL, Halim AX, Brent B, Boden-Albala B, Hauser WA, Sacco RL. Subarachnoid hemorrhage incidence among Whites, Blacks and Caribbean Hispanics: the Northern Manhattan Study. *Neuroepidemiology.* 2006;26(3):147–50.

7. Krings T, Mandell DM, Kiehl TR, Geibprasert S, Tymianski M, Alvarez H, *et al.* Intracranial aneurysms: from vessel wall pathology to therapeutic approach. *Nat Rev Neurol.* 2011;7(10):547–59.

8. Brisman JL, Song JK, Newell DW. Cerebral aneurysms. *N Engl J Med.* 2006;355(9):928–39.

9. Nehls DG, Flom RA, Carter LP, Spetzler RF. Multiple intracranial aneurysms: determining the site of rupture. *J Neurosurg.* 1985;63(3):342–8.

10. Provencio JJ, Vora N. Subarachnoid hemorrhage and inflammation: bench to bedside and back. *Semin Neurol.* 2005;25:435–44.

11. Aoki T, Kataoka H, Ishibashi R, Nozaki K, Hashimoto N. Simvastatin suppresses the progression of experimentally induced cerebral aneurysms in rats. *Stroke.* 2008;39(4):1276–85.

12. Tulamo R, Frosen J, Hernesniemi J, Niemela M. Inflammatory changes in the aneurysm wall: a review. *J Neurointerv Surg.* 2010;2(2):120–30.

13. Kojima M, Nagasawa S, Lee YE, Takeichi Y, Tsuda E, Mabuchi N. Asymptomatic familial cerebral aneurysms. *Neurosurgery.* 1998;43(4):776–81.

14. Mitchell P, Jakubowski J. Estimate of the maximum time interval between formation of cerebral aneurysm and rupture. *J Neurol Neurosurg Psychiatry.* 2000;69(6):760–7.

15. Broderick JP, Brown RD, Jr., Sauerbeck L, Hornung R, Huston J, 3rd, Woo D, *et al.* Greater rupture risk for familial as compared to sporadic unruptured intracranial aneurysms. *Stroke.* 2009;40(6):1952–7.

16. Tiel Groenestege AT, Rinkel GJ, van der Bom JG, Algra A, Klijn CJ. The risk of aneurysmal subarachnoid hemorrhage during pregnancy, delivery, and the puerperium in the Utrecht population: case-crossover study and standardized incidence ratio estimation. *Stroke.* 2009;40(4):1148–51.

17. Connolly ES, Jr., Rabinstein AA, Carhuapoma JR, Derdeyn CP, Dion J, Higashida RT, *et al.* Guidelines for the management of aneurysmal subarachnoid hemorrhage: a guideline for healthcare professionals from the American Heart Association/American Stroke Association. *Stroke.* 2012;43(6):1711–37.

18. Raaymakers TW, Buys PC, Verbeeten B, Jr., Ramos LM, Witkamp TD, Hulsmans FJ, *et al.* MR angiography as a screening tool for intracranial aneurysms: feasibility, test characteristics, and interobserver agreement. *AJR Am J Roentgenol.* 1999;173(6):1469–75.

19. Yanaka K, Nagase S, Asakawa H, Matsumaru Y, Koyama A, Nose T. Management of unruptured cerebral aneurysms in patients with polycystic kidney disease. *Surg Neurol.* 2004;62(6):538–45.

20. de Falco FA. Sentinel headache. *Neurol Sci.* 2004;25 Suppl 3:S215–7.

21. Beck J, Raabe A, Szelenyi A, Berkefeld J, Gerlach R, Setzer M, *et al.* Sentinel headache and the risk of rebleeding after aneurysmal subarachnoid hemorrhage. *Stroke.* 2006;37(11):2733–7.

22. Fisher CM, Roberson GH, Ojemann RG. Cerebral vasospasm with ruptured saccular aneurysm—the clinical manifestations. *Neurosurgery.* 1977;1(3):245–8.

23. Kowalski RG, Claassen J, Kreiter KT, Bates JE, Ostapkovich ND, Connolly ES, *et al.* Initial misdiagnosis and outcome after subarachnoid hemorrhage. *JAMA.* 2004;291(7):866–9.

24. Perry JJ, Stiell IG, Sivilotti ML, Bullard MJ, Emond M, Symington C, *et al.* Sensitivity of computed tomography performed within six hours of onset of headache for diagnosis of subarachnoid haemorrhage: prospective cohort study. *BMJ.* 2011;343:d4277.

25. Fiebach JB, Schellinger PD, Geletneky K, Wilde P, Meyer M, Hacke W, *et al.* MRI in acute subarachnoid haemorrhage; findings with a standardised stroke protocol. *Neuroradiology.* 2004;46(1):44–8.

26. Romijn M, Gratama van Andel HA, van Walderveen MA, Sprengers ME, van Rijn JC, van Rooij WJ, *et al.* Diagnostic accuracy of CT angiography with matched mask bone elimination for detection of intracranial aneurysms: comparison with digital subtraction angiography and 3D rotational angiography. *AJNR Am J Neuroradiol.* 2008;29(1):134–9.

27. Donmez H, Serifov E, Kahriman G, Mavili E, Durak AC, Menku A. Comparison of 16-row multislice CT angiography with conventional angiography for detection and evaluation of intracranial aneurysms. *Eur J Radiol.* 2011;80(2):455–61.

28. Agid R, Andersson T, Almqvist H, Willinsky RA, Lee SK, terBrugge KG, *et al.* Negative CT angiography findings in patients with spontaneous subarachnoid hemorrhage: When is digital subtraction angiography still needed? *AJNR Am J Neuroradiol.* 2010;31(4):696–705.

29. van Gijn J, Rinkel GJ. Subarachnoid haemorrhage: diagnosis, causes and management. *Brain.* 2001;124(Pt 2):249–78.

30. Hunt WE, Hess RM. Surgical risk as related to time of intervention in the repair of intracranial aneurysms. *J Neurosurg.* 1968;28(1):14–20.

31. Report of World Federation of Neurological Surgeons Committee on a Universal Subarachnoid Hemorrhage Grading Scale. *J Neurosurg.* 1988;68(6):985–6.

32. Roitberg BZ, Hardman J, Urbaniak K, Merchant A, Mangubat EZ, Alaraj A, *et al.* Prospective randomized comparison of safety and efficacy of nicardipine and nitroprusside drip for control of hypertension in the neurosurgical intensive care unit. *Neurosurgery.* 2008;63(1):115–20.

33. Liu-Deryke X, Janisse J, Coplin WM, Parker D, Jr., Norris G, Rhoney DH. A comparison of nicardipine and labetalol for acute hypertension management following stroke. *Neurocrit Care.* 2008;9(2):167–76.

34. Diringer MN. Management of aneurysmal subarachnoid hemorrhage. *Crit Care Med.* 2009;37(2):432–40.

35. Suarez-Rivera O. Acute hydrocephalus after subarachnoid hemorrhage. *Surg Neurol.* 1998;49(5):563–5.

36. Hellingman CA, van den Bergh WM, Beijer IS, van Dijk GW, Algra A, van Gijn J, *et al.* Risk of rebleeding after treatment of acute hydrocephalus in patients with aneurysmal subarachnoid hemorrhage. *Stroke.* 2007;38(1):96–9.

37. Hoekema D, Schmidt RH, Ross I. Lumbar drainage for subarachnoid hemorrhage: technical considerations and safety analysis. *Neurocrit Care.* 2007;7(1):3–9.

38. Naidech AM, Janjua N, Kreiter KT, Ostapkovich ND, Fitzsimmons BF, Parra A, *et al.* Predictors and impact of aneurysm rebleeding after subarachnoid hemorrhage. *Arch Neurol.* 2005;62(3):410–6.

39. Roos YB, Rinkel GJ, Vermeulen M, Algra A, van Gijn J. Antifibrinolytic therapy for aneurysmal subarachnoid haemorrhage. *Cochrane Database Syst Rev.* 2003;2:CD001245.

40. Starke RM, Kim GH, Fernandez A, Komotar RJ, Hickman ZL, Otten ML, *et al.* Impact of a protocol for acute antifibrinolytic therapy on aneurysm rebleeding after subarachnoid hemorrhage. *Stroke.* 2008;39(9):2617–21.

41. Molyneux AJ, Kerr RS, Yu LM, Clarke M, Sneade M, Yarnold JA, *et al.* International subarachnoid aneurysm trial (ISAT) of neurosurgical

clipping versus endovascular coiling in 2143 patients with ruptured intracranial aneurysms: a randomised comparison of effects on survival, dependency, seizures, rebleeding, subgroups, and aneurysm occlusion. *Lancet.* 2005;366(9488):809–17.

42. de Oliveira JG, Beck J, Ulrich C, Rathert J, Raabe A, Seifert V. Comparison between clipping and coiling on the incidence of cerebral vasospasm after aneurysmal subarachnoid hemorrhage: a systematic review and meta-analysis. *Neurosurg Rev.* 2007;30(1):22–30.

43. Murayama Y, Nien YL, Duckwiler G, Gobin YP, Jahan R, Frazee J, *et al.* Guglielmi detachable coil embolization of cerebral aneurysms: 11 years' experience. *J Neurosurg.* 2003;98(5):959–66.

44. Piotin M, Blanc R, Spelle L, Mounayer C, Piantino R, Schmidt PJ, *et al.* Stent-assisted coiling of intracranial aneurysms: clinical and angiographic results in 216 consecutive aneurysms. *Stroke.* 2010;41(1):110–15.

45. Uda K, Murayama Y, Gobin YP, Duckwiler GR, Vinuela F. Endovascular treatment of basilar artery trunk aneurysms with Guglielmi detachable coils: clinical experience with 41 aneurysms in 39 patients. *J Neurosurg.* 2001;95(4):624–32.

46. Claassen J, Peery S, Kreiter KT, Hirsch LJ, Du EY, Connolly ES, *et al.* Predictors and clinical impact of epilepsy after subarachnoid hemorrhage. *Neurology.* 2003;60(2):208–14.

47. Ohman J. Hypertension as a risk factor for epilepsy after aneurysmal subarachnoid hemorrhage and surgery. *Neurosurgery.* 1990;27(4):578–81.

48. Choi KS, Chun HJ, Yi HJ, Ko Y, Kim YS, Kim JM. Seizures and Epilepsy following Aneurysmal Subarachnoid Hemorrhage: Incidence and Risk Factors. *J Korean Neurosurg Soc.* 2009;46(2):93–8.

49. Ukkola V, Heikkinen ER. Epilepsy after operative treatment of ruptured cerebral aneurysms. *Acta Neurochir (Wien).* 1990;106(3–4):115–18.

50. Kotila M, Waltimo O. Epilepsy after stroke. *Epilepsia.* 1992;33(3):495–8.

51. Little AS, Kerrigan JF, McDougall CG, Zabramski JM, Albuquerque FC, Nakaji P, *et al.* Nonconvulsive status epilepticus in patients suffering spontaneous subarachnoid hemorrhage. *J Neurosurg.* 2007;106(5):805–11.

52. Claassen J, Hirsch LJ, Frontera JA, Fernandez A, Schmidt M, Kapinos G, *et al.* Prognostic significance of continuous EEG monitoring in patients with poor-grade subarachnoid hemorrhage. *Neurocrit Care.* 2006;4(2):103–12.

53. Rosengart AJ, Huo JD, Tolentino J, Novakovic RL, Frank JI, Goldenberg FD, *et al.* Outcome in patients with subarachnoid hemorrhage treated with antiepileptic drugs. *J Neurosurg.* 2007;107(2):253–60.

54. Chumnanvej S, Dunn IF, Kim DH. Three-day phenytoin prophylaxis is adequate after subarachnoid hemorrhage. *Neurosurgery.* 2007;60(1):99–102.

55. Lanzino G, D'Urso PI, Suarez J, Participants in the International Multi-Disciplinary Consensus Conference on the Critical Care Management of Subarachnoid Hemorrhage. Seizures and anticonvulsants after aneurysmal subarachnoid hemorrhage. *Neurocrit Care.* 2011;15(2):247–56.

56. Rincon F, Gordon E, Starke RM, Buitrago MM, Fernandez A, Schmidt JM, *et al.* Predictors of long-term shunt-dependent hydrocephalus after aneurysmal subarachnoid hemorrhage. *J Neurosurg.* 2010;113(4):774–80.

57. Komotar RJ, Hahn DK, Kim GH, Starke RM, Garrett MC, Merkow MB, *et al.* Efficacy of lamina terminalis fenestration in reducing shunt-dependent hydrocephalus following aneurysmal subarachnoid hemorrhage: a systematic review. Clinical article. *J Neurosurg.* 2009;111(1):147–54.

58. Frontera JA, Fernandez A, Schmidt JM, Claassen J, Wartenberg KE, Badjatia N, *et al.* Defining vasospasm after subarachnoid hemorrhage: what is the most clinically relevant definition? *Stroke.* 2009;40(6):1963–8.

59. Mocco J, Ransom ER, Komotar RJ, Mack WJ, Sergot PB, Albert SM, *et al.* Racial differences in cerebral vasospasm: a systematic review of the literature. *Neurosurgery.* 2006;58(2):305–14.

60. Khurana VG, Sohni YR, Mangrum WI, McClelland RL, O'Kane DJ, Meyer FB, *et al.* Endothelial nitric oxide synthase gene polymorphisms predict susceptibility to aneurysmal subarachnoid hemorrhage and cerebral vasospasm. *J Cereb Blood Flow Metab.* 2004;24(3):291–7.

61. Suzuki H, Muramatsu M, Kojima T, Taki W. Intracranial heme metabolism and cerebral vasospasm after aneurysmal subarachnoid hemorrhage. *Stroke.* 2003;34(12):2796–800.

62. Diringer MN. Subarachnoid hemorrhage: a multiple-organ system disease. *Crit Care Med.* 2003;31(6):1884–5.

63. Vergouwen MD, Vermeulen M, van Gijn J, Rinkel GJ, Wijdicks EF, Muizelaar JP, *et al.* Definition of delayed cerebral ischemia after aneurysmal subarachnoid hemorrhage as an outcome event in clinical trials and observational studies: proposal of a multidisciplinary research group. *Stroke.* 2010;41(10):2391–5.

64. Dhar R, Scalfani MT, Blackburn S, Zazulia AR, Videen TO, Diringer MN. Relationship between angiographic vasospasm and regional hypoperfusion in aneurysmal subarachnoid hemorrhage. *Stroke.* 2012;43(7):1788–94.

65. Vergouwen MD, Ilodigwe D, Macdonald RL. Cerebral infarction after subarachnoid hemorrhage contributes to poor outcome by vasospasm-dependent and -independent effects. *Stroke.* 2011;42(4):924–9.

66. Macdonald RL, Higashida RT, Keller E, Mayer SA, Molyneux A, Raabe A, *et al.* Clazosentan, an endothelin receptor antagonist, in patients with aneurysmal subarachnoid haemorrhage undergoing surgical clipping: a randomised, double-blind, placebo-controlled phase 3 trial (CONSCIOUS-2). *Lancet Neurol.* 2011;10(7):618–25.

67. Vergouwen MD, Vermeulen M, Coert BA, Stroes ES, Roos YB. Microthrombosis after aneurysmal subarachnoid hemorrhage: an additional explanation for delayed cerebral ischemia. *J Cereb Blood Flow Metab.* 2008;28(11):1761–70.

68. Dorhout Mees SM, Rinkel GJ, Feigin VL, Algra A, van den Bergh WM, Vermeulen M, *et al.* Calcium antagonists for aneurysmal subarachnoid haemorrhage. *Cochrane Database Syst Rev.* 2007;3:CD000277.

69. Diringer MN, Bleck TP, Claude Hemphill J, 3rd, Menon D, Shutter L, Vespa P, *et al.* Critical care management of patients following aneurysmal subarachnoid hemorrhage: recommendations from the Neurocritical Care Society's Multidisciplinary Consensus Conference. *Neurocrit Care.* 2011;15(2):211–40.

70. Papavasiliou AK, Harbaugh KS, Birkmeyer NJ, Feeney JM, Martin PB, Faccio C, *et al.* Clinical outcomes of aneurysmal subarachnoid hemorrhage patients treated with oral diltiazem and limited intensive care management. *Surg Neurol.* 2001;55(3):138–46.

71. Shibuya M, Suzuki Y, Enomoto H, Okada T, Ogura K, Sugita K. Effects of prophylactic intrathecal administrations of nicardipine on vasospasm in patients with severe aneurysmal subarachnoid haemorrhage. *Acta Neurochir (Wien).* 1994;131(1–2):19–25.

72. Barth M, Capelle HH, Weidauer S, Weiss C, Munch E, Thome C, *et al.* Effect of nicardipine prolonged-release implants on cerebral vasospasm and clinical outcome after severe aneurysmal subarachnoid hemorrhage: a prospective, randomized, double-blind phase IIa study. *Stroke.* 2007;38(2):330–6.

73. Rinkel GJ, Feigin VL, Algra A, van Gijn J. Circulatory volume expansion therapy for aneurysmal subarachnoid haemorrhage. *Cochrane Database Syst Rev.* 2004;4:CD000483.

74. Amin-Hanjani S, Ogilvy CS, Barker FG, 2nd. Does intracisternal thrombolysis prevent vasospasm after aneurysmal subarachnoid hemorrhage? A meta-analysis. *Neurosurgery.* 2004;54(2):326–34.

75. Kawamoto S, Tsutsumi K, Yoshikawa G, Shinozaki MH, Yako K, Nagata K, *et al.* Effectiveness of the head-shaking method combined with cisternal irrigation with urokinase in preventing cerebral vasospasm after subarachnoid hemorrhage. *J Neurosurg.* 2004;100(2):236–43.

76. Klimo P, Jr., Kestle JR, MacDonald JD, Schmidt RH. Marked reduction of cerebral vasospasm with lumbar drainage of cerebrospinal fluid after subarachnoid hemorrhage. *J Neurosurg.* 2004;100(2):215–24.

77. Sabri M, Macdonald RL. Statins: a potential therapeutic addition to treatment for aneurysmal subarachnoid hemorrhage? *World Neurosurg.* 2010;73(6):646–53.

78. Tseng MY, Czosnyka M, Richards H, Pickard JD, Kirkpatrick PJ. Effects of acute treatment with pravastatin on cerebral vasospasm, autoregulation, and delayed ischemic deficits after aneurysmal subarachnoid hemorrhage: a phase II randomized placebo-controlled trial. *Stroke.* 2005;36(8):1627–32.

79. Lynch JR, Wang H, McGirt MJ, Floyd J, Friedman AH, Coon AL, *et al.* Simvastatin reduces vasospasm after aneurysmal subarachnoid hemorrhage: results of a pilot randomized clinical trial. *Stroke.* 2005;36(9):2024–6.

80. Tseng MY. Summary of evidence on immediate statins therapy following aneurysmal subarachnoid hemorrhage. *Neurocrit Care.* 2011;15(2):298–301.

81. Kramer AH, Fletcher JJ. Statins in the management of patients with aneurysmal subarachnoid hemorrhage: a systematic review and meta-analysis. *Neurocrit Care.* 2010;12(2):285–96.

82. Taccone FS. Vasodilation and neuroprotection: the magnesium saga in subarachnoid hemorrhage. *Crit Care Med.* 2010;38(5):1382–4.

83. Suarez JI, Participants in the International Multidisciplinary Consensus Conference on the Critical Care Management of Subarachnoid Hemorrhage. Magnesium sulfate administration in subarachnoid hemorrhage. *Neurocrit Care.* 2011;15(2):302–7.

84. Muroi C, Terzic A, Fortunati M, Yonekawa Y, Keller E. Magnesium sulfate in the management of patients with aneurysmal subarachnoid hemorrhage: a randomized, placebo-controlled, dose-adapted trial. *Surg Neurol.* 2008;69(1):33–9; discussion 9.

85. Wong GK, Poon WS, Chan MT, Boet R, Gin T, Ng SC, *et al.* Intravenous magnesium sulphate for aneurysmal subarachnoid hemorrhage (IMASH): a randomized, double-blinded, placebo-controlled, multicenter phase III trial. *Stroke.* 2010;41(5):921–6.

86. Rabinstein AA, Lanzino G, Wijdicks EF. Multidisciplinary management and emerging therapeutic strategies in aneurysmal subarachnoid haemorrhage. *Lancet Neurol.* 2010;9(5):504–19.

87. Lanzino G, Kassell NF. Double-blind, randomized, vehicle-controlled study of high-dose tirilazad mesylate in women with aneurysmal subarachnoid hemorrhage. Part II. A cooperative study in North America. *J Neurosurg.* 1999;90(6):1018–24.

88. Zwienenberg-Lee M, Hartman J, Rudisill N, Madden LK, Smith K, Eskridge J, *et al.* Effect of prophylactic transluminal balloon angioplasty on cerebral vasospasm and outcome in patients with Fisher grade III subarachnoid hemorrhage: results of a phase II multicenter, randomized, clinical trial. *Stroke.* 2008;39(6):1759–65.

89. Schmidt JM, Wartenberg KE, Fernandez A, Claassen J, Rincon F, Ostapkovich ND, *et al.* Frequency and clinical impact of asymptomatic cerebral infarction due to vasospasm after subarachnoid hemorrhage. *J Neurosurg.* 2008;109(6):1052–9.

90. Greenberg ED, Gold R, Reichman M, John M, Ivanidze J, Edwards AM, *et al.* Diagnostic accuracy of CT angiography and CT perfusion for cerebral vasospasm: a meta-analysis. *AJNR Am J Neuroradiol.* 2010;31(10):1853–60.

91. Yoon DY, Choi CS, Kim KH, Cho BM. Multidetector-row CT angiography of cerebral vasospasm after aneurysmal subarachnoid hemorrhage: comparison of volume-rendered images and digital subtraction angiography. *AJNR Am J Neuroradiol.* 2006;27(2):370–7.

92. Washington CW, Zipfel GJ, Participants in the International Multi-disciplinary Consensus Conference on the Critical Care Management of Subarachnoid Hemorrhage. Detection and monitoring of vasospasm and delayed cerebral ischemia: a review and assessment of the literature. *Neurocrit Care.* 2011;15(2):312–7.

93. Sviri GE, Ghodke B, Britz GW, Douville CM, Haynor DR, Mesiwala AH, *et al.* Transcranial Doppler grading criteria for basilar artery vasospasm. *Neurosurgery.* 2006;59(2):360–6.

94. Lysakowski C, Walder B, Costanza MC, Tramer MR. Transcranial Doppler versus angiography in patients with vasospasm due to a ruptured cerebral aneurysm: A systematic review. *Stroke.* 2001;32(10):2292–8.

95. Sloan MA, Alexandrov AV, Tegeler CH, Spencer MP, Caplan LR, Feldmann E, *et al.* Assessment: transcranial Doppler ultrasonography: report of the Therapeutics and Technology Assessment Subcommittee of the American Academy of Neurology. *Neurology.* 2004;62(9):1468–81.

96. van der Schaaf I, Wermer MJ, van der Graaf Y, Velthuis BK, van de Kraats CI, Rinkel GJ. Prognostic value of cerebral perfusion-computed tomography in the acute stage after subarachnoid hemorrhage for the development of delayed cerebral ischemia. *Stroke.* 2006;37(2):409–13.

97. Wintermark M, Dillon WP, Smith WS, Lau BC, Chaudhary S, Liu S, *et al.* Visual grading system for vasospasm based on perfusion CT imaging: comparisons with conventional angiography and quantitative perfusion CT. *Cerebrovasc Dis.* 2008;26(2):163–70.

98. Dankbaar JW, de Rooij NK, Velthuis BK, Frijns CJ, Rinkel GJ, van der Schaaf IC. Diagnosing delayed cerebral ischemia with different CT modalities in patients with subarachnoid hemorrhage with clinical deterioration. *Stroke.* 2009;40(11):3493–8.

99. Dankbaar JW, de Rooij NK, Rijsdijk M, Velthuis BK, Frijns CJ, Rinkel GJ, *et al.* Diagnostic threshold values of cerebral perfusion measured with computed tomography for delayed cerebral ischemia after aneurysmal subarachnoid hemorrhage. *Stroke.* 2010;41(9):1927–32.

100. Diringer MN, Bleck TP, Claude Hemphill J, 3rd, Menon D, Shutter L, Vespa P, *et al.* Critical care management of patients following aneurysmal subarachnoid hemorrhage: recommendations from the Neurocritical Care Society's Multidisciplinary Consensus Conference. *Neurocrit Care.* 2011;15(2):211–40.

101. Meixensberger J, Vath A, Jaeger M, Kunze E, Dings J, Roosen K. Monitoring of brain tissue oxygenation following severe subarachnoid hemorrhage. *Neurol Res.* 2003;25(5):445–50.

102. Hanggi D, Participants in the International Multi-Disciplinary Consensus Conference on the Critical Care Management of Subarachnoid Hemorrhage. Monitoring and detection of vasospasm II: EEG and invasive monitoring. *Neurocrit Care.* 2011;15(2):318–23.

103. Mutoh T, Ishikawa T, Suzuki A, Yasui N. Continuous cardiac output and near-infrared spectroscopy monitoring to assist in management of symptomatic cerebral vasospasm after subarachnoid hemorrhage. *Neurocrit Care.* 2010;13(3):331–8.

104. Yokose N, Sakatani K, Murata Y, Awano T, Igarashi T, Nakamura S, *et al.* Bedside assessment of cerebral vasospasms after subarachnoid hemorrhage by near infrared time-resolved spectroscopy. *Adv Exp Med Biol.* 2010;662:505–11.

105. Naidech AM, Bendok BR, Ault ML, Bleck TP. Monitoring with the Somanetics INVOS 5100C after aneurysmal subarachnoid hemorrhage. *Neurocrit Care.* 2008;9(3):326–31.

106. Dankbaar JW, Slooter AJ, Rinkel GJ, Schaaf IC. Effect of different components of triple-H therapy on cerebral perfusion in patients with aneurysmal subarachnoid haemorrhage: a systematic review. *Crit Care.* 2010;14(1):R23.

107. Hoh BL, Carter BS, Ogilvy CS. Risk of hemorrhage from unsecured, unruptured aneurysms during and after hypertensive hypervolemic therapy. *Neurosurgery.* 2002;50(6):1207–11.

108. Raabe A, Beck J, Keller M, Vatter H, Zimmermann M, Seifert V. Relative importance of hypertension compared with hypervolemia for increasing cerebral oxygenation in patients with cerebral vasospasm after subarachnoid hemorrhage. *J Neurosurg.* 2005;103(6):974–81.

109. Jost SC, Diringer MN, Zazulia AR, Videen TO, Aiyagari V, Grubb RL, *et al.* Effect of normal saline bolus on cerebral blood flow in regions with low baseline flow in patients with vasospasm following subarachnoid hemorrhage. *J Neurosurg.* 2005;103(1):25–30.

110. Tseng MY, Al-Rawi PG, Czosnyka M, Hutchinson PJ, Richards H, Pickard JD, *et al.* Enhancement of cerebral blood flow using systemic hypertonic saline therapy improves outcome in patients with poor-grade spontaneous subarachnoid hemorrhage. *J Neurosurg.* 2007;107(2):274–82.

111. Treggiari MM, Participants in the International Multi-disciplinary Consensus Conference on the Critical Care Management of

Subarachnoid Hemorrhage. Hemodynamic management of subarachnoid hemorrhage. *Neurocrit Care.* 2011;15(2):329–35.

112. Tranmer BI, Keller TS, Kindt GW, Archer D. Loss of cerebral regulation during cardiac output variations in focal cerebral ischemia. *J Neurosurg.* 1992;77(2):253–9.

113. Levy ML, Rabb CH, Zelman V, Giannotta SL. Cardiac performance enhancement from dobutamine in patients refractory to hypervolemic therapy for cerebral vasospasm. *J Neurosurg.* 1993;79(4):494–9.

114. Appelboom G, Strozyk D, Hwang BY, Prowda J, Badjatia N, Helbok R, et al. Bedside use of a dual aortic balloon occlusion for the treatment of cerebral vasospasm. *Neurocrit Care.* 2010;13(3):385–8.

115. Ekelund A, Reinstrup P, Ryding E, Andersson AM, Molund T, Kristiansson KA, et al. Effects of iso- and hypervolemic hemodilution on regional cerebral blood flow and oxygen delivery for patients with vasospasm after aneurysmal subarachnoid hemorrhage. *Acta Neurochir.* 2002;144:703–12.

116. Jun P, Ko NU, English JD, Dowd CF, Halbach VV, Higashida RT, et al. Endovascular treatment of medically refractory cerebral vasospasm following aneurysmal subarachnoid hemorrhage. *AJNR Am J Neuroradiol.* 2010;31(10):1911–16.

117. Rosenwasser RH, Armonda RA, Thomas JE, Benitez RP, Gannon PM, Harrop J. Therapeutic modalities for the management of cerebral vasospasm: timing of endovascular options. *Neurosurgery.* 1999;44(5):975–9.

118. Kimball MM, Velat GJ, Hoh BL, Participants in the International Multi-Disciplinary Consensus Conference on the Critical Care Management of Subarachnoid Hemorrhage. Critical care guidelines on the endovascular management of cerebral vasospasm. *Neurocrit Care.* 2011;15(2):336–41.

119. Hoh BL, Ogilvy CS. Endovascular treatment of cerebral vasospasm: transluminal balloon angioplasty, intra-arterial papaverine, and intra-arterial nicardipine. *Neurosurg Clin N Am.* 2005;16(3):501–16.

120. Smith WS, Dowd CF, Johnston SC, Ko NU, DeArmond SJ, Dillon WP, et al. Neurotoxicity of intra-arterial papaverine preserved with chlorobutanol used for the treatment of cerebral vasospasm after aneurysmal subarachnoid hemorrhage. *Stroke.* 2004;35(11):2518–22.

121. Lewis DH, Paul Elliott J, Newell DW, Eskridge JM, Richard Winn H. Interventional endovascular therapy: SPECT cerebral blood flow imaging compared with transcranial Doppler monitoring of balloon angioplasty and intraarterial papaverine for cerebral vasospasm. *J Stroke Cerebrovasc Dis.* 1999;8(2):71–5.

122. Katoh H, Shima K, Shimizu A, Takiguchi H, Miyazawa T, Umezawa H, et al. Clinical evaluation of the effect of percutaneous transluminal angioplasty and intra-arterial papaverine infusion for the treatment of vasospasm following aneurysmal subarachnoid hemorrhage. *Neurol Res.* 1999;21(2):195–203.

123. Coenen VA, Hansen CA, Kassell NF, Polin RS. Endovascular treatment for symptomatic cerebral vasospasm after subarachnoid hemorrhage: transluminal balloon angioplasty compared with intraarterial papaverine. *Neurosurg Focus.* 1998;5(4):e6.

124. Albanese E, Russo A, Quiroga M, Willis RN, Jr., Mericle RA, Ulm AJ. Ultrahigh-dose intraarterial infusion of verapamil through an indwelling microcatheter for medically refractory severe vasospasm: initial experience. Clinical article. *J Neurosurg.* 2010;113(4):913–22.

125. Kilpatrick MM, Lowry DW, Firlik AD, Yonas H, Marion DW. Hyperthermia in the neurosurgical intensive care unit. *Neurosurgery.* 2000;47(4):850–5.

126. Rabinstein AA, Sandhu K. Non-infectious fever in the neurological intensive care unit: incidence, causes and predictors. *J Neurol Neurosurg Psychiatry.* 2007;78(11):1278–80.

127. Diringer MN, Reaven NL, Funk SE, Uman GC. Elevated body temperature independently contributes to increased length of stay in neurologic intensive care unit patients. *Crit Care Med.* 2004;32(7):1489–95.

128. Oddo M, Frangos S, Milby A, Chen I, Maloney-Wilensky E, Murtrie EM, et al. Induced normothermia attenuates cerebral metabolic distress in patients with aneurysmal subarachnoid hemorrhage and refractory Fever. *Stroke.* 2009;40(7):1913–6.

129. Badjatia N, Fernandez L, Schmidt JM, Lee K, Claassen J, Connolly ES, et al. Impact of induced normothermia on outcome after subarachnoid hemorrhage: a case-control study. *Neurosurgery.* 2010;66(4):696–700.

130. Wartenberg KE, Mayer SA. Medical complications after subarachnoid hemorrhage: new strategies for prevention and management. *Curr Opin Crit Care.* 2006;12(2):78–84.

131. van der Bilt IA, Hasan D, Vandertop WP, Wilde AA, Algra A, Visser FC, et al. Impact of cardiac complications on outcome after aneurysmal subarachnoid hemorrhage: a meta-analysis. *Neurology.* 2009;72(7):635–42.

132. Hravnak M, Frangiskakis JM, Crago EA, Chang Y, Tanabe M, Gorcsan J, 3rd, et al. Elevated cardiac troponin I and relationship to persistence of electrocardiographic and echocardiographic abnormalities after aneurysmal subarachnoid hemorrhage. *Stroke.* 2009;40(11):3478–84.

133. Banki NM, Kopelnik A, Dae MW, Miss J, Tung P, Lawton MT, et al. Acute neurocardiogenic injury after subarachnoid hemorrhage. *Circulation.* 2005;112(21):3314–9.

134. Lee VH, Connolly HM, Fulgham JR, Manno EM, Brown RD, Jr., Wijdicks EF. Tako-tsubo cardiomyopathy in aneurysmal subarachnoid hemorrhage: an underappreciated ventricular dysfunction. *J Neurosurg.* 2006;105(2):264–70.

135. Jain R, Deveikis J, Thompson BG. Management of patients with stunned myocardium associated with subarachnoid hemorrhage. *AJNR Am J Neuroradiol.* 2004;25(1):126–9.

136. Bruder N, Rabinstein A, Participants in the International Multi-Disciplinary Consensus Conference on the Critical Care Management of Subarachnoid Hemorrhage. Cardiovascular and pulmonary complications of aneurysmal subarachnoid hemorrhage. *Neurocrit Care.* 2011;15(2):257–69.

137. Kim DH, Haney CL, Van Ginhoven G. Reduction of pulmonary edema after SAH with a pulmonary artery catheter-guided hemodynamic management protocol. *Neurocrit Care.* 2005;3(1):11–5.

138. Diringer MN. Neuroendocrine regulation of sodium and volume following subarachnoid hemorrhage. *Clin Neuropharmacol.* 1995;18(2):114–26.

139. Gress DR, Participants in the International Multi-Disciplinary Consensus Conference on the Critical Care Management of Subarachnoid Hemorrhage. Monitoring of volume status after subarachnoid hemorrhage. *Neurocrit Care.* 2011;15(2):270–4.

140. Hoff R, Rinkel G, Verweij B, Algra A, Kalkman C. Blood volume measurement to guide fluid therapy after aneurysmal subarachnoid hemorrhage: a prospective controlled study. *Stroke.* 2009;40(7):2575–7.

141. Katayama Y, Haraoka J, Hirabayashi H, Kawamata T, Kawamoto K, Kitahara T, et al. A randomized controlled trial of hydrocortisone against hyponatremia in patients with aneurysmal subarachnoid hemorrhage. *Stroke.* 2007;38(8):2373–5.

142. Audibert G, Steinmann G, de Talance N, Laurens MH, Dao P, Baumann A, et al. Endocrine response after severe subarachnoid hemorrhage related to sodium and blood volume regulation. *Anesth Analg.* 2009;108(6):1922–8.

143. Chandy D, Sy R, Aronow WS, Lee WN, Maguire G, Murali R. Hyponatremia and cerebrovascular spasm in aneurysmal subarachnoid hemorrhage. *Neurol India.* 2006;54(3):273–5.

144. Rahman M, Friedman WA. Hyponatremia in neurosurgical patients: clinical guidelines development. *Neurosurgery.* 2009;65(5):925–35.

145. Suarez JI, Qureshi AI, Parekh PD, Razumovsky A, Tamargo RJ, Bhardwaj A, et al. Administration of hypertonic (3%) sodium chloride/acetate in hyponatremic patients with symptomatic vasospasm following subarachnoid hemorrhage. *J Neurosurg Anesthesiol.* 1999;11(3):178–84.

146. Rabinstein AA, Bruder N. Management of hyponatremia and volume contraction. *Neurocrit Care*. 2011;15(2):354–60.

147. Sampson TR, Dhar R, Diringer MN. Factors associated with the development of anemia after subarachnoid hemorrhage. *Neurocrit Care*. 2010;12(1):4–9.

148. Kramer AH, Zygun DA, Bleck TP, Dumont AS, Kassell NF, Nathan B. Relationship between hemoglobin concentrations and outcomes across subgroups of patients with aneurysmal subarachnoid hemorrhage. *Neurocrit Care*. 2009;10(2):157–65.

149. Naidech AM, Jovanovic B, Wartenberg KE, Parra A, Ostapkovich N, Connolly ES, et al. Higher hemoglobin is associated with improved outcome after subarachnoid hemorrhage. *Crit Care Med*. 2007;35(10):2383–9.

150. Oddo M, Milby A, Chen I, Frangos S, MacMurtrie E, Maloney-Wilensky E, et al. Hemoglobin concentration and cerebral metabolism in patients with aneurysmal subarachnoid hemorrhage. *Stroke*. 2009;40(4):1275–81.

151. Le Roux PD. Anemia and transfusion after subarachnoid hemorrhage. *Neurocrit Care*. 2011;15(2):342–53.

152. Dhar R, Zazulia AR, Videen TO, Zipfel GJ, Derdeyn CP, Diringer MN. Red blood cell transfusion increases cerebral oxygen delivery in anemic patients with subarachnoid hemorrhage. *Stroke*. 2009;40(9):3039–44.

153. Kramer AH, Gurka MJ, Nathan B, Dumont AS, Kassell NF, Bleck TP. Complications associated with anemia and blood transfusion in patients with aneurysmal subarachnoid hemorrhage. *Crit Care Med*. 2008;36(7):2070–5.

154. Levi M, van der Poll T. Inflammation and coagulation. *Crit Care Med*. 2010;38(2 Suppl):S26–34.

155. Mack WJ, Ducruet AF, Hickman ZL, Kalyvas JT, Cleveland JR, Mocco J, et al. Doppler ultrasonography screening of poor-grade subarachnoid hemorrhage patients increases the diagnosis of deep venous thrombosis. *Neurol Res*. 2008;30(9):889–92.

156. Helbok R, Schmidt JM, Kurtz P, Hanafy KA, Fernandez L, Stuart RM, et al. Systemic glucose and brain energy metabolism after subarachnoid hemorrhage. *Neurocrit Care*. 2010;12(3):317–23.

157. Naidech AM, Levasseur K, Liebling S, Garg RK, Shapiro M, Ault ML, et al. Moderate hypoglycemia is associated with vasospasm, cerebral infarction, and 3-month disability after subarachnoid hemorrhage. *Neurocrit Care*. 2010;12(2):181–7.

158. Thiele RH, Pouratian N, Zuo Z, Scalzo DC, Dobbs HA, Dumont AS, et al. Strict glucose control does not affect mortality after aneurysmal subarachnoid hemorrhage. *Anesthesiology*. 2009;110(3):603–10.

159. Latorre JG, Chou SH, Nogueira RG, Singhal AB, Carter BS, Ogilvy CS, et al. Effective glycemic control with aggressive hyperglycemia management is associated with improved outcome in aneurysmal subarachnoid hemorrhage. *Stroke*. 2009;40(5):1644–52.

160. Vespa P, Participants in the International Multi-Disciplinary Consensus Conference on the Critical Care Management of Subarachnoid Hemorrhage. SAH pituitary adrenal dysfunction. *Neurocrit Care*. 2011;15(2):365–8.

161. Vergouwen MD, van Geloven N, de Haan RJ, Kruyt ND, Vermeulen M, Roos YB. Increased cortisol levels are associated with delayed cerebral ischemia after aneurysmal subarachnoid hemorrhage. *Neurocrit Care*. 2010;12(3):342–5.

162. Poll EM, Bostrom A, Burgel U, Reinges MH, Hans FJ, Gilsbach JM, et al. Cortisol dynamics in the acute phase of aneurysmal subarachnoid hemorrhage: associations with disease severity and outcome. *J Neurotrauma*. 2010;27(1):189–95.

CHAPTER 19

Intracerebral haemorrhage

Candice Delcourt and Craig Anderson

Of all the different subtypes of acute stroke, intracerebral haemorrhage (ICH) is the most complex and diverse in terms of aetiology. It is also the least treatable and most variable in terms of incidence, investigation, and management (1–3). ICH is the second most common form of stroke (after acute ischaemic stroke) and accounts for approximately 20% of the near 20 million strokes that occur worldwide each year (4). Most cases occur in developing countries where there is a high prevalence of hypertension and other less well-defined predisposing genetic and environmental risk factors (5). ICH is associated with a 30-day mortality of 30–55% and half of the deaths occur within the first few days after the ictus. There has been little change in prognosis over the last decades (3). There is no proven effective medical treatment for ICH and the role of surgery remains controversial. Management is directed at identifying any underlying treatable structural lesion and preventing and treating complications.

Classification

The haemorrhage of ICH arises from within the brain parenchyma. The evolving haematoma may expand substantially and extend into the ventricular system (in up to 30% of cases) and subarachnoid, subdural, and epidural spaces. ICH has traditionally been classified as primary, when it is generally related to hypertension, or secondary to a known cause, most often an underlying structural lesion or anticoagulation therapy. However, as all ICH has an underlying cause it is better defined as either spontaneous or traumatic in nature. Spontaneous ICH is the focus of this chapter.

ICH generally arises from damage to or rupture of the walls of small arterioles. Leakage of blood under pressure dissects through brain tissue to create a haematoma mass which expands along planes of tissue weakness. The most common locations of ICH are the basal ganglia (40–50%), lobar regions (10–20%), thalamus (10–15%), pons (5–10%), cerebellum (5–10%), and brainstem (1–5%).

There are multiple causes of spontaneous ICH (Box 19.1). Small vessel disease from chronic hypertension is by far the most common but antithrombotic agents, such as aspirin and warfarin, and amyloid angiopathy are increasing causes of lobar ICH in older people. ICH secondary to an underlying vascular malformation is more common in children and younger adults. ICH may also occur as a reperfusion injury after ischaemic stroke, either spontaneously (1–2%), following thrombolysis (5–10%), or mechanical clot extraction (5–15%). Uncommon causes of ICH include defects in haemostasis, Moyamoya disease, vasculitis, recreational drug use (e.g. cocaine and amphetamines), and cerebral venous thrombosis.

Clinical presentation

ICH is difficult to differentiate from ischaemic stroke clinically but certain features are highly suggestive of the diagnosis. Rapidly progressing symptoms and signs, including headache, vomiting, seizures, and disturbance of consciousness that is disproportionate to any focal deficit (i.e. paresis) suggest a mass effect from an underlying haematoma. Moreover, neck stiffness (meningism) indicates that blood has breached the subarachnoid space, generally via the ventricular system, causing chemical meningitis with fever and/or coma from hydrocephalus. Drowsiness and disturbances of balance without clear lateralization suggest cerebellar ICH which has a high early mortality from brainstem compression or hydrocephalus. However, the most reliable way to diagnosis ICH is through expedient use of non-contrast computed tomography (NCCT).

Pathophysiology of intracerebral haemorrhage-related brain injury

The most immediate consequence of ICH is direct injury to the brain from the physical disruption and mass effect of the haematoma. Expansion of the haematoma within or near vital structures such as the brainstem has serious consequences. At least one-third of patients with ICH exhibit clinically significant expansion or 'growth' of the haematoma and this is a common cause of early (< 24 hours) neurological deterioration (Figure 19.1) (6). High blood pressure at the time of ICH is associated with a larger initial haematoma and greater likelihood of haematoma expansion (7,8).

Perihaematoma oedema develops in proportion to the size of the underlying haematoma and is a major cause of neurological deterioration after the first 24 hours (9). It increases rapidly over the first 48 hours, peaking towards the end of the second week (10,11). Although the region surrounding the haematoma displays a modest reduction in cerebral blood flow this is not accompanied by significant ischaemia (12). The later consequences of ICH in peri-haematoma tissue are related to cytotoxic and vasogenic oedema secondary to the toxic (inflammatory) effects of thrombin and iron as a consequence of the breakdown of haemoglobin (13).

Major causes of ICH

As noted already, the aetiology of ICH is diverse.

Hypertension

Chronically elevated blood pressure produces a small vessel vasculopathy characterized by lipohyalinosis and deposition of protein material in vessel walls. This predisposes to fibrinoid necrosis and disruption of the endothelium with the production

Box 19.1 Causes of primary intracerebral haemorrhage

- Chronic hypertension
- Amyloid angiopathy
- Antithrombotic agents:
  - warfarin
  - antiplatelet agents (e.g. aspirin, clopidogrel)
  - thrombin inhibitors (e.g. dabigatran)
  - factor Xa inhibitors (e.g. rivaroxaban)
- Vascular abnormalities:
  - arteriovenous malformation
  - intracranial aneurysm
  - cavernoma
- Haemorrhagic conversion of ischaemic stroke:
  - spontaneous
  - complication of thrombolysis
  - complication of mechanical clot retrieval
- Intracranial neoplasm
- Vasculitis
- Moyamoya disease
- Dural venous sinus thrombosis
- Cocaine/amphetamine use.

of micro-aneurysms (Charcot–Bouchard aneurysms) in small penetrating arteries (< 3 mm) in deeper locations of the brain including the putamen, thalamus, pons, and cerebellum. ICH is often associated with clinically silent micro-haemorrhages, often called micro-bleeds, which can be identified by magnetic resonance imaging (MRI). Micro-bleeds have also been associated with ischaemic stroke, vascular dementia and cerebral amyloid angiopathy suggesting that they are a general marker of microvascular brain disease

(14). How micro-haemorrhages are related to chronic hypertension is unclear.

Cerebral amyloid angiopathy

The deposition of amyloid β-peptide in small and middle size vessels can predispose to rupture, most often in lobar locations in the cortex and subcortical white matter. These amyloid deposits are biochemically similar to the material comprising senile plaques in Alzheimer's disease (15).

Cerebral vascular malformation

Congenital cerebral vascular malformations, which occur in 0.1–4.0% of the general population (16), can be categorized into four major subtypes—developmental venous anomalies, capillary telangiectasias, cavernous malformations, and arteriovenous malformations (AVMs).

Developmental venous anomalies and telangiectasia rarely cause ICH whereas cavernous malformations are common causes (17,18). Cavernomas are dilated, thin-walled capillaries with a simple endothelial lining and a thin, fibrous adventitia with no elastic tissue or smooth muscle in the vessel walls. They can be isolated or occur as multiple lesions and in a sporadic or familial context. Cavernomas commonly present in the third or fourth decade of life and although the incidence is similar in both sexes it has been suggested that the risk of bleeding is higher in females (18). Only 25% of cavernomas are located in the posterior fossa but their annual bleeding risk is higher than from supra-tentorial lesions (2–3% versus 0.5–1%). Cavernomas are low blood flow lesions so are often 'silent' on cerebral angiography although they are well visualized on MRI (especially T2-weighted images) which is the preferred diagnostic and screening tool. Because cavernomas contain blood at capillary pressure, bleeding is usually much less destructive than that from an arterial haemorrhage. However, when located within critical sites such as the brainstem they can cause substantial neurological damage and death (19).

AVMs are the most dangerous vascular malformations but a rare cause of ICH accounting for only 0.1% of cases. They are most frequently located in the cerebral hemispheres and are sporadic and rarely inherited. AVMs most commonly manifest between the age of 10 to 40 years and present as an ICH or more commonly with seizures. The overall average annual bleeding rate of an untreated

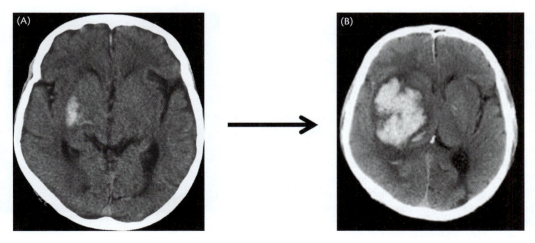

Fig. 19.1 The dynamic nature of intracerebral haemorrhage. Sequential non-contrast computed tomography scans at (A) 3 hours and (B) 24 hours after ictus illustrating a typical site of a hypertension-related intracerebral haemorrhage and rapidly increasing haematoma size.

brain AVM ranges from 2% to 5%. AVMs are high-flow lesions because of their direct arterial to venous connections without an intervening capillary network (20). MRI is the most sensitive diagnostic tool, especially in the setting of a recent ICH.

Anticoagulant-related-ICH

The increasing frequency of ICH is partly related to the increasing use of anticoagulants in an elderly population in association with the earlier-noted additional predisposing factors associated with ageing. A large population-based surveillance study in Finland demonstrated that the use of vitamin K antagonists such as warfarin now accounts for approximately 20% of cases of ICH (21). Mortality from oral anticoagulation-related ICH is high, with studies indicating that over one-half of patients die within 30 days of the ictus (22,23). The risk of ICH appears to be lower with the newer anticoagulants, such as thrombin inhibitors and factor X1 inhibitors, compared to standard-dose warfarin possibly due to their more specific action on the coagulation system. The hazard ratio (95% confidence interval) for dabigatran 150 mg twice a day is 0.4 (0.27–0.6) (24), for apixaban 5 mg twice a day 0.42 (0.3–0.58) (25) and for rivaroxaban 10 mg once daily 0.67 (0.47–0.93) (26).

The increasingly elderly population has also been associated with an increase in the number of patients receiving long-term antiplatelet medication. Aspirin is associated with an absolute increased risk of ICH of 12 events per 10,000 persons, although this is more than offset by its overall benefit in terms of reduced risk of myocardial infarction and ischaemic stroke (27). The risk of ICH is even higher in those taking a combination of aspirin and clopidogrel (28). Antiplatelet therapy is also an independent predictor of haematoma expansion (6).

Investigations

NCCT is the investigation of choice as it is low cost, quick and easy to perform, and highly predictive of confirming blood in the brain. In addition to identifying the location of the ICH, haematoma volume which is the strongest predictor of outcome can quickly be calculated from the initial CT scan using automated CT software algorithms. Alternatively haematoma volume can be calculated manually using the well-established ABC/2 formula which is based on the assumption that the ICH volume can be approximated to an ellipsoid (29). The three perpendicular axes of the haematoma are assessed from the CT images—A is the largest cross-sectional diameter, B a second diameter drawn at right angles to A, and C the height of the ellipsoid estimated from the number and thickness of slices in which the haemorrhage is visible. This simple and reasonably accurate method compares well to automated methods of calculating haematoma volume after ICH (30). As well as providing early prognostic information, assessment of haematoma volume guides acute treatment decisions. A small ICH can resolve rapidly and NCCT can be completely normal 1–2 weeks after the ictus.

The decision to undertake further investigations, such as CT or MR angiography, to identify a causative underlying structural abnormality has generally been based on three principal factors—younger age (< 45 years), location of the ICH (i.e. peripheral), and an absence of premorbid hypertension as the likely cause. MRI is more sensitive than CT in detecting secondary causes of ICH such as aneurysms, AVMs, and cavernomas (31). Although there is little evidence to guide cost-effective clinical decision-making (1), further investigation with CT or MR angiography and subsequent conventional

cerebral angiography is recommended when there are suspicious features such as subarachnoid haemorrhage, an unusual ('non-circular') shape to the haematoma, a disproportionate amount of early cerebral oedema, unusual haematoma location or the presence of an associated mass. MRI with gradient echo sequence (T2) is particularly sensitive for the detection of microbleeds and may confirm the diagnosis of cerebral amyloid angiopathy as the cause of a cortical ICH.

Extravasation of intravenous contrast into the centre or edge of the ICH on CT scan—the so-called spot sign (Figure 19.2)—is indicative of active bleeding. A positive spot sign is highly predictive of haematoma growth and poor outcome (32–34).

A thoughtful and swift approach to establishing the underlying cause of the ICH, particularly in the detection of vascular malformations, including use of conventional cerebral angiography, is important for establishing appropriate treatment and minimizing the risk of recurrent ICH and other complications. Angiography should be considered in all cases of spontaneous ICH involving younger patients (< 45 years), those without pre-existing hypertension, and ICH in atypical locations or with unusual morphology (35).

Management

Spontaneous ICH is a devastating disease at any age and there are no interventions that have been proved beyond doubt to improve outcome. ICH is a neurological emergency and intervention in the first few hours may improve outcome. Indirect evidence supports the value of active, well-coordinated multidisciplinary care in the early stages after ICH.

Acute management

The acute management of the ICH should focus on the following aspects (36):

1. Patient stabilization using standard ABCDE protocols

2. Rapid and accurate diagnosis including neuroimaging

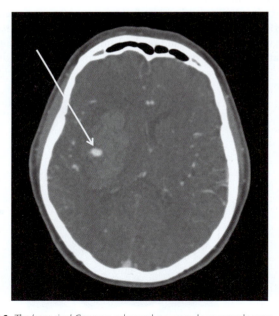

Fig. 19.2 The 'spot sign'. Contrast-enhanced computed tomography scan showing extravasation of intravenous contrast (the 'spot sign') in the centre of the intracerebral haemorrhage. A positive spot sign is predictive of active bleeding and haematoma growth.

3. Rapid clinical assessment including identification of the need for early interventions including:
   a. control of elevated blood pressure
   b. correction of coagulopathy
   c. early surgical intervention
4. Assessment of ongoing management needs including:
   a. anticipation of the risk for early clinical deterioration due to haematoma expansion
   b. requirement for admission to the intensive care unit (ICU)
   c. specific treatment for underlying causes of ICH.

As with all acute medical care initial assessment and management of airway, breathing, and circulation is critical. Until the diagnosis of ICH is confirmed by neuroimaging, airway and haemodynamic management proceeds in a common pathway with other stroke subtypes. However, immediately following the ICH diagnosis, disease-specific treatment can be instituted (36).

Several simple and reliable grading and predictive scores have been developed for ICH (37,38). The ICH score is the most well known and includes age, Glasgow Coma Scale score, haematoma volume and location (supratentorial or infratentorial), and presence of intraventricular haemorrhage (Table 19.1) (37). Each point increase in the total ICH score is associated with an increased risk of mortality and a decreased likelihood of good functional outcome. The ICH score has been shown to be a useful clinical grading scale for 12-month long-term functional outcome (39). However, such simple scoring systems may be difficult to apply in an individual patient and are thus of limited value in determining treatment in the acute phase.

Table 19.1 The ICH score

Component	ICH score points
Glasgow Coma Scale:	
◆ 3–4	2
◆ 5–12	1
◆ 13–15	0
ICH volume:	
◆ ≥ 30 mL	1
◆ < 30 mL	0
Presence of intraventricular haemorrhage:	
◆ Yes	1
◆ No	0
Infratentorial origin of ICH:	
◆ Yes	1
◆ No	0
Age:	
◆ ≥ 80 years	1
◆ < 80 years	0
Total ICH Score	0–6

The lack of effective treatments has clouded the management of ICH, with therapeutic nihilism and low thresholds for withdrawal of active care being common. There is clear evidence that 'do-not-resuscitate' or 'withdrawal of care' orders are independent predictors of early mortality after ICH (40). A policy of active management should initially be applied in all patients to allow time for the critical condition to be stabilized, clarity to be obtained regarding potentially reversible factors (such as early seizure(s) and dehydration) that may have contributed to altered levels of consciousness, and for counselling and discussion with family members regarding ongoing management in the light of the patient's age, pre-existing medical comorbidities, and cultural, religious, and personal beliefs. Ideally, patients should always receive some form of monitored care, either in an ICU or high dependency section of an acute stroke unit. Inevitably though, the management of ICH is largely supportive and expectant.

Surgery

Despite being part of neurosurgical practice for several decades and having undergone evaluation in multiple randomized controlled trials, the role of open craniotomy to decompress the haematoma of supratentorial ICH (and save a patient's life) remains controversial. Decisions to operate are dominated by individuals' clinical judgement and are applied variably around the world. Part of the problem lies in applying the positive results from a meta-analysis of multiple but generally small trials with variable results (41) to an individual patient in whom the potential life-saving benefit of surgery must be weighed against the potential harm involved in cutting into healthy brain and the risks of general anaesthesia in patients with multiple co-morbidities, and postoperative complications such as re-bleeding and infection. The other problem is that the pivotal international Surgical Treatment of Intracerebral Haemorrhage (STICH) trial found no benefit of surgery in terms of 6-month mortality, modified Rankin and Barthal Index scores, although subgroup analysis suggested that patients with haemorrhages closer to the surface had better outcomes with surgery (42). This led to the STICH II trial which randomized 601 conscious patients with small (10–100 mL) superficial (within 1 cm of the cortex) lobar ICH and no intraventricular extension to early surgery or initial conservative management, and also found no benefit of surgery (43). While the potential benefits of open surgery continue to be debated, what is clear is that it offers the greatest potential benefit when applied early (< 8 hours) and before patients develop deep coma (44).

A number of minimally invasive surgical techniques for supratentorial ICH are available. These include endoscopic guidance and/or cranio-puncture, and catheter-insertion techniques with or without the instillation of a lytic to drain the haematoma and/or intraventricular haemorrhage. A recent meta-analysis including several high-quality randomized controlled trials suggested that minimally invasive surgery might be superior to other treatment options including craniotomy and conservative management (45), but the outcome of several ongoing studies is awaited.

Although there have been no randomized trials specifically undertaken in patients with posterior fossa ICH and signs of brainstem compromise, surgical decompression is generally regarded as the standard of care with an acceptable risk because of the high mortality and morbidity if untreated (46). Similarly, the presence of symptomatic obstructive hydrocephalus generally requires drainage of the ventricular system.

There is no evidence that the insertion of an intracranial pressure (ICP) monitor to guide management improves outcome in patients with cerebral oedema after ICH, although ICP monitoring is often undertaken (47).

Surgery is indicated for patients with symptomatic cerebral or cerebellar cavernomas with progressive neurological deficits, intractable epilepsy, or recurrent haemorrhage and also for brainstem cavernomas because of their poor prognosis if untreated (48). There are several approaches to the management of AVMs but the decision to intervene is not straightforward. Factors such as the predicted future risk of re-bleeding, the patient's age, lesion size and location, and prior history of ICH must all be taken into account (49). There are also several treatment approaches including a single procedure or varying combinations of microvascular surgery, endovascular techniques, and radiosurgery (focused radiation). Whether to intervene or adopt a conservative approach, and which intervention is superior, remain highly controversial (50). A large, international, multicentre study, the Randomized Trial of Unruptured Brain Arteriovenous Malformations (ARUBA), showed that medical management alone is superior to medical management with interventional therapy for the prevention of death or stroke in patients with unruptured brain AVMs at 33 months (51).

General supportive treatment

Supportive treatment is aimed at normalizing systemic physiological variables, including airway, breathing, arterial blood gases, circulation, hydration, blood glucose, and temperature, and at preventing systemic and intracranial complications.

Fluid management

Many patients with ICH are dehydrated at the time of presentation. Fluid status requires particularly careful assessment if there has been an unknown or prolonged period of unconsciousness or immobilization. A 0.9% saline or Hartmann's solution should be given as standard intravenous replacement fluid at a rate of approximately 1 mL/kg/h. Hypertonic saline, in the form of a 2% or 3% sodium/chloride-acetate solution (1 mL/kg/h), is a popular alternative to normal saline to reduce perihaematoma oedema causing mass effect, but this treatment is unproven (52).

Seizures

Seizures with variable manifestations occur in up to 8% of cases in the acute phase after ICH, most commonly within the first 24 hours (53). Lobar haemorrhage location is an independent predictor of early seizures (54). Seizures after ICH may not be associated with clinical manifestations and in these circumstances can only be identified by electroencephalogram (EEG) monitoring. In one study, seizures were identified in one-third of patients and over half were not associated with clinical seizures (55). Electrographic seizures were associated with expanding haemorrhages and poor outcome. Non-convulsive seizures may manifest as persistent coma or a fluctuating level of consciousness that is disproportionate to the size of the haematoma and EEG monitoring to exclude seizures is indicated in such circumstances (56). Alternatively the only clinical manifestation of seizures may be only subtle twitches or jerks over the face, trunk, or limbs. EEG monitoring is complicated by sedation, movement artefact, underlying brain injury, and the ability to capture abnormalities only on the surface of the brain.

Despite comatose ICH patients being at high risk of seizures, prophylactic anticonvulsant drugs are not recommended and have been associated with worse outcome (57). Actual seizures must of course be treated aggressively. In unconscious patients, seizures can be treated with phenytoin (loading dose of 20 mg/kg) or levetiracetam as both are available in intravenous formulations. Otherwise, all of the routinely available oral anticonvulsant drugs are useful. The long-term risk of further seizures is higher after ICH than other stroke subtypes but it is uncertain whether seizures have an independent influence on outcome (58).

Fever

Fever (temperature > 38°C) is common after ICH, particularly after intraventricular haemorrhage, and associated with poor outcome in observational studies (59). It should be treated aggressively.

Glycaemic control

Hyperglycaemia is also common and associated with poor outcome (60) but the optimal target for systemic glycaemic control is unknown (61). Aggressively tight glucose control is associated with unacceptably high rates of hypoglycaemia in a general ICU population (62). A recent meta-analysis and systematic review confirmed that intensive insulin therapy (IIT) to achieve tight glycaemic control in critically ill neurological patients is also associated with significantly more frequent episodes of hypoglycaemia, as well as increased mortality and ICU length of stay, compared to standard treatment (63). Until rigorous studies have identified the optimal blood glucose targets after ICH, less tight control seems optimal (see Chapter 28). It is currently suggested that glucose levels should be maintained between 8 and 10 mmol/L (144–180 mg/dL) and that hypoglycaemia and large swings in glucose levels should be avoided (63).

Swallowing dysfunction and aspiration pneumonia

Pulmonary aspiration is a frequent complication in all patients with acute neurological dysfunction and disorders of swallow, including after ICH. It can occur because of disturbance of higher cortical control of swallow in the pharyngeal phase (i.e. dyspraxia) or because of direct involvement of the nerves innervating the bulbar muscles in patients with brainstem lesions. In a critical care environment, the use of simple bedside tests such as the presence of a 'wet' voice, coughing on swallowing 3 mL of water, and cervical auscultation for noisy or wet sound on swallowing jelly have high predictive value as screening tools for swallow dysfunction (64). Patients with swallowing difficulty should be nursed in a head-up position (≥ 30°), be 'nil-by-mouth', and have a nasogastric tube inserted for feeding. They remain at ongoing risk of aspiration and pneumonia for some time by virtue of their disability and potential immune compromise from pre-morbid illness and medications.

Venous thromboembolism prophylaxis

Symptomatic and asymptomatic deep vein thrombosis (DVT) occurs in 3.7% and 40% of ICH patients, respectively, and pulmonary embolism in around 1.0% (65). Low-dose subcutaneous unfractionated heparin, or a low-molecular-weight heparinoid, commenced early in the immobile patient significantly reduces the risk of venous thromboembolism without an excessive increased risk of further ICH or other bleeding complication (66). Consensus guidance recommends that either low-dose heparin or low-molecular-weight heparin should be introduced 1–4 days after ICH onset, once cessation of bleeding is confirmed (56).

Cerebral oedema and raised intracranial pressure

Although randomized evidence is lacking, invasive monitoring of ICP and high-level supportive care should be considered in patients who are comatose, have significant mass effect, intraventricular extension of the haematoma, or hydrocephalus (56). As in other types of brain injury, a simple manoeuvre to reduce increased ICP is to nurse the patient in a head-up position (> 30°). Optimization of oxygenation and blood pressure is essential to maintain adequate cerebral oxygen delivery and minimize the risk of ischaemia-related increases in ICP. Comatose and hypoxaemic patients should be intubated and ventilated to maintain adequate PaO_2. Hypotension is rare and an incidental cause should be identified and treated. In the absence of such a cause, consideration should be given to the administration 0.5–2.0 mL/kg of 23.4% saline solution or pressor agents, administered through a central venous line.

Measures to lower ICP include moderate hyperventilation ($PaCO_2$ 3.5–4.0 kPa (26–30 mmHg)) and 20% mannitol (1.0–1.5 g/kg) by rapid infusion, although the latter can be complicated by a rebound increase in ICP because of its gradual diffusion from the vascular compartment into the brain. Corticosteroids are not beneficial and their use is complicated by hyperglycaemia and dehydration (67). It has been suggested that moderate hypothermia (32–34°C) may be neuroprotective and reduce cerebral oedema after ICH (68), but this is currently an unproven intervention.

Early intensive control of blood pressure

Elevated blood pressure is common after ICH and strongly associated with poor outcome (69,70). The pilot phases of both the Intensive Blood Pressure Reduction in Acute Intracerebral Haemorrhage Trial (INTERACT) (71) and the Antihypertensive Treatment of Acute Cerebral Hemorrhage (ATACH) (72) study demonstrated the feasibility, safety, and potential efficacy of intensive blood pressure lowering after ICH and informed the subsequent main phase studies INTERACT2 and ATACH-2. In particular, further analysis of the original INTERACT dataset is consistent in demonstrating beneficial effects on reducing haematoma growth that are strongly related to both the time to initiation and degree of blood pressure lowering (73,74).

As the largest clinical trial in ICH to date, INTERACT2 has resolved much of the uncertainty regarding the management of elevated blood pressure (75). This study randomly assigned 2839 patients to intensive (target systolic blood pressure < 140 mmHg) or guideline-recommended (target systolic blood pressure < 180 mmHg) blood pressure lowering-treatment within 6 hours of ICH. Data on the primary outcome (death and major disability) was available for 2794 participants of which 719 (52.0%) of the 1382 participants receiving intensive treatment suffered death or major disability compared to 785 (55.6%) of 1412 receiving guideline-recommended treatment (odds ratio (OR) with intensive treatment 0.87, P = 0.06). However, there was significantly better functional recovery according to an ordinal analysis of the modified Rankin scale scores (OR for greater disability 0.87, P = 0.04) in the intensive treatment group and patients receiving intensive blood pressure control reported better physical and mental health-related

quality of life. Moreover, intensive blood pressure control was shown to be safe with no difference in mortality (12.0%) or serious adverse events between the groups. Whilst more randomized data would certainly strengthen these findings, it seems reasonable on the basis of INTERACT2 that all patients with ICH should have elevated blood pressure controlled as early as possible to improve their chances of better functional recovery should they survive.

The most recent guidance from the American Heart Association/American Stroke Association, 'Guidelines for the Management of Intracerebral Hemorrhage', which has been updated since INTERACT 2, is shown in Table 19.2 (56).

The basic principles of blood pressure lowering after ICH are that treatment should be initiated immediately and a titratable agent used to ensure that the target blood pressure is reached quickly and with minimal potential for overshoot to minimize the risk of deleterious hypotension. Intravenous beta blockers and calcium channel blockers are often used in these circumstances in both the emergency department and ICU (36).

Anticoagulant-associated ICH

Whatever the indication for warfarin treatment, the potential benefits of acute reversal after ICH are likely to outweigh the risks. Although randomized data are lacking, all guidelines recommend reversing the effects of warfarin to an international normalized ratio (INR) lower than 1.4 with some combination of vitamin K and clotting factor replacement with fresh frozen plasma (FFP) or prothrombin complex concentrate (PCC) (36,56).

Vitamin K (5–10 mg) has a long duration of action but requires several hours to take effect (76). Unactivated PCC, which contains vitamin K-dependent coagulation factors II, VII, IX, and X offers more rapid reversal of anticoagulation. It can normalize the INR within 30 minutes but is costly. A cheaper and potentially equally effective option is FFP but this exposes the patient to the potential adverse effects of transfusion of a blood product and risk of volume overload (77). There are also delays in treatment associated with the requirement to check blood group compatibility and the time for thawing, in addition to the time taken for normalization of the INR.

Table 19.2 Blood pressure control after ICH

Blood pressure	High ICP suspected	Recommendation
SBP between 150 and 220 mmHg and without contraindication to acute BP treatment	Yes	Acute lowering of SBP to 140 mmHg is safe (Class I; Level of Evidence A) and can be effective for improving functional outcome (Class IIa; Level of Evidence B)
SBP > 220 mmHg	N/A	Consider aggressive reduction of BP with a continuous intravenous infusion and frequent BP monitoring (Class IIb; Level of Evidence C)

BP, blood pressure; ICP, intracranial pressure; SBP, systolic blood pressure.

All recommendations are based only on case studies, consensus expert opinion or standards of care.

Adapted from Morgenstern LB et al., 'Guidelines for the management of spontaneous intracerebral hemorrhage: a guideline for healthcare professionals from the American Heart Association/American Stroke Association', Stroke, 41, pp. 2108–2129, copyright 2010, with permission from American Heart Association.

These problems are avoided with the use of PCCs which are available in smaller volumes than FFP and do not require compatibility testing or thawing. Several non-randomized trials confirm that PCCs correct INR faster than FFP in the setting of warfarin-related ICH, but improvements in outcome have not been demonstrated (23).

Currently there are no antidotes to the new anticoagulants (dabigatran, rivaroxaban, and apixaban), the effects of which take 24–36 hours to clear. More rapid reversal requires dialysis over several hours.

Antiplatelet agents

Although the risk of ICH is increased in patients taking antiplatelet drugs, the benefits of platelet transfusion to reverse their effects are not clear. A recent systematic review concluded that there are no compelling data to support the use of platelet transfusion in the management of patients with ICH who are taking antiplatelet medication and that further studies are required (78).

Recombinant activated factor VII

Despite considerable promise, including strongly positive results from a proof-of-concept phase IIb clinical trial, the pivotal Factor Seven for Acute Hemorrhagic Stroke (FAST) study which investigated standard dose (80 mcg/kg) of the potent pro-thrombotic agent recombinant factor VIIa (rFVIIa) administered within 4 hours of ICH onset, failed to demonstrate any outcome benefits despite attenuation of haematoma growth by approximately 4 mL at 24 hours (79). Moreover, the use of rFVIIa is complicated by increased risks of both venous and arterial thromboembolic complications, the most serious of which are ischaemic stroke and myocardial ischaemia (80). While there is interest in a more focused approach to the use of rFVIIa when administered within 2.5 hours of symptom onset in young patients (i.e. those with a low prevalence of underlying atherosclerotic disease) and a baseline ICH volume less than 60 mL but at high risk of ongoing bleeding (i.e. spot-sign positive) (81), the undeniable fact is that this is an extremely expensive agent with modest effect and clear hazard. It should therefore continue to be considered experimental.

Haemorrhagic transformation of an ischaemic stroke

There is now strong evidence from around 4000 randomized patients that recombinant tissue plasminogen activator (rtPA) provides an overall net outcome benefit after acute ischaemic stroke despite being associated with an increased risk of bleeding (82). ICH is the most feared complication of rtPA and can arise from within the area of cerebral ischaemia/infarction ('haemorrhagic transformation') or elsewhere in the brain. It has variable manifestations ranging from small petechial haemorrhages to overt lobar haematoma with mass effect. Symptomatic haemorrhagic transformation occurs in 5–6% of patients undergoing intravenous rt-PA and intra-arterial recanalization strategies (83), and is more common after intra-arterial compared with intravenous thrombolysis (84).

ICH after acute ischaemic stroke arises in part because rtPA has a prolonged action on thrombi despite having only a short (minutes) half-life in serum but also because of various alterations in blood flow and vessel permeability that occur within and around infarcted brain. Despite this risk, patients who receive rtPA early after ischaemic stroke have a 30% or higher relative increased chance of having

little or no residual disability (see Chapter 20). This equates to one fewer dead or dependent patient for every ten treated, but also to one ICH per 14 treated within 3 hours of stroke onset (85).

Because of this risk of haemorrhage, patients should be monitored for at least 24 hours after receiving rtPA or endovascular mechanical clot-retrieval to allow early detection and management of a subsequent ICH. The decision to monitor patients in an ICU or high dependency area of a stroke unit is determined by clinical status and local resource. Irrespective of care location, it is important that trained nursing and medical staff are available to undertake frequent observations and take appropriate action according to pre-specified protocol(s) if signs of deterioration are detected. ICH should be suspected in any ischaemic stroke patient who develops a sudden deterioration in neurological status, headache, nausea, vomiting, or elevation in blood pressure. An immediate NCCT should be obtained to differentiate ICH from progressive cerebral oedema from the underlying infarction. Checks should also be made of coagulation status. If ICH is confirmed, rtPA should be stopped if the infusion has not been completed, and 6–8 units of cryoprecipitate (containing clotting factor VIII) and 6–8 units of platelets (to correct any residual effect of rtPA) administered. Depending on the size and location, neurosurgical intervention to evacuate the ICH can be undertaken following support with platelets and cryoprecipitate, although the rapidity of neurological deterioration is such that prognosis is often grave irrespective of any treatment.

Conclusion

Although there are few proven therapeutic options for ICH, there is still much that can be done to improve the quality of care of patients and improve outcome. This includes the use of excellent supportive care and an active approach to the surveillance, early detection, and management of complications. Care should be provided in a suitable monitored critical care setting with appropriately trained multidisciplinary staff. Once patients are stable, early rehabilitation is essential to prevent or reduce the risk of further complications and maximize the chances of recovery and return to everyday activities.

References

1. Cordonnier C, Klijn CJ, van BJ, Al-Shahi SR. Radiological investigation of spontaneous intracerebral hemorrhage: systematic review and trinational survey. *Stroke.* 2010;41:685–90.
2. Qureshi AI, Tuhrim S, Broderick JP, Batjer HH, Hondo H, Hanley DF. Spontaneous intracerebral hemorrhage. *N Engl J Med.* 2001;344:1450–60.
3. van Asch CJ, Luitse MJ, Rinkel GJ, van der Tweel I, Algra A, Klijn CJ. Incidence, case fatality, and functional outcome of intracerebral haemorrhage over time, according to age, sex, and ethnic origin: a systematic review and meta-analysis. *Lancet Neurol.* 2010;9:167–76.
4. Strong K, Mathers C, Bonita R. Preventing stroke: saving lives around the world. *Lancet Neurol.* 2007;6:182–7.
5. Feigin VL, Lawes CM, Bennett DA, Barker-Collo SL, Parag V. Worldwide stroke incidence and early case fatality reported in 56 population-based studies: a systematic review. *Lancet Neurol.* 2009;8:355–69.
6. Broderick JP, Diringer MN, Hill MD, Brun NC, Mayer SA, Steiner T, *et al.* Determinants of intracerebral hemorrhage growth: an exploratory analysis. *Stroke.* 2007;38:1072–5.
7. Chen ST, Chen SD, Hsu CY, Hogan EL. Progression of hypertensive intracerebral hemorrhage. *Neurology.* 1989;39:1509–14.

8. Mayer SA, Sacco RL, Shi T, Mohr JP. Neurologic deterioration in noncomatose patients with supratentorial intracerebral hemorrhage. *Neurology*. 1994;44:1379–84.

9. Anderson CS, Huang Y, Arima H, Heeley E, Skulina C, Parsons MW, *et al*. Effects of early intensive blood pressure-lowering treatment on the growth of hematoma and perihematomal edema in acute intracerebral hemorrhage: the Intensive Blood Pressure Reduction in Acute Cerebral Haemorrhage Trial (INTERACT). *Stroke*. 2010;41:307–12.

10. Venkatasubramanian C, Mlynash M, Finley-Caulfield A, Eyngorn I, Kalimuthu R, Snider RW, *et al*. Natural history of perihematomal edema after intracerebral hemorrhage measured by serial magnetic resonance imaging. *Stroke*. 2011;42:73–80.

11. Xi G, Keep RF, Hoff JT. Mechanisms of brain injury after intracerebral haemorrhage. *Lancet Neurol*. 2006;5:53–63.

12. Butcher KS, Baird T, Macgregor L, Desmond P, Tress B, Davis S. Perihematomal edema in primary intracerebral hemorrhage is plasma derived. *Stroke* 2004;35:1879–85.

13. Lou M, Lieb K, Selim M. The relationship between hematoma iron content and perihematoma edema: an MRI study. *Cerebrovasc Dis*. 2009;27:266–71.

14. Provencio JJ, Da Silva IR, Manno EM. Intracerebral hemorrhage: new challenges and steps forward. *Neurosurg Clin N Am*. 2013;24:349–59.

15. Charidimou A, Gang Q, Werring DJ. Sporadic cerebral amyloid angiopathy revisited: recent insights into pathophysiology and clinical spectrum. *J Neurol Neurosurg Psychiatry*. 2012;83:124–37.

16. el-Gohary EG, Tomita T, Gutierrez FA, McLone DG. Angiographically occult vascular malformations in childhood. *Neurosurgery*. 1987;20:759–66.

17. Hon JM, Bhattacharya JJ, Counsell CE, Papanastassiou V, Ritchie V, Roberts RC, *et al*. The presentation and clinical course of intracranial developmental venous anomalies in adults: a systematic review and prospective, population-based study. *Stroke*. 2009;40:1980–5.

18. Pereira VM, Geibprasert S, Krings T, Aurboonyawat T, Ozanne A, Toulgoat F, *et al*. Pathomechanisms of symptomatic developmental venous anomalies. *Stroke*. 2008;39:3201–15.

19. Aiba T, Tanaka R, Koike T, Kameyama S, Takeda N, Komata T. Natural history of intracranial cavernous malformations. *J Neurosurg*. 1995;83:56–9.

20. Stapf C, Mast H, Sciacca RR, Choi JH, Khaw AV, Connolly ES, *et al*. Predictors of hemorrhage in patients with untreated brain arteriovenous malformation. *Neurology*. 2006;66:1350–5.

21. Huhtakangas J, Tetri S, Juvela S, Saloheimo P, Bode MK, Hillbom M. Effect of increased warfarin use on warfarin-related cerebral hemorrhage: a longitudinal population-based study. *Stroke*. 2011;42:2431–5.

22. Cucchiara B, Messe S, Sansing L, Kasner S, Lyden P. Hematoma growth in oral anticoagulant related intracerebral hemorrhage. *Stroke*. 2008;39:2993–6.

23. Sjoblom L, Hardemark HG, Lindgren A, Norrving B, Fahlen M, Samuelsson M, *et al*. Management and prognostic features of intracerebral hemorrhage during anticoagulant therapy: a Swedish multicenter study. *Stroke* 2001;32:2567–74.

24. Connolly SJ, Ezekowitz MD, Yusuf S, Eikelboom J, Oldgren J, Parekh A, *et al*. Dabigatran versus warfarin in patients with atrial fibrillation. *N Engl J Med*. 2009;361:1139–51.

25. Granger CB, Alexander JH, McMurray JJ, Lopes RD, Hylek EM, Hanna M, *et al*. Apixaban versus warfarin in patients with atrial fibrillation. *N Engl J Med*. 2011;365:981–92.

26. Patel MR, Mahaffey KW, Garg J, Pan G, Singer DE, Hacke W, *et al*. Rivaroxaban versus warfarin in nonvalvular atrial fibrillation. *N Engl J Med*. 2011;365:883–91.

27. He J, Whelton PK, Vu B, Klag MJ. Aspirin and risk of hemorrhagic stroke: a meta-analysis of randomized controlled trials. *JAMA*. 1998;280:1930–5.

28. Diener HC, Bogousslavsky J, Brass LM, Cimminiello C, Csiba L, Kaste M, *et al*. Aspirin and clopidogrel compared with clopidogrel alone after recent ischaemic stroke or transient ischaemic attack in high-risk patients (MATCH): randomised, double-blind, placebo-controlled trial. *Lancet*. 2004;364:331–7.

29. Kothari RU, Brott T, Broderick JP, Barsan WG, Sauerbeck LR, Zuccarello M, *et al*. The ABCs of measuring intracerebral hemorrhage volumes. *Stroke*. 1996;27:1304–5.

30. Huttner HB, Steiner T, Hartmann M, Kohrmann M, Juettler E, Mueller S, *et al*. Comparison of ABC/2 estimation technique to computer-assisted planimetric analysis in warfarin-related intracerebral parenchymal hemorrhage. *Stroke*. 2006;37:404–8.

31. Kidwell CS, Chalela JA, Saver JL, Starkman S, Hill MD, Demchuk AM, *et al*. Comparison of MRI and CT for detection of acute intracerebral hemorrhage. *JAMA*. 2004;292:1823–30.

32. Delgado Almandoz JE, Yoo AJ, Stone MJ, Schaefer PW, Goldstein JN, Rosand J, *et al*. Systematic characterization of the computed tomography angiography spot sign in primary intracerebral hemorrhage identifies patients at highest risk for hematoma expansion: the spot sign score. *Stroke*. 2009;40:2994–3000.

33. Demchuk AM, Dowlatshahi D, Rodriguez-Luna D, Molina CA, Blas YS, Dzialowski I, *et al*. Prediction of haematoma growth and outcome in patients with intracerebral haemorrhage using the CT-angiography spot sign (PREDICT): a prospective observational study. *Lancet Neurol*. 2012;11:307–14.

34. Wada R, Aviv RI, Fox AJ, Sahlas DJ, Gladstone DJ, Tomlinson G, *et al*. CT angiography "spot sign" predicts hematoma expansion in acute intracerebral hemorrhage. *Stroke*. 2007;38:1257–62.

35. Zhu XL, Chan MS, Poon WS. Spontaneous intracranial hemorrhage: which patients need diagnostic cerebral angiography? A prospective study of 206 cases and review of the literature. *Stroke*. 1997;28:1406–9.

36. Andrews CM, Jauch EC, Hemphill JC, III, Smith WS, Weingart SD. Emergency neurological life support: intracerebral hemorrhage. *Neurocrit Care*. 2012;17 Suppl 1:S37–S46.

37. Hemphill JC, III, Bonovich DC, Besmertis L, Manley GT, Johnston SC. The ICH score: a simple, reliable grading scale for intracerebral hemorrhage. *Stroke*. 2001;32:891–7.

38. Rost NS, Smith EE, Chang Y, Snider RW, Chanderraj R, Schwab K, *et al*. Prediction of functional outcome in patients with primary intracerebral hemorrhage: the FUNC score. *Stroke*. 2008;39:2304–9.

39. Hemphill JC, III, Farrant M, Neill TA, Jr. Prospective validation of the ICH Score for 12-month functional outcome. *Neurology* 2009;73:1088–94.

40. Zahuranec DB, Morgenstern LB, Sanchez BN, Resnicow K, White DB, Hemphill JC, III. Do-not-resuscitate orders and predictive models after intracerebral hemorrhage. *Neurology* 2010;75:626–33.

41. Prasad K, Mendelow AD, Gregson B. Surgery for primary supratentorial intracerebral haemorrhage. *Cochrane Database Syst Rev*. 2008;4:CD000200.

42. Mendelow AD, Gregson BA, Fernandes HM, Murray GD, Teasdale GM, Hope DT, *et al*. Early surgery versus initial conservative treatment in patients with spontaneous supratentorial intracerebral haematomas in the International Surgical Trial in Intracerebral Haemorrhage (STICH): a randomised trial. *Lancet*. 2005;365:387–97.

43. Mendelow AD, Gregson BA, Rowan EN, Murray GD, Gholkar A, Mitchell PM. Early surgery versus initial conservative treatment in patients with spontaneous supratentorial lobar intracerebral haematomas (STICH II): a randomised trial. *Lancet*. 2013;382:397–408.

44. Gregson BA, Broderick JP, Auer LM, Batjer H, Chen XC, Juvela S, *et al*. Individual patient data subgroup meta-analysis of surgery for spontaneous supratentorial intracerebral hemorrhage. *Stroke*. 2012;43:1496–504.

45. Zhou X, Chen J, Li Q, Ren G, Yao G, Liu M, *et al*. Minimally invasive surgery for spontaneous supratentorial intracerebral hemorrhage: a meta-analysis of randomized controlled trials. *Stroke* 2012;43:2923–30.

46. Dammann P, Asgari S, Bassiouni H, Gasser T, Panagiotopoulos V, Gizewski ER, *et al*. Spontaneous cerebellar hemorrhage—experience with 57 surgically treated patients and review of the literature. *Neurosurg Rev*. 2011;34:77–86.

47. Kirkman MA, Smith M. Supratentorial intracerebral hemorrhage: a review of the underlying pathophysiology and its relevance for multimodality neuromonitoring in neurointensive care. *J Neurosurg Anesthesiol*. 2013;25:228–39.

48. Sandalcioglu IE, Wiedemayer H, Secer S, Asgari S, Stolke D. Surgical removal of brain stem cavernous malformations: surgical indications, technical considerations, and results. *J Neurol Neurosurg Psychiatry* 2002;72:351–5.

49. Hartmann A, Stapf C, Hofmeister C, Mohr JP, Sciacca RR, Stein BM, *et al*. Determinants of neurological outcome after surgery for brain arteriovenous malformation. *Stroke* 2000;31:2361–4.

50. Al-Shahi R, Warlow CP. Interventions for treating brain arteriovenous malformations in adults. *Cochrane Database Syst Rev*. 2006;1:CD003436.

51. Mohr JP, Parides MK, Stapf C, Moquete E, Moy CS, Overbey JR, *et al*. Medical management with or without interventional therapy for unruptured brain arteriovenous malformations (ARUBA): a multicentre, non-blinded, randomised trial. *Lancet*. 2014;383:614–21.

52. Ziai WC, Toung TJ, Bhardwaj A. Hypertonic saline: first-line therapy for cerebral edema? *J Neurol Sci*. 2007;261:157–66.

53. Yang TM, Lin WC, Chang WN, Ho JT, Wang HC, Tsai NW, *et al*. Predictors and outcome of seizures after spontaneous intracerebral hemorrhage. Clinical article. *J Neurosurg*. 2009;111:87–93.

54. Passero S, Rocchi R, Rossi S, Ulivelli M, Vatti G. Seizures after spontaneous supratentorial intracerebral hemorrhage. *Epilepsia* 2002;43:1175–80.

55. Claassen J, Jette N, Chum F, Green R, Schmidt M, Choi H, *et al*. Electrographic seizures and periodic discharges after intracerebral hemorrhage. *Neurology* 2007;69:1356–65.

56. Hemphill JC, Greenberg S, Anderson CS, Becker K, Bendok BR, Cushman M, *et al*., on behalf of the American Heart Association Stroke council, Council on Cardiovascular and Stroke Nursing, and Council on Clinical Cardiology. Guidelines for the management of spontaneous intracerebral hemorrhage: a statement for healthcare professionals from the American Heart Association/American Stroke Association. *Stroke* 2015;46:2032–60.

57. Naidech AM, Garg RK, Liebling S, Levasseur K, Macken MP, Schuele SU, *et al*. Anticonvulsant use and outcomes after intracerebral hemorrhage. *Stroke* 2009;40:3810–5.

58. Balami JS, Buchan AM. Complications of intracerebral haemorrhage. *Lancet Neurol*. 2012;11:101–18.

59. Commichau C, Scarmeas N, Mayer SA. Risk factors for fever in the neurologic intensive care unit. *Neurology* 2003;60:837–41.

60. Godoy DA, Pinero GR, Svampa S, Papa F, Di NM. Early hyperglycemia and intravenous insulin-the rationale and management of hyperglycemia for spontaneous intracerebral hemorrhage patients: is time for change? *Neurocrit Care*. 2009;10:150–3.

61. Fogelholm R, Murros K, Rissanen A, Avikainen S. Admission blood glucose and short term survival in primary intracerebral haemorrhage: a population based study. *J Neurol Neurosurg Psychiatry*. 2005;76:349–53.

62. Finfer S, Chittock DR, Su SY, Blair D, Foster D, Dhingra V, *et al*. Intensive versus conventional glucose control in critically ill patients. *N Engl J Med*. 2009;360:1283–97.

63. Kramer AH, Roberts DJ, Zygun DA. Optimal glycemic control in neurocritical care patients: a systematic review and meta-analysis. *Crit Care*. 2012;16:R203.

64. Caviedes IR, Lavados PM, Hoppe AJ, Lopez MA. Nasolaryngoscopic validation of a set of clinical predictors of aspiration in a critical care setting. *J Bronchology Interv Pulmonol*. 2010;17:33–8.

65. Elliott J, Smith M. The acute management of intracerebral hemorrhage: a clinical review. *Anesth Analg*. 2010;110:1419–27.

66. Boeer A, Voth E, Henze T, Prange HW. Early heparin therapy in patients with spontaneous intracerebral haemorrhage. *J Neurol Neurosurg Psychiatry*. 1991;54:466–7.

67. Poungvarin N, Bhoopat W, Viriyavejakul A, Rodprasert P, Buranasiri P, Sukondhabhant S, *et al*. Effects of dexamethasone in primary supratentorial intracerebral hemorrhage. *N Engl J Med*. 1987;316:1229–33.

68. Kollmar R, Staykov D, Dorfler A, Schellinger PD, Schwab S, Bardutzky J. Hypothermia reduces perihemorrhagic edema after intracerebral hemorrhage. *Stroke*. 2010;41:1684–9.

69. Willmot M, Leonardi-Bee J, Bath PM. High blood pressure in acute stroke and subsequent outcome: a systematic review. *Hypertension*. 2004;43:18–24.

70. Zhang Y, Reilly KH, Tong W, Xu T, Chen J, Bazzano LA, *et al*. Blood pressure and clinical outcome among patients with acute stroke in Inner Mongolia, China. *J Hypertens*. 2008;26:1446–52.

71. Anderson CS, Huang Y, Wang JG, Arima H, Neal B, Peng B, *et al*. Intensive blood pressure reduction in acute cerebral haemorrhage trial (INTERACT): a randomised pilot trial. *Lancet Neurol*. 2008;7:391–9.

72. Antihypertensive Treatment of Acute Cerebral Hemorrhage (ATACH) investigators. Antihypertensive treatment of acute cerebral hemorrhage. *Crit Care Med*. 2010;38:637–48.

73. Arima H, Anderson CS, Wang JG, Huang Y, Heeley E, Neal B, *et al*. Lower treatment blood pressure is associated with greatest reduction in hematoma growth after acute intracerebral hemorrhage. *Hypertension* 2010;56:852–8.

74. Arima H, Huang Y, Wang JG, Heeley E, Delcourt C, Parsons M, *et al*. Earlier blood pressure-lowering and greater attenuation of hematoma growth in acute intracerebral hemorrhage: INTERACT pilot phase. *Stroke* 2012;43:2236–8.

75. Anderson CS, Heeley E, Huang Y, Wang J, Stapf C, Delcourt C, *et al*. Rapid blood-pressure lowering in patients with acute intracerebral hemorrhage. *N Engl J Med*. 2013;368:2355–65.

76. Aguilar MI, Hart RG, Kase CS, Freeman WD, Hoeben BJ, Garcia RC, *et al*. Treatment of warfarin-associated intracerebral hemorrhage: literature review and expert opinion. *Mayo Clin Proc*. 2007;82:82–92.

77. Appelboam R, Thomas EO. Warfarin and intracranial haemorrhage. *Blood Rev*. 2009;23:1–9.

78. Martin M, Conlon LW. Does platelet transfusion improve outcomes in patients with spontaneous or traumatic intracerebral hemorrhage? *Ann Emerg Med*. 2013;61:58–61.

79. Mayer SA, Brun NC, Begtrup K, Broderick J, Davis S, Diringer MN, *et al*. Efficacy and safety of recombinant activated factor VII for acute intracerebral hemorrhage. *N Engl J Med*. 2008;358:2127–37.

80. Yuan ZH, Jiang JK, Huang WD, Pan J, Zhu JY, Wang JZ. A meta-analysis of the efficacy and safety of recombinant activated factor VII for patients with acute intracerebral hemorrhage without hemophilia. *J Clin Neurosci*. 2010;17:685–93.

81. Mayer SA, Davis SM, Skolnick BE, Brun NC, Begtrup K, Broderick JP, *et al*. Can a subset of intracerebral hemorrhage patients benefit from hemostatic therapy with recombinant activated factor VII? *Stroke*. 2009;40:833–40.

82. Wardlaw JM, Murray V, Berge E, del Zoppo G, Sandercock P, Lindley RL, *et al*. Recombinant tissue plasminogen activator for acute ischaemic stroke: an updated systematic review and meta-analysis. *Lancet*. 2012;379:2364–72.

83. Jauch EC, Saver JL, Adams HP, Jr, Bruno A, Connors JJ, Demaerschalk BM, *et al*. Guidelines for the early management of patients with acute ischemic stroke: a guideline for healthcare professionals from the American Heart Association/American Stroke Association. *Stroke*. 2013;44:870–947.

84. Broderick JP. Endovascular therapy for acute ischemic stroke. *Stroke*. 2009;40:S103–S106.

85. Saver JL. Number needed to treat estimates incorporating effects over the entire range of clinical outcomes: novel derivation method and application to thrombolytic therapy for acute stroke. *Arch Neurol*. 2004;61:1066–70.

CHAPTER 20

Acute ischaemic stroke

Barry M. Czeisler, Daniel Sahlein,
and Stephan A. Mayer

Stroke is a rapidly evolving episode of focal or global loss of cerebral function lasting more than 24 hours or leading to death within 24 hours. It represents a collection of devastating clinical syndromes that together are the leading cause of mortality and severe disability worldwide. Acute ischaemic stroke (AIS) is the commonest subtype, accounting for 85% of all strokes, with the remainder being haemorrhagic. Significant advances in the past two decades have resulted in the development of four interventions supported by class I evidence—care on a stroke unit, intravenous (IV) tissue plasminogen activator (tPA) within 4.5 hours of stroke onset, aspirin within 48 hours of stroke onset, and decompressive craniectomy for supratentorial malignant hemispheric cerebral infarction. Expert consensus guidance for the general management of AIS is available from the European Stroke Organisation and the American Stroke Association. In contrast, the evidence base guiding the intensive care unit (ICU) management of AIS is relatively poor despite around 15–20% of stroke patients being admitted to an ICU.

The first stroke unit was described in 1969 and was primarily focused on specialized nursing care (1) but it was the introduction of thrombolysis and endovascular therapies in the 1990s that revolutionized the treatment of AIS. Now considered a true neurological emergency, timely management of AIS has assumed critical importance. Concurrent with the development of new therapies for stroke, the expansion of neurocritical care units (NCCUs) has provided an optimal environment for the neurological monitoring of patients with severe stroke and the management of post-stroke complications. The management of AIS begins prior to admission to the hospital and involves early identification of stroke, notification of emergency medical services (EMS), early IV thrombolysis with tPA and advanced reperfusion techniques on arrival at hospital, as well as targeted management in the post-reperfusion period (Figure 20.1).

Systems of care

The development of acute stroke networks has facilitated timely recognition, diagnosis, and management of AIS and contributed to improved outcomes.

Pre-hospital stroke care

The management of AIS begins with recognition of sudden neurological deficits by the patient or bystanders. Following notification to EMS, dispatchers and EMS personnel must be able to recognize stroke symptoms so that appropriately trained personnel are dispatched to the scene. Pre-hospital stroke scales are available to assist with identification of stroke (2). The Cincinnati Pre-hospital Stroke Scale, also known as the Face Arm Speech Test (FAST), and the Los Angeles Motor Scale (LAMS) are the most widely utilized (Table 20.1) (3,4).

Optimal stroke management requires notification to emergency physicians of when a patient with AIS is en route to hospital, a strategy that has been instituted successfully in several countries (5,6). Pre-hospital notification reduces treatment delays and is recommended in the American Heart Association (AHA)/American Stroke Association (ASA) guidelines (7).

Emergency department stroke care

Coordinated efforts with parallel workflow are necessary for prompt management of the stroke patient on arrival in the emergency department (ED) (8). Longer door-to-needle times for tPA administration are associated with worsened functional outcome and increased rates of symptomatic intracerebral haemorrhage (sICH) after thrombolysis (9). Pre-hospital notification and a single-call activation system to notify all members of the stroke team (stroke physicians, interventional neuroradiology, pharmacy, etc.) is recommended (10).

As soon as the patient arrives at hospital, ED personnel and stroke physicians should obtain a brief history including the neurological deficit and last known normal time, perform a National Institutes for Health (NIH) Stroke Scale (NIHSS) assessment, insert an IV cannula to facilitate computed tomography angiography (CTA), take admission blood tests and check vital signs. When available, point-of-care testing of blood glucose, troponin, international normalized ratio (INR), full blood count, and creatinine testing is desirable. The yield of the prothrombin time (PT), partial thromboplastin time (PTT), or platelet count in identifying unsuspected coagulopathy is extremely low in patients not taking anticoagulation medications or with other reasons to suspect abnormalities, and awaiting such results delays treatment without significant benefit (11). An electrocardiogram (ECG) should be ordered but should not delay computed tomography (CT) scanning unless chest pain is present (7). IV labetalol or nicardipine should be readily available for control of blood pressure that is higher than 185/110 mmHg.

For optimal care of AIS the CT scanning unit should be conceptualized as a resuscitation unit or a far-forward extension of the NCCU. Patients should ideally be taken directly from the ambulance to the CT scanning suite, where initial evaluation is completed and blood tests taken. The availability of trained physicians capable of interpreting CT findings immediately at the patient's bedside is also essential. In Finland, a ten-step protocol initiated over 8 years reduced door-to-needle time from 105 minutes in 1998, to 60

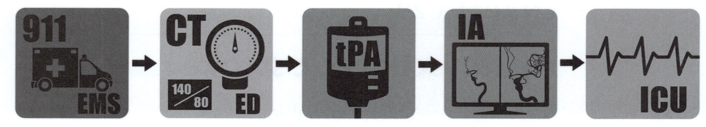

Fig. 20.1 Conceptual framework of the five steps of the stroke chain of survival.
1. Pre-hospital diagnosis
2. Emergency department resuscitation and brain imaging
3. IV thrombolysis
4. IA intervention
5. Intensive care or stroke unit care.
As in all systems, the chain is only as strong as the weakest link.

minutes by 2003, and to 20 minutes by 2011 (Box 20.1) (12). By re-engineering the care pathway in this way it has been possible to administer tPA within accepted time windows to 31% of patients presenting to hospital in Finland, in stark contrast to the 4% of AIS patients who currently receive tPA in the United States (13). Such dramatic improvements highlight the importance of coordinated medical systems management for the successful treatment of AIS.

Neuroimaging

Neuroimaging of acute stroke always begins with non-contrast CT (NCCT) scan. This is the only imaging study required prior to administration of tPA and thrombolysis should never be delayed for further angiographic or perfusion studies. CTA can be considered during the initial imaging study in patients with severe stroke syndromes (NIHSS ≥ 9) or who are ineligible for IV tPA administration; otherwise it should be performed shortly after tPA is given. CTA is currently the optimal imaging modality for the acute identification of large vessel occlusion (LVO) which may be amenable to ultra-early endovascular clot extraction.

Table 20.1 Pre-hospital stroke scales

Cincinnati Pre-hospital Stroke Scale/FAST	Yes	No	
Facial droop?			
Arm drift?			
Speech abnormal?			
Los Angeles Motor Scale	**Points**		
	0	**1**	**2**
Facial strength	Normal	Droop	—
Arms outstretched	Normal	Drifts down	Falls rapidly
Grip strength	Normal	Weak grip	No grip

Defining the infarct

The primary aim of urgent NCCT cranial imaging is to exclude intracerebral haemorrhage (ICH). It is only 40% sensitive for acute

Box 20.1 Ten strategies for reducing door-to-needle time for intravenous thrombolysis after acute ischaemic stroke

- Education of emergency medical services
- Pre-hospital notification for patient registration, ordering of CT and lab tests, and pre-mixing of tPA
- Pre-hospital acquisition of history via cellular phone
- Locating CT scanner in the ED
- Bringing the patient immediately to the CT scanner on hospital arrival
- Obtaining an initial neurological assessment on the CT table
- Immediate interpretation of the CT by a neurologist at the bedside
- Avoiding vascular imaging prior to tPA administration
- Elimination of routine lab testing prior to thrombolysis (can consider point-of-care INR)
- Administration of tPA on the CT table.

Data from Meretoja A *et al.*, 'Reducing in-hospital delay to 20 minutes in stroke thrombolysis', *Neurology*, 2012, 79, 4, pp. 306–313.

infarction and thus will initially be normal in most patients (14), although if early signs of infarction are present they may help guide management. Acute thrombus in a proximal vessel such as the middle cerebral artery (MCA) or basilar artery can appear hyperdense on NCCT (15) and such a finding should trigger mobilization of the neurointerventional team and consideration of suitability for clot extraction.

There are no consistent time-dependent changes in the appearance of brain parenchyma on NCCT within 6 hours of AIS onset, reflecting variation in adequacy of collateral perfusion. Loss of grey–white differentiation from early cytotoxic oedema can be seen in the cortex or deep structures such as the caudate, putamen, or globus pallidus (Figure 20.2). The Alberta Stroke Programme Early CT Score (ASPECTS) was developed to quantify the extent of infarction on initial NCCT and risk of haemorrhagic conversion (16,17), and to predict functional outcome (18). The score consists of seven cortical regions and three subcortical regions in each hemisphere, totalling 10 points for a normal CT scan.

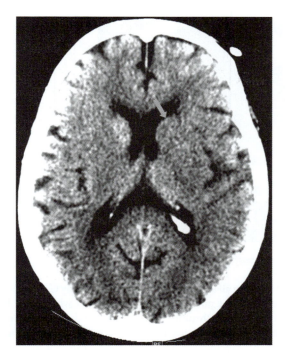

Fig. 20.2 Brain CT scan. Subtle obscuration of grey matter is seen in the left caudate head (arrow) suggesting infarction.

One point is subtracted for each area of visualized infarction (Figure 20.3).

Magnetic resonance (MR) diffusion-weighted imaging (DWI) in conjunction with apparent-diffusion coefficient (ADC) imaging is the most accurate method of detecting infarction within 6 hours of stroke onset. It is 97% sensitive and 100% specific for acute infarction (14). However, MR imaging is not readily available in some centres and it takes substantially longer to obtain MR images than CT, thereby limiting its utility for acute stroke management.

Assessing the vasculature

CTA uses radio-contrast injection to opacify the cervical and cerebral vessels and allow assessment for filling defects or blockages that suggest stenosis and occlusions (Figure 20.4). Patients with an NIHSS of at least 9 have an 86% chance of having an intracranial LVO, making this a good trigger for performing acute vascular imaging with the goal of considering intra-arterial (IA) therapy if LVO is present (19).

MR angiography (MRA) using time-of-flight analysis of flowing blood in the vasculature or contrast for vessel opacification is a well-established technique. However, its utility in AIS is limited by the time necessary for image acquisition. Insonation of proximal cerebral vessels using transcranial Doppler ultrasonography (TCD) can be used to define sites of arterial blockage and guide subsequent therapy. However, substantial technical expertise is required to perform TCD studies, limiting its utility in the acute setting.

Assessing penumbral tissue versus core infarct

ASPECTS may be useful for assessing core infarct that cannot recover with reperfusion. In an analysis of patients successfully recanalized with mechanical thrombectomy in the Penumbra Pivotal Stroke Trial, those with a pre-intervention ASPECTS score of 4 or lower did not benefit from recanalization, those with an ASPECTS score higher than 4 benefited from rapid intervention only, but patients with ASPECTS scores higher than 7 benefited most (20).

CT perfusion (CTP) measures the time for contrast to arrive and the volume of contrast that does arrive in brain regions by repeatedly scanning during a contrast injection (see Chapter 15). By comparing these values to those in the opposite hemisphere an image is created that shows relative amounts of cerebral blood flow (CBF), cerebral blood volume (CBV), and mean transit time (MTT) (Figure 20.5). Low CBF and prolonged MTT suggest impaired perfusion (21). In early states of hypoperfusion, before infarction is established, compensatory distal vasodilation may occur and increase CBV. In

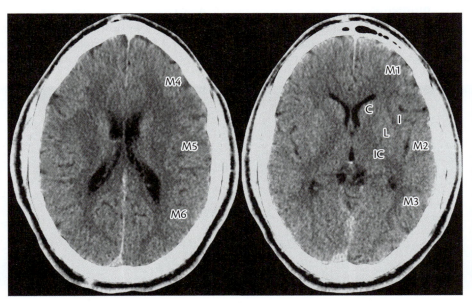

Fig. 20.3 Alberta Stroke Programme Early CT Score (ASPECTS). Two slices of a non-contrast head CT with the 10-point quantitative topographic ASPECTS CT regions overlaid. One point is subtracted from the total of 10 for each area of visualized infarct.

C, caudate head; insular ribbon; IC, internal capsule; L, lentiform nucleus; I, M1, anterior MCA cortex; M2, MCA cortex lateral to insular ribbon; M3, posterior MCA cortex; M4, anterior MCA territory; M5, lateral MCA territory; M6, posterior MCA territory.

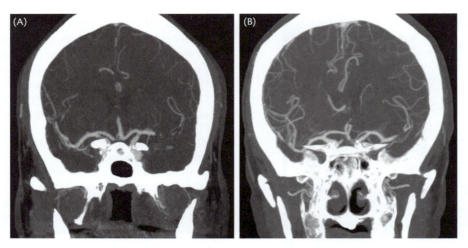

Fig. 20.4 CT angiography, in these examples, confirms blockage of the middle (A) and distal (B) M1 segments of the middle cerebral artery.

contrast, CBV falls in infarcted tissue as blood is shunted away, with low CBV on CTP correlating well with ASPECTS score (22). A large region of low CBF with normal or elevated CBV may represent penumbra that could benefit from reperfusion therapies.

Utilizing a similar technique to CTP, MR perfusion (MRP) imaging obtains similar parameters of CBF, CBV, MTT, and time to peak tracer concentration. Studies suggest that MRP may be able to identify core infarcts and that thrombolysis may prevent large regions with perfusion deficits from progressing to DWI-positive completed infarcts (23,24). MRP has been utilized to select patients with large regions of suspected penumbra to receive thrombolysis beyond the conventional windows for tPA administration, although clinical trials have failed to prove clinical benefit (25,26). MRP is considerably more time consuming to perform than CTP and the delay involved in obtaining and interpreting MRP images may mitigate any benefit of the subsequent intervention.

Summary of imaging recommendations

Ruling out haemorrhage is the primary purpose of brain imaging prior to thrombolysis and therefore, NCCT head, which is widely available, fast, and without contraindications, should be obtained immediately on all suspected stroke patients. Early CTA is indicated in patients with a potential intracranial LVO who might benefit from endovascular thrombectomy. Vessel and perfusion imaging may clarify or confirm sites of vessel occlusion, guide blood pressure (BP) management, guide subsequent treatment location, and establish prognosis (27). However, IV thrombolysis should never be delayed in order to obtain advanced imaging. For patients with severe or fluctuating stroke syndromes presenting beyond 4.5 hours who are not eligible for IV tPA, CTA/CTP or MRA/MRP can be considered as the initial imaging modality (28).

Intravenous thrombolysis

The efficacy of thrombolysis after AIS was established following the publication of the National Institute of Neurological Disorders and Stroke (NINDS) trial in 1995 which confirmed that IV tPA (0.9 mg/kg) administered within 3 hours of stroke onset is associated with an absolute decrease in 3-month functional disability of 13% despite an approximately 6% risk of sICH (29). This outcome benefit remained significant at 1 year post stroke (30). Subsequent large registry studies have confirmed the safety and efficacy of tPA when administered

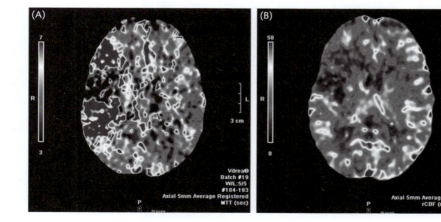
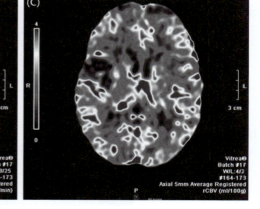

Fig. 20.5 CT perfusion study. The panels show:
(A) Prolonged mean transit time throughout most of the right middle cerebral artery (MCA) territory.
(B) Decreased cerebral blood flow (CBF) in part of the right MCA territory.
(C) Preserved cerebral blood volume (CBV) throughout most of the right MCA territory with small region of low CBV.
Regions of low CBF with preserved CBV may represent salvageable tissue, while regions of low CBV likely represent completed infarct.

within 3 hours of stroke onset (31,32). The European Cooperative Acute Stroke Study (ECASS) III trial showed that IV tPA administered between 3 and 4.5 hours after stroke onset improved outcome compared to placebo in patients age younger than 80 years who were not taking anticoagulation regardless of INR and without comorbid diabetes and prior ischaemic stroke (33). Following these studies the AHA/ASA issued a class I recommendation for use of tPA in in the 3- to 4.5-hour window after AIS onset (34). The third International Stroke Trial (IST-3) was organized in an attempt to expand the treatment window for tPA from 3 to 6 hours, but was unable to show benefit in this extended window (35).

While the utility of tPA up to 4.5 hours after stroke onset is now well established, earlier thrombolysis is always of greater benefit (36). A recent study confirmed that there is a measurable increase in the odds of good recovery for every 15-minute gain in stroke onset-to-needle time (37). Delays in tPA administration decrease its benefit whilst increasing the risk of sICH, with the number need to treat to achieve one functionally independent patient increasing from 4.5 to 15 when tPA is delayed from less than 90 minutes to 4.5 hours after stroke onset (38).

Complications

There are several complications of IV PA and two are worthy of mention. Haemorrhagic conversion of infarcted tissue occurred in 6% of patients in the original NINDS trial (29). Risk factors for haemorrhage include hypertension immediately prior to thrombolysis, advancing age, hyperglycaemia, pre-existing diabetes, more severe stroke, larger infarcts on imaging, early hypo-attenuation on CT, and use of antiplatelet agents other than aspirin (39,40). The presenting symptoms of sICH include headache, nausea, vomiting, worsened neurological deficit, and altered level of consciousness. If a patient develops any of these during thrombolysis, tPA infusion should be discontinued and an urgent CT obtained. Optimal treatment for tPA-related sICH remains undefined but, based on the mechanism of action of tPA, cryoprecipitate and antifibrinolytic therapy with aminocaproic (4 mg IV) or tranexamic (15 mg/kg IV) acid seem reasonable options (41,42). Emergency reversal may not make physiological sense after more than 2 hours after tPA infusion because its half-life is only 5 minutes.

IV tPA has also been associated with orolingual angio-oedema 30–120 minutes after start of the infusion in approximately 1–5% of patients, and the risk is higher in those taking angiotensin-converting enzyme inhibitors. This severe complication carries significant risks of airway compromise, and patients should be treated with diphenhydramine 50 mg IV, methylprednisolone 100 mg IV, and nebulized racemic epinephrine. Endotracheal intubation is required in those with rapidly progressing oedema or evidence of pharyngeal or laryngeal involvement (43).

Interventional therapies

IV tPA has low efficacy for recanalization in LVO and alternative methods of recanalization may be beneficial. Successful recanalization rates of 4% have been reported for internal carotid artery (ICA) occlusion, 32% for proximal MCA (M1) occlusion, 31% for superior or inferior MCA division (M2), occlusion and 4% for basilar artery occlusion (44). Thrombus length of greater than 8 mm is also associated with an extremely low probability of recanalization after IV tPA (45).

Intra-arterial thrombolysis

Early studies showed that IA administration of thrombolytics directly at the site of the thrombus might promote recanalization (46), and prompted the Prolyse in Acute Cerebral Thromboembolism (PROACT) II trial which showed outcome benefit of IA prourokinase (47). In this study, 40% of patients who received IA prourokinase plus heparin achieved a modified Rankin score of 2 or less compared to only 25% of those given heparin alone (P = 0.04), despite a higher rate of sICH in the prourokinase group (10% versus 2%). Recanalization rates were 66% and 18% in the treatment and control groups respectively.

Subsequent studies have been performed using IV tPA as bridging therapy to IA thrombolysis and demonstrated improved recanalization with IA tPA up to 6 hours after stroke onset, but either did not include a control group (48) or demonstrated no definite improvements in clinical outcome (49,50). Increased bleeding risk is a major complication of IA thrombolysis and this may offset some of its potential benefits.

Mechanical thrombectomy

Mechanical thrombectomy became possible after the introduction of the Merci™ device. Early studies demonstrated recanalization rates of 60–70% when the procedure was performed within 8 hours of stroke onset (51). The second approved device, the Penumbra System™, was associated with recanalization rates of 82% within 8 hours of stroke onset (52).

Recent mechanical thrombectomy systems, such as SOLITAIRE™ and TREVO™, incorporate retrievable stents. The SOLITAIRE™ with the intention for thrombectomy (SWIFT) trial compared the Solitaire™ to Merci™ devices within 8 hours of stroke onset and showed recanalization rates of 61% and 24% in the Solitaire™ and Merci™ groups respectively, with lower mortality and improved 3-month outcome in patients treated with Solitaire™ (53). The TREVO™ 2 trial compared the Trevo™ retrievable stent with Merci™ and showed recanalization rates of 68% with Trevo™ compared to only 44% with Merci™ (54). Similar to Solitaire™, Trevo™ was associated with higher rates of long-term functional independence compared with Merci™. In the light of these studies, retrievable stent devices are currently the preferred method for mechanical thrombectomy after AIS. However, in 2013 the Interventional Management of Stroke 3 (IMS 3), Local Versus Systemic Thrombolysis for Acute Ischemic Stroke (SYNTHESIS) and Mechanical Retrieval and Recanalization of Stroke Clots Using Embolectomy (MR-RESCUE) trials were all unable to show benefit for acute endovascular intervention (55–57), even amongst patients with potential salvageable penumbra demonstrated by MRP imaging (57). The results of these trials should be interpreted with caution for several reasons. IV tPA improves outcome only when given within 4.5 hours of stroke onset and endovascular interventions might have a similar window for efficacy. None of these trials adequately addressed this time window, with the angiogram starting after 4.5 hours in 32% of the patients in IMS 3 (55), and endovascular intervention beginning on average 1 hour later than IV tPA in SYNTHESIS (56). In MR-RESCUE the mean time from stroke onset to groin puncture was nearly 6.5 hours, with fewer than 7% of the patients having angiography started within 4.5 hours (57). The degree of recanalization also remains critical to success. In IMS 3, good outcome occurred in 71% of patients with complete recanalization, in 34% of those with less than 50% recanalization and in only 12% with no recanalization. Complete or greater than 50% recanalization occurred in only 23% and 38% of patients in IMS 3 and MR-RESCUE respectively (55,57), with extremely few patients receiving stent retriever devices. In comparison, recanalization rates of 68% to 83% have been reported with the use of stent retrievers in the TREVO 2 and SWIFT trials (53,54).

In 2014 and 2015, numerous subsequent trials reported that endovascular revascularization within 4.5 to 12 hours after stroke onset is effective in improving functional outcome, with one trial showing a benefit in mortality as well (Table 20.2). Recanalization rates in these trials have were high, ranging from 59 to 83%. While the specific inclusion criteria differ amongst the trials, patients were given IV tPA if eligible, and nearly all trials required CT angiography to confirm LVO prior to performing endovascular intervention. For patients presenting with acute ischaemic stroke due to LVO within 6-8 hours, and possibly as far as out as 12 hours from onset, endovascular intervention can be considered as the new standard of care, as stand-alone therapy or as adjunctive therapy with IV tPA.

Complications

Similar to IV tPA, endovascular intervention confers an increased risk of haemorrhagic conversion, with sICH occurring in

approximately 5–10% of patients after IA tPA (47,48) or mechanical intervention (51). Risk factors for haemorrhagic transformation include higher NIHSS score, longer time to recanalization, hyperglycaemia, and low platelet count (58).

Arterial puncture-related complications occurred in 1–2% of patients in the IMS and Merci™ trials (48,59). These took several forms including groin haematoma, retroperitoneal haematoma, pseudoaneurysm formation, arterial dissection, limb ischaemia, and thromboembolism. Frequent groin and distal pulse checks detect problems quickly and should be performed regularly after endovascular intervention. Renal failure secondary to contrast nephropathy is relatively uncommon after endovascular intervention for stroke, occurring in only 3 of 99 patients in one study (60). N-acetylcysteine and hydration with sodium bicarbonate solution have been recommended as preventative strategies in high-risk patients (61,62). Large vessel dissection after interventional therapies is uncommon, occurring in only 0.7% of patients (63). Anticoagulation should be considered to prevent emboli in such cases.

Critical care management

Patients with AIS should be transferred to either a stroke unit or NCCU after initial stabilization and thrombolysis depending on

Table 20.2 Recent trials of intra-arterial therapy for acute ischemic stroke

Trial	N	Imaging selection*	NIHSS	Time window for IAT	TICI 2B-3 for IAT group	mRS 0–2 (%) IAT[†]	mRS 0–2 (%) Control	NNT	OR [95% CI]	Mortality (%) IAT	Mortality (%) Control	OR [95% CI]
MR CLEAN[1]	500	LVO	≥2	≤6 h	59%	33%	19%	7	2.1 [1.4 to 3.4]	21%	22%	NS
EXTEND-IA[2]	70	LVO AND favorable CT perfusion	None	≤6 h	86%	71%	40%	3	4.2 [1.4 to 12]	9%	20%	NS
ESCAPEPE[3]	315	LVO AND favorable collaterals on multiphase CTA	≥6	≤12 h	72%	53%	29%	4	1.7 [1.3 to 2.2]	10%	19%	0.5 [0.3 to 0.8]
REVASCAT[4]	206	LVO	≥6	≤8 h	66%	44%	28%	6	2.0 [1.1 to 3.5]	18%	15%	NS
SWIFT-PRIME[5]	196	LVO AND favorable CT perfusion	10–30	≤6 h	83%	60%	35%	4	1.7 [1.2 to 2.3]	9%	12%	NS
THRACE[6]	395	LVO (including basilar)	10–25	≤5 h	NA	54%	42%	8	NA	13%	13%	NS
THERAPY[‡7]	108	LVO with clot length >8mm on NCHCT	≥8	≤4.5 h	NA	38%	34%	NS	NS	12%	24%	NS

* All studies except for THERAPY used CT angiography for confirmation of LVO.

† Treatment arms were IAT +/– IV tPA (if eligible) vs Best Medical Management except for EXTEND-IA and SWIFT-PRIME which required IV tPA in the interventional group.

‡ THERAPY trial terminated early due to other positive trials (planned enrollment of 692 patients) and was therefore underpowered to show significant results for this outcome.

[1] Berkhemer OA, Fransen PSS, Beumer D, et al. A randomized trial of intraarterial treatment for acute ischemic stroke. N Engl J Med. 2015;372(1):11–20.

[2] Campbell BCV, Mitchell PJ, Kleinig TJ, et al. Endovascular therapy for ischemic stroke with perfusion-imaging selection. N Engl J Med. 2015;372(11):1009–18.

[3] Goyal M, Demchuk AM, Menon BK, et al. Randomized assessment of rapid endovascular treatment of ischemic stroke. N Engl J Med. 2015;372(11):1019–30.

[4] Jovin TG, Chamorro A, Cobo E, et al. Thrombectomy within 8 hours after symptom onset in ischemic stroke. N Engl J Med. 2015. Epub ahead of print. doi: 10.1056/NEJMoa1503780.

[5] Saver JL, Goyal M, Bonafe A, et al. Stent-retriever thrombectomy after intravenous t-PA vs t-PA alone in stroke. N Engl J Med. 2015. Epub ahead of print. doi: 10.1056/NEJMoa1415061.

[6] Trial and Cost Effectiveness Evaluation of Intra-Arterial Thrombectomy in Acute Ischemic Stroke (THRACE). Presented at the meeting of the European Stroke Organisation, April 2015, Glasgow, UK.

[7] Assess the Penumbra System in the Treatment of Acute Stroke (THERAPY). Presented at the meeting of the European Stroke Organisation, April 2015, Glasgow, UK.

CTA, CT angiography; IAT, intra-arterial therapy; LVO, large vessel occlusion; mRS, modified Rankin scale; NA, not available; NCHCT, noncontrast head CT; NS, non-significant; TICI, thrombolysis in cerebral infarction score; tPA, tissue-plasminogen activator.

Reproduced with permission from *Merritt's Textbook of Neurology*, 13th ed. New York: Wolters Kuwer publishers, 2016.

Box 20.2 Indications for admission to a neurocritical care unit

Stroke characteristics

- large MCA infarction
- basilar artery occlusion
- large cerebellar infarction
- capsular-warning syndrome/crescendo TIAs
- blood pressure-dependent symptoms
- rapid neurological worsening

Post-thrombolysis *and*

- need for IV medications to control blood pressure in peri-thrombolysis period
- high bleeding risk after IV tPA

Post-endovascular intervention

Other

- impaired airway, mechanical ventilation
- cardiac infarction or arrhythmia.

various clinical factors (Box 20.2). Transfer should be accomplished quickly as delays are associated with worse outcome (64). Several studies have shown that care by a dedicated neurointensivist-led multidisciplinary team is associated with improved outcomes after AIS (65,66). Based on these data, the AHA/ASA considers NCCUs essential elements of a comprehensive stroke centre (7).

Blood pressure management

The majority of AIS patients are hypertensive at presentation (67), with BP decreasing independently over the subsequent hours and days (68). Studies have shown that both admission hypotension and hypertension are associated with poor outcome (69). Optimal BP management is critical because cerebral autoregulation may be impaired acutely after AIS (70).

Clinical trials to determine optimal BP goals beyond 6 hours after AIS onset have not yielded definitive results (71). Studies of various classes of antihypertensive agents and subsequent meta-analyses of these studies have all failed to show improvement in outcome from antihypertensive therapy after AIS (72–74). In contrast, an acute fall in BP during the acute phase of AIS (< 6 hours) can worsen outcomes. A decrease in systolic BP (SBP) of > 20 mmHg is associated with early neurological deterioration, larger infarcts, and higher mortality (75). In practice, chronic antihypertensive medications are commonly administered at lower dosages or withheld entirely during the acute phase after AIS to minimize the risk of hypotension. Current guidelines recommend avoiding the treatment of hypertension in patients who have not received thrombolytics unless BP is higher than 220/120 mmHg (7). However, severe hypertension may worsen end-organ damage in patients with heart failure, acute coronary syndrome, or accelerated hypertensive nephropathy and may require treatment for this reason. Cautious lowering of BP towards normotension over several days should be considered in patients with stable neurological deficits after the first 24–48 hours.

Specific classes of antihypertensive agents have effects that may be relevant after AIS. Renin–angiotensin–aldosterone system (RAAS) modulators have been well studied and a meta-analysis showed that patients with a recent ischaemic stroke treated with RAAS modulators had a small but significantly lower risk of major vascular events and recurrent stroke (76). If antihypertensive agents are required, angiotensin-converting-enzyme inhibitors or angiotensin-receptor blockers are the preferred first-line agents unless there are contraindications.

There is some weak evidence that a subgroup of patients might benefit from carefully controlled increases in BP after AIS. Retrospective and prospective studies have shown neurological improvement and smaller infarct volumes in selected AIS patients with fluctuating neurological deficits from haemodynamic perfusion failure who were treated with induced hypertension (77,78). In a small prospective study, maintaining SBP greater than 160 mmHg, or 20% higher than baseline, was associated with neurological improvement in seven of 13 patients, and a clear BP threshold below which symptoms again worsened was identified in six (79). Hypertensive therapy was continued for between 1 and 6 days and then successfully weaned in all patients. While some patients in this small study had LVO, others had small vessel infarcts so the potential applicability of this therapy is broad. Induced hypertension is relatively contraindicated in those with a history of coronary artery disease, cardiac arrhythmias, congestive heart failure, or evidence of cardiac ischaemia.

Airway and respiratory management

Stroke patients with large hemispheric infarction, posterior circulation infarction, and history of pulmonary disease may be at risk of airway or respiratory compromise. Among intubated stroke patients, most require intubation within 48 hours of stroke onset and some within the first 6 hours (80). Importantly, once AIS patients deteriorate, up to half require intubation within 1 hour. Close monitoring in a critical care environment is therefore required in the early hours after stroke for those at high risk for this complication.

Oxygen saturations should be maintained between 94% and 100% to optimize oxygen delivery to ischaemic brain tissue (7). Mechanical ventilation is adjusted to maintain normocapnia since hypercapnia can lead to increased ICP in patients with large infarcts and hypocapnia can cause cerebral vasoconstriction and worsen brain ischaemia. BP should be closely monitored when applying higher levels of positive end-expiratory pressure, as increased intrathoracic pressure-associated reductions in BP can worsen cerebral hypoperfusion in some patients (81). Specific modes of mechanical ventilation have not been thoroughly studied after AIS but any ventilator settings necessary to achieve the goals of normoxia and normocapnia whilst minimizing the risk of ventilator-induced lung injury are appropriate (see Chapter 4).

The overall prognosis of patients who require mechanical ventilation after AIS is relatively poor, although approximately 20–40% survive (80,82). Age greater than 65 years, depressed level of consciousness, loss of brainstem reflexes and neurological deterioration after intubation are independent predictors of mortality among intubated stroke patients (83). As many as 50–60% who survive mechanical ventilation have good long-term functional outcomes (83), including up to 25% of those older than 65 years (84). In family surveys, more than 75% report that they would again support a decision to proceed with intubation regardless of whether or not their relatives survived (80).

Specific stroke syndromes

There are different management strategies for ischaemic strokes affecting specific anatomical brain regions.

Malignant middle cerebral artery territory infarction

The malignant MCA infarction syndrome is characterized by massive hemispheric infarction with subsequent oedema. It can lead to brain herniation and death approximately 2–3 days after stroke onset, although neurological worsening can occur anytime between 24 hours and 7 days after stroke onset (85). Up to 30% of deaths related to MCA infarction occur from brain herniation, with others mostly related to infection (86). In patients with space-occupying brain oedema, mortality is as high as 80% despite maximal medical treatment in an ICU (87), raising neurosurgical decompression as a potential treatment option.

Predicting neurological deterioration

Not all patients with large MCA infarction develop oedema severe enough to cause herniation, prompting considerable efforts to identify those who will progress to herniation. Clinical signs of worsening cerebral oedema include drowsiness, asymmetric pupils, periodic breathing patterns, vomiting, and ipsilateral corticospinal tract signs. However, most of these changes occur relatively late, with pupillary abnormalities appearing on average within 4 hours of the onset of drowsiness (88). Clinical signs are therefore unreliable determinants for the development of severe oedema.

Imaging may be of some utility for the prediction of herniation. Studies show that greater than 50% infarction of the MCA territory on CT, or DWI infarct volume of greater than 145 mL, is predictive of progression to 'malignant' infarction (89,90). Clinical trials of hemicraniectomy have therefore usually specified greater than 50–66% involvement of the MCA territory as a trigger for surgical intervention. Elevated ICP does not correlate well with midline shift on imaging and many patients may develop brainstem injury from herniation before ICP becomes critically elevated (91). ICP monitoring is therefore not useful in this setting and may instead provide a false sense of security. Cerebral microdialysis and brain tissue oxygen tension monitoring of non-infarcted brain tissue regions has been attempted to predict malignant changes but these modalities are of uncertain benefit (see Chapters 11 and 12).

Medical management

Various therapies have been used in patients who develop clinical signs of oedema or radiological evidence of midline shift/cisternal effacement, although none have been definitively evaluated in prospective clinical trials. Acute hyperventilation may reverse herniation but this effect is short-lived and prolonged hyperventilation can precipitate cerebral ischaemia (92). Hypertonic saline and mannitol are both effective in the management of elevated ICP or reversal of herniation events (93,94), and theoretical concerns that they might worsen brain shift by more effectively dehydrating the uninvolved hemisphere with intact blood–brain barrier integrity have not been substantiated (94). Hypothermia has been used with some success in patients with malignant MCA infarction. It lowers ICP and cerebral metabolism and possibly improves outcome (95,96), although it is not as effective as hemicraniectomy (97). Moreover, hypothermia is associated with complications such as shivering, thrombocytopenia, bradycardia, and pneumonia (97,98), and slow rewarming is required to prevent rebound cerebral oedema (98).

Barbiturates can potentially lower ICP in the context of malignant MCA infarction but severe side effects prevent any outcome benefit (99). Hyperglycaemia has been associated with worsened cerebral oedema and a higher risk of haemorrhagic conversion (100), and insulin therapy to maintain normoglycaemia is therefore indicated (see Chapter 28).

Surgical management

Case series in the 1990s described lower mortality and higher rates of independence after hemicraniectomy for malignant MCA infarction, with predominant benefit in younger patients (101). Patients older than 55 years had improved survival but worse functional outcomes after surgery. It was also initially supposed that hemicraniectomy might not be useful in dominant hemispheric infarction, although subsequent studies have shown that there can be significant improvement of aphasia over time (102) and similar long-term quality of life compared to those with non-dominant hemispheric infarction undergoing surgical decompression (103).

Some case series evaluating timing of hemicraniectomy have shown survival benefit and improved functional outcome amongst patients treated earlier, usually within the first 24 hours (104,105). One study evaluated hemicraniectomy before and after signs of herniation and confirmed a benefit for survival and ability to perform activities of daily living with early hemicraniectomy (106). However, a systematic review in 2004 found no association between outcome and timing of surgery or presence of signs of herniation prior to surgery (107).

Given the uncertainty in these early data, several clinical trials were initiated. The Decompressive Surgery for the Treatment of Malignant Infarction of the Middle Cerebral Artery (DESTINY) trial included patients aged 18–60 years who were previously independent and had either left or right MCA infarction occupying at least two-thirds of the vascular territory (108). At approximately the same time, the Decompressive Craniectomy in Malignant Middle Cerebral Artery Infarction (DECIMAL) trial recruited patients age 18–55 and with greater than 50% MCA territory infarction (109). Given their similar methodologies, the DESTINY and DECIMAL trials were combined in a pre-planned pooled analysis with the patients already enrolled in the Hemicraniectomy After Middle Cerebral Artery Infarction with Life-Threatening Edema Trial (HAMLET), which was ongoing at the same time (110). The combined analysis included 93 patients aged between 18 and 60 years with surgical intervention within 48 hours of stroke onset and demonstrated that hemicraniectomy was associated with an absolute risk reduction of 51% for death or severe disability (mRS 5 or 6), and a 23% absolute increase in the proportion of patients who were alive and able to walk independently at 6 months (110). These results correspond to an astonishing number needed to treat of two for survival, and four for survival with mild-to-moderate disability (mRS 0–3). In other words, for every ten hemicraniectomies undertaken, five patients would escape death and of these new survivors one would have mild disability, one moderate disability, and three moderate-to-severe disability with an inability to walk. When surveyed, 84% of patients and family members said that they would choose hemicraniectomy again given these outcomes (111). Quality of life after hemicraniectomy has been shown to be satisfactory for most patients even in the face of moderate-to-severe disability or aphasia (112).

More recently, the DESTINY II trial evaluated the benefit of hemicraniectomy for malignant MCA in patients aged over 60 years (113). Surgery reduced mortality from 70% to 33% but at the cost of more survivors with poor neurological outcomes. Of those who survived, nearly all were either bedbound or unable to walk independently and there was no increase in the rate of survival with mild to moderate disability.

Hemicraniectomy should therefore be offered early to all patients under age 60 with large MCA infarctions who had good functional status prior to stroke onset. For older patients, the expected prognosis should be discussed with the patients or family members prior to making treatment decisions.

Cerebellar infarction

Cytotoxic oedema from cerebellar infarction can cause devastating brainstem compression, hydrocephalus from obstruction of the fourth ventricle, and tonsillar or upward brain herniation. Death occurs in up to 85% of untreated cases who deteriorate secondary to worsening oedema (114). Most deterioration occurs between 48 and 96 hours after stroke onset and peaks at 72 hours, although worsening can occur as late as 10 days after infarction (115). Initial clinical signs of worsening oedema include drowsiness, bilateral Babinski's signs, horizontal gaze disturbances, hemiparesis, and respiratory dysrhythmia. These occur on average 24 hours prior to the onset of coma, but in some cases coma can develop within 4 hours of the appearance of the first clinical signs. Patients with large cerebellar infarction should therefore be admitted to an NCCU for close monitoring. As well as clinical observation, serial imaging may also be useful as hydrocephalus, brainstem, or basal cistern compression may herald deterioration (116).

Treatment

In a 1973 review of 36 cases with cerebellar infarction and progressive neurological worsening, 18 of 22 patients who had suboccipital surgical decompression survived while all 14 patients who were managed conservatively died (117). Potential benefit for functional outcome has also been shown after surgical decompression. As many as 40% of cerebellar infarct patients have been reported to live independently after suboccipital craniectomy (118). External ventricular drain placement can be considered as an initial treatment but poses the risk of upward herniation and simply delays decompressive surgery in many cases. Definitive decompressive surgery should be the initial intervention in patients with space-occupying cerebellar infarction, depressed level of consciousness, and clinical signs of corticospinal tract compression.

Basilar artery occlusion

A diagnosis of basilar artery occlusion (BAO) should be considered in patients presenting with vertigo, cranial nerve deficits, horizontal gaze paresis, dysarthria, ataxia, tetraparesis, or sudden alterations in consciousness (119). Some present with progressive mild to moderate symptoms while others are comatose at onset (120). BAO has an extremely poor prognosis. Mortality is as high as 90% without treatment (121), and many survivors are left with functional deficits ranging from ataxia or weakness to locked-in syndrome in severe cases. Similar to strokes in other locations, a penumbral region of salvageable brain tissue may be present after BAO (122) and this warrants consideration of reperfusion. The poor prognosis without treatment has led many to pursue aggressive measures for reperfusion even long after stroke onset.

A high index of suspicion is required for early diagnosis and treatment of BAO. Basilar artery syndromes often begin insidiously, progressing in a stuttering manner over time and are extraordinarily difficult to recognize. Given its wide availability, CTA is the preferred method for confirming the diagnosis of BAO.

Treatment

Recanalization by any means is strongly associated with improved outcome after BAO. A large series of patients treated with IV thrombolysis showed that approximately half were alive at 1 year, and that half of survivors achieved good functional recovery (123). Case series have also demonstrated outcome benefits from IA thrombolysis and mechanical thrombectomy after BAO, even when treated between 12 and 24 hours after stroke onset (124,125). While concerns exist about potential haemorrhage with late recanalization, this is likely outweighed by the extremely poor natural history of untreated BAO. For patients with mild to moderate symptoms, IV tPA and close monitoring may be appropriate, but IV tPA, IA thrombolysis, mechanical thrombectomy or some combination thereof are all appropriate considerations in those with severe syndromes or worsening neurological status.

Crescendo transient ischaemic attacks

There are several causes of crescendo transient ischaemic attacks (TIAs).

Carotid stenosis

Recurrent TIAs or anterior circulation strokes with associated stenosis of the ipsilateral internal carotid artery may result from haemodynamic perfusion failure or artery-to-artery embolus. In the absence of large established infarction, patients with symptomatic carotid stenosis should undergo carotid endarterectomy or carotid stenting as soon as possible after presentation to reduce the risk of recurrent ischaemic strokes (126,127).

Intracranial stenosis

Patients with intracranial stenosis may present with fluctuating symptoms due to hypoperfusion across a fixed stenosis, and haemodynamic support with vasopressors may be required to ensure adequate perfusion until collateral circulation develops. The Stenting and Aggressive Medical Management for Preventing Recurrent stroke in Intracranial Stenosis (SAMMPRIS) study showed that aggressive medical therapy results in a lower risk of stroke or death at 30 days compared to percutaneous angioplasty and intracranial stenting, primarily because of procedural complications (128).

Capsular warning syndrome

The capsular warning syndrome is a complex TIA syndrome characterized by stereotypical recurrent motor or sensorimotor symptoms related to a lesion of a small penetrating artery in the internal capsule, basal ganglia, or pons (129). The underlying pathophysiology may involve occlusion or stenosis of a penetrating artery, or large vessel atherosclerosis at the origin of a perforating vessel (130,131). Capsular warning syndrome is a medical emergency. Sixty per cent of cases progress to permanent infarction within 1 week with dissipation of the stroke risk thereafter (132). Patients with stereotypical recurrent TIAs have been treated with thrombolysis or combination antiplatelet therapy with success (133,134), but anticoagulation with heparin is not efficacious (135). Some patients with capsular warning syndrome have blood pressure dependent symptoms, warranting observation and management, including haemodynamic optimization with vasopressors, in the NCCU (136).

Cervical artery dissection

Carotid and vertebral artery dissections cause 2% of strokes overall, with carotid dissection being twice as common as vertebral dissection. Cervical artery dissection may be the underlying cause of stroke in 10–25% of patients younger than 50 years of age (137). Most strokes result from artery-to-artery embolism and the majority occur within 24 hours of the dissection, although some are delayed by up to 1 week (138,139). Patients may have a history of neck twisting or trauma and commonly present with headache, neck pain and stroke symptoms. Horner's syndrome can also occur after carotid dissection as a result of disruption of the sympathetic fibres surrounding the carotid artery (137).

Concerns of recurrent arterial thrombus with subsequent artery-to-artery emboli have led some to advocate anticoagulation for patients with cervical artery dissection (140). No randomized trial has been completed but clinical studies and meta-analyses have shown no difference in mortality or stroke occurrence in patients treated with antiplatelet agents compared to anticoagulation (141,142). Pending the results of a randomized controlled trial, either treatment seems reasonable. Anticoagulation may be preferred in patients with free-floating thrombus on imaging, recurrent strokes or TIAs, or TCD-demonstrated microemboli, whereas antiplatelet agents are favoured in those with a large established infarct to minimize the risk of haemorrhagic transformation (140).

Prevention of stroke recurrence

Secondary prevention strategies for ischaemic stroke are primarily driven by the mechanistic cause of the infarction determined by diagnostic tests (Boxes 20.3 and 20.4).

Anticoagulation

For much of the twentieth century, heparin was administered after AIS to prevent stroke progression or re-embolization. However,

---

> **Box 20.3** Stroke aetiologies
>
> #### Common aetiologies
>
> - Intracranial small vessel arteriosclerosis
> - Intracranial large vessel atherosclerosis
> - Carotid or vertebral artery atherosclerosis with artery-to-artery embolism
> - Cardioembolism
> - Cryptogenic stroke.
>
> #### Less common aetiologies
>
> - Hypercoagulable state
> - Cervical artery dissection
> - Vasculopathy/vasculitis (numerous infectious and inflammatory aetiologies)
> - Endocarditis
> - Paradoxical embolism.

> **Box 20.4** Diagnostic studies
>
> #### Acute studies
>
> - CT head without contrast—to exclude haemorrhage
> - CT angiogram (if NIHSS ≥ 9)—to confirm/exclude large vessel occlusion
> - Full blood count, urea/electrolytes, PT/PTT, and troponin.
>
> #### Subsequent usual studies
>
> - MRI brain without contrast—evaluate for size and location of infarct
> - MRA brain and neck without contrast—clarify intracranial and extracranial vasculature
> - Transthoracic echocardiogram—evaluate for cardioembolic source
> - Electrocardiogram—monitor for arrhythmia (i.e. atrial fibrillation) as a cardioembolic source
> - HgbA1c—screen for diabetes mellitus
> - Lipid profile—evaluate for hyperlipidaemia
> - Thyroid stimulating hormone—evaluate for hyperthyroidism (could predispose to atrial fibrillation).
>
> #### Other
>
> - Carotid ultrasound or CTA head and neck if contraindication to MRI, poor quality MRI, or otherwise unable to obtain MRI
> - MRI/MRA to exclude neck artery dissection (T1 or proton density fat saturated images, MRA with contrast) if diagnosis is considered
> - Transoesophageal echocardiogram—if cardioembolic source is suspected
> - Lower extremity ultrasound or CT venogram pelvis—evaluate for source of paradoxical embolus in setting of right-to-left cardiac shunt
> - Serum inflammatory markers (e.g. erythrocyte sedimentation rate and C-reactive protein)—evaluate for vasculitis or endocarditis
> - Rheumatological antibody titres
> - Hypercoagulation screen—(homocysteine, antiphospholipid antibody, lupus anticoagulant, factor V Leiden, prothrombin G20210A mutation, protein C/S activity and levels, antithrombin III levels, beta-2 microglobulin).

---

multiple trials have shown that any benefit from unfractionated (UFH) or low-molecular-weight heparin (LMWH) is outweighed by an increased risk of intracranial and systemic haemorrhage (143,144). Moreover, studies in subgroups of patients with atrial fibrillation (AF) (145), cardioembolic strokes in general (146), small infarcts (147) and large artery atherosclerotic disease (148), have also shown no benefit from acute anticoagulation. A non-randomized comparison confirmed that 30% of patients continued to have progressive infarction regardless of whether or not heparin was administered (149).

There were criticisms that early studies enrolled patients too late (24–48 hours) after stroke onset, but the Therapy of Patients with Acute Stroke (TOPAS) trial was also unable to show outcome benefit from treatment with high-dose dalteparin despite administration within 7–8 hours of stroke onset (150). Camerlingo and colleagues studied heparin administration within 3 hours of stroke onset and did demonstrate improved rates of 3 month independence in those receiving heparin compared to placebo (151), but other studies have not yet corroborated these findings. Importantly, the risk of recurrent ischaemic stroke in the IST, Trial of ORG 10172 in Acute Stroke Treatment (TOAST), and Chinese Acute Stroke Trial (CAST) was only 1.4% on average, so there is little potential benefit in preventing recurrent ischaemic stroke during the acute phase of care (152). The majority of evidence suggests that anticoagulation should no longer be routinely administered for this purpose (153). Anticoagulation is important for long-term stroke prevention in patients with AF, but treatment should be delayed for 2–4 weeks in patients with large infarction to minimize the risk of haemorrhagic conversion.

Acute anticoagulation may be warranted for AIS patients with hypercoagulable states, active intracardiac thrombus, large artery dissection, or mechanical prosthetic heart valves, all of which confer significantly higher risk of recurrent emboli (154). However, the risk of haemorrhage with acute anticoagulation must be carefully weighed against potential benefit in such cases.

Antiplatelet agents

Two large trials, IST and CAST, showed that acute aspirin administration has a small but measurable benefit for reducing early recurrent strokes and mortality during the first year after AIS (143,155). Aspirin is therefore routinely recommended after AIS at a dose of 160–326 mg daily in the acute phase (7), decreasing to 75–100 mg at discharge. In patients who received thrombolysis, aspirin administration should be delayed for 24 hours as co-administration with tPA increases the rate of sICH without improving outcome (156).

Acute administration of dual antiplatelet therapy has been evaluated in several studies. One compared early (within 7 days after stroke) or late (after 7 days) aspirin and dipyridamole and showed no difference in functional outcome between the two groups (157). A meta-analysis of patients treated with dual antiplatelet therapy within 72 hours of stroke onset showed significantly reduced stroke recurrence and a non-significant trend to major bleeding, suggesting potential benefit overall (158). Most recently, the Clopidogrel in High-Risk Patients with Acute Non-disabling Cerebrovascular Events (CHANCE) trial showed that the combination of aspirin and clopidogrel given for the first 21 days after minor stroke or TIA reduced recurrent stroke at 90 days compared with aspirin alone, without an increased risk of bleeding (159). Dual antiplatelet therapy may therefore be beneficial when used for a short period after AIS, maximizing benefit while minimizing bleeding risk, but this requires confirmation in further studies.

Statins

Statins have plaque stabilization and potential neuroprotective actions independent of their ability to lower cholesterol (160). The Stroke Prevention by Aggressive Reduction in Cholesterol Levels (SPARCL) trial showed that high-dose atorvastatin reduced overall recurrent AIS and all-cause cardiovascular events when started within several months after AIS (161). Although potential benefit of immediate statin therapy after AIS has been suggested in case series, its efficacy has never been demonstrated in a large clinical trial (162). However, patients taking statins should have their treatment continued in the acute setting as withdrawal has been associated with worse outcome after AIS (163).

Complications after stroke

The neurological and systemic complications of AIS must be treated aggressively to maximize the chances of good recovery.

Neurological complications

The incidence of neurological worsening within the first few days after AIS is variably reported to lie between 13% and 43% (164). Consistently identified predictors of neurological worsening include NIHSS score higher than 7, ICA or M1 occlusion, brainstem infarction, pre-existing or newly diagnosed diabetes mellitus, and early focal hypodensity on CT with cortical and subcortical involvement (164–166). In terms of stroke subtype, neurological worsening is most common after total anterior circulation infarction, followed by small vessel penetrator and posterior circulation infarction, with partial anterior circulation infarction being associated with the lowest risk of deterioration (167).

Treatment should be directed at correcting the underlying cause of the neurological worsening (Table 20.3). Blood pressure should be correlated with previous values to determine whether the neurological deterioration is related to relative hypotension when administration of IV fluids and vasopressors may improve cerebral perfusion and restore neurological function. After initial vital signs assessment and examination an urgent NCCT should be obtained and vessel imaging with either CTA or MRA may also identify a treatable cause. If no other explanation is identified, continuous EEG should be considered to exclude seizure activity.

Haemorrhagic conversion

Haemorrhagic transformation occurs in 9–43% of patients who have not been treated with thrombolysis, although this most often presents as small petechial haemorrhages of little of no clinical consequence (168). Asymptomatic haemorrhagic transformation with no mass effect is not associated with worse outcome and merely requires observation (169). If symptomatic haemorrhagic transformation with associated mass effect is detected, antiplatelet and anticoagulant therapies should be held and reversed.

Seizures

Early seizures (within 1–2 weeks) occur in approximately 3–8% of patients after AIS (170,171). They are most commonly associated with cortical infarcts (172) but can occur after subcortical strokes (171,172).While short-lived post-stroke seizures may not adversely affect outcome, up to 25% of patients who develop seizures progress to status epilepticus which is associated with higher rates of mortality (see Chapter 23) (173,174). Despite this, a 2014 Cochrane review found insufficient evidence to support the routine use of AEDs for primary or secondary seizure prevention after AIS (175), and seizure prophylaxis cannot be recommended.

Delirium

Approximately 10–30% of stroke patients suffer from delirium in the acute setting and this is associated with a fourfold increase in inpatient and 12-month mortality, increased hospital length of stay, and a higher likelihood of discharge to a nursing home or other

Table 20.3 Differential diagnosis and management of neurological worsening after acute ischaemic stroke

Aetiology	Clinical signs/symptoms	Diagnosis	Management
Neurological			
Thrombus propagation or movement	Worsened or new deficits in the same vascular territory	MRA, CTA, TCD, DSA	Heparin, IA intervention if large proximal lesion
Recurrent embolism	New deficits in a different vascular territory	MRI/MRA, CT/CTA	IA intervention if large proximal lesion
Re-occlusion of a recanalized artery	Re-emergence of same deficits after initial improvement	MRA, CTA, TCDs, DSA	IA intervention if large proximal lesion
Hypoperfusion across a fixed lesion	Deficits emerge with relative hypotension	Check blood pressure	Consider BP augmentation
Haemorrhagic conversion	Worsened or new deficits in the same vascular territory. Depressed level of consciousness	Non-contrast CT	Emergency reversal of anticoagulation. Consider neurosurgical intervention if large
Cerebral oedema	Depressed level of consciousness. Respiratory and haemodynamic changes. Posturing. False-localizing signs	Non-contrast CT	ICP management. Consider hemicraniectomy
Seizures	Focal involuntary movements. Eye deviation. Worsened existing deficits. Episodic worsening, stereotypical events	cEEG	Antiepileptic medications
Non-neurological			
Hyperthermia	Worsening correlates with fever	Check temperature	Acetaminophen and/or NSAIDs, consider exogenous cooling to maintain normothermia
Delirium	Waxing and waning level of consciousness	Diagnosis of exclusion	Treat underlying causes, administer antipsychotic agents

cEEG, continuous electroencephalography; CTA, computed tomography angiography; DSA, digital subtraction angiography; IA, intra-arterial; MRA, magnetic resonance angiography; TCD, transcranial Doppler ultrasonography.

institutional care (176). Pre-existing cognitive decline is the primary risk factor for delirium after AIS, although coexisting infection has also been implicated (177). The most effective treatment for delirium is prevention, which involves frequent reorientation, early mobilization, preservation of normal sleep–wake cycles, and minimizing use of unnecessary restraints and monitors (178). If delirium persists despite modification of risk factors, antipsychotic medications should be considered (see Chapter 26).

Non-neurological complications

Non-neurological complications after acute brain injury are discussed in detail in Chapter 27, and only a summary of those issues specific to AIS will be highlighted here.

Hyperglycaemia

Hyperglycaemia occurs in 30–40% of patients in the acute phase after AIS (179) and may occur in those without pre-existing diabetes mellitus. Most non-diabetic stroke patients have no evidence of poor pre-stroke glycaemic control as assessed by HgbA1c values (180). Activation of the hypothalamic–pituitary–adrenal axis causing increased cortisol and catecholamine levels that stimulate glucose production and cause insulin resistance are the likely causes of post-stroke hyperglycaemia (181). Many studies have shown an independent relationship between admission hyperglycaemia and mortality, poor neurological outcome and larger infarct volume or

infarct expansion after AIS (182,183). In a meta-analysis, admission glucose level greater than 7 mmol/L (126 mg/dL) was associated with a threefold increase in 30-day mortality in non-diabetic stroke patients (183). Average glucose values measured over the first several days after AIS are independently associated with higher mortality and worsened outcome (184).

Several studies have attempted to evaluate the safety and efficacy of insulin therapy for hyperglycaemia after AIS. Most have been underpowered to demonstrate efficacy but all have demonstrated a high incidence of hypoglycaemia in patients treated with intensive insulin regimens (185–189). In a cohort study of critically ill neurological patients undergoing intensive insulin therapy (of which 5% had AIS), greater degrees of hypoglycaemia correlated with higher mortality (190). A large trial of intensive glycaemic management in general critical care patients also showed worsened mortality with aggressive glucose control (191), countering previous data suggesting benefit from intensive insulin therapy (192). AHA/ASA guidelines recommend maintaining a target glucose range of 7.5–10.0 mmol/L (140–180 mg/dL) and treating hypoglycaemia when blood glucose is lower than 3.3 mmol/L (60 mg/dL (7).

Cardiovascular

Electrocardiographic abnormalities are identified in around 90% of patients after AIS (193). Elevated serum markers of cardiac injury are seen in up to 34% of patients and are independently associated with increased mortality and impaired post-stroke performance (194). There is a possible association between cardiac troponin elevation and strokes involving the insular or peri-insular cortex (195), suggesting a relationship with autonomic regulation. Most of the changes in serum biomarkers after AIS do not represent cardiac ischaemic events but neurogenic stunned myocardium syndrome (see Chapter 27) (196).

Myocardial infarction (MI) is rare after stroke, occurring in only 0.9% of patients in one large study (195). Importantly, most patients with a true MI in this study were asymptomatic. Cardiology review is indicated in all patients with signs of cardiac ischaemia after AIS, although this may not necessarily be required in the acute inpatient setting.

AF is a strong risk factor for AIS and patients frequently develop AF in the early post-stroke period (197). It is independently associated with higher mortality even after correction for stroke severity (198), and much of this excess mortality is related to cardiac causes (199). Accordingly, patients with AF should be monitored for evidence of developing myocardial ischaemia or worsening heart failure. Ventricular arrhythmias also occur frequently after AIS, and sudden cardiac death has been reported after strokes involving the insula especially on the right side (200). ECG monitoring is warranted for all patients after AIS, both to evaluate for underlying sources of cardioembolism and for the early detection of potentially dangerous arrhythmias.

Decompensated heart failure occurs in approximately 3% of patients within the first week after AIS (201), and both systolic and diastolic failure are associated with worse outcome (202). Heart failure may be precipitated by stroke-related hypertension, post-stroke MI, cardiac arrhythmia or iatrogenic volume overload. Some cases may represent neurogenic stunned myocardium syndrome in the setting of high sympathetic outflow states and insular infarction (see Chapter 27) (203).

Respiratory

Various respiratory dysrhythmias can occur in the setting of AIS. Cheyne–Stokes respiration (see Chapter 4) is by far the most common and occurs in approximately 50% of patients with supratentorial infarction (204). It most commonly resolves after the acute period and does not confer higher mortality. Between 50% and 70% of patients have sleep-disordered breathing in the first 24 hours after AIS and again this commonly improves after a few days (205). Risk factors include elevated body mass index, increasing neck circumference and limb weakness (206). Stroke-associated sleep-disordered breathing is associated with worse functional outcome (207). Continuous positive airway pressure has been shown to improve sleep-disordered breathing patterns and 30-day NIHSS status compared to no respiratory support (208) and should be considered in AIS patients with moderate to severe obstructive sleep apnoea, daytime symptoms, and a high cardiovascular risk profile including therapy-resistant hypertension (205).

Fever

Post-stroke fever occurs in up to 24% of patients (209) and is independently associated with higher mortality and poor neurological outcome in survivors (210,211). One study demonstrated a 2.2 increase in the relative risk of poor outcome for every 1°C rise in body temperature (212).The Paracetamol (Acetaminophen) In Stroke (PAIS) trial evaluated prophylactic administration of acetaminophen 6000 mg/day to stroke patients with admission temperature 36–39°C and found no benefit overall (213). However, a post-hoc analysis identified that acetaminophen was associated with neurological improvement without increased adverse events in patients whose admission temperature was 37–39°C. Although several small studies evaluating physical methods of cooling have demonstrated efficacy in fever reduction and maintenance of normothermia, improvement in neurological outcome using exogenous cooling methods remains unproven (214).

Infection

A period of relative immunosuppression follows AIS resulting in hospital-acquired infections in 30–45% of patients (215). Consistently reported clinical predictors of post-stroke infection include older age, more severe stroke, total anterior circulation infarction, dysphagia, and mechanical ventilation (216). Two meta-analyses suggested that prophylactic antibiotic administration reduces the risk of infection with trends towards benefit for neurological outcome and mortality without major harm or toxicity (217). However, due to the small magnitude of effect and risk of development of multidrug resistant organisms, routine antibiotic prophylaxis is not recommended.

Of all medical complications, pneumonia is associated with the highest proportion of attributable mortality after AIS (218). Post-stroke pneumonia occurs in 6% of patients and is associated with a threefold increase in mortality and, in the United States, with a $15,000 increase in hospitalization cost per patient (219,220). Independent risk factors for the development of pneumonia after stroke include mechanical ventilation, dysphagia, dysarthria, age greater than 65 years, and an abnormal chest X-ray on admission (221,222).

Urinary tract infection (UTI) occurs in 15% of patients in the acute period (223) and is associated with worsened neurological and functional outcome (224). Risk factors include increasing age, female sex, severe disability, post-void residual urinary retention, and, most importantly, urinary catheterization which confers a threefold increase in the risk of UTI (224,225). Vigilance in removing urinary catheters at the earliest opportunity and monitoring post-void residual volumes are crucial in minimizing the risk of UTI in stroke patients.

Dysphagia

Dysphagia occurs in up to 80% of stroke patients and is associated with a threefold increase in the risk of pneumonia (226). Bedside screening methods such as the water test (coughing on administration of a small volume of water) provide sensitive measures for detection of dysphagia (227). Early recognition and nil by mouth orders in those with impaired swallow is important in the prevention of pulmonary aspiration and subsequent pneumonia. Early therapy for dysphagia is associated with significant reductions in swallow-related medical complications, chest infections, and death or long-term institutionalization after AIS (228).

Nutrition

Underfeeding is common after stroke. Malnutrition is reported in 6–60% of patients after AIS (229), is more common in those with dysphagia, and is independently associated with higher mortality (230). One arm of the Feed Or Ordinary Food (FOOD) trial assessed early nutritional support with nasogastric feeding versus withholding feeding for 7 days and demonstrated that early feeding was associated with a non-significant trend toward lower mortality (231). When early feeding was initiated, early percutaneous endoscopic gastrostomy (PEG) placement had no benefit compared to delayed PEG placement. Although patients requiring a PEG do poorly relative to stroke patients overall, those who survive have similar functional recovery and rate of home discharge as case-matched controls (232). Dysphagia improves over several months and around 90% of patients are eventually able to resume full oral nutrition (233). A PEG is therefore indicated in those with persistent dysphagia after stroke unless there are prior wishes to the contrary.

Nutritional protein supplementation was not shown to have any outcome benefit in the third arm of the FOOD trial (234). A Cochrane review also found no benefit of protein supplementation on neurological outcome or mortality after AIS but did identify an associated reduction in pressure ulcers (235).

Gastrointestinal bleeding

Gastrointestinal (GI) haemorrhage occurs in 1–2% of stroke patients during the acute hospitalization episode and is associated with poor outcome (236). Risk factors include worse stroke severity, older age, mechanical ventilation, and a history of peptic ulcer disease and malignancy. Due to the increased risk of pneumonia with acid suppressive therapy, only patients at high risk for GI bleeding should be prescribed proton pump inhibitors or H2-receptor antagonists.

Constipation

Around 7% of bedbound stroke patients become constipated (223) and bowel management regimens with stool softeners and laxatives in association with early mobilization and avoidance of opiates may help limit the development of ileus.

Venous thromboembolism

Stroke patients are at high risk for the development of deep vein thrombosis (DVT) due to paresis and immobility. In the absence of pharmacological prophylaxis, the incidence of DVT is as high as 50% within 2 weeks of stroke onset in hemiplegic patients although most are asymptomatic. DVTs develop as early as the second day after stroke with a peak incidence between 48 hours and 1 week, and around 15% of patients with untreated proximal DVT go on to develop pulmonary embolism (PE) (237).

Subcutaneous UFH is effective for DVT prophylaxis after AIS (238). A dose of 5000 units three times daily is slightly more effective than twice-daily dosing, but with a marginal increased risk of bleeding (239). LMWHs have improved efficacy for DVT prevention over twice-daily subcutaneous UFH (240). A meta-analysis also showed benefit of LMWH over UFH for DVT prevention (241) and cost:benefit analysis suggests that the LMWH enoxaparin may be more cost-effective in stroke patients despite its higher cost compared to UFH (242). Current American College of Physicians guidelines recommend prophylaxis with UFH or LMWH after AIS unless the assessed risk of bleeding outweighs the benefit of treatment (243). Pharmacological prophylaxis should not be started for 24 hours after tPA administration but can usually be instituted thereafter barring other contraindications.

Pneumatic sequential compression devices are effective when used as an adjunctive agent to pharmacological DVT prophylaxis (244) but have unproven efficacy in isolation (245). Graduated compression stockings also do not reduce the risk of DVT when used in isolation and are associated with skin breakdown and development of skin ulcers (246). Below-knee stockings may actually increase the risk of DVT (247). Early mobilization is an effective and safe method for DVT prevention after AIS (248).

References

1. Large H, Tuthill JE, Kennedy FB, Pozen TF. In the first stroke intensive care unit. *Am J Nurs.* 1969;69(1):76–80.
2. Acker JE, Pancioli AM, Crocco TJ, Eckstein MK, Jauch EC, Larrabee H, *et al.* Implementation strategies for emergency medical services within stroke systems of care: a policy statement from the American Heart Association/American Stroke Association Expert Panel on Emergency Medical Services Systems and the Stroke Council. *Stroke.* 2007;38:3097–115.
3. Kothari RU, Pancioli A, Liu T, Brott T, Broderick J. Cincinnati Prehospital Stroke Scale: reproducibility and validity. *Ann Emerg Med.* 1999;33(4):373–8.
4. Kidwell CS, Starkman S, Eckstein M, Weems K, Saver JL. Identifying stroke in the field. Prospective validation of the Los Angeles prehospital stroke screen (LAPSS). *Stroke.* 2000;31(1):71–6.
5. Patel MD, Rose KM, O'Brien EC, Rosamond WD. Prehospital notification by emergency medical services reduces delays in stroke evaluation: findings from the North Carolina stroke care collaborative. *Stroke.* 2011;42(8):2263–8.
6. Kim SK, Lee SY, Bae HJ, Lee YS, Kim SY, Kang MJ, *et al.* Pre-hospital notification reduced the door-to-needle time for IV t-PA in acute ischaemic stroke. *Eur J Neurol.* 2009;16(12):1331–5.
7. Jauch EC, Saver JL, Adams HP, Bruno A, Connors JJB, Demaerschalk BM, *et al.* Guidelines for the early management of patients with acute ischemic stroke: a guideline for healthcare professionals from the American Heart Association/American Stroke Association. *Stroke.* 2013;44(3):870–947.
8. Ford AL, Williams JA, Spencer M, McCammon C, Khoury N, Sampson TR, *et al.* Reducing door-to-needle times using Toyota's lean manufacturing principles and value stream analysis. *Stroke.* 2012;43(12):3395–8.
9. Mikulik R, Kadlecová P, Czlonkowska A, Kobayashi A, Brozman M, Svigelj V, *et al.* Factors influencing in-hospital delay in treatment with intravenous thrombolysis. *Stroke.* 2012;43(6):1578–83.
10. Fonarow GC, Smith EE, Saver JL, Reeves MJ, Hernandez AF, Peterson ED, *et al.* Improving door-to-needle times in acute ischemic stroke: the design and rationale for the American Heart Association/American Stroke Association's Target: Stroke initiative. *Stroke.* 2011;42(10):2983–9.
11. Gottesman RF, Alt J, Wityk RJ, Llinas RH. Predicting abnormal coagulation in ischemic stroke: reducing delay in rt-PA use. *Neurology.* 2006;67(9):1665–7.
12. Meretoja A, Strbian D, Mustanoja S, Tatlisumak T, Lindsberg PJ, Kaste M. Reducing in-hospital delay to 20 minutes in stroke thrombolysis. *Neurology.* 2012;79(4):306–13.
13. Kleindorfer D, de Los Ríos la Rosa F, Khatri P, Kissela B, Mackey J, Adeoye O. Temporal trends in acute stroke management. *Stroke.* 2013;44(6 Suppl 1):S129–31.
14. Mullins ME, Schaefer PW, Sorensen AG, Halpern EF, Ay H, He J, *et al.* CT and conventional and diffusion-weighted MR imaging in acute stroke: study in 691 patients at presentation to the emergency department. *Radiology.* 2002;224(2):353–60.
15. Schuknecht B, Ratzka M, Hofmann E. The "dense artery sign"—major cerebral artery thromboembolism demonstrated by computed tomography. *Neuroradiology.* 1990;32(2):98–103.
16. Dzialowski I, Hill MD, Coutts SB, Demchuk AM, Kent DM, Wunderlich O, *et al.* Extent of early ischemic changes on computed tomography (CT) before thrombolysis: prognostic value of the Alberta Stroke Program Early CT Score in ECASS II. *Stroke.* 2006;37(4):973–8.
17. Hirano T, Sasaki M, Tomura N, Ito Y, Kobayashi S, Japan Alteplase Clinical Trial G. Low Alberta Stroke Program Early Computed Tomography Score within 3 hours of onset predicts subsequent symptomatic intracranial hemorrhage in patients treated with 0.6 mg/kg alteplase. *J Stroke Cerebrovasc Dis.* 2012;21(8):898–902.
18. Barber PA, Demchuk AM, Zhang J, Buchan AM, ASPECTS Study Group. Validity and reliability of a quantitative computed tomography

score in predicting outcome of hyperacute stroke before thrombolytic therapy. *Lancet.* 2000;355(9216):1670–4.

19. Heldner MR, Zubler C, Mattle HP, Schroth G, Weck A, Mono M-L, *et al.* National Institutes of Health stroke scale score and vessel occlusion in 2152 patients with acute ischemic stroke. *Stroke.* 2013;44(4):1153–7.

20. Goyal M, Menon BK, Coutts SB, Hill MD, Demchuk AM, Penumbra Pivotal Stroke Trial Investigators CSP, *et al.* Effect of baseline CT scan appearance and time to recanalization on clinical outcomes in endovascular thrombectomy of acute ischemic strokes. *Stroke.* 2011;42(1):93–7.

21. Röther J, Jonetz-Mentzel L, Fiala A, Reichenbach JR, Herzau M, Kaiser WA, *et al.* Hemodynamic assessment of acute stroke using dynamic single-slice computed tomographic perfusion imaging. *Arch Neurol.* 2000;57(8):1161–6.

22. Lin K, Rapalino O, Law M, Babb JS, Siller KA, Pramanik BK. Accuracy of the Alberta Stroke Program Early CT Score during the first 3 hours of middle cerebral artery stroke: comparison of noncontrast CT, CT angiography source images, and CT perfusion. *AJNR Am J Neuroradiol.* 2008;29(5):931–6.

23. Shih LC, Saver JL, Alger JR, Starkman S, Leary MC, Vinuela F, *et al.* Perfusion-weighted magnetic resonance imaging thresholds identifying core, irreversibly infarcted tissue. *Stroke.* 2003;34(6):1425–30.

24. Parsons MW, Barber PA, Chalk J, Darby DG, Rose S, Desmond PM, *et al.* Diffusion- and perfusion-weighted MRI response to thrombolysis in stroke. *Ann Neurol.* 2002;51(1):28–37.

25. Hacke W, Albers G, Al-Rawi Y, Bogousslavsky J, Davalos A, Eliasziw M, *et al.* The Desmoteplase in Acute Ischemic Stroke Trial (DIAS): a phase II MRI-based 9-hour window acute stroke thrombolysis trial with intravenous desmoteplase. *Stroke.* 2005;36(1):66–73.

26. Hacke W, Furlan AJ, Al-Rawi Y, Davalos A, Fiebach JB, Gruber F, *et al.* Intravenous desmoteplase in patients with acute ischaemic stroke selected by MRI perfusion-diffusion weighted imaging or perfusion CT (DIAS-2): a prospective, randomised, double-blind, placebo-controlled study. *Lancet Neurol.* 2009;8(2):141–50.

27. Lev MH. Acute stroke imaging: what is sufficient for triage to endovascular therapies? *AJNR Am J Neuroradiol.* 2012;33(5):790–2.

28. Latchaw RE, Alberts MJ, Lev MH, Connors JJ, Harbaugh RE, Higashida RT, *et al.* Recommendations for imaging of acute ischemic stroke: a scientific statement from the American Heart Association. *Stroke.* 2009;40(11):3646–78.

29. The National Institute of Neurological Disorders and Stroke rt-PA Stroke Study Group. Tissue plasminogen activator for acute ischemic stroke. *N Engl J Med.* 1995;333(24):1581–7.

30. Kwiatkowski TG, Libman RB, Frankel M, Tilley BC, Morgenstern LB, Lu M, *et al.* Effects of tissue plasminogen activator for acute ischemic stroke at one year. *N Engl J Med.* 1999;340(23):1781–7.

31. Albers GW, Bates VE, Clark WM, Bell R, Verro P, Hamilton SA. Intravenous tissue-type plasminogen activator for treatment of acute stroke: the Standard Treatment with Alteplase to Reverse Stroke (STARS) study. *JAMA.* 2000;283(9):1145–50.

32. Wahlgren N, Ahmed N, Davalos A, Ford GA, Grond M, Hacke W, *et al.* Thrombolysis with alteplase for acute ischaemic stroke in the Safe Implementation of Thrombolysis in Stroke-Monitoring Study (SITS-MOST): an observational study. *Lancet.* 2007;369(9558):275–82.

33. Hacke W, Kaste M, Bluhmki E, Brozman M, Davalos A, Guidetti D, *et al.* Thrombolysis with alteplase 3 to 4.5 hours after acute ischemic stroke. *N Engl J Med.* 2008;359(13):1317–29.

34. Del Zoppo GJ, Saver JL, Jauch EC, Adams HP, American Heart Association Stroke C. Expansion of the time window for treatment of acute ischemic stroke with intravenous tissue plasminogen activator: a science advisory from the American Heart Association/American Stroke Association. *Stroke.* 2009;40:2945–8.

35. Sandercock P, Wardlaw JM, Lindley RI, Dennis M, Cohen G, Murray G, *et al.* The benefits and harms of intravenous thrombolysis with recombinant tissue plasminogen activator within 6 h of acute ischaemic stroke (the third international stroke trial (IST-3)): a randomised controlled trial. *Lancet.* 2012;379(9834):2352–63.

36. Marler JR, Tilley BC, Lu M, Brott TG, Lyden PC, Grotta JC, *et al.* Early stroke treatment associated with better outcome: the NINDS rt-PA stroke study. *Neurology.* 2000;55(11):1649–55.

37. Saver JL, Fonarow GC, Smith EE, Reeves MJ, Grau-Sepulveda MV, Pan W, *et al.* Time to treatment with intravenous tissue plasminogen activator and outcome from acute ischemic stroke. *JAMA.* 2013;309(23):2480–8.

38. Lees KR, Bluhmki E, von Kummer R, Brott TG, Toni D, Grotta JC, *et al.* Time to treatment with intravenous alteplase and outcome in stroke: an updated pooled analysis of ECASS, ATLANTIS, NINDS, and EPITHET trials. *Lancet.* 2010;375(9727):1695–703.

39. Simoons ML, Maggioni AP, Knatterud G, Leimberger JD, de Jaegere P, van Domburg R, *et al.* Individual risk assessment for intracranial haemorrhage during thrombolytic therapy. *Lancet.* 1993;342(8886-8887):1523–8.

40. Tanne D, Kasner SE, Demchuk AM, Koren-Morag N, Hanson S, Grond M, *et al.* Markers of increased risk of intracerebral hemorrhage after intravenous recombinant tissue plasminogen activator therapy for acute ischemic stroke in clinical practice: the Multicenter rt-PA Stroke Survey. *Circulation.* 2002;105(14):1679–85.

41. Rasler F. Emergency treatment of hemorrhagic complications of thrombolysis. *Ann Emerg Med.* 2007;50(4):485.

42. French KF, White J, Hoesch RE. Treatment of intracerebral hemorrhage with tranexamic acid after thrombolysis with tissue plasminogen activator. *Neurocrit Care.* 2012;17(1):107–11.

43. Fugate JE, Kalimullah EA, Wijdicks EFM. Angioedema after tPA: what neurointensivists should know. *Neurocrit Care.* 2012;16(3):440–3.

44. Bhatia R, Hill MD, Shobha N, Menon B, Bal S, Kochar P, *et al.* Low rates of acute recanalization with intravenous recombinant tissue plasminogen activator in ischemic stroke: real-world experience and a call for action. *Stroke.* 2010;41(10):2254–8.

45. Riedel CH, Zimmermann P, Jensen-Kondering U, Stingele R, Deuschl G, Jansen O. The importance of size: successful recanalization by intravenous thrombolysis in acute anterior stroke depends on thrombus length. *Stroke.* 2011;42(6):1775–7.

46. del Zoppo GJ, Higashida RT, Furlan AJ, Pessin MS, Rowley HA, Gent M, *et al.* PROACT: a phase II randomized trial of recombinant pro-urokinase by direct arterial delivery in acute middle cerebral artery stroke. *Stroke.* 1998;29(1):4–11.

47. Furlan A, Higashida R, Wechsler L, Gent M, Rowley H, Kase C, *et al.* Intra-arterial prourokinase for acute ischemic stroke. The PROACT II study: a randomized controlled trial. Prolyse in Acute Cerebral Thromboembolism. *JAMA.* 1999;282(21):2003–11.

48. IMS II Trial Investigators. The Interventional Management of Stroke (IMS) II Study. *Stroke.* 2007;38(7):2127–35.

49. Lewandowski CA, Frankel M, Tomsick TA, Broderick J, Frey J, Clark W, *et al.* Combined intravenous and intra-arterial r-TPA versus intra-arterial therapy of acute ischemic stroke: Emergency Management of Stroke (EMS) Bridging Trial. *Stroke.* 1999;30(12):2598–605.

50. Ogawa A, Mori E, Minematsu K, Taki W, Takahashi A, Nemoto S, *et al.* Randomized trial of intraarterial infusion of urokinase within 6 hours of middle cerebral artery stroke: the middle cerebral artery embolism local fibrinolytic intervention trial (MELT) Japan. *Stroke.* 2007;38(10):2633–9.

51. Smith WS, Sung G, Saver J, Budzik R, Duckwiler G, Liebeskind DS, *et al.* Mechanical thrombectomy for acute ischemic stroke: final results of the Multi MERCI trial. *Stroke.* 2008;39(4):1205–12.

52. The Penumbra Pivotal Stroke Trial Investigators. The penumbra pivotal stroke trial: safety and effectiveness of a new generation of mechanical devices for clot removal in intracranial large vessel occlusive disease. *Stroke.* 2009;40(8):2761–8.

53. Saver JL, Jahan R, Levy EI, Jovin TG, Baxter B, Nogueira RG, *et al.* Solitaire flow restoration device versus the Merci Retriever in patients

with acute ischaemic stroke (SWIFT): a randomised, parallel-group, non-inferiority trial. *Lancet.* 2012;380(9849):1241–9.

54. Nogueira RG, Lutsep HL, Gupta R, Jovin TG, Albers GW, Walker GA, *et al.* Trevo versus Merci retrievers for thrombectomy revascularisation of large vessel occlusions in acute ischaemic stroke (TREVO 2): a randomised trial. *Lancet.* 2012;380(9849):1231–40.

55. Broderick JP, Palesch YY, Demchuk AM, Yeatts SD, Khatri P, Hill MD, *et al.* Endovascular therapy after intravenous t-PA versus t-PA alone for stroke. *N Engl J Med.* 2013;368(10):893–903.

56. Ciccone A, Valvassori L, Nichelatti M, Sgoifo A, Ponzio M, Sterzi R, *et al.* Endovascular treatment for acute ischemic stroke. *N Engl J Med.* 2013;368(10):904–13.

57. Kidwell CS, Jahan R, Gornbein J, Alger JR, Nenov V, Ajani Z, *et al.* A Trial of imaging selection and endovascular treatment for ischemic stroke. *N Engl J Med.* 2013;368(10):914–23.

58. Kidwell CS, Saver JL, Carneado J, Sayre J, Starkman S, Duckwiler G, *et al.* Predictors of hemorrhagic transformation in patients receiving intra-arterial thrombolysis. *Stroke.* 2002;33(3):717–24.

59. Smith WS, Sung G, Starkman S, Saver JL, Kidwell CS, Gobin YP, *et al.* Safety and efficacy of mechanical embolectomy in acute ischemic stroke: results of the MERCI trial. *Stroke.* 2005;36(7):1432–8.

60. Loh Y, McArthur DL, Vespa P, Shi ZS, Liebeskind DS, Jahan R, *et al.* The risk of acute radiocontrast-mediated kidney injury following endovascular therapy for acute ischemic stroke is low. *AJNR Am J Neuroradiol.* 2010;31(9):1584–7.

61. Marenzi G, Assanelli E, Marana I, Lauri G, Campodonico J, Grazi M, *et al.* N-acetylcysteine and contrast-induced nephropathy in primary angioplasty. *N Engl J Med.* 2006;354(26):2773–82.

62. Merten GJ, Burgess WP, Gray LV, Holleman JH, Roush TS, Kowalchuk GJ, *et al.* Prevention of contrast-induced nephropathy with sodium bicarbonate: a randomized controlled trial. *JAMA.* 2004;291(19):2328–34.

63. Cloft HJ, Jensen ME, Kallmes DF, Dion JE. Arterial dissections complicating cerebral angiography and cerebrovascular interventions. *AJNR Am J Neuroradiol.* 2000;21(3):541–5.

64. Rincon F, Mayer SA, Rivolta J, Stillman J, Boden-Albala B, Elkind MSV, *et al.* Impact of delayed transfer of critically ill stroke patients from the emergency department to the neuro-ICU. *Neurocrit Care.* 2010;13(1):75–81.

65. Varelas PN, Schultz L, Conti M, Spanaki M, Genarrelli T, Hacein-Bey L. The impact of a neuro-intensivist on patients with stroke admitted to a neurosciences intensive care unit. *Neurocrit Care.* 2008;9(3):293–9.

66. Bershad EM, Feen ES, Hernandez OH, Suri MFK, Suarez JI. Impact of a specialized neurointensive care team on outcomes of critically ill acute ischemic stroke patients. *Neurocrit Care.* 2008;9(3):287–92.

67. Britton M, Carlsson A, de Faire U. Blood pressure course in patients with acute stroke and matched controls. *Stroke.* 1986;17(5):861–4.

68. Harper G, Castleden CM, Potter JF. Factors affecting changes in blood pressure after acute stroke. *Stroke.* 1994;25(9):1726–9.

69. Leonardi-Bee J, Bath PMW, Phillips SJ, Sandercock PAG, I.S.T. Collaborative Group. Blood pressure and clinical outcomes in the International Stroke Trial. *Stroke.* 2002;33(5):1315–20.

70. Immink RV, van Montfrans GA, Stam J, Karemaker JM, Diamant M, van Lieshout JJ. Dynamic cerebral autoregulation in acute lacunar and middle cerebral artery territory ischemic stroke. *Stroke.* 2005;36(12):2595–600.

71. Geeganage C, Bath PMW. Interventions for deliberately altering blood pressure in acute stroke. *Cochrane Database Syst Rev.* 2008;4:CD000039.

72. Sandset EC, Bath PMW, Boysen G, Jatuzis D, Kõrv J, Lüders S, *et al.* The angiotensin-receptor blocker candesartan for treatment of acute stroke (SCAST): a randomised, placebo-controlled, double-blind trial. *Lancet.* 2011;377(9767):741–50.

73. Potter JF, Robinson TG, Ford GA, Mistri A, James M, Chernova J, *et al.* Controlling hypertension and hypotension immediately post-stroke (CHHIPS): a randomised, placebo-controlled, double-blind pilot trial. *Lancet Neurol.* 2009;8(1):48–56.

74. Barer DH, Cruickshank JM, Ebrahim SB, Mitchell JR. Low dose beta blockade in acute stroke ("BEST" trial): an evaluation. *BMJ.* 1988;296(6624):737–41.

75. Castillo J, Leira R, García MM, Serena J, Blanco M, Davalos A. Blood pressure decrease during the acute phase of ischemic stroke is associated with brain injury and poor stroke outcome. *Stroke.* 2004;35(2):520–6.

76. Lee M, Saver JL, Hong K-S, Hao Q, Chow J, Ovbiagele B. Renin-Angiotensin system modulators modestly reduce vascular risk in persons with prior stroke. *Stroke.* 2012;43(1):113–9.

77. Koenig MA, Geocadin RG, de Grouchy M, Glasgow J, Vimal S, Restrepo L, *et al.* Safety of induced hypertension therapy in patients with acute ischemic stroke. *Neurocrit Care.* 2006;4(1):3–7.

78. Chalela JA, Dunn B, Todd JW, Warach S. Induced hypertension improves cerebral blood flow in acute ischemic stroke. *Neurology.* 2005;64(11):1979.

79. Rordorf G, Koroshetz WJ, Ezzeddine MA, Segal AZ, Buonanno FS. A pilot study of drug-induced hypertension for treatment of acute stroke. *Neurology.* 2001;56(9):1210–3.

80. Grotta J, Pasteur W, Khwaja G, Hamel T, Fisher M, Ramirez A. Elective intubation for neurologic deterioration after stroke. *Neurology.* 1995;45(4):640–4.

81. Georgiadis D, Schwarz S, Baumgartner RW, Veltkamp R, Schwab S. Influence of positive end-expiratory pressure on intracranial pressure and cerebral perfusion pressure in patients with acute stroke. *Stroke.* 2001;32(9):2088–92.

82. Gujjar AR, Deibert E, Manno EM, Duff S, Diringer MN. Mechanical ventilation for ischemic stroke and intracerebral hemorrhage: indications, timing, and outcome. *Neurology.* 1998;51(2):447–51.

83. Mayer SA, Copeland D, Bernardini GL, Boden-Albala B, Lennihan L, Kossoff S, *et al.* Cost and outcome of mechanical ventilation for life-threatening stroke. *Stroke.* 2000;31(10):2346–53.

84. Foerch C, Kessler KR, Steckel DA, Steinmetz H, Sitzer M. Survival and quality of life outcome after mechanical ventilation in elderly stroke patients. *J Neurol Neurosurg Psychiatry.* 2004;75(7):988–93.

85. Qureshi AI, Suarez JI, Yahia AM, Mohammad Y, Uzun G, Suri MFK, *et al.* Timing of neurologic deterioration in massive middle cerebral artery infarction: a multicenter review. *Crit Care Med.* 2003;31(1):272–7.

86. Bounds JV, Wiebers DO, Whisnant JP, Okazaki H. Mechanisms and timing of deaths from cerebral infarction. *Stroke.* 1981;12(4):474–7.

87. Berrouschot J, Sterker M, Bettin S, Köster J, Schneider D. Mortality of space-occupying ('malignant') middle cerebral artery infarction under conservative intensive care. *Intensive Care Med.* 1998;24(6):620–3.

88. Ropper AH, Shafran B. Brain edema after stroke. Clinical syndrome and intracranial pressure. *Arch Neurol.* 1984;41(1):26–9.

89. Krieger DW, Demchuk AM, Kasner SE, Jauss M, Hantson L. Early clinical and radiological predictors of fatal brain swelling in ischemic stroke. *Stroke.* 1999;30(2):287–92.

90. Oppenheim C, Samson Y, Manaï R, Lalam T, Vandamme X, Crozier S, *et al.* Prediction of malignant middle cerebral artery infarction by diffusion-weighted imaging. *Stroke.* 2000;31(9):2175–81.

91. Poca MA, Benejam B, Sahuquillo J, Riveiro M, Frascheri L, Merino MA, *et al.* Monitoring intracranial pressure in patients with malignant middle cerebral artery infarction: is it useful? *J Neurosurg.* 2010;112(3):648–57.

92. Muizelaar JP, Marmarou A, Ward JD, Kontos HA, Choi SC, Becker DP, *et al.* Adverse effects of prolonged hyperventilation in patients with severe head injury: a randomized clinical trial. *J Neurosurg.* 1991;75(5):731–9.

93. Koenig MA, Bryan M, Lewin JL, Mirski MA, Geocadin RG, Stevens RD. Reversal of transtentorial herniation with hypertonic saline. *Neurology.* 2008;70(13):1023–9.

94. Manno EM, Adams RE, Derdeyn CP, Powers WJ, Diringer MN. The effects of mannitol on cerebral edema after large hemispheric cerebral infarct. *Neurology*. 1999;52(3):583–7.

95. Keller E, Steiner T, Fandino J, Schwab S, Hacke W. Changes in cerebral blood flow and oxygen metabolism during moderate hypothermia in patients with severe middle cerebral artery infarction. *Neurosurg Focus*. 2000;8(5):e4.

96. Schwab S, Schwarz S, Spranger M, Keller E, Bertram M, Hacke W. Moderate hypothermia in the treatment of patients with severe middle cerebral artery infarction. *Stroke*. 1998;29(12):2461–6.

97. Georgiadis D, Schwarz S, Aschoff A, Schwab S. Hemicraniectomy and moderate hypothermia in patients with severe ischemic stroke. *Stroke*. 2002;33(6):1584–8.

98. Schwab S, Georgiadis D, Berrouschot J, Schellinger PD, Graffagnino C, Mayer SA. Feasibility and safety of moderate hypothermia after massive hemispheric infarction. *Stroke*. 2001;32(9):2033–5.

99. Schwab S, Spranger M, Schwarz S, Hacke W. Barbiturate coma in severe hemispheric stroke: useful or obsolete? *Neurology*. 1997;48(6):1608–13.

100. Berger L, Hakim AM. The association of hyperglycemia with cerebral edema in stroke. *Stroke*. 1986;17(5):865–71.

101. Curry WT, Sethi MK, Ogilvy CS, Carter BS. Factors associated with outcome after hemicraniectomy for large middle cerebral artery territory infarction. *Neurosurgery*. 2005;56(4):681–92.

102. Kastrau F, Wolter M, Huber W, Block F. Recovery from aphasia after hemicraniectomy for infarction of the speech-dominant hemisphere. *Stroke*. 2005;36(4):825–9.

103. Woertgen C, Erban P, Rothoerl RD, Bein T, Horn M, Brawanski A. Quality of life after decompressive craniectomy in patients suffering from supratentorial brain ischemia. *Acta Neurochir (Wien)*. 2004;146(7):691–5.

104. Schwab S, Steiner T, Aschoff A, Schwarz S, Steiner HH, Jansen O, et al. Early hemicraniectomy in patients with complete middle cerebral artery infarction. *Stroke*. 1998;29(9):1888–93.

105. Cho D-Y, Chen T-C, Lee H-C. Ultra-early decompressive craniectomy for malignant middle cerebral artery infarction. *Surg Neurol*. 2003;60(3):227–32.

106. Mori K, Nakao Y, Yamamoto T, Maeda M. Early external decompressive craniectomy with duroplasty improves functional recovery in patients with massive hemispheric embolic infarction: timing and indication of decompressive surgery for malignant cerebral infarction. *Surg Neurol*. 2004;62(5):420–9.

107. Gupta R, Connolly ES, Mayer S, Elkind MSV. Hemicraniectomy for massive middle cerebral artery territory infarction: a systematic review. *Stroke*. 2004;35(2):539–43.

108. Juttler E, Schwab S, Schmiedek P, Unterberg A, Hennerici M, Woitzik J, et al. Decompressive Surgery for the Treatment of Malignant Infarction of the Middle Cerebral Artery (DESTINY): a randomized, controlled trial. *Stroke*. 2007;38(9):2518–25.

109. Vahedi K, Vicaut E, Mateo J, Kurtz A, Orabi M, Guichard J-P, et al. Sequential-design, multicenter, randomized, controlled trial of early decompressive craniectomy in malignant middle cerebral artery infarction (DECIMAL Trial). *Stroke*. 2007;38(9):2506–17.

110. Vahedi K, Hofmeijer J, Juettler E, Vicaut E, George B, Algra A, et al. Early decompressive surgery in malignant infarction of the middle cerebral artery: a pooled analysis of three randomised controlled trials. *Lancet Neurol*. 2007;6(3):215–22.

111. Kiphuth IC, Köhrmann M, Lichy C, Schwab S, Huttner HB. Hemicraniectomy for malignant middle cerebral artery infarction: retrospective consent to decompressive surgery depends on functional long-term outcome. *Neurocrit Care*. 2010;13(3):380–4.

112. Weil AG, Rahme R, Moumdjian R, Bouthillier A, Bojanowski MW. Quality of life following hemicraniectomy for malignant MCA territory infarction. *Can J Neurol Sci*. 2011;38(3):434–8.

113. Juttler E, Unterberg A, Woitzik J, Bösel J, Amiri H, Sakowitz OW, et al. Hemicraniectomy in older patients with extensive middle-cerebral-artery stroke. *N Engl J Med*. 2014;370(12):1091–100.

114. Edlow JA, Newman-Toker DE, Savitz SI. Diagnosis and initial management of cerebellar infarction. *Lancet Neurol*. 2008;7(10):951–64.

115. Jauss M, Krieger D, Hornig C, Schramm J, Busse O. Surgical and medical management of patients with massive cerebellar infarctions: results of the German-Austrian Cerebellar Infarction Study. *J Neurol*. 1999;246(4):257–64.

116. Koh MG, Phan TG, Atkinson JL, Wijdicks EF. Neuroimaging in deteriorating patients with cerebellar infarcts and mass effect. *Stroke*. 2000;31(9):2062–7.

117. Momose KJ, Lehrich JR. Acute cerebellar infarction presenting as a posterior fossa mass. *Radiology*. 1973;109(2):343–52.

118. Pfefferkorn T, Eppinger U, Linn J, Birnbaum T, Herzog J, Straube A, et al. Long-term outcome after suboccipital decompressive craniectomy for malignant cerebellar infarction. *Stroke*. 2009;40(9):3045–50.

119. Ferbert A, Brückmann H, Drummen R. Clinical features of proven basilar artery occlusion. *Stroke*. 1990;21(8):1135–42.

120. Schonewille WJ, Wijman CAC, Michel P, Rueckert CM, Weimar C, Mattle HP, et al. Treatment and outcomes of acute basilar artery occlusion in the Basilar Artery International Cooperation Study (BASICS): a prospective registry study. *Lancet Neurol*. 2009;8(8):724–30.

121. Brandt T, von Kummer R, Müller-Küppers M, Hacke W. Thrombolytic therapy of acute basilar artery occlusion. Variables affecting recanalization and outcome. *Stroke*. 1996;27(5):875–81.

122. Ostrem JL, Saver JL, Alger JR, Starkman S, Leary MC, Duckwiler G, et al. Acute basilar artery occlusion: diffusion-perfusion MRI characterization of tissue salvage in patients receiving intra-arterial stroke therapies. *Stroke*. 2004;35(2):e30–4.

123. Lindsberg PJ, Soinne L, Tatlisumak T, Roine RO, Kallela M, Happola O, et al. Long-term outcome after intravenous thrombolysis of basilar artery occlusion. *JAMA*. 2004;292(15):1862–6.

124. Wijdicks EF, Nichols DA, Thielen KR, Fulgham JR, Brown RD, Meissner I, et al. Intra-arterial thrombolysis in acute basilar artery thromboembolism: the initial Mayo Clinic experience. *Mayo Clin Proc*. 1997;72(11):1005–13.

125. Favrole P, Saint-Maurice JP, Bousser MG, Houdart E. Use of mechanical extraction devices in basilar artery occlusion. *J Neurol Neurosurg Psychiatry*. 2005;76(10):1462–4.

126. North American Symptomatic Carotid Endarterectomy Trial Collaborators. Beneficial effect of carotid endarterectomy in symptomatic patients with high-grade carotid stenosis. *N Engl J Med*. 1991;325(7):445–53.

127. Mantese VA, Timaran CH, Chiu D, Begg RJ, Brott TG. The Carotid Revascularization Endarterectomy versus Stenting Trial (CREST): stenting versus carotid endarterectomy for carotid disease. *Stroke*. 2010;41(10 Suppl):S31–4.

128. Derdeyn CP, Fiorella D, Lynn MJ, Turan TN, Lane BF, Janis LS, et al. Intracranial stenting: SAMMPRIS. *Stroke*. 2013;44(6 Suppl 1):S41–4.

129. Staaf G, Geijer B, Lindgren A, Norrving B. Diffusion-weighted MRI findings in patients with capsular warning syndrome. *Cerebrovasc Dis*. 2004;17(1):1–8.

130. Lee J, Albers GW, Marks MP, Lansberg MG. Capsular warning syndrome caused by middle cerebral artery stenosis. *J Neurol Sci*. 2010;296(1-2):115–20.

131. Terai S, Hori T, Miake S, Tamaki K, Saishoji A. Mechanism in progressive lacunar infarction: a case report with magnetic resonance imaging. *Arch Neurol*. 2000;57(2):255–8.

132. Paul NLM, Simoni M, Chandratheva A, Rothwell PM. Population-based study of capsular warning syndrome and prognosis after early recurrent TIA. *Neurology*. 2012;79(13):1356–62.

133. Vivanco-Hidalgo RM, Rodríguez-Campello A, Ois A, Cucurella G, Pont-Sunyer C, Gomis M, et al. Thrombolysis in capsular warning syndrome. *Cerebrovasc Dis*. 2008;25(5):508–10.

134. Asil T, Ir N, Karaduman F, Cagli B, Tuncel S. Combined antithrombotic treatment with aspirin and clopidogrel for patients with capsular warning syndrome: a case report. *Neurologist*. 2012;18(2):68–9.

135. Dobkin BH. Heparin for lacunar stroke in progression. *Stroke.* 1983;14(3):421–3.

136. Lim TS, Hong JM, Lee JS, Shin DH, Choi JY, Huh K. Induced-hypertension in progressing lacunar infarction. *J Neurol Sci.* 2011;308(1–2):72–6.

137. Schievink WI. Spontaneous dissection of the carotid and vertebral arteries. *N Engl J Med.* 2001;344(12):898–906.

138. Benninger DH, Georgiadis D, Kremer C, Studer A, Nedeltchev K, Baumgartner RW. Mechanism of ischemic infarct in spontaneous carotid dissection. *Stroke.* 2004;35(2):482–5.

139. Biousse V, D'Anglejan-Chatillon J, Touboul PJ, Amarenco P, Bousser MG. Time course of symptoms in extracranial carotid artery dissections. A series of 80 patients. *Stroke.* 1995;26(2):235–9.

140. Engelter ST, Brandt T, Debette S, Caso V, Lichy C, Pezzini A, *et al.* Antiplatelets versus anticoagulation in cervical artery dissection. *Stroke.* 2007;38(9):2605–11.

141. Lyrer P, Engelter S. Antithrombotic drugs for carotid artery dissection. *Cochrane Database Syst Rev.* 2010;10:CD000255.

142. Georgiadis D, Arnold M, von Buedingen HC, Valko P, Sarikaya H, Rousson V, *et al.* Aspirin vs anticoagulation in carotid artery dissection: a study of 298 patients. *Neurology.* 2009;72(21):1810–5.

143. International Stroke Trial Collaborative Group. The International Stroke Trial (IST): a randomised trial of aspirin, subcutaneous heparin, both, or neither among 19435 patients with acute ischaemic stroke. *Lancet.* 1997;349(9065):1569–81.

144. The Publications Committee for the Trial of ORG 10172 in Acute Stroke Treatment (TOAST) Investigators. Low molecular weight heparinoid, ORG 10172 (danaparoid), and outcome after acute ischemic stroke: a randomized controlled trial. *JAMA.* 1998;279(16):1265–72.

145. Berge E, Abdelnoor M, Nakstad PH, Sandset PM, HAEST Study Group. Low molecular-weight heparin versus aspirin in patients with acute ischaemic stroke and atrial fibrillation: a double-blind randomised study. *Lancet.* 2000;355(9211):1205–10.

146. Paciaroni M, Agnelli G, Micheli S, Caso V. Efficacy and safety of anti-coagulant treatment in acute cardioembolic stroke: a meta-analysis of randomized controlled trials. *Stroke.* 2007;38(2):423–30.

147. Duke RJ, Bloch RF, Turpie AG, Trebilcock R, Bayer N. Intravenous heparin for the prevention of stroke progression in acute partial stable stroke. *Ann Intern Med.* 1986;105(6):825–8.

148. Wong KS, Chen C, Ng PW, Tsoi TH, Li HL, Fong WC, *et al.* Low-molecular-weight heparin compared with aspirin for the treatment of acute ischaemic stroke in Asian patients with large artery occlusive disease: a randomised study. *Lancet Neurol.* 2007;6(5):407–13.

149. Rödén-Jüllig A, Britton M. Effectiveness of heparin treatment for progressing ischaemic stroke: before and after study. *J Intern Med.* 2000;248(4):287–91.

150. Diener HC, Ringelstein EB, von Kummer R, Langohr HD, Bewermeyer H, Landgraf H, *et al.* Treatment of acute ischemic stroke with the low-molecular-weight heparin certoparin: results of the TOPAS trial. *Stroke.* 2001;32(1):22–9.

151. Camerlingo M, Salvi P, Belloni G, Gamba T, Cesana BM, Mamoli A. Intravenous heparin started within the first 3 hours after onset of symptoms as a treatment for acute nonlacunar hemispheric cerebral infarctions. *Stroke.* 2005;36(11):2415–20.

152. Swanson RA. Intravenous heparin for acute stroke: what can we learn from the megatrials? *Neurology.* 1999;52(9):1746–50.

153. Sandercock PAG, Counsell C, Kamal AK. Anticoagulants for acute ischaemic stroke. *Cochrane Database Syst Rev.* 2008;4:CD000024.

154. Yasaka M, Yamaguchi T, Oita J, Sawada T, Shichiri M, Omae T. Clinical features of recurrent embolization in acute cardioembolic stroke. *Stroke.* 1993;24(11):1681–5.

155. CAST (Chinese Acute Stroke Trial) Collaborative Group. CAST: randomised placebo-controlled trial of early aspirin use in 20,000 patients with acute ischaemic stroke. *Lancet.* 1997;349(9066):1641–9.

156. Zinkstok SM, Roos YB, investigators A. Early administration of aspirin in patients treated with alteplase for acute ischaemic stroke: a randomised controlled trial. *Lancet.* 2012;380(9843):731–7.

157. Dengler R, Diener H-C, Schwartz A, Grond M, Schumacher H, Machnig T, *et al.* Early treatment with aspirin plus extended-release dipyridamole for transient ischaemic attack or ischaemic stroke within 24 h of symptom onset (EARLY trial): a randomised, open-label, blinded-endpoint trial. *Lancet Neurol.* 2010;9(2):159–66.

158. Geeganage CM, Diener H-C, Algra A, Chen C, Topol EJ, Dengler R, *et al.* Dual or mono antiplatelet therapy for patients with acute ischemic stroke or transient ischemic attack: systematic review and meta-analysis of randomized controlled trials. *Stroke.* 2012;43(4):1058–66.

159. Wang Y, Wang Y, Zhao X, Liu L, Wang D, Wang C, *et al.* Clopidogrel with aspirin in acute minor stroke or transient ischemic attack. *N Engl J Med.* 2013;369(1):11–19.

160. Willey JZ, Elkind MSV. 3-Hydroxy-3-methylglutaryl-coenzyme A reductase inhibitors in the treatment of central nervous system diseases. *Arch Neurol.* 2010;67(9):1062–7.

161. Amarenco P, Bogousslavsky J, Callahan A, 3rd, Goldstein LB, Hennerici M, Rudolph AE, *et al.* High-dose atorvastatin after stroke or transient ischemic attack. *N Engl J Med.* 2006;355(6):549–59.

162. Ní Chróinín D, Callaly EL, Duggan J, Merwick Á, Hannon N, Sheehan Ó, *et al.* Association between acute statin therapy, survival, and improved functional outcome after ischemic stroke: the North Dublin Population Stroke Study. *Stroke.* 2011;42(4):1021–9.

163. Blanco M, Nombela F, Castellanos M, Rodriguez-Yáñez M, García-Gil M, Leira R, *et al.* Statin treatment withdrawal in ischemic stroke: a controlled randomized study. *Neurology.* 2007;69(9):904–10.

164. Weimar C, Mieck T, Buchthal J, Ehrenfeld CE, Schmid E, Diener H-C, *et al.* Neurologic worsening during the acute phase of ischemic stroke. *Arch Neurol.* 2005;62(3):393–7.

165. DeGraba TJ, Hallenbeck JM, Pettigrew KD, Dutka AJ, Kelly BJ. Progression in acute stroke: value of the initial NIH stroke scale score on patient stratification in future trials. *Stroke.* 1999;30(6):1208–12.

166. Davalos A, Toni D, Iweins F, Lesaffre E, Bastianello S, Castillo J. Neurological deterioration in acute ischemic stroke: potential predictors and associated factors in the European cooperative acute stroke study (ECASS) I. *Stroke.* 1999;30(12):2631–6.

167. Tei H, Uchiyama S, Ohara K, Kobayashi M, Uchiyama Y, Fukuzawa M. Deteriorating ischemic stroke in 4 clinical categories classified by the Oxfordshire Community Stroke Project. *Stroke.* 2000;31(9):2049–54.

168. Paciaroni M, Agnelli G, Corea F, Ageno W, Alberti A, Lanari A, *et al.* Early hemorrhagic transformation of brain infarction: rate, predictive factors, and influence on clinical outcome: results of a prospective multicenter study. *Stroke.* 2008;39(8):2249–56.

169. England TJ, Bath PMW, Sare GM, Geeganage C, Moulin T, O'Neill D, *et al.* Asymptomatic hemorrhagic transformation of infarction and its relationship with functional outcome and stroke subtype: assessment from the Tinzaparin in Acute Ischaemic Stroke Trial. *Stroke.* 2010;41(12):2834–9.

170. Bladin CF, Alexandrov AV, Bellavance A, Bornstein N, Chambers B, Côte R, *et al.* Seizures after stroke: a prospective multicenter study. *Arch Neurol.* 2000;57(11):1617–22.

171. Szaflarski JP, Rackley AY, Kleindorfer DO, Khoury J, Woo D, Miller R, *et al.* Incidence of seizures in the acute phase of stroke: a population-based study. *Epilepsia.* 2008;49(6):974–81.

172. Giroud M, Gras P, Fayolle H, André N, Soichot P, Dumas R. Early seizures after acute stroke: a study of 1,640 cases. *Epilepsia.* 1994;35(5):959–64.

173. Velioğlu SK, Ozmenoğlu M, Boz C, Alioğlu Z. Status epilepticus after stroke. *Stroke.* 2001;32(5):1169–72.

174. Labovitz DL, Hauser WA, Sacco RL. Prevalence and predictors of early seizure and status epilepticus after first stroke. *Neurology.* 2001;57(2):200–6.

175. *Cochrane Database Syst Rev.* 2014 Jan 24;1:CD005398.

176. Shi Q, Presutti R, Selchen D, Saposnik G. Delirium in acute stroke: a systematic review and meta-analysis. *Stroke*. 2012;43(3):645–9.

177. Oldenbeuving AW, de Kort PLM, Jansen BPW, Algra A, Kappelle LJ, Roks G. Delirium in the acute phase after stroke: incidence, risk factors, and outcome. *Neurology*. 2011;76(11):993–9.

178. Oldenbeuving AW, de Kort PLM, Jansen BPW, Roks G, Kappelle LJ. Delirium in acute stroke: a review. *Int J Stroke*. 2007;2(4):270–5.

179. Luitse MJA, Biessels GJ, Rutten GEHM, Kappelle LJ. Diabetes, hyperglycaemia, and acute ischaemic stroke. *Lancet Neurol*. 2012;11(3):261–71.

180. Oppenheimer SM, Hoffbrand BI, Oswald GA, Yudkin JS. Diabetes mellitus and early mortality from stroke. *BMJ*. 1985;291(6501):1014–15.

181. Kruyt ND, Biessels GJ, Devries JH, Roos YB. Hyperglycemia in acute ischemic stroke: pathophysiology and clinical management. *Nat Rev Neurol*. 2010;6(3):145–55.

182. Parsons MW, Barber PA, Desmond PM, Baird TA, Darby DG, Byrnes G, et al. Acute hyperglycemia adversely affects stroke outcome: a magnetic resonance imaging and spectroscopy study. *Ann Neurol*. 2002;52(1):20–8.

183. Capes SE, Hunt D, Malmberg K, Pathak P, Gerstein HC. Stress hyperglycemia and prognosis of stroke in nondiabetic and diabetic patients: a systematic overview. *Stroke*. 2001;32(10):2426–32.

184. Fuentes B, Castillo J, San José B, Leira R, Serena J, Vivancos J, et al. The prognostic value of capillary glucose levels in acute stroke: the GLycemia in Acute Stroke (GLIAS) study. *Stroke*. 2009;40(2):562–8.

185. Scott JF, Robinson GM, French JM, O'Connell JE, Alberti KG, Gray CS. Glucose potassium insulin infusions in the treatment of acute stroke patients with mild to moderate hyperglycemia: the Glucose Insulin in Stroke Trial (GIST). *Stroke*. 1999;30(4):793–9.

186. Kreisel SH, Berschin UM, Hammes H-P, Leweling H, Bertsch T, Hennerici MG, et al. Pragmatic management of hyperglycaemia in acute ischaemic stroke: safety and feasibility of intensive intravenous insulin treatment. *Cerebrovasc Dis*. 2009;27(2):167–75.

187. McCormick M, Hadley D, McLean JR, Macfarlane JA, Condon B, Muir KW. Randomized, controlled trial of insulin for acute poststroke hyperglycemia. *Ann Neurol*. 2010;67(5):570–8.

188. Staszewski J, Brodacki B, Kotowicz J, Stepien A. Intravenous insulin therapy in the maintenance of strict glycemic control in nondiabetic acute stroke patients with mild hyperglycemia. *J Stroke Cerebrovasc Dis*. 2011;20(2):150–4.

189. Gray CS, Hildreth AJ, Sandercock PA, O'Connell JE, Johnston DE, Cartlidge NEF, et al. Glucose-potassium-insulin infusions in the management of post-stroke hyperglycaemia: the UK Glucose Insulin in Stroke Trial (GIST-UK). *Lancet Neurol*. 2007;6(5):397–406.

190. Graffagnino C, Gurram AR, Kolls B, Olson DM. Intensive insulin therapy in the neurocritical care setting is associated with poor clinical outcomes. *Neurocrit Care*. 2010;13(3):307–12.

191. NICE-SUGAR Study Investigators, Finfer S, Chittock DR, Su SY-S, Blair D, Foster D, et al. Intensive versus conventional glucose control in critically ill patients. *N Engl J Med*. 2009;360(13):1283–97.

192. van den Berghe G, Wouters P, Weekers F, Verwaest C, Bruyninckx F, Schetz M, et al. Intensive insulin therapy in critically ill patients. *N Engl J Med*. 2001;345(19):1359–67.

193. Khechinashvili G, Asplund K. Electrocardiographic changes in patients with acute stroke: a systematic review. *Cerebrovasc Dis*. 2002;14(2):67–76.

194. Jensen JK, Atar D, Mickley H. Mechanism of troponin elevations in patients with acute ischemic stroke. *Am J Cardiol*. 2007;99(6):867–70.

195. Lee S-J, Lee K-S, Kim Y-I, An J-Y, Kim W, Kim J-S. Clinical features of patients with a myocardial infarction during acute management of an ischemic stroke. *Neurocrit Care*. 2008;9(3):332–7.

196. Chalela JA, Ezzeddine MA, Davis L, Warach S. Myocardial injury in acute stroke: a troponin I study. *Neurocrit Care*. 2004;1(3):343–6.

197. Norris JW, Froggatt GM, Hachinski VC. Cardiac arrhythmias in acute stroke. *Stroke*. 1978;9(4):392–6.

198. Kimura K, Minematsu K, Yamaguchi T, Japan Multicenter Stroke Investigators C. Atrial fibrillation as a predictive factor for severe stroke and early death in 15,831 patients with acute ischaemic stroke. *J Neurol Neurosurg Psychiatry*. 2005;76(5):679–83.

199. Kaarisalo MM, Immonen-Räihä P, Marttila RJ, Salomaa V, Kaarsalo E, Salmi K, et al. Atrial fibrillation and stroke. Mortality and causes of death after the first acute ischemic stroke. *Stroke*. 1997;28(2):311–15.

200. Abboud H, Berroir S, Labreuche J, Orjuela K, Amarenco P, Investigators G. Insular involvement in brain infarction increases risk for cardiac arrhythmia and death. *Ann Neurol*. 2006;59(4):691–9.

201. Weimar C, Roth MP, Zillessen G, Glahn J, Wimmer MLJ, Busse O, et al. Complications following acute ischemic stroke. *Eur Neurol*. 2002;48(3):133–40.

202. Ois A, Gomis M, Cuadrado-Godia E, Jiménez Conde J, Rodríguez-Campello A, Bruguera J, et al. Heart failure in acute ischemic stroke. *J Neurol*. 2008;255(3):385–9.

203. Yoshimura S, Toyoda K, Ohara T, Nagasawa H, Ohtani N, Kuwashiro T, et al. Takotsubo cardiomyopathy in acute ischemic stroke. *Ann Neurol*. 2008;64(5):547–54.

204. Lee MC, Klassen AC, Resch JA. Respiratory pattern disturbances in ischemic cerebral vascular disease. *Stroke*. 1974;5(5):612–16.

205. Hermann DM, Bassetti CL. Sleep-related breathing and sleep-wake disturbances in ischemic stroke. *Neurology*. 2009;73(16):1313–22.

206. Turkington PM, Bamford J, Wanklyn P, Elliott MW. Prevalence and predictors of upper airway obstruction in the first 24 hours after acute stroke. *Stroke*. 2002;33(8):2037–42.

207. Turkington PM, Allgar V, Bamford J, Wanklyn P, Elliott MW. Effect of upper airway obstruction in acute stroke on functional outcome at 6 months. *Thorax*. 2004;59(5):367–71.

208. Minnerup J, Ritter MA, Wersching H, Kemmling A, Okegwo A, Schmidt A, et al. Continuous positive airway pressure ventilation for acute ischemic stroke: a randomized feasibility study. *Stroke*. 2012;43(4):1137–9.

209. Indredavik B, Rohweder G, Naalsund E, Lydersen S. Medical complications in a comprehensive stroke unit and an early supported discharge service. *Stroke*. 2008;39(2):414–20.

210. Hajat C, Hajat S, Sharma P. Effects of poststroke pyrexia on stroke outcome: a meta-analysis of studies in patients. *Stroke*. 2000;31(2):410–4.

211. Phipps MS, Desai RA, Wira C, Bravata DM. Epidemiology and outcomes of fever burden among patients with acute ischemic stroke. *Stroke*. 2011;42(12):3357–62.

212. Reith J, Jørgensen HS, Pedersen PM, Nakayama H, Raaschou HO, Jeppesen LL, et al. Body temperature in acute stroke: relation to stroke severity, infarct size, mortality, and outcome. *Lancet*. 1996;347(8999):422–5.

213. den Hertog HM, van der Worp HB, van Gemert HMA, Algra A, Kappelle LJ, van Gijn J, et al. The Paracetamol (Acetaminophen) In Stroke (PAIS) trial: a multicentre, randomised, placebo-controlled, phase III trial. *Lancet Neurol*. 2009;8(5):434–40.

214. Kallmünzer B, Kollmar R. Temperature management in stroke—an unsolved, but important topic. *Cerebrovasc Dis*. 2011;31(6):532–43.

215. Vogelgesang A, Dressel A. Immunological consequences of ischemic stroke: immunosuppression and autoimmunity. *J Neuroimmunol*. 2011;231(1–2):105–10.

216. Emsley HCA, Hopkins SJ. Acute ischaemic stroke and infection: recent and emerging concepts. *Lancet Neurol*. 2008;7(4):341–53.

217. Westendorp WF, Vermeij J-D, Vermeij F, den Hertog HM, Dippel DWJ, van de Beek D, et al. Antibiotic therapy for preventing infections in patients with acute stroke. *Cochrane Database Syst Rev*. 2012;1:CD008530.

218. Heuschmann PU, Kolominsky-Rabas PL, Misselwitz B, Hermanek P, Leffmann C, Janzen RWC, et al. Predictors of in-hospital mortality and attributable risks of death after ischemic stroke: the German Stroke Registers Study Group. *Arch Intern Med*. 2004;164(16):1761–8.

219. Katzan IL, Cebul RD, Husak SH, Dawson NV, Baker DW. The effect of pneumonia on mortality among patients hospitalized for acute stroke. *Neurology*. 2003;60(4):620–5.

220. Katzan IL, Dawson NV, Thomas CL, Votruba ME, Cebul RD. The cost of pneumonia after acute stroke. *Neurology.* 2007;68(22):1938–43.

221. Hilker R, Poetter C, Findeisen N, Sobesky J, Jacobs A, Neveling M, et al. Nosocomial pneumonia after acute stroke: implications for neurological intensive care medicine. *Stroke.* 2003;34(4):975–81.

222. Sellars C, Bowie L, Bagg J, Sweeney MP, Miller H, Tilston J, et al. Risk factors for chest infection in acute stroke: a prospective cohort study. *Stroke.* 2007;38(8):2284–91.

223. Ingeman A, Andersen G, Hundborg HH, Svendsen ML, Johnsen SP. In-hospital medical complications, length of stay, and mortality among stroke unit patients. *Stroke.* 2011;42(11):3214–18.

224. Aslanyan S, Weir CJ, Diener HC, Kaste M, Lees KR, Committee GIS, et al. Pneumonia and urinary tract infection after acute ischaemic stroke: a tertiary analysis of the GAIN International trial. *Eur J Neurol.* 2004;11(1):49–53.

225. Ersoz M, Ulusoy H, Oktar MA, Akyuz M. Urinary tract infection and bacteriurua in stroke patients: frequencies, pathogen microorganisms, and risk factors. *Am J Phys Med Rehabil.* 2007;86(9):734–41.

226. Martino R, Foley N, Bhogal S, Diamant N, Speechley M, Teasell R. Dysphagia after stroke: incidence, diagnosis, and pulmonary complications. *Stroke.* 2005;36(12):2756–63.

227. Daniels SK, Anderson JA, Willson PC. Valid items for screening dysphagia risk in patients with stroke: a systematic review. *Stroke.* 2012;43(3):892–7.

228. Carnaby G, Hankey GJ, Pizzi J. Behavioural intervention for dysphagia in acute stroke: a randomised controlled trial. *Lancet Neurol.* 2006;5(1):31–7.

229. Foley NC, Salter KL, Robertson J, Teasell RW, Woodbury MG. Which reported estimate of the prevalence of malnutrition after stroke is valid? *Stroke.* 2009;40(3):e66–74.

230. Food Trial Collaboration. Poor nutritional status on admission predicts poor outcomes after stroke: observational data from the FOOD trial. *Stroke.* 2003;34(6):1450–6.

231. Dennis MS, Lewis SC, Warlow C, Collaboration FT. Effect of timing and method of enteral tube feeding for dysphagic stroke patients (FOOD): a multicentre randomised controlled trial. *Lancet.* 2005;365(9461):764–72.

232. Iizuka M, Reding M. Use of percutaneous endoscopic gastrostomy feeding tubes and functional recovery in stroke rehabilitation: a case-matched controlled study. *Arch Phys Med Rehabil.* 2005;86(5):1049–52.

233. Horner J, Buoyer FG, Alberts MJ, Helms MJ. Dysphagia following brain-stem stroke. Clinical correlates and outcome. *Arch Neurol.* 1991;48(11):1170–3.

234. Dennis MS, Lewis SC, Warlow C, Collaboration FT. Routine oral nutritional supplementation for stroke patients in hospital (FOOD): a multicentre randomised controlled trial. *Lancet.* 2005;365(9461):755–63.

235. Geeganage C, Beavan J, Ellender S, Bath PMW. Interventions for dysphagia and nutritional support in acute and subacute stroke. *Cochrane Database Syst Rev.* 2012;10:CD000323.

236. O'Donnell MJ, Kapral MK, Fang J, Saposnik G, Eikelboom JW, Oczkowski W, et al. Gastrointestinal bleeding after acute ischemic stroke. *Neurology.* 2008;71(9):650–5.

237. Kelly J, Rudd A, Lewis R, Hunt BJ. Venous thromboembolism after acute stroke. *Stroke.* 2001;32(1):262–7.

238. McCarthy ST, Turner J. Low-dose subcutaneous heparin in the prevention of deep-vein thrombosis and pulmonary emboli following acute stroke. *Age Ageing.* 1986;15(2):84–8.

239. King CS, Holley AB, Jackson JL, Shorr AF, Moores LK. Twice vs three times daily heparin dosing for thromboembolism prophylaxis in the general medical population: A metaanalysis. *Chest.* 2007;131(2):507–16.

240. Sherman DG, Albers GW, Bladin C, Fieschi C, Gabbai AA, Kase CS, et al. The efficacy and safety of enoxaparin versus unfractionated heparin for the prevention of venous thromboembolism after acute ischaemic stroke (PREVAIL Study): an open-label randomised comparison. *Lancet.* 2007;369(9570):1347–55.

241. Shorr AF, Jackson WL, Sherner JH, Moores LK. Differences between low-molecular-weight and unfractionated heparin for venous thromboembolism prevention following ischemic stroke: a metaanalysis. *Chest.* 2008;133(1):149–55.

242. Pineo GF, Lin J, Annemans L. The economic impact of enoxaparin versus unfractionated heparin for prevention of venous thromboembolism in acute ischemic stroke patients. *Clinicoecon Outcomes Res.* 2012;4:99–107.

243. Qaseem A, Chou R, Humphrey LL, Starkey M, Shekelle P, Clinical Guidelines Committee of the American College of P. Venous thromboembolism prophylaxis in hospitalized patients: a clinical practice guideline from the American College of Physicians. *Ann Intern Med.* 2011;155:625–32.

244. Kamran SI, Downey D, Ruff RL. Pneumatic sequential compression reduces the risk of deep vein thrombosis in stroke patients. *Neurology.* 1998;50(6):1683–8.

245. Naccarato M, Chiodo Grandi F, Dennis M, Sandercock PA. Physical methods for preventing deep vein thrombosis in stroke. *Cochrane Database Syst Rev.* 2010;8:CD001922.

246. Clots Trials Collaboration, Dennis M, Sandercock PAG, Reid J, Graham C, Murray G, et al. Effectiveness of thigh-length graduated compression stockings to reduce the risk of deep vein thrombosis after stroke (CLOTS trial 1): a multicentre, randomised controlled trial. *Lancet.* 2009;373(9679):1958–65.

247. Clots Trial Collaboration. Thigh-length versus below-knee stockings for deep venous thrombosis prophylaxis after stroke: a randomized trial. *Ann Intern Med.* 2010;153(9):553–62.

248. Bernhardt J, Collaboration AT. Early mobilization testing in patients with acute stroke. *Chest.* 2012;141(6):1641–2.

CHAPTER 21

Traumatic spinal cord injury

Jefferson R. Wilson, Newton Cho, and Michael G. Fehlings

Spinal cord injury (SCI) is a potentially devastating condition that presents significant management challenges in both its acute and chronic stages. This chapter reviews the pathophysiology and the acute and chronic management of SCI, highlighting the importance of an integrated team approach to maximize the chance of good outcome and minimize the long-term consequences of this condition.

Epidemiology

The incidence of traumatic SCI varies between 14.5 and 57.8 per million per year, depending on the world region considered (1,2). In spite of these regional differences in incidence, the characteristics of injured patients are remarkably consistent between countries. SCI is roughly three to four times more common in males than females and typically has a bimodal age distribution, with a peak in the early adult period being largely due to motor vehicle accidents, and the second peak largely related to falls in the elderly (3,4).

The cervical spinal cord is the most common site of injury, accounting for 50–75% of SCI, with thoracic and lumbosacral lesions accounting for 15–30% and 10–20% of injuries respectively (4,5). In recent years, the percentage of cervical injuries, specifically high cervical lesions, has been increasing with a concomitant rise in the number of patients who remain ventilator dependent in the long term (3). The proportion of patients with complete (no motor or sensory function below the level of the lesion) and incomplete (some degree of motor or sensory preservation below the lesion level) injuries has traditionally been approximately equivalent, but there has been a recent trend towards an increase in the proportion of incomplete injuries, most likely as a result of the rising number of fall-related SCI in the elderly, and a decrease in the proportion of complete injuries, possibly because of a decline in gunshot-related injuries (3).

Aside from significant emotional and physical repercussions, SCI has a substantial economic impact at both a personal and societal level. According to the National Spinal Cord Injury Statistical Center, lifetime costs vary according to the level of injury but are nonetheless substantial regardless of the injury characteristics (Table 21.1) (6).

Pathophysiology

The pathobiology of SCI is comprised of two sequential stages. The primary injury results from the immediate compressive force applied to the spinal cord at the time of the trauma (7–10). This causes immediate grey/white matter petechial haemorrhage, axonal severing, and focal tissue destruction (11,12). Within seconds of the primary injury a cascade of secondary injury mechanisms that further exacerbates and extends the initial spinal cord damage is initiated, and continues for several weeks (Table 21.2). These include oedema formation, glutamate-mediated excitotoxicity, disruption of neuronal membrane integrity, and, importantly, neuroinflammation that is characterized by early neutrophil infiltration, subacute macrophage infiltration, and lipid peroxidation (13). In addition, reactive astrocytosis results in the formation of a glial scar around the site of injury that further prevents regeneration of axonal tracts across the lesion site (14). From a vascular perspective, microvascular thrombosis and vasospasm have been shown in animal models to lead to a dramatic reduction in spinal cord blood flow for a minimum of 24 hours post injury, and with variable return of perfusion depending on the severity and nature of the injury (15). Together, these processes collectively increase the volume of neural tissue destruction and negatively impact on an individual's potential for long-term neurological recovery. Currently, extensive research is being conducted targeting neuroprotective and regenerative approaches to ameliorate secondary damage and reconstitute damaged tissue (16,17).

Acute management

Pre-hospital management

The primary focus of the pre-hospital management of trauma patients with a suspected SCI is to expedite transfer to a definitive care unit while optimizing medical status and ensuring immobilization of the craniospinal axis (18,19). Timely transfer to a healthcare facility that can offer appropriate medical and surgical care of SCI is paramount (20). Observational studies have demonstrated that the implementation of improved transport systems, combined with management of patients at centres experienced in the treatment of SCI, result in fewer deaths, reduced complication rates, and shorter hospital lengths of stay (21,22).

Throughout transfer, the craniospinal axis must be maintained in a neutral position to prevent further cord injury (20,23). Typically, this is accomplished at the accident site through the placement of a hard cervical collar and transfer to a rigid spine board through the log roll manoeuvre (20,23). Vigilant monitoring of cardiorespiratory status is essential given the propensity of patients with SCI to

Table 21.1 Annual healthcare and living costs associated with spinal cord injury according to level and severity of injury

Spinal cord injury level and severity	Average annual cost (US $)	
	First year post injury	Subsequent years
High tetraplegia (C1–C4) AIS grade A, B, C	1,023,924	177,808
Low tetraplegia (C5–C8) AIS grade A, B, C	739,874	109,077
Paraplegia AIS grade A, B, C	499,023	66,106
Incomplete injury (any level) AIS grade D	334,170	40,589

AIS, ASIA (American Spinal Injury Association) Impairment Scale.

Reproduced with permission from NSCISC 'Spinal Cord Injury: Facts and Figures at a Glance 2012'. Available from: https://www.nscisc.uab.edu/.

develop pulmonary and haemodynamic complications soon after injury. In view of the potential for systemic deterioration, transporting personnel should be equipped with the capacity to manage the airway as well as provide basic haemodynamic resuscitation (23,24).

Neurological examination

After medical stabilization, a detailed neurological examination should be performed as soon as possible after hospital admission to establish the pattern and severity of the injury. For purposes of standardization, all examinations should be performed in accordance with the International Standards for Neurological Classification of Spinal Cord Injury (ISNCSCI) (25). Now in its fifth iteration, the 2011 version of the ISNCSCI consists of three main components: the American Spinal Injury Association (ASIA) Motor Score (AMS), the ASIA Sensory Score (ASS), and the ASIA Impairment Scale (AIS) grade (26).

The AMS is obtained by quantifying and summating motor function in ten key muscle groups bilaterally. For each muscle group, function is graded on a scale from 0 (total paralysis) to 5 (normal

Table 21.2 Mechanisms of secondary injury after spinal cord injury

Time after injury	Mechanism
Early acute (< 48 hours)	Oedema
	Excitotoxicity
	Haemorrhage
	Necrosis
	Neuronal membrane lipid peroxidation
	Neutrophil infiltration
	Axonal demyelination
	Reactive oxygen species production
Subacute/intermediate (14 days to 6 months)	Macrophage infiltration
	Glial scar and cyst formation
Chronic (> 6 months)	Wallerian degeneration
	Persistent demyelinated axons

active movement, full range of motion against gravity, and sufficient resistance to be considered normal) producing an ordinal score between 0 and 100, reflecting no and perfect motor function respectively. The AMS is often conventionally divided into an upper extremity motor score and lower extremity score, each representing a total of 50 possible points. For the sensory score, pinprick and light touch sensation are assessed in 28 pre-specified dermatomes bilaterally (C2–S5), with each dermatome receiving a score of 0, 1, or 2 depending on whether the sensation is absent, abnormal, or normal respectively. This yields two cumulative sensory scores, one for pinprick and one light touch, both with minimum values of 0 and maximum values of 112. Based on the patient's AMS, ASS, and findings on digital rectal examination to evaluate neurological function in distal sacral segments, an AIS grade is assigned according to the criteria outlined in Table 21.3 and Figure 21.1.

Lastly, the neurological level of injury is assigned by identifying the level with normal motor power (at least a score of 3/5) and sensory function bilaterally. Traditionally, the neurological examination obtained at 72 hours post injury is considered the baseline or 'acute' examination, and is used for purposes of comparison during patient follow-up and to evaluate for neurological improvement over time (27,28).

Radiological evaluation

When evaluating a patient with spinal trauma and suspected SCI, plain radiographs, computed tomography (CT), and magnetic resonance imaging (MRI) all contribute to the diagnostic picture. All patients with a history of trauma and an impaired level of consciousness should undergo a CT of the cervical spine with thin cuts from the occiput to T1 and reformatted images. At hospital admission, all trauma patients should undergo, as a minimum, a cross-table lateral cervical spine plain X-ray as part of the Advanced Trauma Life Support (ATLS) protocol (29–31). Although this modality is somewhat insensitive for identifying occult fractures and injuries, it is useful as a screening tool to identify an overt fractures

Table 21.3 American Spinal Injury Association (ASIA) Impairment Scale grading system

AIS grade	Description
A	Complete lack of motor and sensory function in sacral segments S4 to S5
B	Sensory function is preserved below the neurological level including S4 to S5. Motor function is not preserved, and there is no motor function more than three levels below the neurological level on either side of the body
C	Motor function is preserved below the neurological level with > 50% of the muscles below the neurological level with a grade < 3
D	Motor function is preserved below the neurological level with at least 50% of the muscles below the neurological level with a grade of 3 or higher
E	Normal sensory and motor function in a patient who previously had deficits

AIS, ASIA (American Spinal Injury Association) Impairment Scale.

American Spinal Injury Association: Impairment Scale grading system, revised 2013; Atlanta, GA. Reprinted 2013.

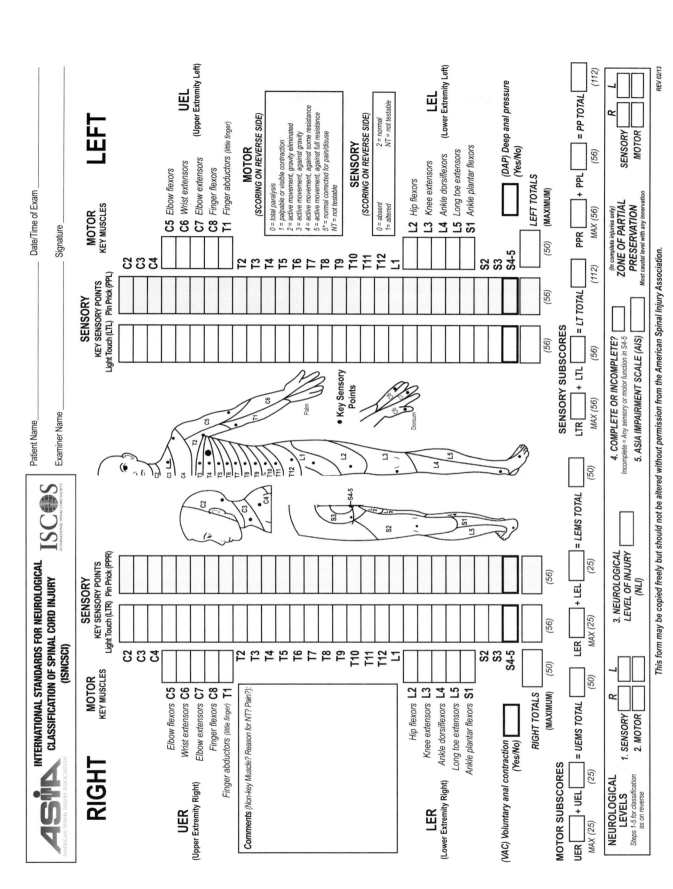

Fig. 21.1 The American Spinal Injury Association (ASIA) score sheet for documenting the severity of spinal cord injury

American Spinal Injury Association: *International Standards for Neurological Classification of Spinal Cord Injury*, revised 2013; Atlanta, GA. Reprinted 2013.

or deformity, and to direct further imaging investigations. If the patient has undergone a total body CT, additional radiographs of the spine can be omitted.

Even in the absence of abnormality on plain radiographs, CT with three-dimensional reconstructions is recommended to definitively exclude the presence of a bony injury (32,33). Soft tissues, such as ligamentous structures, intervertebral discs, spinal cord, and nerve roots, are best visualized by MRI, which can establish the anatomical level of injury as well characterize the nature of the cord lesion itself (31,34). Such information is important not only for diagnosis and surgical treatment planning, but also for counselling the patient on prognosis. At the two extremes, an MRI-confirmed haematoma within the spinal cord portends a poor prognosis for recovery whereas the absence of any abnormal MRI spinal cord signal is associated with the best potential for recovery (34,35). MRI-demonstrated spinal cord contusions and oedema reflect lesions of intermediate severity where individuals' potential for recovery falls in between these two extremes (34,36). Although rare, discontinuity of the spinal cord, spinal cord transection, is associated with the most dismal potential for future recovery (31). In a single-centre study, other MRI variables associated with poor recovery include rostrocaudal lesion length, greater degree of cord compression, and greater degree of canal compromise (34).

MRI is particularly useful for identifying areas of persistent spinal canal compromise and spinal cord compression which are targets for surgical decompression. However, for many years, consensus surrounding the appropriate methodology for assessing these variables was absent, leading to a lack of consistency in defining treatment plans. Recently, Fehlings and colleagues have described two separate measurements, maximum spinal cord compression (MSCC) and maximum canal compromise (MCC), to standardize such assessments (37). These measures are produced from the mid-sagittal image on a T2-weighted MRI and compare the degree of compression and compromise at the site of injury with that at adjacent normal levels (37). Both measures have been shown to be valid and reliable, and have become the basis for the radiological evaluation of SCI in recent surgical trials (38,39). Figure 21.2 depicts the preoperative MRI of a cervical SCI patient and demonstrates the methodology for calculating the MSCC.

Critical care management

Given the often precarious nature of an individual's medical status in the acute period following injury, it is recommended that SCI patients, particularly those with severe cervical lesions, should be managed in an intensive care unit (ICU) for a minimum of 1–2 weeks (40–44). During this critical period, continuous cardiorespiratory monitoring, as well as the option for rapid intervention in the event of deterioration, is essential. This section outlines the approach to the diagnosis and management of the major cardiovascular, haemodynamic, and respiratory issues of concern during the critical acute period following SCI.

Cardiovascular and haemodynamic management

One of the strongest predictors of poor outcome after injury to the central nervous system is the development of hypotension (45). Whilst the majority of the evidence on this topic is extrapolated from the traumatic brain injury literature, there is a strong consensus that hypotension must also be avoided and/or aggressively corrected in the acute phases after SCI to avoid or minimize secondary

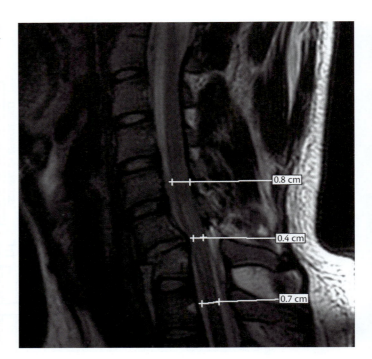

Fig. 21.2 Preoperative T2-weighted cervical spinal MRI scan demonstrating spinal cord compression at level C6–7 with concomitant hyperintense signal changes within the cord. Based on the formula (1 – [corddiam@injury/(corddiam@normalabove + corddiam@normalbelow)/2]) × 100%, the maximal degree of spinal cord compression in this case is (1 – [0.4/(0.8 + 0.7)/2]) × 100% = 53%. Reproduced from Springer and *Neurotheraputics*, 8, 2, 2011, pp. 187–194, 'Emerging Approaches to the Surgical Management of Acute Traumatic Spinal Cord Injury'. With kind permission from Springer Science and Business Media.

injury. As in trauma patients generally, the most common cause of hypotension after SCI is haemorrhage-associated hypovolaemia. In addition to haemorrhage, pneumothorax and cardiac tamponade should be excluded and treated before hypotension is attributed to neurological dysfunction secondary to SCI (46). The diagnosis and treatment of hypotension should follow the standard ATLS protocol.

Whilst there is strong consensus that hypotension should always be avoided, defining a blood pressure target and an optimal time window for maintenance of this target is less clear. Current recommendations are based largely on the results from uncontrolled observational studies which examined the impact on short-term outcomes of invasive blood pressure monitoring and aggressive achievement of physiological targets during the days and weeks following injury (47,48). Summarizing the results of these studies, the 2002 American Association of Neurological Surgeons acute SCI consensus guidelines recommended that mean arterial pressure should be maintained between 85 and 90 mmHg for the first week following injury (49).

Neurogenic shock

Neurogenic shock refers to the loss of sympathetic outflow after a cervical or upper thoracic SCI, leading to decreased systemic vascular resistance, unopposed vagal stimulation (40,50,51), and resultant peripheral vasodilation and bradycardia. These changes are responsible for the classic clinical findings after SCI—hypotension with a wide pulse pressure, slow heart rate, and warm, well-perfused skin and extremities. This is in contrast to the classic clinical picture associated with hypovolaemic hypotension in which low blood pressure is generally associated with a narrow pulse pressure, tachycardia, and cool and pale skin and extremities. Given that the outflow of the sympathetic plexus ends at T4, it is rare for lesions below this level to result in neurogenic shock.

When neurogenic shock is suspected, initial treatment should consist of volume replacement with intravenous crystalloid (49–52). If hypotension persists despite volume resuscitation, vasopressors should be considered (40,50,51). Although there is no evidence to support the use of one vasopressor regimen over another, given that sympathetic output to both the heart and peripheral vasculature is affected, it makes physiological sense to employ agents which possess both alpha and beta adrenergic activity, such as dopamine, norepinephrine (noradrenaline) or epinephrine (adrenaline) (53).

In addition to causing hypotension, cervical and upper thoracic injuries are often associated with cardiac dysrhythmias (40,50,51). Sinus bradycardia secondary to impaired supraspinal sympathetic outflow is the most commonly observed finding, but other abnormalities, such as atrioventricular conduction blocks, supraventricular and ventricular tachycardia, are also reported. The frequency of bradycardia is directly associated with the severity of injury, and the highest incidence is seen in patients with AIS grade A lesions in whom there is complete disruption of sympathetic cardiac outflow (51). In the majority of such cases, bradyarrhythmias can be averted by the administration of the cholinergic receptor antagonist atropine, although a minority of patients require placement of a cardiac pacemaker (40,51). In treating hypotension in this context, it is also recommended that vasopressor medications with pure alpha adrenergic activity, such as phenylephrine, are avoided as they may cause reflex slowing of the heart and exacerbate pre-existing bradycardia. Interestingly, many of the dysrhythmias observed during the first days and weeks after SCI typically become less problematic in the chronic phase (51).

Airway and respiratory management

Airway and pulmonary complications are the leading cause of in-hospital morbidity and mortality after SCI (44,54). The majority are directly related to paralysis of respiratory related musculature including the diaphragm (innervated at spinal level C3–5), thoracic intercostal muscles (spinal level T1–11) and respiratory accessory muscles (predominately cranial nerve XI–XII and upper cervical levels). In addition to muscle paralysis, a variety of changes related to unopposed parasympathetic outflow including bronchospasm, increased bronchial secretions, abdominal distension, and the development of pulmonary oedema, negatively impact on respiratory physiology in patients with cervical and upper thoracic injuries (55,56). Patients with SCI are therefore at high risk of complications such as atelectasis, pneumonia, acute respiratory distress syndrome, and hypoventilation secondary to fatigue. This risk is greatest in those with severe cervical injury (57).

Because of the potential for rapid clinical decompensation from the time of admission onwards, close monitoring of respiratory function is essential. There should be a low threshold for intubation and mechanical ventilation which should be instituted at the first sign of distress or fatigue (44,54,57,58). Prophylactic intubation and ventilation in patients with complete injury and a neurological level rostral to C5 is recommended by some experts because of the invariable requirement for assisted ventilation at

some stage during the acute period of hospitalization (58). When intubation is required, the objective is to secure the airway with as little movement of the neck as possible. In the emergency setting, rapid sequence induction with orotracheal intubation and manual in-line neck stabilization is the standard of care but, in non-urgent situations, consideration should be given to fibreoptic endoscopic intubation techniques to further limit cervical manipulation (59).

For patients who do not require mechanical ventilation, continuous pulse oximetry and frequent bedside respiratory assessments, including evaluation of forced vital capacity (FVC), have been recommended to monitor for evidence of respiratory deterioration (44,54,56–58). In general, signs of physical distress including tachypnoea, desaturation, and decrease in FVC below 15 mL/kg should be treated as evidence of respiratory decompensation that requires intervention (54).

Following intubation and mechanical ventilation, several measures have been recommended to reduce the incidence of respiratory complications after SCI. Notably, aggressive pulmonary toilet and intrapulmonary percussive ventilation combined with the administration of warm humidified air, bronchodilators, and mucolytics can help clear retained secretions, reduce the risk of atelectasis and prevent pneumonia (44,54,56). Early and frequent fibreoptic bronchoscopy and bronchial lavage, as well as adjuncts such as a rotational bed and the use of Trendelenburg position to promote postural lung drainage, may also facilitate the clearance of airway secretions (44,54–56).

Venous thromboembolism

Given the extent of paralysis which typically follows SCI, especially complete cervical injuries, venous thromboembolism (VTE) is a particular concern. In the absence of pharmacological prophylaxis, the incidence of VTE is reported as high as 50%, with the vast majority of events occurring in the first few months after injury (60). As a result, institution of early prophylaxis is a priority. The 2008 Spinal Cord Medicine acute care guidelines recommend commencing treatment with low-molecular-weight heparin or unfractionated heparin, plus pneumatic compression devices, as soon as possible post SCI, in the absence of acute haemorrhage risk (61). Although the optimal duration of prophylaxis remains unclear, 8–12 weeks after complete cervical SCI is often recommended (62). If pharmacological prophylaxis must be delayed beyond 72 hours because of bleeding risk, the insertion of an inferior vena caval filter should be considered to reduce the risk of pulmonary embolus secondary to deep venous thrombosis.

Fever

Fever is frequently observed throughout the acute hospitalization and early discharge periods, and is more common in those with complete injuries or an indwelling urinary catheter (63). Investigation and management of fever after SCI is particularly relevant since animal studies have associated post-traumatic hyperthermia with worsened neurological outcome (64). Whilst pneumonia and urinary tract infections are commonly reported, no aetiology is identified in up to 65% of SCI patients with fever (65) when it is usually attributed to abnormal thermoregulation arising from post-traumatic autonomic dysfunction. After identifying treatable infectious and non-infectious causes of fever and administrating antipyretics, cooling to normothermia should be considered. Recently, endovascular cooling techniques have been described in the management of patients with severe (> 40°C) SCI-related hyperthermia (66).

Pharmacological therapy

Although several different agents have been evaluated in the context of randomized controlled trials, no drug administered at any time point after injury has currently demonstrated definitive evidence of improved neurological or long-term functional recovery after SCI (10).

Steroids

Over 30 years ago, methylprednisolone sodium succinate (MPSS) was the first agent to be evaluated for the treatment of SCI in a large-scale efficacy trial in the first National Acute Spinal Cord Injury Study (NASCIS I) (67). This was undertaken following preclinical evidence that MPSS reduced post-traumatic inflammation and neuronal membrane disruption. Today, the use of steroids continues to galvanize significant controversy amongst clinicians. The main subject of continued debate is the results of the NASCIS II published in 1990 (68). In this study, a 24-hour infusion of high-dose MPSS (30 mg/kg IV bolus followed by 5.4 mg/kg/h IV for 23 hours) was compared to placebo. Considering all time points of administration, there was no significant difference in the primary outcome measure of motor recovery between admission and 6-month follow-up, between the MPSS and placebo groups, although there was a non-significant trends towards a higher incidence of wound infections and gastrointestinal haemorrhage in the MPSS group. However, in an a priori defined subgroup analysis, MPSS was associated with a significantly better motor recovery at follow-up compared to placebo in patients receiving MPSS within eight hours of injury. A recent Cochrane review incorporating the results of NASCIS II in a meta-analysis with two other trials using the same MPSS dose confirmed that 24-hour infusion of MPSS when initiated within 8 hours of injury was associated with an additional 4 points of NASCIS motor score recovery compared to placebo or no treatment (69).

Critics of these studies point to the use of post hoc comparisons to prove effect, as well as increased complications with steroid administration. The subsequent NASCIS III study compared a 48-hour MPSS regimen to the 24-hour infusion in NASCIS II (70) and, although the primary analysis was negative, a pre-planned subgroup analysis demonstrated superior motor recovery in the 48-hour MPSS regimen in patients receiving treatment between 3 and 8 hours after injury. Given that the 48-hour regimen represents the largest dosage of corticosteroids ever studied in human disease, the trend towards increased infectious complications, such as severe pneumonia and sepsis, in in this group is perhaps unsurprising (70,71). Notably, potential confounding effects of steroid induced hyperglycaemia were not accounted for in the steroid trials.

In attempt to summarize the existing evidence on the use of MPSS in SCI, several major bodies, including the American Association of Neurological Surgeons and the Congress of Neurological Surgeons, have recommended that MPSS should not be considered a standard of care but 'a treatment option, the administration of which may lead to serious medical complications' (72,73).

Other agents

Although the NASCIS studies represent the first major therapeutic trials after SCI, the largest clinical trial to date has investigated the efficacy of the purported neuroprotective/neuroregenerative

ganglioside molecule GM-1 (74). In this study, which enrolled 760 subjects, there was no difference in the proportion of patients with good neurological recovery at 6 months between the treatment and placebo groups (74). In addition to MPSS and GM-1, several other putative neuroprotective agents have been studied after SCI. These include nimodipine, the L-type calcium channel blocker (75,76), naloxone, the opioid receptor antagonist, and tirilazad, a synthetic compound designed to reduce neuronal membrane damage (76). Whilst all have been promising in preclinical studies, none have been effective in improving long-term recovery in phase III trials and are not currently routinely used for the treatment of SCI.

As well as pharmacological agents, implantation of stem cells and autologous non-stem cells has been widely investigated as a potential neuroregenerative strategy in preclinical studies of SCI (77). Although several early phase trials are enrolling patients, this therapy is currently considered purely investigational.

Hypothermia

On the basis of preclinical work, local and systemic therapeutic hypothermia (TH) has been hypothesized to improve outcome after SCI by disrupting the secondary injury cascade and reducing tissue metabolism in the post-injury setting (78–82). However, there is a paucity of clinical evidence supporting this hypothesis. In a single-centre phase I study, the use of moderate TH (33°C) was investigated in 14 patients with complete SCI (83). Target temperature was achieved in all patients within 48 hours of injury through placement of a cooling catheter in the femoral vein. Six of the 14 cooled patients (42.8%) were incomplete at final follow-up (50 weeks), three improved to AIS B, two to AIS C, and one patient improved to AIS D.

The complication rates in the TH and normothermic groups were similar. Pending definitive evidence of efficacy, TH cannot currently be recommended in the routine management of SCI.

Surgery

The majority of spinal column injuries that result in injury to the spinal cord itself involve substantial disruption of the bony and ligamentous spinal anatomy, leading to significant biomechanical instability. If this situation remains untreated, there is potential for ongoing dynamic injury to the spinal cord and progressive worsening of neurological status. In this instance, surgery is indicated to restore normal anatomical alignment and re-establish spinal stability, usually with an instrumented fusion procedure (84).

Apart from these biomechanical objectives, the other central goal of surgery is to decompress the spinal cord. Preclinical studies confirm that ongoing cord compression potentiates the secondary injury cascade and results in worsened pathological, electrophysiological, and neurological outcomes (85–90). A multitude of animal studies have also suggested that outcome can be improved by rapid decompression of the spinal cord (91–94). Although this makes intuitive sense, clinical evidence demonstrating the safety and efficacy of early spinal decompression has remained largely absent until recently. In a 1997 randomized controlled trial by Vaccaro and colleagues, 62 patients with traumatic SCI were randomly assigned to undergo early (before 72 hours) or late (after 72 hours) decompressive surgery (95). There was no difference in neurological outcome between early and late surgical intervention, although 20 of the 62 patients were lost to follow-up (95). It was subsequently concluded that a 72-hour time window was too late after injury to positively affect secondary injurious mechanisms and clinical outcome, and that a 24-hour window was more appropriate (96). The Surgical Timing in Acute Spinal Cord Injury Study (STASCIS) was undertaken in the context of the international cooperative Spine Trauma Study Group to investigate this time frame for surgical intervention after SCI (97). STASCIS was a prospective cohort study reporting 6-month outcomes in 222 patients enrolled at 6 North American centres. After adjusting for relevant cohort differences, early surgery was associated with significantly greater odds of neurological recovery at follow-up as defined by a 2 AIS grade improvement, with no differences in acute in-hospital complications between early and late surgery. These findings have subsequently been confirmed in a smaller Canadian cohort study, which demonstrated that decompressive surgery performed within 24 after SCI was associated with superior motor neurological outcomes at 6 months (98).

Based on current evidence, combined with surveys of surgical opinion favouring the practice of early intervention, the authors recommend decompression of the spinal cord within 24 hours of injury whenever possible.

Chronic spinal cord injury management

The management of chronic SCI has been reviewed in detail elsewhere (99) and only key areas are discussed in this chapter.

Autonomic dysreflexia

In the chronic phase of SCI with an injury at or rostral to the T4 neurological level, the presence of a noxious stimulus below the level of injury can lead to a clinical syndrome known as autonomic dysreflexia (AD) (50,51,100–102). AD is characterized by a clinical picture of hypertension, bradycardia, pounding headache, and pale, cold skin below the level of the lesion and pink, well-perfused skin and perspiration above. The pathophysiological basis of these findings is as follows. The stimulus causes a surge in autonomic outflow from the sympathetic centres in the cervical and thoracic spinal cord leading to a rise in blood pressure. This is detected by carotid and aortic baroreceptors resulting in activation of central parasympathetic centres in an attempt to maintain cardiovascular haemostasis by increasing vagal output to reduce heart rate, and rostral inhibition of sympathetic outflow. However, in severe complete SCI the inhibitory impulses cannot be transmitted beyond the lesion site (101) and, as a result, there is dominance of parasympathetic activity above the level of the lesion and of sympathetic activity below.

Recognition and treatment of AD is important because several complications, including intracranial haemorrhage and seizures, have been associated with its hypertensive response (100,102). From a management perspective, the initial step is to move the patient into an upright and seated position which typically results in an orthostatic drop in blood pressure (100,102). The next step is to identify and remove the inciting noxious stimulus (100,102), the most common of which is urinary retention and bladder distension. All patients at risk of AD should therefore have a urinary catheter in place. Other precipitating factors include faecal impaction, decubitus ulcers, and lower extremity spasticity. If blood pressure remains uncontrolled (i.e. systolic blood pressure > 150 mmHg) following the change in posture, pharmacological intervention is required (100). Rapid-onset and short-duration vasodilators such as oral nifedipine or cutaneous nitroglycerine applied above the lesion level have been recommended (100,102).

Chronic urinary dysfunction

The primary cause of urinary complications after SCI is the disrupted communication between central voiding centres and the micturition reflex centre in the sacral spinal cord. In non-injured individuals, the sensation of the bladder filling is transmitted via the spinal cord to regions of the frontal lobe involved in the coordination of voiding. Activation of this frontal voiding region disinhibits the pontine micturition centre which in turn sends a descending message via the spinal cord that coordinates bladder contraction and sphincter relaxation (103,104). In the presence of SCI, the sensation of bladder filling is carried to the sacral spinal cord via the intact peripheral nervous system but is not rostrally conducted to the central voiding centres. This can result in reflective contraction of the detrusor muscles, sometimes without concurrent relaxation of urinary sphincters, a syndrome known as detrusor-sphincter dyssynergia (103,104). Untreated, this condition can lead to vesicoureteral reflux, hydronephrosis, and renal failure (104). To prevent such complications, orally administered anticholinergic drugs, such as oxybutynin and probanthine, that facilitate detrusor relaxation are often used. Injection of botulinum A toxin into detrusor muscle to prevent bladder contraction by blocking presynaptic acetylcholine release is required in some (103,105). To prevent overfilling of the bladder, these treatments must be combined with intermittent self- or caregiver bladder catheterization (106,107). Following the complete return of spinal reflexes, usually several months after injury, patients should undergo urodynamic studies to identify ongoing bladder dysfunction, and assess for the presence of dyssynergia so that long-term complications can be avoided (106).

Pressure ulcers

The development of pressure ulcers is one of the most common, but also one of the most preventable, complications of SCI. The prevalence of pressure ulcers in chronic SCI ranges from 15% to 30%, but specific patient factors are associated with a higher risk. These include motor/sensory complete injuries, male sex, smoking, poor nutritional status, pre-existing peripheral arterial disease and/or diabetes, and excess moisture in dependent regions (108,109). Pressure ulcers are estimated to account for about 25% of hospital admissions in the chronic phase of SCI and have a major adverse impact of an individual's quality of life as well as on healthcare costs (110,111).

Pressure ulcers form as a result of prolonged application of cutaneous pressure, typically at bony anatomical prominences such as the ischial tuberosities, posterior foot/heel, sacral region, and posterior shoulder region. In individuals with a properly functioning nervous system, this sustained pressure would typically evoke discomfort prompting a voluntary change in position. However, many SCI patients are unable to sense or respond to such discomfort and, as a result, the pressure continues and leads to progressive ischaemia and ultimately necrosis of the skin, subcutaneous tissue, and sometimes muscle. Pressure ulcer severity is graded by evaluation of the depth of tissue visible on inspection of the wound according to the National Pressure Ulcer Advisory Panel recommendations (Table 21.4) (112).

Table 21.4 National Pressure Ulcer Advisory Panel pressure ulcer grading system

Grade	Description
I: Non-blanchable erythema	Intact skin Non-blanchable erythema over bony prominence Area may be painful, soft, warmer/cooler
II: Partial thickness	Partial loss of dermis Shallow shiny/dry ulcer without sloughing or bruising
III: Full-thickness skin loss	Full thickness skin loss Fat may be visible but not tendon, muscle, or bone
IV: Full-thickness tissue loss	Exposure tendon, muscle, or bone Slough/eschar may be present

Modified from the National Pressure Ulcer Advisory Panel Pressure Ulcer Stages/Categories (http://www.npuap.org/resources/educational-and-clinical-resources/npuap-pressure-ulcer-stagescategories/). Used with permission of the National Pressure Ulcer Advisory Panel January 2015.

Undoubtedly prevention is the best approach to pressure ulcer management after SCI. A variety of preventive measures have been outlined including daily skin inspection by the patient and/or caregiver for identification of potential problem areas, prevention of excess moisture accumulation in dependent regions, the use of cushions and tilt mechanisms on chairs and beds to redistribute pressure regularly, adequate nutritional support, and smoking cessation. If ulcers do develop, the principles of treatment include basic wound care and dressing, debridement of necrotic tissue, optimization of nutritional state, and treatment of any underlying infection. In addition, a variety of adjunct treatments, including hydrocolloid dressings as well as electrical stimulation and pulsed electromagnetic energy, have been shown to promote wound healing (113). In extreme situations, it may be necessary to perform a diverting colostomy to prevent repeated contamination of serve sacral ulcers with faecal material.

Spasticity

As defined by Lance in 1980, spasticity is a 'motor disorder characterized by a velocity dependent increase in tonic stretch reflexes (muscle tone) with exaggerated tendon jerks, resulting from hyper-excitability of the stretch reflex, as one component of the upper motor neuron syndrome' (114). Approximately 65–78% of patients experience symptoms of spasticity at greater than 1 year after SCI, with the greatest incidence (up to 93%) in patients with AIS grade A injury (115,116). Clinically, spasticity manifests as painful muscle spasms, unpredictable jerking movements of the extremities, and limited range of motion. It not only leads to substantial discomfort, but also makes tending to hygiene and grooming, as well as participation in physiotherapy, a significant challenge.

From a therapeutic perspective, both systemic and local therapies can be used to reduce the burden of spasticity. Oral agents that mimic the effects of GABA (benzodiazepines, baclofen, gabapentin), stimulate central alpha-2 adrenergic activity (tizanidine, clonidine) or directly inhibit skeletal muscle contraction (dantrolene) have been used in the treatment of SCI-related spasticity (117). Local injection of botulinum toxin and chemo-denervating agents such as phenol and ethanol can also be used to treat spasticity in individual muscles groups without the attendant systemic side effects of oral medication (118).

Long-term ventilation and weaning

It is estimated that 2–4% of patients require long-term mechanical ventilation after SCI (119). Patients with a higher level of quadriplegia and reduced level of consciousness are at the highest risk of becoming ventilator dependent in the long term. Quantified from the standpoint of survival, the incentive to successively wean patients from a ventilator is substantial; annual survival rates for ventilated patients have been reported to be as low as 33% whereas rates for non-ventilated patients are dramatically higher at around 84% (120). Respiratory-related conditions, including pneumonia, are the most frequent cause of mortality in ventilator-dependent patients, accounting for 30% of deaths (119).

In spite of the strong imperative to reduce the proportion of patients with SCI who become ventilator dependent, there is a paucity of evidence identifying the optimal strategies to facilitate weaning. In a 1994 study of 52 patients with C3 or C4 level quadriplegia, Peterson and colleagues retrospectively compared the effectiveness of two weaning strategies—intermittent mandatory ventilation (IMV) with a gradual reduction in the set ventilator rate allowing the patient to take increasing spontaneous breaths, and progressive periods of ventilator free breathing (PVFB) in which the patient breathed spontaneously through a T-piece device (121). The rate of complete ventilator weaning was significantly greater with the PVFB (67.6%) compared to the IMV (34.6%) technique, although these findings have yet to be confirmed by other studies. Gutierrez and colleagues evaluated the impact of introducing an evidence based protocol to optimize respiratory status and encourage ventilator weaning in seven tetraplegic ventilator dependent SCI patients (122). This protocol involved pre-training optimization, inspiration/expiration resistance training, and on- and off-ventilator endurance training. Following adoption of the protocol, all patients with a neurological level below C4 were weaned completely, whilst those with injuries above this level had substantial improvement in their off-ventilator capacities. Although the results of this study are promising, larger follow-up studies have not been completed to our knowledge.

There is increasing interest in the use of phrenic nerve or direct diaphragmatic stimulation in ventilator-dependent patients with a high quadriplegia (123,124). This treatment involves surgical placement of electrodes on the cervical or thoracic portion of the phrenic nerve, or in the diaphragmatic muscle itself, and connection to an internal pulse generator implanted in a subcutaneous pocket on the chest wall. Observational studies, mostly of small sample sizes, have demonstrated mechanical ventilation cessation rates of up to 50% with the use of such pacing systems (125). That said, this therapy is only appropriate for selected individuals and has a number of recognized limitations that currently limit its scope.

References

1. Hagen EM, Rekand T, Gilhus NE, Gronning M. Traumatic spinal cord injuries—incidence, mechanisms and course. *Tidsskr Nor Laegeforen.* 2012;132(7):831–7.
2. O'Connor P. Incidence and patterns of spinal cord injury in Australia. *Accid Anal Prev.* 2002;34(4):405–15.
3. Devivo MJ. Epidemiology of traumatic spinal cord injury: trends and future implications. *Spinal Cord.* 2012;50(5):365–72.

4. Pickett GE, Campos-Benitez M, Keller JL, Duggal N. Epidemiology of traumatic spinal cord injury in Canada. *Spine (Phila Pa 1976)*. 2006;31(7):799–805.

5. Couris CM, Guilcher SJ, Munce SE, Fung K, Craven BC, Verrier M, *et al*. Characteristics of adults with incident traumatic spinal cord injury in Ontario, Canada. *Spinal Cord*. 2010;48(1):39–44.

6. National Spinal Cord Injury Statistical Center. *Spinal Cord Injury Facts and Figures at a Glance 2012*. [Online] https://www.nscisc.uab.edu/

7. Hagg T, Oudega M. Degenerative and spontaneous regenerative processes after spinal cord injury. *J Neurotrauma*. 2006;23(3–4):264–80.

8. Profyris C, Cheema SS, Zang D, Azari MF, Boyle K, Petratos S. Degenerative and regenerative mechanisms governing spinal cord injury. *Neurobiol Dis*. 2004;15(3):415–36.

9. Sekhon LH, Fehlings MG. Epidemiology, demographics, and pathophysiology of acute spinal cord injury. *Spine (Phila Pa 1976)*. 2001;26(24 Suppl):S2–12.

10. Rowland JW, Hawryluk GW, Kwon B, Fehlings MG. Current status of acute spinal cord injury pathophysiology and emerging therapies: promise on the horizon. *Neurosurg Focus*. 2008;25(5):E2.

11. Sandler AN, Tator CH. Effect of acute spinal cord compression injury on regional spinal cord blood flow in primates. *J Neurosurg*. 1976;45(6):660–76.

12. Tator C, Fehlings M. Review of the secondary injury theory of acute spinal cord trauma with emphasis on vascular mechanisms. *J Nerosurg*. 1991;75:15–26.

13. Schwartz G, Fehlings M. Secondary injury mechanisms of spinal cord trauma: a novel therapeutic approach for the management of secondary pathophysiology with the sodium channel blocker riluzole. *Prog Brain Res*. 2002;137:177–90.

14. Bradbury EJ, Moon LD, Popat RJ, King VR, Bennett GS, Patel PN, *et al*. Chondroitinase ABC promotes functional recovery after spinal cord injury. *Nature*. 2002;416(6881):636–40.

15. Sandler A, Tator C. Review of the effect of spinal cord trauma on the vessels and blood flow in the spinal cord. *J Nerosurg*. 1976;45:638–46.

16. Baptiste DC, Fehlings MG. Pharmacological approaches to repair the injured spinal cord. *J Neurotrauma*. 2006;23(3–4):318–34.

17. Baptiste DC, Tighe A, Fehlings MG. Spinal cord injury and neural repair: focus on neuroregenerative approaches for spinal cord injury. *Expert Opin Invest Drugs*. 2009;18(5):663–73.

18. Hachen HJ. Emergency transportation in the event of acute spinal cord lesion. *Paraplegia*. 1974;12(1):33–7.

19. Hachen HJ. Idealized care of the acutely injured spinal cord in Switzerland. *J Trauma*. 1977;17(12):931–6.

20. Ahn H, Singh J, Nathens A, MacDonald RD, Travers A, Tallon J, *et al*. Pre-hospital care management of a potential spinal cord injured patient: a systematic review of the literature and evidence-based guidelines. *J Neurotrauma*. 2011;28(8):1341–61.

21. Tator CH, Rowed DW, Schwartz ML, Gertzbein SD, Bharatwal N, Barkin M, *et al*. Management of acute spinal cord injuries. *Can J Surg*. 1984;27(3):289–93, 96.

22. Tator CH, Duncan EG, Edmonds VE, Lapczak LI, Andrews DF. Changes in epidemiology of acute spinal cord injury from 1947 to 1981. *Surg Neurol*. 1993;40(3):207–15.

23. Bernhard M, Gries A, Kremer P, Bottiger BW. Spinal cord injury (SCI)—prehospital management. *Resuscitation*. 2005;66(2):127–39.

24. Transportation of patients with acute traumatic cervical spine injuries. *Neurosurgery*. 2002;50(3 Suppl):S18–20.

25. American Spinal Injury Association. *International Standards for Neurological Classification of Spinal Cord Injury*. ASIA; 2012. [Online] http://www.asia-spinalinjury.org/elearning/ISNCSCI.php

26. Kirshblum SC, Burns SP, Biering-Sorensen F, Donovan W, Graves DE, Jha A, *et al*. International standards for neurological classification of spinal cord injury (revised 2011). *J Spinal Cord Med*. 2011;34(6):535–46.

27. Burns AS, Ditunno JF. Establishing prognosis and maximizing functional outcomes after spinal cord injury: a review of current and future directions in rehabilitation management. *Spine (Phila Pa 1976)*. 2001;26(24 Suppl):S137–45.

28. Wilson JR, Cadotte DW, Fehlings MG. Clinical predictors of neurological outcome, functional status, and survival after traumatic spinal cord injury: a systematic review. *J Neurosurg Spine*. 2012;17(1 Suppl):11–26.

29. American College of Surgeons. *Advanced Trauma Life Support System Program for Physicians*. Chicago, IL: American College of Surgeons; 1993.

30. Mirvis SE, Diaconis JN, Chirico PA, Reiner BI, Joslyn JN, Militello P. Protocol-driven radiologic evaluation of suspected cervical spine injury: efficacy study. *Radiology*. 1989;170(3 Pt 1):831–4.

31. Lammertse D, Dungan D, Dreisbach J, Falci S, Flanders A, Marino R, *et al*. Neuroimaging in traumatic spinal cord injury: an evidence-based review for clinical practice and research. *J Spinal Cord Med*. 2007;30(3):205–14.

32. Gale SC, Gracias VH, Reilly PM, Schwab CW. The inefficiency of plain radiography to evaluate the cervical spine after blunt trauma. *J Trauma*. 2005;59(5):1121–5.

33. Ghaffarpasand F, Paydar S, Foroughi M, Saberi A, Abbasi H, Karimi AA, *et al*. Role of cervical spine radiography in the initial evaluation of stable high-energy blunt trauma patients. *J Orthop Sci*. 2011;16(5):498–502.

34. Bozzo A, Marcoux J, Radhakrishna M, Pelletier J, Goulet B. The role of magnetic resonance imaging in the management of acute spinal cord injury. *J Neurotrauma*. 2011;28(8):1401–11.

35. Miyanji F, Furlan JC, Aarabi B, Arnold PM, Fehlings MG. Acute cervical traumatic spinal cord injury: MR imaging findings correlated with neurologic outcome—prospective study with 100 consecutive patients. *Radiology*. 2007;243(3):820–7.

36. Bondurant FJ, Cotler HB, Kulkarni MV, McArdle CB, Harris JH, Jr. Acute spinal cord injury. A study using physical examination and magnetic resonance imaging. *Spine (Phila Pa 1976)*. 1990;15(3):161–8.

37. Fehlings MG, Rao SC, Tator CH, Skaf G, Arnold P, Benzel E, *et al*. The optimal radiologic method for assessing spinal canal compromise and cord compression in patients with cervical spinal cord injury. Part II: Results of a multicenter study. *Spine (Phila Pa 1976)*. 1999;24(6):605–13.

38. Furlan JC, Kailaya-Vasan A, Aarabi B, Fehlings MG. A novel approach to quantitatively assess posttraumatic cervical spinal canal compromise and spinal cord compression: a multicenter responsiveness study. *Spine (Phila Pa 1976)*. 2011;36(10):784–93.

39. Furlan JC, Fehlings MG, Massicotte EM, Aarabi B, Vaccaro AR, Bono CM, *et al*. A quantitative and reproducible method to assess cord compression and canal stenosis after cervical spine trauma: a study of interrater and intrarater reliability. *Spine (Phila Pa 1976)*. 2007;32(19):2083–91.

40. Lehmann KG, Lane JG, Piepmeier JM, Batsford WP. Cardiovascular abnormalities accompanying acute spinal cord injury in humans: incidence, time course and severity. *J Am Coll Cardiol*. 1987;10(1):46–52.

41. Levi L, Wolf A, Belzberg H. Hemodynamic parameters in patients with acute cervical cord trauma: description, intervention, and prediction of outcome. *Neurosurgery*. 1993;33(6):1007–16.

42. Management of acute spinal cord injuries in an intensive care unit or other monitored setting. *Neurosurgery*. 2002;50(3 Suppl):S51–7.

43. Gschaedler R, Dollfus P, Mole JP, Mole L, Loeb JP. Reflections on the intensive care of acute cervical spinal cord injuries in a general traumatology centre. *Paraplegia*. 1979;17(1):58–61.

44. Reines HD, Harris RC. Pulmonary complications of acute spinal cord injuries. *Neurosurgery*. 1987;21(2):193–6.

45. Chesnut R, Marshall L, Klauber M, Blunt B, Baldwin N, Eisenberg H, *et al*. The role of secondary brain injury in determining outcome from severe head injury. *J Trauma*. 1993;34:216–22.

46. Amar A, Levy M. Pathogenesis and pharmacological strategies for mitigating secondary damage in acute spinal cord injury. *Neurosurgery*. 1999;44:1027–39.

47. Levi L, Wolf A, Belzber H. Hemodynamic parameters in patients with acute cervical cord trauma: Description, intervention, and prediction of outcome. *Neurosurgery*. 1993;33:1007–17.

48. Vale F, Burns J, Jackson A, Hadley M. Combined medical and surgical treatment after acute spinal cord injury: results of a prospective pilot

study to assess the merits of aggressive medical resuscitation and blood pressure management. *J Neurosurg.* 1997;87:239–46.

49. Blood pressure management after acute spinal cord injury. *Neurosurgery.* 2002;50(3 Suppl):S58–62.

50. Furlan JC, Fehlings MG. Cardiovascular complications after acute spinal cord injury: pathophysiology, diagnosis, and management. *Neurosurg Focus.* 2008;25(5):E13.

51. Grigorean VT, Sandu AM, Popescu M, Iacobini MA, Stoian R, Neascu C, *et al.* Cardiac dysfunctions following spinal cord injury. *J Med Life.* 2009;2(2):133–45.

52. Vale FL, Burns J, Jackson AB, Hadley MN. Combined medical and surgical treatment after acute spinal cord injury: results of a prospective pilot study to assess the merits of aggressive medical resuscitation and blood pressure management. *J Neurosurg.* 1997;87(2):239–46.

53. Ploumis A, Yadlapalli N, Fehlings MG, Kwon BK, Vaccaro AR. A systematic review of the evidence supporting a role for vasopressor support in acute SCI. *Spinal Cord.* 2010;48(5):356–62.

54. Berlly M, Shem K. Respiratory management during the first five days after spinal cord injury. *J Spinal Cord Med.* 2007;30(4):309–18.

55. McMichan JC, Michel L, Westbrook PR. Pulmonary dysfunction following traumatic quadriplegia. Recognition, prevention, and treatment. *JAMA.* 1980;243(6):528–31.

56. Mansel JK, Norman JR. Respiratory complications and management of spinal cord injuries. *Chest.* 1990;97(6):1446–52.

57. Berney S, Bragge P, Granger C, Opdam H, Denehy L. The acute respiratory management of cervical spinal cord injury in the first 6 weeks after injury: a systematic review. *Spinal Cord.* 2011;49(1):17–29.

58. Como JJ, Sutton ER, McCunn M, Dutton RP, Johnson SB, Aarabi B, *et al.* Characterizing the need for mechanical ventilation following cervical spinal cord injury with neurologic deficit. *J Trauma.* 2005;59(4):912–16.

59. Ball PA. Critical care of spinal cord injury. *Spine (Phila Pa 1976).* 2001;26(24 Suppl):S27–30.

60. Jones T, Ugalde V, Franks P, Zhou H, White RH. Venous thromboembolism after spinal cord injury: incidence, time course, and associated risk factors in 16,240 adults and children. *Arch Phys Med Rehabil.* 2005;86(12):2240–7.

61. Consortium for Spinal Cord Medicine. Early acute management in adults with spinal cord injury: a clinical practice guideline for health-care professionals. *Spinal Cord Med.* 2008;31(4):403–79.

62. Consortium for Spinal Cord Medicine. *Clinical Practice Guidelines: Prevention of Thromboembolism in Spinal Cord Injury* (2nd edn). Washington, DC: Paralyzed Veterans of America; 1999.

63. Unsal-Delialioglu S, Kaya K, Sahin-Onat S, Kulakli F, Culha C, Ozel S. Fever during rehabilitation in patients with traumatic spinal cord injury: analysis of 392 cases from a national rehabilitation hospital in Turkey. *J Spinal Cord Med.* 2010;33(3):243–8.

64. Yu CG, Jagid J, Ruenes G, Dietrich WD, Marcillo AE, Yezierski RP. Detrimental effects of systemic hyperthermia on locomotor function and histopathological outcome after traumatic spinal cord injury in the rat. *Neurosurgery.* 2001;49(1):152–8.

65. Castillo-Abrego G. Hypothermia in spinal cord injury. *Crit Care.* 2012;16(Suppl 2):A12.

66. Tripathy S, Whitehead CF. Endovascular cooling for severe hyperthermia in cervical spine injury. *Neurocrit Care.* 2011;15(3):525–8.

67. Bracken MB, Collins WF, Freeman DF, Shepard MJ, Wagner FW, Silten RM, *et al.* Efficacy of methylprednisolone in acute spinal cord injury. *JAMA.* 1984;251(1):45–52.

68. Bracken MB, Shepard MJ, Collins WF, Holford TR, Young W, Baskin DS, *et al.* A randomized, controlled trial of methylprednisolone or naloxone in the treatment of acute spinal-cord injury. Results of the Second National Acute Spinal Cord Injury Study. *N Engl J Med.* 1990;322(20):1405–11.

69. Bracken MB. Steroids for acute spinal cord injury. *Cochrane Database Syst Rev.* 2012;1:CD001046.

70. Bracken MB, Shepard MJ, Holford TR, Leo-Summers L, Aldrich EF, Fazl M, *et al.* Administration of methylprednisolone for 24 or 48 hours or tirilazad mesylate for 48 hours in the treatment of acute spinal cord injury. Results of the Third National Acute Spinal Cord Injury Randomized Controlled Trial. National Acute Spinal Cord Injury Study. *JAMA.* 1997;277(20):1597–604.

71. Ito Y, Sugimoto Y, Tomioka M, Kai N, Tanaka M. Does high dose methylprednisolone sodium succinate really improve neurological status in patient with acute cervical cord injury?: a prospective study about neurological recovery and early complications. *Spine (Phila Pa 1976).* 2009;34(20):2121–4.

72. Hugenholtz H, Cass DE, Dvorak MF, Fewer DH, Fox RJ, Izukawa DM, *et al.* High-dose methylprednisolone for acute closed spinal cord injury—only a treatment option. *Can J Neurol Sci.* 2002;29(3):227–35.

73. Pharmacological therapy after acute cervical spinal cord injury. *Neurosurgery.* 2002;50(3 Suppl):S63–72.

74. Geisler FH, Coleman WP, Grieco G, Poonian D, Sygen Study G. The Sygen multicenter acute spinal cord injury study. *Spine (Phila Pa 1976).* 2001;26(24 Suppl):S87–98.

75. Tator CH, Hashimoto R, Raich A, Norvell D, Fehlings MG, Harrop JS, *et al.* Translational potential of preclinical trials of neuroprotection through pharmacotherapy for spinal cord injury. *J Neurosurg Spine.* 2012;17(1 Suppl):157–229.

76. Hawryluk GW, Rowland J, Kwon BK, Fehlings MG. Protection and repair of the injured spinal cord: a review of completed, ongoing, and planned clinical trials for acute spinal cord injury. *Neurosurg Focus.* 2008;25(5):E14.

77. Wilson JR, Forgione N, Fehlings MG. Emerging therapies for acute traumatic spinal cord injury. *CMAJ.* 2013;185(6):485–92.

78. Dietrich WD, Levi AD, Wang M, Green BA. Hypothermic treatment for acute spinal cord injury. *Neurotherapeutics.* 2011;8(2):229–39.

79. Kwon BK, Mann C, Sohn HM, Hilibrand AS, Phillips FM, Wang JC, *et al.* Hypothermia for spinal cord injury. *Spine J.* 2008;8(6):859–74.

80. Batchelor PE, Kerr NF, Gatt AM, Aleksoska E, Cox SF, Ghasem-Zadeh A, *et al.* Hypothermia prior to decompression: buying time for treatment of acute spinal cord injury. *J Neurotrauma.* 2010;27(8):1357–68.

81. Maybhate A, Hu C, Bazley FA, Yu Q, Thakor NV, Kerr CL, *et al.* Potential long-term benefits of acute hypothermia after spinal cord injury: assessments with somatosensory-evoked potentials. *Crit Care Med.* 2012;40(2):573–9.

82. Lo TP, Jr, Cho KS, Garg MS, Lynch MP, Marcillo AE, Koivisto DL, *et al.* Systemic hypothermia improves histological and functional outcome after cervical spinal cord contusion in rats. *J Comp Neurol.* 2009;514(5):433–48.

83. Levi AD, Casella G, Green BA, Dietrich WD, Vanni S, Jagid J, *et al.* Clinical outcomes using modest intravascular hypothermia after acute cervical spinal cord injury. *Neurosurgery.* 2010;66(4):670–7.

84. Amar A, Levy M. Surgical controversies in the management of spinal cord injury. *J Am Coll Surg.* 1999;188:550–66.

85. Brodkey JS, Richards DE, Blasingame JP, Nulsen FE. Reversible spinal cord trauma in cats. Additive effects of direct pressure and ischemia. *J Neurosurg.* 1972;37(5):591–3.

86. Carlson GD, Minato Y, Okada A, Gorden CD, Warden KE, Barbeau JM, *et al.* Early time-dependent decompression for spinal cord injury: vascular mechanisms of recovery. *J Neurotrauma.* 1997;14(12):951–62.

87. Delamarter RB, Sherman J, Carr JB. Pathophysiology of spinal cord injury. Recovery after immediate and delayed decompression. *J Bone Joint Surg Am.* 1995;77(7):1042–9.

88. Dimar JR, 2nd, Glassman SD, Raque GH, Zhang YP, Shields CB. The influence of spinal canal narrowing and timing of decompression on neurologic recovery after spinal cord contusion in a rat model. *Spine (Phila Pa 1976).* 1999;24(16):1623–33.

89. Dolan EJ, Tator CH, Endrenyi L. The value of decompression for acute experimental spinal cord compression injury. *J Neurosurg.* 1980;53(6):749–55.

90. Guha A, Tator CH, Endrenyi L, Piper I. Decompression of the spinal cord improves recovery after acute experimental spinal cord compression injury. *Paraplegia.* 1987;25(4):324–39.

91. Furlan JC, Noonan V, Cadotte DW, Fehlings MG. Timing of decompressive surgery of spinal cord after traumatic spinal cord injury: an evidence-based examination of pre-clinical and clinical studies. *J Neurotrauma*. 2011;28(8):1371–99.

92. Carlson GD, Gorden CD, Oliff HS, Pillai JJ, LaManna JC. Sustained spinal cord compression: part I: time-dependent effect on long-term pathophysiology. *J Bone Joint Surg Am*. 2003;85-A(1):86–94.

93. Kobrine AI, Evans DE, Rizzoli HV. Experimental acute balloon compression of the spinal cord. Factors affecting disappearance and return of the spinal evoked response. *J Neurosurg*. 1979;51(6):841–5.

94. Nystrom B, Berglund JE. Spinal cord restitution following compression injuries in rats. *Acta Neurol Scand*. 1988;78(6):467–72.

95. Vaccaro AR, Daugherty RJ, Sheehan TP, Dante SJ, Cotler JM, Balderston RA, et al. Neurologic outcome of early versus late surgery for cervical spinal cord injury. *Spine (Phila Pa 1976)*. 1997;22(22):2609–13.

96. Fehlings MG, Perrin RG. The timing of surgical intervention in the treatment of spinal cord injury: a systematic review of recent clinical evidence. *Spine (Phila Pa 1976)*. 2006;31(11 Suppl):S28–35.

97. Fehlings MG, Vaccaro A, Wilson JR, Singh A, D WC, Harrop JS, et al. Early versus delayed decompression for traumatic cervical spinal cord injury: results of the Surgical Timing in Acute Spinal Cord Injury Study (STASCIS). *PLoS One*. 2012;7(2):e32037.

98. Wilson JR, Singh A, Craven C, Verrier MC, Drew B, Ahn H, et al. Early versus late surgery for traumatic spinal cord injury: the results of a prospective Canadian cohort study. *Spinal Cord*. 2012;50(11):840–3.

99. Ditunno JF, Jr, Formal CS. Chronic spinal cord injury. *N Engl J Med*. 1994;330(8):550–6.

100. Cragg JJ, Stone JA, Krassioukov AV. Management of cardiovascular disease risk factors in individuals with chronic spinal cord injury: an evidence-based review. *J Neurotrauma*. 2012;29(11):1999–2012.

101. Krassioukov AV, Furlan JC, Fehlings MG. Autonomic dysreflexia in acute spinal cord injury: an under-recognized clinical entity. *J Neurotrauma*. 2003;20(8):707–16.

102. Krassioukov A, Warburton DE, Teasell R, Eng JJ, Spinal Cord Injury Rehabilitation Evidence Research Team. A systematic review of the management of autonomic dysreflexia after spinal cord injury. *Arch Phys Med Rehabil*. 2009;90(4):682–95.

103. del Popolo G, Mencarini M, Nelli F, Lazzeri M. Controversy over the pharmacological treatments of storage symptoms in spinal cord injury patients: a literature overview. *Spinal Cord*. 2012;50(1):8–13.

104. Consortium for Spinal Cord Medicine. Bladder management for adults with spinal cord injury: a clinical practice guideline for health-care providers. *J Spinal Cord Med*. 2006;29(5):527–73.

105. Chen CY, Liao CH, Kuo HC. Therapeutic effects of detrusor botulinum toxin A injection on neurogenic detrusor overactivity in patients with different levels of spinal cord injury and types of detrusor sphincter dyssynergia. *Spinal Cord*. 2011;49(5):659–64.

106. Stohrer M, Blok B, Castro-Diaz D, Chartier-Kastler E, Del Popolo G, Kramer G, et al. EAU guidelines on neurogenic lower urinary tract dysfunction. *Eur Urol*. 2009;56(1):81–8.

107. Sugimura T, Arnold E, English S, Moore J. Chronic suprapubic catheterization in the management of patients with spinal cord injuries: analysis of upper and lower urinary tract complications. *BJU Int*. 2008;101(11):1396–400.

108. Gelis A, Dupeyron A, Legros P, Benaim C, Pelissier J, Fattal C. Pressure ulcer risk factors in persons with spinal cord injury part 2: the chronic stage. *Spinal Cord*. 2009;47(9):651–61.

109. Krause JS, Vines CL, Farley TL, Sniezek J, Coker J. An exploratory study of pressure ulcers after spinal cord injury: relationship to protective behaviors and risk factors. *Arch Phys Med Rehabil*. 2001;82(1):107–13.

110. Jones ML, Mathewson CS, Adkins VK, Ayllon T. Use of behavioral contingencies to promote prevention of recurrent pressure ulcers. *Arch Phys Med Rehabil*. 2003;84(6):796–802.

111. Bogie KM, Reger SI, Levine SP, Sahgal V. Electrical stimulation for pressure sore prevention and wound healing. *Assist Technol*. 2000;12(1):50–66.

112. National Pressure Ulcer Advisory Panel. *NPUAP Pressure Ulcer Stages/Categories*. 2012. [Online] http://www.npuap.org/resources/educational-and-clinical-resources/npuap-pressure-ul cer-stagescategories/

113. Regan MA, Teasell RW, Wolfe DL, Keast D, Mortenson WB, Aubut JA, et al. A systematic review of therapeutic interventions for pressure ulcers after spinal cord injury. *Arch Phys Med Rehabil*. 2009;90(2):213–31.

114. Lance JW. The control of muscle tone, reflexes, and movement: Robert Wartenberg Lecture. *Neurology*. 1980;30(12):1303–13.

115. Maynard FM, Karunas RS, Waring WP, 3rd. Epidemiology of spasticity following traumatic spinal cord injury. *Arch Phys Med Rehabil*. 1990;71(8):566–9.

116. Skold C, Levi R, Seiger A. Spasticity after traumatic spinal cord injury: nature, severity, and location. *Arch Phys Med Rehabil*. 1999;80(12):1548–57.

117. Adams MM, Hicks AL. Spasticity after spinal cord injury. *Spinal Cord*. 2005;43(10):577–86.

118. Kita M, Goodkin DE. Drugs used to treat spasticity. *Drugs*. 2000;59(3):487–95.

119. Shavelle RM, DeVivo MJ, Strauss DJ, Paculdo DR, Lammertse DP, Day SM. Long-term survival of persons ventilator dependent after spinal cord injury. *J Spinal Cord Med*. 2006;29(5):511–19.

120. DeVivo MJ, Ivie CS, 3rd. Life expectancy of ventilator-dependent persons with spinal cord injuries. *Chest*. 1995;108(1):226–32.

121. Peterson W, Charlifue W, Gerhart A, Whiteneck G. Two methods of weaning persons with quadriplegia from mechanical ventilators. *Paraplegia*. 1994;32(2):98–103.

122. Gutierrez CJ, Harrow J, Haines F. Using an evidence-based protocol to guide rehabilitation and weaning of ventilator-dependent cervical spinal cord injury patients. *J Rehabil Res Dev*. 2003;40(5 Suppl 2):99–110.

123. Onders RP, Khansarinia S, Weiser T, Chin C, Hungness E, Soper N, et al. Multicenter analysis of diaphragm pacing in tetraplegics with cardiac pacemakers: positive implications for ventilator weaning in intensive care units. *Surgery*. 2010;148(4):893–7.

124. Onders RP, Dimarco AF, Ignagni AR, Aiyar H, Mortimer JT. Mapping the phrenic nerve motor point: the key to a successful laparoscopic diaphragm pacing system in the first human series. *Surgery*. 2004;136(4):819–26.

125. DiMarco AF. Phrenic nerve stimulation in patients with spinal cord injury. *Respir Physiol Neurobiol*. 2009;169(2):200–9.

CHAPTER 22

Neuromuscular disorders and acquired neuromuscular weakness

Nicola Latronico and Nazzareno Fagoni

Neuromuscular disorders include pathological processes involving one or more components of the motor unit comprising a motor neuron with its axon and myelin sheath, neuromuscular transmission, and all the muscle fibres it innervates. This chapter will discuss the general care of patients with neuromuscular disease and then describe the more common conditions seen in the intensive care setting.

General aspects of care

Neuromuscular disorders have multiple effects on several non-neurological organ systems.

Respiratory system

Respiratory failure is common in patients with neuromuscular disease. It may present acutely in conditions such as botulism or Guillain–Barré syndrome (GBS) or as a gradual progression in patients with chronic condition such as amyotrophic lateral sclerosis (Table 22.1) (1). Many non-neurological conditions, such as chronic obstructive pulmonary disease, congestive heart failure, cancer, and ageing, may contribute to, or precipitate, respiratory and peripheral muscle dysfunction (2). Acute decompensation of chronic respiratory insufficiency may be precipitated by factors that increase respiratory workload, such as respiratory infection, by atelectasis caused by inadequate clearing of tracheobronchial secretions, or a restrictive load, for example, as a consequence of constipation (3). Several drugs may also worsen respiratory muscle weakness by effects on single or multiple components of the motor unit (4–7).

Respiratory failure is the consequence of respiratory muscle weakness when it is sufficiently severe to compromise the generation of normal pressures and airflow during inspiration and expiration, or the ability to maintain airway patency (3,8). Eventually, impaired gas exchange leads to carbon dioxide retention and hypoxaemia.

Weakness of the diaphragm, the principal muscle of inspiration, other chest wall inspiratory muscles, and the accessory muscles results in inadequate lung expansion and microatelectasis, ventilation/perfusion mismatch, and consequent hypoxaemia (Table 22.2) (8). With diaphragmatic paralysis (or fatigue), the flaccid diaphragm moves upwards rather than downwards as the ribcage expands during inspiration, and is passively followed by the abdominal wall resulting in a typical paradoxical inward movement of the abdomen. This is most marked in the supine position because gravity assists the inward movement of the abdominal contents. Consequently, patients with diaphragmatic paralysis use their accessory muscles of respiration, have a smaller supine than erect vital capacity (VC), and often become distressed when lying supine. Reduction of VC and maximal inspiratory pressure (MIP) are commonly observed during inspiratory muscle weakness (2). Although low MIP values may reflect poor technique or patient cooperation, high MIP values (i.e. more negative) exclude clinically significant respiratory muscle weakness.

The muscles of the mouth, uvula, palate, tongue, and larynx are essential for maintaining upper airway patency and therefore airway resistance and airflow (Table 22.2). Weakness of any may result in mechanical obstruction of the airway and increased airway resistance, and this is more likely in the supine position when it is referred to as positional airway obstruction. Weakness of the laryngeal muscles, which play an important role in phonation, respiration, and swallowing, may allow silent aspiration of colonized oropharyngeal secretions into the lungs, a primary cause of pneumonia. In such cases, acute respiratory failure may occur even in the presence of near normal inspiratory muscle strength.

Weakness of expiratory muscles of the chest wall and abdomen (Table 22.2) results in impaired cough and secretion clearance, and increases the risk of pulmonary aspiration and pneumonia. Expiratory muscle weakness results in a reduced maximal expiratory pressure (MEP). Since expiration during normal tidal breathing occurs without direct muscular effort, contraction of the abdominal muscles during expiration can be a sign of respiratory muscle dysfunction.

Clinical signs of respiratory failure

All patients with progressive muscle weakness, especially involving the upper limbs and bulbar muscles, should be considered at risk of respiratory failure. Clinical assessment, combined with respiratory function tests, guides decisions about endotracheal intubation and mechanical ventilation.

There are several warning signs of imminent respiratory failure including bulbar signs such as a hoarse voice, nasal regurgitation of food, cough after swallowing (indicating aspiration), low speech

Table 22.1 Neurological causes of muscle weakness in the critically ill patient

Localization	Pre-existing	Previously undiagnosed/ new onset	ICU complication
Brain cortex and brainstem	Encephalitis Epilepsy Multiple sclerosis Vascular causes (brainstem infarction or haemorrhage; cerebral haemorrhage; ischaemic stroke)	Acute disseminated encephalomyelitis Encephalitis (including paralytic form of rabies) Multiple sclerosis Post-cardiac arrest encephalopathy Status epilepticus Tetanus Vascular causes	Post-cardiac arrest encephalopathy Status epilepticus (including non-epileptic) Vascular causes
Spinal cord (including anterior horn cells)	Amyotrophic lateral sclerosis Ischaemia Malformations (Arnold–Chiari) Poliomyelitis Post-polio syndrome Spinal muscular atrophy Trauma	Compression (tumour, infection, haematoma) Herpes zoster Ischaemia transverse myelitis Surgery Tetanus Trauma West Nile virus poliomyelitis	Hopkins syndrome
Peripheral nerve	Alcohol abuse Chronic inflammatory demyelinating polyneuropathy Drugs* (bortezomib, cisplatin, dichloroacetate epothilone, isoniazid, ixabepilone, leflunomide, linezolid, nitrofurantoin, oxaliplatin, pyridoxine, reverse transcriptase inhibitors, statins, taxanes, thalidomide, tumour necrosis factor-alpha blockers, vincristine) Guillain–Barré syndrome Hormonal disorders (acromegaly, hypothyroidism) Infections (diphtheria, HIV, Lyme disease) Tumours (carcinoma, lymphoma, multiple myeloma) Metabolic (diabetes, porphyria, tyrosinaemia, uraemia) Nutritional (thiamine deficiency) Sarcoidosis Toxic (acrylamide; heavy metals: arsenic, thallium, lead, gold; organophosphates, hexacarbons) Vasculitis (polyarteritis nodosa, lupus erythematous, rheumatoid arthritis, Churg–Strauss)	Acute intermittent porphyria Entrapment neuropathy Guillain–Barré syndrome HIV Tetanus Tick paralysis Toxic Vasculitis	Entrapment neuropathy Critical illness polyneuropathy
Neuromuscular junction	Botulism Lambert–Eaton syndrome Myasthenia gravis Drugs* Anaesthetic agents (desflurane, enflurane, halothane, isoflurane, nitrous oxide, opioids, propofol, sevoflurane) Antibiotics: *aminoglycosides*+ (amikacin, clindamycin, gentamycin, kanamycin, lincomycin, neomycin, streptomycin, tobramycin); *fluoroquinolones* (ciprofloxacin, gemifloxacin, levofloxacin, lomefloxacin, moxifloxacin, norfloxacin, ofloxacin, and trovafloxacin); *macrolides* (azithromycin, erythromycin, telithromycin); *other antibiotics* (ampicillin, bacitarcin, polymyxins, tetracyclin, imipenem/cilastatin, penicillin, vancomycin)	Hypermagnesaemia Myasthenia gravis Snake, scorpion, and spider bites, fish, shellfish, jellyfish, and crab toxins Tetanus	Hypermagnesaemia Prolonged neuromuscular blockade

(continued)

Table 22.1 (Continued)

Localization	Pre-existing	Previously undiagnosed/new onset	ICU complication
	Antiarrhythmic agents (etafenone, peruvoside, procainamide, propafenone) antiepileptics (carbamazepine, gabapentin, phenytoin, trimethadione) Beta blockers** (atenolol, nadolol, oxprenolol, practolol, propranolol, sotalol, ophthalmic timolo1) Calcium channel blockers** (amlodipine, felodipine, nifedipine, verapamil). Corticosteroids*** Chemotherapics (doxorubicin, etoposide, cisplatin) H-2 receptor antagonists (cimetidine, ranitidine, roxatidine). Quinolone derivatives (chloroquine, quinidine, quinine) Non-competitive neuromuscular blocking agents* Psychotropic medications (amitriptyline, chlorpromazine, haloperidol, imipramine, lithium) Other drugs (interferon, penicillamine)		
Muscle	Metabolic/congenital Mitochondrial myopathies Muscular dystrophies Periodic paralyses (muscle channelopathies) Polymyositis	Adult-onset acid maltase deficiency Hypo- and hyperkalaemia Hypophosphataemia Muscular dystrophies Polymyositis Pyomyositis Rhabdomyolysis Tetanus Toxic myopathies	Corticosteroid myopathy Critical illness myopathy Hypo- and hyperkalaemia Hypophosphataemia Propofol infusion syndrome Disuse atrophy Rhabdomyolysis

With the exception of neuromuscular blocking agents, drugs do not directly cause neuromuscular respiratory failure, they potentiate the effect of primary disease of the nerve, neuromuscular transmission or muscle.

For review see references (4–7).

* For several drugs the evidence stems from single case reports or small case series.

** Long-term use of calcium-channel and beta-blockers can be risky in patients with myasthenia gravis.

*** Corticosteroids are considered to be effective treatment for myasthenia gravis; however, they can worsen muscle strength acutely due to a direct blocking effect on the acetylcholine receptor through ionic channels.

+ Indicates drugs that are better avoided in patients with myasthenia gravis; for the other drugs, the suggestion is to use them with caution or no specific indications can be made.

Modified from a previous paper published by one of us: Latronico N, 'European Critical Care & Emergency Medicine', 2010, 2, pp. 61–64, which in turn was based on modification of a previous paper by another author. On the website http://www.touchemergencymedicine.com/articles/muscle-weakness-during-critical-illness, there is no link to ask permission. Dhand UK, 'Clinical approach to the weak patient in the intensive care unit', *Respir Care*, 2006, 51, 9, pp. 1024–40, discussion 40–41.

volume, or breathlessness when swallowing or speaking. An awake, snoring breath in the supine position that is relieved by placing the patient head up or erect suggests positional airway obstruction. The need to pause between words while speaking (staccato speech), exertional or at-rest dyspnoea, rapid shallow breathing, accessory respiratory muscle recruitment, weak cough with inability to clear secretions, abdominal paradox, and orthopnoea are also important warning signs. Although somnolence may indicate severe hypercapnia or hypoxaemia, arterial blood gases are unreliable indicators of respiratory muscle strength or the need for mechanical ventilation. Patients with rapid shallow breathing, or other signs of imminent respiratory failure, should be closely monitored even if blood gases are normal.

Respiratory function tests

Repeated assessment of VC, MIP, MEP, and the rapid shallow breathing index (RSBI) is a useful complement to clinical evaluation, but requires an awake and cooperative patient.

Vital capacity

VC is the maximum volume of air that can be expired after maximum inspiration. It is a global index of inspiratory and expiratory muscle strength. Precise determination of lung volumes requires a spirometer. A rough estimate of VC can be obtained by asking the patient to count to 20 in a single breath, and an inability to do so suggests critical reduction of VC (< 1L). During measurement of forced vital capacity (FVC) the patient takes a maximum inspiration and then blows out all the air as fast and as completely as possible with the nares occluded. During slow vital capacity (SVC) measurement air is expired as completely, but not as fast, as possible (3).

Maximal inspiratory and expiratory pressures

MIP is a global index of inspiratory muscle strength and is measured at functional residual capacity with the patient breathing against an occluded mouthpiece connected to a pressure transducer. Because respiratory effort against an occluded circuit can be uncomfortable

Table 22.2 Muscles groups involved in inspiration, expiration, and maintenance of airway patency

Muscles of inspiration		Innervation
Diaphragm		C3–5
Chest wall	Parasternal intercostal muscles	T1–7
	External intercostal muscles	T1–12
Accessory muscles	Sternocleidomastoids	Cranial nerves XI, C1–2
	Trapezoids	Cranial nerves XI, C2–3
	Scalene muscles	C4–8
	Pectoralis major	C5–7
Muscles maintaining airway patency		
Mouth		Cranial nerves IX, X
Uvula and palate		Cranial nerve XI
Tongue		Cranial nerves IX, XII
Muscles of expiration		
Chest wall	Internal intercostal muscles	Thoracic nerves T1–12
Abdominal	Rectus abdominis	T7–L1
	Transverse abdominis,	T7–L1
	External oblique	T7–L1
	Internal obliques	T7–L1

Table 22.3 Factors that predict respiratory failure requiring mechanical ventilation in patients with neuromuscular disorders

Variable	Normal values	Predictors of the need for mechanical ventilation
Forced vital capacity	60–70 mL/kg	< 20 mL/kg < 50% predicted normal value Rapid decline in FVC
Maximal inspiratory pressure	Males: −110 to −83 cmH$_2$O Females: −110 to −83 cmH$_2$O (age dependent)	> −30 cmH$_2$O
Maximal expiratory pressure	Males: 128–103 cmH$_2$O Females: 84–69 cmH$_2$O (age dependent)	< 40 cmH$_2$O
Maximal sniff nasal inspiratory pressure	Males: 117–91 cmH$_2$O Females: 84–76 cmH$_2$O	> −40 cmH$_2$O

for a dyspnoeic patient, the maximal sniff nasal inspiratory pressure (SNIP) test is often used instead of MIP. During SNIP measurement a plug is placed in one nostril and peak nasal pressure measured by occluding the contralateral nostril whilst the patient performs a number of maximum sniffs.

MEP is an index of global expiratory muscle strength and is measured in the same manner as MIP at total lung capacity. Expiratory muscle strength can also be evaluated using peak cough expiratory flow; normal levels are greater than 6 L/s. The RSBI, calculated as the ratio of respiratory rate to tidal volume, rises as the respiratory rate increases to compensate for reduced tidal volume; normal values are less than 50/min/L.

Intubation and mechanical ventilation

Factors that predict respiratory failure requiring mechanical ventilation in patients with neuromuscular disorders are shown in Table 22.3 (3).

With a need for ventilatory support established, non-invasive ventilation (NIV) may be an option if a short duration of support is anticipated and the airway is patent. However, tracheal intubation with mechanical ventilation and continuous positive pressure is the preferred option in patients with frank respiratory failure, upper airway obstruction, and other contraindications to NIV.

Intubation should be performed in a safe environment, ideally in the intensive care unit (ICU), and is best achieved by the oral route following adequate dose of intravenous anaesthetic or sedative agent, analgesia, and muscle relaxation. Succinylcholine, a competitive neuromuscular blocking agent (NMBA) providing rapid onset neuromuscular block, may lead to a precipitous and large increase in serum potassium in patients with ICU-acquired or pre-existing myopathy, recent lower motor neuron denervation, or after prolonged immobilization, and should be avoided. Cardiac arrest and death after succinylcholine-induced hyperkalaemia has been observed as early as 5 days after immobilization (9). Competitive non-depolarizing, intermediate-acting NMBAs are best suited to these circumstances, and options include benzylisoquinolinium agents such as atracurium and cisatracurium, or amino-steroids such as vecuronium and rocuronium.

The optimal mode of mechanical ventilation in patients with neuromuscular disease is not established, but assisted ventilation with pressure support is commonly used and can be initiated early. When the patient is judged to be ready for extubation based on clinical assessment (i.e. adequate cough, absence of excessive tracheobronchial secretion) and objective measurements (i.e. stable cardiovascular and metabolic status, no evidence of ongoing infection, and adequate oxygenation, pulmonary function, and mentation), a 30-minute spontaneous breathing trial (SBT) should implemented as a test for successful extubation (10). Most patients who develop respiratory failure as a consequence of neuromuscular disorder will require a tracheostomy, and this can be permanent in end-stage disease.

Cardiovascular system

Tachycardia with loss of normal sinus arrhythmia is commonly seen in patients with neuromuscular disorders. Heart rate variability is also often reduced, and can be used to estimate the risk of developing severe arrhythmias. Autonomic dysfunction, presenting with rapid fluctuations in heart rate and blood pressure, and profuse sweating, can also be a prominent feature. These abnormalities may be harbingers of life-threatening tachy- or bradyarrhythmias or unexpected cardiac arrest, particularly in tetanus or GBS. Postural hypotension is common during mobilization, making physiotherapy difficult.

Direct cardiac involvement is often seen in myotonic dystrophy and manifests as conduction defects, fatal arrhythmias, and congestive cardiac failure. The typical clinical triad in Kearns–Sayre syndrome, a rare mitochondrial cytopathy, includes complete heart block, progressive external ophthalmoplegia, and atypical pigmentary retinal degeneration. QT interval prolongation, ventricular tachycardia, and torsade de pointes are also reported in some neuromuscular disorders and may require implantation of an automatic implantable cardioverter–defibrillator.

Gastrointestinal system

Enteral feeding should be initiated as early as possible. Ileus, distended abdomen, large gastric residual volume, and absence of bowel sounds are common and may prevent adequate enteral nutrition in patients with neuromuscular disease. In such cases, parenteral nutrition should be considered pending recovery of gastrointestinal function when conversion to full enteral nutrition can be achieved. Prokinetic agents such as metoclopramide, a dopamine (D2 receptor) antagonist, and erythromycin, a competitive agonist of motilin, can be used alone or in combination to treat gastroparesis. However, metoclopramide may cause drowsiness, agitation, and extrapyramidal effects, and erythromycin can prolong the QT interval. Both should therefore be used with caution in patients with autonomic disturbance.

Constipation is a nearly universal symptom of botulism, but is also common in other neuromuscular disease states including Lambert–Eaton myasthenic syndrome (LEMS) and myasthenia gravis, and may be potentiated by concurrent requirement for opioid analgesia. Bowel hypomotility can be improved by a nutritional regimen that includes increased fibre with a concomitant increase in fluid, stool softeners, and osmotic laxative. Mu-opioid receptor antagonists are safe and effective for the treatment of opioid-induced constipation.

Infection

Pneumonia is the most common infectious complication in patients with neuromuscular disorders because disordered swallow leads to accumulation of oral secretions, and weakness of laryngeal muscles to their aspiration into the tracheobronchial system. Secretions may be increased by treatment with anticholinergic drugs in myasthenia gravis. Inadequacy of cough and secretion clearance because of expiratory muscle weakness also predisposes to atelectasis and pneumonia, which in turn may precipitate respiratory failure and the need for admission to the ICU.

Pain

Pain is a common complaint in patients with neuromuscular disease and should be closely monitored and treated appropriately. Myalgic pain is the most disabling symptom in myotonic dystrophy type 2, whereas abdominal pain is a cardinal feature of the acute neuropathy of acute intermittent porphyria, and a common presenting symptom in rhabdomyolysis and thallium poisoning. The muscle spasms of tetanus are excruciatingly painful. Prolonged immobilization can itself result in pain as well as decubitus ulcers in those with profound muscle weakness and wasting.

Pain is often so severe that opioid analgesia is required. Gabapentin or carbamazepine should be added in those with neuropathic pain. In new-onset disease, anxiety and fear can also have devastating effects once a patient realizes that he/she is paralysed, and intensive psychological support is often needed. Light sedation with propofol or dexmedetomidine may also be helpful in the short term.

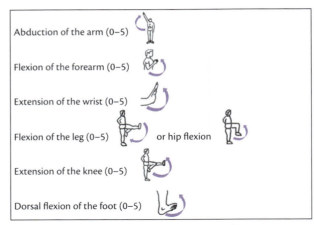

Fig. 22.1 MRC sum score. Muscle groups (right and left) assessed in the measurement of the MRC sum score. Score ranges from 0 (total paralysis) to 60 (normal).
http://besport.org/sportmedicina/muscoli_e_movimento.htm.

Testing muscle strength

Muscle strength can be tested in functional limb muscle groups with the Medical Research Council (MRC) scale. Individual MRC scores can be combined into a sum score, which yields an overall estimation of motor function. A score of less than 48 defines a severe muscle weakness (Figure 22.1).

Guillain–Barré syndrome

GBS is a post-infectious autoimmune polyneuropathy resulting in rapidly progressive, symmetrical weakness in the arms and legs of otherwise healthy individuals (11). Acute inflammatory demyelinating polyradiculoneuropathy (AIDP) is the most common subtype of GBS in Europe and North America. Other variants include acute motor axonal (AMAN), sensory-motor axonal neuropathy (AMSAN), pure dysautonomia and regional variants (Miller–Fisher syndrome which is limited to oropharyngeal), and GBS with unexcitable nerves (12).

The onset of neurological signs is frequently preceded by an infection in the previous 2–4 weeks. This is most often related to gastrointestinal *Campylobacter jejuni* infection with diarrhoea, although fever, cough, sore throat, nasal discharge, and respiratory tract infection are also common preceding events. Importantly, symptoms and signs of infection have often subsided by the time the neurological signs appear. Although there is often public concern about the risk of GBS or GBS recurrence after vaccination, this risk is low and the benefits of inactivated pandemic vaccines greatly outweigh their minimal risks.

Clinical presentation

The usual presentation of GBS is one of ascending, symmetrical limb weakness associated with reduced or absent deep tendon reflexes, paraesthesia, numbness, and sometimes pain. Although the weakness usually begins in the legs, all four limbs are involved simultaneously in one-third of patients, and the progression is from upper to lower limbs in 12%. The facial muscles are frequently involved, in distinction to their sparing in critical illness polyneuropathy (CIP). Respiratory muscles weakness leading to acute respiratory failure is very common in severe GBS, whereas ophthalmoplegia, areflexia, and ataxia, but not muscle weakness, are the dominant signs in the Miller–Fisher variant (13,14). Persistent fever, severe respiratory muscle weakness with limited limb weakness at onset, bladder or bowel dysfunction at onset, a clear sensory level, and persistent asymmetrical weakness call the diagnosis of GBS into doubt.

Diagnosis

In its typical presentation, the diagnosis of GBS is straightforward and based on a careful history and meticulous neurological evaluation.

Cerebrospinal fluid (CSF) examination may show elevated protein with a normal white cell count, although there may be no abnormalities in the early stages of GBS. Diagnostic lumbar puncture is therefore best performed after the first week unless bacterial or viral meningitis is suspected. Increased CSF mononuclear (> 50 cells/mm^3) or polymorphonuclear (> 5 cells/mm^3) cells suggest an alternative diagnosis such as Lyme disease, HIV infection, or malignancy (14).

Electrophysiological investigations are required for diagnostic certainty, to define the GBS subtype, monitor the response to treatment, and for prognosis (15). They should be performed early in the course of the disease but may be normal in the first 7 days following weakness onset. Under such circumstances electrophysiological investigations should be repeated at 1–2 weeks. Nerve-conduction studies are not obligatory in resource-poor environments or in paediatric cases of GBS (15). Diagnosis of AMAN requires serial evaluations and recognition of reversible conduction failure at initial electrophysiological evaluation (16). Imaging is not required for the diagnosis of GBS, although lumbosacral roots may exhibit contrast enhancement on spinal MR imaging.

GBS is often considered in the differential diagnosis of CIP, but distinction is usually obvious. GBS is a (rare) cause of ICU admission, whereas CIP arises as a complication of critical illness *after* ICU admission (17). However, the differential diagnosis can be difficult in cases of rapid progression of respiratory failure in previously undiagnosed GBS (Table 22.1) (18).

Clinical course

Rapidly progressive weakness is the essential clinical feature of GBS. Severe arrhythmias and extreme fluctuations of arterial blood pressure occur in around 20% of patients, and temporary cardiac pacing may be required for severe bradycardia (14). About 25% of patients with severe GBS affecting respiratory muscles progress to acute respiratory failure requiring mechanical ventilation. Demyelinating GBS is associated with an increased risk of respiratory failure compared to other subtypes.

Arterial blood gases are unreliable guides to impending respiratory failure because they may remain normal until shortly before hypercapnia and respiratory arrest supervene. Clinical features, such as symptom onset to admission to hospital of less than 7 days, bulbar/facial involvement, low MRC sum score reflecting reduced limb muscle weakness (Figure 22.1) at admission, and inability to cough, stand, or lift the elbows or head are more reliable predictors

of impending respiratory failure. The Erasmus GBS Respiratory Insufficiency Score (EGRIS) has been proposed as a way to estimate the need for mechanical ventilation based on five categories of the MRC sum score, three categories of time between onset of weakness and admission to hospital, and the presence or absence of facial/bulbar weakness (Table 22.4) (19). Serial measurement of respiratory muscle strength can be useful complements to clinical evaluation in the prediction of respiratory failure (Table 22.2), as is a low ratio of the proximal:distal compound muscle action potential amplitude of the common peroneal nerve (20).

Maximum weakness is usually reached 2–4 weeks after symptom onset. The plateau phase of the disease lasts from days to several weeks or months, and is followed by a much slower recovery period of varying duration. In mechanically ventilated patients, time to weaning is also variable.

Management

Specific treatments with intravenous immunoglobulin (IVIg) 0.4 g/kg daily for 5 consecutive days or plasma exchange (PE), five exchanges over a period of 2 weeks with a total exchange of five plasma volumes, are equally effective in reducing morbidity and mortality after GBS. IVIg has become the standard treatment because it is more rapidly and easily implemented and has fewer side effects than PE. The combination of PE and IVIg does not confer supplemental benefit compared to either treatment alone. Corticosteroids are not indicated after GBS, and may be associated with a worse outcome (12,13).

Regular monitoring of respiratory muscle strength is recommended, with timely institution of mechanical ventilation when critical reductions of FVC, MIP, and MEP are observed. Even in the absence of clinical respiratory distress, mechanical ventilation should be considered in patients with at least one of the following

Table 22.4 Predicting the risk of respiratory failure requiring mechanical ventilation using the Erasmus GBS Respiratory Insufficiency Score (EGRIS)

	Category	EGRIS
MRC Sum Score	60–51	0
	50–41	1
	40–31	2
	30–21	3
	< 20	4
Weakness onset to hospital admission	> 7 days	0
	4–7 days	1
	≤ 3 days	2
Bulbar/facial weakness	Absent	0
	Present	1

EGRIS 0 to 2—low risk (4%) of respiratory failure requiring mechanical ventilation.

EGRIS 3 to 4—intermediate risk (24%) of respiratory failure requiring mechanical ventilation.

EGRIS 5 to 7—high risk (65%) of respiratory failure requiring mechanical ventilation.

Reproduced with permission from Walgaard C, Lingsma HF, Ruts L, Drenthen J, van Koningsveld R, Garssen MJ et al., 'Prediction of respiratory insufficiency in Guillain-Barre syndrome', *Annals of Neurology*, 67, 6, pp. 781–787, Copyright © 2010 John Wiley and Sons.

major criterion—$PaCO_2$ greater than 6.4 kPa (48 mmHg), PaO_2 less than 7.5 kPa (56 mmHg) breathing room air, FVC lower than 15 mL/kg—or two minor criteria including inefficient cough, impaired swallowing, and atelectasis (14,20).

Autonomic dysfunction, pulmonary infection, and deep venous thrombosis should be treated aggressively. Hyponatraemia, most often associated with normovolaemia, may occur and should be treated with fluid restriction in the first instance. If symptoms develop, or the serum sodium concentration falls below 120 mEq/L, 3% intravenous saline solution should be considered. Pain usually responds to gabapentin and carbamazepine, but opioids may occasionally be required.

Prognosis

Despite the demonstrated efficacy of IVIg and PE, GBS remains a disabling disease in about 20% of patients with severe symptoms, and these interventions have not improved mortality. Even when appropriately treated, GBS remains fatal in about 4% of patients, and only 60% recover full motor strength by 1 year (21). Older age, diarrhoea as a preceding symptom, and reduced MRC sum score are independent predictors of persisting disability at 6 months (22).

Myasthenia gravis

Myasthenia gravis (MG) is a rare autoimmune disease with a prevalence of about 20 cases per 100,000 population. The incidence is between 10 to 20 cases per million per year, and MG is more common in men over the age of 50 and in women younger than 40 years. It is extremely rare in children.

There are two main forms of MG in adults—generalized MG and an ocular form in which muscle weakness is limited to eyelid and extraocular eye movements. Classification of MG is based on distinctive clinical features or the severity of disease which may indicate different prognoses or responses to therapy (23).

Pathogenesis

MG is caused by autoantibodies against the acetylcholine receptor (AchR) in the postsynaptic membrane. Serum AchR antibodies (AchR-ab) are IgG type antibodies with a high affinity for the AchR that directly inhibit the binding of acetylcholine to the receptor, and are detected in 80% of patients with MG. AchR-ab also reduces the number of AchRs in two ways. It forms AChR-antibody complexes that become internalized and degraded by the muscle fibre, and also activates the membrane attack complex leading to destruction of the postsynaptic muscle membrane. With a reduced number of available binding sites for acetylcholine, generation of muscle fibre action potentials becomes inconsistent, translating into fatigable muscle weakness on repetitive contraction of affected muscles.

Around 20% of patients with generalized MG are 'seronegative', and do not have AchR-ab. Forty to sixty per cent of such patients have serum antibodies directed against muscle specific tyrosine kinase receptor (MuSK), and these may injure AChR by altering their clustering or causing complement-dependent lysis. Recently, a new class of autoantibodies to postsynaptic low-density lipoprotein receptor-related protein has been identified (24).

Clinical presentation

Fatigable muscle weakness is the cardinal feature of MG (25). It typically worsens with exertion and improves with rest, and the weakness ranges from mild localized muscle weakness in purely ocular forms of MG to severe generalized weakness and respiratory failure in generalized MG.

The extrinsic ocular muscles are initially involved in about two-thirds of patients, with signs at presentation that include ptosis and diplopia without pupillary changes. A minority of patients (15%) present with bulbar weakness and alterations of voice after prolonged speaking, or difficulty with chewing or swallowing. Bulbar and respiratory symptoms are common in patients with MuSK antibodies. Neck flexion is more affected than neck extension, and limb weakness is a rare initial presentation of MG. Paradoxical abdominal movement during inspiration is present if the diaphragm is involved. In poorly controlled generalized MG, a myasthenic crisis, with acute neuromuscular respiratory failure, may occur and this requires urgent treatment (26).

Diagnosis

The history confirms fluctuating muscle weakness, with symptoms that are typically better upon awakening or after rest, and which become progressively worse with prolonged use or later in the day. Clinical examination relies on manual testing of specific muscle groups and confirms reduced power that worsens with repetition (e.g. weakness of forced eyelid or mouth closure) and improves with rest (27).

Tensilon test

Intravenous bolus injection of edrophonium chloride (Tensilon), a short-acting acetylcholinesterase inhibitor that prolongs the duration of action of acetylcholine at the neuromuscular junction, can rapidly (30 seconds) and transiently (< 5 minutes) improve muscle strength in patient with MG. The initial dose of 2 mg may be followed by repeated 2 mg boluses up to a maximum of 10 mg. The test should be performed only if an objective improvement in muscle strength, such as resolution of ptosis, can be shown clinically. Adverse effects of the Tensilol test are rare and usually mild, and include increased sweating, lacrimation, salivation, nausea, abdominal cramps, and diarrhoea. More serious muscarinic side effects, including bronchospasm, bradycardia, and asystole, can occur rarely. Cardiac monitoring and prompt availability of atropine are therefore required during a Tensilon test. MuSK-MG patients may not improve significantly following intravenous edrophonium.

Autoantibodies

Identification of circulating autoantibodies in a patient with compatible clinical features confirms the diagnosis of MG, although negative tests do not exclude the diagnosis because antibodies are not detected in 10–13% of patients with generalized MG. AchR-ab can also be negative in the early stages of the disease and measurement should be repeated within 6–12 months of symptom onset. AchR-ab levels are not correlated with disease severity, nor are they a reliable marker of response to treatment. MuSK antibodies are not present in patients with persistent localized ocular MG.

Electrophysiology

Repetitive nerve stimulation testing involves supra-maximal stimulation of the relevant nerve at 2–5 Hz in a train of six stimulations at rest, and again after a period of exercise. A 10% decrement in the compound muscle action potential (CMAP) amplitude between the first and the fifth evoked CMAP confirms the diagnosis of MG.

The test is abnormal in approximately 70% of patients with generalized MG and 50% of those with ocular MG.

Single-fibre electromyography (SFEMG) is the most sensitive diagnostic test for MG, and has a diagnostic yield of greater than 95%. It is technically demanding and performed using a microelectrode that allows identification of action potentials from individual muscle fibres and measurement of neuromuscular jitter, the variability of the time intervals between adjacent muscle fibre potentials in the same motor unit. SFEMG demonstrates increased jitter in 95–99% of patients with MG patients when appropriate muscles are examined. Abnormal jitter is not specific for MG, although it is diagnostic for a disorder of neuromuscular transmission in the presence of a normal EMG.

Other

Chest computed tomography or magnetic resonance imaging should be performed in all patients with confirmed MG to exclude the presence of a thymoma. MG often coexists with thyroid disease, so baseline testing of thyroid function should be obtained at the time of diagnosis.

Myasthenic crisis

Approximately 10% of patients with MG develop a myasthenic crisis (26), a severe and at times fatal condition resulting in an acute inability to breathe. By definition, all patients with myasthenic crisis are in respiratory failure secondary to severe weakness of respiratory or upper airway muscles, or both. Non-invasive ventilation or tracheal intubation and invasive mechanical ventilation is always necessary. Overtreatment with anticholinesterases can lead to cholinergic crises which are characterized by weakness and ventilatory failure, increased salivation, abdominal colic, diarrhoea, sweating, and small pupils.

Treatment

Treatment of MG involves a two-tiered approach—control of symptoms by acetylcholinesterase inhibitors and modulation of the immune system by immunosuppressants and surgery (28).

Symptom control with acetylcholinesterase inhibitors is the first-line treatment, although these drugs do not alter disease progression or outcome. Pyridostigmine is the most commonly used agent, and an initial oral dose of 15–30 mg 4–6-hourly is titrated against response.

Prednisone (oral 60 mg/day) is first-line immunosuppressant therapy and should be introduced when symptoms of MG are not adequately controlled by acetylcholinesterase inhibitors alone. Strength improves after about 2–3 weeks of therapy and full improvement is achieved after about 3 months. Azathioprine (AZA) reduces nucleic acid synthesis and T-cell proliferation and also has a place in the management of MG. AZA monotherapy takes up to 1 year to reach maximal effect and is better tolerated and more effective when used in combination with prednisone. Mycophenolate mofetil, cyclophosphamide, and tacrolimus should be considered in patients who do not tolerate or respond to AZA. All immunosuppressant therapies, including thymectomy, cannot be considered part of acute care because of their delayed benefits.

Thymectomy is strongly recommended if a thymoma is present, and is also a therapeutic option in young (< 50 years) non-thymomatous patients with generalized MG who are AChR-ab positive. Thymectomy is not recommended for patients over the age of 60 years, in those with antibodies to MuSK or pure ocular MG.

PE and IVIg also have a place in the treatment of MG. Clinical improvement is seen within days, but is a transient. Both agents are used in specific situations such as myasthenic crisis, and before thymectomy or other surgical procedures. PE and IVIg can also be used intermittently to maintain remission in patients with MG who remain poorly controlled despite the use of chronic immunomodulating drugs. PE is performed every other day for a total of four to six exchanges, and IVIg is given in a dose of 0.4 mg/kg/day for 5 days. The two treatments are similar in terms of efficacy, mortality improvements and complications. In myasthenic crisis, there is also no substantive evidence to support the use of one modality over the other.

Treatment of myasthenic crisis

Supportive treatment with airway and ventilator support is vital. PE or IVIg combined with high-dose corticosteroids (prednisolone 1 mg/kg/day) is the cornerstone of treatment for this fully reversible cause of neuromuscular paralysis. Discontinuation of anticholinesterases or any other drugs that act on the neuromuscular junction is also recommended to rule out cholinergic crisis (4,7). Patients with MG have an increased sensitivity to competitive NMBA and, if prolonged neuromuscular blockade following the use of steroidal NMBAs is suspected, sugammadex, a selective binding agent that may fully reverse even profound pharmacological neuromuscular transmission block, can be considered (29).

Prognosis

The natural course of generalized MG is improvement in 57% of patients and remission in 13% at 2 years. Remission is more common in females than in males (30). MG remains unchanged in 20% of patients and becomes worse than at the time of maximal weakness in 4% of those who survive beyond 2 years. Although anticholinesterase drugs usually provide symptomatic improvement, especially of ptosis, they do not effect MG remissions. Overall mortality in MG is 5–9%. Eighty per cent of patients with initial ocular symptoms progress to generalized MG, although if symptoms remain localized to the extraocular muscles for 1 year there is a high probability that muscle weakness will remain localized in the long term.

Lambert–Eaton myasthenic syndrome

LEMS is a rare neuromuscular autoimmune disease affecting the presynaptic neuromuscular junction. Patients with LEMS typically present with muscle weakness, dysautonomia, and areflexia. The prevalence of LEMS is 0.1–0.2 per 100,000. Although 50% of cases of LEMS are associated with small-cell lung carcinoma (SCLC), LEMS is relatively rare among the total SCLC patient population, occurring in only 0.5–3%. Non-tumour LEMS occurs at all ages, but has two peaks of onset at age 35 and 60 years. SCLS-related LEMS has a mean onset age of 60 years. The male to female ratio is 1:1 for non-tumour-LEMS, but SCLC-LEMS predominates in males (31).

Pathogenesis

The muscle weakness in LEMS is caused by autoantibodies to P/Q-type voltage-gated calcium channels (VGCC) in the presynaptic nerve terminals resulting in impaired acetylcholine release at the neuromuscular junction. A similar mechanism is also likely to be responsible for the associated autonomic dysfunction, via impaired transmitter release from parasympathetic and sympathetic neurons. VGCC autoantibodies are present in 85–90% of patients with non-tumour LEMS, and in close to 100% of those with SCLC-LEMS.

Although often described as 'myasthenic', the muscle weakness of LEMS is not fatigable. It is usually more prominent in proximal muscle groups, especially of the legs. Ocular, bulbar, and respiratory muscles weakness is less common and also less severe than in MG, and frequently transient. Muscle strength may improve initially after exercise and then weaken with sustained activity. Reflexes are absent or depressed but can return or increase after 10 seconds of maximal muscle contraction (post-tetanic potentiation). Autonomic neuropathy causes dry eyes, erectile dysfunction, constipation, and a dry mouth in patients with and without SCLC. Serum CK is normal in over 80% of cases.

Diagnosis

Diagnosis should be suspected based on clinical features and particularly the typical triad of proximal muscle weakness, areflexia, and autonomic dysfunction. LEMS may be first discovered when prolonged neuromuscular blockade follows the use of competitive NMBA during surgery.

The diagnosis is confirmed by neurophysiological investigations, and detection of antibody. Neurophysiological studies reveal a presynaptic neuromuscular junction defect with markedly reduced amplitude of the motor response at baseline, with an increase in amplitude (> 25%) after repetitive stimulation at high rates (20 Hz or greater), compared with the 4 Hz rate used in the diagnosis of myasthenia gravis. Post-tetanic potentiation is above 100%, and often reaches 300–400% or more, with a test specificity of around 99% (31).

Antibodies to P/Q-type VGCC are highly specific for LEMS. If LEMS is confirmed, or even suspected, screening for SCLC is mandatory. Antibodies against SOX1 protein represent a specific serological marker for SCLC. The probability of SCLC increases with increasing Dutch-English LEMS Tumor Association Prediction (DELTA-P) score (32), which is based on the following independent predictors: age 50 years or older, smoking behaviour, weight loss of at least 5% of body weight within the first 3 months, Karnofsky performance status 70 or below, bulbar involvement, male sexual impotence, and the presence of SOX1 protein antibodies. All patients with LEMS, even those with a low DELTA-P prediction of SCLC, should be screened for SCLC with chest CT scan and ^{18}F-fluorodeoxyglucose PET. Non-tumour-LEMS diagnosis is concluded if repeated screening is normal.

Treatment

The first-line treatment of LEMS is 3,4-diaminopyridine (3,4-DAP), 20–80 mg in 2–4 divided doses per day. 3,4-DAP increases the duration of the presynaptic action potential by blocking potassium channel efflux in nerve terminals, thereby increasing acetylcholine release (33). It is effective in both the acute and chronic phases of LEMS. If 3,4-DAP treatment is insufficient, immunosuppressive drug therapy should be started with a combination of prednisone/prednisolone and AZA. Rituximab is promising for all auto-antibody-mediated disorders, including LEMS. Effective treatment of an underlying SCLC improves SCLC-related LEMS.

Prognosis

Response to therapy is generally good in non-tumour-LEMS but patients with SCLC-LEMS tend to have progressive disease, a less satisfactory response to treatment, and poor prognosis for survival.

Motor neuron disease

The motor neuron diseases are a heterogeneous group of acquired and hereditary disorders that primarily affect the upper motor neurons (UMNs) in the brain, the lower motor neurons (LMNs) in the spinal cord and brainstem, or both, resulting in voluntary muscle weakness.

Amyotrophic lateral sclerosis (ALS) is the most common acquired motor neuron disease and affects spinal cord and cerebral motor neurons. It usually results in both UMN and LMN signs, although pure LMN and UMN variants are described. The pathological hallmark of ALS is degeneration and loss of motor neurons and astrocytic gliosis. At autopsy, the glial scar confers a feeling of hardness to palpation of the lateral columns of the spinal cord, from which the description 'lateral sclerosis' was derived. The aetiology of ALS is unknown (34).

Clinical features

The LMN features of ALS include muscle wasting, weakness and fasciculation of the tongue, arm, abdominal and paraspinal muscles, reduced muscle tone, and normal or depressed reflexes. UMN features include muscle weakness, increased muscle tone and spasticity, hyperactive deep tendon reflexes, positive Babinski sign, and reappearance of primitive responses such as snout, palmomental, and root reflexes. Focal muscle weakness starting in the arms or legs is the classical presentation of ALS, and there are usually no sensory symptoms, autonomic or sphincter dysfunction, or pain. The involvement of adjacent muscles before those of another region accounts for the asymmetrical distribution of the weakness, which is also most prominent distally. Muscle atrophy, particularly in the intrinsic muscles of the hands, is commonly seen, as implied by the term 'amyotrophic'. Bulbar signs such as dysarthria and dysphagia may also be presenting features. Respiratory failure from insufficiency of the respiratory muscles is the inevitable end stage of ALS, and is the most common cause of death (35).

Diagnosis

The diagnosis of motor neuron disease is clinical and depends on a detailed history and neurological examination which together confirm progressive muscle weakness with asymmetric distribution in multiple segments. Neuromuscular respiratory failure is common and FVC, MIP, and MEP should be assessed at regular intervals irrespective of the presence of clinical symptoms. SNIP measurement can be useful because it obviates the use of a mouthpiece (3).

Sensory and motor nerve conduction studies are mostly normal, although EMG signs of muscle denervation may be present in multiple bulbar/cranial, cervical, thoracic and lumbar regions. MRI is essential to exclude other spinal cord or brain pathology.

Management

Riluzole, a glutamate inhibitor, is the only neuroprotective drug approved for the treatment of ALS. It may slow the disease progression and delay death by an average of 3–4 months.

Table 22.5 Criteria for initiating non-invasive ventilator support in motor neurone disease

	Indications for non-invasive ventilation
FVC	< 50% predicted normal value
	Substantial difference between supine and erect FVC
MIP	< 60% of predicted
	> –60 cmH$_2$O
SNIP	> –40 cmH$_2$O (confirmed in > 10 sniffs)
PaCO$_2$	≥ 6.0 kPa (45 mmHg)
	Orthopnoea

FVC, forced vital capacity; MIP, maximal inspiratory pressure; MEP, maximal expiratory pressure; SNIP, maximal sniff nasal inspiratory pressure.

Non-invasive ventilation is useful to assist inspiratory muscles in maintaining adequate gas exchange, and may improve survival and quality of life by slowing the rate of decline in pulmonary function. Criteria for initiating NIV are shown in Table 22.5 (3) Patients with ALS may also develop inadequate expiratory muscle function making cough inadequate. Mechanical in-ex-sufflators and bronchoscopic toilet of respiratory secretions are useful to allow patients to maintain adequate airway clearance. Pressures of +40 cmH$_2$O for insufflation and –40cm H$_2$O for exsufflation are usually required as +35/–35 cm H$_2$O are the minimum pressures needed to clear airway secretions.

The need for invasive ventilation and tracheostomy should be discussed with the patient early to evaluate personal preferences. It should be considered in those requiring non-invasive ventilation for longer than 12 hours per day, if dyspnoea, altered swallowing and accumulating tracheobronchial secretions persist despite treatment, or if bulbar signs predominate. In the case of dysphagia, placement of a percutaneous gastrostomy tube is associated with prolonged survival and should be offered to patients.

Prognosis

ALS is a progressive, invariably fatal neurodegenerative disease. Most patients die within 3–5 years of diagnosis, although survival for greater than 10 years has been reported. Older age, female gender, and the presence of bulbar symptoms at disease presentation are associated with shorter survival.

Muscular dystrophies

Muscular dystrophies are a heterogeneous group of genetically determined muscle disorders characterized by muscle fibre degeneration and abnormal muscle regeneration (dystrophy), usually associated with an increase in fat and fibrous connective tissue. Other inherited muscle diseases include the hereditary myopathies, muscle ion channel disorders, and metabolic myopathies. Myotonic dystrophy which includes a characteristic muscular dystrophy, myotonic discharges indicating an ion-channel disorder, and mitochondrial skeletal muscle abnormalities with a metabolic component (36), overlaps these categories.

Muscular dystrophies occur at any age and have variable severity and clinical course. Early- or childhood-onset disease is often associated with profound loss of muscle function affecting ambulation,

posture and cardiac and respiratory function, whereas late-onset disease may be associated with relatively mild weakness. Some conditions are rapidly lethal, while others are asymptomatic and present only with increases in serum creatine kinase (CK).

Decrease in muscle strength is the major clinical feature of muscular dystrophies. Limb weakness may be proximal or distal, and can be generalized or selectively affect individual muscle groups depending on disease type. The respiratory and cardiac muscles are frequently involved making respiratory and cardiac failure common causes of death in the muscular dystrophies. Patients may have prolonged respiratory depression after general anaesthesia following even minor surgery, and anaesthesia may also lead to fatal hypotension and sudden death from malignant cardiac arrhythmias. Exposure to inhalational anaesthetic agents may also cause malignant hyperthermia-like reactions and rhabdomyolysis, and should be avoided in favour of total intravenous anaesthesia. Succinylcholine can cause fatal hyperkalaemia and should be avoided (9).

Muscle atrophy can be a prominent feature but may be difficult to assess because of fibrotic and adipose muscle degeneration, tightness of muscles and tendon shortening. Pseudohypertrophy of calf and thigh muscles may be particularly noticeable in boys, and result in them walking on their toes. The sensory nervous system is unaffected. Elevated serum CK and liver enzymes (γ-glutamyltransferase), pain, cramps, and myoglobinuria are also commonly seen.

Diagnosis is suspected on the basis of the history, clinical assessment of the pattern of muscle involvement, and laboratory tests (CK levels). Confirmation may require genetic analyses, such as DNA analysis of the dystrophin gene in the Duchenne muscular dystrophy and its less severe allelic counterpart Becker muscular dystrophy. EMG is useful in confirming the ongoing myopathy. Muscle biopsy demonstrates focal muscle necrosis, regenerative myofibres, mononuclear inflammatory infiltrates and, in chronic cases, increased connective tissue in the form of interstitial fibrosis and fatty replacement.

Periodic paralysis

Periodic paralysis is a disorder of skeletal muscle characterized by attacks of flaccid muscle weakness secondary to abnormal muscle membrane excitability (37). The primary periodic paralyses (PPs) are autosomal dominant disorders characterized by ion channel dysfunction. Several mutations causing muscle membrane voltage-gated ion channel dysfunction have been identified. Primary PPs include hypokalaemic and hyperkalaemic periodic paralysis, Anderson–Tawil syndrome (ATS), and thyrotoxic periodic paralysis. All share the final common mechanism of an aberrant muscle depolarization that inactivates sodium or calcium channels and thereby reduces muscle membrane excitability or renders the muscle electrically unexcitable. Nerve conduction studies demonstrate reduced amplitude of the compound muscle action potential, and EMG reveals myopathic changes and myotonia.

The main clinical feature of PPs is spontaneous muscle weakness, or weakness initiated by a variety of triggers including strenuous physical activity, high-carbohydrate diet, exposure to cold temperature, intercurrent viral infection, stress, menstruation, and many drugs including corticosteroids, epinephrine (adrenaline), and insulin. The severity and duration of symptoms are variable.

Attacks can last from a few minutes to several days, and may involve only one body segment or be generalized. In some cases, myotonia can also be present. In addition to the acute episodes, most patients develop a chronic and significant muscle weakness (38).

Increases or decreases in serum potassium levels are frequently observed during an attack. Even in patients with hyperkalaemic PP, transient episodes of normokalaemia or hypokalaemia may occur during attacks of weakness. Normalization of serum potassium is associated with symptom resolution.

Subtypes

Several subtypes of primary and secondary PPs are identified.

Hypokalaemic periodic paralysis

Hypokalaemic PP (hypoK-PP) is the most common form of PP, with a European prevalence of 0.4–1:100,000. It is sporadic in 10–15% of cases and affects mostly males aged between 5 and 20 years, although onset in the second decade has been described. Genes implicated in familial hypoK-PP include *CACNA1S* which is located on chromosome 1q32 and encodes Cav1.1, the α subunit of the L-type voltage-dependent calcium channels (dihydropyridine receptor), and *SCN4A* which is located on chromosome 17q11.2–24 and encodes the voltage-dependent sodium channel protein Nav 1.4. Mutations of *CACNA1S* (the voltage-gated calcium channel gene) account for the majority of cases, with mutations of *SCN4A* (the voltage-gated sodium channel gene) being responsible fewer than 10% of cases.

Symptoms generally begin in the teenage years with attacks occurring in the morning or upon awakening during the night. They are characterized by flaccid paralysis, either generalized or focal, and absent or reduced tendon reflexes. Consciousness remains clear and, because the cranial nerves are always spared, the patient can open their eyes, speak, and breathe. Weakness of respiratory muscles is rarely reported and myotonia is typically absent. A prodromal phase of vague symptoms, including fatigue, nausea, thirst, and distal paraesthesia, may precede the acute attack by several hours. Hypokalaemia is a constant finding.

Both onset and resolution of symptoms are gradual, and abrupt onset of weakness argues against the diagnosis of hypoK-PP. The crisis rarely lasts longer than 72 hours, although cases of several days' duration have been reported. During the crisis, ECG changes, including prominent U waves, flattening of T waves, and ST depression, may be observed in association with the profound hypokalaemia. Echocardiography demonstrates normal cardiac muscle function. Between attacks the patient is completely asymptomatic in the early stage of disease, although permanent proximal muscle weakness usually develops over time. Myopathy may occur even in the absence of a long-lasting history of frequent attacks.

The frequency of attacks can vary from daily to a few episodes in a lifetime, and often decreases later in life. Attacks can occur spontaneously or be provoked by the triggers highlighted previously.

Hyperkalaemic periodic paralysis

Hyperkalaemic periodic paralysis (hyperK-PP) is a channelopathy caused by mutations in the *SCN4A* gene which encodes the alpha-subunit of the skeletal muscle voltage-gated sodium channel Nav1.4. Attacks begin in the first decade of life, usually occur during the daytime, are short-lived lasting less than 4 hours, and, in most cases, less than an hour. Complete paralysis is unusual,

and involvement of respiratory muscles rare. There are no specific neurological signs other than flaccid paralysis. Serum potassium level can be increased during an attack, but in 50% of cases potassium remains within normal limits. Myoglobin and CK can also be increased during attacks. Between attacks, lid lag (the inability of the eyelid to follow the downward eye movement quickly enough so that the upper sclera is seen), and eyelid myotonia may be the only clinical signs. EMG confirms myotonia in half to two-thirds of patients.

The frequency of attacks and severity decrease with time, but persistent myopathy is almost universal.

Anderson–Tawil syndrome

The ATS is the rarest form of PP, and is caused in most cases by different mutations in the *KCNJ2* gene which encodes the K channel Kir 2.1 (ATS1). The prevalence of ATS is unknown. It presents with episodic spontaneous or triggered weakness in the first or second decade of life. In addition to the general features of other PPs, ATS is characterized by ventricular arrhythmias and skeletal abnormalities.

The frequency, duration and severity of attacks are variable and do not correlate with serum potassium levels, which may be normal, reduced, or elevated. ECG changes, including prominent U waves, premature ventricular contractions, ventricular bigeminy, polymorphic ventricular tachycardia, and prolonged QT interval, occur frequently. Myotonia is not a feature.

Thyrotoxic periodic paralysis

Thyrotoxic periodic paralysis (TPP) is the only non-familial PP. It is often classified as a secondary PP because its expression may be a result of an inherited predisposition that is uncovered by thyrotoxicosis (39). The prevalence of TPP is low in Caucasian populations (0.1–0.2%), but ten times greater in those of Asian origin. It is sporadic in 95% of cases and has a marked male predominance despite a higher incidence of thyrotoxicosis in women. It is mainly associated with autoimmune thyrotoxicosis (Graves' disease), but also with TSH-secreting pituitary tumours, toxic multinodular goitre, amiodarone-induced thyrotoxicosis, lymphocytic thyroiditis, factitious thyrotoxicosis, and toxic adenomas. In fact, any cause of thyrotoxicosis, including excessive thyroid hormone replacement therapy, can trigger paralysis in susceptible patients (40).

Mutation in the *KCNJ18* gene, which encodes the potassium channel Kir 2.6, is thought to result in inability to extrude potassium outside the muscle cell (41). The reduction in potassium efflux, in association with increased sodium-potassium ATPase activity stimulated by thyroid hormone, and/or hyperadrenergic activity and hyperinsulinaemia, results in hypokalaemia and paradoxical depolarization. This in turn inactivates sodium channels and results in muscle non-excitability and paralysis. Hypokalaemia develops without a deficit in total body potassium (41).

TPP is a neurological emergency that usually presents between 20 and 40 years of age. Attacks only develop whilst a patient is thyrotoxic, regardless of the aetiology of the thyrotoxicosis. Symptoms resemble those of hypoK-PP, with flaccid paralysis associated with the hypokalaemia and, typically, with hyperthyroidism. Symptoms present at night, often at weekends, after large carbohydrate meals, alcohol consumption or strenuous exercise. As with other types of PPs, infection, emotional stress, trauma, and corticosteroids may also trigger an attack.

Reduced or absent tendon reflexes is a remarkable feature in a patient with symptoms of thyrotoxicosis, in whom hyperactive reflexes would be expected. Laboratory abnormalities include hypokalaemia, suppressed levels of TSH, increased levels of thyroid hormones (total and free T4 and T3), positive antithyroid antibodies attributed to Graves' disease, and abnormalities in the thyroid gland confirmed by ultrasonography or thyroid scintigraphy.

Secondary periodic paralysis

Muscle symptoms are commonplace in potassium depletion, and include cramp, fasciculation, and weakness. In severe cases, diaphragmatic paralysis and respiratory failure may ensue. Thiazide or loop diuretics are the commonest cause of hypokalaemia in clinical practice, and large amounts of potassium can also be lost with diarrhoea or small intestinal pathology. With severe hypokalaemia there is an associated risk of significant arrhythmias, paralytic ileus, and rhabdomyolysis, in addition to neuromuscular respiratory failure (42).

Paralysis secondary to hyperkalaemia is less common. Excessive potassium intake is an unusual cause of hyperkalaemia unless renal dysfunction is present. In rhabdomyolysis, particularly if myoglobinuria also results in acute kidney injury, life-threatening hyperkalaemia can quickly develop owing to rapid release of cellular potassium stores. Most cases of secondary hyperK-PP are related to administration of drugs that increase serum potassium, usually in combination with overzealous potassium supplementation or in patients with chronic renal failure (43). Succinylcholine may cause severe hyperkalaemia in patients with spinal cord injury, motor neuron disease, muscle dystrophies, or chronic myopathy and should be avoided (9).

Diagnosis

The diagnosis of PP requires a history of transient episodes of flaccid weakness, confirmation of serum potassium levels during an attack, and exclusion of secondary causes. Physical examination identifies typical facial dysmorphism in patients with ATS. ECG, echocardiography and exercise testing can be helpful in patients with ATS. Assessment of thyroid status is essential to differentiate hypoK-PP from TPP. Provocative tests, such as administration of potassium (orally or intravenously), cooling of limbs or exercise (or a combination) in suspected hyperK-PP, and a glucose load with or without additional insulin in hypoK-PP, are used less frequently since the introduction of genetic testing.

Nerve conduction studies during an attack reveal normal conduction velocity, reduced CMAP amplitude, or a completely unexcitable muscle. EMG reveals motor unit potentials of low amplitude and short duration which are highly polyphasic, and typical of a myopathy. Signs of denervation in the form of fibrillation potentials and positive sharp waves may also be seen. EMG may be normal in the interictal period in patients with short disease duration, although changes in CMAP can be evoked by exercise or cold exposure. In patients with persisting myopathy, reduced CMAP amplitude and EMG myopathic changes are constant findings. Myotonic discharges are present in the majority of patients with hyperK-PP, even when myotonia cannot be demonstrated clinically, but absent in hypoK-PP. Such findings may be useful in directing genetic testing. Reduced muscle conduction velocity can be demonstrated with specialized electrophysiological techniques, but is not specific for PPs. DNA testing is now the major diagnostic tool in familial PPs.

Treatment

Correction of an ionic abnormality is of primary importance during an attack. Potassium administration is warranted in hypoK-PP, and 20–30 mEq/L should be administered orally every 15–30 minutes until serum potassium is normalized. The oral route is preferred because of the risk of rebound hyperkalaemia following intravenous administration. If hypokalaemia is severe enough to cause cardiac arrhythmias (values of < 1 mmol/L have been documented in TPP) (44), or the patient is unable to take oral medication, potassium should be administered by slow intravenous infusion (20–40 mmol/L in 2 hours). Whatever the route of administration, regular monitoring of serum potassium levels must be undertaken. If thyrotoxicosis is caused by the overproduction of thyroid hormones, thionamides are first-line therapy. Methimazole 20–60 mg once daily or propylthiouracil 200–600 mg of daily in three divided are suitable. Thionamides block only new thyroid hormone synthesis, so stores of pre-existing hormone must become exhausted before the drug is fully effective. This may take 3–8 weeks in patients with Graves' disease. Therefore, intravenous propranolol is used as a first-line therapy for patients with TPP (20–40 mg every 8 hours, maximal daily dose of 240 mg), and, because it does not induce rebound hyperkalaemia, can be usefully combined with potassium supplementation. Definitive management of TPP involves correcting the thyrotoxic state.

Preventive measures in all PPs include avoidance of excessive exertion, particularly when followed by a long period of rest such as overnight sleep. Gentle physical activity can be helpful in aborting symptoms during an attack. In hypokalaemic attacks, frequent meals with low carbohydrate content and sodium restriction are recommended. Drugs causing hypokalaemia and large carbohydrate-rich meals, particularly late in the evening, should be avoided. The carbonic anhydrase inhibitors acetazolamide (250–1500 mg/day) and dichlorphenamide (50–200 mg/day) may reduce the frequency of attacks. The potassium pool is not depleted since the hypokalaemia is caused by potassium shift into cells. Administration of potassium between attacks does not therefore prevent future attacks, and is not recommended. Propranolol (80–160 mg per day) can also be used as preventive treatment.

Mild attacks in hyperK-PP do not require treatment, but severe hyperkalaemia warrants urgent treatment. Acetazolamide and dichlorphenamide are also effective prevention as in hypokalaemic PPs. Dietary preventive measures include regular meals, and avoidance of potassium rich foods and medications that increase serum potassium (e.g. spironolactone). Continued mild activity and ingestion of carbohydrate-containing drinks or foods may be helpful to prevent or shorten attacks. Beta-agonist inhalers attenuate hyperkalaemic attacks. Acetazolamide and dichlorphenamide are also effective in ATS, and beta blockers are frequently used to reduce the risk of ventricular tachycardia. In cases of syncope or cardiac arrest, an implantable cardioverter–defibrillator should be considered.

Flaccid paralysis may rarely involve the respiratory muscles and precipitate admission to the ICU for ventilatory support, although non-invasive ventilation and rapid correction of the underlying ionic abnormality usually resolve the condition.

Prognosis

The highest frequency of attacks in familial PPs is in the first decades of life, with a decreasing attack frequency with increasing age.

Chronic myopathy is common in patients with familial PP. In TPP, remission is the usual outcome after thyrotoxicosis is corrected.

Rarer conditions

There are many hundreds of rarer disorders that may cause muscle weakness, and some are so rare that the average intensivist working in the developed world will never encounter one in their working life (Table 22.1). However, an awareness of them is crucial to allow prompt diagnosis and treatment when such cases do present.

Tetanus

Tetanus is a toxin-mediated acute neurological disorder characterized by increased muscle spasms and rigidity. It is caused by tetanospasmin, a potent exotoxin with absolute neurospecificity, produced by *Clostridium tetani* (45). The genus *Clostridium* is a group of anaerobic Gram-positive bacilli capable of forming spores which are widely distributed in the environment, particularly in soil, and in the gastrointestinal tract and faeces of animals and humans. The spores are resistant to environmental extremes, allowing the organism to survive for years. There are more than 100 distinct species of bacteria in the *Clostridium* genus but, among pathogens, *C. tetani* and *C. botulinum* are the most important causing toxin-mediated diseases. Tetanus and botulinum neurotoxins are highly homologous in their amino acid structure and share the ability to inhibit neurotransmitter release. However, whereas tetanus is transported to the central nervous system, botulinum toxin remains at the periphery where it inhibits the release of acetylcholine. This explains the differences in clinical symptoms between the two diseases (see later) (45).

Contamination of wounds with *C. tetani* spores is common, but germination into mature bacilli releasing the tetanospasmin occurs only when local conditions favour anaerobiosis. *C. tetani* does not cause local inflammation and the portal of entry often appears innocuous. Furthermore, germination may begin after the wound has healed so many cases of tetanus have no identifiable source. Once released, the toxin attaches to GD1b and GT1b gangliosides on peripheral nerves, and is subsequently internalized and transported from the peripheral to the central nervous system by retrograde axonal transport and trans-synaptic spread. Tetanospasmin preferentially blocks inhibitory (i.e. GABAergic and glycinergic) synapse afferent to motor neurons in the spinal cord and brainstem, but toxin acts also on peripheral nerves, neuromuscular junctions, and directly on muscles. This leads to the characteristic muscle rigidity and spasms of tetanus, although a flaccid paralysis can sometimes occur in cases of cephalic tetanus (46).

Tetanus is a rare disease in high-income countries, but still represents a major health problem in developing countries. Eighty per cent of the 1 million tetanus-related deaths per year occur in Africa and south-east Asia, and 400,000 of these deaths are due to neonatal tetanus. Clusters of infections have recently occurred after tsunamis and earthquakes in countries where tetanus immunization coverage is low or non-existent (47).

Clinical presentation

Generalized tetanus accounts for 80–90% of cases in Europe and the United States. Trismus ('lockjaw' secondary to masseter muscle spasm), back pain and muscle stiffness are the initial complaints in most cases, and may be associated with restlessness, sweating, and dysphagia. Risus

sardonicus, secondary to facial muscle contraction and tonic neck spam, may also be the presenting feature. Rigidity spreads to affect all muscle groups as the disease progresses. Opisthotonus, a position of extreme hyperextension of the body in which the head, neck, and spine are arched backwards, is a classic manifestation of severe tetanus. Autonomic disturbance, include labile blood pressure, heart rate, and hyperpyrexia, may also occur. Cardiovascular instability is a particular cause for concern as it may lead to cardiac arrest. Ileus, diarrhoea, salivation, profuse sweating, increased bronchial secretions, and fever are also common features of dysautonomia.

Localized tetanus leads to muscle rigidity adjacent to the wound and may resolve without sequelae. However, cephalic tetanus, an uncommon variant of local tetanus related to craniofacial wounds, may involve the vocal cords and lead to life-threatening laryngospasm. In neonatal tetanus, the portal of spore entry is the freshly cut umbilical cord and subsequent umbilical stump infection. In addition to classical muscle spasms and rigidity, seizures and an ability to suckle are common presenting feature of neonatal tetanus.

Diagnosis

The diagnosis of tetanus is clinical, based on history and physical examination. There are no confirmatory tests, although culture of *C. tetani* from a wound supports the diagnosis (48). The differential diagnosis of tetanus includes strychnine poisoning, hypocalcaemic tetany, trismus due to orofacial infection, drug (phenothiazine)-induced dystonia, rabies, malignant neuroleptic syndrome, and stiff-person syndrome. In neonates, hypoglycaemia, meningitis, and seizures should also be considered.

Clinical course

Following wound contamination there is usually an incubation period of 7–10 days prior to symptom onset. However, the incubation period can be as short as 1 day or as long as several months, reflecting the distance the toxin must travel within the nervous system. The time from the onset of signs and symptoms to the appearance of muscle spasms is also variable. Although symptoms and signs usually progress for up to 2 weeks after disease onset, the clinical course is unpredictable and patients should be closely monitored throughout this period. Muscle spasms are extremely painful and often induced by minor stimuli. Autonomic disturbances are the leading cause of death from tetanus in Western countries. They usually present after the onset of muscle spasms and peak during the second week of the disease. Rigidity may extend beyond the duration of both spasms and autonomic disturbance, and treatment may sometimes be required for prolonged periods. Recovery may take up to 4–6 weeks.

Management

C. tetani spores are ubiquitous and cannot be eliminated from the environment. As such, immunization and proper treatment of wounds are essential for tetanus prevention (49).

Intramuscular human tetanus immunoglobulin, given as a single dose of 500 IU, neutralizes circulating toxin. Any benefit from higher doses or intrathecal administration has not been demonstrated. Wound debridement, where one exists, decreases the anaerobic environment and reduces spore germination, but should be performed after immunoglobulin administration because of the risk of further toxin release during the procedure. Despite antibiotics having only a minor role in the management of tetanus, intravenous metronidazole (500 mg IV every 6 hours) or penicillin G is usually recommended. Active immunization with tetanus toxoid should be given to all patients with tetanus (using a separate site of injection from human tetanus immunoglobulin) because the active infection does not confer immunity following recovery from acute illness. Neonatal tetanus can be prevented by immunization of women during pregnancy.

Control of muscle spasm is of primary importance because they can lead to respiratory and cardiovascular failure. The associated pain is often described as excruciating. Diazepam, midazolam, and lorazepam are equally effective at controlling spasms, and may be required for prolonged periods and at high doses. Diazepam has the advantage of being cheap and available in most parts of the world. Propofol and non-competitive neuromuscular blocking agents are indicated if benzodiazepines alone are insufficient at controlling the spasms. Under such circumstances, tracheal intubation and artificial ventilation are required. Intrathecal baclofen can be considered in countries where access to ICU facilities and mechanical ventilation is limited. Maintaining serum magnesium concentrations at 2–4 mmol/L reduces muscle spasms. As none of the above-mentioned drugs have analgesic properties, the concurrent use of opioids to cannot be overemphasized.

Magnesium also reduces cardiovascular instability (50), and benzodiazepines and opioids are also useful to control the effects of the dysautonomia. Rapid swings in blood pressure make treatment of hypertension difficult, and a continuous intravenous infusion of short-acting agents is preferred. Labetalol is often used because of its dual alpha- and beta-blocking effect, but its duration of action is 3–6 hours. Intravenous esmolol, a pure beta blocker with a half-life of 10–30 minutes, has therefore been recommended. Whatever agent is used, periods of hypotension requiring vasopressor support may still occur.

Supportive care has greatly reduced the morbidity and mortality from tetanus, and is the mainstay of treatment. Tracheal intubation and mechanical ventilation are invariably required in severe cases, and tracheostomy should be planned early to facilitate prolonged mechanical ventilation, secretion clearance, and weaning from the ventilator. Mechanical and pharmacological venous thromboembolism prophylaxis and nutritional support with enteral feeding should be started as soon as possible. Percutaneous gastrostomy is required if the need for prolonged enteral feeding is anticipated. Physical rehabilitation should be started soon after the resolution of spams.

Prognosis

The severity of the disease is related to the duration of the incubation period and interval from symptom onset to the appearance of muscle spasms; the shorter the interval, the more severe the disease and the risk of permanent disability. Despite modern intensive care, mortality in generalized tetanus remains high at around 20–25%. Mortality is higher in low-income countries where artificial ventilation may not be available for every case, in neonatal tetanus, and in older patients. In high-income countries, autonomic instability, pneumonia, and sepsis are the predominant cause of death after tetanus. Survivors may recover completely, but prolonged drug-induced paralysis and immobilization may lead to persistent muscle weakness and disability.

Botulism

Botulism is characterized by acute, symmetric, descending, flaccid paralysis caused by potent neurotoxins produced by C. botulinum,

a spore-forming obligate anaerobe with natural soil and water sediment as its habitat. Different strains produce one of eight exotoxin types (A, B, C1, C2, D, E, F, or G), of which toxin types A, B, E, and rarely F, cause human disease. Type A is the most potent exotoxin known (51). By impeding fusion of acetylcholine-containing vesicles it blocks the presynaptic release of acetylcholine and neuromuscular transmission of the motor nerve action potential, resulting in flaccid paralysis (45).

The toxin can contaminate food (food-borne botulism), whereas the spores usually contaminate wounds although they can also be introduced as a result of soil contamination of drugs of abuse such as 'black tar heroin' injected into subcutaneous or muscle tissue (52). Infant botulism follows the absorption of toxin produced in situ by C. botulinum colonization of the intestine of infants before bowel florae fully mature. Inhalation botulism is not a naturally occurring disease but has been planned by bioterrorists. A single gram of crystalline botulinum toxin evenly dispersed and inhaled would kill more than 1 million people. Botulism has also occurred accidentally in laboratory workers. Iatrogenic botulism can be related to injection of unlicensed, highly concentrated botulinum toxin for cosmetic purposes (53).

The ingested toxin is pre-formed in food-borne botulism, and the delay before appearance of symptoms shorter (2 hours to 8 days) than in wound contamination (4–18 days) where the toxin must be synthesized and released. In contrast to the spore, toxin is readily inactivated by heat ($\geq 85°C$ for 5 minutes), and hence foodborne botulism is always a consequence of foods that are not heated, or not heated thoroughly, before eating. The toxin enters the bloodstream and is primarily transported to the presynaptic cholinergic motor nerve endings. The autonomic nervous system can also be affected, but usually without significant consequence. The central nervous system is not involved.

Clinical presentation

All forms of human botulism are clinically similar, with presenting symptoms that include visual disturbance and difficulty in speaking and swallowing secondary to cranial nerve palsies (51). Neurological examination confirms the '6 Ds' of botulism—ptosis, dilated pupils, diplopia, dry mouth, dysarthria, dysphagia, and dysphonia.

Respiratory failure and arrest are the most feared complications, particularly because patients do not appear distressed. Indeed they usually appear tranquil and comfortable because of generalized facial and limb skeletal muscle paralysis. Positional airway obstruction secondary to pharyngeal collapse may compromise airway patency in the supine position and necessitate tracheal intubation even in the absence of inspiratory muscle insufficiency. With descending paralysis, the muscles of the neck, shoulders, proximal and then distal upper limbs, and proximal followed by distal lower limbs are involved sequentially. Paralysis of the respiratory muscles results in respiratory failure. Tendon reflexes progressively disappear. Abdominal symptoms may be early signs in foodborne botulism. Signs of autonomic dysfunction include anhydrosis with severe dry mouth and throat, and postural hypotension. Constipation is almost invariably present in the later stages of the disease.

Diagnosis

Diagnosis is based on a careful history and neurological evaluation (54). A combination of cranial nerve palsy and descending, symmetric, flaccid muscle paralysis in association with an unaffected sensory system, maintained mental function, and absence of fever is virtually pathognomonic of botulism. Gag and cough reflexes, FVC and respiratory muscle strength, adequacy of clearing of oropharyngeal secretions, and airway patency in the supine position should be assessed repeatedly to identify pharyngeal and respiratory muscle insufficiency at an early stage.

Laboratory investigations include anaerobic cultures and toxin assays of serum, gastric secretions, vomitus, stool, wound material, and the implicated food in original containers. The standard test for toxin identification is the mouse bioassay which involves intraperitoneal injection of toxin into mice and observation for the subsequent development of botulism-specific symptoms. The sensitivity of laboratory tests of clinical specimens is high in the early phase after inoculation, but declines later. Accordingly, when syndromes other than infant botulism are suspected, serum should be obtained immediately and prior to the administration of antitoxin, because antitoxin will neutralize all circulating toxin and render the test meaningless (55).

Neurophysiological studies demonstrate a presynaptic neuromuscular junction defect, although post-tetanic potentiation is less pronounced in botulism than in the LEMS. Sensory nerve action potentials and motor nerve conduction velocities remain normal.

Clinical course

The rapidity of onset and the severity of paralysis depend on the amount of toxin absorbed into the circulation. Some patients may be mildly affected with cranial nerve palsy but no evidence of descending muscle paralysis whereas in others, flaccid paralysis may be generalized and involve the facial, limb, and respiratory muscles, with ptosis, complete ophthalmoplegia, dilated unreactive pupils, facial palsy, and flaccid tetraplegia, often to such a degree that it may mimic areflexic deep coma. Patients retain mental competency, although cognition can be impaired in cases of secondary infection, sepsis and delirium. Months of ventilatory support and extended physical rehabilitation are required in such cases (56).

Management

Patients with suspected botulism should be admitted immediately to the ICU (55). Intravenous administration of botulinum antitoxin is the mainstay of treatment; the earlier it is administrated the better the prognosis. Penicillin G or metronidazole is widely prescribed, even though the efficacy is unproven. Supportive care with head-up positioning and prompt institution of tracheal intubation and mechanical ventilation in cases of positional airway obstruction or neuromuscular respiratory failure is essential. In severe cases, early tracheostomy should be considered. Venous thromboembolism prophylaxis, enteral feeding, pain control, use of protocol-driven light sedation, and early physical rehabilitation are also important aspects of treatment. Drugs (including antibiotics) interfering with neuromuscular transmission should be avoided (Table 22.1).

Prognosis

The overall mortality rate of botulism is around 3–8%, but less than 1% in infant botulism. Recovery of muscle strength results from motor axon regeneration, and this may take weeks or months to be complete. Data on long-term outcome are scarce and persistent disability is likely to be an under-recognized problem, particularly in older patients or those with a protracted clinical course who require long-term mechanical ventilation. Fatigue, generalized weakness,

dizziness, dry mouth, difficulty lifting things, and difficulty breathing caused by moderate exertion may persist years after the acute illness, whereas ocular and bulbar signs and symptoms which may have been prominent during the acute attack, resolve more quickly (56).

Acute intermittent porphyria

Porphyrias are caused by altered activity of specific enzymes of the haem biosynthetic pathway and, when clinically expressed, lead to accumulation of haem pathway intermediates. Acute intermittent porphyria (AIP) is characterized by intermittent, acute attacks lasting for several days or longer, usually followed by complete recovery (57). Severe abdominal pain is the most common presenting symptom and often accompanied by nausea, vomiting, constipation and signs of ileus mimicking a surgical emergency. Signs of sympathetic overactivity are also common. Acute attacks are precipitated by hormonal fluctuations during the menstrual cycle, fasting, smoking, infections, and exposure to porphyrinogenic drugs such as ketamine, thiopental, nifedipine, nicardipine, diltiazem, clonidine, propafenone, carbamazepine, phenytoin, clonazepam, ketorolac, quetiapine, fluconazole, clindamycin, amiodarone, and spironolactone (http://www.drugs-porphyria.org).

Peripheral neuropathy in AIP is mostly motor in nature and resembles GBS. It develops when porphyrinogenic drugs are used during an attack. The muscle weakness is symmetrical and begins in the proximal muscles of the arms. As the syndrome progresses, tetraparesis, or tetraplegia develops in most patients. Worsening neuropathy may lead to respiratory and bulbar paralysis requiring immediate tracheal intubation and mechanical ventilation. The cranial nerves are usually spared. Nerve conduction studies demonstrate axonal neuropathy. Changes in urine colour occur when the urine is exposed to light, and increased urinary excretion of D-aminolevulinic acid and porphobilinogen during an acute attack of AIP establishes the diagnosis.

The specific treatment of AIP is daily intravenous human haemin, 4 mg/kg per day for 3–4 consecutive days, and carbohydrate loading (58). Supportive treatment consists of stopping porphyrinogenic drugs, and institution of mechanical ventilation in cases of severe respiratory muscle weakness. Maintenance of fluid and calorie intake, and treatment of hyponatraemia are also important. Limb, abdominal, and back pain often requires high-dose opioids.

Intensive care unit-acquired neuromuscular weakness

Patients in the ICU may suffer from several complications that can cause muscle weakness and paralysis (see Table 22.1). Among them, critical illness polyneuropathy (CIP) and critical illness myopathy (CIM) are the most prevalent, affecting between one-third and one-half of the most severely ill patients (17). CIP and CIM most often coexist and, in that circumstance, are called critical illness neuromyopathy (CINM) or critical illness myopathy and neuropathy (CRIMYNE).

Definition and clinical presentation

CIP is a distal axonal sensory-motor polyneuropathy causing generalized, symmetrical limb and respiratory muscles weakness, with sparing of the facial muscles. Reflexes are usually reduced or absent, but can be preserved. In severe cases, a flaccid tetraplegia can develop. CIP is strongly associated with failure to wean patients from mechanical ventilation and this is often the presenting feature. The MRC scale is used clinically to test strength in functional limb muscle groups, and individual MRC scores can be combined into a sum score to yield an overall estimate of motor function (Figure 22.1) (59). A score of less than 48 identifies ICU-acquired weakness (ICUAW). Grip dynamometry of the dominant hand correlates well with MRC scores and is a rapid alternative to a comprehensive MRC evaluation of muscle strength (60). However, both assessments require a fully cooperative patient, making them worthless in many ICU patients (61). CIP alone, or in association with CIM, is likely to occur in 33–50% of critically ill patients overall (62,63), although an incidence up to 100% has been reported in those with septic shock, severe sepsis, or coma (64).

CIM is an acute myopathy causing muscle dysfunction and disruption of normal muscle fibre structure. It is a primary myopathy and therefore not related to denervation. CIM encompasses a variety of histological pictures including thick-filament (myosin) myopathy, and acute myopathy with scattered or diffuse necrosis (necrotizing myopathy) (17). In some cases the muscle can be completely electrically unexcitable (Figure 22.2) (65,66). The clinical features are the same as for CIP, except that sensation is normal.

Diagnosis

The first indication of CIP or CIM is the identification of weak and flaccid limbs when sedation is withdrawn, or difficulty with weaning from mechanical ventilation. In patients who are comatose, a painful stimulus will induce facial grimacing but little limb movement. The differential diagnosis mostly relies on appearance of muscle weakness after the onset of critical illness (Figure 22.3).

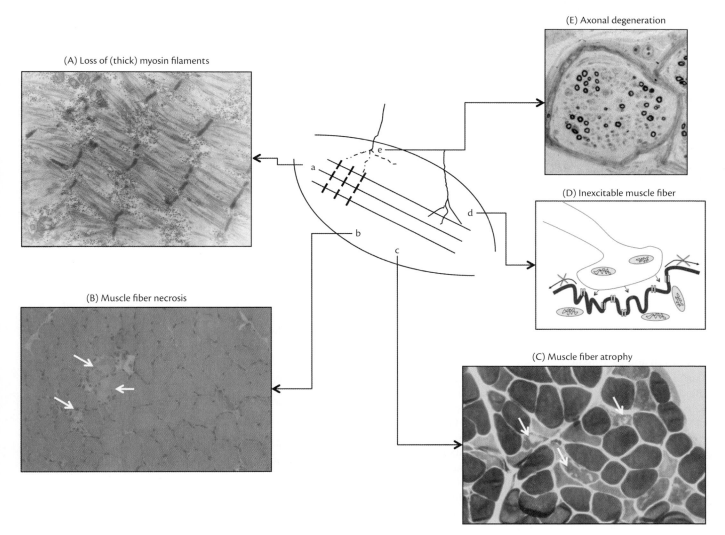

Fig. 22.2 Major histopathologic features of critical illness myopathy.
(A) Electron microscopy: myofibrils devoid of thick filaments with preserved Z lines (original magnification 12,000×).
(B) Haematoxylin eosin: necrotic muscle fibres (arrows) (original magnification 20×).
(C) ATPase pH 4.6: muscle fibre atrophy (mainly type II) and focal loss of reactivity indicating loss of myofilaments (arrows) (original magnification 40×).
(D) Schematic representation of inexcitable muscle with preserved neuromuscular transmission.
(E) Light microscopic image, toluidine blue stain, sural nerve biopsy: nerve axon degeneration with decreased density of myelinated fibres, magnification 150×. CIM, critical illness myopathy.

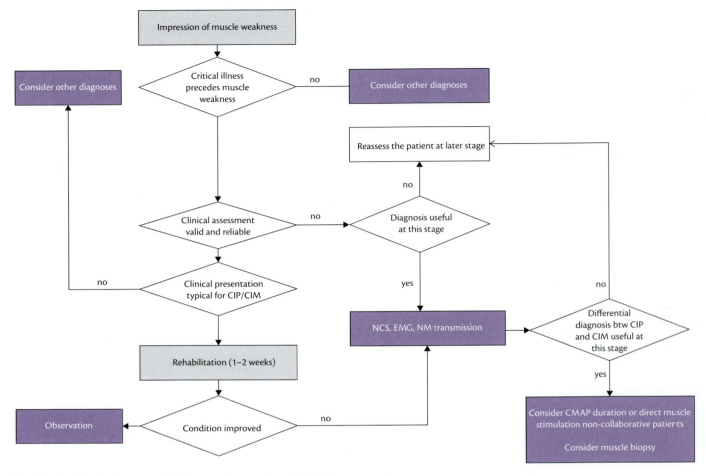

Fig. 22.3 Algorithm for diagnosing critical illness polyneuropathy and critical illness myopathy.
CIM, critical illness myopathy; CIP, critical illness polyneuropathy, CMAP, compound muscle action potential; EMG, electromyography; NCS, nerve conduction study; NM, neuromuscular.
Reprinted from *The Lancet Neurology*, 10, Latronico N and Bolton CF, 'Critical illness polyneuropathy and myopathy: a major cause of muscle weakness and paralysis', pp. 931–941, Copyright 2011, with permission from Elsevier.

The definitive diagnosis of CIP and CIM requires a combined clinical and electrophysiological evaluation (Tables 22.6 and 22.7) (17).

Prevention and treatment

There are many risk factors for CIP and CIM (Box 22.1), but no specific treatments. Strict glycaemic control during the ICU episode may reduce the incidence and severity of electrophysiologically-proven CIM and CIP (67), but intensive insulin treatment targeting normoglycaemia increases mortality (68) and the optimal level of blood glucose remains unclear. Electrical muscle stimulation remains of unproven benefit in preventing CIP and CIM and, although passive stretching preserves muscle structure in the sedated paralysed patient, it does not preserve protein content. Minimizing the use of sedation with an integrated early mobilization programme may reduce ventilator dependency and ICU length of stay, and improve functional outcome (69,70).

Prognosis

Delayed weaning from mechanical ventilation with increased ICU and hospital stay, higher hospital costs, increased mortality and protracted disability are common consequences of CIP and CIM.

Box 22.1 Risk factors for the development of critical illness polyneuropathy and myopathy

- Sepsis, systemic inflammatory response syndrome
- Multiorgan dysfunction/failure
- Hyperglycaemia
- Chronic corticosteroid use
- Neuromuscular blocking drugs
- Bed rest and immobility due to sedation
- Severe electrolyte abnormalities (CIM only):
  - hypokalaemia
  - hyperkalaemia
  - hypophosphataemia
  - hypomagnesaemia
  - hypermagnesaemia
  - hypercalcaemia.

Table 22.6 Diagnostic criteria for critical illness polyneuropathy. A definite diagnosis of critical illness polyneuropathy is established if all four criteria are fulfilled, and a probable diagnosis if criteria 1, 3, and 4 are fulfilled. A diagnosis of intensive care unit-acquired weakness is established if only criteria 1 and 2 are fulfilled

Criteria	Description
1	The patient is critically ill (multiple organ dysfunctions and failures)
2	Limb weakness or difficulty weaning patient from ventilator after non-neuromuscular causes such as heart and lung disease have been excluded
3	Electrophysiological evidence of axonal motor and sensory polyneuropathy
4	Absence of a decremental response on repetitive nerve stimulation

Reprinted from *The Lancet Neurology*, 10, Latronico N and Bolton CF, 'Critical illness polyneuropathy and myopathy: a major cause of muscle weakness and paralysis', pp. 931–941, Copyright 2011, with permission from Elsevier.

Although prognosis is better in CIM than CIP, nearly one-third of patients with CIP, CIM, or both do not recover independent walking or spontaneous ventilation (71,72). Patients with muscle-biopsy proven thick filament myopathy have a much better prognosis than those with necrotizing myopathy, and a precise pathological diagnosis is therefore important in prognostication.

Table 22.7 Diagnostic criteria for critical illness myopathy. A definite diagnosis of critical illness myopathy is established if all seven criteria are fulfilled, and a probable diagnosis if criteria 1 and 3–6 are fulfilled. A diagnosis of ICU-acquired weakness is established if only criteria 1 and 2 are fulfilled

Criteria	Description
1	The patient is critically ill (multiple organ dysfunction and failures)
2	Limb weakness or difficulty weaning patient from ventilator after non-neuromuscular causes such as heart and lung disease have been excluded
3	Compound muscle action potential amplitudes < 80% of the lower limit of normal in two or more nerves without conduction block
4	Sensory nerve action potential amplitudes > 80% of the lower limit of normal
5	Needle EMG with short-duration, low-amplitude motor unit potentials with early or normal full recruitment, with or without fibrillation potentials in conscious and collaborative patients or Increased CMAP duration or reduced muscle membrane excitability on direct muscle stimulation in non collaborative patients
6	Absence of a decremental response on repetitive nerve stimulation
7	Muscle histopathologic findings of primary myopathy (e.g. myosin loss or muscle necrosis)

CMAP, compound muscle action potential.

Reprinted from *The Lancet Neurology*, 10, Latronico N and Bolton CF, 'Critical illness polyneuropathy and myopathy: a major cause of muscle weakness and paralysis', pp. 931–941, Copyright 2011, with permission from Elsevier.

References

1. Dhand UK. Clinical approach to the weak patient in the intensive care unit. *Respir Care*. 2006;51(9):1024–40.
2. Doorduin J, van Hees HW, van der Hoeven JG, Heunks LM. Monitoring of the respiratory muscles in the critically ill. *Am J Respir Crit Care Med*. 2013;187(1):20–7.
3. Gruis KL, Lechtzin N. Respiratory therapies for amyotrophic lateral sclerosis: a primer. *Muscle Nerve*. 2012;46(3):313–31.
4. Mor A, Wortmann RL, Mitnick HJ, Pillinger MH. Drugs causing muscle disease. *Rheum Dis Clin North Am*. 2011;37(2):219–31.
5. Mor A, Mitnick HJ, Pillinger MH, Wortmann RL. Drug-induced myopathies. *Bull NYU Hosp Jt Dis*. 2009;67(4):358–69.
6. Ahmed A, Simmons Z. Drugs which may exacerbate or induce myasthenia gravis: a clinician's guide. *Internet J Neurol*. 2009;10(2).
7. Dalakas MC. Toxic and drug-induced myopathies. *J Neurol Neurosurg Psychiatry*. 2009;80(8):832–8.
8. Kelly BJ, Luce JM. The diagnosis and management of neuromuscular diseases causing respiratory failure. *Chest*. 1991;99(6):1485–94.
9. Martyn JA, Richtsfeld M. Succinylcholine-induced hyperkalemia in acquired pathologic states: etiologic factors and molecular mechanisms. *Anesthesiology*. 2006;104(1):158–69.
10. Boles JM, Bion J, Connors A, Herridge M, Marsh B, Melot C, et al. Weaning from mechanical ventilation. *Eur Respir J*. 2007;29(5):1033–56.
11. Winer JB. Guillain-Barre syndrome. *BMJ*. 2008;337:a671.
12. Hughes RA, Cornblath DR. Guillain-Barre syndrome. *Lancet*. 2005;366(9497):1653–66.
13. van Doorn PA, Ruts L, Jacobs BC. Clinical features, pathogenesis, and treatment of Guillain-Barre syndrome. *Lancet Neurol*. 2008;7(10):939–50.
14. Yuki N, Hartung HP. Guillain-Barre syndrome. *N Engl J Med*. 2012;366(24):2294–304.
15. Sejvar JJ, Kohl KS, Gidudu J, Amato A, Bakshi N, Baxter R, et al. Guillain-Barre syndrome and Fisher syndrome: case definitions and guidelines for collection, analysis, and presentation of immunization safety data. *Vaccine*. 2011;29(3):599–612.
16. Uncini A, Manzoli C, Notturno F, Capasso M. Pitfalls in electrodiagnosis of Guillain-Barre syndrome subtypes. *J Neurol Neurosurg Psychiatry*. 2010;81(10):1157–63.
17. Latronico N, Bolton CF. Critical illness polyneuropathy and myopathy: a major cause of muscle weakness and paralysis. *Lancet Neurol*. 2011;10(10):931–41.
18. Cabrera Serrano M, Rabinstein AA. Causes and outcomes of acute neuromuscular respiratory failure. *Arch Neurol*. 2010;67(9):1089–94.
19. Walgaard C, Lingsma HF, Ruts L, Drenthen J, van Koningsveld R, Garssen MJ, et al. Prediction of respiratory insufficiency in Guillain-Barre syndrome. *Ann Neurol*. 2010;67(6):781–7.
20. Durand MC, Porcher R, Orlikowski D, Aboab J, Devaux C, Clair B, et al. Clinical and electrophysiological predictors of respiratory failure in Guillain-Barre syndrome: a prospective study. *Lancet Neurol*. 2006;5(12):1021–8.
21. Rajabally YA, Uncini A. Outcome and its predictors in Guillain-Barre syndrome. *J Neurol Neurosurg Psychiatry*. 2012;83(7):711–18.
22. Walgaard C, Lingsma HF, Ruts L, van Doorn PA, Steyerberg EW, Jacobs BC. Early recognition of poor prognosis in Guillain-Barre syndrome. *Neurology*. 2011;76(11):968–75.
23. Cavalcante P, Bernasconi P, Mantegazza R. Autoimmune mechanisms in myasthenia gravis. *Curr Opin Neurol*. 2012;25(5):621–9.
24. Higuchi O, Hamuro J, Motomura M, Yamanashi Y. Autoantibodies to low-density lipoprotein receptor-related protein 4 in myasthenia gravis. *Ann Neurol*. 2011;69(2):418–22.
25. Spillane J, Higham E, Kullmann DM. Myasthenia gravis. *BMJ*. 2012;345:e8497.
26. Sakaguchi H, Yamashita S, Hirano T, Nakajima M, Kimura E, Maeda Y, et al. Myasthenic crisis patients who require intensive care unit management. *Muscle Nerve*. 2012;46(3):440–2.

27. Vincent A, Palace J, Hilton-Jones D. Myasthenia gravis. *Lancet.* 2001;357(9274):2122–8.

28. Hilton-Jones D. When the patient fails to respond to treatment: myasthenia gravis. *Pract Neurol.* 2007;7(6):405–11.

29. Blichfeldt-Lauridsen L, Hansen BD. Anesthesia and myasthenia gravis. *Acta Anaesthesiol Scand.* 2012;56(1):17–22.

30. Grob D, Brunner N, Namba T, Pagala M. Lifetime course of myasthenia gravis. *Muscle Nerve.* 2008;37(2):141–9.

31. Titulaer MJ, Lang B, Verschuuren JJ. Lambert-Eaton myasthenic syndrome: from clinical characteristics to therapeutic strategies. *Lancet Neurol.* 2011;10(12):1098–107.

32. Titulaer MJ, Maddison P, Sont JK, Wirtz PW, Hilton-Jones D, Klooster R, *et al.* Clinical Dutch-English Lambert-Eaton Myasthenic syndrome (LEMS) tumor association rediction score accurately predicts small-cell lung cancer in the LEMS. *J Clin Oncol.* 2011;29(7):902–8.

33. Keogh M, Sedehizadeh S, Maddison P. Treatment for Lambert-Eaton myasthenic syndrome. *Cochrane Database Syst Rev.* 2011;2:CD003279.

34. Mitchell JD, Borasio GD. Amyotrophic lateral sclerosis. *Lancet.* 2007;369(9578):2031–41.

35. Yoshii Y, Hadano S, Otomo A, Suzuki K, Ikeda K, Ikeda JE, *et al.* Natural history of young-adult amyotrophic lateral sclerosis. *Neurology.* 2009;73(8):648–9; author reply 9–50.

36. Emery AE. The muscular dystrophies. *Lancet.* 2002;359(9307):687–95.

37. Venance SL, Cannon SC, Fialho D, Fontaine B, Hanna MG, Ptacek LJ, *et al.* The primary periodic paralyses: diagnosis, pathogenesis and treatment. *Brain.* 2006;129(Pt 1):8–17.

38. Fialho D, Hanna MG. Myopathies. Periodic paralysis. In Aminoff MJ, Boller F, Swaab DF, Mastaglia FL, Hilton-Jones D (eds) *Handbook of Clinical Neurology.* Amsterdam: Elsevier; 2007:77–106.

39. Ryan DP, da Silva MR, Soong TW, Fontaine B, Donaldson MR, Kung AW, *et al.* Mutations in potassium channel Kir2.6 cause susceptibility to thyrotoxic hypokalemic periodic paralysis. *Cell.* 2010;140(1):88–98.

40. Maciel RM, Lindsey SC, Dias da Silva MR. Novel etiopathophysiological aspects of thyrotoxic periodic paralysis. *Nat Rev Endocrinol.* 2011;7(11):657–67.

41. Lin SH, Huang CL. Mechanism of thyrotoxic periodic paralysis. *J Am Soc Nephrol.* 2012;23(6):985–8.

42. Seifter JL. Potassium disorders. In Goldman L, Schaefer AI (eds) *Godman's Cecil Medicine* (24th edn). Philadelphia: Elsevier Saunders; 2012:734–41.

43. Nyirenda MJ, Tang JI, Padfield PL, Seckl JR. Hyperkalaemia. *BMJ.* 2009;339:b4114.

44. Chen DY, Schneider PF, Zhang XS, He ZM, Chen TH. Fatality after cardiac arrest in thyrotoxic periodic paralysis due to profound hypokalemia resulting from intravenous glucose administration and inadequate potassium replacement. *Thyroid.* 2012;22(9):969–72.

45. Lalli G, Bohnert S, Deinhardt K, Verastegui C, Schiavo G. The journey of tetanus and botulinum neurotoxins in neurons. *Trends Microbiol.* 2003;11(9):431–7.

46. Cook TM, Protheroe RT, Handel JM. Tetanus: a review of the literature. *Br J Anaesth.* 2001;87(3):477–87.

47. Afshar M, Raju M, Ansell D, Bleck TP. Narrative review: tetanus-a health threat after natural disasters in developing countries. *Ann Intern Med.* 2011;154(5):329–35.

48. Farrar JJ, Yen LM, Cook T, Fairweather N, Binh N, Parry J, *et al.* Tetanus. *J Neurol Neurosurg Psychiatry.* 2000;69(3):292–301.

49. Thwaites CL, Farrar JJ. Preventing and treating tetanus. *BMJ.* 2003;326(7381):117–18.

50. Thwaites CL, Yen LM, Loan HT, Thuy TT, Thwaites GE, Stepniewska K, *et al.* Magnesium sulphate for treatment of severe tetanus: a randomised controlled trial. *Lancet.* 2006;368(9545):1436–43.

51. Arnon SS, Schechter R, Inglesby TV, Henderson DA, Bartlett JG, Ascher MS, *et al.* Botulinum toxin as a biological weapon: medical and public health management. *JAMA.* 2001;285(8):1059–70.

52. Sheridan EA, Cepeda J, De Palma R, Brett MM, Nagendran K. A drug user with a sore throat. *Lancet.* 2004;364:1286.

53. Chertow DS, Tan ET, Maslanka SE, Schulte J, Bresnitz EA, Weisman RS, *et al.* Botulism in 4 adults following cosmetic injections with an unlicensed, highly concentrated botulinum preparation. *JAMA.* 2006;296(20):2476–9.

54. Sobel J. Diagnosis and treatment of botulism: a century later, clinical suspicion remains the cornerstone. *Clin Infect Dis.* 2009;48(12):1674–5.

55. Sobel J. Botulism. *Clin Infect Dis.* 2005;41(8):1167–73.

56. Gottlieb SL, Kretsinger K, Tarkhashvili N, Chakvetadze N, Chokheli M, Chubinidze M, *et al.* Long-term outcomes of 217 botulism cases in the Republic of Georgia. *Clin Infect Dis.* 2007;45(2):174–80.

57. Lin CS, Krishnan AV, Lee MJ, Zagami AS, You HL, Yang CC, *et al.* Nerve function and dysfunction in acute intermittent porphyria. *Brain.* 2008;131(Pt 9):2510–19.

58. Puy H, Gouya L, Deybach JC. Porphyrias. *Lancet.* 2010; 375(9718): 924–37.

59. Stevens RD, Marshall SA, Cornblath DR, Hoke A, Needham DM, de Jonghe B, *et al.* A framework for diagnosing and classifying intensive care unit-acquired weakness. *Crit Care Med.* 2009;37 Suppl. (10):299–308.

60. Ali NA, O'Brien JM, Jr., Hoffmann SP, Phillips G, Garland A, Finley JC, *et al.* Acquired weakness, handgrip strength, and mortality in critically ill patients. *Am J Respir Crit Care Med.* 2008;178(3):261–8.

61. Hough CL, Lieu BK, Caldwell ES. Manual muscle strength testing of critically ill patients: feasibility and interobserver agreement. *Crit Care.* 2011;15(1):R43.

62. Stevens RD, Dowdy DW, Michaels RK, Mendez-Tellez PA, Pronovost PJ, Needham DM. Neuromuscular dysfunction acquired in critical illness: a systematic review. *Intensive Care Med.* 2007;33(11):1876–91.

63. Latronico N, Bertolini G, Guarneri B, Botteri M, Peli E, Andreoletti S, *et al.* Simplified electrophysiological evaluation of peripheral nerves in critically ill patients: the Italian multi-centre CRIMYNE study. *Crit Care.* 2007;11(1):R11.

64. Latronico N, Fenzi F, Recupero D, Guarneri B, Tomelleri G, Tonin P, *et al.* Critical illness myopathy and neuropathy. *Lancet.* 1996;347(9015):1579–82.

65. Rich MM, Bird SJ, Raps EC, McCluskey LF, Teener JW. Direct muscle stimulation in acute quadriplegic myopathy. *Muscle Nerve.* 1997;20(6):665–73.

66. Latronico N, Tomelleri G, Filosto M. Critical illness myopathy. *Curr Opin Rheumatol.* 2012;24(6):616–22.

67. Van den Berghe G, Schoonheydt K, Becx P, Bruyninckx F, Wouters PJ. Insulin therapy protects the central and peripheral nervous system of intensive care patients. *Neurology.* 2005;64(8):1348–53.

68. Qaseem A, Humphrey LL, Chou R, Snow V, Shekelle P. Use of intensive insulin therapy for the management of glycemic control in hospitalized patients: a clinical practice guideline from the American College of Physicians. *Ann Intern Med.* 2011;154(4):260–7.

69. Schweickert WD, Pohlman MC, Pohlman AS, Nigos C, Pawlik AJ, Esbrook CL, *et al.* Early physical and occupational therapy in mechanically ventilated, critically ill patients: a randomised controlled trial. *Lancet.* 2009;373(9678):1874–82.

70. Mehta S, Burry L, Cook D, Fergusson D, Steinberg M, Granton J, *et al.* Daily sedation interruption in mechanically ventilated critically ill patients cared for with a sedation protocol: a randomized controlled trial. *JAMA.* 2012;308(19):1985–92.

71. Latronico N, Shehu I, Seghelini E. Neuromuscular sequelae of critical illness. *Current Opin Crit Care.* 2005;11(4):381–90.

72. Guarneri B, Bertolini G, Latronico N. Long-term outcome in patients with critical illness myopathy or neuropathy: the Italian multicentre CRIMYNE study. *J Neurol Neurosurg Psychiatry.* 2008;79(7):838–41.

CHAPTER 23

Status epilepticus in adults

Jan Novy and Andrea O. Rossetti

Status epilepticus (SE) is a medical emergency with high morbidity and mortality. It requires urgent treatment as it quickly leads to life-threatening intracranial and systemic disturbances, especially in its generalized convulsive form. This chapter will discuss the pathophysiology, diagnosis, and treatment of SE and the pharmacology of antiepileptic drugs (AEDs).

Definition

SE is a condition in which an epileptic seizure(s) does not stop spontaneously and where acute treatment is required for its control. It is classically defined as the continuous occurrence of prolonged seizures for at least 30 minutes, or seizure recurrence without full recovery between them. This timescale was chosen primarily because 30 minutes of seizure activity is associated with systemic metabolic disturbances (1) and neuronal loss in animal studies (2). However, in clinical practice, 30 minutes should not be used to decide when to start treatment, and a more pragmatic definition of 5 minutes was suggested at the end of the last century. This is based on the observation that discrete seizures mostly subside within a couple of minutes (3) and, if lasting longer than 5 minutes, cease spontaneously within 30 minutes in only 40% of cases (4).

Refractory SE is classically defined as failure of first-line and second-line treatments (see later sections), although some studies additionally incorporate into the definition a time frame of 60 minutes of failed treatment (5,6). Twenty-two to forty-three per cent of cases of SE become refractory (5,7–9). Some authors also describe the concept of extremely treatment-resistant SE, defined as 'malignant' (10) or 'super-refractory' SE (11), in which SE responds only transiently to course(s) of treatment with anaesthetic agents (third-line therapy). A subset of patients with SE require treatment on an intensive care unit (ICU) (9), primarily those admitted for induction of pharmacological coma during an uncontrolled SE episode, and those admitted with severe medical or surgical conditions who subsequently develop SE (most frequently non-convulsive forms).

Epidemiology

SE is an epileptic phenomenon that can occur in patients with chronic epilepsy; 39% (12) to 50% (13) of those presenting with SE already have an epilepsy diagnosis. However, half of cases SE present *de novo* as an acute neurological event. Its annual incidence is variably reported between 6 (14) and 41 (15) per 100,000 population, and its overall mortality in Europe and North America is between 6% (16) and 39% (12). Similar to epilepsy, the incidence of SE has a U-shaped relationship with age, being most common in young children and the elderly (15). Nevertheless, mortality in the paediatric population is lower (< 10%) than in adults (17,18).

The aetiology of SE can be categorized in acute symptomatic, remote symptomatic (i.e. due to a remote cause, which is stable over time), progressive symptomatic, and cryptogenic/idiopathic (19). Acute or chronic cerebrovascular disease, encephalitis and other brain infections, brain tumours, head trauma, substance abuse, drug withdrawal, metabolic disturbances, cerebral anoxia, and AED blood level in known epileptics are the major causes (12–14,16,20,21). More rarely, SE can be part of autoimmune or paraneoplastic syndrome, or related to chromosomal, genetic, or mitochondrial disorders, inborn metabolic diseases, and degenerative conditions (22,23). In particular, autoimmune disorders causing SE, associated with autoantibodies against N-methyl-D-aspartate (NMDA), α-amino-3-hydroxy-5-methyl-4-isoxazolepropionic acid (AMPA), and γ-aminobutyric acid $(GABA)_B$ receptors, voltage-gated potassium channels (VGKC), and glutamic acid decarboxylase (GAD), are increasingly reported and likely to account for a considerable proportion of previously labelled 'cryptogenic' cases (24–28).

Diagnosis

The diagnosis of SE relies on four main criteria:

1. Duration of the episode

2. Clinical manifestations

3. Electroencephalogram (EEG) findings

4. Response to treatment.

Whilst seemingly straightforward, these factors can sometimes be difficult to assess. There is still some controversy about the exact electrophysiological criteria of SE, clinical observation may be incomplete, the SE episode may start with a build-up of discrete seizures merging progressively in continuous activity (29), and the response to treatment can be difficult to interpret. Moreover, these four criteria can also interact with, and modify, each other. For example, the duration of the SE episode can modify the clinical manifestations (typically in generalized convulsive SE), as can the treatment. Generally, the diagnosis of SE is clinical although it may in addition rely on any of the aforementioned criteria. In cases of non-convulsive SE, an EEG is of course required to confirm the diagnosis.

Clinical manifestations

SE can present with different clinical manifestations and these are often subdivided into convulsive and non-convulsive types, and into generalized and focal (or partial) forms (Table 23.1).

Table 23.1 Classification of status epilepticus

	Focal	Generalized
Convulsive	Simple partial	Tonic–clonic
		Myoclonic
Non-convulsive	Simple/complex partial	Absence (typical/atypical/*de novo* in the elderly)
		'Subtle' (non-convulsive SE in coma (NCSEC))

Generalized convulsive status epilepticus

Generalized convulsive SE, where motor symptoms are bilateral, is the most severe form of SE and has been shown to induce cerebral lesions in clinical (30,31) and experimental (2,32) studies. Generalized convulsive SE most frequently has a focal onset and/or a focal underlying lesion (20). After the convulsive phase it may evolve into a non-convulsive form in which the motor manifestations significantly decrease or disappear, and is eventually manifest as only subtle jerking, twitching, or blinking in the presence of continuous seizure activity on the EEG. This electromechanical dissociation has been called 'subtle SE' (33), and, in comatose patients, may also be designated as 'non-convulsive SE in coma'. It may occur if SE continues for prolonged periods or as a result of insufficient treatment (29), and is a sign of poor prognosis.

In myoclonic SE, another subtype of generalized SE, motor manifestations take the form of multifocal continuous brisk muscular jerks. It can be associated with different conditions such as genetic (idiopathic) myoclonic epilepsies, and anoxic encephalopathy. Absence SE can be the manifestation of a genetic (idiopathic) epilepsy and is characterized by typical absences in association with greater than 2.5 Hz generalized spike and waves on the EEG. It may also occur in patients with mental retardation as atypical absences with lower than 2.5 Hz spike and waves, and can occur *de novo* in the elderly, typically as a consequence of drug (usually benzodiazepine) withdrawal. It presents with various cognitive signs, ranging from complete loss of contact to barely noticeable clouding of consciousness. Absence SE has an almost invariable excellent prognosis following treatment with broad-spectrum AEDs, and should never require admission to an ICU.

Partial (or focal) status epilepticus

Partial SE encompasses several forms that can occur with or without movements (convulsions) and altered consciousness. Focal motor SE, also referred to a Kozewnikow syndrome or epilepsia partialis continua, involves continuous but somewhat irregular clonic or myoclonic movements in a discrete part of the body. Although originally associated with Russian spring–summer tick-borne viral encephalitis (34), partial SE is most frequently a sign of an underlying structural cerebral abnormality. Focal SE can involve virtually any part of the cortex and produces long-lasting focal neurological signs, with loss of function or sensory or visual symptoms, sometimes referred to as *aura continua*.

Complex partial SE is the most frequent form of SE (9), and manifests with variable alteration of consciousness and some behavioural motor activity. Temporal lobe foci typically present with motor automatisms, orofacial stereotypias and/or autonomic changes (35), whereas frontal lobe associated forms lead to variable

disturbances of consciousness, affective changes, and neuropsychological impairment including dysexecutive symptoms, typically with cyclic fluctuations (36). Around 19% of critically ill patients have seizures identified on long-term EEG monitoring (37), and 8% of comatose patients are in non-convulsive SE (38). However, this incidence may be considerably higher in those with severe, acute brain injury, particularly cerebral anoxia (39).

Electroencephalography

The EEG criteria for the diagnosis of SE are the subject of some debate, although it is widely agreed that epileptic activity in SE can present either with discrete electrographic seizures or with continuous periodic/rhythmical epileptiform discharges. The EEG identification of ongoing seizure activity in a patient with compatible clinical changes is usually straightforward, but the interpretation of periodic/rhythmical discharges more difficult and may reflect an ictal–interictal continuum (40,41). Continuous discharges occurring at a low frequency (< 2–3Hz) are also described as periodic and can be seen in the presence of acute structural lesions in the absence of symptoms of seizures (42). To be diagnostic of SE, periodic discharges should show some dynamic change, specifically evolution in voltage, field, frequency, and respond to treatment alongside resolution of clinical symptoms (43,44). Triphasic waves are frequently seen in metabolic encephalopathies, but may also represent epileptiform elements of SE, especially if occurring with focal predominance. Absence of reactivity to external stimulation, sharply contoured shape with a prominent first (negative) phase, absence of phase lag throughout the discharges, and frequency greater than 2 Hz suggest that these EEG elements are signs of epileptic rather than encephalopathic processes (45). Examples of some typical EEG patterns consistent with SE are shown in Figure 23.1.

Simple partial SE may not be associated with epileptiform activity on the EEG in at least one-third of cases, and in up to one-sixth the EEG may be completely normal (44,46). In simple partial seizures, detection of ictal discharges is mostly dependent on source localization (more easily recorded from the convexity) and the degree of cortical involvement (47). For example, simple partial motor SE with clonic movements involving only a limited part of the body is relatively unlikely to be associated with EEG epileptiform correlates. Back-averaging to detect subtle changes time-locked with clinical manifestations can be useful in such circumstances, but EEG abnormalities are not usually specific for a particular SE aetiology. Interestingly, it has recently been suggested that 'extreme delta brushes' in adults, that is, rhythmical delta waves with superimposed fast activity, are specific for anti-NMDA antibodies encephalitis and identified in up to one-third of patients (48).

Response to treatment

A treatment trial is the final criterion that can be used to diagnose SE. This is performed by administrating a benzodiazepine intravenously, often at a lower dose than standard first line of treatment (see 'Specific Treatment'), during EEG monitoring. A significant clinical and electrophysiological improvement is strongly supportive of the diagnosis of SE, although this therapeutic test can take several hours to be effective. Moreover, improvement of EEG only is not supportive of a diagnosis of SE. Triphasic waves found in Creutzfeldt–Jakob disease or metabolic encephalopathies, for example, can disappear after administration of benzodiazepines (49), despite the patient becoming more somnolent. In complex

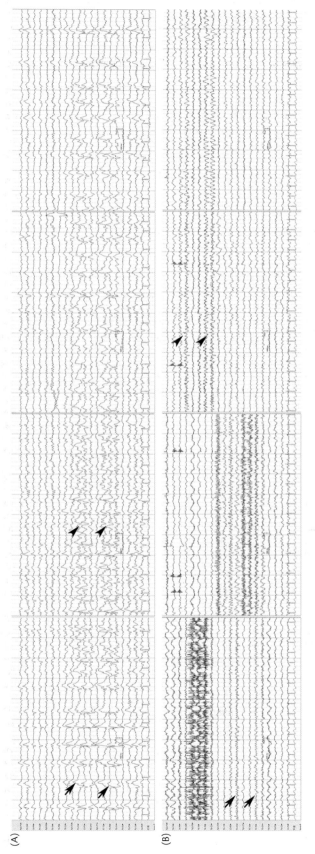

Fig. 23.1 Examples of EEG patterns seen in status epilepticus. Four sequential EEG recordings (bipolar longitudinal montage, scale included) in two people with status epilepticus.

(A) A 73-year-old female with intermittent aphasia showing left hemisphere slow periodic discharges (arrows) evolving dynamically into a seizure (arrow heads).

(B) A 17-year-old male with seizure over the left hemisphere starting in posterior regions (arrows) with contralateral muscular artefacts. One minute later another seizure is seen over the right hemisphere (arrow heads).

situations, a longer treatment trial with non-sedating AEDs, such as phenytoin or valproate, and regular EEG reassessments may be needed.

Pathophysiology

SE represents an extreme pathophysiological condition. A very large number of neurons are firing synchronously at high frequencies and for prolonged periods of time, with massive release of neurotransmitters. The pathophysiology of SE has mainly been studied in animal models of generalized convulsive SE, and is primarily believed to represent an imbalance between increased excitation and decreased neuronal inhibition, although this is likely to be a gross over-simplification (50).

Both animal models and human data suggest that there are several stages in the development, maintenance, and termination of generalized SE (1,29). Clinically, initial recurrent discrete seizures (< 30 minutes) merge progressively together (30–60 minutes), and generalized convulsions are then progressively replaced by myoclonic jerks that progressively fade away. In parallel, the EEG initially shows discrete seizures merging into continuous ictal discharges, followed by the appearance of increasing intermixed flat periods of activity, and finally electromechanical dissociation with periodic discharges against a flat background activity. These stages are associated with major changes in systemic and cerebral physiology (Table 23.2). In seminal experiments in baboons carried out 40 years ago, it was shown that compensatory mechanisms come into play in the early stages of SE (2,32), but then follows a general increase in systemic blood pressure, cerebral blood flow, blood glucose, blood and brain lactate levels, and cerebral glucose consumption. In the later stages of SE, compensatory systemic mechanisms progressively fail, resulting in low blood pressure, blood glucose, and lactate, and progressive decreases in brain lactate and cerebral blood flow suggesting a mismatch between metabolic demand and substrate delivery (51). Such data suggest that the transition to the late phase of SE, which occurs when discrete seizures merge after 30 minutes, may prove crucial for the occurrence of SE-related brain damage. Importantly, brain damage is not linked exclusively to systemic factors, and can occur when convulsive movements and compromised breathing are controlled through muscle paralysis and mechanical ventilation (52), and when cerebral energy supply is maintained (53). There is likely to be a wide variability in the anatomical spreading of SE, dependent on the location of the initiating insult and the point of 'least resistance' to seizure propagation. However, rodent studies have demonstrated that limbic structures are involved early (54), and this might explain why generalized convulsive SE-related brain damage is frequently seen in the hippocampi (55).

Many efforts have been made to identify the mechanisms underpinning SE self-sustainment, and multiple, probably parallel pathways, are implicated. Dysfunction or exhaustion of inhibitory circuits has received most attention. Animal models have shown that recurrent seizures can decrease the response to the neurotransmitter GABA by internalization (56) and loss of phosphorylation (57) of GABA$_A$ receptors, possibly because of a GABA-saturated extracellular environment (58). A reversed intra- and extracellular chloride gradient may also decrease, or even reverse, the effect of GABAergic transmission (59,60), similarly to that which occurs physiologically in newborns before 'maturation' of this gradient.

Table 23.2 Cerebral and systemic changes in early (< 30 minutes) and late (> 30 minutes) phase generalized convulsive status epilepticus

Early phase = physiological stress	Late phase = deregulation
Arterial hypertension	Arterial hypotension
Hyperthermia	Hyper-/hypothermia
Tachycardia	Tachy-/bradycardia
Hyperglycaemia	Hypoglycaemia
Lactic acidosis	Lactic and respiratory acidosis
	Rhabdomyolysis
	Diffuse intravascular coagulation
	Oedema

Data from Lothman E, 'The biochemical basis and pathophysiology of status epilepticus', *Neurology*, 40, 5 Suppl 2, pp. 13–23, Copyright © 1990 American Academy of Neurology.

Loss of inhibitory interneurons has also been demonstrated during SE (61), and regional factors such as elevated extracellular potassium might play an important initiating role in this regard (62). Dysfunction of other endogenous anticonvulsant pathways, such as adenosinergic, cannabinoid, and peptidergic inhibitory mechanisms, might play an aggravating role (59). Simultaneous to GABA$_A$ receptors internalization, excitatory NMDA receptors are increasingly externalized to synapses after 60 minutes of SE (63), thereby allowing influx of intracellular calcium and the potential for mitochondrial dysfunction and apoptotic neuronal death. Furthermore, inflammatory changes of the microglia have been observed in electrical stimulation models of SE (64), with release of inflammatory cytokines such as interleukin 1b that shift further the balance towards excitability (65). These effects might also play a role in neuronal death. GABA$_A$ receptor trafficking is considered to be the major mechanism underlying resistance to benzodiazepines. Although it is not entirely clear why SE might become resistant to other drug therapies, molecular and functional changes in sodium and other channels have been suggested as the reason for resistance to phenytoin (66). Further, increased expression of multidrug transporters (P-glycoproteins) at the blood–brain barrier might prevent accumulation of AEDs in neuron (66). It is unclear if AEDs in general are substrates of P-glycoproteins; phenytoin and phenobarbital appear to be, whereas carbamazepine does not (67).

It is widely recognized that generalized convulsive SE induces brain damage independently of systemic factors and the underlying cause. There is neuroradiological evidence of early hippocampal oedema with subsequent atrophy (31,68,69), and neuropathological studies confirming neuronal loss in CA1 and CA3 hippocampal regions, the dentate gyrus, and the Purkinje cells of the cerebellum (70,71). Neuronal death is believed to be the end result of overwhelming neuronal excitation (excitotoxicity), which triggers cellular necrosis and apoptosis (72) that is already apparent after 30 minutes of SE (73). It is far less clear how some forms of non-convulsive or partial SE can result in such severe brain damage. Absence SE is widely regarded as harmless (74,75), but the major confounder in assessing neuronal loss in focal SE is how much the SE leads to the brain insult independently from the underlying cause of the SE. Animal models of SE using techniques less prone to cause brain damage directly, such as repeated electrical stimulation, have shown that limbic SE does indeed cause neuronal loss in CA1 hippocampal regions (76). Increased serum neuron-specific enolase levels, a marker of neuronal injury, have been found after complex partial SE in humans occurring with no identifiable acute cause (77), but how this correlates with neuronal death in this context is unclear (72). There are very conflicting clinical and radiological data regarding non-convulsive and/or partial SE-related brain damage that is independent from the underlying cause of the SE (78–83). Overall, it seems reasonable to postulate that complex partial SE does not invariably lead to significant brain damage, and that absence SE is definitely not harmful. The ability to confidently predict focal SE-induced brain damage is important in determining how aggressive the treatment should be.

Treatment

SE is a medical emergency with high mortality and morbidity that should be terminated as quickly as possible. Indeed SE becomes progressively less responsive to treatment, especially with benzodiazepines, over time (66); first-line treatment with benzodiazepines is much more successful earlier than in the later stages of SE (55% versus 15%) (84). Furthermore, escalation of treatment bring little gain (7–10% response) when first-line treatment has failed (85), emphasizing the need for a prompt treatment on the one hand but, on the other, raising the possibility that the responsiveness of SE to treatment is predetermined by the underlying aetiology.

Vital functions should be stabilized urgently. Ventilation may be compromised by convulsive movements and decreased consciousness may interfere with airway protection, so endotracheal intubation and mechanical ventilation may be required. Cardiovascular function may also be disturbed. Therefore, and as with all emergencies, airway, breathing, and circulation (ABC) should be assessed and treated immediately.

Whilst vital parameters are being stabilized, specific SE treatment should begin without delay, even in the pre-hospital setting (86). An operational time definition of 5 minutes should be used to initiate first-line treatment (3). It has recently been shown that the ease of intramuscular administration of anticonvulsant medication results in more rapid time to treatment and improved outcome in comparison with intravenous administration in a pre-hospital environment, although only midazolam is available via this route. Second-line treatments with long action AEDs are usually administered in hospital with careful cardiorespiratory monitoring. Treatment of SE (see 'Specific Treatment') should be conducted alongside investigation of its cause.

An important, but often forgotten, early task is the collection of circumstantial information about the aetiology of the SE. In particular, evidence of substance or alcohol abuse, withdrawal (or non-compliance) of antiepileptic medications (reportedly one of the most common causes of SE (20)), new neurological or systemic symptoms preceding SE, as well as the duration of the episode, should be sought. Blood samples, including electrolytes (particularly sodium, calcium, and magnesium), glucose, liver and renal function, inflammatory markers, albumin, blood levels of chronic AEDs, and full blood count, should be taken early. In parallel, EEG (if available) should be performed in order to confirm the diagnosis and rule out SE imitators or psychogenic, non-epileptic, seizures. A correct electrophysiological diagnosis is impossible once the patient is in a pharmacological coma, potentially leading to dangerous iatrogenic complications.

Acute movement disorders, such as dystonias, tremors, and choreiform movements, can sometimes be confused with SE (87). Clonus, a sign of spasticity being triggered by passive movements, shivering in a sedated patient, and jerking movements related to incomplete neuromuscular blockade can also be mistaken for SE. Psychogenic, non-epileptic seizure (PNES)-SE is probably the most frequent SE imitator (88). Several clinical signs, including resistance of eye opening in apparently unconscious patients, and ongoing breathing during prolonged generalized convulsions, are suggestive of PNES-SE (89). Absence of elevation of creatine kinase (CK) and lactate elevation in an apparently generalized convulsive case of SE should also prompt consideration of a non-epileptic aetiology. Administration of thiamine (100 mg intravenously) has been recommended as a routine (90), although this should arguably be reserved for cases of hypoglycaemia, severe malnutrition, and/or in alcohol abuse (91).

With few exceptions, all pre-hospital patients and most inpatients should have emergency brain imaging. The main exceptions are inpatients with known severe epilepsy, and recurrent episodes of SE following confirmed substance abuse and AED withdrawal in the absence of evidence of trauma. Although brain magnetic resonance imaging is the most informative study, it is rarely available in emergency settings and computed tomography is most frequently used. Plain and contrast-enhanced images should be obtained to identify inflammatory, infectious, or neoplastic processes. If a focal neurological deficit preceded the onset of SE, or if a clear focal deficit is present between seizures, the search for a cause should include investigation of vascular processes with perfusion/diffusion and vessel imaging. In cases where the diagnosis of SE cannot be confirmed clinically (especially for non-convulsive forms), it is advisable to perform EEG before brain imaging if the patient's condition allows. Prolonged continuous video EEG monitoring significantly increases the diagnostic pick-up of non-convulsive SE (of up to 8%) in the ICU when compared with conventional, intermittent EEG monitored over 20–30 minutes (92). In one study, the seizure detection yield in the critically ill was 56% in the first hour of recording and 88% in the first 24 hours (37).

If no clear cause of SE can be identified with these investigations, lumbar puncture and CSF analysis should be performed in order to explore further the potential of an inflammatory, infectious or neoplastic aetiology. Lumbar puncture should be preceded by brain imaging to avoid the risk of downward brain herniation secondary to undiagnosed elevations in intracranial pressure. Not uncommonly, patients may need to be intubated and/or sedated to perform the lumbar puncture. If an infectious/meningitic process is suspected, empirical treatment should begin immediately, even before imaging and lumbar puncture (see Chapter 24).

The specific treatment of SE is discussed in detail later in this chapter but in summary should follow a sequential approach of first- (benzodiazepines), second- (long acting AEDs) and third- (drug-induced coma) line drug therapies (Figure 23.2). The effects of each stage of treatment should be assessed clinically and, if possible, electrographically. If no response is observed to one treatment, the next line of treatment should be administered. It is however important to note that first- and second-line treatments are often administered almost simultaneously. There is no evidences to guide how long a patient should be observed after administration of one line of treatment before progression to the next, although it seems reasonable to wait no longer than 5 minutes after first-line treatment and 5–10 minutes after second line, so that pharmacological coma, if required, is not delayed. Generalized convulsive SE should

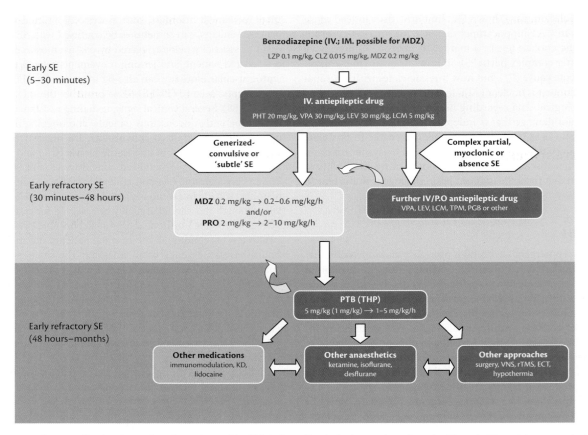

Fig. 23.2 Treatment of status epilepticus. Increasing refractoriness of the SE is indicated by the background grey intensity. The early SE panel shows standard first-line drugs, the early refractory SE panel standard second-line drugs, and the late refractory SE panel third-line drugs. Other medications and approaches represent options for consideration when other interventions have failed.

CLZ, clonazepam; ECT, electroconvulsive therapy; KD, ketogenic diet; LCM, lacosamide; LEV, levetiracetam; LZP, lorazepam; MDZ, midazolam; PGB, pregabalin; PHT, phenytoin; PRO, propofol; PTB, pentobarbital; rTMS, repetitive transcranial magnetic stimulation; SE, status epilepticus; THP, thiopental; TPM, topiramate; VNS, vagus nerve stimulation; VPA, valproate.

Adapted from *The Lancet Neurology*, 10, 10, Rossetti AO and Lowenstein DH, 'Management of refractory status epilepticus in adults: still more questions than answers', pp. 922–930, Copyright 2011, with permission from Elsevier.

be treated the most aggressively and, to minimize the early cerebral damage that will inevitably occur if SE is not terminated, pharmacological (drug-induced) coma should be initiated without delay if there is no response to the first two lines of treatment.

The optimal speed and aggressiveness of treatment for complex partial SE is less widely agreed, primarily because of the controversy regarding the severity of potential brain damages induced by it. Whilst there is a general consensus that the initial treatment of complex partial SE should be as urgent and follow the same sequential procedure as for generalized convulsive SE, the use of pharmacological coma after failure of the first two lines of treatment is less widely accepted. The good overall outcome of some episodes of complex partial SE must be balanced against the risks of drug-induced coma in an ICU environment (93,94). These include, amongst other, hypotension, neuromuscular complications, thrombosis, infections, and ileus. Surveys have confirmed that it is not uncommon in this situation for clinicians to use additional antiepileptic medication, and to observe for longer periods of time, before deciding to induce pharmacological coma (95). Indeed, such patients are probably best treated relatively conservatively by second-line treatment for 12–36 hours, before considering drug-induced coma (9,96–98). Absence and myoclonic SE occurring in the context of genetic (idiopathic) epilepsy almost never

require pharmacological coma, and can usually be treated outside an ICU with benzodiazepines and broad-spectrum AEDs, especially valproate (74). Treatment with anaesthetic agents should also be avoided in simple partial SE, which frequently proves resistant to several lines of treatment. In these cases, addressing the underlying structural abnormality/metabolic disturbance is paramount.

Treatment should preferably be individually tailored. The validated Status Epilepticus Severity Score (STESS), which includes age, seizure semiology, severity of consciousness impairment, and history of previous seizures, reliably identifies those at lower mortality risk who do not require the most aggressive treatments (99). It can be easily and quickly assessed prior to the start of treatment.

The role of therapeutic drug monitoring is not established in SE. However, serum drug levels can be used to assess the absorption of oral medication administered via a gastric tube, to detect clinically relevant interactions affecting AED levels, and to guide dosage in medications with complicated kinetics such as phenytoin.

There is very little evidence available to guide third-line treatment of SE with anaesthetic agents. Although there is no evidence to determine how long it should be continued, it is common practice to maintain drug-induced coma for 24 hours before weaning the anaesthetic agent over 6–12 hours under EEG monitoring. If SE recurs, a second course of pharmacological coma should consider in association with optimization of the dosage of concomitant AEDs or introduction of additional AEDS. Pharmacological coma should always be monitored with continuous EEG to assess its depth.

The importance of a multidisciplinary approach to the management of SE, with neurological, neurophysiological, ICU and emergency teams, cannot be overemphasized, and the availability of treatment protocols has also been shown to significantly minimize the delay to treatment (100).

Specific treatment

This section provides a more in depth overview of the agents used to treat SE. It should be noted that the treatment lines are not mutually exclusive, but should be used synergistically to maximize a combined pharmacological approach to management. Only first-line treatments have a firm evidence base.

First-line treatments

Two seminal randomized controlled trials have confirmed the role of benzodiazepines, which act on $GABA_A$ receptors, in generalized SE (84,101). In these studies, lorazepam effectively controlled SE in 59% (101) to 65% (84) of cases and was statistically superior to phenytoin and placebo, but not to phenobarbital or to phenytoin and diazepam combined. Recently, intramuscular midazolam has been shown to be at least as efficacious as intravenous lorazepam in the pre-hospital setting, controlling SE in 73% and 63% of cases respectively (86). Occurrence of cardiorespiratory complications, including hypotension, cardiac arrhythmia, and respiratory dysfunction, was significantly lower with benzodiazepines compared to placebo (10% and 22% respectively) (101). In a recent study, 14% of patients required endotracheal intubation, but it was unclear whether this was related to uncontrolled SE or because of respiratory depression following treatment (86).

Recurrence of SE after an initial response can be a concern because some first-line agents have a short half-life. Recurrence of seizures within the first 12 hours after first-line treatment with both midazolam and lorazepam has been reported in around 10% of cases (86). A theoretical concern, but rather exceptional in clinical practice, is the fact that benzodiazepines have very been occasionally reported to worsen Lennox–Gastaut syndrome (102).

Lorazepam, diazepam, clonazepam, and midazolam are the most commonly used benzodiazepines for first-line treatment of SE (Table 23.3).

Lorazepam

Lorazepam is best given intravenously as it is erratically absorbed rectally and relatively slowly absorbed when administered intramuscularly, with peak plasma levels being reached only at 75 minutes (103). An initial intravenous dose of 0.1 mg/kg is recommended, although a 4 mg bolus is preferred by some (104), administered at a rate of 2 mg/min. A serum peak level is reached within 5–10 minutes and brain levels peak within 20 minutes after intravenous administration (105). The latency of action is 3–10 minutes after administration (106). The blood half-life of lorazepam ranges from 8 to 24 hours (mean 15 hours), explaining why it can have a long lasting effect (up to 24 hours) (107). Lorazepam has a small distribution volume, with limited diffusion into fatty tissues. It is metabolized by hepatic microsomal enzymes, primarily by glucuronidation, and has no active metabolite. Its elimination is not significantly affected even in moderate to severe hepatic insufficiency

(104), although co-administration with valproate can decrease its clearance by 40% (108). Lorazepam clearance is increased by liver enzyme inducers, such as phenytoin, phenobarbital, carbamazepine, and rifampicin, although its bioavailability is less affected after intravenous administration because of the absence of a first-pass effect (109). It is highly protein bound (> 90%). Side effects of lorazepam include sedation, hypotension, and respiratory depression which is reported in up to 10% of the cases (106). Lorazepam should not be used for longer-term maintenance management as tolerance can develop after 24 hours (104).

Diazepam

Diazepam is preferentially administered intravenously as is slowly absorbed via the intramuscular route, where a significant proportion of the drug precipitates (110). It is occasionally given rectally. The dose of diazepam is 0.3 mg/kg intravenously, and 10–30 mg rectally. Intravenous diazepam is administered at a rate of 5 mg/min, and peak blood and brain levels are reached almost simultaneously after 10 minutes (111). After rectal administration, the blood peak concentration is not reached until 20 minutes after administration (112). The latency of action is less than 5 minutes for intravenous administration (113) and between 5 and 15 minutes for rectal use (114).

The pharmacokinetics of diazepam is complicated by its high affinity for fatty tissues. Blood and brain levels decrease bi-exponentially after peak levels are reached because of the large volume of redistribution. Repeated boluses continue to redistribute to fatty tissues leading, after about three bolus doses, to a late increase in blood concentration and a steady brain level that surpasses the initial peak (111). Repeated administration of diazepam should thus be avoided because of the risk of delayed overdose and respiratory depression. Diazepam's extensive redistribution also explains its short effect duration (< 1 hour) after a single dose (115). Diazepam is metabolized in the liver, via cytochrome P450 (CYP)-2C19 and CYP3A4 pathways, and has several active metabolites. Its elimination half-life is highly variable (between 18 and 100 hours) and, for some of its active metabolites, even longer (108). Inhibitors of CYP3A4, such as erythromycin, ketoconazole, diltiazem, verapamil, and cimetidine, and of CYP2C19 (omeprazole), reduce diazepam clearance (108). As with other benzodiazepines, its clearance is increased by liver enzyme inducers. Diazepam is highly protein bound (> 97%). As with lorazepam, the side effects of diazepam include sedation, respiratory depression, and, occasionally, hypotension. Intravenous administration can lead to local irritation and thrombophlebitis. Because of its pharmacokinetics, diazepam should not be used as maintenance treatment.

Midazolam

Unlike most other benzodiazepines used in SE, midazolam is quickly absorbed via the intramuscular route, and its water solubility also allows buccal and intranasal administration. The usual dose of midazolam is 0.2 mg/kg, although some recommend a standard 10 mg dose (86). Peak blood levels are reached within 5 minutes after intravenous administration, within 20–30 minutes after intramuscular administration, within 10–15 minutes after intranasal administration, and 15–90 minutes after buccal administration (108). Midazolam becomes lipophilic at a physiological pH. The latency to action is 5–10 minutes after intramuscular administration and 5 minutes after intranasal administration using a spray (116). These characteristics of absorption make midazolam a useful

Table 23.3 Pharmacokinetic properties of commonly used intravenous treatments of status epilepticus

Line of treatment	Substance	Usual bolus dose	Latency of action	Redistribution in fatty tissues	Blood half-life	Protein binding	Interactions as substrate	Interactions induced
First	Lorazepam	0.1 mg/kg	3–10 min (IV)	+	8–24 h	> 90%	Clearance decreased by glucuronization inhibitor, increased by inducers	—
First	Diazepam	0.3 mg/kg	< 5 min (IV)	++	20–40 h	> 97%	Clearance decreased by inhibitors of CYP3A4, CYP2C19, increased by inducers	—
First	Midazolam	0.2 mg/kg	5–10 min (IM)	+	1.5–4 h	> 94%	Clearance decreased by inhibitors of CYP3A4, increased by inducers	—
First	Clonazepam	0.015 mg/kg	< 1 min (IV)	++	19–60 h	60–80%	Clearance increased by liver enzyme inducers	—
Second	Phenytoin	20 mg/kg	10–30 min (IV)	—	20 h	> 90%	Clearance decreased by CYP2C9 and CYP2C19 inhibitors, increased by inducers	Liver enzyme induction
Second	Valproate	20–40 mg/kg	< 30 min (IV)	—	8–19 h	> 90%	Clearance increased by liver enzyme inducers	Liver enzyme inhibition
Second	Phenobarbital	15 mg/kg	5–30 min (IV)	++	Up to 100 h	40–60%	Clearance decreased by CYP2C9 inhibitors, increased by inducers	Liver enzyme induction
Second	Levetiracetam	20–30 mg/kg	?	—	6–8 h[a]	< 10%	—	—
Second	Lacosamide	400 mg	?	—	12–16 h	15%	—	—
Third	Midazolam	0.2 mg/kg then 0.2–0.6 mg/kg/h	< 1 min (IV)	+	1 h (up to 20 h)	> 94%	Clearance decreased by inhibitors of CYP3A4, increased by inducers	—
Third	Propofol	2 mg/kg then 2–10 mg/kg/h	< 1 min (IV)	+	30–60 min	98%	Clearance potentially decreased by some glucuronidation inhibitors	Potential competitive inhibition of CYP3A4
Third	Thiopental pentobarbital	1–2 (5) mg/kg then 1–5 mg/kg/h	< 1 min (IV)	++	27–36 h	80%	Clearance decreased by CYP2C9 inhibitors, increased by inducers	Liver enzyme induction

[a] Central nervous system half-life of levetiracetam may be longer.

option in the pre-hospital setting where it is replacing the use of rectal diazepam. Moreover, buccal and intranasal administrations are more convenient and socially acceptable than rectal. Midazolam has a short half-life (1.5–4 hours) which explains its short duration of action (1–3 hours) (90). Despite this, a recent study did not find a higher proportion of relapse of SE within 12 hours after pre-hospital use of midazolam compared to other agents, although the subsequent hospital treatment was not described in detail in this study (86). Like diazepam, midazolam also undergoes extensive liver metabolism via CYP3A4 and CYP3A5 pathways. Its active metabolite has an even shorter half-life than the parent drug (108). Inhibitors of CYP3A4 reduce midazolam clearance, and liver enzyme inducers increase its clearance. Midazolam is highly protein bound. The most frequent side effects of midazolam are sedation and respiratory depression. As well as being a first-line therapy

in SE, midazolam can be also be used as third-line treatment (see 'Third-Line Treatment').

Clonazepam

Although several case series underscore the efficacy of clonazepam in SE, there are no comparative studies with other agents. It has similar pharmacological properties to lorazepam, and is administered intravenously at doses of 0.015 mg/kg, with some advocating boluses of 1–4 mg (117). Clonazepam reaches the brain less than 1 minute after intravenous injection and this rapid action is clearly recognizable on EEG monitoring (117). Clonazepam has a slightly longer half-life of 19–60 hours (mean 24 hours) than lorazepam but a higher volume of redistribution in fatty tissue (104), which may explain its relatively shorter duration of action (109). Clonazepam is eliminated by hepatic metabolism, and enzyme inducers increase its clearance. Its protein binding is between 60% and 80% (117). As with other benzodiazepines, the most frequent side effects are sedation and respiratory depression. The initial intravenous bolus may be followed by maintenance treatment, with infusion or additional intravenous or oral boluses, of 1–8 mg daily that is tapered progressively. Of note, clonazepam is not licensed by the Food and Drug Administration in the United States for the treatment of SE, and is most widely used in Europe.

Second-line treatments

Second-line treatment of SE is administered when first-line treatment has failed, or in conjunction with it, to prevent mid- or long-term seizure recurrence. Second-line treatments are AEDs available in intravenous formulations including phenytoin, fosphenytoin, valproate, levetiracetam, lacosamide, and phenobarbital. In generalized convulsive SE, administering second-line intravenous treatment after failure of a first-line treatment results in control of fewer than 7% of episodes, and treating subtle SE with second-line agents is even less successful, with fewer than 3% of episodes controlled (85).

There is little evidence base for second-line treatments (118). There are no adequately controlled studies comparing the efficacy of individual second-line treatment agents, and the use of some newer AEDs has only been reported in small cases series (119). A retrospective observational study suggested that phenytoin was not significantly different from valproate and levetiracetam at controlling SE, and that levetiracetam may be less effective than valproate (120). Furthermore, the increasing use of the newer AEDs, such as levetiracetam and lacosamide, does not appear to have changed the overall prognosis of SE (121). Strict adherence to treatment guidelines, particularly in terms of drug dosage, has also not been shown to improve the overall outcome (122). Together, these observations suggest that the specific treatment may not be a major factor in the outcome of SE, highlighting the central role of the underlying biological background, including SE aetiology and patient age.

Commonly used second-line therapies include phenytoin, valproate, phenobarbital, levetiracetam, and lacosamide (Table 23.3).

Phenytoin

Phenytoin acts by enhancing the fast inactivation of voltage-gated sodium channels. It has been available for the treatment of SE for more than four decades and this very long experience is often cited to justify its use. However, phenytoin has several disadvantages. It is poorly water-soluble, and the solution in which it is diluted contains alcohol and is alkaline, and is thus highly irritant at the injection site. Rapid administration can induce cardiac arrhythmia, and the recommended loading dose of 20 mg/kg intravenously should be administered at a maximum rate of 50 mg/min. A lower infusion rate of 20 mg/min is recommended in those at high risk of arrhythmias, such as the elderly and those with a cardiac history. Such infusion rates can result in total administration times of up to 1 hour. Regardless of the rate of administration, intravenous phenytoin loading should always be performed under ECG monitoring.

The duration of action of phenytoin is up to 12 hours. It has non-linear hepatic metabolism, via CYP2C9 and CYP2C19 pathways, and substances inhibiting this metabolism, such as fluconazole, metronidazole, omeprazole, and fluoxetine, can decrease its clearance. Phenytoin is itself a potent metabolism inducer and can increase the clearance of multiple substances including several

AEDs, chemotherapeutic agents, steroids, and statins, as well as its own metabolism through auto-induction (123). The mean half-life of phenytoin is 20 hours, but this is extremely variable because of the variability in its elimination half-life. After a loading dose, plasma levels should be checked to ensure that the therapeutic target blood concentration of 40–80 μmol/L or 10–20 mg/L, has been achieved. Phenytoin has a high protein binding rate (90%), which is responsible for further complicated pharmacokinetic interactions with other highly protein-bound agents including valproate. In such cases, monitoring of free drug levels may be of great help. The loading dose of phenytoin is followed by maintenance therapy of 5 mg/kg/24 h, but often pragmatically at 300 mg daily. This can be given in three divided doses to decrease the risk of toxicity linked with peak levels. Phenytoin is contraindicated in patients with unstable cardiac function and known arrhythmia. It should also be avoided in myoclonic or absence SE as it has the potential to worsen these seizure types. In addition to the cardiac problems, the most common side effects after the acute use of phenytoin are sleepiness, ataxia, and cutaneous rash. An extreme but rare complication of local toxicity after injection is the 'purple glove' syndrome comprising extensive cutaneous inflammation and local venous thrombosis.

Fosphenytoin, a pro-drug of phenytoin, has better water solubility and is less irritating locally, allowing a faster injection rate. It is, however, much more expensive than phenytoin. Equivalent doses of fosphenytoin are 50% higher than phenytoin and, to avoid confusion, are reported in 'phenytoin equivalents'. Fosphenytoin can be administered at rates up to 150 mg phenytoin equivalent/min, but some of the benefit of more rapid infusion is lost because of the time required for conversion into phenytoin (the conversion half-time is 8–15 minutes) (90). Fosphenytoin increases the proportion of free phenytoin by displacing its protein binding. Unlike phenytoin, fosphenytoin can also be administered intramuscularly. Peak blood concentration of fosphenytoin is reached within 10 minutes of completing intravenous administration and, in animal models, its antiepileptic effect starts within 3 minutes (124). Other studies have suggested, however, that phenytoin and fosphenytoin have very similar latencies of action (10–30 minutes) (125,126). Fosphenytoin is not entirely devoid of cardiac side effects and can induce bradyarrhythmias (127).

Valproate

Intravenous valproate has been available for more than 15 years. It is water-soluble and devoid of arrhythmogenic effects and can therefore be administered much more rapidly than phenytoin. The usual dose is 20–40 mg/kg over 5–10 minutes, and the latency to action less than 30 minutes (128). The loading dose is usually followed by a maintenance dose of 600–2000 mg daily.

Valproate acts through multiple mechanisms including increased GABAergic transmission, reduced release and/or effects of excitatory amino acids, and modulation of voltage-gated sodium channels (129). It is highly protein bound (> 90%), and has a half-life of 8–19 hours. Valproate is almost entirely eliminated by the liver through multiple metabolic pathways, and its clearance is increased by enzyme-inducing drugs such as phenytoin and phenobarbital. It is an inhibitor of liver metabolism and therefore can significantly decrease the clearance a wide range of medications including other AEDs undergoing hepatic metabolism. Some drugs, such as imipenem antibiotics and ritonavir, markedly decrease valproate levels (130). The target range for blood valproate levels is 50–100 mg/L, but higher targets were reported in acute SE treatment (131). Common side effects include sedation and tremor. Over the longer term, valproate-related encephalopathy may develop and, although this is usually associated with high ammonium, persistence of a markedly slow EEG pattern after SE resolution should raise the possibility of valproate encephalopathy even in the presence of a normal ammonia level. Levocarnitine (up to 3 g daily) has been reported to improve the symptoms of valproate encephalopathy and reduce ammonium levels, although valproate should always be decreased or discontinued (132).

Valproate is increasingly used as a second-line treatment especially when cardiorespiratory monitoring is not available, and is the first choice in absence or myoclonic SE. It is also contraindicated in mitochondriopathies where it may lead to severe, at times fatal, hepatic failure (133).

Phenobarbital

Phenobarbital is one of the oldest treatments of epilepsy. It turned 100 years old in 2012 and has been used for decades in the treatment of SE. The initial dose is 15 mg/kg administered at a rate of 100 mg/min. Peak brain levels are reached within 3 minutes, and its latency of action is 5–30 minutes (90,134). It acts primarily by increasing GABAergic transmission. Phenobarbital redistributes rapidly into fat, with a redistribution half-life of 5–15 minutes (104), but its elimination half-life is very long (up to 100 hours). It is eliminated by hepatic metabolism (CYP2C9) and is a very potent enzyme inducer. Valproate increases phenobarbital levels by inhibition of its metabolism. It is only moderately protein bound (40–60%) (135). Common side effects include sedation and respiratory depression, but the extensive redistribution of phenobarbital can delay their occurrence and make then long lasting because of the long half-life. Hypotension occurs in a significant minority (up to 34%) of cases (84). Because of these issues, phenobarbital is now rarely used in the treatment of SE.

Levetiracetam

An intravenous formulation of levetiracetam has been available since 2006. Its efficacy in SE has been reported only in case series, apart from a recent study in India finding it equivalent to lorazepam as a first-line treatment (136). The loading dose is 20–30 mg/kg over 5–15 minutes, although some suggest up to 4000 mg. Maintenance doses are between 1000 and 3000 mg daily. Peak blood concentration is reached in 15 minutes (137), but it is not clear how quickly levetiracetam crosses the blood–brain barrier. Its mechanism of action is also not completely understood, although it does bind to the synaptic vesicle protein SV2A. Levetiracetam has no significant protein binding and no redistribution. Its half-life is 6–8 hours, but it is probably retained longer in the brain (138). It is mostly eliminated unchanged through renal clearance, but up to a third undergoes extrahepatic hydrolysis (139). Importantly, levetiracetam has no significant drug interactions. It is well tolerated with minimal sedation and no reported cardiovascular effects, although thrombocytopenia has been rarely reported (140). In the longer term, psychiatric and behavioural side effects are the most important issues.

Lacosamide

Lacosamide has recently been licensed in an intravenous form, currently only in the United States, Canada, Europe, Russia, Australia, and some South American countries. Its use in SE has been reported

in case series only (119,141). The usual dose is 400 mg, commonly administered over 5–10 minutes. Maintenance dose is 400 mg daily. Lacosamide acts on voltage-gated sodium channels, where it enhances their slow inactivation. Its half-life is 12–16 hours, and it undergoes partial hepatic metabolism (CYP2C19), but this does not seem to be relevant clinically as it has not been shown to induce any major drug interactions (142). The most common side effects are moderate sedation and ataxia. Lacosamide can prolong the PQ interval, but extremely rarely with significant consequences.

Third-line treatments

When the first two lines of treatment have failed, pharmacological coma is the final line of treatment in generalized convulsive SE. As discussed earlier, in partial SE where the prognosis is better, further trials with other (non-sedating) second-line treatments should be considered first. In some cases, additional oral AEDs, such as pregabalin (143) and topiramate (144) can be tried relatively quickly (within 2–3 days) as additional second-line treatment.

When pharmacological coma induction is indicated, three drugs are commonly used as initial options—midazolam, propofol, and the barbiturates thiopental and pentobarbital (Table 23.3). These agents share the same principal mechanism of action of modulation of $GABA_A$ receptors, although each acts on specific sites. A meta-analysis completed more than 10 years ago comparing barbiturates with propofol and midazolam did not show any significant difference in short-term mortality, although efficacy was somewhat better but tolerability somewhat worse for barbiturates (145). There is so far only one small randomized study (of 24 patients) comparing propofol and barbiturates in SE (146), reflecting the marked difficulty of organizing clinical trials in this area. This study showed no difference between propofol and barbiturates in terms of adverse effects or efficacy, but, unsurprisingly, barbiturates were associated with a significantly longer duration of mechanical ventilation. The rates of complications were high in both groups, with a 50–66% rate of infections and a 50% rate of hypotension requiring treatment. Overall, midazolam seems to represent the safest third-line treatment option but it often needs to be combined with propofol to achieve seizure control. Regardless of the agent, drug-induced coma is usually maintained for 24–36 hours after which the anaesthetic is weaned off. The period of pharmacological coma can also be used to introduce further antiepileptic treatments.

Midazolam

The properties of midazolam have been described earlier (see 'First-Line Treatments'). As third-line therapy, a bolus of 0.2 mg/kg is generally followed by maintenance dose of 0.2–0.6 mg/kg/h. Tachyphylaxis may develop within 24–48 hours (147), so the dose needs to be constantly increased to achieve and maintain a constant therapeutic effect. Adjunct drugs, commonly propofol, may also be needed to maintain clinical effect. As discussed earlier, the half-life of midazolam can be significantly increased after prolonged administration (148), and its effects are substantially prolonged in patients with hepatic or renal dysfunction. Of note, an antagonist (flumazenil) is available.

Propofol

Propofol is an intravenous general anaesthetic formulated in a white 'milky emulsion' because of its lipid solubility (see Chapter 6). A bolus of 2 mg/kg is administered followed by a maintenance dose of 2–10 mg/kg/h. In addition to modulation of $GABA_A$ receptors, propofol modulates sodium and calcium channels and possibly also NMDA receptors (149). It rapidly redistributes in fatty tissues (distribution half time 2–4 minutes) and has an elimination half-life of 30–60 minutes. It can decrease midazolam clearance possibly by competitively inhibiting CYP3A4 (150), and its clearance can theoretically be decreased by glucuronidation inhibitors (151). Propofol has the advantage of a short-lived sedation, but its main disadvantage is the risk of hypotension and the propofol infusion syndrome (see Chapter 6).

Barbiturates

The barbiturate thiopental (mostly used in Europe; presently not available in the United States), or its metabolite pentobarbital (mostly used in North America), are the oldest compounds used as third-line treatments of SE. In addition to $GABA_A$ receptor modulation, barbiturates have NMDA-antagonist actions which might be relevant in view of the pathophysiology of late SE. The initial bolus dose of thiopental is 1–2 mg/kg and of pentobarbital 5 mg/kg, with a maintenance dose of 1–5 mg/kg per hour for both. Barbiturates have a high affinity for fatty tissues and redistribute very rapidly (initial half-time 2.5 minutes for thiopental) (104). Repeated boluses, administered with EEG monitoring, are thus needed to saturate fatty tissues before obtaining a sustained response. Both compounds eventually saturate fatty tissues leading to a long elimination half-life that may be as high as 27–36 hours after continuous administration. These results in prolonged and deep sedation after the drugs are stopped, and long periods of mechanical ventilation and ICU length of stay. Significant hypotension is a very common feature of barbiturate treatment and is seen more frequently than with midazolam and propofol (145). This can be challenging to manage especially in the elderly and those with pre-existing cardiovascular disease. As barbiturates are formulated as sodium salts, they can also lead to hypernatraemia during prolonged use.

Other pharmacological treatments

Other agents have anecdotally been reported in the treatment of SE, mostly in small selected case series with mitigated outcome. These drugs should only be tried after failure of more conventional options.

Isoflurane is an inhalation anaesthetic that has been reported to control SE at expired concentrations between 0.8% and 2% (104,152). It can accumulate in fatty tissues but is usually rapidly cleared by exhalation and therefore has a short effective half-life. It is less hepatotoxic than other halogenated anaesthetic agents such as halothane (90,153). Gas scavenging is a concern that must be addressed during clinical use on the ICU, and a closed system administration system has recently been described (154). End-tidal agent concentration provides real-time information on dose and blood level and correlates with the degree of EEG suppression.

Ketamine is an anaesthetic acting primarily though inhibition of NMDA receptors at which it binds to the phencyclidine site. This makes it a conceptually interesting option in the treatment of refractory SE. Bolus doses of 0.9–3 mg/kg, with maintenance doses up to 10 mg/kg/h, have been reported (155–157). In these series, when ketamine was used after 8 days following the onset of SE (156,157) or with infusion dosage lower than 0.9 mg/kg/h, no response was observed (156). With low concentration solutions, care should be taken not to fluid overload the patient given the important quantities needed. Tachyphylaxis when initiating the treatment has been

rarely reported (158). To avoid possible neurotoxicity, it is usually combined with a GABAergic medication such as a benzodiazepine. Ketamine has minimal effects on blood pressure.

Etomidate, an anaesthetic agent whose exact mechanism of action is unclear, has also been used to treat refractory SE. Bolus doses of 0.3 mg/kg, and maintenance dose up to 7.2 mg/kg/h, have been reported (155). It has a relatively favourable cardiovascular profile but a reversible inhibition of cortisol synthesis represents an important concern during prolonged treatment, essentially precluding its use (156). Moreover, dose can be also limited by the propylene glycol vehicle which can cause lactic acidosis (157).

Verapamil has also been reported in SE as an inhibitor of P-glycoprotein (multidrug transporter) to reduce the egress of antiepileptic medication from the brain. As discussed earlier, it is unclear which AEDs are substrates of P-glycoproteins so the relevance of this is unclear. Verapamil is relatively safe up to doses of 360 mg daily (158), but as it is a CYP3A4 inhibition it can potentially increase the blood level of drugs such as carbamazepine (159).

Lidocaine, a class Ib antiarrhythmic, modulates sodium channels and has also been used in SE. Initial boluses up to 5 mg/kg, and infusions of up to 6 mg/kg/h, have been reported (160) with treatment effects within 1 hour. Lidocaine should be used with cardiac monitoring, and blood levels should be maintained below 5 mg/L to avoid pro-convulsant effects (161).

Magnesium has occasionally been used in SE, at doses similar to those recommended in eclampsia, that is, 4 g intravenous loading dose followed by an infusion of 1 g/h for 24 hours (162). The recommended target blood magnesium level is 3.5 mmol/L (163). Its mechanism of action is unclear, but it might enhance NMDA receptor blockade. However, magnesium's beneficial effects in eclampsia might in fact be related to its antivasospastic properties, and it has been suggested that it has little antiepileptic effect (164). At high dose, magnesium can induce neuromuscular blockade masking the symptoms of convulsions.

Anti-inflammatory treatments, such as corticosteroids, plasma exchanges, intravenous immunoglobulin, and immunosuppressants, are the treatment of choice for autoimmune causes of SE and should be started as soon as the diagnosis is confirmed. These treatments may also be considered once an infectious aetiology has been ruled out, as inflammatory mechanisms are often involved in the pathogenesis of SE (see above) (165).

Non-pharmacological treatments

Several case reports and small case series report non-pharmacological treatments of SE.

Mild therapeutic hypothermia (32–36°C) for 24–48 hours has efficacy in animal models of SE. Concomitant barbiturates should be avoided because of the risk of paralytic ileus, favouring the use of midazolam or propofol in these circumstances (93). Close monitoring of cardiovascular function, coagulation, and blood lactate, to detect metabolic acidosis secondary severe infections or intestinal necrosis, are mandatory.

A ketogenic diet is increasingly reported in SE mostly, but not only, in paediatric populations. A 4:1 proportion of fat/sugar (with no additional glucose) administered through a nasogastric tube forms the basis of this treatment (166,167). Blood glucose should be monitored closely (several times daily) to avoid hypoglycaemia. Ketone bodies level can be checked in urine, and a plasma β-hydroxybutyrate level above 4 mmol/L (in children) is optimal (167). Defects in oxidative metabolism, such as pyruvate carboxylase or beta oxidation deficiencies, are contraindications to this mode of treatment. Latency of action is a few days and treatment is usually maintained in the long term (at least several weeks). Side effects include hyperlipidaemia and renal calculi.

Resective surgery is an option in cases where there is a clear single causative lesion in a non-eloquent brain region (168). Several stimulation therapies represent further possible options in the treatment of refractory SE. Vagus nerve stimulation (169) and electroconvulsive therapy have been described (170), with some suggesting that decreasing antiepileptic medication may increase the chance of a response (171). Transcranial magnetic stimulation has also been used in partial SE (169,171).

Electroencephalography monitoring

Drug-induced coma should always be conducted under EEG monitoring to assess its efficacy and depth. Automated EEG analysis techniques, such as seizure detection algorithms, are increasingly available and may be useful during prolonged monitoring. However, their sensitivity and specificity in the context of SE are unproven and they should not replace regular EEG review by a neurophysiologist (44). The bispectral index (BIS), developed as a depth of anaesthesia monitor, is an automated, amplitude-integrated measure of a two-channel EEG derivation that includes a burst-suppression ratio (172). This device uses a single commercial sensor, encompassing several electrodes, over the forehead, and has been used to guide drug-induced coma treatment in SE. If the BIS is between 0 and 30, the number of EEG bursts per minute is usually between 0 and 10, and a BIS of 15 is equivalent to one burst every 10 seconds (172). Although BIS can be used as a rough guide, it should not replace EEG monitoring during drug-induced coma because it does have the comprehensive coverage of the EEG, and the difference between pharmacologically induced burst-suppression and seizure-suppression patterns can be very difficult to detect.

The optimum proportion of EEG suppression, ranging from seizure suppression, burst-suppression pattern, to flat (isoelectric) recording, has not been assessed in prospective studies of SE and is thus not known. Retrospective studies have not found a clear difference between these patterns in terms of guiding management (8,173). It is usual to practically aim for an EEG burst-suppression pattern with a burst every 10 seconds. This is an easily recognizable pattern for untrained staff and ensures that distinct seizures are suppressed. There is also no clear evidence for how long the pharmacological EEG suppression should continue or how the anaesthetic should be weaned. An initial drug-induced coma targeting EEG burst suppression with an interburst interval of about 10 seconds for 24 hours, followed by progressive tapering of the drug over 6–12 hours under EEG monitoring, seems a reasonable initial option. The appearance of isolated 'spike-like' transients upon anaesthetic withdrawal should not be a cause of major concern as triphasic waves, reflecting the underlying encephalopathy (either pharmacological, postictal, or of other cause), can be difficult to differentiate from true epileptiform transients. Moreover, the aim of the treatment at that point should be the suppression of epileptic seizures, and not of isolated EEG transients.

Invasive EEG recordings have recently been used and can detect seizures and SE that are not apparent on scalp EEG (174). Invasive electroencephalographic monitoring in combination with other modalities, such as microdialysis, might in the future allow more accurate assessment of when SE should be treated and how aggressively, depending on its potential to generate secondary neuronal injury. Practical points like the position of focal monitors, the relevance of the findings in terms of overall outcome, and the balance between benefit and risks of invasive procedures are yet to be assessed.

Outcome

SE, mostly generalized convulsive types, can induce systemic complications, as shown in Table 23.2. Metabolic disturbances such as acidosis and hyperthermia can occur independently of convulsive movements (52). Rhabdomyolysis, rarely leading to acute kidney injury, can also occur as can cardiorespiratory complications.

SE has a significant mortality (6–39%) and high morbidity from the underlying condition and the SE itself. Independent mortality predictors include the underlying cause, patient age and the extent of consciousness impairment (reflecting the underlying brain dysfunction) (9,175–177), as well as the duration of the episode in generalized forms (especially in the first 10 hours) (178). Along with the underlying aetiology, co-morbid conditions also have an effect on the overall outcome (179). In most cases, death occurs after the episodes of SE have resolved, underscoring the importance of the underlying biological background (9). Severe aetiologies, such as acute large vessel ischaemic stroke, acute central nervous system infection, severe systemic infection, malignant brain tumour, acquired immunodeficiency syndrome with central nervous system complications, chronic renal failure requiring dialysis, systemic vasculitis, marked metabolic disturbances, or acute intoxication sufficient to cause coma in the absence of SE and eclampsia, are more likely to present with refractory SE and have poor outcome (9,173,180). There may also be a synergistic effect between the underlying cause and SE. For example, short- (181) and longer-term (182) mortality is markedly higher in SE and stroke than in stroke alone. The role of the duration of the episode may be also linked to the type of SE; duration is a clear prognostic factor in convulsive SE but not in absence seizure. The STESS score has been validated to allow an estimation of prognosis before treatment is started (99).

Although long-lasting refractory SE generally heralds a poor prognosis, there are exceptions to this rule. Some patients who have had SE for several weeks, or even months, can recover with a good functional outcome (183–187), possibly because in those with an infectious or autoimmune cause the underlying disease process subsides after some time. Therefore, if imaging shows no major lesion, and if no underlying condition with an invariable poor prognosis is identified, supportive treatment, including repetitive courses of anaesthetics if necessary, should be continued. This is particularly the case in young patients who are better able to tolerate side effects of long-term anaesthetic treatments.

SE in the setting of cerebral anoxia after cardiac arrest deserves a particular mention. Despite being widely regarded as synonymous with very poor outcome, this is not invariably the case. Electrographic seizures or SE during therapeutic hypothermia and sedation probably do reflect extreme brain damage and very poor outcome (188). However, SE arising after rewarming can sometimes be successfully treated with AEDs particularly if the EEG background is reactive to stimuli, early cortical somatosensory evoked potentials are present, and brainstem reflexes are preserved. In these selected cases, representing about 3% of all comatose patients after cardiac arrest, survival with reasonable functional outcome is possible (189). AEDs with antimyoclonic effects, such as valproate, levetiracetam, and benzodiazepines are preferred in this situation.

Another important point is the increased risk of developing epilepsy after a *de novo* SE episode. This risk appears to be related to the refractoriness of the episode, as the vast majority (88%) of people with refractory SE develop epilepsy compared to only 22% with non-refractory SE (7,190). The occurrence of SE should thus be considered a major epileptogenic insult and antiepileptic treatment continued, at least initially, after resolution of the episode.

References

1. Lothman E. The biochemical basis and pathophysiology of status epilepticus. *Neurology*. 1990;40(5 Suppl 2):13–23.
2. Meldrum BS, Horton RW. Physiology of status epilepticus in primates. *Arch Neurol*. 1973;28(1):1–9.
3. Lowenstein DH, Bleck T, Macdonald RL. It's time to revise the definition of status epilepticus. *Epilepsia*. 1999;40(1):120–2.
4. DeLorenzo RJ, Garnett LK, Towne AR, Waterhouse EJ, Boggs JG, Morton L, et al. Comparison of status epilepticus with prolonged seizure episodes lasting from 10 to 29 minutes. *Epilepsia*. 1999;40(2):164–9.
5. Mayer SA, Claassen J, Lokin J, Mendelsohn F, Dennis LJ, Fitzsimmons BF. Refractory status epilepticus: frequency, risk factors, and impact on outcome. *Arch Neurol*. 2002;59(2):205–10.
6. Hanley DF, Kross JF. Use of midazolam in the treatment of refractory status epilepticus. *Clin Ther*. 1998;20(6):1093–105.
7. Holtkamp M, Othman J, Buchheim K, Meierkord H. Predictors and prognosis of refractory status epilepticus treated in a neurological intensive care unit. *J Neurol Neurosurg Psychiatry*. 2005;76(4):534–9.
8. Rossetti AO, Logroscino G, Bromfield EB. Refractory status epilepticus: effect of treatment aggressiveness on prognosis. *Arch Neurol*. 2005;62(11):1698–702.
9. Novy J, Logroscino G, Rossetti AO. Refractory status epilepticus: a prospective observational study. *Epilepsia*. 2010;51(2):251–6.
10. Holtkamp M, Othman J, Buchheim K, Masuhr F, Schielke E, Meierkord H. A 'malignant' variant of status epilepticus. *Arch Neurol*. 2005;62(9):1428–31.
11. Shorvon S. Super-refractory status epilepticus: an approach to therapy in this difficult clinical situation. *Epilepsia*. 2011;52:53–6.
12. Vignatelli L, Tonon C, D'Alessandro R, Bologna Group for the Study of Status Epilepticus. Incidence and Short-term Prognosis of Status Epilepticus in Adults in Bologna, Italy. *Epilepsia*. 2003;44(7):964–8.
13. Knake S, Rosenow F, Vescovi M, Oertel WH, Mueller HH, Wirbatz A, et al. Incidence of status epilepticus in adults in Germany: a prospective, population-based study. *Epilepsia*. 2001;42(6):714–8.
14. Wu YW, Shek DW, Garcia PA, Zhao S, Johnston SC. Incidence and mortality of generalized convulsive status epilepticus in California. *Neurology*. 2002;58(7):1070–6.
15. DeLorenzo RJ, Pellock JM, Towne AR, Boggs JG. Epidemiology of status epilepticus. *J Clin Neurophysiol*. 1995;12(4):316–25.
16. Coeytaux A, Jallon P, Galobardes B, Morabia A. Incidence of status epilepticus in French-speaking Switzerland: (EPISTAR). *Neurology*. 2000;55(5):693–7.
17. Maytal J, Shinnar S, Moshe SL, Alvarez LA. Low morbidity and mortality of status epilepticus in children. *Pediatrics*. 1989;83(3):323–31.
18. Kravljanac R, Jovic N, Djuric M, Jankovic B, Pekmezovic T. Outcome of status epilepticus in children treated in the intensive care unit: A study of 302 cases. *Epilepsia*. 2011;52(2):358–63.
19. Commission on Epidemiology and Prognosis, International League Against Epilepsy. Guidelines for epidemiologic studies on epilepsy. *Epilepsia*. 1993;34(4):592–6.
20. DeLorenzo RJ, Hauser WA, Towne AR, Boggs JG, Pellock JM, Penberthy L, et al. A prospective, population-based epidemiologic study of status epilepticus in Richmond, Virginia. *Neurology*. 1996;46(4):1029–35.
21. Hesdorffer DC, Logroscino G, Cascino G, Annegers JF, Hauser WA. Incidence of status epilepticus in Rochester, Minnesota, 1965–1984. *Neurology*. 1998;50(3):735–41.
22. Tan RYL, Neligan A, Shorvon SD. The uncommon causes of status epilepticus: a systematic review. *Epilepsy Res*. 2010;91(2–3):111–22.
23. Trinka E, Höfler J, Zerbs A. Causes of status epilepticus. *Epilepsia*. 2012;53:127–38.
24. Lancaster E, Lai M, Peng X, Hughes E, Constantinescu R, Raizer J, et al. Antibodies to the GABA(B) receptor in limbic encephalitis with seizures: case series and characterisation of the antigen. *Lancet Neurol*. 2010;9(1):67–76.
25. Vincent A, Buckley C, Schott JM, Baker I, Dewar BK, Detert N, et al. Potassium channel antibody-associated encephalopathy: a potentially immunotherapy-responsive form of limbic encephalitis. *Brain*. 2004;127(Pt 3):701–12.
26. Dalmau J, Lancaster E, Martinez-Hernandez E, Rosenfeld MR, Balice-Gordon R. Clinical experience and laboratory investigations in patients with anti-NMDAR encephalitis. *Lancet Neurol*. 2011;10(1):63–74.
27. Lai M, Hughes EG, Peng X, Zhou L, Gleichman AJ, Shu H, et al. AMPA receptor antibodies in limbic encephalitis alter synaptic receptor location. *Ann Neurol*. 2009;65(4):424–34.
28. Malter MP, Helmstaedter C, Urbach H, Vincent A, Bien CG. Antibodies to glutamic acid decarboxylase define a form of limbic encephalitis. *Ann Neurol*. 2010;67(4):470–8.
29. Treiman DM, Walton NY, Kendrick C. A progressive sequence of electroencephalographic changes during generalized convulsive status epilepticus. *Epilepsy Res*. 1990;5(1):49–60.
30. Salmenpera T, Kalviainen R, Partanen K, Mervaala E, Pitkanen A. MRI volumetry of the hippocampus, amygdala, entorhinal cortex, and perirhinal cortex after status epilepticus. *Epilepsy Res*. 2000;40(2–3):155–70.
31. Tien RD, Felsberg GJ. The hippocampus in status epilepticus: demonstration of signal intensity and morphologic changes with sequential fast spin-echo MR imaging. *Radiology*. 1995;194(1):249–56.
32. Meldrum BS, Brierley JB. Prolonged epileptic seizures in primates. Ischemic cell change and its relation to ictal physiological events. *Arch Neurol*. 1973;28(1):10–7.
33. Treiman DM. Electroclinical features of status epilepticus. *J Clin Neurophysiol*. 1995;12(4):343–62.
34. Vein AA, van Emde Boas W. Kozhevnikov epilepsy: The disease and its eponym. *Epilepsia*. 2011;52(2):212–18.
35. Treiman DM, Delgado-Escueta AV. Complex partial status epilepticus. *Adv Neurol*. 1983;34:69–81.
36. Thomas P, Zifkin B, Migneco O, Lebrun C, Darcourt J, Andermann F. Nonconvulsive status epilepticus of frontal origin. *Neurology*. 1999;52(6):1174–83.
37. Claassen J, Mayer SA, Kowalski RG, Emerson RG, Hirsch LJ. Detection of electrographic seizures with continuous EEG monitoring in critically ill patients. *Neurology*. 2004;62(10):1743–8.
38. Towne AR, Waterhouse EJ, Boggs JG, Garnett LK, Brown AJ, Smith JR, et al. Prevalence of nonconvulsive status epilepticus in comatose patients. *Neurology*. 2000;54(2):340–5.
39. Rossetti AO, Oddo M, Logroscino G, Kaplan PW. Prognostication after cardiac arrest and hypothermia: a prospective study. *Ann Neurol*. 2010;67(3):301–7.
40. Chong DJ, Hirsch LJ. Which EEG patterns warrant treatment in the critically ill? Reviewing the evidence for treatment of periodic epileptiform discharges and related patterns. *J Clin Neurophysiol*. 2005;22(2):79–91.
41. Sutter R, Kaplan PW. Electroencephalographic criteria for nonconvulsive status epilepticus: synopsis and comprehensive survey. *Epilepsia*. 2012;53:1–51.

42. Westmoreland BF, Klass DW, Sharbrough FW. Chronic periodic lateralized epileptiform discharges. *Arch Neurol*. 1986;43(5):494–6.

43. Young GB, Jordan KG, Doig GS. An assessment of nonconvulsive seizures in the intensive care unit using continuous EEG monitoring: an investigation of variables associated with mortality. *Neurology*. 1996;47(1):83–9.

44. Herman ST. The electroencephalogram in status epilepticus. In Drislane FW (ed) *Status Epilepticus: A Clinical Perspective*. New York: Humana Press; 2005:77–124.

45. Boulanger JM, Deacon C, Lecuyer D, Gosselin S, Reiher J. Triphasic waves versus nonconvulsive status epilepticus: EEG distinction. *Can J Neurol Sci*. 2006;33(2):175–80.

46. Mameniskiene R, Bast T, Bentes C, Canevini MP, Dimova P, Granata T, et al. Clinical course and variability of non-Rasmussen, nonstroke motor and sensory epilepsia partialis continua: a European survey and analysis of 65 cases. *Epilepsia*. 2011;52(6):1168–76.

47. Bare MA, Burnstine TH, Fisher RS, Lesser RP. Electroencephalographic changes during simple partial seizures. *Epilepsia*. 1994;35(4):715–20.

48. Schmitt SE, Pargeon K, Frechette ES, Hirsch LJ, Dalmau J, Friedman D. Extreme delta brush, A unique EEG pattern in adults with anti-NMDA receptor encephalitis. *Neurology*. 2012;79(11):1094–100.

49. Fountain NB, Waldman WA. Effects of benzodiazepines on triphasic waves: implications for nonconvulsive status epilepticus. *J Clin Neurophysiol*. 2001;18(4):345–52.

50. Fountain NB, Lothman EW. Pathophysiology of status epilepticus. *J Clin Neurophysiol*. 1995;12(4):326–42.

51. Siesjo BK, Ingvar M, Folbergrova J, Chapman AG. Local cerebral circulation and metabolism in bicuculline-induced status epilepticus: relevance for development of cell damage. *Adv Neurol*. 1983;34:217–30.

52. Meldrum BS, Vigouroux RA, Brierley JB. Systemic factors and epileptic brain damage. Prolonged seizures in paralyzed, artificially ventilated baboons. *Arch Neurol*. 1973;29(2):82–7.

53. Siesjo BK, Wieloch T. Epileptic brain damage: pathophysiology and neurochemical pathology. *Adv Neurol*. 1986;44:813–47.

54. Handforth A, Treiman DM. Functional mapping of the late stages of status epilepticus in the lithium-pilocarpine model in rat: a 14C-2-deoxyglucose study. *Neuroscience*. 1995;64(4):1075–89.

55. Shinnar S, Bello JA, Chan S, Hesdorffer DC, Lewis DV, Macfall J, et al. MRI abnormalities following febrile status epilepticus in children: the FEBSTAT study. *Neurology*. 2012;79(9):871–7.

56. Goodkin HP, Joshi S, Mtchedlishvili Z, Brar J, Kapur J. Subunit-specific trafficking of GABA(A) receptors during status epilepticus. *J Neurosci*. 2008;28(10):2527–38.

57. Terunuma M, Xu J, Vithlani M, Sieghart W, Kittler J, Pangalos M, et al. Deficits in phosphorylation of GABA(A) receptors by intimately associated protein kinase C activity underlie compromised synaptic inhibition during status epilepticus. *J Neurosci*. 2008;28(2):376–84.

58. Naylor DE. Glutamate and GABA in the balance: convergent pathways sustain seizures during status epilepticus. *Epilepsia*. 2010;51 Suppl 3:106–9.

59. Walker MC. Basic physiology of limbic status epilepticus. *Epilepsia*. 2009;50:5–6.

60. Rivera C, Voipio J, Thomas-Crusells J, Li H, Emri Z, Sipila S, et al. Mechanism of activity-dependent downregulation of the neuron-specific K-Cl cotransporter KCC2. *J Neurosci*. 2004;24(19):4683–91.

61. Sloviter RS, Zappone CA, Harvey BD, Bumanglag AV, Bender RA, Frotscher M. 'Dormant basket cell' hypothesis revisited: relative vulnerabilities of dentate gyrus mossy cells and inhibitory interneurons after hippocampal status epilepticus in the rat. *J Comp Neurol*. 2003;459(1):44–76.

62. Hope O, Blumenfeld H. Cellular physiology of status epilepticus. In Drislane FW (ed) *Status Epilepticus: A Clinical Perspective*. New York: Humana Press; 2005:159–80.

63. Wasterlain CG, Liu H, Naylor DE, Thompson KW, Suchomelova L, Niquet J, et al. Molecular basis of self-sustaining seizures and pharmacoresistance during status epilepticus: the receptor trafficking hypothesis revisited. *Epilepsia*. 2009;50 Suppl 12:16–18.

64. Vezzani A, Balosso S, Aronica E, Ravizza T. Basic mechanisms of status epilepticus due to infection and inflammation. *Epilepsia*. 2009;50:56–7.

65. Bernardino L, Xapelli S, Silva AP, Jakobsen B, Poulsen FR, Oliveira CR, et al. Modulator effects of interleukin-1beta and tumor necrosis factor-alpha on AMPA-induced excitotoxicity in mouse organotypic hippocampal slice cultures. *J Neurosci*. 2005;25(29):6734–44.

66. Loscher W. Molecular mechanisms of drug resistance in status epilepticus. *Epilepsia*. 2009;50 Suppl 12:19–21.

67. Liu JY, Thom M, Catarino CB, Martinian L, Figarella-Branger D, Bartolomei F, et al. Neuropathology of the blood-brain barrier and pharmaco-resistance in human epilepsy. *Brain*. 2012;135 Pt 10:3115–33.

68. Nohria V, Lee N, Tien RD, Heinz ER, Smith JS, DeLong GR, et al. Magnetic resonance imaging evidence of hippocampal sclerosis in progression: a case report. *Epilepsia*. 1994;35(6):1332–6.

69. Wieshmann UC, Woermann FG, Lemieux L, Free SL, Bartlett PA, Smith SJ, et al. Development of hippocampal atrophy: a serial magnetic resonance imaging study in a patient who developed epilepsy after generalized status epilepticus. *Epilepsia*. 1997;38(11):1238–41.

70. Corsellis JAN, Bruton CJ. Neuropathology of status epilepticus in humans. In Delgado-Escueta AV, Wasterlain CG, Treiman DM, Porter RJ (eds) *Status Epilepticus*. New York: Raven Press; 1983:129–40.

71. DeGiorgio CM, Tomiyasu U, Gott PS, Treiman DM. Hippocampal pyramidal cell loss in human status epilepticus. *Epilepsia*. 1992;33(1):23–7.

72. Fountain NB. Cellular damage and the neuropathology of status epilepticus. In Drislane FW (eds) *Status Epilepticus: A Clinical Perspective*. New York: Humana Press; 2005:181–93.

73. Towfighi J, Kofke WA, O'Connell BK, Housman C, Graybeal JM. Substantia nigra lesions in mercaptopropionic acid induced status epilepticus: a light and electron microscopic study. *Acta Neuropathol*. 1989;77(6):612–20.

74. Genton P, Ferlazzo E, Thomas P. Absence status epilepsy: Delineation of a distinct idiopathic generalized epilepsy syndrome. *Epilepsia*. 2008;49(4):642–9.

75. Thomas P, Lebrun C, Chatel M. De novo absence status epilepticus as a benzodiazepine withdrawal syndrome. *Epilepsia*. 1993;34(2):355–8.

76. Bertram EH, Lothman EW, Lenn NJ. The hippocampus in experimental chronic epilepsy: a morphometric analysis. *Ann Neurol*. 1990;27(1):43–8.

77. DeGiorgio CM, Heck CN, Rabinowicz AL, Gott PS, Smith T, Correale J. Serum neuron-specific enolase in the major subtypes of status epilepticus. *Neurology*. 1999;52(4):746.

78. Bauer G, Gotwald T, Dobesberger J, Embacher N, Felber S, Bauer R, et al. Transient and permanent magnetic resonance imaging abnormalities after complex partial status epilepticus. *Epilepsy Behav*. 2006;8(3):666–71.

79. Fernandez-Torre JL, Figols J, Martinez-Martinez M, Gonzalez-Rato J, Calleja J. Localisation-related nonconvulsive status epilepticus: further evidence of permanent cerebral damage. *J Neurol*. 2006;253(3):392–5.

80. Engel J, Jr., Ludwig BI, Fetell M. Prolonged partial complex status epilepticus: EEG and behavioral observations. *Neurology*. 1978;28(9 Pt 1):863–9.

81. Williamson PD, Spencer DD, Spencer SS, Novelly RA, Mattson RH. Complex partial status epilepticus: a depth-electrode study. *Ann Neurol*. 1985;18(6):647–54.

82. Dodrill CB, Wilensky AJ. Intellectual impairment as an outcome of status epilepticus. *Neurology*. 1990;40 Suppl 2:23–7.

83. Adachi N, Kanemoto K, Muramatsu R, Kato M, Akanuma N, Ito M, et al. Intellectual prognosis of status epilepticus in adult epilepsy patients: analysis with Wechsler Adult Intelligence Scale–Revised. *Epilepsia*. 2005;46(9):1502–9.

84. Treiman DM, Meyers PD, Walton NY, Collins JF, Colling C, Rowan AJ, et al. A comparison of four treatments for generalized convulsive status epilepticus. Veterans Affairs Status Epilepticus Cooperative Study Group. *N Engl J Med*. 1998;339(12):792–8.

85. Treiman DM, Walton NY, Collins JF. Treatment of status epilepticus if first treatment fails. *Epilepsia*. 1999;40 (s7):243.

86. Silbergleit R, Durkalski V, Lowenstein D, Conwit R, Pancioli A, Palesch Y, et al. Intramuscular versus intravenous therapy for prehospital status epilepticus. *New Engl J Med*. 2012;366(7):591–600.

87. Poston KL, Frucht SJ. Movement disorder emergencies. *J Neurol*. 2008;255 Suppl 4:2–13.

88. Holtkamp M, Othman J, Buchheim K, Meierkord H. Diagnosis of psychogenic nonepileptic status epilepticus in the emergency setting. *Neurology*. 2006;66(11):1727–9.

89. Dworetzky BA, Bromfield EB. Differential diagnosis of status epilepticus, pseudostatus epilepticus. In Drislane FW (ed) *Status Epilepticus: A Clinical Perspective*. New York: Humana Press; 2005:33–54.

90. Shih T, Bazil CW. Treatment of generalised convulsive status epilepticus. In Drislane FW (ed) *Status Epilepticus: A Clinical Perspective*. New York: Humana Press; 2005:265–88.

91. Slovis CM, Wrenn KD. Treatment of status epilepticus. *JAMA*. 1994;271(13):980.

92. Sutter R, Fuhr P, Grize L, Marsch S, Rüegg S. Continuous video-EEG monitoring increases detection rate of nonconvulsive status epilepticus in the ICU. *Epilepsia*. 2011;52(3):453–7.

93. Cereda C, Berger MM, Rossetti AO. Bowel ischemia: a rare complication of thiopental treatment for status epilepticus. *Neurocrit Care*. 2009;10(3):355–8.

94. Sutter R, Tschudin-Sutter S, Grize L, Fuhr P, Bonten MJM, Widmer AF, et al. Associations between infections and clinical outcome parameters in status epilepticus: a retrospective 5-year cohort study. *Epilepsia*. 2012;53(9):1489–97.

95. Holtkamp M, Masuhr F, Harms L, Einhaupl KM, Meierkord H, Buchheim K. The management of refractory generalised convulsive and complex partial status epilepticus in three European countries: a survey among epileptologists and critical care neurologists. *J Neurol Neurosurg Psychiatry*. 2003;74(8):1095–9.

96. Meierkord H, Holtkamp M. Non-convulsive status epilepticus in adults: clinical forms and treatment. *Lancet Neurol*. 2007;6(4):329–39.

97. Outin H, Blanc T, Vinatier I. [Emergency and intensive care unit management of status epilepticus in adult patients and children (newborn excluded). Societe de reanimation de langue francaise experts recommendations]. *Rev Neurol (Paris)*. 2009;165(4):297–305.

98. Miller LC, Drislane FW. Treatment of status epilepticus. *Expert Rev Neurother*. 2008;8(12):1817–27.

99. Rossetti AO, Logroscino G, Milligan TA, Michaelides C, Ruffieux C, Bromfield EB. Status Epilepticus Severity Score (STESS): a tool to orient early treatment strategy. *J Neurol*. 2008;255(10):1561–6.

100. Gilbert KL. Evaluation of an algorithm for treatment of status epilepticus in adult patients undergoing video/EEG monitoring. *J Neurosci Nurs*. 2000;32(2):101–7.

101. Alldredge BK, Gelb AM, Isaacs SM, Corry MD, Allen F, Ulrich S, et al. A comparison of lorazepam, diazepam, and placebo for the treatment of out-of-hospital status epilepticus. *N Engl J Med*. 2001;345(9):631–7.

102. Tassinari CA, Daniele O, Michelucci R, Burea M, Dravet CM, Roger R. Benzodiazepines: efficacy in status epilepticus. In Delgado-Escueta AV, Wasterlain CG, Treiman DM, Porter RJ (eds) *Advances in Neurology*. New York: Raven Press; 1983:465–76.

103. Greenblatt DJ, Divoll M, Harmatz JS, Shader RI. Pharmacokinetic comparison of sublingual lorazepam with intravenous, intramuscular, and oral lorazepam. *J Pharm Sci*. 1982;71(2):248–52.

104. Shorvon SD. *Status Epilepticus: Its Clinical Features and Treatment in Children and Adults*. Cambridge: Cambridge University Press; 1994.

105. Walton NY, Treiman DM. Lorazepam treatment of experimental status epilepticus in the rat: relevance to clinical practice. *Neurology*. 1990;40(6):990–4.

106. Leppik IE, Derivan AT, Homan RW, Walker J, Ramsay R, Patrick B. Double-blind study of lorazepam and diazepam in status epilepticus. *JAMA*. 1983;249(11):1452–4.

107. Walker JE, Homan RW, Vasko MR, Crawford IL, Bell RD, Tasker WG. Lorazepam in status epilepticus. *Ann Neurol*. 1979;6(3):207–13.

108. Trinka E. Benzodiazepines used primarily for emergency treatment (diazepam, lorazepam and midazolam. In Shorvon SD, Perucca E, Engel J Jr (eds) *The Treatment of Epilepsy*. Oxford: Wiley-Blackwell; 2011:431–46.

109. Camfield P, Camfield C. Benzodiazepines used primarily for chronic epilepsy (clobazam, clonazepam, clorazepate and nitrazepam). In Shorvon SD, Perucca E, Engel J, Jr (eds) *The Treatment of Epilepsy*. Oxford: Wiley-Blackwell; 2011:421–30.

110. Towne AR, DeLorenzo RJ. Use of intramuscular midazolam for status epilepticus. *J Emerg Med*. 1999;17(2):323–8.

111. Walker MC, Tong X, Brown S, Shorvon SD, Patsalos PN. Comparison of single- and repeated-dose pharmacokinetics of diazepam. *Epilepsia*. 1998;39(3):283–9.

112. Remy C, Jourdil N, Villemain D, Favel P, Genton P. Intrarectal diazepam in epileptic adults. *Epilepsia*. 1992;33(2):353–8.

113. Ramsay RE, Hammond EJ, Perchalski RJ, Wilder BJ. Brain uptake of phenytoin, phenobarbital, and diazepam. *Arch Neurol*. 1979;36(9):535–9.

114. Cloyd JC, Lalonde RL, Beniak TE, Novack GD. A single-blind, crossover comparison of the pharmacokinetics and cognitive effects of a new diazepam rectal gel with intravenous diazepam. *Epilepsia*. 1998;39(5):520–6.

115. Ramsay RE. Treatment of status epilepticus. *Epilepsia*. 1993;34 Suppl 1:S71–81.

116. Knoester PD, Jonker DM, Van Der Hoeven RT, Vermeij TA, Edelbroek PM, Brekelmans GJ, et al. Pharmacokinetics and pharmacodynamics of midazolam administered as a concentrated intranasal spray. A study in healthy volunteers. *Br J Clin Pharmacol*. 2002;53(5):501–7.

117. Treiman DM. Pharmacokinetics and clinical use of benzodiazepines in the management of status epilepticus. *Epilepsia*. 1989;30:S4–S10.

118. Trinka E. What is the relative value of the standard anticonvulsants: phenytoin and fosphenytoin, phenobarbital, valproate, and levetiracetam? *Epilepsia*. 2009;50:40–3.

119. Kellinghaus C, Berning S, Immisch I, Larch J, Rosenow F, Rossetti AO, et al. Intravenous lacosamide for treatment of status epilepticus. *Acta Neurol Scand*. 2011;123(2):137–41.

120. Alvarez V, Januel J-M, Burnand B, Rossetti AO. Second-line status epilepticus treatment: Comparison of phenytoin, valproate, and levetiracetam. *Epilepsia*. 2011;52(7):1292–6.

121. Jaques L, Rossetti AO. Newer antiepileptic drugs in the treatment of status epilepticus: impact on prognosis. *Epilepsy Behav*. 2012;24(1):70–3.

122. Rossetti AO, Novy J, Ruffieux C, Olivier P, Foletti GB, Hayoz D, et al. Management and prognosis of status epilepticus according to hospital setting: a prospective study. *Swiss Med Wkly*. 2009;139(49–50):719–23.

123. Chetty M, Miller R, Seymour MA. Phenytoin auto-induction. *Ther Drug Monit*. 1998;20(1):60–2.

124. Leppik IE, Sherwin AL. Intravenous phenytoin and phenobarbital: anticonvulsant action, brain content, and plasma binding in rat. *Epilepsia*. 1979;20(3):201–7.

125. Knapp LE, Kugler AR. Clinical experience with fosphenytoin in adults: pharmacokinetics, safety, and efficacy. *J Child Neurol*. 1998;13(1 Suppl):S15–S8.

126. Cranford RE, Leppik IE, Patrick B, Anderson CB, Kostick B. Intravenous phenytoin: clinical and pharmacokinetic aspects. *Neurology*. 1978;28(9 Pt 1):874–80.

127. Adams BD, Buckley NH, Kim JY, Tipps LB. Fosphenytoin may cause hemodynamically unstable bradydysrhythmias. *J Emerg Med*. 2006;30(1):75–9.

128. Sinha S, Naritoku DK. Intravenous valproate is well tolerated in unstable patients with status epilepticus. *Neurology*. 2000;55(5):722–4.

129. Perucca E. Pharmacological and therapeutic properties of valproate: a summary after 35 years of clinical experience. *CNS Drugs*. 2002;16(10):695–714.

130. Bourgeois BFD. Valproate. In Shorvon SD, Perucca E, Engel J Jr (eds) *The Treatment of Epilepsy*. Oxford: Wiley-Blackwell; 2011:685–97.

131. Hirsch LJ, Claassen J. The current state of treatment of status epilepticus. *Curr Neurol Neurosci Rep*. 2002;2(4):345–56.

132. Mock CM, Schwetschenau KH. Levocarnitine for valproic-acid-induced hyperammonemic encephalopathy. *Am J Health Syst Pharm*. 2012;69(1):35–9.

133. Finsterer J, Zarrouk Mahjoub S. Mitochondrial toxicity of antiepileptic drugs and their tolerability in mitochondrial disorders. *Expert Opin Drug Metab Toxicol*. 2012;8(1):71–9.

134. Fischer JH, Patel TV, Fischer PA. Fosphenytoin: clinical pharmacokinetics and comparative advantages in the acute treatment of seizures. *Clin Pharmacokinet*. 2003;42(1):33–58.

135. Michelucci R, Pasini E, Tassinari CA. Phenobarbital, primidone and others barbiturates. In Shorvon SD, Perucca E, Engel J Jr (eds) *The Treatment of Epilepsy*. Oxford: Wiley-Blackwell; 2011:585–605.

136. Misra U, Kalita J, Maurya P. Levetiracetam versus lorazepam in status epilepticus: a randomized, open labeled pilot study. *J Neurol*. 2012;259(4):645–8.

137. Ramael S, Daoust A, Otoul C, Toublanc N, Troenaru M, Lu Z, et al. Levetiracetam intravenous infusion: a randomized, placebo-controlled safety and pharmacokinetic study. *Epilepsia*. 2006;47(7):1128–35.

138. Edwards KR, Glantz MJ. The pharmacokinetics of levetiracetam in human cerebrospinal fluid and serum: a controlled dose-ranging study in malignant brain-tumor patients. *Epilepsia*. 2004;45 Suppl 7:121.

139. French JA, Tonner F. Levetiracetam. In Shorvon SD, Perucca E, Engel J Jr (eds) *The Treatment of Epilepsy*. Oxford: Wiley-Blackwell; 2011:559–73.

140. Ruegg S, Naegelin Y, Hardmeier M, Winkler DT, Marsch S, Fuhr P. Intravenous levetiracetam: treatment experience with the first 50 critically ill patients. *Epilepsy Behav*. 2008;12(3):477–80.

141. Hofler J, Unterberger I, Dobesberger J, Kuchukhidze G, Walser G, Trinka E. Intravenous lacosamide in status epilepticus and seizure clusters. *Epilepsia*. 2011;52(10):e148–52.

142. Doty P, Rudd GD, Stoehr T, Thomas D. Lacosamide. *Neurotherapeutics*. 2007;4(1):145–8.

143. Novy J, Rossetti AO. Oral pregabalin as an add-on treatment for status epilepticus. *Epilepsia*. 2010;51(10):2207–10.

144. Stojanova V, Rossetti AO. Oral topiramate as an add-on treatment for refractory status epilepticus. *Acta Neurol Scand*. 2012;125(2):e7–e11.

145. Claassen J, Hirsch LJ, Emerson RG, Mayer SA. Treatment of refractory status epilepticus with pentobarbital, propofol, or midazolam: a systematic review. *Epilepsia*. 2002;43(2):146–53.

146. Rossetti AO, Milligan TA, Vulliémoz S, Michaelides C, Bertschi M, Lee J. A randomized trial for the treatment of refractory status epilepticus. *Neurocrit Care*. 2011;14(1):4–10.

147. Claassen J, Hirsch LJ, Emerson RG, Bates JE, Thompson TB, Mayer SA. Continuous EEG monitoring and midazolam infusion for refractory nonconvulsive status epilepticus. *Neurology*. 2001;57(6):1036–42.

148. Naritoku DK, Sinha S. Prolongation of midazolam half-life after sustained infusion for status epilepticus. *Neurology*. 2000;54(6):1366–8.

149. Marik PE. Propofol: therapeutic indications and side-effects. *Curr Pharm Res*. 2004;10(29):3639–49.

150. Hamaoka N, Oda Y, Hase I, Mizutani K, Nakamoto T, Ishizaki T, et al. Propofol decreases the clearance of midazolam by inhibiting CYP3A4: an in vivo and in vitro study. *Clin Pharmacol Ther*. 1999;66(2):110–17.

151. Le Guellec C, Lacarelle B, Villard PH, Point H, Catalin J, Durand A. Glucuronidation of propofol in microsomal fractions from various tissues and species including humans: effect of different drugs. *Anesth Analg*. 1995;81(4):855–61.

152. Kofke WA, Young RS, Davis P, Woelfel SK, Gray L, Johnson D, et al. Isoflurane for refractory status epilepticus: a clinical series. *Anesthesiology*. 1989;71(5):653–9.

153. Ropper AH, Kofke WA, Bromfield EB, Kennedy SK. Comparison of isoflurane, halothane, and nitrous oxide in status epilepticus. *Ann Neurol*. 1986;19(1):98–9.

154. Kofke WA, Snider MT, Young RS, Ramer JC. Prolonged low flow isoflurane anesthesia for status epilepticus. *Anesthesiology*. 1985;62(5):653–6.

155. Yeoman P, Hutchinson A, Byrne A, Smith J, Durham S. Etomidate infusions for the control of refractory status epilepticus. *Intensive Care Med*. 1989;15(4):255–9.

156. Beyenburg S, Bauer J, Elger CE. [Therapy of generalized tonic-clonic status epilepticus in adulthood]. *Nervenarzt*. 2000;71:65–77.

157. International Programme on Chemical Safety Poisons Information. *Propylene Glycol*. Monograph 443. [Online] http://www.inchem.org/documents/pims/chemical/pim443.htm.

158. Iannetti P, Spalice A, Parisi P. Calcium-channel blocker verapamil administration in prolonged and refractory status epilepticus. *Epilepsia*. 2005;46(6):967–9.

159. Macphee GJA, Thompson GG, McInnes GT, Brodie MJ. Verapamil potentiates carabamazepine neurotoxocity: a clinically important inhibitory interaction. *Lancet*. 1986;327(8483):700–3.

160. Walkes LA, Slovis CM. Lidocaine in the treatment of status epilepticus. *Acad Emerg Med*. 1997;4(9):918–25.

161. Hamano S, Sugiyama N, Yamashita S, Tanaka M, Hayakawa M, Minamitani M, et al. Intravenous lidocaine for status epilepticus during childhood. *Dev Med Child Neurol*. 2006;48(3):220–2.

162. The Eclampsia Trial Collaborative Group. Which anticonvulsant for women with eclampsia? Evidence from the Collaborative Eclampsia Trial. *Lancet*. 1995;345(8963):1455–63.

163. Visser NA, Braun KP, Leijten FS, van Nieuwenhuizen O, Wokke JH, van den Bergh WM. Magnesium treatment for patients with refractory status epilepticus due to POLG1-mutations. *J Neurol*. 2011;258(2):218–22.

164. Kaplan PW. The neurologic consequences of eclampsia. *Neurologist*. 2001;7(6):357–63.

165. Robakis TK, Hirsch LJ. Literature review, case report, and expert discussion of prolonged refractory status epilepticus. *Neurocrit Care*. 2006;4(1):35–46.

166. Wusthoff CJ, Kranick SM, Morley JF, Christina Bergqvist AG. The ketogenic diet in treatment of two adults with prolonged nonconvulsive status epilepticus. *Epilepsia*. 2010;51(6):1083–5.

167. Nabbout R, Mazzuca M, Hubert P, Peudennier S, Allaire C, Flurin V, et al. Efficacy of ketogenic diet in severe refractory status epilepticus initiating fever induced refractory epileptic encephalopathy in school age children (FIRES). *Epilepsia*. 2010;51(10):2033–7.

168. Lhatoo SD, Alexopoulos AV. The surgical treatment of status epilepticus. *Epilepsia*. 2007;48 Suppl 8:61–5.

169. Rossetti AO. Novel anesthetics and other treatment strategies for refractory status epilepticus. *Epilepsia*. 2009;50:51–3.

170. Lambrecq V, Villéga F, Marchal C, Michel V, Guehl D, Rotge J-Y, et al. Refractory status epilepticus: electroconvulsive therapy as a possible therapeutic strategy. *Seizure*. 2012; 21(9):661–4.

171. Walker MC. The potential of brain stimulation in status epilepticus. *Epilepsia*. 2011;52:61–3.

172. Musialowicz T, Mervaala E, Kälviäinen R, Uusaro A, Ruokonen E, Parviainen I. Can BIS monitoring be used to assess the depth of propofol anesthesia in the treatment of refractory status epilepticus? *Epilepsia*. 2010;51(8):1580–6.

173. Krishnamurthy KB, Drislane FW. Depth of EEG suppression and outcome in barbiturate anesthetic treatment for refractory status epilepticus. *Epilepsia*. 1999;40(6):759–62.

174. Waziri A, Claassen J, Stuart RM, Arif H, Schmidt JM, Mayer SA, et al. Intracortical electroencephalography in acute brain injury. *Ann Neurol*. 2009;66(3):366–77.

175. Towne AR, Pellock JM, Ko D, DeLorenzo RJ. Determinants of mortality in status epilepticus. *Epilepsia*. 1994;35(1):27–34.

176. Logroscino G, Hesdorffer DC, Cascino G, Annegers JF, Hauser WA. Short-term mortality after a first episode of status epilepticus. *Epilepsia.* 1997;38(12):1344–9.

177. Lowenstein DH, Alldredge BK. Status epilepticus at an urban public hospital in the 1980s. *Neurology.* 1993;43(3 Pt 1):483–8.

178. Drislane FW, Blum AS, Lopez MR, Gautam S, Schomer DL. Duration of refractory status epilepticus and outcome: loss of prognostic utility after several hours. *Epilepsia.* 2009;50(6):1566–71.

179. Alvarez V, Januel J-M, Burnand B, Rossetti AO. Role of comorbidities in outcome prediction after status epilepticus. *Epilepsia.* 2012;53(5):e89–e92.

180. Rossetti AO, Hurwitz S, Logroscino G, Bromfield EB. Prognosis of status epilepticus: role of aetiology, age, and consciousness impairment at presentation. *J Neurol Neurosurg Psychiatry.* 2006;77(5):611–15.

181. Waterhouse EJ, Vaughan JK, Barnes TY, Boggs JG, Towne AR, Kopec-Garnett L, *et al.* Synergistic effect of status epilepticus and ischemic brain injury on mortality. *Epilepsy Res.* 1998;29(3):175–83.

182. Knake S, Rochon J, Fleischer S, Katsarou N, Back T, Vescovi M, *et al.* Status epilepticus after stroke is associated with increased long-term case fatality. *Epilepsia.* 2006;47(12):2020–6.

183. Standley K, Abdulmassih R, Benbadis S. Good outcome is possible after months of refractory convulsive status epilepticus: lesson learned. *Epilepsia.* 2012;53(1):e17–e20.

184. Bausell R, Svoronos A, Lennihan L, Hirsch LJ. Recovery after severe refractory status epilepticus and 4 months of coma. *Neurology.* 2011;77(15):1494–5.

185. Drislane FW, Lopez MR, Blum AS, Schomer DL. Survivors and nonsurvivors of very prolonged status epilepticus. *Epilepsy Behav.* 2011;22(2):342–5.

186. Maeder-Ingvar M, Prior JO, Irani SR, Rey V, Vincent A, Rossetti AO. FDG-PET hyperactivity in basal ganglia correlating with clinical course in anti-NDMA-R antibodies encephalitis. *J Neurol Neurosurg Psychiatry.* 2011;82(2):235–6.

187. Dara SI, Tungpalan LA, Manno EM, Lee VH, Moder KG, Keegan MT, *et al.* Prolonged coma from refractory status epilepticus. *Neurocrit Care.* 2006;4(2):140–2.

188. Rossetti AO, Urbano LA, Delodder F, Kaplan PW, Oddo M. Prognostic value of continuous EEG monitoring during therapeutic hypothermia after cardiac arrest. *Crit Care.* 2010;14(5):R173.

189. Rossetti AO, Oddo M, Liaudet L, Kaplan PW. Predictors of awakening from postanoxic status epilepticus after therapeutic hypothermia. *Neurology.* 2009;72(8):744–9.

190. Hesdorffer DC, Logroscino G, Cascino G, Annegers JF, Hauser WA. Risk of unprovoked seizure after acute symptomatic seizure: effect of status epilepticus. *Ann Neurol.* 1998;44(6):908–12.

CHAPTER 24

Central nervous system infection and inflammation

Erich Schmutzhard, Ronny Beer,
Raimund Helbok, and Bettina Pfausler

Infections and inflammatory disorders of the central nervous system (CNS) are a distinct group of clinical syndromes that include encephalitis, meningitis, and acute para- or post-infectious demyelinating diseases. Although CNS infections are relatively rare, they can lead to life-threatening emergencies because of significant destruction of CNS structures and the complications thereof. An extraordinarily high index of suspicion is therefore essential to diagnose and treat CNS infections in a timely and appropriate manner. Effective management, with the prompt introduction of symptomatic and specific therapies, has a dramatic influence on survival and reduces the degree of permanent neurological disability in survivors (1–6).

CNS infections are caused by a wide range of microorganisms including bacteria, viruses, fungi, protozoa, helminths, and arthropods, all of which are capable of invading the CNS leading to inflammation of the meninges, subarachnoid space, and brain parenchyma. The pattern of aetiological agents varies in different geographical and climatic settings, and also depends on the presence of specific vectors, transmission routes, virulence factors, and the immunological state of the host (7–9). In addition, community-acquired CNS infections must be distinguished from post-traumatic, post-neurosurgical, or other healthcare associated causes because of the different spectra of causative microorganisms and the evolving problem of multidrug resistance (10–12).

Patients with CNS infection frequently require admission to a neurocritical care unit (NCCU) for monitoring and management, and often have a long hospital length of stay (LOS). Specific therapy and supportive and symptomatic treatments are essential for optimal outcome. Timely recognition or prevention of the wide range of neurological and systemic complications may result in shorter NCCU and hospital LOS, and reduce acute and long-term mortality and morbidity (2,4,13–16).

From the neurocritical care perspective, standard therapies may be difficult to apply in patients with acute CNS infections. For example, antiepileptic drugs with potential pro-arrhythmic activity (e.g. phenytoin) should be avoided in patients with viral encephalitis and coexistent viral myocarditis (17). Similarly, significant liver dysfunction precludes the administration of potential hepatotoxic anticonvulsants such as sodium valproate (18). Furthermore, recent evidence suggests that hyperosmotic agents such as mannitol should be used with caution in patients with severe CNS infections because of concomitant capillary leakage secondary to the systemic inflammatory response syndrome (19–21).

This chapter provides an overview of infectious and non-infectious causes of encephalitis, acute bacterial meningitis, and external ventricular drain (EVD)/shunt infections, highlighting the epidemiology, clinical and diagnostic features, and NCCU management.

Encephalitis

Encephalitis is defined by the presence of an inflammation in brain parenchyma and can be related to an infective or non-infective process. In many cases, some degree of inflammatory meningeal involvement is also present and therefore the term meningoencephalitis is commonly used. Encephalitis must be differentiated from encephalopathy, a syndrome characterized by disruption of brain function caused by metabolic derangements, toxins, hypoxia, or systemic infection (2,22–24).

Infectious causes of encephalitis include a variety of viruses and bacteria, especially intracellular pathogens such as *Mycoplasma* and *Chlamydia* species, and certain parasites and fungi. A significant proportion of cases of acute encephalitis have an immune-mediated pathogenesis (25,26) of which acute disseminated encephalomyelitis (ADEM) is the most common subtype. This demyelinating inflammatory disease typically follows an infection or vaccination usually after a 2–30-day latency period, although longer delays have been reported. It occurs predominantly in children with an incidence of approximately 0.5 per 100,000, but is also seen in adults. Viral agents commonly associated with ADEM include enteroviruses, influenza, measles, mumps, and hepatitis A. Vaccinations against measles, hepatitis B, influenza, and Japanese encephalitis have also been reported as triggers of ADEM (27,28). Other immune-mediated encephalitic syndromes are associated with antineuronal antibodies such as those specific for the *N*-methyl-D-aspartate (NMDA) receptor or voltage-gated potassium channels, and may or may not be paraneoplastic (29,30). Despite recent advances in diagnosis, neither a pathogenic mechanism nor microbial aetiology is identifiable in a significant proportion (up to 65%) of cases of suspected encephalitis (25,31,32).

Whereas the incidence of acute bacterial meningitis has decreased over the last decade (33–36), the incidence of viral meningoencephalitis has remained fairly static at approximately 0.7–13.8 per 100,000 in all age groups in industrialized nations (7,23,31).

Table 24.1 Important causes of viral infections of the central nervous system

Viral meningitis	Viral (meningo-) encephalitis
Enteroviruses: ◆ Enterovirus 71 ◆ Coxsackieviruses ◆ Echoviruses	Herpes viruses: ◆ Herpes simplex virus type 1 and 2 ◆ Varicella zoster virus ◆ Epstein–Barr virus
Tick-borne encephalitis virus and other arthropod-borne viruses (e.g. _West Nile virus, Toscana virus, Tahyna virus_)	Paramyxoviruses: ◆ _Mumps virus_ ◆ _Measles virus_
Paramyxoviruses: ◆ _Mumps virus_ ◆ _Measles virus_	Arthropod-borne viruses: ◆ _West Nile virus_ ◆ Tick-borne encephalitis virus ◆ Others (e.g. _Japanese encephalitis virus_, Western and Eastern equine encephalitis viruses, _Chikungunya virus, La Crosse virus_)
Herpes viruses	
Human immunodeficiency virus	
Influenza viruses	
Rotaviruses	
Lymphocytic choriomeningitis virus	Human immunodeficiency virus

Data from Solomon T Hart IJ, Beeching NJ, 'Viral Encephalitis: a Clinician's Guide', _Practical Neurology_, 7, pp. 288–305, Copyright © 2007 John Wiley & Sons and Domingues RB, 'Viral Encephalitis: Current Treatments and Future Perspectives', _Central Nervous System Agents in Medicinal Chemistry_, 12, pp. 277–285, Copyright 2012 Bentham Science.

In immune competent individuals, herpes simplex virus (HSV) and enteroviruses are responsible for most cases of viral CNS infections whereas varicella zoster virus (VZV) is common in the immunocompromised (Table 24.1). Viral aetiology is dependent on environmental factors. In Central, Eastern, and Northern European countries, _Tick-borne encephalitis virus_ (TBEV) is a frequent cause of viral meningoencephalitis and _West Nile virus_ (WNV) has recently become an important cause of encephalitis in the United States and in certain European countries (37–39). Other vector-borne zoonotic neuroinvasive diseases caused by, amongst others, Hantaan virus, _Chikungunya virus_, Crimean-Congo haemorrhagic fever virus, and _Dengue virus_, have also been introduced into new regions as a result of travel-related pathogen movement. Exposure to vectors is further affected by climate. Higher temperatures are associated with increased vector development, biting rate, and pathogen replication (40).

Public health factors are also important in the prevalence of encephalitis. CNS infections caused by vaccine-preventable viruses are less common in developed countries. Several poliomyelitis epidemics with high rates of mortality have occurred worldwide but no infections with wild-type poliovirus have been reported in Europe or the United States in the last decade (41). Reduced immunization uptake in high-income countries has been linked to a resurge of viral diseases previously thought to have been controlled.

Clinical features

Irrespective of the causative agent, the diagnosis of an invasive CNS infection should be suspected in the context of an acute or recent febrile ('flu'-like) illness with headache, nausea and vomiting, altered level of consciousness, and other symptoms and signs of cerebral

irritation. Early clinical findings may also relate to meningeal irritation and disruption of brain function and include cognitive dysfunction presenting as acute memory and orientation disturbances, behavioural changes, and focal neurological deficits such as dysphasia and hemiparesis, myoclonus, and seizures. Autonomic and hypothalamic disturbances, with loss of temperature and vasomotor control, and electrolyte imbalances, may also occur (2,14,16,22–24,42).

The pattern of neurological deficits may provide clues to the aetiological agent (Table 24.2) (14,23,24,39,42). Movement disorders with myoclonus, chorea, or tremor are related to involvement of the thalamus and other basal ganglia and are often seen in _Flavivirus_ infections, such as TBEV, WNV, and _Japanese encephalitis virus_ (JEV), as well as CNS toxoplasmosis. Autonomic dysfunction and cranial nerve palsies indicating brainstem involvement are associated with HSV, _Flavivirus_, and enterovirus 71 infections, and also with listeriosis, brucellosis, and neurotuberculosis. Cerebellitis is associated with Epstein–Barr virus (EBV), VZV, mumps, and some _Flavivirus_ infections. Involvement of the spinal cord, with weakness or acute flaccid paralysis, is characteristic of enteroviruses, such as poliovirus, enterovirus 71, WNV, and flaviviruses. Encephalitis associated with radiculitis is seen in EBV and _Cytomegalovirus_ (CMV) infections. Seizures and non-convulsive status epilepticus may occur in encephalitis that involves the cerebral cortex and is often related to HSV infection. A complex neurological syndrome of behavioural changes, cognitive dysfunction, and focal neurological deficits may suggest 'limbic' encephalitis due to HSV infection or immune-mediated encephalitis of either paraneoplastic or non-paraneoplastic aetiology (29,43).

In contrast to infectious causes of encephalitis, the course of immune-mediated disease is usually less acute and develops as a multistage illness progressing from psychosis, memory deficits, seizures, and language disintegration to a state of unresponsiveness, abnormal movements, and autonomic instability (29,30). These features are not exclusive to antibody-mediated disease and may also be present in subacute or chronic viral encephalitis.

ADEM differs from acute infectious encephalitis by a predominance of inflammation and demyelination, and failure to isolate pathogens from neural tissue. Its clinical course is rapidly progressive and usually develops over hours, with maximum deficits established within days. The typical symptoms and signs of ADEM are acute-onset encephalopathy and multifocal central and peripheral neurological deficits (26–28).

Diagnosis

The diagnostic approach to suspected encephalitis includes a detailed history, general and neurological examination, blood and cerebrospinal fluid (CSF) microbiological analysis, neuroimaging, and electroencephalography (EEG) (22–24).

History and clinical examination

The history should examine contact with an individual afflicted by an infective condition, recent travel, seasonal occurrence, geographic location, occupation, and contact with animals. A history of insect or animal bite, or outdoor activity in an infested area, is particularly suggestive of arthropod-borne infections. Assessment of immune status is relevant because certain pathogens cause encephalitis more frequently in immunocompromised individuals.

The clinical examination may also provide clues to aetiology. Skin rashes are common in viral and some bacterial infections,

Table 24.2 Clinical features and preferential involvement of intracranial and extracranial structures of selected causes of encephalitis

Clinical feature(s)/ structures involved	Common aetiology
Autonomic dysfunction, cranial nerve involvement	Herpes simplex virus
	Flaviviruses, e.g. *Tick-borne encephalitis virus, West Nile virus, Japanese encephalitis virus*
	Enterovirus 71
	Listeria monocytogenes
	Brucella spp.
	Mycobacterium tuberculosis
Cerebellitis	Epstein–Barr virus
	Varicella zoster virus
	Mumps virus
	(Some) flaviviruses
Encephalitis plus radiculitis	Epstein–Barr virus
	Cytomegalovirus
'Limbic encephalitis'	Herpes simplex virus
	Immune mediated
Movement disorders/ thalamus and other basal ganglia	Flaviviruses, e.g. *Tick-borne encephalitis virus, West Nile virus, Japanese encephalitis virus*
	Toxoplasma gondii
'Poliomyelitis-like' paralysis/ spinal cord	Enteroviruses
	Flaviviruses, e.g. *Tick-borne encephalitis virus, West Nile virus, Japanese encephalitis virus*
Seizures and/or status epilepticus	Herpes simplex virus

Adapted from Kennedy PG, 2005, 'Viral Encephalitis', *Journal of Neurology*, 252, pp. 268–272; Solomon T *et al.*, 2012, 'Management of Suspected Viral Encephalitis in Adults – Association of British Neurologists and British Infection Association National Guidelines', *Journal of Infection*, 64, pp. 347–373; Steiner I *et al.*, 2010, 'Viral Meningoencephalitis: a Review of Diagnostic Methods and Guidelines for Management', *European Journal of Neurology*, 17, pp. 999–e57; Turtle L *et al.*, 2012, 'Encephalitis Caused by Flaviviruses', *QJM: An International Journal of Medicine*, 105, pp. 219–223; and Sips *et al.*, 2012, 'Neuroinvasive Flavivirus Infections', *Reviews in Medical Virology*, 22, pp. 69–87.

and other organs may also be involved prior to or in parallel with neurological manifestations of the disease. For example, a vesicular rash may be suggestive of VZV infection, parotitis of mumps, gastrointestinal signs of enteroviral disease, and respiratory symptoms of HSV and influenza virus infections (2,22–24).

Cerebrospinal fluid analysis

CSF analysis is an essential investigation in all patients with suspected CNS infection or inflammation to confirm the diagnosis and rule out other disease states. Lumbar puncture should be performed as soon as possible after admission unless there are contraindications such as focal neurological symptoms or signs or impairment of consciousness, in which case neuroimaging is required to exclude contraindications to the spinal tap such as raised intracranial pressure (ICP). Lumbar puncture should also be delayed until coagulation disturbances have been excluded or corrected. CSF investigations include measurement of opening pressure, total red and white cell count with differential, microscopy and culture, and protein and glucose measurement (Table 24.3) (22). CSF chemistry should be compared with contemporaneous serum samples. CSF and other samples should also be sent for microbiological and serological examination (Table 24.4) (2,23,24,44), and a sample should be stored for further analysis as necessary.

Nucleic acid detection by CSF polymerase chain reaction (PCR) has high sensitivity and specificity for some viral CNS infections, making it the most reliable diagnostic test (24,44). Serological tests for antibodies in CSF and serum should also be performed. The detection of pathogen-specific immunoglobulin M (IgM) in CSF is strong evidence for aetiology because IgM does not normally cross the blood–brain barrier (BBB). If BBB breakdown is suspected, the ratio of CSF to serum antibodies can be compared and, if the IgM level in CSF is higher than in serum, an intrathecal origin is confirmed. Diagnoses confirmed with antibody testing include EBV, flaviviruses, borreliosis, brucellosis, rickettsioses, ehrlichioses, *Mycoplasma pneumoniae*, and *Chlamydophilia pneumoniae* (23). In cases of diagnostic uncertainty, PCR should be repeated after 3-7 days and serological tests after 2–4 weeks to monitor for possible seroconversion or increase in antibody titres (24). Ancillary tests that establish systemic infection may be supportive (Table 24.4) but are not necessarily confirmatory of CNS involvement.

Table 24.3 Characteristic cerebrospinal fluid findings in viral meningoencephalitis and acute bacterial meningitis

	Normal	Viral meningoencephalitis	Acute bacterial meningitis
Opening pressure	10–20 cm	Normal or elevated	High
Colour	Clear	'Gin' clear	Cloudy
Cells (/mm³)[a]	< 5	Slightly increased (i.e. < 1000)	High to very high (i.e. > 1000)
Differential[b]	Mononuclear cells	Predominantly lymphocytes	Neutrophils
CSF/serum glucose ratio	> 0.5	> 0.5	< 0.4
Protein (mg/dL)[a]	< 50	Normal to high (i.e. < 100)	High (i.e. > 100)
Lactate (mmol/L)	1.5–2.5	< 3.5	> 3

[a] A 'bloody' lumbar puncture will falsely elevate the CSF white count and protein. For correction, subtraction of 1 leucocyte for every 700 erythrocytes per mm³ in the CSF, and 10 mg/dL of protein for every 1000 erythrocytes per mm³ in the CSF has been suggested (22).
[b] In viral CNS infections, an early CSF analysis may give predominantly neutrophils, or there may be no cells in early or late lumbar punctures. In patients with partially pre-treated acute bacterial meningitis, the CSF cell count may not be very high with lymphocytic preponderance.
Adapted by permission from BMJ Publishing Group Limited. *Practical Neurology*, 'Viral Encephalitis: a Clinician's Guide', Solomon T Hart IJ, Beeching NJ, 2007, 7, pp. 288–305.

Table 24.4 A suggested approach to microbiological investigations of patients with suspected encephalitis

Cerebrospinal fluid PCR		
All patients	HSV-1, HSV-2, VZV	
	Enteroviruses, parechoviruses	
If indicated	EBV, CMV	Especially if immunocompromised
	HHV-6, HHV-7	Especially if immunocompromised, or children
	Adenoviruses, influenza viruses, rotaviruses	Children
	Measles virus, Mumps virus	If clinically suspected
	Erythrovirus (parvovirus) B19	
	Chlamydia spp.	If clinically suspected
Special circumstances	Rabies virus, WNV, TBEV	If appropriate exposure
	Human polyomavirus (JC, BK)	If immunosuppressed
Antibody testing (when indicated)—IgM and IgG in CSF and serum (acute and covalescent)[a]		
Viruses	HSV-1, HSV-2, VZV, CMV, HHV-6, HHV-7, enteroviruses, RSV, erythrovirus B19, adenoviruses, influenza viruses	
If associated with 'atypical' pneumonia	Mycoplasma pneumoniae serology and cold agglutinins	
	Chlamydia spp. (especially Chlamydophilia pneumoniae) serology	
	Legionella pneumophila serology	
Brain biopsy		
PCR, culture, electron microscopy, and immunohistochemistry	Various infective agents causing encephalitis	
Ancillary investigations[b]		
Throat swab	PCR and culture for enteroviruses	
	PCR for Mycoplasma pneumoniae, Chlamydophilia pneumoniae	
Nasopharyngeal aspirate	PCR and antigen detection for respiratory viruses, influenza viruses, adenoviruses (especially children)	
Vesicle fluid (e.g. herpetic lesions)	Electron microscopy, PCR and culture for HSV, VZV	
Urine	Antigen detection for Legionella pneumophila	
	PCR and culture for Measles virus, Mumps virus, Rubella virus	
Rectal swab	PCR and culture for enteroviruses	

CNS, central nervous system; CSF, cerebrospinal fluid; PCR, polymerase chain reaction.

[a] Antibody detection in the serum identifies infection (past or recent depending on type of antibodies), but does not necessarily indicate CNS disease.

[b] These tests establish carriage or systemic infection, but do not necessarily indicate CNS disease.

Virus taxonomy: CMV, Cytomegalovirus; EBV, Epstein–Barr virus; HHV, human herpes virus; HSV, herpes simplex virus; RSV, respiratory syncytial virus; TBEV, Tick-borne encephalitis virus; VZV, varicella zoster virus; WNV, West Nile virus.

Reprinted from Journal of Infection, 64, 4, Solomon T, Michael BD, Smith PE et al., 'Management of Suspected Viral Encephalitis in Adults – Association of British Neurologists and British Infection Association National Guidelines', pp. 347–373, Copyright (2012) with permission from Elsevier.

Oligoclonal bands in CSF are a non-specific indicator of a CNS inflammatory process. They may be helpful in the diagnosis of acute demyelinating disorders such as ADEM in which CSF PCR and serological tests are negative because they are not related to primary tissue invasion by an infectious agent (26–28). In patients with suspected antibody-mediated encephalitis, specific antibody studies including those against the NMDA, α-amino-3-hydroxy-5-methyl-4-isoxazolepropionic acid (AMPA), and γ-aminobutyric acid (GABA)-B receptors should be performed in both serum and CSF. In cases of autoimmune encephalitis an underlying tumour, particularly ovarian teratoma or a testicular germ cell tumour, should be excluded (29).

Imaging

Magnetic resonance imaging (MRI) is the preferred modality in patients with suspected encephalitis and should be performed as soon as possible, including when there is diagnostic uncertainty (23,24,45,46). Contrast-enhanced MRI is more sensitive in demonstrating brain parenchymal lesions and additional information can be gained from MR diffusion-weighted (DWI) and diffusion tensor (DTI) imaging. If MRI is not readily available, or if the patient's condition precludes MRI, a computed tomography (CT) scan will rule out structural causes of increased ICP and possibly reveal alternative diagnoses.

Different encephalitic aetiologies have distinctive neuroimaging features and these can guide confirmatory tests (2,14,23,24,47–50). MRI changes in the cingulate gyrus and medial temporal lobe are frequently seen in the early phase of HSV encephalitis (Figure 24.1a), whereas patients with *Flavivirus* encephalitis, such as TBV, WNV, and JEV, often have characteristic lesions in the thalamus, basal ganglia, and midbrain (Figure 24.1b).

In ADEM, MRI generally reveals multiple focal or confluent areas of signal abnormality in the subcortical white matter and sometimes in subcortical grey matter (Figure 24.2). The lesions are often enhancing and display similar stages of evolution, a feature that helps distinguish them from the subcortical white matter lesions of multiple sclerosis and progressive multifocal leucoencephalopathy in which the lesions rarely enhance and uncommonly affect grey matter (26–28).

In autoantibody-mediated encephalitis, the neuroimaging findings are often unremarkable despite the severity and duration of symptoms. MRI-delineated lesions have been reported in the limbic structures, cerebral cortex, basal ganglia, brainstem, and occasionally the spinal cord (29,30). Although some appear demyelinating, they do not usually enhance and are transient.

Electroencephalography

Although EEG is often considered a non-specific investigation in the diagnosis of encephalitis, it is useful in identifying subtle epileptic seizures and non-convulsive status epilepticus (see Chapter 14) (51,52). Diffuse generalized slowing and rhythmic slow activity are prevalent EEG abnormalities. There are also pathognomonic EEG changes including periodic lateralized epileptiform discharges (PLEDs) in HSV encephalitis (Figure 24.3) (53), viral encephalitides, and non-infectious conditions (see Chapter 14).

Brain biopsy

Brain biopsy is reserved for unusual cases or those of diagnostic difficulty when it can exclude other causes such as vasculitis in patients with progressive deterioration despite adequate treatment.

Stereotactic guidance should be used to target the biopsy site to a specific area of the brain identified by neuroimaging (23,46).

Management

Patients with suspected encephalitis can deteriorate rapidly so early diagnosis and treatment is essential. In those with a decreasing level of consciousness, urgent assessment of the need for intubation and mechanical ventilation, and management of increased ICP, is required. Autonomic dysfunction resulting in hypotension and cardiac arrhythmias can occur early. Patients should be monitored and managed in a high dependency area or NCCU with access to neuroimaging and continuous EEG recording facilities until clinically stable (2,14,23,24).

Anti-infective agents

Despite the many causes of infectious encephalitis, specific therapy is limited to selected pathogens. Aciclovir is indicated for the treatment of HSV encephalitis and may also be effective in VZV encephalitis. The earlier that treatment is started for herpes encephalitis the more likely there will be a favourable outcome. Intravenous aciclovir (10 mg/kg every 8 hours in children and adults with normal renal function) should be commenced in all patients with suspected encephalitis as soon as possible, pending results of diagnostic studies (23,24,46,54). Ganciclovir and foscarnet can be used to treat CMV encephalitis and pleconaril should be considered in patients with severe enterovirus encephalitis. Antiviral therapy with oseltamivir and rimantadine has been successful in the treatment of encephalitis associated with seasonal influenza virus (24). Empirical antimicrobial agents, including therapy for presumed bacterial meningitis, should be initiated on the basis of specific epidemiological or clinical factors. For example, doxycycline should be administered to patients with suspected rickettsial or ehrlichial infection (46). Once the aetiology of encephalitis is confirmed, therapy should be rationalized to the identified infectious agent and empirical antiviral therapy discontinued if specific treatment is not available.

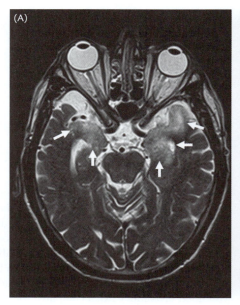 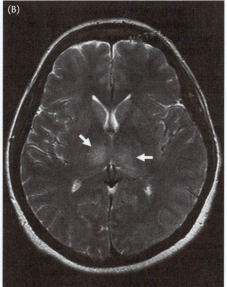

Fig. 24.1 Magnetic resonance imaging abnormalities associated with viral encephalitis.
(A) Herpes simplex virus type 1 encephalitis showing increased T2-weighted signal in both temporal lobes.
(B) Tick-borne encephalitis showing increased T2-weighted signal of both thalami (arrows).

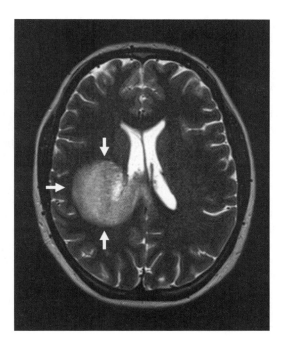

Fig. 24.2 Magnetic resonance imaging in a patient with acute disseminated encephalomyelitis (ADEM) 3 weeks after influenza vaccination. Note that this T2 sequence shows a large, hyperintense lesion (arrows) extending from the periventricular to the peripheral white matter of the right hemisphere.

Steroids

The use of corticosteroids as adjunct treatment for acute infectious encephalitis is controversial. Although not generally effective, corticosteroids in combination with antiviral agents may have a role in the presence of progressive cerebral oedema or in the context of a major vasculitic component of the disease (23,24,55). Corticosteroid therapy should be limited to only a few days.

Adjuvant therapies

Continuous ICP monitoring and aggressive ICP management are indicated in patients with diffuse encephalitis who develop brain oedema and increased ICP (see Chapters 7 and 9). Therapeutic hypothermia or surgical decompression has been shown to improve outcome in individual cases of acute viral encephalitis with refractory intracranial hypertension (47,56,57), but is not routinely recommended.

Other complications of viral encephalitis, including seizures, cerebral venous thrombosis, cerebral infarction, and metabolic disturbance, are common. Patients are also at risk of general critical care complications such as aspiration pneumonia, urinary tract and other infections, and coagulopathy. The management of the various non-neurological complications is discussed in detail in Chapter 27.

Specific treatment of immune-mediated encephalitis

In the absence of randomized controlled trials, the optimal treatment of immune-mediated encephalitis is uncertain. High-dose

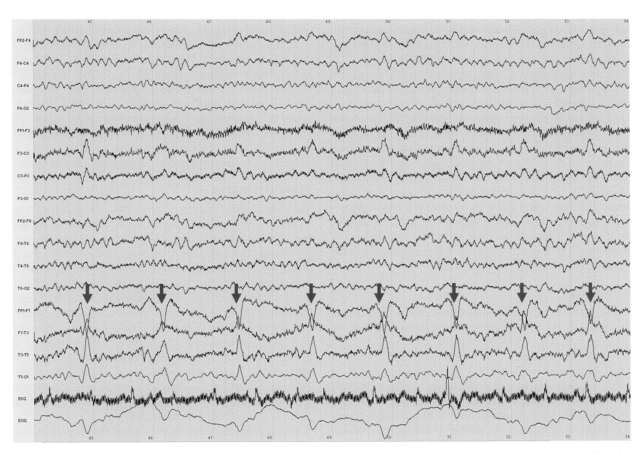

Fig. 24.3 Digital 16-channel electroencephalogram in a patient with herpes simplex encephalitis. Note the periodic lateralized epileptiform discharges (PLEDs) over the left hemisphere (best seen in FP1–F7, T3–T5, and T5–O1, arrows) and predominant left temporal lobe involvement.

Courtesy of Iris Unterberger, MD, EEG laboratory, Department of Neurology, Innsbruck Medical University.

intravenous corticosteroids are widely used as first-line therapy in ADEM, and other non-specific immunomodulatory therapies, including co-administration of cyclophosphamide, plasma exchange, or intravenous immunoglobulins, are often recommended in patients who do not respond to steroids (26–28). Most patients with anti-NMDA receptor encephalitis are also treated with corticosteroids in addition to intravenous immunoglobulin or plasma exchange. Second-line immunotherapy with rituximab, cyclophosphamide, or azathioprine may be helpful in non-responders. As noted earlier, all patients with autoantibody-associated encephalitis should be investigated for an associated tumour because tumour resection with immunotherapy is associated with a faster response making second-line therapy less likely (29).

Isolation

Isolation of immunocompetent patients with community-acquired infective encephalitis is not mandatory for infection control purposes, but is required for immunosuppressed patients and for those with exanthematous encephalitis and contagious viral haemorrhagic fever (2).

Acute bacterial meningitis

Meningitis refers to an inflammation of the membranes surrounding the brain and spinal cord and the interposed CSF, and is classified into bacterial and aseptic subtypes. Aseptic meningitis is defined as meningeal inflammation without evidence of pyogenic (usually bacterial) infection of the CSF, and can be further subdivided into infectious (mainly non-bacterial) and non-infectious causes. In contrast, acute bacterial meningitis is a pyogenic infection characterized by a pronounced polymorphonuclear response in the CSF.

Acute bacterial meningitis remains an important cause of CNS infection worldwide. It is associated with substantial morbidity and mortality despite the availability of vaccines for immunoprophylaxis and antibiotics for treatment (9,58–62). The incidence of community-acquired bacterial meningitis is 2–5 per 100,000 population per year in developed countries and up to ten times higher in other parts of the world (4,8,33,63). Acute bacterial meningitis is among the top ten causes of infection-related death worldwide, and 25–50% of survivors suffer permanent neurological sequelae including hearing loss (in up to one-third), cognitive impairment, and focal neurological deficits (9,13,36). Acute bacterial meningitis can occur at any age and in previously healthy immune competent individuals, although is more comment in the immune-compromised and at extremes of age.

Infective agents

The causative organism of bacterial meningitis can be reliably predicted by the age of the patient, predisposing factors, underlying diseases, and immunological competence (Table 24.5).

Streptococcus pneumoniae (pneumococci) and *Neisseria meningitidis* (meningococci) are the predominant causes of community-acquired bacterial meningitis, followed by *Haemophilus influenzae* type b (Hib), group B streptococci and *Listeria monocytogenes* (4,34,36). The relative contribution of these infective agents differs according to time, location, access to healthcare, and age group. In developed countries, meningitis epidemiology has changed significantly since the introduction of conjugate vaccines against Hib and several serotypes of *Streptococcus pneumoniae*. As a consequence, the age-specific incidence of bacterial meningitis has decreased in

children in high-income countries, thereby increasing the proportion of adult patients contracting the disease. There is an emerging trend of *Haemophilus influenzae* meningitis caused by serotype a and uncapsulated strains (34). The introduction of immunoprophylaxis for meningococci which offers protection against serogroups A, C, Y, and W135 has led to reduced rates of meningococcal disease in developed countries. Recently, a meningococcal vaccine against the serogroup B of *Neisseria meningitidis* has been approved in the United States and Europe. Whether this vaccine works sufficiently well in protecting from disease has to be determined; however, results from trials show that this vaccine indeed triggers a strong immune response in infants and adolescents. In low-income countries, *Neisseria meningitidis* causes regular epidemics predominantly in a well-defined region of sub-Saharan Africa known as the 'meningitis belt'. In Southeast Asia, *Streptococcus suis* is an important cause of meningitis. Immunocompromised individuals, including asplenic patients and those receiving immunosuppressive medications, have increased rates of infection with *Listeria monocytogenes* and Gram-negative bacteria such as *Enterobacteriaceae* and *Pseudomonas aeruginosa* (2,4,8,9,36,64).

Differential diagnosis

The differential diagnosis of pyogenic CNS infections includes eosinophilic meningitis and parameningeal infections such as brain abscess, subdural empyema, and epidural abscess (2,4). Eosinophilic meningitis is characterized by a significant percentage (> 10%) of eosinophils in the CSF and is frequently caused by a parasitic infection of the CNS by helminths and protozoa. Pyogenic parameningeal infections occur because of direct spread from a contiguous site or by haematogenous seeding (65). Common causes of parameningeal infection include dental infections, sinusitis, otitis media, and mastoiditis. Primary infections that cause brain abscess by haematogenous spread include endocarditis, and (chronic) pulmonary, intra-abdominal, skin, and soft tissue infections. There is a wide range of parameningeal infection-causing pathogens including anaerobes, aerobic Gram-positive cocci, and Gram-negative rods. In contrast to community-acquired bacterial meningitis, parameningeal infections are frequently of poly-microbial origin (65–67).

Clinical features

The clinical presentation of acute bacterial meningitis is highly variable. Symptoms and signs include headache, nausea and vomiting, neck pain, focal neurological deficits, and impairment of consciousness. The diagnosis is more straightforward in the presence of the so-called meningitis syndrome comprising fever, signs of meningeal irritation such as neck stiffness, and altered mental status (2,4,9,58,59). In a retrospective study, this classic triad of meningitis was present in only 44% of microbiologically proven cases, but 95% of episodes were characterized by at least two of the four signs and symptoms of headache, fever, neck stiffness, and altered mental state (9,58). The diagnosis of meningitis can be difficult in some groups, such as immunocompromised individuals or those at extremes of age, because they may not present with typical symptoms and signs. This is also the case in patients with previously or partially treated bacterial meningitis.

Seizures have been reported in about 25% of patients with acute bacterial meningitis and are associated with a higher risk of unfavourable outcome. They are more likely in patients with focal abnormalities on neuroimaging, and in pneumococcal rather than meningococcal disease (2,4,64). A petechial skin rash or purpura

Table 24.5 Bacterial organisms causing meningitis in specific age groups and immunization states

Age group	Immunization status	Predominant bacterial organisms
< 1 month	Not applicable	Group B streptococci, *Escherichia coli*, *Listeria monocytogenes* (so-called neonatal pathogens)
1–3 months	Not applicable or first dose of 'primary immunization'	'Neonatal pathogens' plus *Streptococcus pneumoniae*, *Neisseria meningitidis*, *Haemophilus influenzae* type b
3–6 months	No immunization	*Streptococcus pneumoniae*, *Neisseria meningitidis*, *Haemophilus influenzae* type b
	More than two doses of primary immunization with Hib conjugate vaccine (PRP-OMP or HbOC)	*Streptococcus pneumoniae*, *Neisseria meningitidis*
7 months to 5 years	No immunization	*Streptococcus pneumoniae*, *Neisseria meningitidis*, *Haemophilus influenzae* type b
	Primary immunization completed	*Streptococcus pneumoniae* (non-PCV serotypes), *Neisseria meningitidis*
6–50 years	Primary immunization completed	*Streptococcus pneumoniae*, *Neisseria meningitidis*
> 50 years	Primary immunization completed	*Streptococcus pneumoniae*, *Neisseria meningitidis*
Very elderly patients or immunocompromised state		*Streptococcus pneumoniae*, *Listeria monocytogenes*, and other bacteria, e.g. Gram-negative rods

Hib, *H. influenzae* type b; PCV, pneumococcal conjugate vaccine.

Data from Beckham JD and Tyler KL, 2012, 'Neuro-Intensive Care of Patients With Acute CNS Infections', *Neurotherapeutics*, 9, pp. 124–138; Chaudhuri A *et al.*, 2008, 'EFNS Guideline on the Management of Community-Acquired Bacterial Meningitis: Report of an EFNS Task Force on Acute Bacterial Meningitis in Older Children and Adults', *European Journal of Neurology*, 15, pp. 649–659; Scarborough M and Thwaites GE, 2008, 'The Diagnosis and Management of Acute Bacterial Meningitis in Resource-Poor Settings', *The Lancet Neurology*, 7, pp. 637–648; and Thigpen MC *et al.*, 2011, 'Bacterial Meningitis in the United States, 1998–2007', *New England Journal of Medicine*, 364, pp. 2016–2025.

is highly suggestive of meningococcal meningitis but can also be associated with other bacterial or viral causes. Because patients with acute bacterial meningitis may suffer from predisposing disorders including head and neck infections, pneumonia, or endocarditis, additional appropriate diagnostic studies must be instituted dependent on the history and findings of the clinical examination.

Investigations

The primary purpose of the investigation of suspected acute bacterial meningitis is confirmation of the diagnosis and identification of the causative microorganism. Without doubt, CSF analysis by lumbar puncture is the essential part of the assessment and should be performed as soon as is safely possible (2,4,58,59). Lumbar puncture is contraindicated in patients with uncorrected coagulopathy, those receiving anticoagulation therapy (prior to reversal), or in those with symptoms and signs of raised ICP (68,69). Neuroimaging prior to lumbar puncture is advised in patients with new-onset seizures, focal neurological signs, a history of a CNS lesion, signs suggesting space-occupying lesions, immunocompromised state, and moderate to severe impairment of consciousness. Non-contrast CT findings are mostly unremarkable in the early phase of acute bacterial meningitis. Contrast-enhanced CT is superior and will identify abnormal meningeal enhancement over the cerebral convexity, in the basal cisterns and deep within the cortical sulci (70,71).

Importantly, if lumbar puncture is delayed or postponed, empirical antibiotic treatment should be commenced immediately after obtaining blood samples for culture. An algorithm based on international expert recommendations for the fast-track assessment and initial treatment of patients with suspected acute bacterial meningitis is summarized in Figure 24.4 (2,4,8,72,73).

CSF findings

Characteristic CSF findings supporting the diagnosis of community-acquired bacterial meningitis include polymorphonuclear pleocytosis, raised CSF protein concentration, and low CSF glucose concentration resulting in a decreased CSF to blood glucose ratio (Table 24.2). Low CSF glucose concentration in association with elevated CSF lactate confirms bacterial meningitis even in the absence of CSF pleocytosis. This is often referred to as 'status bacillosus' and is likely related to an insufficient cellular immune response in the CSF.

Gram stain and culture of the CSF are the current gold standards for diagnosis, and positive in 80–90% of patients with community-acquired bacterial meningitis when samples are obtained prior to the commencement of antibiotics. Pre-treatment with antibiotics reduces the sensitivity of CSF culture to approximately 50% but Gram stain sensitivity is not substantially reduced (2,4,58). CSF bacterial antigen measurement has limited sensitivity and is not recommended for routine use, although it may be helpful in patients who have received prior antibiotic therapy (4,74). PCR assays may identify the causative microorganisms in cases with negative Gram stain and culture findings (44).

CSF analysis should be repeated during the course of acute bacterial meningitis if the diagnosis is uncertain or if there is a poor clinical response to treatment. Of note, Gram stain and CSF culture should become negative after 48 hours of appropriate antibiotic therapy. Patients without clinical improvement after 24–48 hours of treatment should undergo further neuroimaging to rule out cerebral ischaemia/infarction, brain abscess, subdural empyema, cerebral venous thrombosis, hydrocephalus, or ventriculitis (4,59,64).

Management

Acute bacterial meningitis is a neurological emergency and clinical outcome is directly related to the immediate institution of appropriate therapy. The main therapeutic strategy is antibiotics, possibly in association with mitigation of the intrathecal inflammatory response with adjunctive agents such as dexamethasone.

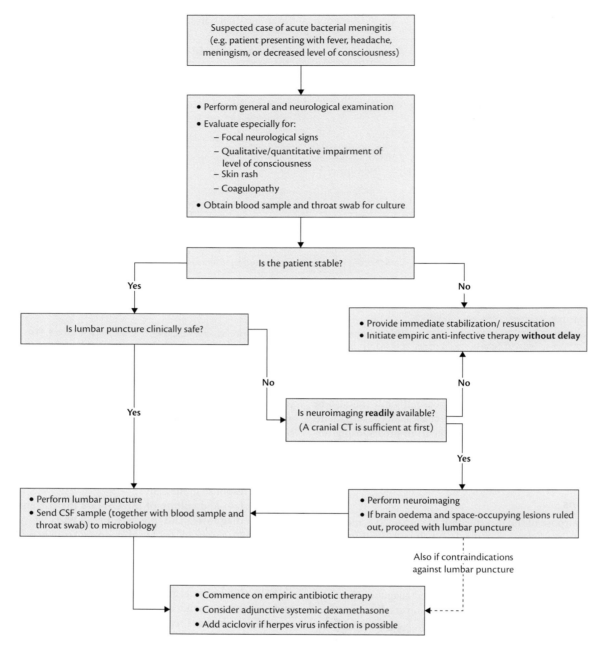

Fig. 24.4 Management algorithm for suspected acute bacterial meningitis.

Data from Beckham JD and Tyler KL, 2012, 'Neuro-Intensive Care of Patients With Acute CNS Infections', *Neurotherapeutics*, 9, pp. 124–138; Chaudhuri A *et al.*, 2008, 'EFNS Guideline on the Management of Community-Acquired Bacterial Meningitis: Report of an EFNS Task Force on Acute Bacterial Meningitis in Older Children and Adults', *European Journal of Neurology*, 15, pp. 649–659; Scarborough M and Thwaites GE, 2008, 'The Diagnosis and Management of Acute Bacterial Meningitis in Resource-Poor Settings', *The Lancet Neurology*, 7, pp. 637–648; Shin SH and Kim KS, 2012, 'Treatment of Bacterial Meningitis: an Update', *Expert Opinion in Pharmacotherapy*, 13, pp. 2189–2206; and van de Beek D *et al.*, 2006, 'Community-Acquired Bacterial Meningitis in Acults', *New England Journal of Medicine*, 354, pp. 44–53.

Antibiotics

The importance of early antibiotic administration cannot be over-estimated. A delay in starting treatment by more than 3 hours after presentation to hospital is independently associated with increased mortality (1,5,6). While some experts advocate antibiotic admin-istration to patients with suspected bacterial meningitis before or during transportation to hospital, consensus exists on rapid insti-tution of antibiotic therapy in the emergency department (2,4). Practice guidelines recommend broad-spectrum therapy until the

causative agent is confirmed. The choice of initial antibiotic should be based on local epidemiology, patterns of antimicrobial suscep-tibility, patient age, clinical setting, and the presence of underlying disease or risk factors (Table 24.6).

For suspected pneumococcal and meningococcal meningitis, third-generation cephalosporins such as cefotaxime, ceftriaxone, or ceftazidime are the established empirical agents of choice in Europe and North America in both children and adults (2,4,63,64,73,75). In areas with a high prevalence of cephalosporin-resistant pneumococci,

Table 24.6 Empirical antibiotic therapy for bacterial meningitis according to age group and suspected microorganisms

Age group/predisposing factor	Recommended antibiotics	Standard intravenous dosage[a]
< 1 month	Ampicillin plus gentamicin or ampicillin plus cefotaxime (can be used in the setting of suspected Gram-negative bacilli)	Ampicillin 50–100 mg/kg every 6–8 h; gentamicin 2.5 mg/kg every 12 h; cefotaxime 50 mg/kg every 6–8 h
1–3 months	Ampicillin plus third-generation cephalosporin (cefotaxime or ceftriaxone) or vancomycin (can be added in the setting of suspected pneumococcal meningitis based on Gram stain)	Ampicillin 50–100 mg/kg every 6–8 h; cefotaxime 50 mg/kg every 6–8 h; ceftriaxone 50 mg/kg every 12 h; vancomycin 20 mg/kg every 6 h
3 months to 5 years	Third-generation cephalosporin (cefotaxime or ceftriaxone) plus—if indicated to cover for resistant *S. pneumoniae*—vancomycin or rifampicin (dexamethasone[b] should be administered before or at the same time as the first antibiotic dosage)	Cefotaxime 50–75 mg/kg every 6–8 h (max. 12 g/day); ceftriaxone 50 mg/kg every 12 h (max. 4 g/day); vancomycin 20 mg/kg every 6–8 h (max. 2 g/day); rifampicin 10 mg/kg every 12 h (max. 600 mg/day)
6–50 years	Third-generation cephalosporin (cefotaxime or ceftriaxone) plus—if indicated to cover for resistant *S. pneumoniae*—vancomycin or linezolid or rifampicin (dexamethasone[b] should be administered before or at the same time as the first antibiotic dosage)	Cefotaxime 50–75 mg/kg every 6–8 h (max. 12 g/day); ceftriaxone 50 mg/kg every 12 h (max. 4 g/day); vancomycin 20 mg/kg every 6–8 h (max. 2 g/day); linezolid 600 mg every 12 h; rifampicin 10 mg/kg every 12 h (max. 600 mg/day)
> 50 years	Third-generation cephalosporin (cefotaxime or ceftriaxone) plus ampicillin plus vancomycin or linezolid	Cefotaxime 50–75 mg/kg every 6–8 h (max. 12 g/day); ceftriaxone 50 mg/kg every 12 h (max. 4 g/day); ampicillin 50–100 mg/kg every 6 h (max. 10–12 g/day), vancomycin 20 mg/kg every 6–8 h (max. 2 g/day); linezolid 600 mg every 12 h
Immunocompromised state	Vancomycin or linezolid plus meropenem or ceftazidime (alternatively cefepime)	Vancomycin 20 mg/kg every 6–8 h (max. 2 g/day); linezolid 600 mg every 12 h; meropenem 1–2 g every 8 h; ceftazidime 2 g every 8 h; cefepime 1–2 g every 8–12 h

[a] Antibiotic dosage adjustments may be necessary in patients with kidney and/or liver dysfunction.

[b] Adjunctive systemic steroid therapy (see text) with dexamethasone 10 mg every 6 h over the first 4 days of treatment.

Adapted from Tunkel AR *et al.*, 'Practice Guidelines for the Management of Bacterial Meningitis', *Clinical Infectious Diseases*, 2004, 39, 9, pp. 1267–1284, by permission of Oxford University Press. Data from Chaudhuri A *et al.*, 'EFNS guideline on the management of community-acquired bacterial meningitis: report of an EFNS Task Force on acute bacterial meningitis in older children and adults', *European Journal of Neurology*, 2008, 15, 7, pp. 649–659.

patients should receive vancomycin in addition to a third-generation cephalosporin (4,76). Alternative agents in these settings include rifampicin (in combination with vancomycin), a fluoroquinolone with antipneumococcal activity such as moxifloxacin or the oxazolidinone linezolid (63,77). *Listeria monocytogenes* is intrinsically resistant to cephalosporins, and an aminopenicillin or high-dose trimethoprim-sulfamethoxazole should be used in adults older than 50 years and immunosuppressed patients because of the higher risk of listerial meningitis in these groups. In severe cases, addition of an aminoglycoside should be considered. Fourth-generation cephalosporins or carbapenems should be administered to patients with suspected Gram-negative bacilli-related meningitis (4).

Once the bacterial pathogen is identified and antibiotic sensitivities confirmed, antimicrobial therapy should be modified accordingly. An overview of the recommended standard and alternative antibiotic regimes based on the results of CSF culture is shown in Table 24.7.

The global emergence of multidrug resistant bacteria has led to the consideration of newer antimicrobial agents such as daptomycin, tigecycline, moxifloxacin, cefepime, and ceftaroline for the treatment of acute bacterial meningitis. However, data on the use of these agents are limited to extrapolations from experimental studies, anecdotal reports, and small case series (63,78,79,80,81).

The optimum duration of therapy in community-acquired bacterial meningitis is a matter of debate. In high-income countries, consensus guidance recommends at least 7 days of treatment for *Neisseria meningitidis* and *Haemophilus influenzae* infections, and 10–14 days for *Streptococcus pneumoniae* meningitis. *Listeria monocytogenes* and Gram-negative bacilli meningitis should be treated for 3–4 weeks (4,64).

Steroids

Acute bacterial meningitis is characterized by an intense inflammatory response within the subarachnoid space which may be aggravated by bacterial disruption after the institution of antibiotic therapy. Experimental data suggest that outcome is related to the severity of this inflammatory response and that it can potentially be modified by anti-inflammatory therapies, but clinical studies investigating the potential benefit of adjuvant dexamethasone in children and adults with acute bacterial meningitis have yielded conflicting results (82,83). However, international consensus guidelines recommend adjuvant dexamethasone in non-immunocompromised patients with suspected or proven community-acquired bacterial meningitis in high-income countries (2,4,58). It should be given for 4 days at a dose of 10 mg intravenously every 6 hours in adults and 0.15 mg per kg bodyweight every 6 hours in children (2,4,58). Steroids should be discontinued if the patient is discovered not to have bacterial meningitis caused by *Streptococcus pneumoniae* or *Haemophilus influenzae*. If steroids are indicated, dexamethasone should be given shortly before or with the first parenteral dose of

Table 24.7 Antibiotic therapy of acute bacterial meningitis based on isolated pathogen and susceptibility testing

Microorganism (susceptibility)	Standard treatment	Alternative therapies
Streptococcus pneumoniae Penicillin-susceptible (MIC ≤ 0.06 mg/L) Penicillin-resistant (MIC ≥ 0.12 mg/L)	Penicillin G or ampicillin Cefotaxime or ceftriaxone plus vancomycin	Cefotaxime or ceftriaxone, cefepime, meropenem Fluoroquinolone (e.g. moxifloxacin) plus rifampicin (if MIC of ceftriaxone ≥ 2 mg/L)
Neisseria meningitidis Penicillin-susceptible (MIC < 0.1 mg/L) Penicillin-intermediate (MIC 0.1–1 mg/L)	Penicillin G or ampicillin Cefotaxime or ceftriaxone	Cefotaxime or ceftriaxone, chloramphenicol Meropenem, chloramphenicol, fluoroquinolone (e.g. moxifloxacin)
Haemophilus influenzae type b	Cefotaxime or ceftriaxone	Cefepime, fluoroquinolone (e.g. moxifloxacin), chloramphenicol
Listeria monocytogenes	Penicillin G or ampicillin (plus aminoglycoside)	Meropenem, trimethoprim-sulfamethoxazole
Group B streptococci (*S. agalactiae*)	Penicillin G or ampicillin (plus aminoglycoside)	Cefotaxime or ceftriaxone
Staphylococci Methicillin-susceptible Methicillin-resistant	Flucloxacillin (plus rifampicin) Vancomycin (plus rifampicin)	Clindamycin, vancomycin Linezolid, daptomycin, trimethoprim-sulfamethoxazole
Enterobacteriaceae (*E. coli* and others)	Cefotaxime or ceftriaxone	Meropenem, fluoroquinolone
Pseudomonas aeruginosa	Ceftazidime or cefepime (plus aminoglycoside)	Meropenem, ciprofloxacin (plus aminoglycoside)

MIC, minimal inhibitory concentration.

Data from Beckham JD and Tyler KL, 2012, 'Neuro-Intensive Care of Patients With Acute CNS Infections', *Neurotherapeutics*, 9, pp. 124–138; Chaudhuri A *et al.*, 2008, 'EFNS Guideline on the Management of Community-Acquired Bacterial Meningitis: Report of an EFNS Task Force on Acute Bacterial Meningitis in Older Children and Adults', *European Journal of Neurology*, 15, pp. 649–659; Scarborough M and Thwaites GE, 2008, 'The Diagnosis and Management of Acute Bacterial Meningitis in Resource-Poor Settings', *The Lancet Neurology*, 7, pp. 637–648; van de Beek D *et al.*, 2006, 'Community-Acquired Bacterial Meningitis in Adults', *New England Journal of Medicine*, 354, pp. 44–53; and Sinner SW and Tunkel AR, 2004, 'Antimicrobial Agents in the Treatment of Bacterial Meningitis', *Infectious Disease Clinics of North America*, 18, pp. 581–602.

antibiotic. High-dose corticosteroids are associated with a small increase in the risk of delayed cerebral thrombosis but a recent meta-analysis showed that the survival benefit in patients with pneumococcal meningitis outweighs this risk (83).

Other adjuvant therapies

Other adjunctive therapeutic strategies currently under investigation include antipyretic therapy with targeted temperature management (63). Despite some reported beneficial effects of reducing ICP in patients with bacterial meningitis (84), there is currently insufficient evidence to justify routine administration of hyperosmolar agents (19,20). Nevertheless, all measures for immediate ICP reduction must be taken in patients with intracranial hypertension and impending brain herniation (see Chapter 7).

Complications

Acute bacterial meningitis may result in obstructive hydrocephalus requiring external ventricular drainage. Electrolyte imbalances, particularly sodium disturbances, are also common. Hyponatraemia may be iatrogenic or related to the syndrome of inappropriate antidiuretic hormone secretion or cerebral salt wasting (see Chapter 28), but most episodes are benign and resolve spontaneously within a few days without specific treatment. Hypernatraemia on the other hand is associated with more severe disease and independently predicts unfavourable outcome (64).

A wide range of serious complications with adverse effects on outcome may be seen in patients with pneumococcal and meningococcal meningitis (4). The triad of *Streptococcus pneumoniae*-related

meningitis, endocarditis, and pneumonia is associated with high mortality, as is the development of septic shock secondary to pyogenic CNS infection. The most severe clinical course is seen in meningococcal sepsis presenting as purpura fulminans (Figure 24.5A) (85), or in asplenic patients in whom pneumococci can lead to an overwhelming pneumococcal sepsis syndrome and disseminated intravascular coagulopathy (Figure 24.5B).

Bacterial meningitis may also cause vascular complications. Ischaemia due to arterial occlusion or vasculitis occurs in up to 15% of patients, and cerebral venous infarction secondary to septic venous thrombosis in 3–5% (64). Experience with therapeutic anticoagulation is limited and treatment should only be considered in patients who experience rapid neurological deterioration because of brain swelling associated with venous outflow obstruction (4).

Public health issues

Given the substantial morbidity and mortality associated with acute bacterial meningitis, healthcare providers must not only be familiar with current treatment recommendations but also with prophylaxis guidelines to prevent outbreaks of contagious meningitis. All cases of suspected meningococcal or Hib meningitis should be reported urgently to local public health authorities. Patients suffering from meningitis, as well as asymptomatic carriers of Hib and meningococci, may pass the microorganisms via droplet or close contact spread to others who may in turn become carriers or develop invasive disease. Secondary cases in close contacts occur in 2–4 per 1000 population (4,72), and there are a number of settings with an established increased risk of secondary meningitis cases due to

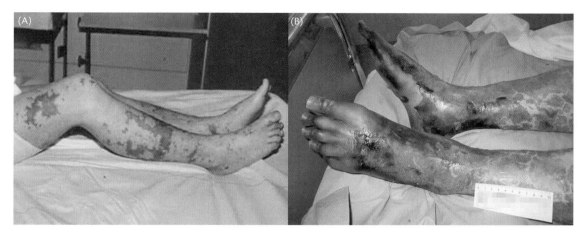

Fig. 24.5 The result of coagulation abnormalities in patients with Gram-negative and Gram-positive sepsis.
(A) Meningococcal septicaemia in a young male patient with confluent petechial and purpuric lesions (also referred to as 'purpura fulminans') propagating to suffusions on both lower extremities.
(B) Disseminated intravascular coagulopathy in an asplenic patient with overwhelming pneumococcal infection presenting with haemorrhagic necrosis and ischaemia of both distal lower extremities.

close and prolonged contact with the patient or carrier in the 7 days prior to their symptom onset. These include household, sexual, and travel contacts, as well as childcare, school, university, and health-care environments. The risk to healthcare workers is estimated to be 25 times that of the general population, but this excess risk is small and inappropriate use of chemoprophylaxis should be avoided. Only clinical personnel directly exposed to respiratory secretions of an index case, such as during 'unprotected' airway management without a facemask or mouth-to-mouth resuscitation, require chemoprophylaxis. Other healthcare staff members involved in routine patient management do not. Recommended chemoprophylaxis for haemophilus influenzae type b is oral rifampicin for 4 days, although this drug should be avoided in pregnant women. For *Neisseria meningitidis* the alternatives are oral rifampicin for 2 days, a single dose of intravenous/intramuscular ceftriaxone, or a single oral dose of either ciprofloxacin or azithromycin (72).

External ventricular drain and shunt infections

EVDs and ventricular shunts provide a reliable means of controlling elevated ICP secondary to acute or chronic hydrocephalus, and are commonly encountered in the NCCU. Bacterial colonization of the indwelling intracranial catheter is a major complication of external or internal CSF drainage and may result in ventriculitis, encephalitis, brain abscess, subdural empyema, and even systemic sepsis. Established EVD/shunt-associated ventriculitis is a potentially life-threatening condition which may lead to permanent neurological deficits in survivors.

The reported incidence of ventricular catheter-associated infection ranges from 2% to 45% (10,12), with an average rate of 9.5% in the last decade (86). A meta-analysis of 23 retrospective studies reported a cumulative rate of positive CSF cultures of 8.8% per patient and 8.1% per ventricular catheter episode (87). It has been suggested that the majority of catheter-associated ventriculitis occur within the first week after catheter insertion, but recent studies identified a later peak of infection at around 2 weeks, particularly in patients with severe intracranial pathology (87,88). Other

relevant predisposing factors for ventriculostomy-related infections are the frequency of CSF sampling and catheter irrigation, intraventricular and subarachnoid haemorrhage, surgical technique, and other infections (10,12,88). However, risk profiles have been inconsistently reported in the literature (89,90,91).

Aetiology

It is important to differentiate clinically relevant infections of the subarachnoid space that require immediate treatment from contamination and colonization by microorganisms of the catheter surface (87,88). Contamination constitutes an isolated positive CSF culture in the absence of abnormal CSF findings. In patients with a catheter *in situ*, colonization is defined by at least two positive CSF cultures with minor associated CSF changes and a lack of clinical signs other than fever. Of note, some experts consider positive CSF cultures in conjunction with any change in CSF cell count and chemistry as evidence of infection and advise antibiotic therapy even if the patient is classified as being colonized. Definite EVD/shunt infection is defined by positive CSF culture and abnormal CSF findings in association with clinical symptoms and signs, whereas pathological CSF findings in the absence of positive CSF cultures suggests device-related ventriculitis (Table 24.8). In addition, aseptic inflammation resulting from tissue response to brain injury or stimulation by non-infectious agents such as blood breakdown products should be distinguished from infection (92).

The microorganisms most frequently involved in catheter-associated ventriculitis are shown in Table 24.9. Gram-positive organisms such as coagulase-negative staphylococci and *Staphylococcus aureus* consistent with a skin flora source are the most common pathogens causing EVD/shunt-associated infections, and account for approximately two-thirds of nosocomial CSF infections (12,86–88,93). Other Gram-positive bacteria causing ventricular catheter-related infections include *Propionibacterium acnes* and enterococci. Despite the predominance of Gram-positive species, an increasing proportion of Gram-negative catheter-related ventriculitis is reported (93,94). The spectrum of potentially causative Gram-negative organisms is broad and includes Enterobacteriaceae such as *Escherichia coli, Klebsiella, Serratia,* and

Table 24.8 Definition of cerebrospinal fluid infections in patients with external ventricular drains or ventricular shunts

Contamination	Isolated positive CSF culture and/or Gram stain
	Expected CSF chemistry profile
	Expected CSF cell count
Colonization	Multiple positive CSF cultures and/or Gram stains
	Expected CSF chemistry profile
	Expected CSF cell count
	Lack of clinical signs and symptoms other than fever
Suspected ventricular catheter-related infection	Absence of positive CSF cultures or Gram stains
	Progressively declining CSF chemistry (i.e. decrease of glucose, increase of protein)
	Advancing CSF pleocytosis
Ventricular catheter-related infection	One or more positive CSF culture(s) or Gram stain(s)
	Low CSF glucose, increasing levels of CSF protein and lactate
	CSF pleocytosis
	Clinical signs of meningitis other than fever

Adapted from Lozier AP, Sciacca RR, Romagnoli MF, Connolly ES, Jr., 'Ventriculostomy-Related Infections: a Critical Review of the Literature', *Neurosurgery*, 2002, 51, pp. 170–181, with permission from Wolters Kluwer Health and the Congress of Neurological Surgeons. Springer and *Journal of Neurology*, 255, 2008, pp. 1617–1624, 'Nosocomial Ventriculitis and Meningitis in Neurocritical Care Patients', Beer R *et al.*, with kind permission from Springer Science and Business Media.

Enterobacter species and non-fermenters such as *Pseudomonas aeruginosa* and *Acinetobacter baumanii*. Anaerobes and fungi, primarily *Candida* species, are rarely implicated. Risk factors for fungal nosocomial CSF infections include broad-spectrum anti-infective therapy and compromised immune status (90). Poly-microbial infections have been reported in patients with ventriculoperitoneal (VP) shunts (95), and are serious complications of shunt tip-related intestinal perforation. Other intestinal diseases such as diverticulitis or (spontaneous) bacterial peritonitis have also been reported as

Table 24.9 Typical microorganisms causing ventricular catheter-associated infections

Microorganism	Percentage causation
Coagulase-negative staphylococci	47–65%
Staphylococcus aureus	12–29%
Propionibacterium acnes	1–14%
Gram-negative bacteria (e.g. *Enterobacteriaceae*, *Pseudomonas aeruginosa*)	6–20%
Polymicrobial infections	~ 15%
Anaerobes (e.g. *Bacteroides* spp.)	Rare
Candida spp.	Very rare

Adapted from Lozier AP, Sciacca RR, Romagnoli MF, Connolly ES, Jr., 'Ventriculostomy-Related Infections: a Critical Review of the Literature', *Neurosurgery*, 2002, 51, pp. 170–181. Springer and *Journal of Neurology*, 255, 2008, pp. 1617–1624, 'Nosocomial Ventriculitis and Meningitis in Neurocritical Care Patients', Beer R, Lackner P, Pfausler B, Schmutzhard E, figure number(s), with kind permission from Springer Science and Business Media.

causes of ascending catheter-infections in patients with VP shunts *in situ* (96). Differences in microbiological profiles between studies are likely related to differences in antibiotic usage and local flora.

Clinical features and diagnosis

Any suspected catheter-related infection must prompt an immediate diagnostic workup and, pending definitive diagnosis, the initiation of empirical antimicrobial therapy. Fever and deterioration in the level of consciousness or an increase in ICP in the comatose or sedated patient are important early indicators of intracranial infection (97). Neuroimaging (Figure 24.6) and CSF analysis are the cornerstones of the diagnosis. CT and MRI findings are similar and include identification of irregular ventricular debris and choroid plexitis confirmed by a poorly defined margin of a swollen choroid plexus and enhancement on contrast study (71).

Again it should be emphasized that diagnostic workup must not delay the initiation of appropriate antimicrobial therapy. In many cases lumbar puncture may be contraindicated because of intracranial hypertension, but CSF recovery may be possible through the EVD or via aspiration from the cranial end of a ventricular shunt. Analysis of ventricular CSF does not always confirm the diagnosis of ventriculitis because CSF circulation and therefore spread of the infecting organism can be impeded by blood or expanding mass lesions. A focal collection, such as a brain abscess or empyema, warrants immediate neurosurgical evacuation to reduce ICP and allow microbiological analysis of the purulent collection. In addition, samples from blood and other body fluids, such as secretions from paranasal sinuses, must be obtained (12,67). CSF cultures may require prolonged incubation times and negative results are not uncommon in patients receiving prior antibiotic therapy. A study comparing the results from Gram stain and CSF

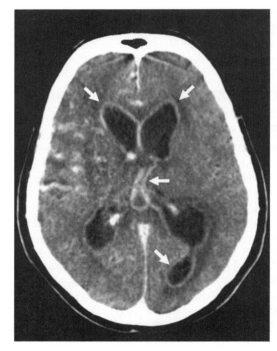

Fig. 24.6 Contrast-enhanced cranial computed tomography scan of a patient with fulminant ventriculitis. Note the choroid plexitis with massive ependymal enhancement (arrows).

culture demonstrated that Gram staining had a very high specificity but an unacceptably low sensitivity (18%) in screening for EVD/shunt-associated infections (98).

Management

An algorithm for the management of suspected EVD/shunt-associated ventriculitis is shown in Figure 24.7.

The empirical antimicrobial therapy of nosocomial ventriculitis must take into account the most likely pathogens, local resistance patterns, underlying disease processes, and patient factors as age, comorbidities, and immune status. The agents used must adequately penetrate the blood–brain and blood–CSF barriers. Initial therapy with an antistaphylococcal agent with good CSF penetration such as rifampicin or fosfomycin and a cephalosporin is often recommended as first-line therapy because of the high incidence of staphylococci-associated EVD/shunt-related ventriculitis. Initial empirical treatment with the glycopeptide antibiotic vancomycin, in combination with a cephalosporin with antipseudomonal activity or a carbapenem, is increasingly recommended in high-risk settings because of the risk that nosocomial intracranial infections might be caused by multidrug resistant Gram-positive and Gram-negative pathogens (10,12,67). In patients with a contraindication to systemic vancomycin administration (e.g. acute kidney injury) in whom an EVD is in place, vancomycin can safely be administered intrathecally with daily doses ranging from 10 to 20 mg (see 'Intrathecal antibiotics') (99). In terms of carbapenems, meropenem is the agent of choice in patients with CNS infections because the combination of imipenem and cilastatin has been associated with neurotoxicity and seizures (100). For patients with allergy to beta-lactam antibiotics, intravenous moxifloxacin is an alternative (101). The efficacy of linezolid and daptomycin for the treatment of Gram-positive ventriculitis has recently been confirmed (102–104). EVD/shunt infections due to antibiotic resistant *Acinetobacter* species is increasingly common and combination therapy with systemic and intrathecally administered polymyxins plus removal of infected devices is recommended (105). For the treatment of CNS fungal infections the triazole antifungal agent voriconazole and the polyene amphotericin B are promising options, but the use of echinocandins such as caspofungin remains controversial (88).

Intrathecal antibiotics

Management of device-associated CNS infections has become increasingly complex with the emergence of bacteria with reduced antibiotic sensitivity. Intraventricular administration of antibiotics represents an alternative strategy to the systemic route to optimize anti-infective drug delivery to the CSF (99). However, the use of intrathecal antimicrobials is challenging and there are limited clinical data to support this route of administration in adults which is potentially toxic and requires careful preparation and delivery of drugs to avoid infection. Some experts therefore recommend that intrathecal administration should be reserved for circumstances in which intravenous therapy has failed. However, it should be considered in the presence of severe ventriculitis, persistently positive CSF cultures despite appropriate intravenous drug dosing, multidrug resistant pathogen requiring a specific antimicrobial agent that does not achieve target concentrations in the CSF when given by another route, adverse reaction or comorbidities leading to intolerance of systemic administration, and in the rare cases when

device removal is not feasible (106). There is no standard approach to intrathecal antimicrobial dosing, although targeting a CSF concentration ten times the minimal inhibitory concentration of the drug for the isolated pathogen is believed to be adequate to achieve rapid eradication. Calculation of this 'inhibitory quotient' prior to subsequent doses of intrathecal therapy ensures optimal dosing. The greatest clinical experience is with vancomycin (usually a 10–20 mg dose per day) and gentamicin (usual daily dose in adults is 4–8 mg), and there is very limited literature on the intrathecal administration of other antimicrobial agents (99,106).

Drug therapy should always be rationalized when pathogen sensitivity results are available. Recommendations on the duration of antimicrobial therapy for catheter-associated ventriculitis have not been studied rigorously. Treatment is usually continued for 10–14 days but some experts suggest shorter duration therapy if repeated CSF cultures are negative and the CSF white cell count is low. It is crucially important that therapy of nosocomial CSF infections is individualized because some patients with prior or concurrent anti-infective therapy may need continued empirical antimicrobial treatment despite negative CSF Gram stain or culture (10). Of note, in the setting of a delayed or incomplete clinical response, longer courses of antimicrobial therapy may be warranted until resolution of local and/or systemic symptoms and signs such as meningeal irritation and fever.

Recurrence of nosocomial CSF infections is reported in 25% of cases (107), and a high level of suspicion must therefore be maintained after termination of antimicrobial therapy.

Catheter removal

The routine prophylactic exchange of non-infected EVDs remains controversial (108), but consensus does exist on the timely removal of catheters infected with pathogens capable of forming a biofilm (109). Importantly, catheter removal requires concomitant antimicrobial therapy (67). There are few data addressing optimal timing of device replacement or conversion of an EVD to a ventricular shunt after an episode of ventriculitis. However, it is generally agreed that, prior to shunt (re-) placement, the CSF should be sterile for 3 days in the setting of colonization and up to 10 days in infections with more virulent pathogens (106).

Prevention of ventricular catheter infections

Because of the potential pitfalls in the early diagnosis of catheter-related ventriculitis and subsequent delay in the initiation of appropriate antimicrobial therapy, prevention is of paramount importance. Preventive measures include meticulous surgical technique and possibly the prophylactic administration of antibiotics during catheter insertion, although the potential benefits of periprocedural antibiotics may be outweighed by predisposition to subsequent infection with more resistant pathogens and associated increased mortality (90,110).

An important strategy in the infection control process is microbiological surveillance of the CSF. Although surveillance CSF samples are taken routinely from an EVD there is no consensus on the optimal sampling frequency. Routine CSF sampling has been recommended daily, every 3–5 days, only at EVD insertion or removal and only when clinically indicated (98). Minimizing disruption of the EVD system for CSF sampling is itself likely to minimize the risk of device-associated infection, and a recent study suggested that it is safe and cost effective to reduce surveillance sampling to every

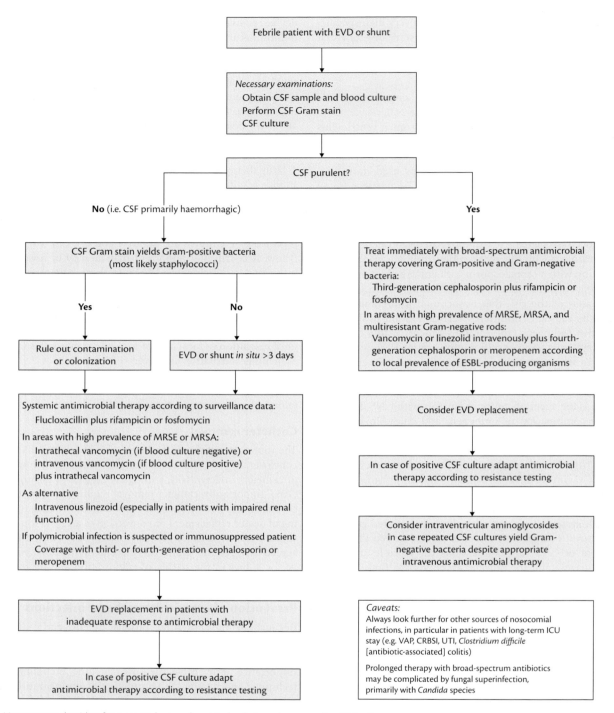

Fig. 24.7 Management algorithm for suspected external ventricular drain or shunt-associated infection.
CRBSI, catheter-related bloodstream infection; ESBL, extended spectrum beta-lactamases; MRSA, methicillin-resistant *Staphylococcus aureus*; MRSE, methicillin-resistant *Staphylococcus epidermidis*;
UTI, urinary tract infection; VAP, ventilator-associated pneumonia.
Adapted from Beer R, Pfausler B, Schmutzhard E, 'Infectious Intracranial Complications in the Neuro-ICU Patient Population', *Current Opinion in Critical Care*, 16, pp. 117–122, Copyright © 2010
Wolters Kluwer Health.

third day (111). In addition, routine exchange of indwelling devices does not significantly reduce the incidence of catheter-associated ventriculitis because infection may be acquired by introduction of bacteria during insertion of a new catheter (107).

The use of antimicrobial-impregnated ventriculostomy catheters has been reported to reduce bacterial colonization along the catheter surface and the risk of device-related ventriculitis (112), but the potential for induction of antimicrobial resistance is a concern (113). Catheters impregnated with silver nanoparticles are also associated with reduced infection rates but do not have the disadvantage of the development of antibiotic resistance (114).

References

1. Auburtin M, Wolff M, Charpentier J, Varon E, Le Tulzo Y, Girault C, et al. Detrimental role of delayed antibiotic administration and penicillin-nonsusceptible strains in adult intensive care unit patients with pneumococcal meningitis: the PNEUMOREA Prospective Multicenter Study. Crit Care Med. 2006;34:2758–65.

2. Beckham JD, Tyler KL. Neuro-intensive care of patients with acute CNS infections. Neurotherapeutics. 2012;9:124–38.

3. Brun R, Blum J. Human African trypanosomiasis. Infect Dis Clin North Am. 2012;26:261–73.

4. Chaudhuri A, Martinez-Martin P, Kennedy PG, Andrew Seaton R, Portegies P, Bojar M, et al. EFNS guideline on the management of community-acquired bacterial meningitis: report of an EFNS Task Force on acute bacterial meningitis in older children and adults. Eur J Neurol. 2008;15:649–59.

5. Køster-Rasmussen R, Korshin A, Meyer CN. Antibiotic treatment delay and outcome in acute bacterial meningitis. J Infect. 2008;57:449–54.

6. Proulx N, Fréchette D, Toye B, Chan J, Kravcik, S. Delays in the administration of antibiotics are associated with mortality from adult acute bacterial meningitis. QJM. 2005;98:291–8.

7. Jmor F, Emsley HC, Fischer M, Solomon T, Lewthwaite P. The incidence of acute encephalitis syndrome in western industrialised and tropical countries. Virol J. 2008;5:134.

8. Scarborough M, Thwaites GE. The diagnosis and management of acute bacterial meningitis in resource-poor settings. Lancet Neurol. 2008;7:637–48.

9. van de Beek D, de Gans J, Spanjaard L, Weisfelt M, Reitsma JB, Vermeulen M. Clinical features and prognostic factors in adults with bacterial meningitis. N Engl J Med. 2004;351:1849–59.

10. Beer R, Pfausler B, Schmutzhard E. Infectious intracranial complications in the neuro-ICU patient population. Curr Opin Crit Care. 2010;16:117–22.

11. Kim HI, Kim SW, Park, GY, Kwon EG, Kim HH, Jeong JY, et al. The causes and treatment outcomes of 91 patients with adult nosocomial meningitis. Korean J Intern Med. 2012;27:171–9.

12. van de Beek D, Drake JM, Tunkel AR. Nosocomial bacterial meningitis. N Engl J Med. 2010;362:146–54.

13. Edmond K, Clark A, Korczak VS, Sanderson C, Griffiths UK, Rudan I. Global and regional risk of disabling sequelae from bacterial meningitis: a systematic review and meta-analysis. Lancet Infect Dis. 2010;10:317–28.

14. Kennedy PG. Viral encephalitis. J Neurol. 2005;252:268–72.

15. Koedel U, Klein M, Pfister HW. New understandings on the pathophysiology of bacterial meningitis. Curr Opin Infect Dis. 2010;23:217–23.

16. Parikh V, Tucci V, Galwankar S. Infections of the nervous system. Int J Crit Illn Inj Sci. 2012;2:82–97.

17. Craig S. Phenytoin poisoning. Neurocrit Care. 2005;3:161–70.

18. Chitturi S, George J. Hepatotoxicity of commonly used drugs: non-steroidal anti-inflammatory drugs, antihypertensives, antidiabetic agents, anticonvulsants, lipid-lowering agents, psychotropic drugs. Semin Liver Dis. 2002;22:169–83.

19. Ajdukiewicz KM, Cartwright KE, Scarborough M, Mwambene JB, Goodson P, Molyneux ME, et al. Glycerol adjuvant therapy in adults with bacterial meningitis in a high HIV seroprevalence setting in Malawi: a double-blind, randomised controlled trial. Lancet Infect Dis. 2011;11:293–300.

20. Mohanty S, Mishra SK, Patnaik R, Dutt AK, Pradhan S, Das B, et al. Brain swelling and mannitol therapy in adult cerebral malaria: a randomized trial. Clin Infect Dis. 2011;53:349–55.

21. Solomon T, Dung NM, Kneen R, Thao le TT, Gainsborough M, Nisalak A, et al. Seizures and raised intracranial pressure in Vietnamese patients with Japanese encephalitis. Brain. 2002;125:1084–93.

22. Solomon T, Hart IJ, Beeching NJ. Viral encephalitis: a clinician's guide. Pract Neurol. 2007;7:288–305.

23. Solomon T, Michael BD, Smith PE, Sanderson F, Davies NW, Hart IJ, et al. Management of suspected viral encephalitis in

adults—Association of British Neurologists and British Infection Association National Guidelines. J Infect. 2012;64:347–73.

24. Steiner I, Budka H, Chaudhuri A, Koskiniemi M, Sainio K, Salonen O, et al. Viral meningoencephalitis: a review of diagnostic methods and guidelines for management. Eur J Neurol. 2010;17:999-e57.

25. Granerod J, Tam CC, Crowcroft NS, Davies NW, Borchert M, Thomas SL. Challenge of the unknown. A systematic review of acute encephalitis in non-outbreak situations. Neurology. 2010;75:924–32.

26. Sonneville R, Klein IF, Wolff M. Update on investigation and management of postinfectious encephalitis. Curr Opin Neurol. 2010;23:300–4.

27. Tenembaum S, Chitnis T, Ness J, Hahn JS, International Pediatric MS Study Group. Acute disseminated encephalomyelitis. Neurol. 2007;68(Suppl 2):S23–36.

28. Wender M. Acute disseminated encephalomyelitis (ADEM). J Neuroimmunol. 2011;231:92–9.

29. Dalmau J, Lancaster E, Martinez-Hernandez E, Rosenfeld MR, Balice-Gordon R. Clinical experience and laboratory investigations in patients with anti-NMDAR encephalitis. Lancet Neurol. 2011;10:63–74.

30. Vincent A, Buckley C, Schott JM, Baker I, Dewar BK, Detert N, et al. Potassium channel antibody-associated encephalopathy: a potentially immunotherapy-responsive form of limbic encephalitis. Brain. 2004;127:701–12.

31. Child N, Croxson MC, Rahnama F, Anderson NE. A retrospective review of acute encephalitis in Adults in Auckland over a five-year period (2005–2009). J Clin Neurosci. 2012;19:1483–5.

32. Huppatz C, Durrheim DN, Levi C, Dalton C, Williams D, Clements MS, et al. Etiology of encephalitis in Australia, 1990–2007. Emerg Infect Dis. 2009;15:1359–65.

33. Centers for Disease Control and Prevention (CDC). Comparison of meningococcal disease surveillance systems—United States, 2005–2008. MMWR Morbid Mortal Wkly Rep. 2012;61:306–8.

34. McIntyre PB, O'Brien KL, Greenwood B, van de Beek D. Effect of vaccines on bacterial meningitis worldwide. Lancet. 2012;380:1703–11.

35. Ojo LR, O'Loughlin RE, Cohen AL, Loo JD, Edmond KM, Shetty SS, et al. Global use of Haemophilus influenzae type b conjugate vaccine. Vaccine. 2010;28:7117–22.

36. Thigpen MC, Whitney CG, Messonnier NE, Zell ER, Lynfield R, Hadler JL, et al. Bacterial meningitis in the United States, 1998–2007. N Engl J Med. 2011;364:2016–25.

37. Denizot M, Neal JW, Gasque P. Encephalitis due to emerging viruses: CNS innate immunity and potential therapeutic targets. J Infect. 2012;65:1–16.

38. Donoso Mantke O, Escadafal C, Niedrig M, Pfeffer M, on behalf of the Working Group For Tick-Borne Encephalitis Virus. Tick-borne encephalitis in Europe, 2007 to 2009. Eurosurveillance. 2011;16:pii:19976.

39. Turtle L, Griffiths MJ, Solomon T. Encephalitis caused by flaviviruses. QJM. 2012;105:219–23.

40. Kilpatrick AM, Randolph SE. Drivers, dynamics, and control of emerging vector-borne zoonotic diseases. Lancet. 2012;380:1946–55.

41. Gregory CJ, Ndiaye S, Patel M, Hakizamana E, Wannemuehler K, Ndinga E, et al. Investigation of elevated case-fatality rate in poliomyelitis outbreak in Pointe Noire, Republic of Congo, 2010. Clin Infect Dis. 2012;55: 1299–306.

42. Sips GJ, Wilschut J, Smit JM. Neuroinvasive flavivirus infections. Rev Med Virol. 2012;22:69–87.

43. Meyding-Lamadé U, Strank C. Herpesvirus infections of the central nervous system in immunocompromised patients. Ther Adv Neurol Disord. 2012;5:279–96.

44. Steiner I, Schmutzhard E, Sellner J, Chaudhuri A, Kennedy PG. EFNS-ENS guidelines for the use of PCR technology for the diagnosis of infections of the nervous system. Eur J Neurol. 2012;19:1278–91.

45. Rath TJ, Hughes M, Arabi M, Shah GV. Imaging of cerebritis, encephalitis, and brain abscess. Neuroimaging Clin N Am. 2012;22:585–607.

46. Tunkel AR, Glaser CA, Bloch KC, Sejvar JJ, Marra CM, Roos KL, et al. The management of encephalitis: clinical practice guidelines by the Infectious Diseases Society of America. Clin Infect Dis. 2008;47:303–27.

47. Domingues RB. Viral encephalitis: current treatments and future perspectives. *Cent Nerv Syst Agents Med Chem.* 2012;12:277–85.
48. Gupta RK, Soni N, Kumar S, Khandelwal N. Imaging of central nervous system viral diseases. *J Magn Reson Imaging.* 2012;35:477–91.
49. Marchbank ND, Howlett DC, Sallomi DF, Hughes DV. Magnetic resonance imaging is preferred in diagnosing suspected cerebral infections. *BMJ.* 2000;320:187–8.
50. Siguier M, Sellier P, Bergmann JF. BK-virus infections: a literature review. *Med Mal Infect.* 2012;42:181–7.
51. Kalita J, Nair PP, Misra UK. Status epilepticus in encephalitis: a study of clinical findings, magnetic resonance imaging, and response to antiepileptic drugs. *J Neurovirol.* 2008;14:412–17.
52. Misra UK, Kalita J, Nair PP. Status epilepticus in central nervous system infections: an experience from a developing country. *Am J Med.* 2008;121:618–23.
53. Whitley RJ. Herpes simplex encephalitis: adolescents and adults. *Antiviral Res.* 2006;71:141–8.
54. Raschilas F, Wolff M, Delatour F, Chaffaut C, De Broucker T, Chevret S, et al. Outcome of and prognostic factors for herpes simplex encephalitis in adult patients: results of a multicenter study. *Clin Infect Dis.* 2002;35:254–60.
55. Martinez-Torres F, Menon S, Pritsch M, Victor N, Jenetzky E, Jensen K, et al. Protocol for German trial of acyclovir and corticosteroids in herpes-simplex-virus-encephalitis (GACHE): a multicenter, multinational, randomized, double-blind, placebo-controlled German, Austrian and Dutch Trial [ISRCTN45122933]. *BMC Neurol.* 2008;8:40.
56. Kutleša M, Baršić B, Lepur D. Therapeutic hypothermia for adult viral meningoencephalitis. *Neurocrit Care.* 2011;15:151–5.
57. Pérez-Bovet J, Garcia-Armengol R, Buxó-Pujolràs M, Lorite-Díaz N, Narváez-Martínez Y, Caro-Cardera JL, et al. Decompressive craniectomy for encephalitis with brain herniation: case report and review of the literature. *Acta Neurochir (Wien).* 2012;154:1717–24.
58. Brouwer MC, Thwaites GE, Tunkel AR, van de Beek D. Dilemmas in the diagnosis of acute community-acquired bacterial meningitis. *Lancet.* 2012;380:1684–92.
59. Fitch MT, van de Beek D. Emergency diagnosis and treatment of adult meningitis. *Lancet Infect Dis.* 2007;7:191–200.
60. Lu CH, Huang CR, Chang WN, Chang CJ, Cheng BC, Lee PY, et al. Community-acquired bacterial meningitis in adults: the epidemiology, timing of appropriate antimicrobial therapy, and prognostic factors. *Clin Neurol Neurosurg.* 2002;104:352–8.
61. Viner RM, Booy R, Johnson H, Edmunds WJ, Hudson L, Bedford H, et al. Outcomes of invasive Meningococcal Serogroup B Disease in Children and Adolescents (MOSAIC): a case-control study. *Lancet Neurol.* 2012;11:774–83.
62. Vyse A, Wolter JM, Chen J, Ng T, Soriano-Gabarro M. Meningococcal disease in Asia: an under-recognized public health burden. *Epidemiol Infect.* 2011;139:967–85.
63. van de Beek D, Brouwer MC, Thwaites GE, Tunkel AR. Advances in treatment of bacterial meningitis. *Lancet,* 2012;380:1693–702.
64. Schut ES, de Gans J, van de Beek D. Community-acquired bacterial meningitis in adults. *Pract Neurol.* 2008;8:8–23.
65. Mace SE. Central nervous system infections as a cause of an altered mental status? What is the pathogen growing in your central nervous system? *Emerg Med Clin N Am.* 2010;28:535–70.
66. Nau R, Sörgel F, Eiffert H. Penetration of drugs through the blood-cerebrospinal fluid/blood-brain barrier for treatment of central nervous system infections. *Clin Microbiol Rev.* 2010;23:858–83.
67. Ziai WC, Lewin JJ, 3rd Advances in the management of central nervous system infections in the ICU. *Crit Care Clin.* 2006;22:661–94.
68. Joffe AR. Lumbar puncture and brain herniation in acute bacterial meningitis: a review. *J Intens Care Med.* 2007;22:194–207.
69. van Crevel H, Hijdra A, de Gans J. Lumbar puncture and the risk of herniation: when should we first perform CT? *J Neurol.* 2002;249:129–37.
70. Hegde AN, Mohan S, Pandya A, Shah GV. Imaging in infections of the head and neck. *Neuroimaging Clin N Am.* 2012;22:727–54.
71. Mohan S, Jain KK, Arabi M, Shah GV. Imaging of meningitis and ventriculitis. *Neuroimaging Clin N Am.* 2012;22:557–83.
72. Shin SH, Kim KS. Treatment of bacterial meningitis: an update. *Expert Opin Pharmacother.* 2012;13:2189–206.
73. van de Beek D, de Gans J, Tunkel AR, Wijdicks EF. Community-acquired bacterial meningitis in adults. *N Engl J Med.* 2006;354:44–53.
74. Nigrovic LE, Kuppermann N, McAdam AJ, Malley R. Cerebrospinal latex agglutination fails to contribute to the microbiologic diagnosis of pretreated children with meningitis. *Pediatr Infect Dis J.* 2004;23:786–8.
75. Sinner SW, Tunkel AR. Antimicrobial agents in the treatment of bacterial meningitis. *Infect Dis Clin North Am.* 2004;18:581–602.
76. Whitney CG, Farley MM, Hadler J, Harrison LH, Lexau C, Reingold A, et al. Increasing prevalence of multidrug-resistant streptococcus pneumoniae in the United States. *N Engl J Med.* 2000;343:1917–24.
77. Corti G, Cinelli R, and Paradisi F. Clinical and microbiologic efficacy and safety profile of linezolid, a new oxazolidinone antibiotic. *Int J Antimicrob Agents.* 2000;16:527–30.
78. Cottagnoud P, Pfister M, Acosta F, Cottagnoud M, Flatz L, Kühn F, et al. Daptomycin is highly efficacious against penicillin-resistant and penicillin- and quinolone-resistant pneumococci in experimental meningitis. *Antimicrob Agents Chemother.* 2004;48:3928–33.
79. Grandgirard D, Oberson K, Bühlmann A, Gäumann R, Leib SL. Attenuation of cerebrospinal fluid inflammation by the nonbacteriolytic antibiotic daptomycin versus that by ceftriaxone in experimental pneumococcal meningitis. *Antimicrob Agents Chemother.* 2010;54:1323–6.
80. Sipahi OR, Turhan T, Pullukcu H, Calik S, Tasbakan M, Sipahi H, et al. Moxifloxacin versus ampicillin plus gentamicin in the therapy of experimental Listeria monocytogenes meningitis. *J Antimicrob Chemother.* 2008;61:670–3.
81. Zhanel GG, Yachison C, Nichol K, Adam H, Noreddin AM, Hoban DJ, et al. Assessment of the activity of ceftaroline against clinical isolates of penicillin-intermediate and penicillin-resistant Streptococcus pneumoniae with elevated MICs of ceftaroline using an in vitro pharmacodynamic model. *J Antimicrob Chemother.* 2012;67:1706–11.
82. de Gans J, van de Beek D, European Dexamethasone in Adulthood Bacterial Meningitis Study Investigators. Dexamethasone in adults with bacterial meningitis. *N Engl J Med.* 2002;347:1549–56.
83. van de Beek D, Farrar JJ, de Gans J, Mai NT, Molyneux EM, Peltola H, et al. Adjunctive dexamethasone in bacterial meningitis: a meta-analysis of individual patient data. *Lancet Neurol.* 2010;9:254–63.
84. Glimåker M, Johansson B, Halldorsdottir H, Wanecek M, Elmi-Terander A, Ghatan PH, et al. Neuro-intensive treatment targeting intracranial hypertension improves outcome in severe bacterial meningitis: an intervention-control study. *PLoS One.* 2014;25:e91976.
85. Schoeller T, Schmutzhard E. Waterhouse-Friderichsen syndrome. *N Engl J Med.* 2001;344:1372.
86. Kim JH, Desai NS, Ricci J, Stieg PE, Rosengart AJ, Härtl R, et al. Factors contributing to ventriculostomy infection. *World Neurosur.* 2012;77:135–40.
87. Lozier AP, Sciacca RR, Romagnoli MF, Connolly ES, Jr. Ventriculostomy-related infections: a critical review of the literature. *Neurosurgery.* 2002;51:170–81.
88. Beer R, Lackner P, Pfausler B, Schmutzhard E. Nosocomial ventriculitis and meningitis in neurocritical care patients. *J Neurol.* 2008;255:1617–24.
89. Korinek AM, Baugnon T, Golmard JL, van Effenterre R, Coriat P, Puybasset L. Risk factors for adult nosocomial meningitis after craniotomy: role of antibiotic prophylaxis. *Neurosurgery.* 2006;59:126–33.
90. Korinek AM, Golmard JL, Elcheick A, Bismuth R, van Effenterre R, Coriat P, et al. Risk factors for neurosurgical site infections after craniotomy: a critical reappraisal of antibiotic prophylaxis on 4,578 patients. *Br J Neurosurg.* 2005;19:155–62.
91. Park P, Garton HJ, Kocan MJ, Thompson BG. Risk of infection with prolonged ventricular catheterization. *Neurosurgery.* 2004;55:594–9.

92. Zarrouk V, Vassor I, Bert F, Bouccara D, Kalamarides M, Bendersky N, et al. Evaluation of the management of postoperative aseptic meningitis. Clin Infect Dis. 2007;44:1555–9.

93. Conen A, Walti LN, Merlo A, Fluckiger U, Battegay M, Trampuz A. Characteristics and treatment outcome of cerebrospinal fluid shunt-associated infections in adults: a retrospective analysis over an 11-year period. Clin Infect Dis. 2008;47:73–82.

94. Camacho EF, Boszczowski I, Basso M, Jeng BC, Freire MP, Guimarães T, et al. Infection rate and risk factors associated with infections related to external ventricular drain. Infection. 2011;39:47–51.

95. Vinchon M, Baroncini M, Laurent T, Patrick D. Bowel perforation caused by peritoneal shunt catheters: diagnosis and treatment. Neurosurgery. 2006;58 (Suppl 1):ONS76–ONS82.

96. Chung JJ, Yu, JS, Kim JH, Nam SJ, Kim MJ. Intraabdominal complications secondary to ventriculoperitoneal shunts: CT findings and review of the literature. AJR Am J Roentgenol. 2009;193:1311–17.

97. Beer R, Pfausler B, Schmutzhard E. Management of nosocomial external ventricular drain-related ventriculomeningitis. Neurocrit Care. 2009;10:363–7.

98. Schade RP, Schinkel J, Roelandse FW, Geskus RB, Visser LG, van Dijk JM, et al. Lack of value of routine analysis of cerebrospinal fluid for prediction and diagnosis of external drainage-related bacterial meningitis. J Neurosurg. 2006;104:101–8.

99. Ziai WC, Lewin JJ, 3rd. Improving the role of intraventricular antimicrobial agents in the management of meningitis. Curr Opin Neurol. 2009;22:277–82.

100. Linden P. Safety profile of meropenem: an updated review of over 6,000 patients treated with meropenem. Drug Saf. 2007;30:657–68.

101. Kanellakopoulou K, Pagoulatou A, Stroumpoulis K, Vafiadou M, Kranidioti H, Giamarellou H, et al. Pharmacokinetics of moxifloxacin in non-inflamed cerebrospinal fluid of humans: implication for a bactericidal effect. J Antimicrob Chemother. 2008;61:1328–31.

102. Beer R, Engelhardt KW, Pfausler B, Broessner G, Helbok R, Lackner P, et al. Pharmacokinetics of intravenous linezolid in cerebrospinal fluid and plasma in neurointensive care patients with staphylococcal ventriculitis associated with external ventricular drains. Antimicrob Agents Chemother. 2007;51:379–82.

103. Elvy J, Porter D, Brown E. Treatment of external ventricular drain-associated ventriculitis caused by Enterococcus faecalis with intraventricular daptomycin. J Antimicrob Chemother. 2008;61:461–2.

104. Myrianthefs P, Markantonis SL, Vlachos K, Anagnostaki M, Boutzouka E, Panidis D, et al. Serum and cerebrospinal fluid concentrations of linezolid in neurosurgical patients. Antimicrob Agents Chemother. 2006;50:3971–6.

105. Kim BN, Peleg AY, Lodise TP, Lipman J, Li J, Nation R, et al. Management of meningitis due to antibiotic-resistant Acinetobacter species. Lancet Infect Dis. 2009;9:245–55.

106. Tunkel AR, Hartman BJ, Kaplan SL, Kaufman BA, Roos KL, Scheld WM, et al. Practice guidelines for the management of bacterial meningitis. Clin Infect Dis. 2004;39:1267–84.

107. Kestle JR, Garton HJ, Whitehead WE, Drake JM, Kulkarni AV, Cochrane DD, et al. Management of shunt infections: a multicenter pilot study. J Neurosurg. 2006;105:177–81.

108. Lo CH, Spelman D, Bailey M, Cooper, DJ, Rosenfeld JV, Brecknell JE. External ventricular drain infections are independent of drain duration: an argument against elective revision. J Neurosurg. 2007;106:378–83.

109. Vajramani GV, Jones G, Bayston R, Gray WP. Persistent and intractable ventriculitis due to retained ventricular catheters. Br J Neurosurg. 2005;19:496–501.

110. Barker FG, 2nd. Efficacy of prophylactic antibiotics against meningitis after craniotomy: a meta-analysis. Neurosurgery. 2007;60:887–94.

111. Williams TA, Leslie GD, Dobb GJ, Roberts B, van Heerden PV. Decrease in proven ventriculitis by reducing the frequency of cerebrospinal fluid sampling from extraventricular drains. J Neurosurg. 2011;115:1040–6.

112. Thomas R, Lee S, Patole S, Rao S. Antibiotic-impregnated catheters for the prevention of CSF shunt infections: a systematic review and meta-analysis. Br J Neurosurg. 2012;26:175–84.

113. Pople I, Poon W, Assaker R, Mathieu D, Iantosca M, Wang E, et al. Comparison of infection rate with the use of antibiotic-impregnated versus standard extraventricular drainage devices: a prospective, randomized controlled trial. Neurosurgery. 2012;71:6–13.

114. Keong NC, Bulters DO, Richards HK, Farrington M, Sparrow OC, Pickard JD, et al. The SILVER (Silver Impregnated Line Versus EVD Randomized trial): a double-blind, prospective, randomized, controlled trial of an intervention to reduce the rate of external ventricular drain infection. Neurosurgery. 2012;71:394–403.

CHAPTER 25

Post-cardiac arrest syndrome

Jerry P. Nolan

The annual incidence of emergency medical service-treated out-of-hospital cardiac arrest (OHCA) is 0.5 per 1000 population (1) and, based on unpublished data from the UK National Cardiac Arrest Audit, the annual incidence of in-hospital cardiac arrest (IHCA) to which a resuscitation team is called is 2 per 1000 admissions. Unless the period of cardiac arrest has been very brief, most of those patients in whom return of spontaneous circulation (ROSC) has been achieved will remain comatose for a variable period, and will require further treatment on an intensive care unit (ICU). Data from the UK Intensive Care National Audit and Research Centre indicate that approximately 6350 patients each year are admitted to UK ICUs after cardiac arrest (2); these are estimated to represent 13% of the total 48,000 treated cardiac arrests (in and out of hospital) annually in the United Kingdom. Mechanically ventilated survivors of cardiac arrest account for 6% of all admissions to UK ICUs (2).

Interventions applied after ROSC impact significantly on the quality of survival. However, there is considerable variation in post-cardiac arrest treatment and patient outcome between hospitals (3). Approximately 30–40% of patients admitted to an ICU after cardiac arrest will survive to be discharged from hospital, and most of these will have a good neurological outcome (2,4,5).

This chapter will review the pathophysiology of the post-cardiac arrest syndrome (PCAS), therapeutic strategies to improve outcome among post-cardiac arrest patients, and approaches to prognostication in those patients remaining comatose after initial treatment.

Post-cardiac arrest syndrome

Systemic ischaemia during cardiac arrest, and the subsequent reperfusion response after ROSC, causes PCAS (Figure 25.1) (6,7). The severity of PCAS is determined by the cause and duration of cardiac arrest, and has four key clinical components (Box 25.1).

Post-cardiac arrest brain injury

Post-cardiac arrest brain injury is a common cause of morbidity and mortality. In patients surviving to ICU admission but subsequently dying in-hospital, brain injury or, more precisely, withdrawal of care because of brain injury, is the cause of death in two-thirds of cases after OHCA and in approximately 25% after IHCA (8,9). Clinical manifestations of post-cardiac arrest brain injury include coma, seizures, myoclonus, varying degrees of neurocognitive dysfunction, and brain death (10).

The pathophysiology of hypoxic-ischaemic injury caused by cardiac arrest is complex (11). Anoxic depolarization occurs 1–3 minutes after the onset of cardiac arrest. Brain glucose, glycogen, and adenosine triphosphate are depleted by 10 minutes, the intracellular concentration of calcium increases by 25%, and there is a profound intracellular acidosis. Cell protein synthesis is depressed by ischaemia but can recover over 12–48 hours if oxygen delivery is restored in time. After resuscitation, ischaemic cell death (by necrosis, apoptosis, or autophagocytosis) can be delayed for hours to up to 4 days (11), which theoretically provides a therapeutic window for the delivery of neuroprotective strategies. The CA1 pyramidal neurons of the hippocampus are the most vulnerable to hypoxic-ischaemic injury (11).

Several post-arrest factors can potentially exacerbate post-cardiac arrest brain injury. Impairment of the cerebral microcirculation is caused by endothelial swelling, leucocyte adherence to endothelium, and red blood cell sludging, which collectively cause the 'no reflow' phenomenon (6,12). Other secondary factors that may contribute to post-resuscitation brain injury include hypotension (cerebral autoregulation is impaired) (13,14), hyperoxia (15), hypocapnia (16), pyrexia (17), hyperglycaemia (2), blood glucose variability (18), and seizures (19). Therapeutic strategies to limit these potential causes of secondary brain injury are discussed later in this chapter. Although brain oedema occurs transiently during the first 15 minutes after ROSC, it is rarely associated with a significant increase in intracranial pressure (ICP), except after asphyxial cardiac arrest (6). This brief period of hyperaemia is typically followed by cerebral hypoperfusion for 24–72 hours (20,21).

Post-cardiac arrest myocardial dysfunction

Post-cardiac arrest myocardial dysfunction is another significant cause of morbidity and mortality after both IHCA and OHCA (8,9). Animal data indicate that 30 minutes after ROSC, ejection fraction decreases to about 20% (22). In a series of OHCA patients who were monitored with a pulmonary artery catheter, cardiac index values reached a nadir 8 hours after ROSC, but then returned gradually to normal by 72 hours (23). More sustained depression of ejection fraction among in- and out-of-hospital post-cardiac arrest patients has been reported with continued recovery over weeks to months (24).

Systemic ischaemia/reperfusion response

During cardiac arrest and in the absence of cardiopulmonary resuscitation (CPR) ('no flow') there is no delivery of oxygen and metabolic substrates, and metabolites are not removed. CPR reverses this process only partially because it achieves a cardiac output of only 25% of normal. Inadequate tissue oxygen delivery can persist even following ROSC because of myocardial dysfunction and microcirculatory failure. Restoration of tissue oxygenation leads to

Phases of Post-Cardiac Arrest Syndrome

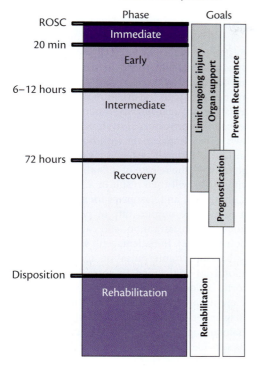

Fig. 25.1 Phases of the post-cardiac arrest syndrome.
Reprinted from *Resuscitation*, 79, 3, JP Nolan *et al.*, 'Post-cardiac arrest syndrome: Epidemiology, pathophysiology, treatment, and prognostication A Scientific Statement from the International Liaison Committee on Resuscitation; the American Heart Association Emergency Cardiovascular Care Committee; the Council on Cardiovascular Surgery and Anesthesia; the Council on Cardiopulmonary, Perioperative, and Critical Care; the Council on Clinical Cardiology; the Council on Stroke', pp. 350–379, Copyright 2008, with kind permission from Elsevier.

the generation of reactive oxygen species and the development of reperfusion injury.

The whole-body ischaemia/reperfusion associated with cardiac arrest activates immunological and coagulation pathways causing multiple organ failure and increased risk of infection (25). Thus, this condition resembles sepsis with high concentrations of inflammatory mediators (26) and activation of coagulation and fibrinolysis (27). Hydroxyl radicals generated during perfusion cause substantial endothelial damage (28). Procalcitonin values are increased in post-cardiac arrest patients and are associated with the severity of the ischaemia-reperfusion injury and outcome (29,30). Clinical manifestations of this systemic ischaemic-reperfusion response

---

Box 25.1 Key components of the post-cardiac arrest syndrome

- Post-cardiac arrest brain injury—this manifests as coma and seizures.
- Post-cardiac-arrest myocardial dysfunction—this can be severe and usually recovers after 48–72 hours.
- Systemic ischaemia/reperfusion response—tissue reperfusion can cause programmed cell death (apoptosis) effecting all organ systems.
- Persisting precipitating pathology—coronary artery disease is the commonest precipitating cause after OHCA.

---

include intravascular volume depletion, impaired vasoregulation, impaired oxygen delivery and utilization, and increased susceptibility to infection (31).

Persisting precipitating pathology

The commonest cause of OHCA is ischaemic heart disease and many of these cases will be associated with acute myocardial infarction (32). Following ST-elevation myocardial infarction (STEMI), urgent coronary reperfusion is essential and discussed later (see 'Circulation'). Other potential precipitating causes that also need treatment include:

- cardiovascular disease (acute myocardial infarction/acute coronary syndrome, cardiomyopathy)
- respiratory disease (chronic obstructive pulmonary disease, asthma)
- central nervous system disease (cerebrovascular accident)
- thromboembolic disease (pulmonary embolism)
- toxicological issues(overdose, poisoning)
- infection (sepsis, pneumonia)
- hypovolaemia

Treatment of the post-cardiac arrest patient

All components of the PCAS must be addressed if outcome is to be optimized. Post-cardiac arrest care should start immediately after ROSC has been achieved, irrespective of location. An 'ABCDE' (Airway, Breathing, Circulation, Disability, Exposure) systems approach is used to identify and treat physiological abnormalities and organ injury.

Airway and breathing with controlled reoxygenation

After a brief period of cardiac arrest (e.g. single successful shock for witnessed ventricular fibrillation (VF) arrest) patients usually recover consciousness, maintain their airway safely, and breathe adequately without the need for tracheal intubation. Those who remain comatose or agitated with a decreased conscious level, and those with breathing difficulties, will require sedation, tracheal intubation, and mechanical ventilation. The duration of ventilation is determined by the need for targeted temperature management (see 'Targeted Temperature Management'), and the extent of the neurological injury.

It is postulated that exposing ischaemic brain tissue to significant hyperoxaemia at the time of reperfusion increases the formation of reactive oxygen species and increases post-ischaemic oxidative injury and cellular death (33). This hypothesis has been confirmed in several laboratory studies, which have shown increased neurological injury in animals exposed to variable periods of 100% oxygen compared with air or oxygen titrated to achieve normal arterial oxygen saturation after ROSC (15).

In a very small pilot study, OHCA patients who achieved ROSC were randomized to be ventilated with 100% oxygen or 30% oxygen (34). In a subgroup of patients who were not cooled, neuron-specific enolase (NSE) values were higher at 24 hours in the 100% oxygen group. Although there were very few patients in this study, it remains the only randomized controlled trial on this intervention in humans. Two observational studies of hyperoxia after cardiac arrest that comprised analyses of large ICU databases reached different conclusions (35,36). In the first, 6326 post-cardiac arrest patients were divided into three groups based on the PaO_2 of their first arterial blood gas after admission to the ICU; the hypoxic group had a PaO_2 less than 60 mmHg or a PaO_2/FiO_2 ratio of less than 300, the hyperoxia group a PaO_2 greater than 300 mmHg, and the remainder formed the normoxia group (35). The in-hospital mortality in the hyperoxia group (63%; 95% confidence interval (CI) 60–66%) was significantly higher than both the normoxia (45%; 95% CI 43–48%) and hypoxia groups (57%; 95% CI 56–59%). On further analysis, the relationship between supranormal oxygen tension and mortality was linear (37). In the other, an analysis of over 12,000 post-cardiac arrest patients in the Australia and New Zealand Intensive Care Society (ANZICS) database adopted similar methodology, except it used the worst PaO_2 value in the first 24 hours after admission (36). In this analysis, crude mortality in the hyperoxia and hypoxia groups was the same, although this was significantly higher than the normoxia group. However, after adjustment for sickness severity, for FiO_2 and for relevant covariates, PaO_2 was no longer predictive of hospital mortality. Aside from better adjustment for confounders, the much greater use of therapeutic hypothermia among the patients in the ANZICS database might account for the different findings. In particular, hypothermia might have mitigated any harm caused by hyperoxia.

There are numerous weaknesses in these observational studies (e.g. timing of PaO_2 value in relation to ROSC is unknown but is certainly beyond the initial critical period of reperfusion after ROSC, and duration of hyperoxia is unknown) and a prospective trial is essential. In the meantime, current guidance recommends adjusting the inspired oxygen concentration immediately after ROSC to achieve normal arterial oxygen saturation (94–98%) when it can be measured reliably by pulse oximetry or arterial blood gas analysis (38). Clearly, hypoxaemia must be avoided.

Ventilation should also be adjusted to achieve normocapnia, and monitored using end-tidal CO_2 with waveform capnography, and arterial blood gas analysis. Hyperventilation should be avoided since this will cause cerebral vasoconstriction and possible cerebral ischaemia (16). A recent analysis of the ANZICS cardiac arrest dataset, using methodology similar to the hyperoxia study above, showed that, in comparison with the normocapnia group ($PaCO_2$ 35–45 mmHg; n = 6705), the hypocapnia group ($PaCO_2$ < 35 mmHg; n = 3010) had a higher risk-adjusted in-hospital mortality (odds ratio 1.2; 95% CI 1.00–1.24, p = 0.04) (39). In contrast, the hypercapnia group ($PaCO_2$ > 45 mmHg; n = 6827) had similar in-hospital mortality to the normocapnia group but a higher rate of discharge home among survivors, implying better neurological outcome.

Circulation

About 80% of sudden OHCAs are caused by coronary artery disease (32). Early coronary reperfusion therapy is indicated for STEMI and this is achieved most effectively with primary percutaneous intervention (PCI) as long as a first medical contact-to-balloon time of less than 120 minutes can be achieved; if not, fibrinolysis (thrombolysis) may be preferable (40). In the past, patients in coma after a cardiac arrest were often denied PCI in the expectation that few would make a good neurological recovery. There is now a trend towards considering immediate coronary artery angiography in all OHCA patients without an obvious non-cardiac cause of arrest, regardless of ECG changes. This is because the early post-resuscitation 12-lead electrocardiogram (ECG) is less reliable

for diagnosing acute coronary occlusion than in non-arrest patients (41). About 25% of patients without an obvious non-cardiac cause for their cardiac arrest and no evidence of STEMI on the initial 12-lead ECG will have a coronary lesion on angiography that is amenable to stenting (42).

Haemodynamic instability and arrhythmias associated with reversible myocardial dysfunction often occur after cardiac arrest. The severity increases with the duration of the arrest and in those with pre-existing myocardial dysfunction. Echocardiography enables the extent of myocardial dysfunction to be quantified; it usually shows global impairment with both systolic and diastolic dysfunction (24). Although systematic vascular resistance (SVR) may be high initially, the release of inflammatory cytokines associated with the PCAS will then result in a low SVR (6). Treatment with fluids, inotropes, and vasopressors is guided by blood pressure, heart rate, urine output, rate of plasma lactate clearance, central venous oxygen saturation, and cardiac output monitoring (typically non-invasive). In patients with severe cardiogenic shock, intra-aortic balloon counterpulsation may be used, although a recent randomized trial failed to show mortality benefit from the intra-aortic balloon pump in patients with cardiogenic shock (43). There are no proven evidence-based haemodynamic targets for the management of patients in the post-cardiac arrest period, although maintaining a mean arterial pressure (MAP) greater than 65 mmHg is sensible given the likely cerebral hypoperfusion in the early post-cardiac arrest period (44).

Patients who survive a cardiac arrest caused by VF/pulseless ventricular tachycardia and who have no evidence of a disease that can be effectively treated (e.g. coronary revascularization) should be considered for an implantable cardioverter-defibrillator before leaving hospital.

Brain (disability)

The incidence of neurological causes of OHCA has been reported with a wide range of 3.3% to 20%, but a recent large French study documented an incidence of around 4%, which is probably much more consistent with the experience in the United Kingdom (45). It is becoming common practice for all OHCA patients to have an immediate computed tomography (CT) brain scan even when there are clear indications for immediate coronary angiography. This is predicated on the desire to eliminate the presence of intracerebral bleeding before powerful antiplatelet drugs are given during PCI. However, there are no robust data to support this practice and the disadvantage is that PCI could be delayed significantly by undertaking a CT brain scan first. A French group with considerable experience in the treatment of OHCA patients has advocated early brain and chest CT (45).

Their protocol directs the patient to immediate coronary angiography unless there was a neurological or respiratory prodrome, in which case brain and chest CT is undertaken first; CT scanning is undertaken secondarily in those patients in whom no culprit lesion is found on immediate coronary angiography (45).

Neurological injury is the commonest cause of death, or precipitant for withdrawal of care, among patients admitted to ICU after OHCA (8). Strategies for improving neurological outcome in the comatose post-cardiac arrest patient include:

♦ controlled reoxygenation
♦ controlled ventilation to normocapnia

♦ maintenance of an adequate cerebral perfusion pressure (MAP > 65 mmHg)

♦ targeted temperature management

♦ adequate sedation

♦ control of seizures

♦ glycaemic control.

The first three of these have been discussed earlier in the chapter and the remaining four are discussed in detail below.

Targeted temperature management

Pyrexia associated with a systemic inflammatory response is common in the first 72 hours after cardiac arrest, and associated with worse neurological outcome (46). Mild hypothermia improves outcome after a period of global cerebral hypoxia-ischaemia (47,48). Cooling suppresses many of the pathways associated with ischaemia-reperfusion injury, including apoptosis (programmed cell death) and the harmful release of excitatory amino acids and free radicals (47,49). Hypothermia also decreases cerebral oxygen requirements (6% for each 1°C reduction in temperature), although this is not thought to be a primary mechanism for its impact on outcome.

Indications for post arrest cooling

Several animal studies have shown that mild hypothermia applied after ROSC improves neurological outcome (50). Two randomized studies in humans demonstrated improved neurological outcome at hospital discharge and at 6 months in comatose patients after out-of-hospital VF cardiac arrest (51,52). Cooling was initiated within hours after ROSC and a target temperature of 32–34°C was maintained for 12–24 hours. Notably, fever occurred in untreated patients. The use of hypothermia for non-shockable rhythms and after IHCA is supported mainly by observational data, which have a substantial risk of bias (53). Despite this, many centres use hypothermia irrespective of the initial cardiac arrest rhythm or location. In the Targeted Temperature Management (TTM) trial, 950 all-rhythm OHCA patients were randomized to 24 hours of temperature control at either 33°C or 36°C (64). Strict protocols were followed for assessing prognosis and for withdrawal of life-sustaining treatment. There was no difference in the primary outcome—all cause mortality—and neurological outcome at 180 days was also similar in the two groups. Importantly, patients in both arms of this trial had their temperature well controlled, so fever was prevented even in the 36°C group. Pending an international consensus on the optimal target temperature, clinicians will need to decide locally which target temperature to adopt in their post-resuscitation protocol. Clearly, if there are problems with attaining a target of 33°C it is rational to aim for 36°C instead. In any case, the TTM trial does not support abandoning temperature control.

Cooling techniques, timing, and duration

Targeted temperature management comprises induction of hypothermia, maintenance at 32–34°C, gradual rewarming while preventing hyperthermia, and, finally, maintaining normothermia until the patient recovers consciousness. Methods for inducing and maintaining hypothermia are listed in Box 25.2.

Infusion of 30 mL/kg of 4°C 0.9% sodium chloride or Hartmann's solution decreases core temperature by approximately 1.5°C and, until recently, was thought to be well tolerated even in patients with post-cardiac arrest myocardial dysfunction

---

Box 25.2 Methods for inducing and maintaining hypothermia

♦ Ice-cold fluids are effective for starting the cooling process but used alone cannot maintain hypothermia; however, even the addition of simple ice packs may control the temperature adequately. Use of IV cold fluid is being investigated for cooling *during* cardiac arrest.

♦ Intranasal cooling by evaporating perflurocarbon through intranasal cannulae is available but further clinical data are awaited.

♦ Simple ice packs and/or wet towels (inexpensive but may be more time consuming for nursing staff, may result in greater temperature fluctuations, and do not enable controlled rewarming).

♦ Cooling blankets or pads.

♦ Water or air circulating blankets.

♦ Water circulating gel-coated pads.

♦ Cold water immersion.

♦ Intravascular heat exchanger (catheter with balloons with circulating fluid or a metal catheter), placed usually in the femoral or subclavian veins.

♦ Cardiopulmonary bypass, for example, during extracorporeal life support.

---

(47). A randomized controlled trial in which post-cardiac arrest patients were assigned to either 2 L of 4°C normal saline prehospital or standard care showed no difference in survival to hospital discharge (55). Patients who received prehospital cold intravenous (IV) fluid were more likely than the control group to re-arrest during transport and to have pulmonary oedema on initial chest X-ray. The use of prehospital IV cold fluid must be reviewed in the light of this study, but careful use (with close monitoring) in hospital remains routine.

Following induction with cold IV fluids, ice packs and/or wet towels can be used to maintain hypothermia although fluctuations in temperature are common when using techniques that do not include temperature feedback control and automatic temperature regulation (56). Several surface cooling devices that include temperature feedback control are available (47,57), and core temperature is monitored from the bladder or oesophagus. There are several intravascular cooling systems that provide tight temperature control via a cooling catheter in a large vein (usually femoral) but there is no evidence that they produce better neurological outcome than external cooling systems. Initial cooling is facilitated by concomitant neuromuscular blockade with sedation to prevent shivering, although continuous infusion of neuromuscular blocking drugs is usually unnecessary. Addition of magnesium (e.g. 5 g IV over 5 hours) will help to reduce the shivering threshold.

Animal evidence indicates that outcomes are better the earlier cooling is started but, so far, this has not been demonstrated in clinical trials (58). By starting cooling in the prehospital phase, it is possible to achieve the target temperature more rapidly. A confounder in clinical trials of early cooling is the possibility that patients with more severe hypoxic-ischaemic brain injury, and therefore worse outcome, cool spontaneously more rapidly than those with less severe brain injury (59). Nasopharyngeal cooling, achieved by instilling perflurocarbon via nasal prongs (cooling is produced by evaporation), enables induction of hypothermia during cardiac arrest (60). Several trials of intra-arrest cooling are ongoing (61).

The optimal duration of induced hypothermia is unknown. Although current guidelines suggest 12–24 hours, some experts apply longer periods of hypothermia (at least 24 hours and sometimes up to 72 hours), especially when there has been a long duration of cardiac arrest. Rewarming should always be controlled at 0.25–0.5°C per hour and potentially harmful rebound hyperthermia avoided.

The complications of therapeutic hypothermia are listed in Box 25.3 (57); many of these are more accurately described as normal physiological responses to mild hypothermia. Pneumonia occurs in about two-thirds of patients admitted to ICU after OHCA and is more common in those treated with mild hypothermia (62). There are few absolute contraindications to the use of mild hypothermia in the post-cardiac arrest patient. Severe sepsis (hypothermia depresses immune function) and pre-existing coagulopathy (use of thrombolysis is not a contraindication) are the main contraindications. High-risk surgery where haemorrhage due to hypothermic coagulopathy would be an unacceptable risk (e.g. intracranial surgery) is a relative contraindication. Cardiogenic shock was previously considered to be a contraindication, but mild hypothermia reduces heart rate, and increases stroke volume and cardiac index in patients in severe cardiogenic shock (63,64). Animal data also indicate that mild hypothermia improves myocardial salvage, reduces infarct size and results in better long-term left ventricular function (65). There are ongoing trials of inducing mild hypothermia before establishing coronary reperfusion after myocardial infarction.

Sedation

Patients are sedated during treatment with therapeutic hypothermia because this reduces oxygen consumption, prevents shivering, and facilitates cooling (57). Short-acting sedatives and opioids (e.g. propofol, alfentanil, and remifentanil) enable earlier neurological assessment after rewarming. In one randomized trial, post-cardiac arrest patients sedated with propofol and remifentanil were able to be extubated earlier following discontinuation of sedation than those sedated with midazolam and fentanyl, but there were no important differences in other clinical outcomes (66). Clearance of many drugs is reduced by about one-third at 34°C and this must be considered carefully before making decisions about prognosis (see 'Prognostication') (67).

Control of seizures

Seizures, myoclonus, or both occur in about 20–30% of patients who remain comatose and are cooled after cardiac arrest (19,68,69). Many of these cases will have non-convulsive status epilepticus, which requires electroencephalography (EEG) for reliable detection. Continuous EEG monitoring should be used in patients receiving neuromuscular blocking drugs to ensure that seizures are not missed. Although seizures are associated with a fourfold increase in mortality, good neurological recovery has been documented in up to 17% of those who develop seizures (19,68). Seizures are treated with benzodiazepines, phenytoin, levetiracetam, sodium valproate, propofol, or a barbiturate (see Chapter 23).

Box 25.3 Complications associated with therapeutic hypothermia

- Shivering—reduced with sedation, neuromuscular blockers, and magnesium
- Dysrhythmias—bradycardia is the most common
- Diuresis—may cause hypovolaemia and electrolyte abnormalities
- Electrolyte abnormalities:
  - hypophosphataemia
  - hypokalaemia
  - hypomagnesaemia
  - hypocalcaemia
- Decreased insulin sensitivity and insulin secretion—hyperglycaemia
- Impaired coagulation and increased bleeding
- Impairment of the immune system—increased infection rates, for example, pneumonia
- Increased plasma amylase concentration
- Reduced drug clearance—clearance of sedative and neuromuscular blocking drugs is reduced by up to 30% at a temperature of 34°C.

Post-hypoxic myoclonus can be very difficult to control, and neurological advice should be sought. Cortical myoclonus may be best treated with levetiracetam but subcortical myoclonus is usually treated with clonazepam. Propofol is often effective but phenytoin is relatively ineffective.

Glucose control

Both hyperglycaemia and hypoglycaemia after ROSC are associated with poor neurological outcome (2,68). Glucose variability may be more harmful than its absolute value (18). Based on the available data and expert consensus, blood glucose should be maintained between 4 and 10 mmol/L following ROSC.

Prognostication

A post-cardiac arrest patient is generally considered to have a good outcome if a Cerebral Performance Category (CPC) score of 1 or 2 (Box 25.4) is achieved by 6 months. Some prognostication studies include a CPC score of 3 as a good outcome but this is partly because these outcomes are often documented at hospital discharge and many patients will improve their CPC score by 6 months (70).

In patients who remain comatose after cardiac arrest, reliable prediction of those who will not achieve a good neurological outcome allows withdrawal of futile therapy and informs discussion with families. Unfortunately, predicting outcome in comatose patients post-cardiac arrest is challenging, and guidance is changing rapidly as more data become available (71–73). Until recently, the American Academy of Neurology (AAN) guidelines, published in 2006, were considered to be the gold standard (74), but these were developed using data collected before the introduction of therapeutic hypothermia. The other important limitation of virtually all prognostication studies is a self-fulfilling prophecy. In the

Box 25.4 The Cerebral Performance Category scale

1. Good Cerebral Performance (*normal life*):

- Conscious, alert, able to work and lead a normal life.

- May have minor psychological or neurologic deficits (mild dysphasia, non-incapacitating hemiparesis, or minor cranial nerve abnormalities).

2. Moderate Cerebral Disability (*disabled but independent*):

- Conscious. Sufficient cerebral function for part-time work in sheltered environment or independent activities of daily life (dress, travel by public transportation, food preparation).

- May have hemiplegia, seizures, ataxia, dysarthria, dysphasia, or permanent memory or mental changes.

3. Severe Cerebral Disability (*conscious but disabled and dependent*):

- Conscious; dependent on others for daily support (in an institution or at home with exceptional family effort).

- Has at least limited cognition.

- This category includes a wide range of cerebral abnormalities, from patients who are ambulatory but have severe memory disturbances or dementia precluding independent existence to those who are paralysed and can communicate only with their eyes, as in the locked-in syndrome.

4. Coma/Vegetative State (*unconscious*):

- Unconscious, unaware of surroundings, no cognition.

- No verbal or psychological interaction with environment.

5. Brain Death (*certified brain dead or dead by traditional criteria*).

Box 25.5 Potential methods for predicting outcome in the comatose post-cardiac arrest patient

- Clinical examination:
  - brainstem reflexes:
    - corneal reflex
    - pupillary light reflex
    - vestibular-ocular reflex
  - Glasgow Coma Scale score and its components
  - seizures
- Electrophysiology:
  - EEG:
    - alpha coma
    - burst suppression pattern
    - suppression (low voltage)
    - reactivity
    - status epilepticus
  - somatosensory evoked potentials (SSEP):
    - N20—bilaterally absent
    - N70—bilaterally absent
- Biomarkers:
  - neuron specific enolase (NSE)—various thresholds
  - S-100 protein—various thresholds
- Imaging:
  - CT scan:
    - brain swelling
    - loss of grey/white differentiation
  - MRI—diffuse abnormalities.

---

vast majority of studies, clinicians were not blinded to the results of the investigations and, in many cases, at least some of the results were used to make treatment withdrawal decisions. Prevention of self-fulfilling prophecy bias would require blinding of test results to the treating team, as well as providing prolonged life support to patients who do not recover consciousness after resuscitation and rewarming; both of these would be very difficult to achieve.

Methods that have been investigated for predicting outcome in the comatose post-cardiac arrest patients are categorized and listed in Box 25.5.

Recent evidence from patients treated with hypothermia indicates that the AAN prognostication guidelines are unreliable (10,75). This may reflect a direct effect of hypothermia on the progress of neurological recovery and/or the residual effects of sedatives and opioids, which tend to be used in larger doses and take longer to clear (67), confounding neurological assessment.

Clinical examination

Several studies have shown that a Glasgow Coma Scale motor score of 1 or 2 on day 3, which was previously documented by the AAN guidelines to have a false positive rate (FPR) of 0% (95% CI 0–3%), is a highly unreliable predictor of poor outcome in patients who have been cooled (10,75). Amongst these studies, there are some examples of good outcomes despite absent pupil or absent corneal reflexes

on day 3. There are also reports of good outcome in patients with myoclonic status (19,69,76). Hypothermia, and the sedation used during this treatment, tend to supress myoclonic activity. Myoclonic status arising within the first 24 hours after cardiac arrest and during hypothermia, usually, but not always, indicates severe brain injury. Seizure activity that arises after rewarming and stopping of sedative drugs may also be compatible with a good recovery (72).

Electrophysiology

Somatosensory evoked potentials (SSEPs) involving electrical stimulation of the median nerve at the wrist and recording of the N20 response over the contralateral sensory cerebral cortex can provide valuable prognostic information (see Chapter 13). The 2006 AAN guidelines indicated that bilaterally absent N20 responses on days 1–3 predicted a poor outcome with a FPR of 0.7% (95% CI 0–3.7%) (74). In recent studies of patients treated with hypothermia, bilateral absence of N20 responses when recorded after return to normothermia continue to be associated with high prognostic specificity (10).

In most centres, the EEG is recorded for 30 minutes using 20 scalp electrodes, but some specialist neurological centres also have the ability to record the EEG continuously (77,78). Stimuli, such as manual eye opening, sound (speech or a loud clap), pain, or, perhaps best, tracheal suction, are used to assess EEG reactivity. The absence of EEG background reactivity is a strong predictor of a poor outcome. In one study, none of 25 patients showing an unreactive EEG made a good recovery (75). In contrast, development of electroencephalographic status epilepticus from a continuous and reactive background indicates a potential for recovery (72,75). Status epilepticus in post-cardiac arrest patients is a heterogeneous condition that includes different clinical or EEG variants associated with different implications on prognosis. Expert advice from neurologists is essential.

Biomarkers

NSE is a cytoplasmic glycolytic enzyme found in neurons, cells, and tumours of neuroendocrine origin; concentrations increase in serum a few hours after neurological injury. The biochemical marker S100β is a calcium-binding protein from astroglial and Schwann cells. Both NSE and S100β have been studied for their potential to predict outcome after cardiac arrest but these tests are not widely available. Serum NSE values >33 mcg/L (the threshold recommended by AAN in 2006) do not reliably predict poor outcome among patients who have been treated with hypothermia (10). Further, haemolysis may increase plasma values for NSE, and renal impairment increases plasma concentrations of S100β. Low values of these biomarkers in a comatose post-cardiac arrest patient might indicate a potentially treatable condition (72).

Imaging

On CT imaging, hypoxic-ischaemic brain injury may appear as loss of grey–white differentiation visible within 24 hours of cardiac arrest, indicating cerebral oedema. An MRI scan is more sensitive for the detection of hypoxic-ischaemic brain injury but is also more laborious and difficult to acquire in critically ill patients. Neither of these imaging modalities have sufficient specificity to be used alone for prognostication but they do add value as part of a multimodal approach (71,72).

Multimodal approach to prognostication

The current consensus is that a multimodal approach should be used for prognostication in comatose patients after cardiac arrest; this means a combination of neurological examination and electrophysiological and imaging investigations (71,72). Reliable neurological examination, CT and MRI imaging, and EEG should therefore be available for all post-cardiac arrest patients treated in an ICU. Although SSEPs are not widely available in the United Kingdom, most experts consider this to be a very valuable investigation for prognostication and it is likely SSEP monitoring will become more widely available in the near future. Most importantly, the delayed clearance of sedation and modification of neurological recovery by hypothermia means that in most cases prognostication should be delayed until at least 72 hours after restoration of normothermia (72,79).

Organ donation

Up to 16% of patients who achieve sustained ROSC after cardiac arrest fulfil criteria for brain death and can be considered for organ donation (80). Transplant outcomes for organs from brain-dead donors who have suffered a cardiac arrest are similar to those achieved with organs from other beating-heart donors (81). Controversially, some countries that use non-conventional resuscitation procedures after standard CPR has failed have begun to incorporate techniques aimed solely at organ preservation to maximize the potential for uncontrolled donation after circulatory death (82).

Cardiac arrest centres

Post-cardiac arrest patients are likely to have improved outcomes if they are cared for in a hospital that offers a comprehensive package of care that includes PCI, therapeutic hypothermia, and a strong and responsive neurology service (83). In some observational studies, hospitals that offer a post-cardiac arrest 'care bundle' have shown improved good quality survival (44). Although these findings may represent a volume effect, whereby hospitals treating the most post-cardiac arrest patients achieve the best outcomes, studies on this topic have reached a variety of conclusions.

References

1. Atwood C, Eisenberg MS, Herlitz J, Rea TD. Incidence of EMS-treated out-of-hospital cardiac arrest in Europe. *Resuscitation*. 2005;67:75–80.
2. Nolan JP, Laver SR, Welch CA, Harrison DA, Gupta V, Rowan K. Outcome following admission to UK intensive care units after cardiac arrest: a secondary analysis of the ICNARC Case Mix Programme Database. *Anaesthesia*. 2007;62:1207–16.
3. Carr BG, Kahn JM, Merchant RM, Kramer AA, Neumar RW. Inter-hospital variability in post-cardiac arrest mortality. *Resuscitation*. 2009;80:30–4.
4. Lund-Kordahl I, Olasveengen TM, Lorem T, Samdal M, Wik L, Sunde K. Improving outcome after out-of-hospital cardiac arrest by strengthening weak links of the local Chain of Survival; quality of advanced life support and post-resuscitation care. *Resuscitation*. 2010;81:422–6.
5. Elliott VJ, Rodgers DL, Brett SJ. Systematic review of quality of life and other patient-centred outcomes after cardiac arrest survival. *Resuscitation*. 2011;82:247–56.
6. Nolan JP, Neumar RW, Adrie C, Aibiki M, Berg RA, Bottiger BW, *et al*. Post-cardiac arrest syndrome: epidemiology, pathophysiology, treatment, and prognostication. A Scientific Statement from the International Liaison Committee on Resuscitation; the American Heart Association Emergency Cardiovascular Care Committee; the Council on Cardiovascular Surgery and Anesthesia; the Council on Cardiopulmonary, Perioperative, and Critical Care; the Council on Clinical Cardiology; the Council on Stroke. *Resuscitation*. 2008;79:350–79.
7. Negovsky VA. The second step in resuscitation—the treatment of the 'post-resuscitation disease'. *Resuscitation*. 1972;1:1–7.
8. Laver S, Farrow C, Turner D, Nolan J. Mode of death after admission to an intensive care unit following cardiac arrest. *Intensive Care Med*. 2004;30:2126–8.
9. Dragancea I, Rundgren M, Englund E, Friberg H, Cronberg T. The influence of induced hypothermia and delayed prognostication on the mode of death after cardiac arrest. *Resuscitation*. 2013;84:337–42.
10. Bouwes A, Binnekade JM, Kuiper MA, Bosch FH, Zandstra DF, Toornvliet AC, *et al*. Prognosis of coma after therapeutic hypothermia: a prospective cohort study. *Ann Neurol*. 2012;71:206–12.
11. Busl KM, Greer DM. Hypoxic-ischemic brain injury: pathophysiology, neuropathology and mechanisms. *NeuroRehabilitation*. 2010;26:5–13.
12. Bottiger BW, Krumnikl JJ, Gass P, Schmitz B, Motsch J, Martin E. The cerebral 'no-reflow' phenomenon after cardiac arrest in rats—influence of low-flow reperfusion. *Resuscitation*. 1997;34:79–87.
13. Nishizawa H, Kudoh I. Cerebral autoregulation is impaired in patients resuscitated after cardiac arrest. *Acta Anaesthesiol Scand*. 1996;40:1149–53.

14. Sundgreen C, Larsen FS, Herzog TM, Knudsen GM, Boesgaard S, Aldershvile J. Autoregulation of cerebral blood flow in patients resuscitated from cardiac arrest. *Stroke*. 2001;32:128–32.

15. Pilcher J, Weatherall M, Shirtcliffe P, Bellomo R, Young P, Beasley R. The effect of hyperoxia following cardiac arrest—a systematic review and meta-analysis of animal trials. *Resuscitation*. 2012;83:417–22.

16. Curley G, Kavanagh BP, Laffey JG. Hypocapnia and the injured brain: more harm than benefit. *Crit Care Med*. 2010;38:1348–59.

17. Langhelle A, Tyvold SS, Lexow K, Hapnes SA, Sunde K, Steen PA. In-hospital factors associated with improved outcome after out-of-hospital cardiac arrest. A comparison between four regions in Norway. *Resuscitation*. 2003;56:247–63.

18. Cueni-Villoz N, Devigili A, Delodder F, Cianferoni S, Feihl F, Rossetti AO, et al. Increased blood glucose variability during therapeutic hypothermia and outcome after cardiac arrest. *Crit Care Med*. 2011;39:2225–31.

19. Bouwes A, van Poppelen D, Koelman JH, Kuiper MA, Zandstra DF, Weinstein HC, et al. Acute posthypoxic myoclonus after cardiopulmonary resuscitation. *BMC Neurol*. 2012;12:63.

20. Buunk G, van der Hoeven JG, Frolich M, Meinders AE. Cerebral vasoconstriction in comatose patients resuscitated from a cardiac arrest? *Intensive Care Med*. 1996;22:1191–96.

21. Lemiale V, Huet O, Vigue B, Mathonnet A, Spaulding C, Mira JP, et al. Changes in cerebral blood flow and oxygen extraction during post-resuscitation syndrome. *Resuscitation*. 2008;76:17–24.

22. Kern KB, Hilwig RW, Rhee KH, Berg RA. Myocardial dysfunction after resuscitation from cardiac arrest: an example of global myocardial stunning. *J Am Coll Cardiol*. 1996;28:232–40.

23. Laurent I, Monchi M, Chiche JD, Joly LM, Spaulding C, Bourgeois B, et al. Reversible myocardial dysfunction in survivors of out-of-hospital cardiac arrest. *J Am Coll Cardiol*. 2002;40:2110–16.

24. Ruiz-Bailen M, Aguayo de Hoyos E, Ruiz-Navarro S, Diaz-Castellanos MA, Rucabado-Aguilar L, Gomez-Jimenez FJ, et al. Reversible myocardial dysfunction after cardiopulmonary resuscitation. *Resuscitation*. 2005;66:175–81.

25. Cerchiari EL, Safar P, Klein E, Diven W. Visceral, hematologic and bacteriologic changes and neurologic outcome after cardiac arrest in dogs. The visceral post-resuscitation syndrome. *Resuscitation*. 1993;25:119–36.

26. Adrie C, Adib-Conquy M, Laurent I, Monchi M, Vinsonneau C, Fitting C, et al. Successful cardiopulmonary resuscitation after cardiac arrest as a "sepsis-like" syndrome. *Circulation*. 2002;106:562–68.

27. Adrie C, Monchi M, Laurent I, Um S, Yan SB, Thuong M, et al. Coagulopathy after successful cardiopulmonary resuscitation following cardiac arrest: implication of the protein C anticoagulant pathway. *J Am Coll Cardiol*. 2005;46:21–8.

28. Huet O, Dupic L, Batteux F, Matar C, Conti M, Chereau C, et al. Postresuscitation syndrome: potential role of hydroxyl radical-induced endothelial cell damage. *Crit Care Med*. 2011;39:1712–20.

29. Annborn M, Dankiewicz J, Erlinge D, Hertel S, Rundgren M, Smith JG, et al. Procalcitonin after cardiac arrest—an indicator of severity of illness, ischemia-reperfusion injury and outcome. *Resuscitation*. 2013;84(6):782–7.

30. Engel H, Ben Hamouda N, Portmann K, Delodder F, Suys T, Feihl F, et al. Serum procalcitonin as a marker of post-cardiac arrest syndrome and long-term neurological recovery, but not of early-onset infections, in comatose post-anoxic patients treated with therapeutic hypothermia. *Resuscitation*. 2013;84(6):776–81.

31. Mongardon N, Perbet S, Lemiale V, Dumas F, Poupet H, Charpentier J, et al. Infectious complications in out-of-hospital cardiac arrest patients in the therapeutic hypothermia era. *Crit Care Med*. 2011;39:1359–64.

32. Myerburg RJ, Junttila MJ. Sudden cardiac death caused by coronary heart disease. *Circulation*. 2012;125:1043–52.

33. Neumar RW. Optimal oxygenation during and after cardiopulmonary resuscitation. *Curr Opin Crit Care*. 2011;17:236–40.

34. Kuisma M, Boyd J, Voipio V, Alaspaa A, Roine RO, Rosenberg P. Comparison of 30 and the 100% inspired oxygen concentrations during early post-resuscitation period: a randomised controlled pilot study. *Resuscitation*. 2006;69:199–206.

35. Kilgannon JH, Jones AE, Shapiro NI, Angelos MG, Milcarek B, Hunter K, et al. Association between arterial hyperoxia following resuscitation from cardiac arrest and in-hospital mortality. *JAMA*. 2010;303:2165–71.

36. Bellomo R, Bailey M, Eastwood GM, Nichol A, Pilcher D, Hart GK, et al. Arterial hyperoxia and in-hospital mortality after resuscitation from cardiac arrest. *Crit Care*. 2011;15:R90.

37. Kilgannon JH, Jones AE, Parrillo JE, Dellinger RP, Milcarek B, Hunter K, et al. Relationship between supranormal oxygen tension and outcome after resuscitation from cardiac arrest. *Circulation*. 2011;123:2717–22.

38. Deakin CD, Nolan JP, Soar J, Sunde K, Koster RW, Smith GB, et al. European Resuscitation Council Guidelines for Resuscitation 2010 Section 4. Adult advanced life support. *Resuscitation*. 2010;81:1305–52.

39. Schneider AG, Eastwood GM, Bellomo R, Bailey M, Lipcsey M, Pilcher D, et al. Arterial carbon dioxide tension and outcome in patients admitted to the intensive care unit after cardiac arrest. *Resuscitation*. 2013;84(7):927–34.

40. O'Gara PT, Kushner FG, Ascheim DD, Casey DE, Jr., Chung MK, de Lemos JA, et al. 2013 ACCF/AHA guideline for the management of ST-elevation myocardial infarction: executive summary: a report of the American College of Cardiology Foundation/American Heart Association Task Force on Practice Guidelines. *Circulation*. 2013;127:529–55.

41. Sideris G, Voicu S, Dillinger JG, Stratiev V, Logeart D, Broche C, et al. Value of post-resuscitation electrocardiogram in the diagnosis of acute myocardial infarction in out-of-hospital cardiac arrest patients. *Resuscitation*. 2011;82:1148–53.

42. Dumas F, Cariou A, Manzo-Silberman S, Grimaldi D, Vivien B, Rosencher J, et al. Immediate percutaneous coronary intervention is associated with better survival after out-of-hospital cardiac arrest: insights from the PROCAT (Parisian Region Out of hospital Cardiac ArresT) registry. *Circ Cardiovasc Interv*. 2010;3:200–7.

43. Thiele H, Zeymer U, Neumann FJ, Ferenc M, Olbrich HG, Hausleiter J, et al. Intraaortic balloon support for myocardial infarction with cardiogenic shock. *N Engl J Med*. 2012;367:1287–96.

44. Tomte O, Andersen GO, Jacobsen D, Draegni T, Auestad B, Sunde K. Strong and weak aspects of an established post-resuscitation treatment protocol. A five-year observational study. *Resuscitation*. 2011;82(9):1186–93.

45. Chelly J, Mongardon N, Dumas F, Varenne O, Spaulding C, Vignaux O, et al. Benefit of an early and systematic imaging procedure after cardiac arrest: insights from the PROCAT (Parisian Region Out of Hospital Cardiac Arrest) registry. *Resuscitation*. 2012;83:1444–50.

46. Zeiner A, Holzer M, Sterz F, Schorkhuber W, Eisenburger P, Havel C, et al. Hyperthermia after cardiac arrest is associated with an unfavorable neurologic outcome. *Arch Intern Med*. 2001;161:2007–12.

47. Holzer M. Targeted temperature management for comatose survivors of cardiac arrest. *N Engl J Med*. 2010;363:1256–64.

48. Walters JH, Morley PT, Nolan JP. The role of hypothermia in post-cardiac arrest patients with return of spontaneous circulation: A systematic review. *Resuscitation*. 2011;82:508–16.

49. Polderman KH. Induced hypothermia and fever control for prevention and treatment of neurological injuries. *Lancet*. 2008;371:1955–69.

50. Sterz F, Safar P, Tisherman S, Radovsky A, Kuboyama K, Oku K. Mild hypothermic cardiopulmonary resuscitation improves outcome after prolonged cardiac arrest in dogs. *Crit Care Med*. 1991;19:379–89.

51. Mild therapeutic hypothermia to improve the neurologic outcome after cardiac arrest. *N Engl J Med*. 2002;346:549–56.

52. Bernard SA, Gray TW, Buist MD, Jones BM, Silvester W, Gutteridge G, et al. Treatment of comatose survivors of out-of-hospital cardiac arrest with induced hypothermia. *N Engl J Med*. 2002;346:557–63.

53. Kim YM, Yim HW, Jeong SH, Klem ML, Callaway CW. Does therapeutic hypothermia benefit adult cardiac arrest patients presenting with

non-shockable initial rhythms?: A systematic review and meta-analysis of randomized and non-randomized studies. *Resuscitation.* 2012;83:188–96.

54. Nielsen N, Wetterslev J, Cronberg T, Erlinge D, Gasche Y, Hassanger C, et al. Targeted temperature management at 33 degrees C versus 36 degrees C after cardiac arrest. *N Engl J Med.* 2013;369:2197–206.

55. Kim F, Nichol G, Maynard C, Hallstrom A, Kudenchuk PJ, Rea T, et al. Effect of prehospital induction of mild hypothermia on survival and neurological status among adults with cardiac arrest: a randomized clinical trial. *JAMA.* 2014;311:45–52.

56. Gillies MA, Pratt R, Whiteley C, Borg J, Beale RJ, Tibby SM. Therapeutic hypothermia after cardiac arrest: a retrospective comparison of surface and endovascular cooling techniques. *Resuscitation.* 2010;81:1117–22.

57. Polderman KH, Herold I. Therapeutic hypothermia and controlled normothermia in the intensive care unit: practical considerations, side effects, and cooling methods. *Crit Care Med.* 2009;37:1101–20.

58. Bernard SA, Smith K, Cameron P, Masci K, Taylor DM, Cooper DJ, et al. Induction of therapeutic hypothermia by paramedics after resuscitation from out-of-hospital ventricular fibrillation cardiac arrest: a randomized controlled trial. *Circulation.* 2010;122:737–42.

59. Haugk M, Testori C, Sterz F, Uranitsch M, Holzer M, Behringer W, et al. Relationship between time to target temperature and outcome in patients treated with therapeutic hypothermia after cardiac arrest. *Crit Care.* 2011;15:R101.

60. Castren M, Nordberg P, Svensson L, Taccone F, Vincent JL, Desruelles D, et al. Intra-arrest transnasal evaporative cooling: a randomized, prehospital, multicenter study (PRINCE: Pre-ROSC IntraNasal Cooling Effectiveness). *Circulation.* 2010;122:729–36.

61. Scolletta S, Taccone FS, Nordberg P, Donadello K, Vincent JL, Castren M. Intra-arrest hypothermia during cardiac arrest: a systematic review. *Crit Care.* 2012;16:R41.

62. Perbet S, Mongardon N, Dumas F, Bruel C, Lemiale V, Mourvillier B, et al. Early-onset pneumonia after cardiac arrest: characteristics, risk factors and influence on prognosis. *Am J Respir Crit Care Med.* 2011;184:1048–54.

63. Schmidt-Schweda S, Ohler A, Post H, Pieske B. Moderate hypothermia for severe cardiogenic shock (COOL Shock Study I & II). *Resuscitation.* 2013;84:319–25.

64. Zobel C, Adler C, Kranz A, Seck C, Pfister R, Hellmich M, et al. Mild therapeutic hypothermia in cardiogenic shock syndrome. *Crit Care Med.* 2012;40:1715–23.

65. Kelly FE, Nolan JP. The effects of mild induced hypothermia on the myocardium: a systematic review. *Anaesthesia.* 2010;65:505–15.

66. Bjelland TW, Dale O, Kaisen K, Haugen BO, Lydersen S, Strand K, et al. Propofol and remifentanil versus midazolam and fentanyl for sedation during therapeutic hypothermia after cardiac arrest: a randomised trial. *Intensive Care Med.* 2012;38:959–67.

67. Tortorici MA, Kochanek PM, Poloyac SM. Effects of hypothermia on drug disposition, metabolism, and response: A focus on hypothermia-mediated alterations on the cytochrome P450 enzyme system. *Crit Care Med.* 2007;35:2196–204.

68. Nielsen N, Sunde K, Hovdenes J, Riker RR, Rubertsson S, Stammet P, et al. Adverse events and their relation to mortality in out-of-hospital cardiac arrest patients treated with therapeutic hypothermia. *Crit Care Med.* 2011;39:57–64.

69. Legriel S, Hilly-Ginoux J, Resche-Rigon M, Merceron S, Pinoteau J, Henry-Lagarrigue M, et al. Prognostic value of electrographic postanoxic status epilepticus in comatose cardiac-arrest survivors in the therapeutic hypothermia era. *Resuscitation.* 2013;84:343–50.

70. Arrich J, Zeiner A, Sterz F, Janata A, Uray T, Richling N, et al. Factors associated with a change in functional outcome between one month and six months after cardiac arrest: a retrospective cohort study. *Resuscitation.* 2009;80:876–80.

71. Sandroni C, Cariou A, Cavallaro F, Cronberg T, Friberg H, Hoedemaekers C, et al. Prognostication in comatose survivors of cardiac arrest: An advisory statement from the European Resuscitation Council and the European Society of Intensive Care Medicine. *Resuscitation* 2014;85:1779–89.

72. Cronberg T, Brizzi M, Liedholm LJ, Rosen I, Rubertsson S, Rylander C, et al. Neurological prognostication after cardiac arrest-Recommendations from the Swedish Resuscitation Council. *Resuscitation.* 2013; 84: 867–72.

73. Stevens RD, Sutter R. Prognosis in Severe Brain Injury. *Crit Care Med.* 2013;41:1104–23.

74. Wijdicks EF, Hijdra A, Young GB, Bassetti CL, Wiebe S. Practice parameter: prediction of outcome in comatose survivors after cardiopulmonary resuscitation (an evidence-based review): report of the Quality Standards Subcommittee of the American Academy of Neurology. *Neurology.* 2006;67:203–10.

75. Rossetti AO, Oddo M, Logroscino G, Kaplan PW. Prognostication after cardiac arrest and hypothermia: a prospective study. *Ann Neurol.* 2010;67:301–7.

76. Lucas JM, Cocchi MN, Salciccioli J, Stanbridge JA, Geocadin RG, Herman ST, et al. Neurologic recovery after therapeutic hypothermia in patients with post-cardiac arrest myoclonus. *Resuscitation.* 2012;83:265–9.

77. Rundgren M, Westhall E, Cronberg T, Rosen I, Friberg H. Continuous amplitude-integrated electroencephalogram predicts outcome in hypothermia-treated cardiac arrest patients. *Crit Care Med.* 2010;38:1838–44.

78. Cloostermans MC, van Meulen FB, Eertman CJ, Hom HW, van Putten MJ. Continuous electroencephalography monitoring for early prediction of neurological outcome in postanoxic patients after cardiac arrest: a prospective cohort study. *Crit Care Med.* 2012;40:2867–75.

79. Kamps MJA, Horn J, Oddo M, Fugate JE, Storm C, Cronberg T, et al. Prognostication of neurologic outcome in cardiac arrest patients after mild therapeutic hypothermia: a meta-analysis of the current literature. *Intensive Care Med* 2013;39(10):1671–82.

80. Adrie C, Haouache H, Saleh M, Memain N, Laurent I, Thuong M, et al. An underrecognized source of organ donors: patients with brain death after successfully resuscitated cardiac arrest. *Intensive Care Med.* 2008;34:132–7.

81. Sandroni C, Adrie C, Cavallaro F, Marano C, Monchi M, Sanna T, et al. Are patients brain-dead after successful resuscitation from cardiac arrest suitable as organ donors? A systematic review. *Resuscitation.* 2010;81:1609–14.

82. Rodriguez-Arias D, Deballon IO. Protocols for uncontrolled donation after circulatory death. *Lancet.* 2012;379:1275–6.

83. Nichol G, Aufderheide TP, Eigel B, Neumar RW, Lurie KG, Bufalino VJ, et al. Regional systems of care for out-of-hospital cardiac arrest: A policy statement from the American Heart Association. *Circulation.* 2010;121:709–29.

CHAPTER 26

Disorders of consciousness

Olivier Bodart, Aurore Thibaut,
Steven Laureys, and Olivia Gosseries

Disorders of consciousness occurring after coma present a major challenge in clinical practice. Neuroscientists have brought new insights into brain function and neural correlates of the pathological states of consciousness which have permitted the differentiation of various conscious states after severe brain injury. Some patients in coma will die, others recover full consciousness, whilst others can suffer from a chronic alteration of consciousness, namely the unresponsive wakefulness syndrome (UWS) and minimally conscious state (MCS). Some in these intermediate states will continue to improve, but others will have altered consciousness for several years or even permanently. Neuroscientists now focus on the validation of neuroimaging and electrophysiological modalities to improve the diagnosis, prognosis, treatment, and quality of life in patients with disorders of consciousness. Such modalities may also assist in resolving some of the ethical issues that arise in patients who are likely to survive with little chance of regaining consciousness. Delirium is another state of altered consciousness that may occur in patients as they awaken from coma, or which may itself lead to coma. It may also occur in the setting of any acute illness, particularly in critically ill patients. This chapter will outline disorders of consciousness following a period of coma, and discuss their investigation and diagnosis.

Aetiology of disorders of consciousness

Acute coma

Coma is defined as an acute state of unresponsiveness which lasts for at least 1 hour in which a patient who cannot be aroused lies with their eyes closed (1). This state rarely lasts longer than 2–4 weeks (2), thus the term 'acute' in the definition. With the airway secured and stable clinical parameters, determining the aetiology of the loss of consciousness should be the primary aim so that appropriate management can be planned. Clinical examination may provide clues to the cause of the loss of consciousness. For example, specific respiratory patterns, temperature changes, increased or decreased blood pressure, skin lesions, and abnormalities in the neurological examination may all point to the cause of the coma.

Coma has numerous causes (Table 26.1), but can be divided clinically into two major categories—traumatic and non-traumatic. Whilst the former is usually suspected from the history, presentation, or clinical examination, the latter may be harder to delineate because its causes are many. The underlying cause of coma of all types is interruption and/or global impairment of the arousal system.

Traumatic brain injury (TBI) can induce coma because of the initial brain damage (as in diffuse axonal injury or extensive bilateral hemisphere lesions) or the strategic location of a lesion (e.g. of the brainstem or bilateral lesion of the thalami), but the cause of the coma is the same in both, consisting of disruption of the arousal system. Even when a primary lesion does not itself result in coma, patients can suffer secondary complications, including brain swelling, haemorrhage, or herniation, which can lead to loss of consciousness. Anoxic and ischaemic insults also induce coma, depending on the extent of the brain damage or its location. However, they are less easy to diagnose than TBI, particularly in patients with no known cardiovascular risk factors in whom the diagnosis may not be suspected, or if computed tomography (CT) of the brain is performed early when little or no hypodensity will be observed. In metabolic or toxic aetiologies, coma usually follows severe encephalopathy which may initially manifest as delirium. In these conditions the underlying pathophysiology is more variable, and alterations in excitatory–inhibitory amino acid balance may be implicated (3) in addition to impairment of the arousal system (1). To be more specific, electrolyte disturbances modify neuronal excitability, certain drugs may prevent physiological activity of neuronal membrane ion channels or receptors, and toxins and nutritional disorders may lead to cellular death and severe brain damage (1,4).

The unresponsive wakefulness syndrome and minimally conscious state

Coma, as discussed in the previous paragraphs, is an acute state where patients lay with their eyes closed, showing no signs of voluntary reactions to stimuli (1). As coma persists, patients will either die or recover some consciousness, but usually altered, such as the UWS (5) or MCS (Figure 26.1) (6). Unresponsive wakefulness syndrome is now preferred to the term 'vegetative state' (7,8) because it has no pejorative connotations and is a more precise description of the clinical state, referring to patients unable to react to stimuli in a non-reflexive way (unresponsive), whilst showing periods of time with eyes opened (wakefulness). Indeed, patients with an UWS do not show any signs of voluntary or purposeful responses to sensory stimuli but they can open their eyes during the day, mimicking a normal sleep–wake cycle (9). Although recovery of the sleep–wake cycle is part of the definition of the UWS, recent studies have demonstrated an absence of electrophysiological characteristics of normal sleep (10,11). When patients in the UWS begin to show reproducible signs of awareness, such as command following, visual pursuit, or intelligible verbalizations, they enter the MCS. The authors

Table 26.1 Common causes of coma

Structural causes	Functional and other non-structural causes
Compressive	*Toxins and drugs*
Bilateral epidural or subdural empyema, haematomas	Alcohol
	Amphetamines
	Anticholinergics
Cerebellum abscess, haemorrhage, tumour	Barbiturates
	Benzodiazepines
Pituitary tumour	Ethylene glycol
Pontine haemorrhage	Lithium
Subarachnoid haemorrhage	LSD
	Monoamine oxidase inhibitors
Thalamus haemorrhage	Opiates
Uncal herniation	Tricyclic antidepressants
Destructive	*Metabolic*
Acute anoxic injury	Acidosis
Basilar occlusion	Addison's disease
Bilateral carotid occlusion	Alkalosis
	Cushing's disease
Brainstem haemorrhage	Hepatic encephalopathy
	Hypercapnia
Central pontine myelinolysis	Hypertensive encephalopathy and posterior reversible leucoencephalopathy syndrome
Concussion and traumatic brain injuries	Hypoglycaemia
	Hypothermia
Midbrain infarct	Hypothyroidism
Thalamus infarct	Ionic disturbances (Na^+, Ca^{2+}, Mg^{2+}, hyper- and hypo-, PO_4^{3-}, hypo-)
Venous sinus thrombosis	Sepsis
	Severe hyperglycaemia, with or without ketoacidosis
	Severe hyperthermia
	Uraemic encephalopathy
	Wernicke's encephalopathy (thiamine deficiency)
Infections	*Oxygen-related*
Acute disseminated encephalomyelitis	Carbon monoxide intoxication
	Cyanide intoxication
Bacterial meningitis	Diffuse ischaemia
Viral encephalitis	Disseminated intravascular coagulation
	Hyperviscosity
	Hypoxia
	Other
	Adrenoleucodystrophy
	Creutzfeldt–Jakob disease
	Non convulsive status epilepticus
	Postictal seizure
	Vasculitis

recently proposed that the MCS should be subcategorized into MCS+ for those who show high-level behavioural responses, such as following commands, and MCS– for those who show low-level behavioural responses, such as visual pursuit (Figure 26.1) (12). Such

classification is supported by neuroanatomical data that demonstrate better preservation of language-related networks in MCS+ compared to MCS– patients (Figure 26.2), even though MCS+ patients cannot communicate reliably (13). Emergence from MCS is characterized by the recovery of the ability to communicate or the functional use of objects (6). Further recovery is then possible, although residual cognitive and/or functional disabilities of various severities are likely.

Locked-in syndrome

Disorders of consciousness must be differentiated from the locked-in syndrome which usually results from lesions of the mid pons and a complete disruption of the pyramidal tract and most of the cranial nerves. In this condition, usually following a period of coma, patients appear unresponsive. However, they are actually fully conscious but lack the ability to react to stimuli because of complete paralysis of voluntary muscle action except for eye movements and blinking (14). Patients with the locked-in syndrome can only communicate using vertical eye movements or by closing their eyelids (14,15). Whilst it is vital to make the correct diagnosis, this is unfortunately often delayed.

Clinical assessment

Evaluation of coma and related states is primarily clinical. As discussed earlier, a general examination can often give clues to the causes of the underlying brain injury. Multiple scales have been developed in an attempt to bring uniformity to the neurological examination, and to standardize communication between clinicians about the level of consciousness (Table 26.2).

The most widely used scale to assess depth of coma is the Glasgow Coma Scale (GCS) (16). It was initially developed to assess patients after TBI and measures the best response to three parameters: eye opening which assesses the arousal level (from 1 to 4), verbal responses which evaluates the integrity of the nervous system (from 1 to 5), and motor responses which assesses the integrity of the motor system (from 1 to 6) (17). Thus the total score ranges from 3 to 15, and brain damage is described as severe if the GCS is less than or equal to 8, moderate if the score is between 9 and 12, and mild if greater than or equal to 13. The short-term evolution of a patient's status is best predicted by the score of the motor subset (18). The GCS has considerable limitations, including inconsistent interobserver reliability (19), inability to test verbal responses in intubated patients (20,21), lack of assessment of brainstem reflexes (22), and inability to detect subtle or focal changes in neurological examination. In 1982, Born et al. suggested adding an assessment of brainstem reflexes to the GCS to improve its prognostic value (22). However, this scale, called the Glasgow Liège Scale (GLS), did not gain widespread international acceptance.

More recently, Wijdicks and colleagues (23) proposed a new coma scale named the Full Outline of UnResponsiveness (FOUR), as an alternative to the GCS in the evaluation of consciousness in severely brain-injured patients of both traumatic and non-traumatic causes. As its name suggests, the FOUR scale consists of four components—eye and motor responses, brainstem reflexes, and respiration (Table 26.2). In contrast to the GCS and GLS, it avoids assessment of verbal function. This is an advantage in the acute care setting as most patients are intubated or tracheotomized. It also offers the advantage of being able to identify subtle non-verbal signs of consciousness by evaluating visual pursuit, which is not

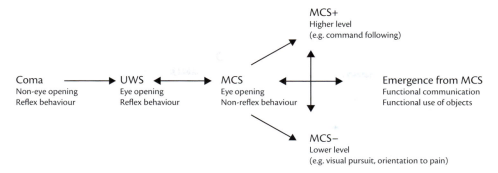

Fig. 26.1 Nosology of disorders of consciousness. The nosology of disorders of consciousness is rapidly changing. As new diagnostic tools are developed, new conditions are described, each with its own prognosis for outcome and survival. However, the boundaries between each of these more precisely defined conditions are less and less clear-cut. MCS, minimally conscious state; UWS, unresponsive wakefulness syndrome.

assessed by the GCS or GLS scales (24,25). The assessment of visual pursuit is particularly important because it can be a behavioural marker signifying transition from the UWS to MCS (26).

In the setting of chronic coma, the use of the Coma Recovery Scale—Revised (CRS-R) is advised (27). This scale was specifically developed to differentiate between conscious and unconscious patients and incorporates the diagnostic criteria of MCS, including assessment of visual pursuit (28). The CRS-R contains six subscales (auditory, visual, motor, oromotor, communication, and arousal), each with several components. However, its use is limited in intensive care units because it takes up to 1 hour to perform and training in its application is required.

Investigation of impaired consciousness

Despite the best clinical assessment, patients with disorders of consciousness are often poorly evaluated in terms of residual brain function and conscious awareness. Severe motor deficits, language and cognitive impairments, as well as arousal fluctuations, can all lead to high rates of misdiagnosis (29). Various electrophysiological

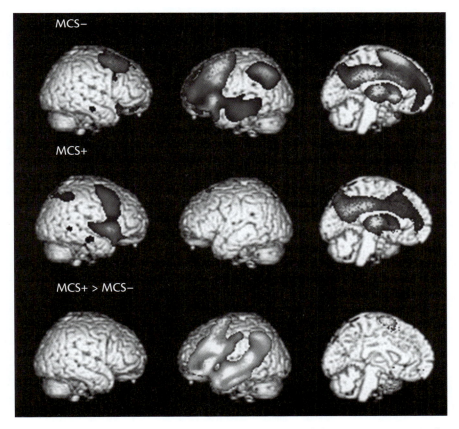

Fig. 26.2 Differentiation between minimally conscious plus and minus states. Areas with impaired metabolism in patients in a minimally conscious state (MCS) are shaded in the top two panels. The top panel illustrates MCS− (showing non-reflex behaviour) and the middle panel MCS+ (showing command following). The lowest panel illustrates areas with higher metabolism in MCS+ compared to MCS− (shaded). These areas are predominantly the associative frontal, temporal, and parietal cortices. All results are shown on a 3D MRI template and thresholded at false discovery rate corrected P <0.05.
Reproduced from Springer and the *Journal of Neurology*, 2011, 258, 7, pp. 1373–1384, 'From unresponsive wakefulness to minimally conscious PLUS and functional locked-in syndromes: recent advances in our understanding of disorders of consciousness', Bruno MA *et al*. With kind permission from Springer Science and Business Media.

Table 26.2 Scales validated for the evaluation of disorders of consciousness

GCS/GLS	FOUR	CRS-R	
Eye response	**Eye response**	**Auditory function**	**Communication**
4. Eyes open spontaneously	4. Eyelids open or opened, tracking or blinking to command	4. Consistent movement to command*	2. Functional: accurate[+]
3. Eye opening to verbal command	3. Eyelids open but not tracking	3. Reproducible movement to command*	1. Non-functional: intentional*
2. Eye opening to pain	2. Eyelids closed but opens to loud voice	2. Localization to sound	0. None
1. No eye opening	1. Eyelids closed but opens to pain	1. Auditory startle	
	0. Eyelids remain closed with pain	0. None	**Arousal**
Verbal response			3. Attention
5. Oriented	**Motor response**	**Visual function**	2. Eye opening w/o stimulation
4. Confused	4. Thumbs up, fist, or peace sign to command	5. Object recognition*	1. Eye opening with stimulation
3. Inappropriate words	3. Localizing pain	4. Object localization: reaching*	0. Unarousable
2. Incomprehensible sounds	2. Flexion response to pain	3. Visual pursuit*	
1. No verbal response	1. Extensor posturing	2. Fixation*	
	0. No response to pain or generalized myoclonus status epilepticus	1. Visual startle	
Motor response		0. None	
6. Obeys commands	**Brainstem reflexes**		
5. Localizing pain	4. Pupil and corneal reflexes present	**Motor function**	
4. Withdrawal from pain	3. One pupil wide and fixed	6. Functional object use[+]	
3. Stereotyped flexion to pain	2. Pupil or corneal reflexes absent	5. Automatic motor response*	
2. Stereotyped extension to pain	1. Pupil and corneal reflexes absent	4. Object manipulation*	
1. No motor response	0. Absent pupil, corneal, and cough reflex	3. Localization to noxious stimulation*	
		2. Flexion withdrawal	
Brainstem reflexes (only in GLS)	**Respiration**	1. Abnormal posturing	
5. Fronto-orbicular reflex	4. Not intubated, regular breathing pattern	0. None/flaccid	
4. Vertical oculocephalic reflex	3. Not intubated, Cheyne–Stokes breathing pattern		
3. Pupillary light reflex	2. Not intubated, irregular breathing pattern	**Oromotor/verbal function**	
2. Horizontal oculocephalic reflex	1. Breathes above ventilator	3. Intelligible verbalization*	
1. Oculocardiac reflex	0. Breathes at ventilator rate or apnoea	2. Vocalization/oral movement	
0. No brainstem reflex		1. Oral reflexive movement	
		0. None	

CRS-R, Coma Recovery Scale-Revised; EMCS, Emergence from the Minimally Conscious State; FOUR, Full Outline of UnResponsiveness; GCS, Glasgow Coma Scale; GLS, Glasgow Liege Coma Scale; MCS, Minimally Conscious State; UWS, Unresponsive Wakefulness Syndrome.

The GCS is composed of three subscales (eye, verbal, and motor responses) and can score from 3 to 15. GLS is the addition of a fourth subscale to the GCS (the brainstem reflexes) and can score from 3 to 20. The FOUR is composed of four subscales (eye, motor, brainstem and respiration) each composed of 4 items. The CRS-R is composed of six subscales (auditory, visual, motor, oromotor/verbal, communication, and arousal). It can score from 0 to 23. * denotes MCS, and [+] denotes EMCS.

GCS: Reprinted from *The Lancet*, 1, 7968, Jennett B , Teasdale G, Braakman R, Minderhoud J, Knill-Jones R, 'Predicting outcome in individual patients after severe head injury', pp. 1031–1034, Copyright 1976, with permission from Elsevier. FOUR: Reproduced from Wijdicks EF *et al.*, 'Validation of a new coma scale: The FOUR score', *Annals of Neurology*, 58, 4, pp. 585–593, Copyright 2005, John Wiley and Sons CRS-R: Reprinted from *Archives of Physical Medicine and Rehabilitation*, 85, 12, Giacino J , Kalmar K, Whyte J, 'The JFK Coma Recovery Scale-Revised: measurement characteristics and diagnostic utility', pp. 2020–2029, Copyright 2004, with permission from Elsevier.

techniques, as well as new neuroimaging tools that allow direct measurement of brain activity without a motor interface (neuroimaging with active paradigm) or without patient participation (resting state studies), may inform the assessment of the patient's conscious state.

Electrophysiology

A standard clinical electroencephalogram (EEG) recorded in patients at rest is a routine examination in the neurocritical care unit. Visual inspection of EEG traces can give insights into the origin and severity of the underlying brain damage (Figure 26.3). In healthy awake subjects at rest, the EEG displays a posterior and symmetric alpha rhythm that oscillates between 8 and 12 Hz. An irregular beta rhythm (13–30 Hz) of smaller amplitude may be superimposed on this alpha rhythm, especially if the eyes are opened, if the subject is attentive to the environment, and also if benzodiazepines have been taken. After severe brain injury, EEG activity is slower, often in proportion to the severity of the injury. In diffuse brain damage, the normal posterior alpha rhythm is usually replaced by diffuse theta or delta activity (30), and in severe brain injury, a variant of alpha activity, known as alpha-coma, can be observed (31). In contrast to normal alpha rhythm, alpha-coma activity is frontally distributed and non-reactive to stimuli such as eye opening/closing, or auditory

stimulation. With supratentorial lesions, polymorphic focal delta rhythm may be observed over the damaged areas (32). In asymmetric brain injury, the EEG will likely also be asymmetric. The electrophysiological activity of one hemisphere can be nearly normal whilst being severely abnormal in the other. EEG activity may be normal in infratentorial lesions, as it is in patients with the locked-in syndrome (33,34). Burst suppression, where bursts of slow waves mingled with high-frequency transients are followed by periods of electrophysiological inactivity, is an EEG pattern that may also be observed in patients with disorders of consciousness. It reflects neuronal exhaustion and is a sign of very poor prognosis. A flat or isoelectric EEG represents a state of cerebral electrical inactivity, and is one of the confirmatory criteria for the diagnosis of brain death in some jurisdictions (35). Under such circumstances repeated assessments are necessary because an inactive EEG may be reversible, for example, after drug (e.g. barbiturate) intoxication. EEG recordings are also used to identify various epileptic activities, although a precise location of a lesion or seizure focus cannot be determined from scalp EEG because of its low spatial resolution.

Establishing a diagnosis based solely on a standard EEG may be difficult because the observed patterns are not necessarily specific for any coma aetiology, and EEG patterns may vary in the same patient within short time intervals (36).

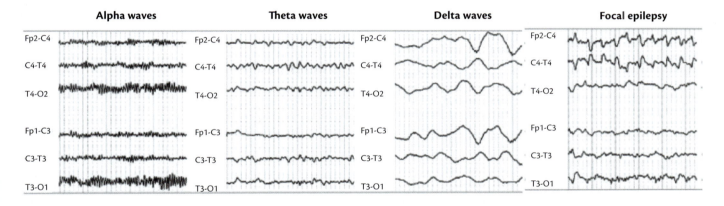

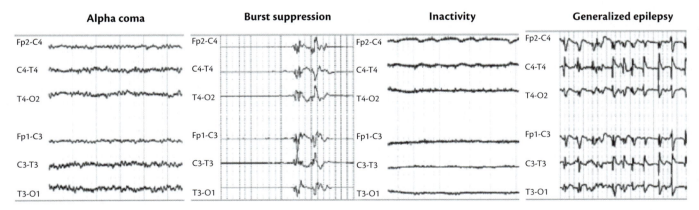

Fig. 26.3 EEG patterns. The three upper lines (even numbers) in each EEG panel refer to the right hemisphere while the three bottom ones (odd numbers) the left hemisphere. From alpha waves to delta waves, the EEG shows a progressive slowing. Alpha waves have a frequency between 8 and 13 Hz, theta between 4 and 7 Hz, and delta below 4 Hz. Alpha coma can appear very similar to normal alpha rhythm but is not reactive. The panel showing focal epilepsy illustrates sharp elements on the right hemisphere, while the generalized epilepsy panel shows a more diffuse spread of these paroxysmal elements. Burst suppression shows a period of global isoelectric recording followed suddenly by a global discharge of neuronal electric activity. This illustrates the progressive exhaustion of the neurons, and rapidly leads to the next figure, inactivity, which can be one sign of a brain death.

C, central; Fp, fronto-parietal; O, occipital; T, temporal.

Other investigations include quantitative analysis of the EEG and event-related potentials (ERPs). Various quantitative EEG techniques are available and most use EEG derived numerical parameters that can be computed to analyse entropy, power spectrum or connectivity. ERPs are based on the averaging of sensory or motor stimulus time-locked events (see Chapter 14). Although encouraging results have demonstrated differences between conscious and unconscious patients using these techniques, both at the diagnostic and prognostic level (30), it is currently not possible to identify a single parameter that will provide an accurate diagnosis and prognosis in an individual patient.

Imaging

Cranial CT and magnetic resonance imaging (MRI) scans provide additional information in the acute phase about the nature and extent of brain lesions. The purpose of imaging is different for traumatic and non-traumatic injury. Patients with TBI-related coma require rapid exclusion of any condition that requires urgent surgery or neuromonitoring and, for this reason, CT remains the gold standard to detect both primary and secondary intracranial events in the acute phase (37). CT is also more widely available, easier to perform in critically ill patients, and quicker than MRI, although MRI is able to detect more subtle brain injuries, such as diffuse axonal injury, cortical contusions, and acute subdural haematoma (38). Although MRI findings rarely change patient management in the acute phase (39), they can lead to improved prognostication (40,41). In non-TBI patients, CT may be diagnostic in certain pathologies such as intracerebral and subarachnoid haemorrhage, and allow localization of pathological findings. However, CT changes are delayed and less sensitive than MRI in conditions such as acute ischaemic stroke, encephalitis, and encephalopathy (37). MRI is therefore increasingly being used as an acute diagnostic tool in comatose patients.

Assessment of prognosis

Probably the most common question posed to clinicians by a family of a patient in a coma is whether he/she will wake up and make a meaningful recovery. Clinicians and scientists have searched for ways to predict accurately awakening and recovery from coma in an attempt to answer such fundamental questions.

Clinical indicators

Younger age and the absence of important comorbidities, such as alcoholism, drug use, or mental illness, are usually associated with a better outcome (42,43). Further, increased length of time spent in an unconscious state, as well as the cause of the coma, also have major impacts on prognosis. Traumatic aetiology is usually associated with a better prognosis than non-traumatic causes of coma. Patients with an UWS following TBI may continue to improve for up to 12 months after the original insult, whereas significant improvement beyond 3 months is rarely observed in non-traumatic causes of coma (42). Patients in the MCS tend to show greater improvements than those with an UWS, even into the chronic stage, that is, beyond 1 year (44).

Accurate diagnosis of the current state of consciousness is crucial for the accurate estimation of prognosis because each of the subacute to chronic states of altered consciousness is associated with its own prognosis. A Belgian study demonstrated that half of patients in the MCS diagnosed 1 month after a traumatic insult had emerged from this state by 12 months, compared to only 23% of those with an UWS (45). There are reported cases of UWS (46) and MCS (44) patients who have improved long after 3 months in non-traumatic causes of coma and after 12 months for traumatic causes, but functional outcome is usually very poor.

In summary, UWS of non-traumatic aetiology has the worst prognosis, with 90% of patients either dead or still unconscious at 12 months, whereas the MCS of traumatic origin has the best prognosis, with 50% of patients emerging from that state by 1 year (45).

Laboratory investigations

Two serum biomarkers—neuron-specific enolase (NSE) and protein S-100B—have been widely studied as predictors of outcome in patients with disorders of consciousness. NSE is a marker of neuronal death, and considered to be an indicator of hypoxic brain damage. S-100B release on the other hand is related to glial cell damage, and a high level of serum NSE is a marker of poor prognosis in anoxic (47) and traumatic (48) brain injuries. A serum NSE level greater than 33 mcg/L is often considered as a relevant prognostic threshold, although this varies markedly between studies. A rise in S-100B level in the cerebrospinal fluid is also an indicator of poor outcome after TBI (48). A recent meta-analysis confirmed the difficulty in setting an accurate cut-off value for both biomarkers (49), thus limiting their clinical value in isolation. However, their use in combination with other markers of prognosis, such as electrophysiology, is often recommended.

Electrophysiology

Notwithstanding the limited diagnostic value of EEG in patients with disorders of consciousness, it does have some prognostic utility. Alpha coma or burst suppression patterns are usually associated with poor prognosis whereas an EEG that is reactive to stimulation, or has varying patterns, is indicative of a better prognosis (50).

ERPs also have some predictive ability and can be divided in two categories—short and long latency. The absence of short-latency ERPs, such as somatosensory or brainstem auditory-evoked potentials (where the response is elicited between 0 and 100 ms after the presentation of the external stimulation), is associated with a poor outcome. N20 is an early component of the somatosensory ERP recorded at the scalp following electric stimulation of the median nerve at the wrist, and its absence has almost a 100% prognostic value for death or poor neurological outcome after anoxic brain injury in certain coma types (50). However, the presence of an intracranial lesion in a strategic location may be the reason for the absence of this negative wave, thereby limiting its prognostic value after TBI and other cases of coma presenting with intracranial mass lesions (50). Further, the presence of short-latency ERPs does not necessarily indicate that the outcome will be good.

Long-latency ERPs, which are elicited more than 100 ms after external stimulation, have also been used to assess prognosis after coma. These include cognitive ERPs, such as the mismatch negativity (MMN) which is an early negative waveform potential elicited by a deviant tone in a repetitive series of auditory stimuli, and the P300 which is a positive wave potential occurring 300 ms after the stimulus. Using several auditory stimulations, such as different tones, words or names, the MMN and P300 reflect sound discrimination since the patient has to differentiate between the different sounds for these waveforms to be elicited. The presence of these components is usually a marker of good prognosis, although they can be present in both conscious and unconscious patients. In a recent meta-analysis, the presence of a P300 and MMN was predictive of awakening after coma (51). In a tree-based design, Fischer and colleagues described an algorithm that is able to predict awakening when MMN is present, or non-awakening when MMN and either pupillary reflexes or somatosensory N20 are absent, with good accuracy in post-anoxic unconscious patients (52).

Imaging

More recently, assessment of residual consciousness has been conducted using imaging techniques, such as active functional MRI paradigms, positron emission tomography, and combined transcranial magnetic stimulation and EEG, but these still require validation at the single-patient level.

Delirium

Delirium is a condition linked to coma since it is also a state of altered consciousness. It can precede the progression to coma, and complicate its resolution, especially in the intensive care setting. Delirium is characterized by a sudden, often transient and fluctuating impairment of the level of consciousness, an alteration in the ability to sustain attention, cognitive deterioration, and/or disturbances in environmental perception manifesting as temporal and spatial disorientation and hallucinations. It is often associated with a modification of the sleep–wake cycle, including reversal of the sleep cycle, and changes (both increases and decreases) in sleep time. Motor agitation and inappropriate emotional reactions may also be present (53). The reported incidence of delirium in patients in intensive care units varies from 20% in non-intubated patients to 80% in mechanically ventilated patients (54). In patients in general medical wards, the incidence of delirium is around 30%, and up to 60% in the perioperative period (55). The median duration of delirium is 3 days, although this is extremely variable.

Classification

Three categories of delirium can be identified—hyperactive, hypoactive, and mixed. Hyperactive delirium is characterized by hallucinations, psychomotor agitation, and decreased sleep time, whereas the hypoactive type is associated with temporospatial disorientation and increased sleepiness (56). Patients suffering from mixed delirium fluctuate between hyperactive and hypoactive subtypes.

Outcome

Delirium is a major health issue despite being regarded by many clinicians as an annoying condition, and is reversible when the causes are withdrawn. A recent meta-analysis found that delirium is associated with higher inpatient and 12-month mortality after stroke, as well as with longer hospital stay and a higher degree of dependence at discharge (57). Delirium is also associated with mortality increases in postoperative patients managed in general wards (56). Hypoactive delirium, which is the most common form of delirium in older patients, is associated with worse prognosis than other delirium types (56). The duration of delirium is also a major mortality risk. Patients who suffer from delirium in the intensive care unit have a higher risk of long-term cognitive impairment than those who do not (58).

Risk factors

There are many risk factors for the development of delirium and they are usually split into predisposing and precipitating factors. In the neurocritical care unit, predisposing factors include advanced age, severity of presenting illness, history of alcoholism, dementia, hypertension, coma, and the use of benzodiazepines. Common precipitating factors include acute illness, sleep deprivation, metabolic disturbance, immobilization, infection, dopaminergic, anticholinergic or benzodiazepines drugs, and environmental factors such as lack of daylight and increased background noise levels (53,58).

Pathophysiology

The exact pathophysiology of delirium remains unclear, although it is hypothesized that it is precipitated by an imbalance in neurotransmitter levels. More precisely, a decrease in acetylcholinergic activity and an increase in dopaminergic, serotoninergic, and GABAergic activities are believed to be causative factors. This is compatible with the actions on these neurotransmitters of drugs, including benzodiazepines, dopaminergic agonists, and anticholinergics (including the side effects of tricyclic antidepressants), that are known to precipitate delirium. Inflammatory markers such as interleukin (IL)-6, IL-8, C-reactive protein, and procalcitonin have also been proposed as causes of delirium, but these findings are inconsistent between studies, possibly because of the rapid variation in the serum levels of these markers, as well as other confounding factors (58).

Assessment of delirium

In the intensive care unit, the most reliable and validated scales to assess delirium are the Confusion Assessment Method for the Intensive Care Unit (CAM-ICU) and the Intensive Care Delirium Screening Checklist (ICDSC). Up to 75% of delirious patients are misdiagnosed if these validated scales are not used (58). The CAM-ICU has four components assessing respectively fluctuation of the baseline mental status, inattention, disorganized thinking, and altered level of consciousness. It is positive, confirming the diagnosis of delirium, if items one, two, and either three or four are present (59).

A number of other conditions can be mistaken for delirium and should be excluded. Patients suffering from Wernicke aphasia may be misdiagnosed as delirious because they do not understand a simple order. However, their deficit concerns only language processing and other cognitive functions remain intact. Patients with bifrontal lesions, leading to frontal dementia, may also appear delirious because they are apathic, have memory and attentional disturbance, as well as inappropriate emotional reactions, but the chronic nature of this condition distinguishes it from delirium. However, it is important to note that patients with pre-existing dementia may develop delirium when acutely ill. Non-convulsive status epilepticus can mimic some of the features of hypoactive delirium, and an EEG should be performed in all patients with a suspected diagnosis of delirium to exclude seizures.

Treatment

As the proverb says, prevention is better than cure. This is especially true for delirium because of the multiple predisposing and precipitating factors. In the neurocritical care unit, early mobilization and sleep hygiene (noise suppression, dimmed lights at night, and daytime clustering of clinical interventions) can lower the incidence and duration of delirium, although such manoeuvers can be difficult to achieve in this acute care setting. In general medical wards, non-pharmacological measures such as promotion of sleep, decreases in noise level, early mobilization, and repeated reorientation lower the incidence of delirium by as much as 40% (58), and also reduce the duration of the delirious state and length of hospital stay (60).

The most efficient treatment for delirium is to prevent or treat its cause; with the resolution of precipitating factors, delirium is more likely to disappear. When the cause of delirium is unknown, or unlikely to resolve within a reasonable time, management may rely on pharmacological treatments, although there is no consensus on the ideal drug. Antipsychotic agents lower the duration of delirium in critically ill patients, although there is currently no evidence to support the use of pharmacological agents to prevent delirium in the intensive care unit. Agents such as intravenous haloperidol, oral olanzapine, quetiapine, and ziprasidone have all been used to treat delirium. Atypical antipsychotics are no better than haloperidol, but are associated with fewer extrapyramidal symptoms. It was believed that a cholinesterase inhibitor such as rivastigmine might be an effective therapy as it would act on the hypothesized lowered cholinergic activity in a delirious patient's brain. However, studies have reported mixed results, and there are currently no recommendations for its use in this setting. Alpha-2 agonists, such as dexmedetomidine, might have advantages over haloperidol in reducing the duration of delirium in intensive care patients (61). Benzodiazepines may precipitate delirium and should be avoided at all costs, unless the precipitating factor for delirium is alcohol or benzodiazepine withdrawal where this class of drug is first choice.

Conclusion

Acute coma has many different causes and lies at one end of a spectrum of disordered consciousness that includes UWS, MCS, and delirium. Clinical examination alone is insufficient to confirm the causes of an altered state of consciousness in most cases and confirmatory investigations, such as imaging, EEG, and serum biomarkers can assist physicians in clarifying the neurological status and in prognostication. Nevertheless, the exact mechanisms underlying chronic disorders of consciousness remain poorly understood and further studies are needed to identify the best diagnostic and prognostic modalities in these patients. Delirium occurs most often in frail and/or elderly patients and can lead to several complications, of which coma is the most extreme. Studying patients who recover from abnormal conscious states might assist in understanding the mechanisms underlying the recovery of consciousness in post-comatose patients.

Acknowledgements

This work was supported by the Belgian National Funds for Scientific Research (FNRS), Fonds Léon Frédericq, James S. McDonnell Foundation, Mind Science Foundation, European Commission (Mindbridge, DISCOS, DECODER & COST), Concerted Research Action (ARC 06/11-340), Public Utility Foundation 'Université Européenne du Travail', 'Fondazione Europea di Ricerca Biomedica' and the University of Liège. OB is a research fellow, OG is a post-doctoral researcher and SL is the research director at the FNRS.

References

1. Posner JB, Saper CB, Schiff ND, Plum F. *Plum and Posner's Diagnosis of Stupor and Coma* (4th edn). Oxford: Oxford University Press; 2007.
2. Laureys S. Eyes open, brain shut. *Sci Am.* 2007;296(5):84–9.
3. Lipton SA, Rosenberg PA. Excitatory amino acids as a final common pathway for neurologic disorders. *N Engl J Med.* 1994;330(9):613–22.
4. Young GB, Ropper AH, Bolton CF. *Coma and Impaired Consciousness: A Clinical Perspective.* New York: McGraw-Hill; 1998.
5. Laureys S, Celesia GG, Cohadon F, Lavrijsen J, León-Carrión J, Sannita WG, et al. Unresponsive wakefulness syndrome: a new name for the vegetative state or apallic syndrome. *BMC Med.* 2010;8,68.
6. Giacino JT, Ashwal S, Childs N, Cranford R, Jennett B, Katz DI, et al. The minimally conscious state: definition and diagnostic criteria. *Neurology.* 2002;58(3):349–53.
7. Plum F, Posner JB. The diagnosis of stupor and coma. *Contemp Neurol Ser.* 1972;10:1–286.
8. Gosseries O, Bruno MA, Chatelle C, Vanhaudenhuyse A, Schnakers C, Soddu A, et al. Disorders of consciousness: what's in a name? *NeuroRehabilitation.* 2011;28(1):3–14.
9. The Multi-Society Task Force on PVS. Medical aspects of the persistent vegetative state (1). The Multi-Society Task Force on PVS. *N Engl J Med.* 1994;330(21):1499–508.
10. Cologan V, Drouot X, Parapatics S, Delorme A, Gruber G, Moonen G, et al. Sleep in the unresponsive wakefulness syndrome and minimally conscious state. *J Neurotrauma.* 2013;30(5):339–46.
11. Landsness E, Bruno MA, Noirhomme Q, Riedner B, Gosseries O, Schnakers C, et al. Electrophysiological correlates of behavioural changes in vigilance in vegetative state and minimally conscious state. *Brain.* 2011;134(Pt 8):2222–32.
12. Bruno MA, Vanhaudenhuyse A, Thibaut A, Moonen G, Laureys S. From unresponsive wakefulness to minimally conscious PLUS and functional locked-in syndromes: recent advances in our understanding of disorders of consciousness. *J Neurol.* 2011;258(7):1373–84.
13. Bruno MA, Majerus S, Boly M, Vanhaudenhuyse A, Schnakers C, Gosseries O, et al. Functional neuroanatomy underlying the clinical subcategorization of minimally conscious state patients. *J Neurol.* 2012;259(6):1087–98.
14. Gosseries O, Bruno MA, Vanhaudenhuyse A, Laureys S, Schnakers C. Consciousness in the locked-in syndrome. In Steven L, Giulio T (eds) *The Neurology of Consciousness.* San Diego, CA: Academic Press; 2009:191–203.
15. Schnakers C, Perrin F, Schabus M, Hustinx R, Majerus S, Moonen G, et al. Detecting consciousness in a total locked-in syndrome: an active event-related paradigm. *Neurocase.* 2009;15(4):271–7.
16. Jennett B, Teasdale G, Braakman R, Minderhoud J, Knill-Jones R. Predicting outcome in individual patients after severe head injury. *Lancet.* 1976;1(7968):1031–4.
17. Prasad K. The Glasgow Coma Scale: a critical appraisal of its clinimetric properties. *J Clin Epidemiol.* 1996;49(7):755–63.
18. Jagger J, Jane JA, Rimel R. The Glasgow coma scale: to sum or not to sum? *Lancet.* 1983;2(8341):97.
19. Rowley G, Fielding K. Reliability and accuracy of the Glasgow Coma Scale with experienced and inexperienced users. *Lancet.* 1991;337(8740):535–8.
20. Marion DW, Carlier PM. Problems with initial Glasgow Coma Scale assessment caused by prehospital treatment of patients with head injuries: results of a national survey. *J Trauma.* 1994;36(1):89–95.
21. Murray GD, Teasdale GM, Braakman R, Cohadon F, Dearden M, Iannotti F, et al. The European Brain Injury Consortium survey of head injuries. *Acta Neurochir (Wien).* 1999;141(3):223–36.
22. Born JD, Hans P, Dexters G, Kalangu K, Lenelle J, Milbouw G, et al. Practical assessment of brain dysfunction in severe head trauma. *Neurochirurg.* 1982;28(1):1–7.
23. Wijdicks EF, Bamlet WR, Maramattom BV, Manno EM, McClelland RL. Validation of a new coma scale: the FOUR score. *Ann Neurol.* 2005;58(4):585–93.

24. Bruno MA, Ledoux D, Lambermont B, Damas F, Schnakers C, Vanhaudenhuyse A, et al. Comparison of the Full Outline of UnResponsiveness and Glasgow Liege Scale/Glasgow Coma Scale in an intensive care unit population. *Neurocrit Care*. 2011;15(3):447–53.

25. Schnakers C, Giacino J, Kalmar K, Piret S, Lopez E, Boly M, et al. Does the FOUR score correctly diagnose the vegetative and minimally conscious states? *Ann Neurol*. 2006;60(6):744–5.

26. Giacino J, Whyte J. The vegetative and minimally conscious states: current knowledge and remaining questions. *J Head Trauma Rehabil*. 2005;20(1):30–50.

27. Giacino J, Kalmar K, Whyte J. The JFK Coma Recovery Scale-Revised: measurement characteristics and diagnostic utility. *Arch Phys Med Rehabil*. 2004;85(12):2020–9.

28. American Congress of Rehabilitation Medicine, Brain Injury-Interdisciplinary Special Interest Group, Disorders of Consciousness Task Force, Seel RT, Sherer M, Whyte J, et al. Assessment scales for disorders of consciousness: evidence-based recommendations for clinical practice and research. *Arch Phys Med Rehabil*. 2010;91(12):1795–813.

29. Schnakers C, Vanhaudenhuyse A, Giacino J, Ventura M, Boly M, Majerus S, et al. Diagnostic accuracy of the vegetative and minimally conscious state: clinical consensus versus standardized neurobehavioral assessment. *BMC Neurol*. 2009;9,35.

30. Lehembre R, Gosseries O, Lugo Z, Jedidi Z, Chatelle C, Sadzot B, et al. Electrophysiological investigations of brain function in coma, vegetative and minimally conscious patients. *Arch Ital Biol*. 2012;150(2–3):122–39.

31. Kaplan PW, Genoud D, Ho TW, Jallon P. Etiology, neurologic correlations, and prognosis in alpha coma. *Clin Neurophysiol*. 1999;110(2):205–13.

32. Brenner RP. The interpretation of the EEG in stupor and coma. *Neurologist*. 2005;11(5):271–84.

33. Bassetti C, Mathis J, Hess CW. Multimodal electrophysiological studies including motor evoked potentials in patients with locked-in syndrome: report of six patients. *J Neurol Neurosurg Psychiatry*. 1994;57(11):1403–6.

34. Gutling E, Isenmann S, Wichmann W. Electrophysiology in the locked-in-syndrome. *Neurology*. 1996;46(4):1092–101.

35. Husain AM. Electroencephalographic assessment of coma. *J Clin Neurophysiol*. 2006;23(3):208–20.

36. Kulkarni VP, Lin K, Benbadis SR. EEG findings in the persistent vegetative state. *J Clin Neurophysiol*. 2007;24(6):433–7.

37. Le TH, Gean AD. Neuroimaging of traumatic brain injury. *Mt Sinai J Med*. 2009;76(2):145–62.

38. Morais DF, Spotti AR, Tognola WA, Gaia FF, Andrade AF. Clinical application of magnetic resonance in acute traumatic brain injury. *Arq Neuropsiquiatr*. 2008;66(1):53–8.

39. Manolakaki D, Velmahos GC, Spaniolas K, de Moya M, Alam HB. Early magnetic resonance imaging is unnecessary in patients with traumatic brain injury. *J Trauma*. 2009;66(4):1008–12.

40. Firsching R, Woischneck D, Diedrich M, Klein S, Rückert A, Wittig H, et al. Early magnetic resonance imaging of brainstem lesions after severe head injury. *J Neurosurg*. 1998;89(5):707–12.

41. Kampfl A, Schmutzhard E, Franz G, Pfausler B, Haring HP, Ulmer H, et al. Prediction of recovery from post-traumatic vegetative state with cerebral magnetic-resonance imaging. *Lancet*. 1998;351(9118):1763–7.

42. The Multi-Society Task Force on PVS. Medical aspects of the persistent vegetative state (2). The Multi-Society Task Force on PVS. *N Engl J Med*. 1994;330(22):1572–9.

43. Laureys S, Berré J, Goldman S. Cerebral function in coma, vegetative state, minimally conscious state, locked-in syndrome, and brain death.

In Vincent J-L (ed) *2001 Yearbook of Intensive Care and Emergency Medicine*. Berlin: Springer; 2001:386–96.

44. Luaute J, Maucort-Boulch D, Tell L, Quelard F, Sarraf T, Iwaz J, et al. Long-term outcomes of chronic minimally conscious and vegetative states. *Neurology*. 2010;75(3):246–52.

45. Ledoux D, Bruno M, Schnakers C, Giacino J, Ventura M, Vanopdenbosch L, et al. Outcome of vegetative and minimally conscious states: results from the Belgian Federal expertise network. In *Eighteenth Meeting of the European Neurological Society*. Nice, France; 2008:24.

46. Estraneo A, Moretta P, Loreto V, Lanzillo B, Santoro L, Trojano L. Late recovery after traumatic, anoxic, or hemorrhagic long-lasting vegetative state. *Neurology*. 2010;75(3):239–45.

47. Daubin C, Quentin C, Allouche S, Etard O, Gaillard C, Seguin A, et al. Serum neuron-specific enolase as predictor of outcome in comatose cardiac-arrest survivors: a prospective cohort study. *BMC Cardiovasc Disord*. 2011;11,48.

48. Bohmer AE, Oses JP, Schmidt AP, Perón CS, Krebs CL, Oppitz PP, et al. Neuron-specific enolase, S100B, and glial fibrillary acidic protein levels as outcome predictors in patients with severe traumatic brain injury. *Neurosurgery*. 2011;68(6):1624–30.

49. Shinozaki K, Oda S, Sadahiro T, Nakamura M, Hirayama Y, Abe R, et al. S-100B and neuron-specific enolase as predictors of neurological outcome in patients after cardiac arrest and return of spontaneous circulation: a systematic review. *Crit Care*. 2009;13(4):R121.

50. Oddo M, Rossetti AO. Predicting neurological outcome after cardiac arrest. *Curr Opin Crit Care*. 2011;17(3):254–9.

51. Daltrozzo J, Wioland N, Mutschler V, Kotchoubey B. Predicting coma and other low responsive patients outcome using event-related brain potentials: a meta-analysis. *Clin Neurophysiol*. 2007;118(3):606–14.

52. Fischer C, Luaute J, Nemoz C, Morlet D, Kirkorian G, Mauguiere F. Improved prediction of awakening or nonawakening from severe anoxic coma using tree-based classification analysis. *Crit Care Med*. 2006;34(5):1520–4.

53. Barr J, Fraser GL, Puntillo K, Ely EW, Gélinas C, Dasta JF, et al. Clinical practice guidelines for the management of pain, agitation, and delirium in adult patients in the intensive care unit. *Crit Care Med*. 2013;41(1):278–80.

54. Cavallazzi R, Saad M, Marik PE. Delirium in the ICU: an overview. *Ann Intensive Care*. 2012;2(1):49.

55. Stevens RD, Nyquist PA. Coma, delirium, and cognitive dysfunction in critical illness. *Crit Care Clin*. 2006;22(4):787–804.

56. Robinson TN, Raeburn CD, Tran ZV, Brenner LA, Moss M. Motor subtypes of postoperative delirium in older adults. *Arch Surg*. 2011;146(3):295–300.

57. Shi Q, Presutti R, Selchen D, Saposnik G. Delirium in acute stroke: a systematic review and meta-analysis. *Stroke*. 2012;43(3):645–9.

58. Zaal IJ, Slooter AJ. Delirium in critically ill patients: epidemiology, pathophysiology, diagnosis and management. *Drugs*. 2012;72(11):1457–71.

59. Ely EW, Margolin R, Francis J, May L, Truman B, Dittus R, et al. Evaluation of delirium in critically ill patients: validation of the Confusion Assessment Method for the Intensive Care Unit (CAM-ICU). *Crit Care Med*. 2001;29(7):1370–9.

60. Lundstrom M, Edlund A, Karlsson S, Brannstrom B, Bucht G, Gustafson Y. A multifactorial intervention program reduces the duration of delirium, length of hospitalization, and mortality in delirious patients. *J Am Geriatr Soc*. 2005;53(4):622–8.

61. Bledowski J, Trutia A. A review of pharmacologic management and prevention strategies for delirium in the intensive care unit. *Psychosomatics*. 2012;53(3):203–11.

CHAPTER 27

Non-neurological complications of acquired brain injury

Derek J. Roberts and David A. Zygun

Acquired brain injury is commonly associated with several extracranial, or non-neurological, complications (1–4). In a prospective cohort study of 209 consecutive mechanically ventilated adults admitted to an intensive care unit (ICU) after severe traumatic brain injury (TBI), 185 (88.5%) developed dysfunction of at least one non-neurological organ system (2). Non-neurological complications include disturbance of the immune or autonomic nervous system (ANS) and dysfunction of cardiovascular, pulmonary, haematological, endocrine, renal, and gastrointestinal organ systems. The occurrence of non-neurological complications is often linked with significant morbidity and mortality, possibly because many increase the risk of hypotension, hypoxaemia, and/or coagulopathy, all of which are known associates of poor outcome after acquired brain injury. Moreover, as several of these complications present acutely (neurogenic pulmonary oedema has been reported at the scene of a motor vehicle collision in patients with TBI) (5), interdisciplinary collaboration between emergency medicine physicians, trauma and neurological surgeons, cardiologists, neurologists, neurointensivists, and other specialists is likely to be required to achieve optimal outcomes.

This chapter provides an evidence-based overview of the pathophysiology, epidemiology, clinical manifestations, prevention, and diagnosis of non-neurological complications of acquired brain injury. Each section also reviews potential management considerations and strategies, although evidence for the treatment of these complications is limited.

Autonomic nervous system dysfunction

Two different types of episodic ANS overactivity may occur after acquired brain injury (6). Paroxysmal sympathetic hyperactivity (PSH) is characterized by increased activation of the sympathetic division of the ANS alone (7), whereas mixed autonomic hyperactivity involves both the sympathetic and parasympathetic divisions of the ANS (Table 27.1) (6). While PSH is the most accurate term used to describe the sympathetic overactivity, at least 31 different synonyms exist. Dysautonomia, sympathetic or autonomic storming, and paroxysmal autonomic instability with dystonia are the most common (6,8).

Although the outcome of patients with mixed autonomic hyperactivity has not been well studied, the development of PSH has been associated with poor neurological outcomes, prolonged post-traumatic amnesia, protracted ICU and hospital lengths of stay, and greater likelihood of the need for tracheostomy (6,9–11).

Patients with PSH may also exhibit hypermetabolism with resultant body weight loss, and may be at an increased risk of hyperthermia, cardiovascular dysfunction, and even heterotopic ossification (6,12–14).

Pathophysiology

The pathophysiology of mixed autonomic hyperactivity has not yet been clarified, but two general hypotheses have been proposed to explain the development of PSH after acquired brain injury (15). It was previously believed that PSH results from a brain injury-induced epileptic focus, but attempts to identify or treat seizures in patients with PSH have largely been unsuccessful (16–21). Thus, many now argue that it results from a 'disconnection syndrome' along the brain/brainstem/spinal cord axis, leading to release from higher inhibitory control of one or more central nervous system (CNS) excitatory centres (15). Mechanical factors, particularly increased intracranial pressure (ICP), also likely contribute to the development of increased sympathetic activity (see 'Cardiovascular dysfunction') (22).

Conventional disconnection theories suggest that brain injury cranial to the diencephalic or brainstem sympatho-excitatory preganglionic neurons release these cells from higher CNS inhibitory control and allow adrenergic paroxysms to occur (15). However, computed tomography (CT) and magnetic resonance (MR) studies have failed to demonstrate a single brain lesion consistently associated with hyperadrenergic activity (15,22). As PSH has been linked with diffuse axonal injury as well as brainstem, focal parenchymal, and deep brain lesions, it is possible that deep lesions are more common among those with PSH (11,22,23). Conversely, hyperadrenergic activity may simply relate to the severity of acquired brain injury (22).

Another disconnection theory, the excitatory:inhibitory ratio model, argues that brainstem and diencephalic structures are inhibitory in nature and that damage to them results in activation of excitatory spinal cord processes and leads to PSH (15,24). Interestingly, this model also suggests that noxious and non-noxious peripheral inputs may modulate hyperadrenergic activity by stimulating afferents that converge on these excitatory spinal cord centres (15,24). Some support for this hypothesis is afforded by reports of autonomic paroxysms among brain-injured patients during or after exposure to pain, blocked urinary catheters, endotracheal suctioning, turning/repositioning, and even loud environmental noise (6,15,17–20,25,26).

Table 27.1 Characteristics of autonomic overactivity syndromes after acquired brain injury

Autonomic overactivity syndrome	Pathophysiology	Clinical manifestations		Diagnosis	Aetiology	Estimated incidence	Prognosis
		Autonomic	Non-autonomic				
PSH	Disconnection syndrome; ↑ ICP	Paroxysms of sympathetic hyperactivity	Paroxysms of abnormal motor function	Most sets of diagnostic criteria require ↑ HR, BP, RR, and temperature; abnormal motor activity; and diaphoresis	TBI (79%), hypoxic brain injury, and likely all other CNS diseases	8–33% among ICU patients with brain injury; 8–14% later after TBI	Resolution during ICU stay or acute recovery phase (short duration variant) versus persistence into rehabilitation period (prolonged variant)
Mixed autonomic hyperactivity	Unknown	Paroxysms of sympathetic and parasympathetic hyperactivity	Intermittent hiccups, lacrimation, sighing, and yawning	No diagnostic criteria exist; syndrome was only recently proposed as separate from PSH	Intracranial tumours and congenital CNS conditions; only one reported case after TBI	Unknown	Unknown

BP, blood pressure; CNS, central nervous system; HR, heart rate; ICP, intracranial pressure; ICU, intensive care unit; PSH, paroxysmal sympathetic hyperactivity; RR, respiratory rate; TBI, traumatic brain injury.

Clinical manifestations and diagnosis

In addition to the signs and symptoms associated with episodic hyperactivity of the sympathetic and parasympathetic nervous systems, patients with paroxysmal autonomic overactivity may also display several other abnormal clinical manifestations (6). Increased sympathetic activity may manifest as tachycardia, tachypnoea, hypertension, hyperthermia, sweating, and mydriasis (6), whereas increased parasympathetic tone presents with decreases in heart rate (HR), respiratory rate (RR), blood pressure (BP), body temperature, and miosis (6). In addition to episodically increased sympathetic tone, patients with PSH may also exhibit paroxysms of abnormal motor function, including decerebrate or decorticate posturing, spasticity, hypertonia and/or dystonia, teeth-grinding, and agitation (6). In contrast, those with mixed autonomic hyperactivity have variable motor abnormalities, but may develop intermittent hiccups, lacrimation, sighing and yawning in addition to mixed sympathetic/parasympathetic activity (6).

No consensus set of diagnostic criteria exists to define either type acquired brain injury related paroxysmal autonomic overactivity. A recent systematic review by Perkes and colleagues identified nine sets of related, but unique, diagnostic criteria for PSH (8), but none for mixed autonomic hyperactivity (7,9,11,13,27–32). As expected, most of the diagnostic criteria for PSH include descriptions of increased HR, BP, RR and temperature, as well as abnormal motor activity and diaphoresis (8). Moreover, paroxysms of episodic activity and feature severity (e.g. HR >120 beats/min, RR >30 breaths/min, or systolic BP >160 mmHg during a paroxysm) were used for the diagnosis of PSH by at least five of these sets of criteria. Other characteristics, including episode frequency (≥ one or two per day), duration (≥ 3 or 14 days), and aetiology (increased ICP), as well as exclusion of differential diagnoses, were less commonly described (8).

Aetiology, epidemiology, natural history, and prognosis

PSH and mixed autonomic hyperactivity are associated with disparate types of brain injury (6). A recent systematic review found that the majority of reported cases of PSH (79%) are associated with TBI, but it has also been described after hypoxic brain injury, stroke, hydrocephalus, brain tumours, autoimmune encephalitis, and other CNS diseases (6). PSH appears to be more common after hypoxic brain injury than TBI in children (6,30). In contrast, only one case of mixed autonomic hyperactivity has been reported after TBI (33), with most being associated with intracranial tumours and congenital CNS conditions such as agenesis of the corpus callosum (6).

The incidence of mixed autonomic hyperactivity has not yet been established. The estimated incidence of PSH varies widely across individual studies, and a systematic review reported PSH in 8–33% of patients with acute brain injury admitted to the ICU, and in 8–14% later after TBI (6). This incidence variability is likely to be related to several factors including use of explicit PSH diagnostic criteria in some studies but not others, variation in the diagnostic criteria in studies that applied them, comparisons of patients with different causes and severity of acquired brain injury, and variations in the time that patients were studied post brain injury.

As PSH appears to persist for variable lengths of time, some have proposed that it may actually exist as two different temporal variants (6). The first is a transitory, short duration variant that occurs largely during the ICU stay or in the acute phase of recovery, whereas in the second, more prolonged variant, PSH may last for weeks to months and thus extend into the rehabilitation/convalescence period. As mixed autonomic hyperactivity has only recently been considered a different disorder from PSH (6), it is unknown whether this temporal variant classification scheme can also be applied to this condition.

Management

Treatment of PSH has only been described in case reports or series, with its effectiveness defined as improvements in sympathetic or motor hyperactivity rather than patient outcome (6). As such, treatment recommendations are largely opinion rather than evidence based.

Potential pharmacological treatment options fall within three broad categories—analgesia (e.g. opioids), sedation (e.g. benzodiazepines), and symptom control (e.g. α-adrenergic agonists, β-adrenergic antagonists, and gabapentin) (22). A 2010 systematic review suggested orally administered opioids, gabapentin, benzodiazepines, α-agonists, and β-antagonists as first-line therapy, and bromocriptine in combination with other agents as second line (6). Intravenous opioids are associated with transient but large increases in ICP and decreases in cerebral perfusion pressure (CPP) in patients with severe TBI (34), and high-dose boluses should be avoided in patients with reduced intracranial compliance.

In addition to pharmacological therapy, it is important to identify and treat pain, investigate for and (if necessary) treat heterotopic ossification, consider CSF drainage for hydrocephalus, improve limb positioning, and avoid unnecessary bathing, turning, and endotracheal tube suctioning, or offer pharmacological prophylaxis against a paroxysm during such manoeuvres (6,13,35,36).

Cardiovascular dysfunction

Cardiovascular dysfunction may develop immediately after brain injury or after several hours (22), and manifest as arterial hypertension, elevated cardiac biomarkers, cardiac arrhythmias, electrocardiographic (ECG) changes without arrhythmias, and neurogenic 'stunned' myocardium (37,38). Although most evidence of cardiovascular dysfunction derives from patients with neurovascular disorders, particularly aneurysmal subarachnoid haemorrhage (SAH) and other forms of stroke, it has also been described after nearly every form of brain injury or insult including TBI (2,5,39). In one cohort study, cardiovascular dysfunction occurred in 18% of 209 mechanically ventilated ICU patients with severe TBI, suggesting a higher incidence than previously appreciated (2).

Pathophysiology of cardiovascular dysfunction

At least four theories—epicardial coronary artery spasm, myocardial microvascular dysfunction, catecholamine hypothesis, and parasympathetic nervous system dysfunction with unchecked inflammation—have been proposed to explain the link between cardiovascular dysfunction and acquired brain injury and have been reviewed in detail elsewhere (37,40,41). The complex inter-relationships between these possible causes, the disconnection syndrome theory of PSH development, and the subsequent development of cardiac pathology are shown in Figure 27.1 (15,40,41). The majority of the evidence for cardiovascular dysfunction derives from animal and patient studies of aneurysmal SAH, but is likely to apply to all acquired brain injury types (40).

Epicardial coronary artery spasm

Patients who develop cardiac injury after aneurysmal SAH usually have normal coronary arteries, so early pathophysiological theories suggested that the associated cardiac dysfunction was related to coronary artery spasm secondary to catecholamine release from myocardial sympathetic nerve terminals (42–44). However, case reports of myocardial dysfunction after SAH have failed to demonstrate angiographic evidence of coronary artery spasm, even in the presence of ST-segment elevation (37,45,46). Similarly, although regional wall motion abnormalities (RWMAs) were identified in eight of nine dogs with experimental SAH, this was not associated with angiographic evidence of coronary artery spasm (37,47). Given the lack of supporting data, the coronary artery spasm hypothesis has largely been abandoned (37).

Myocardial microvascular dysfunction

Another theory suggests that cardiovascular dysfunction after acquired brain injury may be caused by myocardial microvascular dysfunction as a result of catecholamine-induced small vessel spasm, platelet aggregation, or other mechanisms (37,47,48). However, very little evidence exists to support this hypothesis, with most clinical and animal studies failing to demonstrate an association between cardiac dysfunction and reduced myocardial perfusion (45,47,49). Although there was a high proportion (32%) of abnormal myocardial thallium perfusion scans in one observational study of 19 patients with aneurysmal SAH, this study lacked a control group and several of the patients with abnormal scans had risk factors for coronary artery disease, and one had a previous history of heart disease (37,49). In a case report of a patient who developed ST elevation and marked left ventricular (LV) apical asynergy after SAH, there was no abnormality on a technetium-99m PYP myocardial infarct scan performed on the fourth hospital day (45). Finally, no evidence of significant myocardial hypoperfusion was observed by either regional myocardial blood flow or myocardial contrast echocardiography in an experimental model of SAH despite the presence of RWMAs in many of the animals (37,47).

The catecholamine hypothesis

Possibly the most widely accepted theory explaining SAH-associated cardiovascular dysfunction is the catecholamine hypothesis (37). This asserts that elevated catecholamines after aneurysmal SAH induce cardiovascular dysfunction through prolonged catecholamine-induced myocardial contraction, cardiac myocyte adenosine triphosphate (ATP) depletion, and mitochondrial dysfunction, ultimately culminating in myocardial cell death (22,37,41). This results in typical histological findings including myocardial mononuclear infiltrates and contraction band necrosis (CBN) (37). One study demonstrated a high incidence of functional cardiac denervation after SAH among patients with LV RMWAs (extending beyond a single coronary artery distribution), suggesting that excessive catecholamine release into the myocardium may also damage sympathetic nerve terminals (50). Moreover, an animal study of intracranial hypertension demonstrated that abnormal cardiac haemodynamics and cardiomyocyte injury could be prevented by total cardiac denervation, suggesting that the final common path of brain injury-induced cardiovascular dysfunction is likely to be intracranial hypertension-induced local release of catecholamines onto the myocardium by sympathetic nerve endings (37,51). Despite this, plasma concentrations of epinephrine (adrenaline) and norepinephrine (noradrenaline) are also commonly increased after SAH, and are significantly higher among patients with poorer grades of SAH (52).

Interestingly, animals with experimental SAH have also been shown to demonstrate cardiac hypersensitivity to adrenergic stimulation. In an in situ perfused, innervated rat heart model of SAH, higher frequency sympathetic nerve stimulation, or increasing

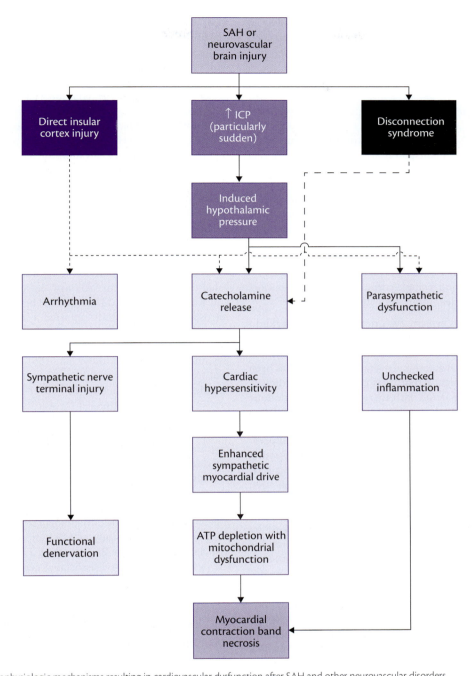

Fig. 27.1 Proposed pathophysiologic mechanisms resulting in cardiovascular dysfunction after SAH and other neurovascular disorders.
ATP, adenosine triphosphate; ICP, intracranial pressure; SAH, subarachnoid haemorrhage.
Adapted from Springer and the *Current Neurology and Neuroscience Reports*, 2009, 9, 6, pp. 486–491, 'Neurogenic stunned myocardium', Hoang Nguyen. With kind permission from Springer Science and Business Media; and Mashaly HA and Provencio JJ, 'Inflammation as a link between brain injury and heart damage: The model of subarachnoid hemorrhage', *Cleveland Clinic Journal of Medicine*, 2008, 75, Suppl 2, p.S2630.

doses of norepinephrine, were associated with greater increases in LV pressure and a higher incidence of arrhythmias compared to sham controls (53). As there was no difference in plasma norepinephrine, LV norepinephrine content, or β-adrenergic receptor density between SAH and control animals, the authors hypothesized that this observation might have been related to enhanced β-adrenergic receptor G-protein coupling to adenylyl cyclase.

Although the exact central mechanism by which intracranial hypertension or acute brain injury increases catecholamine release

into peripheral blood and thence onto the myocardium is largely unknown, at least one theory has been described (22,40). This purports that brain injury may damage the insular cortex and/or result in increased central hypothalamic pressure (likely through increased ICP), thereby leading to increased catecholamine outflow into the systemic circulation and at nerve terminals throughout the myocardium (22,40). Importantly, sudden rather than gradual increases in ICP produce a larger catecholamine response and thereby a greater degree of myocardial injury (54). One animal study reported that whereas a sudden increase in ICP resulted in a 1000-fold increase in circulating catecholamines, an associated hyperdynamic response and severe cardiac ischaemia, when ICP was increased more gradually there was only a 200-fold increase in circulating catecholamine levels and only mild ischaemic changes in the myocardium (54).

Other support for the catecholamine hypothesis derives from its similarity with takotsubo cardiomyopathy which characterized by severe, reversible LV dysfunction after exposure to acute emotional distress (37,55–57). Takotsubo is also known as myocardial stunning, stress-induced cardiomyopathy, transient LV apical ballooning, and 'broken heart syndrome'. Patients with takotsubo cardiomyopathy have increased levels of circulating catecholamines and frequently normal coronary arteries, so excessive sympathetic stimulation is also hypothesized to be its cause (57). Other similarities with SAH-associated myocardial dysfunction include the predilection toward postmenopausal women (suggesting that oestrogen deficiency may play a pathogenetic role), ECG changes, LV RWMAs that extend beyond a single coronary artery distribution, and myocardial mononuclear infiltrates with CBN (37,57).

Parasympathetic nervous system dysfunction with unchecked inflammation

As aneurysmal SAH can be associated with increased parasympathetic tone in addition to sympathetic overactivity (58), it has been proposed that increased vagal activity may contribute to cardiovascular dysfunction in association with increased sympathetic tone (41). One cohort study analysing HR variability suggested that increased parasympathetic activity occurred early after the onset of SAH (58). As outlined by Tracey, whilst the sympathetic and parasympathetic nervous systems are usually thought to have opposing organ-level effects, this is not always true (59). Simultaneous activation of both sympathetic and vagus nerves in animals has been shown to result in higher cardiac output than sympathetic stimulation alone (59,60).

Through the 'neuroinflammatory reflex' (also described by Tracey), the vagus nerve may also be capable of modulating the evolving inflammatory response in the heart and other organs after SAH (41,59). Inflammatory mediators produced in injured organs, such as the heart, activate cardiac afferents that relay signals to the nucleus tractus solitarius which in turn activates vagal efferent activity (59). This then activates nicotinic cholinergic receptors on macrophages within organ systems, including the heart, and reduces inflammatory mediator synthesis and release. Mashaly and Provencio recently proposed that parasympathetic dysfunction, coupled with hyperadrenergic activity, may allow unchecked cardiac inflammation and subsequent cardiac myocyte death and that this is another potential mechanism of cardiac injury after SAH (41).

Clinical manifestations of neurogenic cardiovascular dysfunction

An overview of the manifestations of cardiovascular dysfunction after SAH, their associated risk factors, and prognostic implications are summarized in Table 27.2 and discussed in detail below.

Elevated cardiac biomarkers

Serum levels of the cardiac biomarkers troponin I and creatine kinase-MB (CK-MB) are frequently elevated after aneurysmal SAH (37,61,62). The overall incidence of elevated biomarkers is 33–34%

(63), with higher rates in those with poor grade SAH (61,62). In one prospective observational study, the adjusted odds ratio of troponin I elevation was approximately nine times higher in patients with Hunt–Hess grade higher than 2 SAH compared to those with SAH grades of 2 or lower (62). Troponin I concentration usually peaks on the first or second day after ictus, and declines thereafter (37,61,62).

Elevated cardiac biomarkers are an important prognostic marker after aneurysmal SAH. A 2009 systematic review and meta-analysis reported that troponin I elevation was significantly associated with higher mortality, worse neurological outcome, and the development of delayed cerebral ischaemia (DCI) (63). These findings are supported by a subsequent cohort study of 910 SAH patients in whom cardiac injury (defined as elevated cardiac enzymes or a diagnostic code for acute coronary syndrome) was significantly associated with heart failure and increased all-cause and cardiac mortality (64).

Acute myocardial infarction is typically associated with higher values of troponin I than SAH-associated myocardial dysfunction, and this might allow differentiation between the two (65). One retrospective cohort study reported a tenfold lower rise in peak troponin I concentration in patients with SAH compared to those with myocardial infarction, despite a similar extent of ventricular dysfunction on echocardiography (66). These authors suggested that troponin I values less than 2.8 ng/mL in patients with a left ventricular ejection fraction (EF) lower than 40% were more suggestive of neurogenic stressed myocardium than acute myocardial infarction (66).

Brain (B-type) natriuretic peptide (BNP) is synthesized in the myocardium and released into the circulation in proportion to the degree of right ventricular (RV) dilatation or LV dysfunction/pressure overload (63,67). The plasma concentration of BNP is elevated in 9–100% of patients with aneurysmal SAH and, like troponin I, associated with adverse clinical outcomes (63), including higher mortality and the development of DCI (37,61–63). A recent retrospective cohort study of 119 patients reported a significant association between a BNP level of 276 pg/mL or greater and the development of SAH-associated cerebral infarction, with the strongest association in patients with mild to absent angiographic vasospasm (68).

ECG changes

A number of ECG abnormalities are associated with acute brain injury, most commonly with SAH (37,63,69–71). These include T-wave changes (22%), a new or prominent U wave (20%), signs of LV hypertrophy (LVH) (19%), QT-interval prolongation (18%), ST-segment depression (12%) or elevation (7%), wandering P waves (10%), and bundle branch blocks (9%) (63). Other less commonly reported abnormalities include short and long PR intervals, extrasystoles, P mitrale, or peaked P waves. Brain injury-associated ST-segment and T-wave changes can be differentiated from acute coronary syndromes in many cases as they usually traverse multiple epicardial coronary arterial territories in neurogenic stressed myocardium syndrome (37).

In a meta-analysis of observational studies of SAH, the prevalence of any ECG abnormality ranged from 1% (pathological Q waves) to 22% (T wave changes) (63). However, ECG abnormalities are often transient or intermittent, and studies using continuous ECG monitoring have identified them in up to 100% of patients

Table 27.2 Summary of the incidence, potential risk factors, and reported prognostic implications of cardiovascular dysfunction after aneurysmal subarachnoid haemorrhage

Manifestation	Findings (estimated incidence)	Potential risk factors	Reported prognostic implications	Comment
Elevated cardiac biomarkers	↑ troponin I (33%), CK-MB (34%), and BNP (9–100%) (63)	↑ troponin I and CK-MB: high Hunt–Hess score/ ↑ severity of brain injury (61,62)	↑ troponin I associated with ↑ risk of mortality, poor neurological outcome, delayed cerebral ischaemia, and heart failure (63,64); ↑ BNP associated with ↑ risk of mortality and delayed cerebral ischaemia/infarction (61–63,68)	Troponin I values < 2.8 ng/mL in conjunction with EF < 40% more suggestive of neurogenic stressed myocardium than AMI (66)
ECG changes	T wave changes (22%), new or prominent U wave (20%), LVH (19%), QT prolongation (18%), ST depression (12%) or elevation (7%), wandering P waves (10%), and BBBs (9%) (63)	NA	Q waves, ST depression, and T wave abnormalities associated with ↑ risk of mortality; ST depression associated with ↑ risk of delayed cerebral ischaemia (63,73)	ST/T-wave changes can often be differentiated from AMI/coronary ischaemia as they traverse multiple coronary vascular territories on ECG
Arrhythmias	Sinus bradycardia (13%) or tachycardia (9%) and atrial fibrillation, among others, including ventricular flutter/fibrillation and asystole (63,75–77)	ECG changes, past history of arrhythmia, myocardial ischaemia, hyperglycaemia, and brainstem compression (75); ventricular arrhythmias associated with older age, high Hunt–Hess score, lower HR, absence of ACEI/ARB use during ictus, troponin I ≥ 0.3 ng/mL, and possibly therapeutic hypothermia (76–78)	Sinus bradycardia and tachycardia associated with decreased and ↑ risk of death, respectively (63); clinically significant arrhythmias associated with ↑ risk of mortality and severe disability or death (75)	Arrhythmias may recur, their prognostic implications have been questioned, and the value of ECG monitoring is uncertain (38,74)
Echocardiographic changes	RWMAs not confined to vascular territory of single coronary artery, global hypokinesis with reduced EF, or diastolic dysfunction (74)	↑ troponin I, female gender, postmenopausal status, and poor clinical condition (37,62,65,81)	Wall motion abnormalities associated with ↑ risk of mortality and delayed cerebral ischaemia (63)	Most commonly affected myocardial regions include the basal and middle portions of the anteroseptal and anterior walls and the middle portions of the inferoseptal and anterolateral walls (81)

ACEI/ARB, angiotensin-converting enzyme/angiotensin receptor blocker; AMI, acute myocardial infarction; BBB, bundle branch block; BNP, brain (B-type) natriuretic peptide; CK-MB, creatine-kinase MB; ECG, electrocardiogram; EF, ejection fraction; LVH, left ventricular hypertrophy; NA, not available or well defined; RWMAs, regional wall motion abnormalities.

after SAH (37,72). ECG changes have also been reported in studies from the 1970s in 80–92% of patients after ischaemic, haemorrhagic (including SAH), and embolic stroke (69,70).

Similar to the occurrence of elevated cardiac biomarkers, ECG abnormalities may have significant adverse prognostic implications after brain injury. A systematic review and meta-analysis of observational studies of patients with aneurysmal SAH reported that Q waves, ST-segment depression, and T-wave abnormalities were significantly associated with mortality, while ST-segment depression was associated with development of DCI (63). In a recent post hoc analysis of data from the Intraoperative Hypothermia for Aneurysm Surgery Trial, investigators similarly found a significant association between mortality and non-specific ST- and T-wave abnormalities in a subset of 588 patients in whom a preoperative ECG was conducted (73).

Cardiac arrhythmias

Cardiac arrhythmias, often recurrent, also occur frequently after many acquired brain injury types, but particularly after

aneurysmal SAH, intracerebral haemorrhage, and ischaemic stroke (39,63,74,75). Sinus bradycardia and tachycardia have been reported in 13% and 9% of patients respectively after SAH, and atrial fibrillation in 8% (63). Other brain injury-related arrhythmias include atrial flutter, junctional rhythms, supraventricular tachycardia, second- (including Mobitz types I and II) and third-degree atrioventricular block, ventricular flutter and fibrillation, and asystole leading to sudden cardiac death (75–77).

Arrhythmias occur more frequently in patients with other brain injury-induced ECG changes or a previous history of arrhythmia (75). Other factors that may predict the development of arrhythmias include myocardial ischaemia, hyperglycaemia, brainstem compression from cerebral herniation syndromes, and seizures. Ventricular arrhythmias were reported in 14% of SAH patients in one study, and were more common in older patients, those with poor grade SAH, lower HR, and in the absence of angiotensin-converting enzyme inhibitor or angiotensin II receptor antagonist use during the ictus (77). A higher blood troponin I level (≥ 0.3 ng/mL) has also been significantly associated with ventricular fibrillation and flutter, although largely of a non-sustained form (76). Finally, one prospective cohort study of 16 children with severe TBI reported a non-significantly higher incidence of arrhythmias during moderate therapeutic hypothermia (78).

Similar to other cardiac abnormalities, arrhythmias have been associated with clinical outcome in observational studies (75,77). A systematic review and meta-analysis reported that while brady-cardia was associated with a reduced risk of death after aneurysmal SAH, tachycardia was associated with an increased risk (63). A recent prospective observational study observed clinically significant arrhythmias, defined as any rhythm disturbance other than sinus bradycardia/tachycardia or sinus rhythm with premature atrial or ventricular complexes, to be significantly associated with a higher risk of severe disability and death after adjustment for clinically relevant covariates (75).

Neurogenic stressed myocardium

The development of systolic or diastolic LV dysfunction after acquired brain injury, especially in the absence of a history of coronary artery disease, LV dysfunction or congestive heart failure, and without convincing evidence of acute coronary ischaemia or hypoperfusion, is known as neurogenic 'stressed' myocardium (22). Although many authors have long used the term myocardial 'stunning' to describe this disorder, stunning implies reversible myocardial dysfunction caused by epicardial coronary artery occlusion followed by spontaneous or therapeutic recanalization and reperfusion (37). As myocardial dysfunction after acquired brain injury is due to catecholamine excess rather than transient coronary occlusion, Lee and colleagues suggested that the term neurogenic 'stressed' myocardium is a more accurate descriptor (37). The authors support this modified definition.

Pathophysiology and echocardiographic findings

As outlined above, the pathophysiology of neurogenic stressed myocardium is likely to be due, at least in part, to excessive catecholamine release onto the heart by myocardial sympathetic nerve terminals (37), which are relatively absent at the human LV apex (79). This hypothesis is supported by an echocardiographic study in which RWMAs after SAH were correlated with the distribution of sympathetic nerve terminals; LV apex systolic function was frequently preserved relative to that of basal and mid-ventricular segments (80).

Whereas the majority of patients with aneurysmal SAH present with hyperdynamic LV function, with a mean EF of 68% (81), those with neurogenic stressed myocardium may develop RWMAs alone, global hypokinesia with reduced EF, or diastolic dysfunction (74). Similar to the observations of T-wave and ST-segment abnormalities on ECG, RWMAs are usually not confined to the vascular territory of a single epicardial coronary artery (37,82). A large prospective serial echocardiography study found that the most commonly affected LV regions in aneurysmal SAH-associated myocardial dysfunction are the basal and middle segments of the anteroseptal and anterior walls, and the middle of the inferoseptal and anterolateral walls (81). As expected, the prevalence of RMWAs involving the LV apex was also relatively low in this study.

Cardiac histology

A number of post-mortem studies have described the cardiac pathology after SAH (Figure 27.2) (83–86). Myocardial contraction band necrosis (CBN), also referred to as coagulative myocytolysis and myofibrillar degeneration, is the classic pathological lesion in animal and human studies of SAH (22,37,87). This multifocal lesion extends beyond the supply territory of a single coronary artery and has also been observed in a variety of other conditions associated with excessive sympathetic discharge, including TBI, takotsubo cardiomyopathy, phaeochromocytoma, and fatal status asthmaticus or epilepticus (37,87).

CBN is characterized by disruption of the linear arrangement of myofibrils in cardiac myocytes, and formation of densely eosinophilic transverse bands (37,87). As outlined by Karch and Billingham, the pathological changes within these transverse bands represent a continuum of injury severity that may correlate with the reversibility of cardiovascular dysfunction (87). Hypercontraction represents the reversible end of the spectrum whilst rupture or dehiscence of the intercalated disc the irreversible end (87). Although the exact pathogenesis of CBN is largely unknown, it may be prevented by cardiac sympathectomy or denervation, but not bilateral adrenalectomy, supporting the hypothesis that it is the local release of catecholamines onto the myocardium that is causative (37,51).

An interstitial inflammatory infiltrate is commonly reported after SAH, although myocardial inflammation may be absent for the first 30 minutes after the index cardiac injury (37,83,85–87). Other relevant pathological findings in autopsy studies include normal-appearing coronary arteries without significant atheroma, extensive haemorrhage within the myocardium, and subendocardial haemorrhage or infarction (83,85,86).

Clinical manifestations and diagnostic criteria

Neurogenic stressed myocardium may present in a variety of ways, but often with signs of predominantly left-sided heart failure, including haemodynamic abnormalities and pulmonary oedema (38,40). Associated clinical manifestations include one or more of the echocardiographic abnormalities described earlier, elevated plasma cardiac biomarkers, ECG changes, and cardiac arrhythmias (37,38,40). All patients presenting with acute brain injury should be assessed for risk factors for, or a past history of, coronary artery disease, as well as for factors associated with an increased risk of neurogenic stressed myocardium including postmenopausal females, elevated troponin I, poor grade SAH, and loss of consciousness during the ictus (37).

Initial diagnostic tests include measurement of plasma troponin I and CK-MB, a 12-lead ECG, and a chest X-ray (37). Transthoracic echocardiography should be considered in those with abnormalities of any of these initial investigations (37). Lee and colleagues suggest that cardiac catheterization should be considered to rule out acute coronary syndrome in patients with RWMAs in a single vascular territory and atypical features for neurogenic stressed myocardium, including good grade SAH, male gender, extremely elevated troponin, and failure of cardiac enzymes to normalize in the days after the ictus (37).

Although expert consensus diagnostic criteria for neurogenic stressed myocardium have not yet been proposed, Stevens and Nyquest recently suggested the criteria outlined in Box 27.1 (38). Interestingly, these appear to suggest that if the patient has a history of congestive heart failure, LV dysfunction, or coronary artery disease, a myocardial perfusion scan or coronary angiogram is required to make the diagnosis (38).

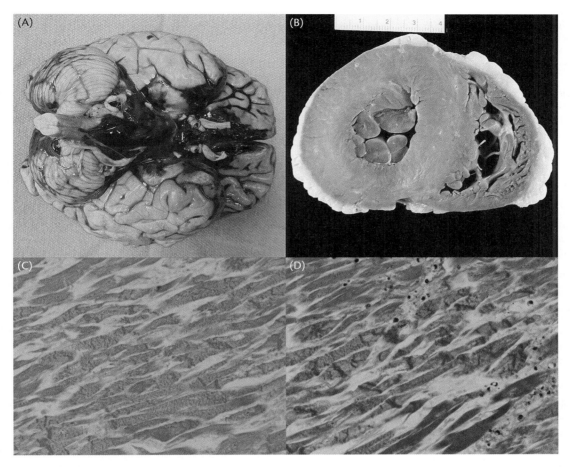

Fig. 27.2 Cardiac pathology after acquired brain injury.
(A) A gross view of the brain at autopsy from a man who died approximately 36 hours after rupture of a posterior cerebral artery berry aneurysm.
(B) A gross view of the cardiac ventricles from this patient. No macroscopic abnormalities are apparent.
(C) A photomicrograph of myocardium exhibiting classic contraction band necrosis (5a H&E, 200× 5b Gomori trichrome, 200×).
(D) A photomicrograph of myocardium at higher magnification exhibiting classic contraction band necrosis (6a H&E, 400× 6b Gomori trichrome, 400×).
Images provided courtesy of Amy B. Bromley, MD, FRCPC.

Epidemiology, natural history, and prognosis

A systematic review and meta-analysis confirmed that the mean prevalence of RWMAs after aneurysmal SAH is 22%, with a range of 13–31% across observational studies (63). One study included in this systematic review also reported diastolic dysfunction in 71% of its study population. In support of the these estimates, a large prospective cohort study of 173 adults with aneurysmal SAH reported regional LV dysfunction in 28% (52% of whom had global LV dysfunction and reduced EF), with the remainder presenting with RWMAs and normal EF (81).

An important clinical characteristic of neurogenic stressed myocardium is that the myocardial dysfunction often improves with time. Normal systolic function is frequently restored within 5–10 days after aneurysmal SAH (37,38) and, in one observational study of 44 patients with hypokinetic, akinetic, or dyskinetic LV systolic function, 25% had complete normalization and a further 41% partial improvement of systolic function over time (81). Another case series that included three patients with TBI and global LV hypokinesia reported complete recovery of LV function on echocardiography performed at 7 and 90 days after the initial investigation (5).

Although neurogenic stressed myocardium has the potential for improvement over time (37,38), its development does have

significant prognostic implications. RWMAs have been significantly associated with mortality and the development of DCI in many studies (63). An observational study also reported that the absolute risk of mortality after SAH was 30% higher in patients with neurogenic stressed myocardium in whom ventricular function did not improve compared to those in whom LV function did, suggesting that the lack of ventricular recovery is a poor prognostic sign (81).

Prevention of myocardial injury after acquired brain injury

As sympathetic hyperactivity is believed to be the key driver of cardiac injury after acquired brain injury, some have suggested that inhibition of the effects of catecholamines on the myocardium might prevent subsequent cardiovascular dysfunction (22,37,38,74,84,88–91). In a randomized controlled trial (RCT) conducted between 1976 and 1978, Neil-Dwyer and colleagues randomly allocated 90 patients with SAH to receive a combination of propranolol and phentolamine or placebo (84). Among those patients who died, myocardial lesions were identified in all six who received placebo and in none of six who received propranolol and phentolamine. These authors subsequently reported that treatment with oral propranolol and phentolamine (or propranolol alone)

Box 27.1 Proposed diagnostic criteria for neurogenic stunned myocardium

1. Acute structural or functional brain disorder

2. New onset of systolic and/or diastolic left ventricular dysfunction. Systolic dysfunction can include regional and/or global wall-motion abnormalities. Regional wall-motion abnormalities should extend beyond a single epicardial vascular distribution

3. Partial or complete resolution of left ventricular dysfunction in less than 4 weeks

4. At least one of the following:

   a. No history of congestive heart failure, left ventricular dysfunction, or coronary artery disease

   b. No evidence of myocardial ischaemia on myocardial perfusion scan

   c. Absence of angiographic evidence of obstructive coronary disease or of acute plaque rupture.

Reprinted from *Journal of the Neurological Sciences*, 261, 1–2, RD Stevens and PA Nyquist, 'The systemic implications of aneurysmal subarachnoid haemorrhage', pp. 143–156, Copyright 2007, with permission from Elsevier.

was associated with a reduction in death and severe disability at 1 year in women (89). Another observational study examined the effects of intravenous clonidine after SAH, but reported no reduction in spillover of norepinephrine into plasma (91). However, as was noted by Hinson and Sheth, the dosage of clonidine did not reduce arterial BP in this study, suggesting that it may have been inadequate (22). Thus, although of theoretical benefit, the role of prophylactic α- and β-adrenergic antagonists after SAH has not been defined (37,92).

Management of arrhythmias and neurogenic stressed myocardium

As there are no specific studies examining the management of arrhythmias after SAH or other forms of acquired brain injury (74), they should be managed according to current Advanced Cardiac Life Support guidelines. Further, although no evidence exists to support this claim, low potassium and magnesium should be corrected to prevent or possibly treat brain injury-induced arrhythmias (74).

A key paradigm in the management of patients with acquired brain injury is the prevention of hypotension and low CPP, since this significantly predicts poor neurological outcome (93). Similarly, hypoxaemia is an independent predictor of poor outcome, and episodes of in-hospital hypoxaemia and hypotension are associated with a graded increase in mortality after TBI (94). As such, the 2007 Brain Trauma Foundation guideline recommends avoidance of hypotension (systolic BP < 90 mmHg) and hypoxaemia (PaO_2 < 8 kPa (< 60 mmHg) or oxygen saturation < 90%) and maintenance of CPP > 60 mmHg after TBI (94,95).

As cardiovascular dysfunction may normalize with time, management of neurogenic stressed myocardium is largely supportive (37). Patients who develop cardiogenic shock may require complex

haemodynamic support guided by echocardiography, non-invasive cardiac output monitoring or, in cases of severe instability, a pulmonary artery catheter (96). Temporary inotropic support may also be required in severe cases (37), including for maintenance of blood pressure in the management of DCI after SAH and CPP after TBI. Although this is often managed with vasopressors such as norepinephrine and phenylephrine, inotropes such as dobutamine or milrinone may represent better alternatives in patients with neurogenic stressed myocardium given that catecholamines are integral to its pathogenesis (37). Furthermore, pure arterial vasoconstrictors increase LV afterload and, in the context of diminished LV function, may decrease cardiac output. Small studies have reported that dobutamine may improve myocardial function, increase cardiac output, improve cerebral blood flow, and reverse symptoms of cerebral ischaemia after SAH (74,97). Similar improvements in cardiac output or CPP after the use of levosimendan or intra-aortic balloon counterpulsation have also been described in case reports (74). As milrinone may decrease vascular resistance and systolic BP, and increase cardiac output and stroke volume more effectively than dobutamine, some have suggested that it may be more effective when increased cardiac output is the goal in patients with decreased systolic function but normal vascular resistance and BP (98).

Pulmonary dysfunction

Pulmonary dysfunction is the most common non-neurological complication after severe TBI and aneurysmal SAH (65,74). Its manifestations include neurogenic pulmonary oedema (NPO), aspiration, hospital-acquired (HAP), and ventilator-associated (VAP) pneumonia, ventilator-induced lung injury, acute lung injury (ALI)/acute respiratory distress syndrome (ARDS), and pulmonary embolism (2,38,65,99,100). Rib fractures, flail chest, and other extracranial injuries may further complicate management in trauma patients. In one cohort study, respiratory failure occurred in 23% of consecutive ICU admissions of patients with severe TBI (2). Pulmonary dysfunction contributes substantially to mortality after brain injury (2,100). In a large nested prospective cohort study, pneumonia, ARDS and pulmonary emboli were responsible for 50% of all deaths from non-neurological causes after aneurysmal SAH (101). Table 27.3 summarizes the characteristics of the more common forms of pulmonary dysfunction after acquired brain injury.

Acute lung injury/acute respiratory distress syndrome

ARDS, defined by the American-European Consensus Conference (AECC) as the acute onset of hypoxaemia (arterial partial pressure of oxygen (PaO_2)/fraction of inspired oxygen (FIO_2) ≤ 26.6 kPa (≤ 200 mmHg)) in association with bilateral infiltrates on chest X-ray and no evidence of left atrial hypertension (102–104), frequently affects patients with acquired brain injury (2,38,74). The Berlin definition of ARDS published in 2012 removes the term ALI and instead classifies ARDS as mild, moderate, or severe. It may be superior to the AECC definition (104), but has not yet been used in studies of patients with acquired brain injury.

The incidence of ALI/ARDS among patients with acute neurological injury varies widely as a result of inclusion of patients with varying degrees of injury severity and differences in definition across studies (105). In observational studies, ARDS has been

Table 27.3 Characteristics of types of pulmonary dysfunction after acquired brain injury

Pulmonary dysfunction	Clinical manifestations/diagnosis	Aetiology	Estimated incidence	Comment
ALI/ARDS	Diagnosed using the AECC [PaO$_2$/FIO$_2$ ≤ 26.6 kPa (200 mmHg) (ARDS) or 39.9 kPa (300 mmHg) (ALI) with bilateral pulmonary infiltrates and no evidence of LA hypertension) (103) or Berlin definitions/criteria (104)	Aspiration pneumonia, non-aspiration pneumonia, and neurogenic pulmonary oedema likely the most important causes (2,38,74)	Aneurysmal SAH (ARDS: 4–8%) and severe TBI (ALI: 20–30%; ARDS: 5–10%) (74,105)	Reported risk factors among those with TBI may include diffuse brain injury with midline shift, non-evacuated intracranial mass lesions, and mechanical ventilation with high RRs or TVs (107,108)
Neurogenic pulmonary oedema	Diagnostic criteria have been suggested by Davison and colleagues (see Box 27.2) (100)	TBI, aneurysmal SAH, intracranial haemorrhage, status epilepticus, meningitis, and many other CNS conditions (100)	SAH (2–43%, with severe pulmonary oedema possibly occurring in 6%) and TBI (up to 20%) (100,101)	An early (which presents within minutes) and a more delayed type (which presents within 12–24 hours) of neurogenic pulmonary oedema may exist (100)
VAP	'New or persistent radiographic infiltrate plus fever, leucocytosis, change in the volume or colour of sputum, or isolation of a new pathogen' (125)	Early-onset frequently due to oropharyngeal flora. Frequent organisms include *Staphylococcus aureus* (MSSA) (46–85%) (126,129), Enterobacteriaceae (20%), *Streptococcus pneumoniae* (9%), *Pseudomonas aeruginosa* (9%), and *Haemophilus influenzae* (7%) Late-onset frequently due to more-resistant/virulent organisms such as *Pseudomonas aeruginosa* (16–66%), *Xanthomonas maltophilia* (28%), or methicillin-resistant *S. aureus* (MRSA) (11%) (126,129)	45% overall (186), including early-onset (52%) and late-onset (48%) pneumonia (126)	Reported risk factors among those with TBI include immunosuppression, barbiturate use, and therapeutic hypothermia (126)

AECC, American-European Consensus Conference; ALI, acute lung injury; ARDS, acute respiratory distress syndrome; CNS, central nervous system; LA, left atrial; RR, respiratory rate; TV, tidal volume; VAP, ventilator-associated pneumonia.

Data from various sources (see References).

reported in 4–8% of patients after aneurysmal SAH and in 2–30% after TBI overall, with higher incidences of both ALI (20–30%) and ARDS (5–10%) after severe TBI (74,105). In one study, ALI was significantly associated with higher Injury Severity Score, greater number of ventilator days and worse neurologic outcome in TBI patients who survived to hospital discharge (106). However, there was no correlation between ALI and the severity of the initial head injury as assessed by the Glasgow Coma Scale (GCS), Marshall Score or intracranial abnormality. However, diffuse brain injury, midline shift, and non-evacuated intracranial mass lesions have been reported as independent predictors for ALI in one study (107). An association between ventilation with relatively high respiratory rate or tidal volumes and ALI has also been reported after severe brain injury (see Chapter 4) (108). In patients with aneurysmal SAH, risk factors for development of ALI include higher Hunt–Hess grades, severe sepsis and transfusion of packed red blood cells (109).

The occurrence of ALI/ARDS has consistently been associated with worse outcome after brain injury (105–109). Patients who develop ALI after TBI have higher mortality and increased risk of poor neurological outcomes, as well as longer length of ICU stay and fewer ventilator-free days, compared to those who do not develop ALI (106–108). In one study, mortality was 38% in patients who developed ALI after TBI and 15% in those who did not, although only 19% of the deaths in the ALI group were directly related to the lung injury (106). Similarly, development of ALI after

aneurysmal SAH has been linked with significant increases in the risk of in-hospital mortality and longer ICU stay (109).

Neurogenic pulmonary oedema

NPO is acute pulmonary oedema following a CNS insult, frequently associated with a substantial increase in ICP and decrease in CPP (100,110). It was first reported by Francis Moutier in patients with penetrating head wounds during World War I (100), and subsequently in autopsies of several Vietnam War soldiers who died shortly after isolated gunshot wounds to the head (111). NPO may occur after TBI, SAH, intracranial haemorrhage, status epilepticus, and meningitis, as well as a myriad of other CNS conditions (100). Although some forms of NPO might partly or completely be related to a cardiogenic aetiology, the term 'neurogenic' in this chapter to refers to all types of brain injury-associated pulmonary oedema.

Pathophysiology

Davison and colleagues recently reviewed the literature and described four main hypotheses that may explain the development of brain injury-related NPO—the neuro-cardiac, neurohaemodynamic, 'blast', and pulmonary venule hypersensitivity theories (100). The neurocardiac and neurohaemodynamic hypotheses largely relate to brain injury-associated alterations in Starling forces, whereas the 'blast' and venule hypersensitivity theories consider the contribution of alveolar–capillary barrier damage, with or without changes in pulmonary hydrostatic pressure to the development of

NPO. Many of these mechanisms are substantially related to development of a hyperadrenergic state after acquired brain injury (37), the pathogenesis of which has been described earlier in the chapter.

Neurocardiac theory

Although NPO has traditionally been considered non-cardiogenic in origin, the neurocardiac theory asserts that excessive catecholamine release onto the myocardium by sympathetic nerve endings results in direct cardiac myocyte injury, myocardial dysfunction, elevated left atrial pressure, and transudative pulmonary oedema (100). In a retrospective observational study of 72 patients with aneurysmal SAH, patients with elevated CK-MB and reduced LV stroke volume and work indices also developed elevated pulmonary artery wedge pressures, and five of these developed pulmonary oedema with 6 hours of ictus (112). In a case series of seven patients with NPO after TBI, elevated pulmonary artery wedge pressures were confirmed in all but one and three developed global myocardial hypokinesia, suggesting a predominantly cardiogenic origin of the pulmonary oedema (5).

Neuro-haemodynamic theory

The neuro-haemodynamic theory purports that myocardial dysfunction results indirectly from increased cardiac afterload secondary to catecholamine-induced increases in peripheral arterial resistance (100,113). One animal study confirmed that the brain-injury associated rise in systemic arterial pressure and cardiac afterload, decreased ventricular compliance, and left heart strain were associated with increased left atrial and pulmonary venous pressures and the development of pulmonary oedema (114). A subsequent study by Ducker and Simmons demonstrated that the mechanisms leading to these cardiovascular changes might be mediated through an acute increase in ICP (113), and could therefore be considered to constitute a pulmonary component of the Cushing reflex (115). In an animal model of intracranial hypertension, an acute increase in ICP was followed by an increase in systemic arterial and pulmonary venous pressures, and subsequently by an increase in pulmonary arterial pressure; pulmonary oedema occurred when pulmonary venous pressure exceeded pulmonary arterial pressure (113).

Blast theory

As opposed to the neurocardiac and neuro-haemodynamic hypotheses which suggest that transudative NPO develops primarily because of alterations in Starling forces, the blast theory suggests that pulmonary oedema results from a combination of acute hydrostatic forces and alveolar–capillary barrier damage (100,116). In this theory, which was originally proposed by Theodore and Robin in 1976 (116), a sudden increase in pulmonary hydrostatic pressure during the sympathetic surge early after TBI is presumed to result in barotrauma-induced increases in pulmonary capillary permeability and an exudative effusion within the pulmonary interstitium and alveoli (100). Similar to the neuro-haemodynamic hypothesis, blast theory also proposes that catecholamine-induced increases in arterial afterload result in a net shift of fluid into the pulmonary circulation, increased pulmonary pressures, and transudative pulmonary oedema (100). The degree of elevation of pulmonary pressures is related to the degree of alveolar–capillary barrier injury, and the resultant increased vascular permeability is therefore pressure dependent (100,117,118).

Although this theory purports that the sympathetic surge and pulmonary hypertension occur early after TBI and may resolve, the resultant alveolar–capillary barrier damage and exudative pulmonary oedema may persist (100). Several experimental and observational human studies provide support for this contention (117–119). Case reports of patients with acquired brain injury have described pulmonary oedema fluid containing red blood cells and protein (which would be unexpected without an increase in pulmonary vascular permeability), whilst others have reported pulmonary oedema after abrupt and significant rises in systemic arterial and pulmonary pressures (100). Maron also reported that transiently raising the pulmonary vascular pressure above 70 mmHg in an animal model resulted in a linear increase in pulmonary vascular permeability, but that no increase in permeability occurred at lower levels of pulmonary venous pressure (117). This suggests that a significant degree of transient pulmonary hypertension may be required to produce NPO, and that this could explain the association between NPO and brain injury severity.

Pulmonary venule adrenergic hypersensitivity

As many case reports of patients with NPO fail to demonstrate marked arterial hypertension or increases in left atrial pressure, an alternate theory suggests that pulmonary sympathetic efferents may directly modulate the permeability of the capillary endothelium after acquired brain injury (100). The lung is richly innervated by sympathetic nerve terminals and pulmonary capillaries contain both α- and β-adrenoceptors (100,120,121). A study by van der Zee and coworkers demonstrated that the induction of intracranial hypertension in sheep was associated with an increase in pulmonary permeability (as measured by lymph-to-plasma protein ratios), but could not be explained by an alteration in pulmonary haemodynamics (122). Moreover, pre-treatment with the α-adrenergic receptor antagonist phentolamine prevented increases in lymph flow and lymph-to-plasma protein concentration ratios, suggesting interruption of the intracranial hypertension-associated increases in pulmonary vascular permeability by alpha blockade (122).

A subsequent study in dogs by McClellan and colleagues provided convincing evidence that the development of NPO cannot solely be explained by systemic haemodynamic alterations (123). In this study, increases in mean arterial and pulmonary arterial pressures induced by an increase in ICP led to a significant increase in pulmonary vascular permeability as measured by the protein leak index, only a moderate elevation of pulmonary artery wedge pressure (< 10 mmHg) and an increase in extravascular lung water. Moreover, increasing left atrial pressure did not increase protein leak index, even in the presence of higher pulmonary vascular pressures.

Clinical manifestations, natural history, and diagnosis

Two types of NPO—early and delayed—can develop after acquired brain injury (100). The early type is characterized by acute onset of respiratory deterioration, whereas delayed NPO manifests clinically after 12–24 hours (100).

Tachypnoea, dyspnoea, a cough productive of pink frothy sputum, and profound hypoxaemia may develop within minutes (100). One small study reported that all seven TBI patients who were subsequently observed to have NPO developed respiratory distress at the scene of injury and required intubation before ICU admission (5). In addition to acute respiratory distress, patients with NPO may also show signs of excessive sympathetic nervous system activation, including tachycardia, arterial hypertension, and fever (100). Auscultation of the chest may reveal bilateral crackles and rales

---

Box 27.2 Diagnostic criteria for neurogenic pulmonary oedema

1. Bilateral infiltrates (on chest imaging)

2. PaO_2/FIO_2 ratio < 200 mmHg (26.6 kPa)

3. No evidence of left atrial hypertension

4. Presence of CNS injury (severe enough to have caused significantly increased ICP)

5. Absence of other common causes of acute respiratory distress or ARDS (e.g. aspiration, massive blood transfusion, sepsis).

ARDS, acute respiratory distress syndrome; CNS, central nervous system; ICP, intracranial pressure; PaO_2/FIO_2, partial of inspired oxygen/fraction of inspired oxygen.

With kind permission from Springer Science+Business Media: *Critical Care*, 'Neurogenic Pulmonary Edema', 16, 2, 2012, p. 212, DL Davison *et al.*

---

while laboratory investigations may confirm leucocytosis. Chest X-ray classically shows bilateral, centrally distributed pulmonary infiltrates, and pulmonary vascular redistribution, while CT scan of the thorax reveals alveolar oedema (5,100). Although NPO often resolves within 24–48 hours, it may persist in patients with evolving or ongoing brain injury and intracranial hypertension (100).

As cardiogenic and non-cardiogenic pulmonary oedema are managed differently, differentiating between them is the crucial first step in determining treatment. For this reason, and in an attempt to facilitate and standardize future epidemiological and interventional research, Davison and colleagues have suggested diagnostic criteria for the non-cardiogenic form of NPO, that is, without detectable LV dysfunction (Box 27.2) (100). These authors also suggest that measurement of serum catecholamines might be helpful in patients who meet these diagnostic criteria, with consideration of administration of an α-adrenergic receptor blocking agent if the BP safely permits (100).

Epidemiology and outcome

As most of the information regarding NPO is derived from case reports or small case series, its exact incidence is unknown (100,110). However, a recent review suggests that it lies between 2% and 43% after SAH and might be as high as 20% following TBI (100). In a prospective cohort study, pulmonary oedema was reported in 23% of adults with aneurysmal SAH, with severe oedema occurring in 6% (101). Rogers and colleagues conducted a retrospective analysis of all-fatal and non-fatal head injuries reported in an American autopsy database and two trauma registries (97,110), and confirmed pulmonary oedema in 32% of patients who died at the scene and in 50% of those who died within 96 hours of injury (110). It is less common in patients who survive TBI (97). Among adults admitted to hospital for isolated severe TBI, Rogers et al. reported that only 8% met the criteria for the diagnosis of NPO (110). The mortality associated with NPO is around 10% (97,100,124).

Pneumonia

The pathophysiology, microbiology, associated risk factors, and diagnosis of pneumonia in patients with acute neurological injury will be discussed in this section, and its incidence and associated outcomes later in the chapter under infectious complications.

Classification, pathophysiology, and microbiology

Patients with severe acquired brain injury commonly develop aspiration pneumonia, HAP, and VAP, the latter being defined as a new or persistent radiographic infiltrates plus fever, leucocytosis, change in the volume or colour of sputum or the isolation of a new pathogen (125). Reported risk factors for development of pneumonia after TBI include immunosuppression and use of therapeutic hypothermia and barbiturates (126,127). VAP may be further subclassified by its temporal presentation relative to the time of initiation of mechanical ventilation into early onset and late onset, with the chronological threshold distinguishing these subtypes varying between 3 and 6 days across studies (128).

The pathophysiology and microbiology of early- and late-onset pneumonia differ significantly and this has implications for choice of antimicrobial therapy (129). Early-onset pneumonia results from aspiration of commensal oropharyngeal flora, such as *Staphylococcus aureus,* into the lungs (128,129). After endotracheal intubation, airway colonization with largely Gram-negative aerobic bacteria begins and is likely to be complete after approximately 48–72 hours (129), and late-onset pneumonia occurs as a result of aspiration of these colonized Gram-negative organisms around the cuff of the endotracheal tube (129).

A retrospective cohort study of 161 adults with severe TBI reported VAP in 65 patients (40%), with just over one-half of the pneumonia episodes presenting as early onset (126). In this study, methicillin-sensitive *S. aureus* (MSSA) was the most common pathogen, occurring in 43% of pneumonia episodes. In contrast methicillin-resistant *S. aureus* (MRSA) and *Pseudomonas aeruginosa* were common infecting organisms in late-onset infections. Similar findings were also reported by Cazzadori and colleagues who observed Gram-positive and Gram-negative organisms to be significantly more common in early- and late-onset HAP respectively in patients with isolated head injury (129). In this study, common organisms in early-onset pneumonia included *Staphylococcus* species (85%), and *P. aeruginosa* and *Xanthomonas maltophilia* were present in 78% of patients with late-onset pneumonia (129).

Diagnosis

Although invasive techniques of VAP diagnosis have not been shown to be superior to non-invasive techniques in mixed ICU populations (125), prompt diagnosis from samples obtained using bronchoalveolar lavage and/or specimen brush samples may prevent or minimize the risk of secondary brain injury in critically ill neurological patients (97). In addition to aiding pulmonary bacterial diagnosis, fibreoptic bronchoscopy may also be useful in optimizing pulmonary toilet, which is often suboptimal in patients with acquired brain injury because of deep sedation or poor cough (97). However, fibreoptic bronchoscopy and endotracheal suctioning/aspiration have been associated with increases in ICP in patients with acute brain injury (130–132). Peerless and colleagues studied 15 sedated and mechanically ventilated adults with severe TBI and reported mean increases in ICP from baseline of 13.5 mmHg during fibreoptic bronchoscopy for the diagnosis of pneumonia or treatment of lobar collapse (132). However, as MAP also increased, CPP was maintained above 60 mmHg throughout the procedure in all patients except one, and ICP returned to pre-procedure levels soon after bronchoscopy. Another study also reported increases in ICP in 81% of 26 patients with severe TBI, and no changes in MAP and CPP, during fibreoptic bronchoscopy, with no effect on neurological status (130). Notwithstanding these observations, there are insufficient data to confirm with certainty that bronchoscopy-related increases in ICP have no detrimental effects, and there is also no convincing evidence that sedative agents effectively prevent cerebral haemodynamic changes during airway manipulation (34,133). Therefore endotracheal aspirates or empirical antimicrobial therapy should be considered instead of bronchoscopy in unstable patients with critically elevated ICP.

Management of pulmonary dysfunction

Strategies to manage pulmonary dysfunction frequently conflict with brain-directed therapies (97). Use of arterial vasopressors and excessive fluid resuscitation to maintain CPP may exacerbate pulmonary oedema (97,134). Lung protective ventilation with low tidal volumes and permissive hypercapnia may lead to increases in ICP and decreases in CPP because of cerebral vasodilatation and increased intracranial blood volume (97). As discussed previously, endotracheal suctioning or therapeutic bronchoscopy may also increase ICP and this cannot be adequately prevented by prophylactic administration of intravenous sedative agents (34,131). Thus, the influence of pulmonary interventions on ICP and CPP must be considered carefully in patients with acquired brain injury (97). Potential benefits must always be weighed against the potential risks of performing, or not performing, interventions.

Intubation and ventilation

In order to prevent secondary brain injury, the Brain Trauma Foundation recommends avoidance of hypoxia after TBI (94). Thus, patients with GCS score less than 9 and inadequate airway reflexes should undergo endotracheal intubation to protect the airway and control ventilation to maintain adequate oxygenation (134). The potential for difficult airway management after TBI should always be considered as patients may present with coincidental face and neck trauma, reduced gastric emptying and/or a full/distended stomach, and cervical spine injuries, each of which may require different airway management techniques (see Chapter 4) (135).

After intubation, a target PaO_2 and $PaCO_2$ should be determined (134). Although the exact PaO_2 target in critically ill brain injured adults is poorly defined, a PaO_2 higher than the ARDSnet recommendation of 7.3–10.6 kPa (55–80 mmHg) is often recommended because hypoxia may increase ICP and is itself a significant negative prognostic indicator (134). Moreover, although the ARDSnet trial reported improved mortality and reduced ventilator-days during low tidal volume (6 mL/kg) ventilation, patients with severe TBI are often ventilated to target a normal $PaCO_2$ because of the risk of increased ICP secondary to hypercapnia during low tidal volume ventilation (134). However, in the setting of brain injury-associated ALI/ARDS, physicians must achieve an appropriate balance between CO_2 control and lung protection, with some experts suggesting that multimodal brain monitoring may be useful to guide therapy in such cases (134).

Many patients with acquired brain injury can be managed with relatively conventional ventilation strategies. Moderate levels of positive end-expiratory pressure (PEEP) are generally well tolerated, but the influence of high levels of PEEP on ICP should be considered in patients with reduced intracranial compliance. Some patients require rescue procedures for failing oxygenation, including high-frequency oscillation and prone positioning ventilation and these issues, as well as the effects of PEEP on ICP, are covered in detail in Chapter 4.

Haematological dysfunction

Haemocoagulative disorders, including coagulopathy, fibrinolysis, and platelet dysfunction, occur frequently after acquired brain injury (136). One in three TBI patients has signs of coagulopathy, with a higher incidence in those with the most severe injury (137). Immune system dysfunction may also be a manifestation of haematological dysfunction.

Pathophysiology

The pathophysiology of disordered haemostasis after brain injury is multifactorial and not yet fully elucidated. Although most data derives from adult TBI studies, it is likely that it is also relevant to other acquired brain injury types. Maegele suggested that development of coagulopathy after TBI involves both hypo- and hypercoagulable states, the severity of which is related to the magnitude and extent of injured brain tissue (136). Laroche and colleagues further reviewed the pathogenesis of coagulopathy after TBI and identified several contributing mechanisms, including (1) alterations in local and systemic coagulation and fibrinolytic pathways secondary to the release of tissue factor, (2) disseminated intravascular coagulation (DIC), (3) thrombocytopenia and platelet dysfunction, and (4) activation of protein C pathways secondary to brain trauma and hypoperfusion (138).

Tissue factor release

Tissue factor is a transmembrane procoagulant protein highly expressed in cells of the CNS as well as perivascular smooth muscle cells, pericytes and fibroblasts associated with the cerebral vasculature (136). After its release into the systemic circulation following cerebrovascular injury during TBI, tissue factor may result in activation of the extrinsic coagulation pathway and development of a consumptive coagulopathy through thrombin activation (139,140). As TBI may also result in blood-brain barrier (BBB) breakdown lasting hours to days, it has been suggested that the temporal release of tissue factor following brain injury may be dependent on BBB integrity, and may thus resolve following restoration of barrier function (139). After release into the systemic circulation, tissue factor binds with microparticles derived from activated platelets which contain receptor sites for procoagulant factors, resulting in initiation of coagulation (136). High levels of procoagulant microparticles have been reported in cerebrospinal fluid (CSF) and blood following TBI (141).

The protein C response

Activated protein C (APC) is an anticoagulant protein that limits thrombin generation (142). It acts by promoting fibrinolysis and inhibiting thrombosis through proteolytic cleavage of clotting factors Va and VIIa (142). Laroche suggested that a maladaptive protein C response to tissue trauma and hypoperfusion together might cause an immediate APC-mediated coagulopathy, as well as a chronic protein C depletion-mediated susceptibility to thromboembolic events (138).

Hyperfibrinolysis

The fibrinolytic system acts as a negative feedback system to the haemostatic cascade, preventing unregulated intravascular coagulation. Hyperfibrinolysis can result in dissolution of newly formed fibrin in local clot, or DIC leading to widespread haemorrhage. It may result from excessive activation of the extrinsic coagulation pathway by tissue factor, elevation of tissue-type plasminogen activator or activated protein C, or depletion of plasmin inhibitor after TBI (138).

Thrombocytopenia and platelet dysfunction

A reduction in the overall number of platelets (thrombocytopenia) has been reported in 3–33% of patients after TBI (138), and associated with progression of intracranial haemorrhage and increased mortality (143). In addition to a reduction in their numbers after TBI, platelets may also become dysfunctional because of decreased aggregability (144). This may result from involvement of the cyclooxygenase pathway, the presence of a platelet inhibitor, or the exhaustion of intracellular platelet mediators involved in haemostasis (138,145). In support of this, Davis and colleagues reported that TBI patients had early platelet dysfunction with a significantly increased percentage of platelet adenosine diphosphate and arachidonic acid receptor inhibition (146).

Clinical manifestations and diagnosis

Abnormal coagulation parameters have been associated with expansion or progression of intracranial haematoma and occurrence of new intracranial lesions. In a review of 253 patients with serial cranial CT scans after TBI, the risk of delayed haemorrhagic insults was 31% if coagulation studies were normal and 85% if at least one clotting test or platelet count was abnormal (147). Neuropathological studies of surgical specimens of human cerebral contusions have demonstrated intravascular coagulation in arterioles and venules of all sizes, and associated ischaemic injury locally and at more distant sites from the injury (148).

The literature is inconsistent in the definition of coagulopathy after brain injury. In many studies coagulopathy is defined as at least one abnormality of prothrombin time (PT), activated partial thromboplastin time (aPTT) or platelet count (149), but a DIC panel (PT, PTT, platelets, D-dimer, and fibrinogen) or thromboelastography (TEG) have been used to confirm the diagnosis in others (150,151). Utilization of point-of-care TEG and platelet mapping has been suggested as a way to guide blood component therapy in a more goal-directed fashion after brain injury (152). Although TEG correlates well with the results of conventional coagulation tests after isolated TBI (153), the authors are not aware of any convincing evidence that a coagulation management strategy using TEG versus conventional testing improves mortality or neurological outcome after acquired brain injury.

Epidemiology, natural history, and prognosis

A meta-analysis of 34 studies reported an overall prevalence of disturbed haemostasis of 33% (range 10–97%) after TBI (137). Early coagulopathy in the emergency department has been reported in 24% of TBI patients, with the incidence increasing to 54% in the first 24 hours post-injury (154). Coagulopathy onset is earlier in patients with more severe head injury (155). Lustenberger reported that coagulopathy developed within 23 hours (range 0.1–108 hours or 0–4.5 days) of admission for TBI, and continued for 68 hours (range 2.6–531.4 hours or 0.1–22.1 days) (155).

Development of coagulopathy has been associated with adverse outcomes after TBI, including with a significantly increased risk of mortality and unfavourable neurological outcome (137). Wafaisade retrospectively studied 706 patients with blunt TBI and reported that coagulopathy was associated with higher rates of the need for craniotomy, single and multiple organ failure and fewer intubation-free days (149). ICU and hospital lengths of stay were also significantly longer in survivors with coagulopathy at admission compared to non-coagulopathic patients, and in-hospital mortality was higher (50% versus 17% respectively). In this study, multivariate analysis identified head Abbreviated Injury Severity (AIS) scale score, GCS score of 8 or less at the scene, hypotension at the scene and/or in the emergency department, pre-hospital intravenous fluid volume of at least 2000 mL, and age 75 or older years as independent risk factors for development of coagulopathy. Early coagulation abnormalities (within < 12 hours) along with head AIS scores of 5, penetrating injury mechanism, subdural haematoma, and low GCS score have also been reported to be independent risk factors for mortality (155).

Management

Fresh frozen plasma (FFP) administration has traditionally been an integral component of the management of coagulopathic trauma patients irrespective of the presence of concomitant head trauma. However, in a study in which 90 patients with severe TBI were randomized to receive FFP or normal saline, empirical use of FFP was associated with the development of a higher number of new intracerebral haematomas (156). Furthermore, although both groups had a similar frequency of poor neurological outcome in survivors, mortality was significantly higher in the FFP group (63% versus 35%) (156). Only 2% of the patients in this study had an abnormal international normalized ratio or PTT (156), suggesting that FFP should be reserved for use only when there is documented evidence of coagulopathy.

Tranexamic acid and recombinant factor VIIa (rFVIIa) have also been studied in the treatment of coagulopathy after acquired brain injury. The CRASH-2 collaborators performed a nested study within a large multicentre RCT (157). A total of 270 patients with (or at risk for) significant extracranial bleeding within 8 hours of injury, who had also sustained TBI, were randomized to receive tranexamic acid or placebo. There were non-significant trends toward reduced haematoma expansion (5.9 versus 8.1 mL), new focal cerebral ischaemic lesions (5% versus 9%), and mortality (11% versus 18%) with tranexamic acid. A RCT also reported a non-significant trend for rFVIIa (80–200 mcg/kg) to limit haemorrhage volume progression in patients with traumatic intracerebral haemorrhage (158). However, this was not associated with improved mortality but with an increased risk of deep vein thrombosis (8% versus 3%).

Platelets have commonly been employed to correct thrombocytopenia or reverse the effects of antiplatelet therapy after TBI. A database multicentre study of patients receiving platelet transfusion in the first 24 hours after trauma reported that a high platelet:red blood cell ratio was associated with improved survival after TBI (159). In patients with known or suspected aspirin usage, the Aspirin Response Test, which allows for an assessment of platelet inhibition, may be used to target and guide platelet transfusions (160).

Electrolyte disorders

Electrolyte disorders, including hyponatraemia, hypernatraemia, hypokalaemia, hyperkalaemia, hypophosphataemia, and hypomagnesaemia, are common after acquired brain injury (161–165). Two of the common causes of hyponatraemia in patients with acute CNS injury are the syndrome of inappropriate antidiuretic hormone secretion and cerebral salt wasting (161), while hypernatraemia may occur as a result of central diabetes insipidus (DI). These topics are discussed in detail in Chapter 28.

Infectious complications

Nosocomial infections affect approximately 30% of patients admitted to ICUs generally and are associated with substantial morbidity and mortality (166). Importantly, when compared to general or mixed populations of ICU patients, critically ill brain injured patients experience significantly higher rates of infection.

Incidence of infection after acquired brain injury

Approximately one-third of patients develop infectious complications after stroke, the most common being pneumonia and urinary tract infection (UTI) (167–170). A meta-analysis reported that the overall pooled infection risk among hospitalized patients after stroke (wherever their care location) was 30%, with the incidence of pneumonia and UTI being approximately 10% (170). However, in the subgroup of patients admitted to the ICU the overall risk of infection generally, pneumonia and UTI was substantially higher at 45%, 28% and 20% respectively. Stroke severity and lower levels of consciousness were associated with a higher risk of infection in this meta-analysis, and the development of pneumonia was associated with a threefold increase in mortality risk.

The incidence of infection in TBI patients admitted to ICU is even higher. In 82 patients with severe TBI, Helling and coworkers found that 50% developed at least one infectious complication (171). Piek and colleagues reviewed 734 patients from the Traumatic Coma Data Bank and reported a 41% incidence of pulmonary infections, and confirmed that its development was a significant independent predictor of unfavourable neurological outcome (172). Backward-elimination, stepwise logistic regression confirmed that the estimated reduction of unfavourable outcome was 2.9% for the elimination of pneumonia.

Pneumonia is particularly common in mechanically ventilated TBI patients. On one study, Zygun and coworkers reported that 45% developed VAP, with an incidence density of 42.7/1000 ventilator days (173). Development of VAP was associated with a significantly greater degree of non-neurological organ dysfunction, a longer duration of mechanical ventilation (15 versus 8 days), and increased ICU (17 versus 9 days) and hospital (60 versus 28 days) lengths of stay. Further, patients who developed VAP were at a significantly greater risk of requiring tracheostomy compared to those who did not (35% versus 18%). Others have also shown that critically ill neurological patients have a significantly higher risk of ICU-acquired sepsis compared to general ICU patients, and that this is associated with increased ICU and in-hospital mortality rates (174). As in stroke, there is a higher incidence of infection, sepsis, severe sepsis, and septic shock, as well as a greater risk of ICU and in-hospital mortality, in patients with severe TBI compared to those with milder degrees of brain injury (171,174,175).

Brain injury-induced immunosuppression

Primarily through release of cytokines, the CNS and immune system are extensively interconnected through neural pathways, hormonal cascades, and cell-to-cell interactions (176). These brain-immune interactions are highly relevant in terms of susceptibility to infection and functional outcome after brain injury (177). In a mouse model of focal cerebral ischaemia, all animals suffered spontaneous bacterial infections within three days of ischaemia (178).

The balance between pro- and anti-inflammatory cytokines determines the overall immunological response to brain injury, and may also influence the fate of injured brain tissue and the threshold for the development of complications including systemic infection (176). In human stroke, the balance between pro- and anti-inflammatory cytokines is an important prognostic factor. Recent data suggest that the development of early infection could be a manifestation of a stroke-induced immunodepression syndrome characterized by adrenergic overactivity and excessive anti-inflammatory drive (176). Chamorro demonstrated that stroke patients might have a low ratio of pro-inflammatory tumour necrosis factor alpha (TNF-α) to anti-inflammatory interleukin 10 (IL-10) concentration, suggesting a stroke-induced immunosuppression via a decrease in systemic T-helper cell (Th)-1 to Th2 ratio (179). Importantly, these immune effects can be long lasting. In an investigation examining causes of death one year post-TBI, patients were 12 times more likely to die from septicaemia than matched individuals from the general population (180).

Wong and colleagues recently reported an increased ratio of Th2-type over Th1-type cytokines in post-ischaemic wild-type mice, highlighting a switch in systemic immunity from Th1 to Th2 type in the early stages of reperfusion after stroke (181). They suggested that inactivation of hepatic invariant natural killer T (iNKT) cells may be responsible for these cytokine changes, as well as the resultant immunosuppression. Importantly, these effects were likely to be mediated by a noradrenergic neurotransmitter, given that local norepinephrine administration induced behavioural changes in hepatic iNKT cells and their release of IL-10. Further, administration of propranolol, a non-specific β-adrenergic receptor blocker, reversed the stroke-induced iNKT cell phenotype, and selective immunomodulation of iNKT cells with a specific activator (α-galactosylceramide) promoted pro-inflammatory cytokine production and prevented infections after stroke.

Prevention of infectious complications

As early tracheal colonization has been identified as a risk factor for the development of pneumonia after TBI (173), it has been suggested that prophylactic systemic antibiotic administration may prevent brain injury-associated infectious complications. Sirvent and colleagues demonstrated lower ICU and hospital lengths of stay in intubated, comatose patients who received prophylactic cefuroxime compared to controls (182). However, early exposure to short-term antibiotics increases the risk of subsequent colonization with Gram-negative enteric bacilli and *Pseudomonas* species, and this might outweigh the potential benefits of protection against early tracheal colonization (183). In a randomized, double-blind, placebo-controlled trial in 80 patients with severe, non-lacunar, ischaemic stroke in the middle cerebral artery territory, Harms and colleagues reported that intravenous moxifloxacin (400 mg daily) was superior to placebo in reducing infections (184).

Pathogen-targeted topical eradication has been suggested as an alternative to systemic antibiotics for the prevention of infection. *S. aureus* is a leading cause of pneumonia in brain-injured patients, and its nasal carriage has been reported to be a significant risk factor for the subsequent development of pulmonary infection (185,186). However, topical mupirocin therapy has not been shown to reduce the risk of infection even though it is highly effective for eradication of the nasal carriage *S. aureus* (187), possibly because of a long term re-setting of immunity after acquired brain injury, that is, one that will not be cured with short-term antibiotic intervention (180). Wong and colleagues have suggested that selective immunomodulation of hepatic iNKT cells is possible and may result in the prevention of infections after stroke (181).

As late-onset pneumonia, bacteraemia, and other types of ICU-acquired infections are likely to occur secondary to colonization of the digestive tract with pathogenic bacteria, a number of RCTs have examined the effect of selective decontamination of the oropharynx or stomach on various infectious and non-infectious outcomes (188–190). The goal of selective decontamination is to eradicate these organisms and prevent VAP (189), and includes selective digestive decontamination (SDD) which is the application of antimicrobial agents to the oropharynx and stomach, often in combination with systemic antibiotic administration, and selective oropharyngeal decontamination (SOD) which is limited to decontamination of the oropharynx. Meta-analyses of RCTs of mixed ICU populations have reported that SDD combined with antibiotics reduces VAP and hospital-acquired infections (188,189), and that it might also decrease overall mortality (190). Although this intervention has not been widely adopted because of concerns that it might lead to increased ICU pathogen resistance rates, a recent meta-analysis reported no association between the use of selective decontamination and development of antimicrobial resistance in common ICU pathogens (188). If this is confirmed by future studies, especially in areas where MRSA and/or vancomycin-resistant *Enterococcus* are endemic (191), selective decontamination may develop a significant role in prevention of VAP and other infections in ICU patients (188).

Gastrointestinal dysfunction

Delayed gastric emptying is common in critically ill patients generally, and there is a considerably higher risk in patients with TBI or multisystem trauma (192). Kao and colleagues reported that gastric emptying was significantly delayed (by 57 minutes) in 80% of patients with moderate to severe TBI patients compared to healthy matched controls (193), possibly related to increased ICP (194).

Although the early use of post-pyloric feeding has not been associated with improved outcome compared to gastric feeding in mixed populations of critically ill patients (195,196), some data indicate that these findings are not be transferable to patients with severe TBI (197). A recent single-centre RCT randomly allocated 104 patients with severe TBI to post-pyloric versus gastric feeding within 24 hours of ICU admission, and reported reduced gastric residuals and a significantly decreased odds of pneumonia, particularly late-onset pneumonia in those who received post-pyloric feeding (197). These findings require confirmation in further studies.

Acknowledgements

Dr Roberts is supported by an Alberta Innovates—Health Solutions Clinician Fellowship Award, a Knowledge Translation Canada Strategic Training in Health Research Fellowship, and funding from the Canadian Institutes of Health Research. We thank Mr Kevin O'Reilly for technical assistance with creation of the figures.

References

1. Zygun DA, Doig CJ, Gupta AK, Whiting G, Nicholas C, Shepherd E, et al. Non-neurological organ dysfunction in neurocritical care. *J Crit Care*. 2003;18(4):238–44.
2. Zygun DA, Kortbeek JB, Fick GH, Laupland KB, Doig CJ. Non-neurologic organ dysfunction in severe traumatic brain injury. *Crit Care Med*. 2005;33(3):654–60.
3. Zygun D. Non-neurological organ dysfunction in neurocritical care: impact on outcome and etiological considerations. *Curr Opin Crit Care*. 2005;11(2):139–43.
4. Zygun D, Berthiaume L, Laupland K, Kortbeek J, Doig C. SOFA is superior to MOD score for the determination of non-neurologic organ dysfunction in patients with severe traumatic brain injury: a cohort study. *Crit Care*. 2006;10(4):R115.
5. Bahloul M, Chaari AN, Kallel H, Khabir A, Ayadi A, Charfeddine H, et al. Neurogenic pulmonary edema due to traumatic brain injury: evidence of cardiac dysfunction. *Am J Crit Care*. 2006;15(5):462–70.
6. Perkes I, Baguley IJ, Nott MT, Menon DK. A review of paroxysmal sympathetic hyperactivity after acquired brain injury. *Ann Neurol*. 2010;68(2):126–35.
7. Rabinstein AA. Paroxysmal sympathetic hyperactivity in the neurological intensive care unit. *Neurol Res*. 2007;29(7):680–2.
8. Perkes IE, Menon DK, Nott MT, Baguley IJ. Paroxysmal sympathetic hyperactivity after acquired brain injury: a review of diagnostic criteria. *Brain Inj*. 2011;25(10):925–32.
9. Baguley IJ, Nicholls JL, Felmingham KL, Crooks J, Gurka JA, Wade LD. Dysautonomia after traumatic brain injury: a forgotten syndrome? *J Neurol Neurosurg Psychiatry*. 1999;67(1):39–43.
10. Baguley IJ, Slewa-Younan S, Heriseanu RE, Nott MT, Mudaliar Y, Nayyar V. The incidence of dysautonomia and its relationship with autonomic arousal following traumatic brain injury. *Brain Inj*. 2007;21(11):1175–81.
11. Fernandez-Ortega JF, Prieto-Palomino MA, Munoz-Lopez A, Lebron-Gallardo M, Cabrera-Ortiz H, Quesada-Garcia G. Prognostic influence and computed tomography findings in dysautonomic crises after traumatic brain injury. *J Trauma*. 2006;61(5):1129–33.
12. Ryan JB, Hicks M, Cropper JR, Garlick SR, Kesteven SH, Wilson MK, et al. Functional evidence of reversible ischemic injury immediately after the sympathetic storm associated with experimental brain death. *J Heart Lung Transplant*. 2003;22(8):922–8.
13. Hendricks HT, Geurts AC, van Ginneken BC, Heeren AJ, Vos PE. Brain injury severity and autonomic dysregulation accurately predict heterotopic ossification in patients with traumatic brain injury. *Clin Rehabil*. 2007;21(6):545–53.
14. Mehta NM, Bechard LJ, Leavitt K, Duggan C. Severe weight loss and hypermetabolic paroxysmal dysautonomia following hypoxic ischemic brain injury: the role of indirect calorimetry in the intensive care unit. *JPEN J Parenter Enteral Nutr*. 2008;32(3):281–4.
15. Baguley IJ, Heriseanu RE, Cameron ID, Nott MT, Slewa-Younan S. A critical review of the pathophysiology of dysautonomia following traumatic brain injury. *Neurocrit Care*. 2008;8(2):293–300.
16. Penfield W. Diencephalic autonomic epilepsy. *Arch Neurol Psychiatry*. 1929;22:358–74.
17. Bullard DE. Diencephalic seizures: responsiveness to bromocriptine and morphine. *Ann Neurol*. 1987;21(6):609–11.
18. Boeve BF, Wijdicks EF, Benarroch EE, Schmidt KD. Paroxysmal sympathetic storms ("diencephalic seizures") after severe diffuse axonal head injury. *Mayo Clin Proc*. 1998;73(2):148–52.
19. Goh KY, Conway EJ, DaRosso RC, Muszynski CA, Epstein FJ. Sympathetic storms in a child with a midbrain glioma: a variant of diencephalic seizures. *Pediatr Neurol*. 1999;21(4):742–4.
20. Tong C, Konig MW, Roberts PR, Tatter SB, Li XH. Autonomic dysfunction secondary to intracerebral hemorrhage. *Anesth Analg*. 2000;91(6):1450–1.
21. Baguley IJ, Heriseanu RE, Gurka JA, Nordenbo A, Cameron ID. Gabapentin in the management of dysautonomia following severe

traumatic brain injury: a case series. *J Neurol Neurosurg Psychiatry*. 2007;78(5):539–41.

22. Hinson HE, Sheth KN. Manifestations of the hyperadrenergic state after acute brain injury. *Curr Opin Crit Care*. 2012;18(2):139–45.

23. Lv LQ, Hou LJ, Yu MK, Qi XQ, Chen HR, Chen JX, et al. Prognostic influence and magnetic resonance imaging findings in paroxysmal sympathetic hyperactivity after severe traumatic brain injury. *J Neurotrauma*. 2010;27(11):1945–50.

24. Baguley IJ. The excitatory:inhibitory ratio model (EIR model): an integrative explanation of acute autonomic overactivity syndromes. *Med Hypotheses*. 2008;70(1):26–35.

25. Cuny E, Richer E, Castel JP. Dysautonomia syndrome in the acute recovery phase after traumatic brain injury: relief with intrathecal Baclofen therapy. *Brain Inj*. 2001;15(10):917–25.

26. Lemke DM. Riding out the storm: sympathetic storming after traumatic brain injury. *J Neurosci Nurs*. 2004;36(1):4–9.

27. Dolce G, Quintieri M, Leto E, Milano M, Pileggi A, Lagani V, et al. Dysautonomia and clinical outcome in vegetative state. *J Neurotrauma*. 2008;25: 1079–108.

28. Blackman JA, Patrick PD, Buck ML, Rust RS Jr. Paroxysmal autonomic instability with dystonia after brain injury. *Arch Neurol*. 2004;61(3):321–8.

29. Turner MS. Early use of intrathecal baclofen in brain injury in pediatric patients. *Acta Neurochir Suppl*. 2003;87:81–3.

30. Krach LE, Kriel RL, Morris WF, Warhol BL, Luxenberg MG. Central autonomic dysfunction following acquired brain injury in children. *J Neurol Rehabil*. 1997;11:41–5.

31. Fearnside MR, Cook RJ, McDougall P, McNeil RJ. The Westmead Head Injury Project outcome in severe head injury. A comparative analysis of pre-hospital, clinical and CT variables. *Br J Neurosurg*. 1993;7(3):267–79.

32. Blackman JA, Patrick PD, Buck ML, Rust RS. Jr. Correction: Paroxysmal autonomic instability with dystonia after brain injury. *Arch Neurol*. 2004;61:980.

33. De Tanti A, Gasperini G, Rossini M. Paroxysmal episodic hypothalamic instability with hypothermia after traumatic brain injury. *Brain Inj*. 2005;19(14):1277–83.

34. Roberts DJ, Hall RI, Kramer AH, Robertson HL, Gallagher CN, Zygun DA. Sedation for critically ill adults with severe traumatic brain injury: a systematic review of randomized controlled trials. *Crit Care Med*. 2011;39(12):2743–51.

35. Lu CS, Ryu SJ. Neuroleptic malignant-like syndrome associated with acute hydrocephalus. *Mov Disord*. 1991;6(4):381–3.

36. Lemke DM. Sympathetic storming after severe traumatic brain injury. *Crit Care Nurse*. 2007;27(1):30–7.

37. Lee VH, Oh JK, Mulvagh SL, Wijdicks EF. Mechanisms in neurogenic stress cardiomyopathy after aneurysmal subarachnoid hemorrhage. *Neurocrit Care*. 2006;5(3):243–9.

38. Stevens RD, Nyquist PA. The systemic implications of aneurysmal subarachnoid hemorrhage. *J Neurol Sci*. 2007;261(1–2):143–56.

39. Kopelnik A, Zaroff JG. Neurocardiogenic injury in neurovascular disorders. *Crit Care Clin*. 2006;22(4):733–52.

40. Nguyen H, Zaroff JG. Neurogenic stunned myocardium. *Curr Neurol Neurosci Rep*. 2009;9(6):486–91.

41. Mashaly HA, Provencio JJ. Inflammation as a link between brain injury and heart damage: the model of subarachnoid hemorrhage. *Cleve Clin J Med*. 2008;75 Suppl 2:S26–30.

42. Goldman MR, Rogers EL, Rogers MC. Subarachnoid hemorrhage. Association with unusual electrocardiographic changes. *JAMA*. 1975;234(9):957–8.

43. Toyama Y, Tanaka H, Nuruki K, Shirao T. Prinzmetal's variant angina associated with subarachnoid hemorrhage: a case report. *Angiology*. 1979;30(3):211–18.

44. Yuki K, Kodama Y, Onda J, Emoto K, Morimoto T, Uozumi T. Coronary vasospasm following subarachnoid hemorrhage as a cause of stunned myocardium. Case report. *J Neurosurg*. 1991;75(2):308–11.

45. Chang PC, Lee SH, Hung HF, Kaun P, Cheng JJ. Transient ST elevation and left ventricular asynergy associated with normal coronary artery

46. de Chazal I, Parham WM 3rd, Liopyris P, Wijdicks EF. Delayed cardiogenic shock and acute lung injury after aneurysmal subarachnoid hemorrhage. *Anesth Analg*. 2005;100(4):1147–9.

47. Zaroff JG, Rordorf GA, Titus JS, Newell JB, Nowak NJ, Torchiana DF, et al. Regional myocardial perfusion after experimental subarachnoid hemorrhage. *Stroke*. 2000;31(5):1136–43.

48. Masuda T, Sato K, Yamamoto S, Matsuyama N, Shimohama T, Matsunaga A, et al. Sympathetic nervous activity and myocardial damage immediately after subarachnoid hemorrhage in a unique animal model. *Stroke*. 2002;33(6):1671–6.

49. Szabo MD, Crosby G, Hurford WE, Strauss HW. Myocardial perfusion following acute subarachnoid hemorrhage in patients with an abnormal electrocardiogram. *Anesth Analg*. 1993;76(2):253–8.

50. Banki NM, Kopelnik A, Dae MW, Miss J, Tung P, Lawton MT, et al. Acute neurocardiogenic injury after subarachnoid hemorrhage. *Circulation*. 2005;112(21):3314–9.

51. Novitzky D, Wicomb WN, Cooper DK, Rose AG, Reichart B. Prevention of myocardial injury during brain death by total cardiac sympathectomy in the Chacma baboon. *Ann Thorac Surg*. 1986;41(5):520–4.

52. Ogura T, Satoh A, Ooigawa H, Sugiyama T, Takeda R, Fushihara G, et al. Characteristics and prognostic value of acute catecholamine surge in patients with aneurysmal subarachnoid hemorrhage. *Neurol Res*. 2012;34(5):484–90.

53. Lambert E, Du XJ, Percy E, Lambert G. Cardiac response to norepinephrine and sympathetic nerve stimulation following experimental subarachnoid hemorrhage. *J Neurol Sci*. 2002;198(1–2):43–50.

54. Shivalkar B, Van Loon J, Wieland W, Tjandra-Maga TB, Borgers M, Plets C, et al. Variable effects of explosive or gradual increase of intracranial pressure on myocardial structure and function. *Circulation*. 1993;87(1):230–9.

55. Ako J, Honda Y, Fitzgerald PJ. Tako-tsubo-like left ventricular dysfunction. *Circulation*. 2003;108(23):e158.

56. Ako J, Sudhir K, Farouque HM, Honda Y, Fitzgerald PJ. Transient left ventricular dysfunction under severe stress: brain-heart relationship revisited. *Am J Med*. 2006 Jan;119(1):10–7.

57. Wittstein IS, Thiemann DR, Lima JA, Baughman KL, Schulman SP, Gerstenblith G, et al. Neurohumoral features of myocardial stunning due to sudden emotional stress. *N Engl J Med*. 2005;352(6):539–48.

58. Kawahara E, Ikeda S, Miyahara Y, Kohno S. Role of autonomic nervous dysfunction in electrocardio-graphic abnormalities and cardiac injury in patients with acute subarachnoid hemorrhage. *Circ J*. 2003;67(9):753–6.

59. Tracey KJ. The inflammatory reflex. *Nature*. 2002;420(6917):853–9.

60. Koizumi K, Terui N, Kollai M, Brooks CM. Functional significance of coactivation of vagal and sympathetic cardiac nerves. *Proc Natl Acad Sci U S A*. 1982;79(6):2116–20.

61. Parekh N, Venkatesh B, Cross D, Leditschke A, Atherton J, Miles W, et al. Cardiac troponin I predicts myocardial dysfunction in aneurysmal subarachnoid hemorrhage. *J Am Coll Cardiol*. 2000;36(4):1328–35.

62. Tung P, Kopelnik A, Banki N, Ong K, Ko N, Lawton MT, et al. Predictors of neurocardiogenic injury after subarachnoid hemorrhage. *Stroke*. 2004;35(2):548–51.

63. van der Bilt IA, Hasan D, Vandertop WP, Wilde AA, Algra A, Visser FC, et al. Impact of cardiac complications on outcome after aneurysmal subarachnoid hemorrhage: a meta-analysis. *Neurology*. 2009;72(7):635–42.

64. Zaroff JG, Leong J, Kim H, Young WL, Cullen SP, Rao VA, et al. Cardiovascular predictors of long-term outcomes after non-traumatic subarachnoid hemorrhage. *Neurocrit Care*. 2012;17(3):374–81.

65. Schuiling WJ, Dennesen PJ, Rinkel GJ. Extracerebral organ dysfunction in the acute stage after aneurysmal subarachnoid hemorrhage. *Neurocrit Care*. 2005;3(1):1–10.

66. Bulsara KR, McGirt MJ, Liao L, Villavicencio AT, Borel C, Alexander MJ, et al. Use of the peak troponin value to differentiate myocardial

and Tc-99m PYP myocardial infarct scan in subarachnoid hemorrhage. *Int J Cardiol*. 1998;63(2):189–92.

infarction from reversible neurogenic left ventricular dysfunction associated with aneurysmal subarachnoid hemorrhage. *J Neurosurg.* 2003;98(3):524–8.

67. de Lemos JA, Morrow DA, Bentley JH, Omland T, Sabatine MS, McCabe CH. et al. The prognostic value of B-type natriuretic peptide in patients with acute coronary syndromes. *N Engl J Med.* 2001;345(14):1014–21.

68. Taub PR, Fields JD, Wu AH, Miss JC, Lawton MT, Smith WS, et al. Elevated BNP is associated with vasospasm-independent cerebral infarction following aneurysmal subarachnoid hemorrhage. *Neurocrit Care.* 2011;15(1):13–18.

69. Dimant J, Grob D. Electrocardiographic changes and myocardial damage in patients with acute cerebrovascular accidents. *Stroke.* 1977;8(4):448–55.

70. Goldstein DS. The electrocardiogram in stroke: relationship to pathophysiological type and comparison with prior tracings. *Stroke.* 1979;10(3):253–9.

71. Oppenheimer SM, Cechetto DF, Hachinski VC. Cerebrogenic cardiac arrhythmias. Cerebral electrocardiographic influences and their role in sudden death. *Arch Neurol.* 1990;47(5):513–19.

72. Brouwers PJ, Wijdicks EF, Hasan D, Vermeulen M, Wever EF, Frericks H, *et al.* Serial electrocardiographic recording in aneurysmal subarachnoid hemorrhage. *Stroke.* 1989;20(9):1162–7.

73. Coghlan LA, Hindman BJ, Bayman EO, Banki NM, Gelb AW, Todd MM, *et al.* Independent associations between electrocardiographic abnormalities and outcomes in patients with aneurysmal subarachnoid hemorrhage: findings from the intraoperative hypothermia aneurysm surgery trial. *Stroke.* 2009;40(2):412–18.

74. Bruder N, Rabinstein A, Participants in the International Multi-Disciplinary Consensus Conference on the Critical Care Management of Subarachnoid Hemorrhage. Cardiovascular and pulmonary complications of aneurysmal subarachnoid hemorrhage. *Neurocrit Care.* 2011;15(2):257–69.

75. Frontera JA, Parra A, Shimbo D, Fernandez A, Schmidt JM, Peter P, *et al.* Cardiac arrhythmias after subarachnoid hemorrhage: risk factors and impact on outcome. *Cerebrovasc Dis.* 2008;26(1):71–8.

76. Hravnak M, Frangiskakis JM, Crago EA, Chang Y, Tanabe M, Gorcsan J,3rd, *et al.* Elevated cardiac troponin I and relationship to persistence of electrocardiographic and echocardiographic abnormalities after aneurysmal subarachnoid hemorrhage. *Stroke.* 2009;40(11):3478–84.

77. Frangiskakis JM, Hravnak M, Crago EA, Tanabe M, Kip KE, Gorcsan J 3rd, *et al.* Ventricular arrhythmia risk after subarachnoid hemorrhage. *Neurocrit Care.* 2009;10(3):287–94.

78. Bourdages M, Bigras JL, Farrell CA, Hutchison JS, Lacroix J, Canadian Critical Care Trials Group. Cardiac arrhythmias associated with severe traumatic brain injury and hypothermia therapy. *Pediatr Crit Care Med.* 2010;11(3):408–14.

79. Kline RC, Swanson DP, Wieland DM, Thrall JH, Gross MD, Pitt B, et al. Myocardial imaging in man with I-123 meta-iodobenzylguanidine. *J Nucl Med.* 1981;22(2):129–32.

80. Zaroff JG, Rordorf GA, Ogilvy CS, Picard MH. Regional patterns of left ventricular systolic dysfunction after subarachnoid hemorrhage: evidence for neurally mediated cardiac injury. *J Am Soc Echocardiogr.* 2000;13(8):774–9.

81. Banki N, Kopelnik A, Tung P, Lawton MT, Gress D, Drew B, et al. Prospective analysis of prevalence, distribution, and rate of recovery of left ventricular systolic dysfunction in patients with subarachnoid hemorrhage. *J Neurosurg.* 2006;105(1):15–20.

82. Kono T, Morita H, Kuroiwa T, Onaka H, Takatsuka H, Fujiwara A. Left ventricular wall motion abnormalities in patients with subarachnoid hemorrhage: neurogenic stunned myocardium. *J Am Coll Cardiol.* 1994;24(3):636–40.

83. Doshi R, Neil-Dwyer G. Hypothalamic and myocardial lesions after subarachnoid haemorrhage. *J Neurol Neurosurg Psychiatry.* 1977;40(8):821–6.

84. Neil-Dwyer G, Walter P, Cruickshank JM, Doshi B, O'Gorman P. Effect of propranolol and phentolamine on myocardial necrosis after subarachnoid haemorrhage. *Br Med J.* 1978;2(6143):990–2.

85. Doshi R, Neil-Dwyer G. A clinicopathological study of patients following a subarachnoid hemorrhage. *J Neurosurg.* 1980;52(3):295–301.

86. Pollick C, Cujec B, Parker S, Tator C. Left ventricular wall motion abnormalities in subarachnoid hemorrhage: an echocardiographic study. *J Am Coll Cardiol.* 1988;12(3):600–5.

87. Karch SB, Billingham ME. Myocardial contraction bands revisited. *Hum Pathol.* 1986;17(1):9–13.

88. Cruickshank JM, Neil-Dwyer G, Lane J. The effect of oral propranolol upon the ECG changes occurring in subarachnoid haemorrhage. *Cardiovasc Res.* 1975;9(2):236–45.

89. Walter P, Neil-Dwyer G, Cruickshank JM. Beneficial effects of adrenergic blockade in patients with subarachnoid haemorrhage. *Br Med J (Clin Res Ed).* 1982;284(6330):1661–4.

90. Neil-Dwyer G, Walter P, Cruickshank JM. Beta-blockade benefits patients following a subarachnoid haemorrhage. *Eur J Clin Pharmacol.* 1985;28 Suppl:25–9.

91. Lambert G, Naredi S, Eden E, Rydenhag B, Friberg P. Sympathetic nervous activation following subarachnoid hemorrhage: influence of intravenous clonidine. *Acta Anaesthesiol Scand.* 2002;46(2):160–5.

92. Macmillan CS, Grant IS, Andrews PJ. Pulmonary and cardiac sequelae of subarachnoid haemorrhage: time for active management? *Intensive Care Med.* 2002;28(8):1012–23.

93. Gruber A, Reinprecht A, Illievich UM, Fitzgerald R, Dietrich W, Czech T, *et al.* Extracerebral organ dysfunction and neurologic outcome after aneurysmal subarachnoid hemorrhage. *Crit Care Med.* 1999;27(3):505–14.

94. Brain Trauma Foundation, American Association of Neurological Surgeons, Congress of Neurological Surgeons, Joint Section on Neurotrauma and Critical Care, AANS/CNS, Bratton SL, Chestnut RM, *et al.* Guidelines for the management of severe traumatic brain injury. I. Blood pressure and oxygenation. *J Neurotrauma.* 2007;24 Suppl 1:S7–13.

95. Brain Trauma Foundation, American Association of Neurological Surgeons, Congress of Neurological Surgeons, Joint Section on Neurotrauma and Critical Care, AANS/CNS, Bratton SL, Chestnut RM, *et al.* Guidelines for the management of severe traumatic brain injury. IX. Cerebral perfusion thresholds. *J Neurotrauma.* 2007;24 Suppl 1:S59–64.

96. Mutoh T, Ishikawa T, Nishino K, Yasui N. Evaluation of the FloTrac uncalibrated continuous cardiac output system for perioperative hemodynamic monitoring after subarachnoid hemorrhage. *J Neurosurg Anesthesiol.* 2009;21(3):218–25.

97. Berthiaume L, Zygun D. Non-neurologic organ dysfunction in acute brain injury. *Crit Care Clin.* 2006;22(4):753–66.

98. Naidech A, Du Y, Kreiter KT, Parra A, Fitzsimmons BF, Lavine SD, *et al.* Dobutamine versus milrinone after subarachnoid hemorrhage. *Neurosurgery.* 2005;56(1):21–61.

99. Lowe GJ, Ferguson ND. Lung-protective ventilation in neurosurgical patients. *Curr Opin Crit Care.* 2006;12(1):3–7.

100. Davison DL, Terek M, Chawla LS. Neurogenic pulmonary edema. *Crit Care.* 2012;16(2):212.

101. Solenski NJ, Haley EC,Jr, Kassell NF, Kongable G, Germanson T, Truskowski L, *et al.* Medical complications of aneurysmal subarachnoid hemorrhage: a report of the multicenter, cooperative aneurysm study. Participants of the Multicenter Cooperative Aneurysm Study. *Crit Care Med.* 1995;23(6):1007–17.

102. Ware LB, Matthay MA. The acute respiratory distress syndrome. *N Engl J Med.* 2000;342(18):1334–49.

103. Bernard GR, Artigas A, Brigham KL, Carlet J, Falke K, Hudson L, *et al.* The American-European Consensus Conference on ARDS. Definitions, mechanisms, relevant outcomes, and clinical trial coordination. *Am J Respir Crit Care Med.* 1994;149(3 Pt 1):818–24.

104. ARDS Definition Task Force, Ranieri VM, Rubenfeld GD, Thompson BT, Ferguson ND, Caldwell E, *et al.* Acute respiratory distress syndrome: the Berlin Definition. *JAMA.* 2012;307(23):2526–33.

105. Mascia L. Acute lung injury in patients with severe brain injury: a double hit model. *Neurocrit Care.* 2009;11(3):417–26.

106. Holland MC, Mackersie RC, Morabito D, Campbell AR, Kivett VA, Patel R, *et al.* The development of acute lung injury is associated with worse neurologic outcome in patients with severe traumatic brain injury. *J Trauma.* 2003;55(1):106–11.

107. Bratton SL, Davis RL. Acute lung injury in isolated traumatic brain injury. *Neurosurgery.* 1997;40(4):707–12.

108. Mascia L, Zavala E, Bosma K, Pasero D, Decaroli D, Andrews P, *et al.* High tidal volume is associated with the development of acute lung injury after severe brain injury: an international observational study. *Crit Care Med.* 2007;35(8):1815–20.

109. Kahn JM, Caldwell EC, Deem S, Newell DW, Heckbert SR, Rubenfeld GD. Acute lung injury in patients with subarachnoid hemorrhage: incidence, risk factors, and outcome. *Crit Care Med.* 2006;34(1):196–202.

110. Rogers FB, Shackford SR, Trevisani GT, Davis JW, Mackersie RC, Hoyt DB. Neurogenic pulmonary edema in fatal and nonfatal head injuries. *J Trauma.* 1995;39(5):860–6.

111. Simmons RL, Martin AM,Jr, Heisterkamp CA 3rd, Ducker TB. Respiratory insufficiency in combat casualties. II. Pulmonary edema following head injury. I. 1969;170(1):39–44.

112. Mayer SA, Lin J, Homma S, Solomon RA, Lennihan L, Sherman D, *et al.* Myocardial injury and left ventricular performance after subarachnoid hemorrhage. *Stroke.* 1999;30(4):780–6.

113. Ducker TB, Simmons RL. Increased intracranial pressure and pulmonary edema. 2. The hemodynamic response of dogs and monkeys to increased intracranial pressure. *J Neurosurg.* 1968;28(2):118–23.

114. Sarnoff SJ, Sarnoff LC. Neurohemodynamics of pulmonary edema. II. The role of sympathetic pathways in the elevation of pulmonary and stemic vascular pressures following the intracisternal injection of fibrin. *Circulation.* 1952;6(1):51–62.

115. Cushing H. Concerning a definite regulatory mechanism of the vasomotor centre which controls blood pressure during cerebral compression. *Bull Johns Hopkins Hosp.* 1901;126:289–92.

116. Theodore J, Robin ED. Speculations on neurogenic pulmonary edema (NPE). *Am Rev Respir Dis.* 1976;113(4):405–11.

117. Maron MB. Effect of elevated vascular pressure transients on protein permeability in the lung. *J Appl Physiol.* 1989;67(1):305–10.

118. Bosso FJ, Lang SA, Maron MB. Role of hemodynamics and vagus nerves in development of fibrin-induced pulmonary edema. *J Appl Physiol.* 1990;69(6):2227–32.

119. Carlson RW, Schaeffer RC Jr, Michaels SG, Weil MH. Pulmonary edema following intracranial hemorrhage. *Chest.* 1979;75(6):731–4.

120. Richardson JB. The innervation of the lung. *Eur J Respir Dis Suppl.* 1982;117:13–31.

121. Richardson JB. Recent progress in pulmonary innervation. *Am Rev Respir Dis.* 1983;128(2 Pt 2):S65–8.

122. van der Zee H, Malik AB, Lee BC, Hakim TS. Lung fluid and protein exchange during intracranial hypertension and role of sympathetic mechanisms. *J Appl Physiol.* 1980;48(2):273–80.

123. McClellan MD, Dauber IM, Weil JV. Elevated intracranial pressure increases pulmonary vascular permeability to protein. *J Appl Physiol.* 1989;67(3):1185–91.

124. Fontes RB, Aguiar PH, Zanetti MV, Andrade F, Mandel M, Teixeira MJ. Acute neurogenic pulmonary edema: case reports and literature review. *J Neurosurg Anesthesiol.* 2003;15(2):144–50.

125. Muscedere J, Dodek P, Keenan S, Fowler R, Cook D, Heyland D, *et al.* Comprehensive evidence-based clinical practice guidelines for ventilator-associated pneumonia: diagnosis and treatment. *J Crit Care.* 2008;23(1):138–47.

126. Lepelletier D, Roquilly A, Demeure dit latte D, Mahe PJ, Loutrel O, Champin P, *et al.* Retrospective analysis of the risk factors and pathogens associated with early-onset ventilator-associated pneumonia in surgical-ICU head-trauma patients. *J Neurosurg Anesthesiol.*2010;22(1):32–7.

127. Peterson K, Carson S, Carney N. Hypothermia treatment for traumatic brain injury: a systematic review and meta-analysis. *J Neurotrauma.* 2008;25(1):62–71.

128. Giard M, Lepape A, Allaouchiche B, Guerin C, Lehot JJ, Robert MO, *et al.* Early- and late-onset ventilator-associated pneumonia acquired in the intensive care unit: comparison of risk factors. *J Crit Care.* 2008;23(1):27–33.

129. Cazzadori A, Di Perri G, Vento S, Bonora S, Fendt D, Rossi M, *et al.* Aetiology of pneumonia following isolated closed head injury. *Respir Med.* 1997;91(4):193–9.

130. Kerwin AJ, Croce MA, Timmons SD, Maxwell RA, Malhotra AK, Fabian TC. Effects of fiberoptic bronchoscopy on intracranial pressure in patients with brain injury: a prospective clinical study. *J Trauma.* 2000;48(5):878–82.

131. White PF, Schlobohm RM, Pitts LH, Lindauer JM. A randomized study of drugs for preventing increases in intracranial pressure during endotracheal suctioning. *Anesthesiology.* 1982;57(3):242–4.

132. Peerless JR, Snow N, Likavec MJ, Pinchak AC, Malangoni MA. The effect of fiberoptic bronchoscopy on cerebral hemodynamics in patients with severe head injury. *Chest.* 1995;108(4):962–5.

133. Roberts DJ, Zygun DA. Comparative efficacy and safety of sedative agents in severe traumatic brain injury. In Vincent J (ed) *Annual Update in Intensive Care and Emergency Medicine 2012.* Berlin Heidelberg: Springer-Verlag; 2012:771–82.

134. Young N, Rhodes JK, Mascia L, Andrews PJ. Ventilatory strategies for patients with acute brain injury. *Curr Opin Crit Care.* 2010;16(1):45–52.

135. Johnson VE, Huang JH, Pilcher WH. Special cases: mechanical ventilation of neurosurgical patients. *Crit Care Clin.* 2007;23(2):275–90.

136. Maegele M. Coagulopathy after traumatic brain injury: incidence, pathogenesis, and treatment options. *Transfusion.* 2013;53 Suppl 1:28S–37S.

137. Harhangi BS, Kompanje EJ, Leebeek FW, Maas AI. Coagulation disorders after traumatic brain injury. *Acta Neurochir (Wien).* 2008;150(2):165–75.

138. Laroche M, Kutcher ME, Huang MC, Cohen MJ, Manley GT. Coagulopathy after traumatic brain injury. *Neurosurgery.* 2012;70(6):1334–45.

139. Halpern CH, Reilly PM, Turtz AR, Stein SC. Traumatic coagulopathy: the effect of brain injury. *J Neurotrauma.* 2008;25(8):997–1001.

140. Keimowitz RM, Annis BL. Disseminated intravascular coagulation associated with massive brain injury. *J Neurosurg.* 1973;39(2):178–80.

141. Morel N, Morel O, Petit L, Hugel B, Cochard JF, Freyssinet JM, *et al.* Generation of procoagulant microparticles in cerebrospinal fluid and peripheral blood after traumatic brain injury. *J Trauma.* 2008;64(3):698–704.

142. Bernard GR, Vincent JL, Laterre PF, LaRosa SP, Dhainaut JF, Lopez-Rodriguez A, *et al.* Efficacy and safety of recombinant human activated protein C for severe sepsis. *N Engl J Med.* 2001;344(10):699–709.

143. Allard CB, Scarpelini S, Rhind SG, Baker AJ, Shek PN, Tien H, *et al.* Abnormal coagulation tests are associated with progression of traumatic intracranial hemorrhage. *J Trauma.* 2009;67(5):959–67.

144. Vecht CJ, Minderhoud JM, Sibinga CT. Platelet aggregability in relation to impaired consciousness after head injury. *J Clin Pathol.* 1975;28(10):814–20.

145. Nekludov M, Bellander BM, Blomback M, Wallen HN. Platelet dysfunction in patients with severe traumatic brain injury. *J Neurotrauma.* 2007;24(11):1699–706.

146. Davis PK, Musunuru H, Walsh M, Cassady R, Yount R, Losiniecki A, *et al.* Platelet dysfunction is an early marker for traumatic brain injury-induced coagulopathy. *Neurocrit Care.* 2013;18(2):201–8.

147. Stein SC, Young GS, Talucci RC, Greenbaum BH, Ross SE. Delayed brain injury after head trauma: significance of coagulopathy. *Neurosurgery.* 1992;30(2):160–5.

148. Stein SC, Chen XH, Sinson GP, Smith DH. Intravascular coagulation: a major secondary insult in nonfatal traumatic brain injury. *J Neurosurg.* 2002;97(6):1373–7.

149. Wafaisade A, Lefering R, Tjardes T, Wutzler S, Simanski C, Paffrath T, *et al.* Acute coagulopathy in isolated blunt traumatic brain injury. *Neurocrit Care.* 2010;12(2):211–19.

150. Levi M, Toh CH, Thachil J, Watson HG. Guidelines for the diagnosis and management of disseminated intravascular coagulation. British Committee for Standards in Haematology. *Br J Haematol.* 2009;145(1):24–33.

151. Kaufmann CR, Dwyer KM, Crews JD, Dols SJ, Trask AL. Usefulness of thromboelastography in assessment of trauma patient coagulation. *J Trauma.* 1997;42(4):716–20.

152. Walsh M, Thomas SG, Howard JC, Evans E, Guyer K, Medvecz A, *et al.* Blood component therapy in trauma guided with the utilization of the perfusionist and thromboelastography. *J Extra Corpor Technol.* 2011;43(3):162–7.

153. Holcomb JB, Minei KM, Scerbo ML, Radwan ZA, Wade CE, Kozar RA, *et al.* Admission rapid thromblestography can replace conventional coagulation tests in the emergency department: experience with 1974 consecutive trauma patients. *Ann Surg.* 2012;256(3):476–86.

154. Greuters S, van den Berg A, Franschman G, Viersen VA, Beishuizen A, Peerdeman SM, *et al.* Acute and delayed mild coagulopathy are related to outcome in patients with isolated traumatic brain injury. *Crit Care.* 2011;15(1):R2.

155. Lustenberger T, Talving P, Kobayashi L, Inaba K, Lam L, Plurad D, *et al.* Time course of coagulopathy in isolated severe traumatic brain injury. *Injury.* 2010;41(9):924–8.

156. Etemadrezaie H, Baharvahdat H, Shariati Z, Lari SM, Shakeri MT, Ganjeifar B. The effect of fresh frozen plasma in severe closed head injury. *Clin Neurol Neurosurg.* 2007;109(2):166–71.

157. CRASH-2 trial collaborators, Shakur H, Roberts I, Bautista R, Caballero J, Coats T, *et al.* Effects of tranexamic acid on death, vascular occlusive events, and blood transfusion in trauma patients with significant haemorrhage (CRASH-2): a randomised, placebo-controlled trial. *Lancet.* 2010;376(9734):23–32.

158. Narayan RK, Maas AI, Marshall LF, Servadei F, Skolnick BE, Tillinger MN, *et al.* Recombinant factor VIIA in traumatic intracerebral hemorrhage: results of a dose-escalation clinical trial. *Neurosurgery.* 2008;62(4):776–86.

159. Brasel KJ, Vercruysse G, Spinella PC, Wade CE, Blackbourne LH, Borgman MA, *et al.* The association of blood component use ratios with the survival of massively transfused trauma patients with and without severe brain injury. *J Trauma.* 2011;71(2 Suppl 3):S343–52.

160. Bachelani AM, Bautz JT, Sperry JL, Corcos A, Zenati M, Billiar TR, *et al.* Assessment of platelet transfusion for reversal of aspirin after traumatic brain injury. *Surgery.* 2011;150(4):836–43.

161. Rabinstein AA, Wijdicks EF. Hyponatremia in critically ill neurological patients. *Neurologist.* 2003;9(6):290–300.

162. Rahman M, Friedman WA. Hyponatremia in neurosurgical patients: clinical guidelines development. *Neurosurgery.* 2009;65(5):925–35.

163. Moritz ML. Syndrome of inappropriate antidiuresis and cerebral salt wasting syndrome: are they different and does it matter? *Pediatr Nephrol.* 2012;27(5):689–93.

164. Adler SM, Verbalis JG. Disorders of body water homeostasis in critical illness. *Endocrinol Metab Clin North Am.* 2006;35(4):873–94.

165. Tisdall M, Crocker M, Watkiss J, Smith M. Disturbances of sodium in critically ill adult neurologic patients: a clinical review. *J Neurosurg Anesthesiol.* 2006;18(1):57–63.

166. Vincent JL. Nosocomial infections in adult intensive-care units. *Lancet.* 2003;361(9374):2068–77.

167. Davenport RJ, Dennis MS, Wellwood I, Warlow CP. Complications after acute stroke. *Stroke.* 1996;27(3):415–20.

168. Fassbender K, Dempfle CE, Mielke O, Rossol S, Schneider S, Dollman M, *et al.* Proinflammatory cytokines: indicators of infection in high-risk patients. *J Lab Clin Med.* 1997;130(5):535–9.

169. Hilker R, Poetter C, Findeisen N, Sobesky J, Jacobs A, Neveling M, *et al.* Nosocomial pneumonia after acute stroke: implications for neurological intensive care medicine. *Stroke.* 2003;34(4):975–81.

170. Westendorp WF, Nederkoorn PJ, Vermeij JD, Dijkgraaf MG, van de Beek D. Post-stroke infection: a systematic review and meta-analysis. *BMC Neurol.* 2011;11:110.

171. Helling TS, Evans LL, Fowler DL, Hays LV, Kennedy FR. Infectious complications in patients with severe head injury. *J Trauma.* 1988;28(11):1575–7.

172. Piek J, Chesnut RM, Marshall LF, van Berkum-Clark M, Klauber MR, Blunt BA, *et al.* Extracranial complications of severe head injury. *J Neurosurg.* 1992;77(6):901–7.

173. Zygun DA, Zuege DJ, Boiteau PJ, Laupland KB, Henderson EA, Kortbeek JB, *et al.* Ventilator-associated pneumonia in severe traumatic brain injury. *Neurocrit Care.* 2006;5(2):108–14.

174. Mascia L, Sakr Y, Pasero D, Payen D, Reinhart K, Vincent JL, *et al.* Extracranial complications in patients with acute brain injury: a post-hoc analysis of the SOAP study. *Intensive Care Med.* 2008;34(4):720–7.

175. Croce MA, Tolley EA, Fabian TC. A formula for prediction of posttraumatic pneumonia based on early anatomic and physiologic parameters. *J Trauma.* 2003;54(4):724–9.

176. Urra X, Obach V, Chamorro A. Stroke induced immunodepression syndrome: from bench to bedside. *Curr Mol Med.* 2009;9(2):195–202.

177. Dirnagl U, Klehmet J, Braun JS, Harms H, Meisel C, Ziemssen T, *et al.* Stroke-induced immunodepression: experimental evidence and clinical relevance. *Stroke.* 2007;38(2 Suppl):770–3.

178. Prass K, Meisel C, Hoflich C, Braun J, Halle E, Wolf T, *et al.* Stroke-induced immunodeficiency promotes spontaneous bacterial infections and is mediated by sympathetic activation reversal by poststroke T helper cell type 1-like immunostimulation. *J Exp Med.* 2003;198(5):725–36.

179. Chamorro A, Amaro S, Vargas M, Obach V, Cervera A, Torres F, *et al.* Interleukin 10, monocytes and increased risk of early infection in ischaemic stroke. *J Neurol Neurosurg Psychiatry.* 2006;77(11):1279–81.

180. Harrison-Felix C, Whiteneck G, Devivo MJ, Hammond FM, Jha A. Causes of death following 1 year postinjury among individuals with traumatic brain injury. *J Head Trauma Rehabil.* 2006;21(1):22–33.

181. Wong CH, Jenne CN, Lee WY, Leger C, Kubes P. Functional innervation of hepatic iNKT cells is immunosuppressive following stroke. *Science.* 2011;334(6052):101–5.

182. Sirvent JM, Torres A, El-Ebiary M, Castro P, de Batlle J, Bonet A. Protective effect of intravenously administered cefuroxime against nosocomial pneumonia in patients with structural coma. *Am J Respir Crit Care Med.* 1997;155(5):1729–34.

183. Ewig S, Torres A, El-Ebiary M, Fabregas N, Hernandez C, Gonzalez J, *et al.* Bacterial colonization patterns in mechanically ventilated patients with traumatic and medical head injury. Incidence, risk factors, and association with ventilator-associated pneumonia. *Am J Respir Crit Care Med.* 1999;159(1):188–98.

184. Harms H, Prass K, Meisel C, Klehmet J, Rogge W, Drenckhahn C, *et al.* Preventive antibacterial therapy in acute ischemic stroke: a randomized controlled trial. *PLoS One.* 2008;3(5):e2158.

185. Bronchard R, Albaladejo P, Brezac G, Geffroy A, Seince PF, Morris W, *et al.* Early onset pneumonia: risk factors and consequences in head trauma patients. *Anesthesiology.* 2004;100(2):234–9.

186. Campbell W, Hendrix E, Schwalbe R, Fattom A, Edelman R. Head-injured patients who are nasal carriers of Staphylococcus aureus are at high risk for Staphylococcus aureus pneumonia. *Crit Care Med.* 1999;27(4):798–801.

187. Laupland KB, Conly JM. Treatment of Staphylococcus aureus colonization and prophylaxis for infection with topical intranasal mupirocin: an evidence-based review. *Clin Infect Dis.* 2003;37(7):933–8.

188. Daneman N, Sarwar S, Fowler RA, Cuthbertson BH; on behalf of the SuDDICU Canadian Study Group. Effect of selective decontamination on antimicrobial resistance in intensive care units: a systematic review and meta-analysis. *Lancet Infect Dis.* 2013;13(4):328–41.

189. Pileggi C, Bianco A, Flotta D, Nobile CGA, Pavia M. Prevention of ventilator-associated pneumonia, mortality and all intensive care unit acquired infections by topically applied antimicrobial or antiseptic agents: a meta-analysis of randomized controlled trials in intensive care units. *Crit Care.* 2011;15:R155.

190. D'Amico R, Pifferi S, Torri V, Brazzi L, Parmelli E, Liberati A. Antimicrobial prophylaxis to reduce respiratory tract infections and mortality in adults receiving intensive care. *Cochrane Database Syst Rev.* 2009;4:CD000022.

191. van Essen EH, de Jonge E. Selective decontamination of the digestive tract (SDD): is the game worth the candle? *Semin Respir Crit Care Med.* 2011;32(2):236–42.

192. Nguyen NQ, Ng MP, Chapman M, Fraser RJ, Holloway RH. The impact of admission diagnosis on gastric emptying in critically ill patients. *Crit Care.* 2007;11(1):R16.

193. Kao CH, ChangLai SP, Chieng PU, Yen TC. Gastric emptying in head-injured patients. *Am J Gastroenterol.* 1998;93(7):1108–12.

194. McArthur CJ, Gin T, McLaren IM, Critchley JA, Oh TE. Gastric emptying following brain injury: effects of choice of sedation and intracranial pressure. *Intensive Care Med.* 1995;21(7):573–6.

195. Marik PE, Zaloga GP. Gastric versus post-pyloric feeding: a systematic review. *Crit Care.* 2003;7(3):R46–51.

196. Ho KM, Dobb GJ, Webb SA. A comparison of early gastric and post-pyloric feeding in critically ill patients: a meta-analysis. *Intensive Care Med.* 2006;32(5):639–49.

197. Acosta-Escribano J, Fernandez-Vivas M, Grau Carmona T, Caturla-Such J, Garcia-Martinez M, Menendez-Mainer A, *et al.* Gastric versus transpyloric feeding in severe traumatic brain injury: a prospective, randomized trial. *Intensive Care Med.* 2010;36(9):1532–9.

CHAPTER 28

Electrolyte and endocrine disturbances

Adikarige Haritha Dulanka Silva,
Antonio Belli, and Martin Smith

Metabolic and acute phase responses are evolutionary mechanisms that serve to preserve organ and tissue perfusion, maintain cellular homeostasis, prevent secondary tissue damage, and couple the delivery of substrates and oxygen with metabolic demand in response to stress. They include acute phase inflammation, and vascular endothelial, sympathetic nervous system, and hormonal/endocrine responses. Acute brain injury (ABI) triggers a complex cascade of stress responses involving metabolic and neurohumoral mechanisms that lead to a variety of derangements in electrolyte and endocrine homeostasis. The resultant clinical picture is a rapidly evolving interplay between failed homeostatic mechanisms, physiological compensatory responses, and intracranial and systemic (non-neurological) complications. A knowledge-based approach to the early identification, timely evaluation, and effective management of metabolic and endocrine derangements is required to normalize and maintain physiological homeostasis and improve patient outcome after ABI.

This chapter will review the pathophysiology, treatment, and outcome effects of important electrolyte and endocrine abnormalities encountered in critically ill neurological patients. For details of the management of chronic and acute electrolyte and endocrine problems generally, the reader is referred elsewhere (1).

Glucose

Hyperglycaemia is common in critically ill patients and may be related to pre-existing diabetes mellitus or the metabolic response to stress. There is a particularly high prevalence of hyperglycaemia after ABI and this is associated with increased morbidity and mortality (2). It is uncertain whether it is hyperglycaemia per se that is responsible for the adverse outcome effects or whether high blood glucose is simply a marker of hormonal and inflammatory dysregulation reflecting the severity of the underlying brain injury (3). Fluctuations in blood glucose concentrations, particularly rapid reductions, may trigger adverse events beyond those related to hyperglycaemia (4,5). Similarly, hypoglycaemia can lead to significant neurological damage and this is a particular concern in the already injured brain (2) in which it causes characteristic neuronal injuries (6,7). Glycaemic control is crucially important during neurocritical care, although actual blood glucose targets are not clearly defined (2).

Management of glucose within pre-specified limits requires frequent and accurate measurement of blood glucose levels to guide therapy and allow prompt recognition of hyper- or hypoglycaemia. Blood glucose values vary with measurement technique, although point-of-care testing (POCT) is the only practical method given the frequency at which samples must be analysed on the neurocritical care unit (NCCU). Modern POCT devices correlate well with laboratory measurements in stable patients (8). Importantly, the same method of measurement should be used to guide glucose management in an individual patient.

Glycaemic control in general critical care

Multiple studies have evaluated the efficacy and safety of glycaemic control with intensive insulin therapy (ITT) in critically ill patients. Early enthusiasm for tight control of blood glucose followed a study published by van den Berge and colleagues in 2001 that demonstrated outcome benefits of ITT to maintain blood glucose between 4.4 and 6.1 mmol/L in 1548 patients admitted to a surgical intensive care unit (ICU) (9). Compared to standard therapy, ITT was associated with a reduction in mortality and decreased incidence of bloodstream infections, acute kidney injury requiring renal replacement therapy, or duration of mechanical ventilation. However, the more recent Normoglycaemia in Intensive Care Evaluation Survival Using Glucose Algorithm (NICE-SUGAR) study came to very different conclusions (10). This large and well-designed study randomized more than 6000 adults requiring treatment on the ICU for at least 3 days to intensive glucose control with IIT (to maintain blood glucose between 4.5 mmol/L and 6.0 mmol/L) or conventional glycaemic control with a glucose target of 10.0 mmol/L or lower. There was a significantly higher 90 day mortality rate in the intensive compared to conventional treatment group (27.5% versus 24.9% respectively, odds ratio (OR) 1.14), and no difference in ICU or hospital length of stay (LOS), duration of mechanical ventilation, or need for renal replacement therapy. Furthermore, severe hypoglycaemia (defined as blood glucose $\leq$ 2.2 mmol/L) occurred much more frequently in patients receiving intensive compared to conventional insulin therapy (6.8% and 0.5% respectively). Subsequent meta-analyses have confirmed a lack of mortality benefit from tight glycaemic control in critical illness, and a high incidence of ITT-related hypoglycaemia is a common theme in all studies (11–13).

Glycaemic control in critically ill neurological patients

Brain metabolism is highly dependent on a constant supply of glucose. Patients with ABI have a heightened susceptibility to hypo- and hyperglycaemia, which are both associated with worse outcome (see Chapter 2).

The deleterious effects of hyperglycaemia on the injured brain are many. Oxidative stress provoked by increased free radical formation and impaired scavenging leads to lipid peroxidation, protein carbonylation, and DNA damage (14). Neutralization of nitric oxide by superoxide and subsequent impairment of vasodilatory mechanisms results in cerebral microcirculatory dysfunction, and inflammatory responses cause destabilization of the blood–brain barrier (BBB) and increase the risk of cerebral oedema. Hyperglycaemia may also result in the development of intracellular acidosis from anaerobic glycolysis and production of lactate, which in turn leads to mitochondrial dysfunction and cellular energy crisis (15). Hyperglycaemia is associated with adverse outcomes in a variety of conditions including traumatic brain injury (TBI) (16,17), aneurysmal subarachnoid haemorrhage (SAH) (18,19), intracerebral haemorrhage (ICH) (20,21), and acute ischaemic stroke (AIS) (22,23).

Hypoglycaemia is also detrimental to the injured brain (see Chapter 2). The brain has limited reserves to protect itself against low glucose concentration and, when these are exhausted, energy failure supervenes leading to glutamate-mediated excitotoxicity, oxygen free radical overload, and activation of apoptotic pathways (24). Even modest systemic hypoglycaemia can lead to low brain glucose levels after ABI (4). A recent microdialysis study has demonstrated that cerebral glucose delivery may become limited when oxidative metabolism is impaired and that brain glucose concentrations might fall below critical thresholds even when systemic glucose is within a generally accepted 'normal' range (25). Amongst its many adverse effects, cerebral hypoglycaemia may precipitate spreading depolarizations which further deplete local glucose levels resulting in a vicious cycle of worsening brain damage (26).

There is substantial interest in the management of blood glucose after ABI because of the adverse effects of both hyper- and hypoglycaemia. A recent study compared IIT (target blood glucose 4.4–6.1 mmol/L) with conventional insulin treatment (to maintain blood glucose < 8.4 mmol/L) in a cohort of 81 critically ill patients with stroke and TBI (27). There was no difference in mortality, ICU or hospital LOS, or neurological outcome between the two groups, although episodes of hypoglycaemia (blood glucose concentration < 3.3 mmol/L) and severe hypoglycaemia (blood glucose < 2.2 mmol/L) were more frequent in the IIT group. However, other studies have demonstrated a significant association between IIT and increased mortality in critically ill neurological patients (28). A recent meta-analysis has confirmed the increased risk of hypoglycaemia and poor outcome with IIT but also demonstrated that very loose control, allowing high blood glucose concentrations, is similarly detrimental (12). Intermediate level control, maintaining blood glucose levels between 7.0 and 10.0 mmol/L and avoiding large swings in glucose concentration, appears to be optimal after ABI.

Traumatic brain injury

The adverse effects of high blood glucose on neurological outcome after human TBI have been recognized for decades (16). More recent studies have confirmed that even relatively modest early hyperglycaemia (> 9.4 mmol/L) is associated with adverse outcome (29,30).

In a subgroup analysis of 63 patients with isolated brain injury in the original van den Berg study, IIT was associated with lower mean and maximal intracranial pressure, an eightfold reduction in vasopressor requirements to maintain adequate cerebral perfusion pressure, a significant reduction in seizures, shorter ICU LOS, and a trend towards improved long-term outcomes (31). However, early enthusiasm for tight glycaemic control after brain injury waned as subsequent studies reached very different conclusions. A randomized study in 97 patients with severe TBI compared IIT (target glucose concentrations 4.4–6.7 mmol/L) with conventional insulin therapy administered only when glucose concentration exceeded 12.2 mmol/L, and found no benefit from IIT on mortality or functional outcome in survivors (32). As in other studies, episodes of hypoglycaemia (defined as blood glucose concentration < 4.4 mmol/L) were significantly higher in patients receiving IIT compared to conventional therapy—the median (range) number of hypoglycaemic episodes was 15 (6–33) and 7 (0–11) in the ITT and conventional groups respectively. IIT can be associated with cerebral hypoglycaemia, energy failure, and metabolic crisis, even in the presence of relatively 'normal' plasma glucose concentration. In one study, cerebral glucose was significantly lower in non-survivors than in survivors, and brain energy crisis (defined as low brain glucose in association with elevated lactate:pyruvate ratio) was associated with significantly increased hospital mortality (4).

Whilst hyperglycaemia should be avoided after severe TBI, further studies are required to confirm the optimal target glucose level being mindful of the absolute need to avoid the deleterious effects of hypoglycaemia. Thus, based on current data, the risks of IIT appear to outweigh any benefits, and moderate level glucose control (between 7.0 and 11.0 mmol/L) is recommended.

Acute ischaemic stroke

A systematic review of 33 studies of AIS reported an 8–63% incidence of admission hyperglycaemia (blood glucose > 6.1 mmol/L) in non-diabetic patients and a 39–83% incidence in diabetics (33). Several studies have shown that admission hyperglycaemia increases short- and long-term mortality after AIS (34,35). In non-diabetics, 30-day mortality is three times higher in those whose admission serum glucose concentration is greater than 7.0 mmol/L (33). Importantly though, it is the persistence of hyperglycaemia beyond the first 4 hours after AIS, and not just admission blood glucose level, that is strongly associated with worse outcome (36,37). Interestingly, the association between hyperglycaemia and poor outcome is stronger in non-diabetic than diabetic patients (34).

Hyperglycaemia is associated with a range of adverse cerebral and systemic effects after AIS including higher rates of infection and post-thrombolysis ICH (38), and attenuation of the benefits of intra-arterial thrombolysis (39). Persisting hyperglycaemia is an independent determinant of infarct volume expansion and worse functional outcome (36). There is also an association between admission hyperglycaemia (blood glucose concentration > 7.8 mmol/L) and worse outcome, including a 25% symptomatic haemorrhagic conversion rate, in patients receiving thrombolytic agents when serum glucose concentration is greater than 11.1 mmol/L (40).

Randomized controlled trials have been inconclusive in terms of identifying outcome benefits of IIT after AIS. The UK Glucose Insulin in Stroke Trial (GIST-UK) randomized 933 patients with admission plasma glucose concentration between 6 and 17 mmol/L presenting within 24 hours of stroke onset to receive either variable-dose glucose-potassium-insulin (GKI) infusions (intervention) or saline (control) (41). GKI infusion titrated to maintain normoglycaemia (capillary glucose 4–7 mmol/L) for 24 hours was not associated with reduced mortality or functional outcome benefits compared to control. However, GKI had a significant blood pressure lowering effect and was associated with an increased incidence of hypoglycaemia, both of which may have offset any potential benefits. Another multicentre randomized pilot trial compared IIT (target glucose < 7.2 mmol/L) with conservative subcutaneous insulin to maintain glucose at less than 11.1 mmol/L continued for 72 hours in 46 AIS patients with mild hyperglycaemia (baseline glucose ≥ 8.3 mmol/L) presenting within 12 hours of stroke onset (42). Outcome was similar in the two groups but 35% (11/31) of patients in the IIT group developed hypoglycaemia (glucose < 3.3 mmol/L), and four of these (13%) had transient associated symptoms including one who developed neurological changes. A recent Cochrane meta-analysis of 11 randomized controlled trials including 1583 patients found no difference in death or final neurological outcome between those receiving IIT to maintain serum glucose between 4.0 and 7.5 mmol/L in the first 24 hours after AIS (n = 791) compared to standard care (n = 792), although the rate of symptomatic hypoglycaemia was substantially higher in the intervention group (OR 14.6) (43).

Meticulous glycaemic control is essential after AIS but the optimal blood glucose target is unknown and varies between guidelines (44). The Stroke Hyperglycaemia Insulin Network Effort (SHINE) randomized, blinded, efficacy trial will recruit 1400 patients to receive either standard sliding scale subcutaneous insulin or continuous intravenous insulin started within 12 hours of stroke symptom onset and continued for at least 72 hours (45). It is hoped that this study will clarify the optimal glycaemic target, method of glycaemic control, and duration of treatment, and quantify the potential risks and benefits of IIT after AIS. In the meantime, the American Stroke Association guidance for initiating glycaemic treatment should be followed (46). This recommends maintaining plasma glucose between 8.0 and 10.0 mmol/L with intravenous insulin infusion whilst avoiding large swings in glucose concentration (46).

Intracerebral haemorrhage

A study of 764 patients noted that both diabetes mellitus and admission hyperglycaemia in non-diabetic patients were predictors of poor outcome after supratentorial ICH (47). An increase in blood glucose concentration of only 1.0 mmol/L has been associated with a 33% increase in early mortality, with a cut-off glucose concentration for optimal outcome prediction of 9.1 mmol/L (21).

Subarachnoid haemorrhage

A 2009 meta-analysis confirmed an association between hyperglycaemia and poor clinical outcome after SAH (48). Hyperglycaemia is independently associated with increased risk of death and disability, and a higher incidence of other early complications including pneumonia, cerebral oedema, and delayed cerebral ischaemia. Further, glucose variability is a significant predictor of cerebral infarction after SAH (49).

Sodium disturbances

Disorders of sodium balance can lead to serious complications and adverse outcomes after ABI. An understanding of the normal physiological control of sodium and water is essential to allow a structured approach to the diagnosis and management of dysnatraemia.

Regulation of sodium and water balance

Sodium is the major extracellular electrolyte, the most osmotically active cation, and the major contributor to plasma osmolality. The control of sodium is inextricably linked with that of water which moves freely in and out of cells along concentration gradients. The body regulates serum sodium concentration within a narrow normal range (135–145 mmol/L) by adjusting the water content of the extracellular fluid via renal mechanisms that control the excretion of water.

Total body water is primarily controlled by renal manipulation of sodium with resulting water adjustment to maintain tonicity (50). The principal regulator of total body water content and plasma osmolality is arginine vasopressin (AVP), also known as antidiuretic hormone (ADH). AVP is a peptide hormone which is synthesized in the supraoptic and paraventricular nuclei of the magnocellular neurons of the hypothalamus. It is stored in the posterior pituitary gland from where it is released in response to various osmotic and non-osmotic stimuli (51). The primary action of AVP is to inhibit renal water excretion by modulation of water re-absorption in the renal tubules and collecting duct, leading to the production of concentrated urine (Figure 28.1). Of three vasopressin receptor subtypes, V_2 receptors in the collecting ducts of the kidney are responsible for the inhibitory effect of AVP on renal water excretion (52). Binding of AVP to V_2 receptors activates adenylate cyclase which leads to increases in intracellular cyclic adenosine monophosphate (cAMP). This in turn stimulates protein kinase A and phosphorylation of aquaporin-2 (AQP-2) channels resulting in reabsorption of free water. Over the ensuing hours, increased AQP-2 expression in the renal collecting ducts further enhances water reabsorption. The V_{1A} AVP receptor subtype is located in vascular smooth muscle and responsible for the vasoconstrictive effects of AVP.

Total body sodium is controlled by renal excretion. Sodium is freely filtered at the glomerulus with the majority being reabsorbed at the proximal tubule under the control of sympathetic nerves and atrial (ANP) and brain (BNP) natriuretic peptides (53). BNP causes natriuresis by several mechanisms including inhibition of sodium transport in the medullary collecting duct, increased glomerular filtration rate and inhibition of renin and aldosterone release. Two other peptides, C- and D-type natriuretic peptides, are also implicated in sodium regulation (54). The central effects of natriuretic peptides include reduction of sympathetic outflow from the brainstem and inhibition of thirst and salt appetite.

Like sodium, plasma osmolality is also normally maintained within a narrow range (285–295 mOsm/kg) primarily via osmoreceptors in the hypothalamus that control AVP synthesis and release. AVP is released when serum osmolality rises above 280 mOsm/kg and this leads to reduced renal water excretion, production of more concentrated urine, and increased plasma osmolality (55). At 295 mOsm/kg thirst prompts increased water intake in conscious patients. AVP release is suppressed when serum osmolality falls below 280 mOsm/kg. The osmotic mechanisms controlling body

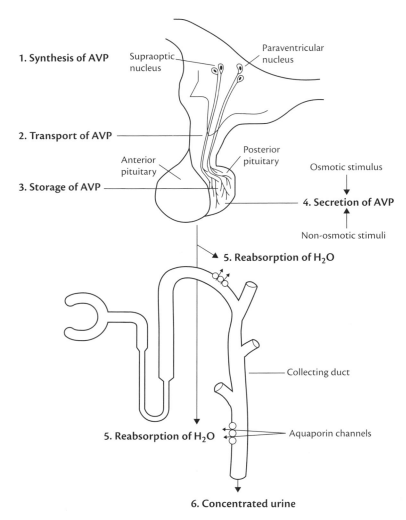

Fig. 28.1 The role of arginine vasopressin (AVP) in the regulation of water and sodium balance.
1. Synthesis of AVP in paraventricular and supraoptic nuclei of the hypothalamus.
2. Transport of AVP via neurophysin carrier proteins along the axons.
3. Storage of AVP in posterior pituitary (neurohypophysis).
4. Secretion of AVP in response to osmotic (e.g. increased plasma osmolality) or non-osmotic (e.g. decreased arterial blood pressure, pain, and nausea) stimuli.
5. Binding of AVP to V_2 receptors in the basolateral membrane of renal collecting duct cells results in the translocation of aquaporin channels from intracellular vesicles to the apical plasma membrane, which leads to water permeability and water reabsorption.
6. Formation of concentrated urine.
Reproduced from Bhardwaj A, 'Neurological impact of vasopressin dysregulation and hyponatremia', *Annals of Neurology*, 2006, 59, pp. 229–236.

water content are exquisitely sensitive, and changes in plasma osmolality as small as 1% result in changes in AVP levels (55). AVP is also released in response to reductions in blood pressure and intravascular volume that are detected by low pressure baroreceptors in the right atrium and great veins, and high pressure baroreceptors in the carotid sinus. Unlike the high sensitivity of osmoreceptors, baroreceptors require changes in pressure or volume greater than 10% to trigger AVP release (55). Hypovolaemia and hypotension also result in increased sympathetic activity and activation of the renin–angiotensin–aldosterone (RAA) axis. Aldosterone is a mineralocorticoid which promotes sodium and water retention at the distal convoluted tubule, as well as being a potent vasoconstrictor.

Given that sodium and water balance are intricately linked, derangements of sodium are usually associated with derangements of water and vice versa. Thus, reduced plasma sodium concentration (hyponatraemia) can be related to water excess or sodium (and secondarily water) depletion, and increased plasma sodium concentration (hypernatraemia) to water depletion or sodium excess.

Hyponatraemia

Hyponatraemia is arbitrarily defined as plasma sodium concentration lower than 135 mmol/L although the clinically significant level of hyponatraemia varies (see later) (56). Hyponatraemia is the most common electrolyte abnormality in the general hospital population and particularly so in critically ill brain-injured patients (54). Hypotonic (dilutional) hyponatraemia is the most common type, especially in patients with central nervous system (CNS) disorders, although hypertonic and isotonic hyponatraemia can occur (57). Hypotonic hyponatraemia is usually associated with low plasma osmolality (54).

Table 28.1 Common causes of hypotonic hyponatraemia

Hypovolaemic hyponatraemia	Normovolaemic hyponatraemia	Hypervolaemic hyponatraemia
CSWS	SIADH:	SIADH
	◆ TBI	
	◆ SAH	
	◆ CNS infection	
	◆ brain tumours	
	◆ drug induced	
	◆ pulmonary pathology	
Diuretics (including osmotic)	Thiazide diuretics	Congestive cardiac failure
Ketonuria	Adrenal insufficiency	Nephrotic syndrome
Diarrhoea/vomiting	Hypothyroidism	Cirrhosis
Sweating	Iatrogenic	Acute kidney injury
Blood loss		Iatrogenic
Adrenal insufficiency		

CNS, central nervous system; CSW, cerebral salt wasting; SAH, subarachnoid haemorrhage; SIADH, syndrome of inappropriate antidiuretic hormone; TBI, traumatic brain injury.

The water retention that leads to hypotonic hyponatraemia is most commonly related to impaired water excretion, although excessive intake may occur in conditions such as in psychogenic polydipsia. Hypotonic hyponatraemia occurs in a number of conditions (Table 28.1) but after ABI is most often related to the syndrome of inappropriate ADH secretion (SIADH) or cerebral salt wasting (CSW) (57–59). Iatrogenic hyponatraemia may be related to inappropriate administration of hypotonic fluids, often in the postoperative period when AVP levels are raised as part of the stress response to surgery (60).

Symptoms and signs of hyponatraemia

In most cases hyponatraemia is associated with hypotonicity and this creates an osmotic gradient across the BBB promoting entry of water into the brain and the development of cerebral oedema (61,62). The symptoms and signs of hyponatraemia are therefore primarily neurological (Table 28.2) and related to both the absolute serum sodium concentration and its rate of reduction (63). In general terms, patients are usually asymptomatic until serum sodium is reduced below 125 mmol/L, although acute onset hyponatraemia (< 48 hours) can be associated with significant symptoms and morbidity at higher serum sodium levels.

Table 28.2 Symptoms and signs of hyponatraemia

Moderate hyponatraemia (serum sodium 120–125 mmol/L)	Severe or rapid onset hyponatraemia (serum sodium < 115 mmol/L or onset < 48 h)
Headache	Drowsiness/confusion
Confusion	Depressed reflexes
Lethargy	Seizures
Irritability/agitation	Coma
Nausea/vomiting	Brainstem herniation
Muscle weakness/cramps	Death

Effects of hyponatraemia on the brain

If hyponatraemia develops slowly, adaptive mechanisms aimed at reducing brain volume minimize cerebral oedema and the risk of neurological sequelae even if serum sodium falls to very low levels (54,64). This adaptive process is known as regulatory volume reserve and has two phases (51,65). In the first few hours after the onset of acute hyponatraemia, sodium, chloride, and potassium ions are lost from cells leading to associated extracellular outflow of water (63,65). A second, adaptive, phase comes into play after 48 hours. Osmolytes such as myoinositol are generated within neurons and, as they leave the cells, water follows allowing cellular volume to return to normal and cerebral oedema to resolve despite the ongoing hypotonic state (50). During correction of hyponatraemia this process is reversed and the organic osmolytes must re-enter neurons to allow water to follow. If this process occurs too rapidly, dehydration of the brain may occur because electrolytes and organic osmolytes are not present in sufficient concentration, nor can they be reintroduced into brain cells sufficiently rapidly (66). This can lead to central pontine and extra-pontine myelinolysis which are often fatal demyelinating syndromes characterized by lethargy, pseudobulbar palsy (e.g. dysphagia, dysarthria), and quadriparesis (67–69).

If hyponatraemia is corrected early (< 48 hours), the risk of treatment-related complications is low. However, once the brain's adaptive responses are in place the risk of myelinolysis during rapid changes in serum sodium concentration is greatly increased. Thus, whilst untreated hyponatraemia can lead to cerebral oedema and severe neurological complications, including permanent neurological damage or death (57,65), there is a risk of myelinolysis if serum sodium is corrected excessively or too quickly (68,69).

Diagnosis

True hyponatraemia is diagnosed by low serum sodium concentration in the presence of low serum osmolality after exclusion of 'pseudo-' or artefactual hyponatraemia. In pseudohyponatraemia, a spuriously low sodium concentration is measured because of increases in the non-aqueous components of plasma, such as that associated with hypertriglyceridaemia or hyperproteinaemia (when serum osmolality is normal), or because of hyperosmolality secondary to severe hyperglycaemia (70).

Figure 28.2 provides a schema to guide clinicians in the investigation of hyponatraemia. This requires a structured assessment of both clinical and biochemical parameters, which can also be used when assessing the response to treatment.

An important issue to consider in causation and assessment of hyponatraemia in patients with ABI is excessive administration of salt containing intravenous fluids. This affects blood and extracellular volumes and makes the presentation of a 'classic' SIADH or CSW picture less likely (71). It also drives salt loss through activation of natriuretic peptides, suppression of aldosterone, and involution of renal tubular membrane sodium transporting receptors (72).

General principles of the treatment of hyponatraemia

The need for treatment of hyponatraemia, and the rapidity of its correction, depends on the presence or absence of neurological symptoms or signs, the chronicity of the hyponatraemia, its rate of development, and associated volume status (59,73). Although various treatment guidelines have been published, there is no evidence-based consensus on the management of hyponatraemia (74). Sodium

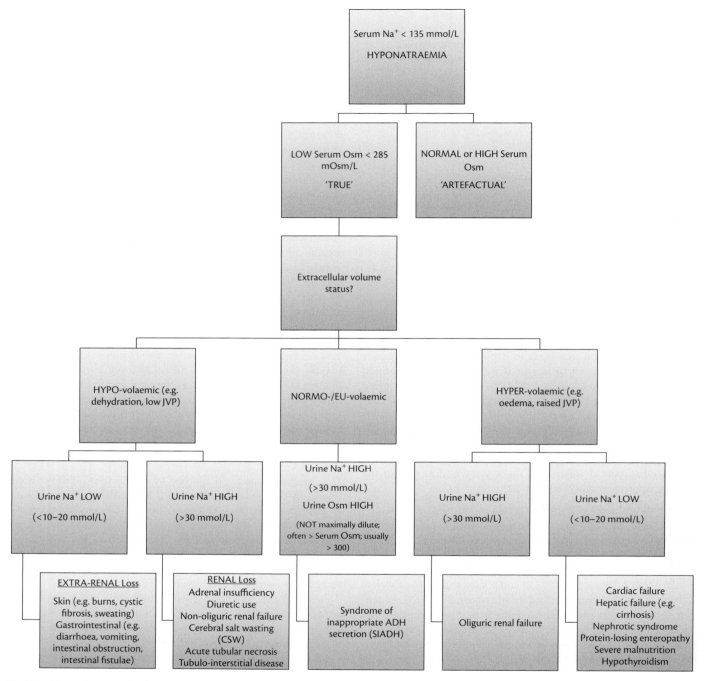

Fig. 28.2 Diagnostic approach to hyponatraemia.
ADH, antidiuretic hormone; JVP, jugular venous pressure.

disturbances are often transient and self-limiting after ABI so an expectant and supportive treatment strategy is appropriate in asymptomatic patients unless the sodium concentration is very low. Prompt treatment is essential in acute symptomatic hyponatraemia, whereas chronic hyponatraemia rarely requires rapid correction.

When treatment is required, serum sodium concentration should generally be increased by no more than 0.5 mmol/L/h or 8–10 mmol/L/day (56), although in symptomatic patients, including those with seizures or acute cerebral oedema, a 1.5–2.0 mmol/L/h increase for 2–4 hours may be appropriate (59,69,75). These recommendations are based on data from case series rather than

randomized trials, but are widely accepted (63). Treatment of hyponatraemia should be targeted to the point of alleviation of symptoms rather than to an arbitrary serum sodium value, and should be monitored and managed in a NCCU to minimize the risk of over-rapid sodium correction (59).

Hyponatraemia in critically ill neurological patients

Hyponatraemia is common in patients with TBI, SAH, and intracranial infection (57), and is also associated with certain antiepileptic drugs including carbamazepine (76), valproate, and lamotrigine (77). Hyponatraemia is associated with increased mortality and morbidity in all brain injury types (56), and with higher rates of delayed cerebral ischaemia (78) and worse functional outcome after SAH (79).

SIADH and CSWS are common causes of hyponatraemia after ABI and both are characterized by hypotonic hyponatraemia and inappropriately high urine sodium concentration (54). It can be difficult to differentiate between them but it is crucial to make the distinction because their management is very different (59,80). SIADH is a dilutional hyponatraemia associated with a hyper- or normovolaemic state, whereas CSW is a volume-deplete (hypovolaemic) condition (59,65). Assessment of intravascular and extracellular volume status is key to the differentiation of SIADH and CSW as clinical and laboratory criteria cannot reliably distinguish between them (Table 28.3) (81) Although it is important to make the correct diagnosis so that appropriate treatment can be applied, the two syndromes may coexist (73).

Syndrome of inappropriate antidiuretic hormone secretion

SIADH was first described in two patients with bronchogenic carcinoma in whom a physiological stimulus for the release of AVP was lacking, and the level of secretion of AVP therefore deemed 'inappropriate' (82). Early reports suggested that release of AVP in SIADH was independent of plasma osmolality although this appears to be the case in only about one-third of patients who fulfil standard diagnostic criteria for SIADH (83). In others, AVP secretion is fully suppressed leading to dilute urine at a serum sodium concentration which is lower than normal and, less commonly, plasma AVP levels can be low or undetectable even in the presence of hyponatraemia (84). Because not all patients with SIADH have elevated circulating levels of AVP, the term syndrome of inappropriate antidiuresis (SIAD) has been proposed as a more accurate descriptor (84). However, in critically ill brain-injured patients, the most common cause of SIAD is 'inappropriate' secretion of AVP, so the term SIADH continues to be used.

Although its exact pathophysiology is not fully understood, SIADH is characterized by release of AVP in the absence of elevated plasma osmolality or non-osmotic stimuli (54). It is the most common cause of dilutional hyponatraemia and associated with a variety of disease states and drug therapy. In the NCCU, SIADH is most commonly encountered in patients with TBI, SAH, brain tumours, and intracranial infections (54,57). Certain drugs can also induce

Table 28.3 Differentiating between the syndrome of inappropriate antidiuretic hormone secretion and cerebral salt wasting

	SIADH	CSW
Serum sodium concentration	Low	Low
Serum osmolality	Decreased	Normal or increased
Volume status	Normo- or euvolaemia	Hypovolaemia
Urine sodium concentration	High (> 25 mmol/L)	Very high (> 40 mmol/L)
Urine osmolality	High	High or normal
Haematocrit	Normal	High

CSW, cerebral salt wasting syndrome; SIADH, syndrome of inappropriate antidiuretic hormone secretion.

Table 28.4 Drugs associated with the syndrome of inappropriate hormone secretion

Diuretics	Thiazides
	Indapamide
Anticonvulsants	Carbamazepine
	Valproate
	Oxcarbazepine
Antidepressants	Selective serotonin release inhibitors
	Serotonin–norepinephrine reuptake inhibitors
	Tricyclics
Antipsychotics	Phenothiazines
	Butyrophenones
Vasopressin (V_2) agonists	Desmopressin
	Vasopressin
Cancer chemotherapy	Vincristine
	Cyclophosphamide
Miscellaneous	Non-steroidal anti-inflammatory agents
	Methylenedioxymethyl-amphetamine (ecstasy)

release of AVP (Table 28.4), as can physiological stimuli, such as pain, nausea, hypovolaemia, and stress.

Diagnosis
Key to the diagnosis of SIADH is the presence of hypotonic hyponatraemia and impaired urinary dilution in the absence of renal disease or a non-osmotic stimulus for AVP release. Although patients with SIADH exist in a water-expanded state, they may not display signs of intravascular volume expansion because two-thirds of the total retained water remains in the intracellular compartment.

The diagnostic criteria of SIADH are (51,85):

- hypo-osmolar hyponatraemia (serum osmolality < 280 mmol/kg and serum sodium < 135 mmol/L)
- continued renal excretion of sodium leading to 'inappropriately' high urine sodium concentration
- 'inappropriate' urine osmolality (i.e. less than maximally diluted)
- absence of clinical evidence of volume depletion
- normal adrenal and renal function.

Whilst these criteria are widely accepted, they are not universally reliable in distinguishing between SIADH and CSW (56,86).

Treatment
As with other forms of hypotonic hyponatraemia, the most important factors directing the management of SIADH are the severity of the hyponatraemia, its duration, and presence or absence of symptoms (84). Since SIADH is often a self-limiting disease after ABI, treatment should be initiated only if the patient is symptomatic or the serum sodium concentration significantly low or falling rapidly. Any precipitating aetiological factor should be identified and treated.

Electrolyte-free water restriction, initially to 800–1000 mL/day, forms the mainstay of treatment of SIADH and usually results in a slow rise in serum sodium of 1.5 mmol/L/day (57). However, free water restriction is contraindicated in many critically ill brain-injured patients as it may worsen cardiovascular instability and increase the risk of cerebral ischaemia. Infusion of hypertonic saline (1.8% or 3%) is indicated in symptomatic acute hyponatraemia or after SAH when fluid restriction is contraindicated. Hypertonic saline infusion should be discontinued when serum sodium reaches 120–125 mmol/L. Enteral salt tablets via a nasogastric tube is an alternative method of sodium replacement in some patients.

Pharmacological treatment is an option when the diagnosis of SIADH is certain and unresponsive to first-line treatments. Demeclocycline (150–300 mg twice daily) inhibits the action of AVP at the renal collecting duct by impairing the generation and action of cyclic adenosine monophosphate. Vasopressin-receptor antagonists, also called vaptans, inhibit the binding of AVP at V_2 receptors in the renal collecting ducts thereby inducing aquaresis, the electrolyte-sparing excretion of free water (50). Vasopressin-receptor antagonists such as conivaptan have been successfully used in the treatment of euvolaemic or hypervolaemic hyponatraemia, although experience in critically ill neurological patients is limited (87). However, recent case series have suggested that vaptans might be a safe and effective alternative to other therapies in selected neurological patients with refractory hyponatraemia (50,88).

Cerebral salt wasting

CSW is a hypovolaemic hyponatraemia caused by a primary natriuresis and associated water loss in patients with any brain injury type, although it is seen most commonly after SAH. The aetiology of CSW is incompletely understood but likely related to the presence of circulating natriuretic factors, such as ANP and BNP, and/or a decreased sympathetic input to the kidney (65).

Treatment

The management of CSW involves correction of precipitating factors and volume repletion initially with 0.9% saline. Hypertonic saline solutions are often required and always indicated in severe hyponatraemia in the presence of neurological symptoms. Fludrocortisone, a synthetic adrenocortical steroid with mineralocorticoid properties which limits sodium loss by increasing its re-absorption from the renal tubule, has been used to reduce sodium and water loss in CSW (51). Fluid restriction is inappropriate since it will worsen the hypovolaemic state of CSW (59). Vasopressin receptor antagonists are contraindicated in hypovolaemic hyponatraemia as they can lead to further volume depletion (89).

Hypernatraemia

Hypernatraemia is arbitrarily defined as serum sodium concentration greater than 145 mmol/L and is associated with hypertonic hyperosmolality. It can result from insufficient water intake, hypotonic fluid loss, or solute excess (90). Hypotonic fluid losses in the critically ill can occur secondary to central diabetes insipidus (DI), nephrogenic DI, osmotic diuresis, diuretic drugs, or the diuretic phase of acute kidney injury. In addition, hypotonic fluids may be lost during vomiting, diarrhoea, nasogastric suction, sweating, burns, and hyperventilation. Iatrogenic solute excess resulting from overzealous infusion of sodium chloride or bicarbonate must also be considered in the differential diagnosis of hypernatraemia. The causes of hypernatraemia are shown in Box 28.1.

> **Box 28.1** Causes of hypernatraemia
>
> **Free water depletion (decreased extracellular fluid volume)**
>
> - Renal water loss:
>   - diabetes insipidus (central or nephrogenic)
>   - osmotic diuresis
>   - diuretic drugs
> - Extrarenal water loss:
>   - respiratory tract (e.g. hyperventilation)
>   - gastrointestinal tract (e.g. vomiting, diarrhoea, nasogastric aspiration)
>   - skin (e.g. fever, burns)
> - Reduced water intake/poor thirst.
>
> **Sodium excess**
>
> - Iatrogenic—administration of sodium containing fluids
> - Mineralocorticoid excess:
>   - primary hyperaldosteronism (Conn's syndrome)
>   - Cushing's syndrome (glucocorticoids have some mineralocorticoid activity)
>   - secondary hyperaldosteronism (relative renal hypoperfusion stimulates renin–angiotensin–aldosterone axis)
>   – cardiac failure
>   – hepatic failure
>   – renal failure
>   - exogenous.

Clinical features

The symptoms of hypernatraemia include thirst, lethargy, irritability, restlessness, muscle weakness, and confusion, although they do not usually manifest in adults until serum sodium concentration rises above 160 mmol/L (50). In cases of severe hypernatraemia, ataxia, seizures, coma, and death can supervene. Rupture of cerebral veins secondary to brain shrinkage may also occur.

Diagnosis

Clinical examination allows differentiation between hypovolaemic hypernatraemia occurring secondary to water loss (e.g. due to dehydration or central DI) and the rarer normo- or hypervolaemic types that are related to excess sodium intake. It is then necessary to differentiate between simple dehydration and central DI on the basis of urine output which is low in dehydration (in the absence of renal failure) and high in DI.

General principles of the treatment of hypernatraemia

The general management of hypernatraemia involves correction of aetiological factors and, if the primary deficit is free water depletion, replenishment with enteral water or relatively hypotonic intravenous fluids. If excessive volumes of hypotonic intravenous fluids are used, or the hypernatraemia is corrected too rapidly, acute cerebral oedema can develop (91). Cautious rehydration with 0.9% saline to correct the volume depletion usually leads to correction of the plasma sodium concentration.

Central diabetes insipidus

In the NCCU, hypernatraemia is most often related to water depletion secondary to central DI. This is a pathological syndrome associated with excessive solute free water excretion as a result of failure of AVP homeostasis. It is characterized by loss of urinary concentrating ability and consequent polyuria, dehydration, hypernatraemia, and serum hyperosmolality. Central DI is related to dysfunction of the hypothalamic-pituitary–adrenal (HPA) axis with failure of production of AVP. It is most commonly associated with severe TBI, pituitary surgery or apoplexy, or brain death. Severe hypernatraemia secondary to central DI is an independent risk factor for poor outcome and associated with an extremely high rate of death in patients with TBI (92).

Nephrogenic DI is caused by insensitivity of renal system to the effects of AVP because of genetic, metabolic, and drug-induced causes, and will not be considered further here.

Diagnosis

In conscious patients, the classic symptoms of polyuria, polydipsia, and thirst make the diagnosis of DI straightforward, although in brain-injured patients thirst is often an unreliable or absent sign. Hyperglycaemia has similar symptomatology and should be excluded as should other causes of high urine volume including excess fluid administration or the use of osmotic diuretics and hypertonic saline.

A pragmatic approach to the diagnosis of central DI is usually taken. The diagnosis is confirmed in the appropriate clinical context with supportive evidence from the following parameters (59):

- hypernatraemia (> 145 mmol/L)
- increased plasma osmolality (> 305 mmol/kg)
- polyuria (> 3 L/day)
- polydipsia in awake patients
- inappropriately dilute urine (< 350 mmoL/kg).

A urine specific gravity (SG) less than 1.005 in the setting of increasing serum sodium suggests DI and is a useful bedside test pending the results of definitive investigations (59). In severe cases of central DI it is reasonable to start treatment based on high urine volumes, low urine SG, and high serum sodium concentration without waiting for the results of formal tests.

Treatment

The underlying cause of central DI should be identified and treated where possible, but the priority is to correct the hyperosmolar state by restoration of intravascular volume over 24–48 hours (91). In conscious patients with intact thirst mechanisms and tolerance of enteral replacement, free access to oral water intake guided by thirst is usually sufficient to replace the water deficit in mild central DI. In unconscious patients, enteral (nasogastric tube) or intravenous fluid replacement is necessary but this should be carefully monitored to avoid over-rapid correction of serum sodium concentration which should not be reduced by more than 1–2 mmol/L/h or 10–12 mmol/L/day (59).

In patients with severe DI and large urinary losses, or those unable to drink, administration of 1-deamino-8-D-arginine vasopressin (DDAVP), a two-amino acid substitute of AVP also called

desmopressin, may be required. In the acute setting it is usually given intravenously (preferred) or subcutaneously in doses of 0.4–1.0 mcg. Small doses, repeated as necessary, can be titrated to the desired clinical effect (59). Intranasal and oral forms of DDAVP can be used in the non-acute setting for patients who require chronic replacement.

The polyuria of central DI may lead to other electrolyte derangements, particularly hypokalaemia, hypomagnesaemia, and hypophosphataemia.

Other electrolyte disturbances

While the most common electrolyte disturbances encountered in the NCCU involve sodium and water balance, other abnormalities do occur. These include disturbances of potassium, calcium, magnesium, and phosphate. The aetiology is usually multifactorial and related to ABI, systemic dysregulation because of multiorgan failure, and iatrogenic causes such as administration of incorrect electrolyte concentrations or fluid volumes. Early identification and management is critical as disorders of potassium, calcium, and magnesium may cause cardiovascular and neurological complications, while phosphate abnormalities affect conscious level and may precipitate diffuse neuromuscular weakness. The reader is referred elsewhere for a comprehensive review of electrolyte abnormalities in the critically ill (93) and their neurological consequences (94).

Endocrine disturbances

Almost any endocrine complication can occur in critically ill patients but thyroid, mineralocorticoid, and glucocorticoid hormone dysfunction are the most clinically relevant in the acute phase after ABI (95). Hormone dysfunction in the NCCU may be identified in patients with pre-existing endocrine disease or as a direct consequence of various CNS disorders including TBI, SAH, pituitary surgery/apoplexy, and brain death.

Pathophysiology of neuroendocrine dysfunction

The anterior pituitary gland produces several peptide hormones including adrenocorticotropic (ACTH), thyroid-stimulating (TSH), and growth (GH) hormones. Pituitary hormone secretion is regulated by hypothalamic-releasing and inhibitory factors and by negative feedback from peripheral hormones. The HPA axis controls secretion of all adrenal cortical hormones except mineralocorticoids. Corticotrophin-releasing factor stimulates ACTH secretion from the anterior pituitary gland which in turn stimulates cortisol production by the adrenal cortex. Failure of the HPA axis therefore leads to secondary adrenal insufficiency or failure. It may also result in under production of TSH leading to 'central' hypothyroidism. This is characterized by low TSH and tetraiodothyronine (T_4) blood concentrations (95) and should be differentiated from the 'euthyroid sick syndrome', a common response to critical illness in which TSH remains normal. GH levels and those of the several gonadal hormones produced by the pituitary gland may also be low after ABI but this is rarely of clinical relevance in the acute phase after injury.

The posterior pituitary stores the hypothalamic hormones oxytocin and AVP and, following ABI, posterior hypopituitarism may lead to central DI (see 'Central Diabetes Insipidus').

Aetiology of endocrine failure after brain injury

Endocrine failure after brain injury is related to multiple mechanisms including direct injury to the HPA axis in TBI, or intracranial hypertension-related hypothalamic and brainstem ischaemia (95). Post-mortem studies have demonstrated structural abnormalities of the HPA axis in a large proportion of patients dying from severe TBI (96). The anterior lobe of the pituitary gland is particularly vulnerable, and ischaemia or haemorrhage has been identified in the hypothalamus and/or anterior pituitary in 40–60% of post-mortem studies of patients dying from severe TBI (95,97). The blood supply to the HPA axis is the site of a watershed phenomenon and imaging studies have identified vascular insults to the HPA axis in up to 50% of brain-injured patients, although no abnormalities are present in 6% of those with proven pituitary dysfunction (98). Spasm of small arteries supplying the HPA axis may be a contributory factor after SAH (99). Reduced neuronal input from cortical and brainstem sites may also adversely affect the HPA axis, and brain injury-induced release of various substances, including somatomedin and catecholamines, may further alter HPA axis hormone release (100). As well as being related to direct HPA axis injury, an accentuated sympathetic nervous system discharge may be implicated in central hypothyroidism (101). Diffuse axonal injury, basal skull fracture, and older age are major risk factors for the development post-TBI hypopituitarism (102).

Primary failure of the adrenal gland, usually related to a systemic inflammatory response, may also complicate the management of ABI (103,104).

Incidence of endocrine failure after brain injury

In a systematic review of 19 studies including 1137 patients, the pooled prevalence of pituitary dysfunction after TBI and SAH was 27.5% and 40.0% respectively (96). However, the incidence in individual studies varied widely, ranging from 15% to 68% after TBI and from 37.5% to 55% after SAH. This likely reflects different methodologies, particular whether or not hormone stimulation tests were used, and variable follow-up times.

There is also great variability in the relative frequency and number of hormone axes affected after ABI. In a prospective study, single hormone deficiency was identified in 21% of patients, multiple hormone defects in another 5.7%, and panhypopituitarism in 5.7% (105). The incidence of pituitary dysfunction is related to the severity of TBI and has been reported in 37.5%, 57.1%, and 59.3% of patients with mild, moderate, and severe injury respectively (106). Conversely, endocrine dysfunction after SAH does not appear to be related to severity of the initial brain injury (107).

Posterior pituitary dysfunction is less common than anterior pituitary failure. Central DI has been reported in 26% of patients in the acute phase after TBI (108) and persists in up to 7% of long-term survivors (109). After SAH, studies have variably reported the incidence of central DI between zero and 3% at 12 months after the ictus (96).

Endocrine dysfunction can persist after brain injury and is sometimes first diagnosed in the rehabilitation phase. A recent review of ten studies including 749 patients identified some degree of hypopituitarism in 27.5% and 47% of patients in the chronic (> 6 months) phase after TBI and SAH respectively (110). In most individuals only a single pituitary axis was affected. Endocrine status improves over time in most patients but, in one study, 5.5% of those whose endocrine profile was normal at 3 months had developed an abnormality by 1 year (105).

Diagnosis of endocrine failure after brain injury

It is important to consider the possibility of endocrine insufficiency or failure after ABI (95), and early assessment of all patients after moderate-to-severe TBI has been recommended (111,112). However, this approach is not universally supported as there is no evidence that endocrine replacement in the acute phase after injury affects outcome, except for replacement of cortisol and AVP in clinically relevant adrenal insufficiency and central DI respectively. Imaging studies confirming direct injury or oedema in the area of the hypothalamus or pituitary gland, or fractures into the sella turcica, should prompt endocrine assessment but treatment is not recommended based on radiological findings alone because of their variable correlation with gland function (113).

A practical approach to investigation of endocrine dysfunction after ABI recommends that hormone assessment should be considered in patients with the following 'warning' signs (95):

- prolonged unresponsiveness not predicted by the severity of the underlying brain injury
- ongoing hypotension requiring vasopressor support
- hyponatraemia
- hypoglycaemia
- polyuria
- imaging evidence of oedema, haemorrhage or infarction in the region of the hypothalamus
- skull base fracture and cranial nerve defects.

To avoid missing endocrine dysfunction, it has been suggested that routine screening might be appropriate in all sedated brain-injured patients requiring high-dose vasopressor support (114).

Post-traumatic hypopituitarism, particularly GH deficiency, is associated with greater functional dependency and worse cognitive function after TBI (115). Routine screening of endocrine status during rehabilitation is recommended after an individual assessment that takes into account ongoing signs suggestive of endocrine dysfunction, severity of original brain injury and likely therapeutic benefits of hormone replacement therapy (116).

Adrenal failure

There are many causes of adrenal insufficiency and failure (Table 28.5) but secondary adrenal failure because of HPA axis dysfunction is most common after ABI. It occurs more frequently in younger patients with more severe injury and is associated with more episodes of hypotension and increased vasopressor requirements (114). A recent study found that 78% of TBI patients developed inappropriately low plasma cortisol levels, and that this was predictive of mortality (117). In this study, 39% of patients had at least one persisting pituitary hormone deficit at follow-up and all of them had low plasma cortisol or central DI during the acute phase after injury. ABI-related adrenal dysfunction usually resolves over time. In one study, 24.6% of patients failed to respond to an ACTH stimulation test at 3 months after brain injury, but only 12.9% were unresponsive at one year (118). Of note, failure to respond to ACTH could not be predicted from basal serum cortisol concentration.

Table 28.5 Causes of adrenal insufficiency and failure

	Primary	Secondary
Site of dysfunction	Adrenal glands	Hypothalamic–pituitary–adrenal (HPA) axis
Causes	Addison's disease (commonest cause in developed countries)	Abrupt withdrawal of chronic steroid therapy
	Infection affecting adrenal glands (e.g. Tuberculosis—commonest cause worldwide)	Damage to HPA (e.g. trauma, radiation therapy, intracranial tumours)
	Severe overwhelming generalized infection and septic shock	Pituitary surgery with inadequate steroid replacement
	Infiltration of adrenal glands (e.g. sarcoidosis, amyloidosis, malignancy)	Pituitary apoplexy
	Adrenal haemorrhage/infarction (e.g. Waterhouse–Friderichsen syndrome, antiphospholipid syndrome)	
	Congenital adrenal hyperplasia	
	Bilateral adrenalectomy	

Adrenal dysfunction can uncommonly develop in the rehabilitation phase of ABI (95,105,119).

Primary adrenal failure and insufficiency has been reported in 13–28% of patients within the first 10 days after severe TBI (120).

Diagnosis

Measurement of baseline serum cortisol is the primary investigation for assessing adrenal status and, in association with measurement of serum ACTH and thyroid hormones, should been performed before steroid replacement is considered. Although a morning cortisol assay is usually recommended, a random measurement is as useful after ABI because of stress-related disruption of the diurnal variation of cortisol (95,114). Serum cortisol is reduced in both primary and secondary adrenal failure but the actual concentration for diagnosis in the context of ABI is not clear. A random cortisol concentration less than 415 nmol/L is generally recommended as the diagnostic threshold for adrenal failure but thresholds of less than 690–990 nmol/L might be more appropriate after ABI because of the 'stress' of brain injury (95).

The serum cortisol response to stimulation by ACTH is widely used in the diagnosis of adrenal dysfunction. Patients are defined as 'responders' or 'non-responders' depending on their cortisol response to a 250 mcg dose of ACTH. A 30-minute cortisol concentration greater than 600 nmol/L (or > 700 nmol/L at 60 min), or an incremental rise greater than 250 nmol/L, indicates adrenal responsiveness (121), although the exact criteria for diagnosis after brain injury are controversial. In a study in which 78% of 113 TBI patients were diagnosed with adrenal insufficiency based on basal cortisol concentrations, only 13% failed to increase serum cortisol concentration less than 250 nmol/L after ACTH stimulation (120).

Treatment

Despite overwhelming evidence that high-dose steroids have adverse effects after TBI (122), proven adrenal failure with symptoms such as hypotension, hyponatraemia, and hypoglycaemia requires steroid replacement (95,121). Hydrocortisone 50–100 mg three times a day is recommended in the acute phase after injury (123), but the dose should be reduced to maintenance levels of 10–20 mg 8-hourly as soon as clinical status allows. A mineralocorticoid should be added in primary adrenal insufficiency or if severe hyponatraemia is a feature (95). Whilst these treatment recommendations are widely accepted, they are not supported by good evidence. There is also no evidence linking treatment of adrenal insufficiency with improved outcome after ABI.

Thyroid dysfunction

There are multiple causes of hypothyroidism (Table 28.6), but central hypothyroidism is most relevant after ABI. It is reported in 10–15% of patients after TBI (106). Hypothyroidism is associated with prolonged coma and, in most studies, with higher mortality and worse functional outcome after ABI (101,124). Assessment of thyroid hormone status is therefore an essential element of the evaluation of coma. The long-term (2–10-year) consequences of post-traumatic hypopituitarism have recently been evaluated in 51 patients with severe TBI and, in contrast to other reports, this study found no correlation between hypopituitarism and patient-reported quality of life and daily functioning (125).

Treatment

Central hypothyroidism after ABI is often diagnosed late or mistaken for the sick euthyroid syndrome. Treatment is not usually indicated although it may be required in the presence of coexisting adrenal insufficiency (126).

Growth hormone

A reduced human GH response has been reported in approximately 18% of patients after severe TBI (127), but the independent outcome effects of low GH are unclear (100). Most studies

Table 28.6 Causes of hypothyroidism

	Primary	Secondary
Site of dysfunction	Thyroid gland	Hypothalamic–pituitary–adrenal (HPA) axis
Causes	Thyroiditis (e.g. Hashimoto's disease)	Pituitary adenoma with absence of TSH production
	Simple colloid goitre (e.g. iodine deficiency, inborn errors of metabolism, congenital agenesis/atrophy of thyroid gland)	Damage to HPA axis (e.g. trauma, radiation therapy, intracranial tumours)
	Iatrogenic causes (e.g. thyroidectomy or radio-iodine ablation with inadequate thyroid replacement therapy)	Pituitary surgery with inadequate steroid replacement
	Drugs (e.g. carbimazole, propyl-thiouracil)	Pituitary apoplexy
		Brain death

confirming early GH deficiency have demonstrated improvement in the first year of follow-up (96), although more recent studies suggest long-term prevalence rates up to 25% (125). GH deficiency and insufficiency in the rehabilitation phase after TBI is associated with increased disability, worse quality of life, and a greater likelihood of depression compared with GH-sufficient patients (128). There is some evidence that GH replacement might have a positive impact in patients with mild TBI, particularly in terms of improving cognition and reducing the feeling of fatigue (129), but this requires confirmation in prospective outcome studies.

Pituitary apoplexy

Sudden haemorrhage into a pituitary mass can lead to pituitary apoplexy. This most commonly occurs into a non-functioning pituitary adenoma, although it can be a complication of elective pituitary surgery (130). Pituitary apoplexy presents with sudden-onset severe headache, visual defects, and oculomotor paralysis, and is characterized by pan-hormone deficiency including secondary adrenal failure, central hypothyroidism, and (often) central DI. It is a medical emergency and treatment of acute adrenal insufficiency and cardiovascular support are of critical importance (131).

Brain death

Brain death is frequently accompanied by substantial disruption of neuroendocrine function (see Chapter 29) (132). Early depletion of AVP and central DI occurs in almost 80% of brain dead organ donors, and a rapid decline in free triiodothyronine (T_3) occurs as a result of impaired TSH secretion and peripheral conversion of T_4. There is also a significant decrease in cortisol levels as a result of HPA axis failure which, in association with reduced T_3 levels, contributes to cardiovascular instability. The use of hormone replacement regimens during the care of brain dead organ donors has been recommended (133), although a recent meta-analysis showed limited efficacy of such interventions on post-transplant organ function (134).

References

1. Hall G, Hunter J, Cooper S (eds). *Core Topics in Endocrinology in Anaesthesia and Critical Care.* Oxford: Oxford University Press; 2010.
2. Godoy DA, Di NM, Rabinstein AA. Treating hyperglycemia in neuro-critical patients: benefits and perils. *Neurocrit Care.* 2010;13:425–38.
3. Fahy BG, Sheehy AM, Coursin DB. Glucose control in the intensive care unit. *Crit Care Med.* 2009;37:1769–76.
4. Oddo M, Schmidt JM, Carrera E, Badjatia N, Connolly ES, Presciutti M, *et al.* Impact of tight glycemic control on cerebral glucose metabolism after severe brain injury: a microdialysis study. *Crit Care Med.* 2008;36:3233–8.
5. Vespa P, Boonyaputthikul R, McArthur DL, Miller C, Etchepare M, Bergsneider M, *et al.* Intensive insulin therapy reduces microdialysis glucose values without altering glucose utilization or improving the lactate/pyruvate ratio after traumatic brain injury. *Crit Care Med.* 2006;34:850–6.
6. Auer RN, Wieloch T, Olsson Y, Siesjo BK. The distribution of hypoglycemic brain damage. *Acta Neuropathol.* 1984;64:177–91.
7. Fujioka M, Okuchi K, Hiramatsu KI, Sakaki T, Sakaguchi S, Ishii Y. Specific changes in human brain after hypoglycemic injury. *Stroke.* 1997;28:584–7.
8. Finkielman JD, Oyen LJ, Afessa B. Agreement between bedside blood and plasma glucose measurement in the ICU setting. *Chest.* 2005;127:1749–51.
9. Van den Berghe G, Wouters P, Weekers F, Verwaest C, Bruyninckx F, Schetz M, *et al.* Intensive insulin therapy in critically ill patients. *N Engl J Med.* 2001;345:1359–67.
10. Finfer S, Chittock DR, Su SY, Blair D, Foster D, Dhingra V, *et al.* Intensive versus conventional glucose control in critically ill patients. *N Engl J Med.* 2009;360:1283–97.
11. Griesdale DE, de Souza RJ, van Dam RM, Heyland DK, Cook DJ, Malhotra A, *et al.* Intensive insulin therapy and mortality among critically ill patients: a meta-analysis including NICE-SUGAR study data. *CMAJ.* 2009;180:821–7.
12. Kramer AH, Roberts DJ, Zygun DA. Optimal glycemic control in neurocritical care patients: a systematic review and meta-analysis. *Crit Care.* 2012;16:R203.
13. Marik PE, Preiser JC. Toward understanding tight glycemic control in the ICU: a systematic review and metaanalysis. *Chest.* 2010;137:544–51.
14. Tomlinson DR, Gardiner NJ. Glucose neurotoxicity. *Nat Rev Neurosci.* 2008;9:36–45.
15. Clausen T, Khaldi A, Zauner A, Reinert M, Doppenberg E, Menzel M, *et al.* Cerebral acid-base homeostasis after severe traumatic brain injury. *J Neurosurg.* 2005;103:597–607.
16. Lam AM, Winn HR, Cullen BF, Sundling N. Hyperglycemia and neurological outcome in patients with head injury. *J Neurosurg.* 1991;75:545–51.
17. Salim A, Hadjizacharia P, Dubose J, Brown C, Inaba K, Chan LS, *et al.* Persistent hyperglycemia in severe traumatic brain injury: an independent predictor of outcome. *Am Surg.* 2009;75:25–9.
18. Badjatia N, Topcuoglu MA, Buonanno FS, Smith EE, Nogueira RG, Rordorf GA, *et al.* Relationship between hyperglycemia and symptomatic vasospasm after subarachnoid hemorrhage. *Crit Care Med.* 2005;33:1603–9.
19. Frontera JA, Fernandez A, Claassen J, Schmidt M, Schumacher HC, Wartenberg K, *et al.* Hyperglycemia after SAH: predictors, associated complications, and impact on outcome. *Stroke.* 2006;37:199–203.
20. Fogelholm R, Murros K, Rissanen A, Avikainen S. Admission blood glucose and short term survival in primary intracerebral haemorrhage: a population based study. *J Neurol Neurosurg Psychiatry.* 2005;76:349–53.
21. Godoy DA, Pinero GR, Svampa S, Papa F, Di Napoli M. Hyperglycemia and short-term outcome in patients with spontaneous intracerebral hemorrhage. *Neurocrit Care.* 2008;9:217–29.
22. Gray CS, Hildreth AJ, Alberti GK, O'Connell JE. Poststroke hyperglycemia: natural history and immediate management. *Stroke.* 2004;35:122–6.
23. Scott JF, Robinson GM, French JM, O'Connell JE, Alberti KG, Gray CS. Prevalence of admission hyperglycaemia across clinical subtypes of acute stroke. *Lancet.* 1999;353:376–77.
24. Suh SW, Hamby AM, Swanson RA. Hypoglycemia, brain energetics, and hypoglycemic neuronal death. *Glia.* 2007;55:1280–6.
25. Magnoni S, Tedesco C, Carbonara M, Pluderi M, Colombo A, Stocchetti N. Relationship between systemic glucose and cerebral glucose is preserved in patients with severe traumatic brain injury, but glucose delivery to the brain may become limited when oxidative metabolism is impaired: implications for glycemic control. *Crit Care Med.* 2012;40:1785–91.
26. Feuerstein D, Manning A, Hashemi P, Bhatia R, Fabricius M, Tolias C, *et al.* Dynamic metabolic response to multiple spreading depolarizations in patients with acute brain injury: an online microdialysis study. *J Cereb Blood Flow Metab.* 2010;30:1343–55.
27. Green DM, O'Phelan KH, Bassin SL, Chang CW, Stern TS, Asai SM. Intensive versus conventional insulin therapy in critically ill neurologic patients. *Neurocrit Care.* 2010;13:299–306.
28. Graffagnino C, Gurram AR, Kolls B, Olson DM. Intensive insulin therapy in the neurocritical care setting is associated with poor clinical outcomes. *Neurocrit Care.* 2010;13:307–12.
29. Jeremitsky E, Omert LA, Dunham CM, Protetch J, Rodriguez A. The impact of hyperglycemia on patients with severe brain injury. *J Trauma.* 2005;58:47–50.
30. Van Beek JG, Mushkudiani NA, Steyerberg EW, Butcher I, McHugh GS, Lu J, *et al.* Prognostic value of admission laboratory parameters in traumatic brain injury: results from the IMPACT study. *J Neurotrauma.* 2007;24:315–28.

31. Van den BG, Schoonheydt K, Becx P, Bruyninckx F, Wouters PJ. Insulin therapy protects the central and peripheral nervous system of intensive care patients. *Neurology*. 2005;64:1348–53.

32. Bilotta F, Caramia R, Cernak I, Paoloni FP, Doronzio A, Cuzzone V, et al. Intensive insulin therapy after severe traumatic brain injury: a randomized clinical trial. *Neurocrit Care*. 2008;9:159–66.

33. Capes SE, Hunt D, Malmberg K, Pathak P, Gerstein HC. Stress hyperglycemia and prognosis of stroke in nondiabetic and diabetic patients: a systematic overview. *Stroke*. 2001;32:2426–32.

34. Stead LG, Gilmore RM, Bellolio MF, Mishra S, Bhagra A, Vaidyanathan L, et al. Hyperglycemia as an independent predictor of worse outcome in non-diabetic patients presenting with acute ischemic stroke. *Neurocrit Care*. 2009;10:181–6.

35. Williams LS, Rotich J, Qi R, Fineberg N, Espay A, Bruno A, et al. Effects of admission hyperglycemia on mortality and costs in acute ischemic stroke. *Neurology*. 2002;59:67–71.

36. Baird TA, Parsons MW, Phanh T, Butcher KS, Desmond PM, Tress BM, et al. Persistent poststroke hyperglycemia is independently associated with infarct expansion and worse clinical outcome. *Stroke*. 2003;34:2208–14.

37. Fuentes B, Castillo J, San JB, Leira R, Serena J, Vivancos J, et al. The prognostic value of capillary glucose levels in acute stroke: the GLycemia in Acute Stroke (GLIAS) study. *Stroke*. 2009;40:562–8.

38. Kruyt ND, Biessels GJ, Devries JH, Roos YB. Hyperglycemia in acute ischemic stroke: pathophysiology and clinical management. *Nat Rev Neurol*. 2010;6:145–55.

39. Leigh R, Zaidat OO, Suri MF, Lynch G, Sundararajan S, Sunshine JL, et al. Predictors of hyperacute clinical worsening in ischemic stroke patients receiving thrombolytic therapy. *Stroke*. 2004;35:1903–7.

40. Bruno A, Williams LS, Kent TA. How important is hyperglycemia during acute brain infarction? *Neurologist*. 2004;10:195–200.

41. Gray CS, Hildreth AJ, Sandercock PA, O'Connell JE, Johnston DE, Cartlidge NE, et al. Glucose-potassium-insulin infusions in the management of post-stroke hyperglycaemia: the UK Glucose Insulin in Stroke Trial (GIST-UK). *Lancet Neurol*. 2007;6:397–406.

42. Bruno A, Kent TA, Coull BM, Shankar RR, Saha C, Becker KJ, et al. Treatment of hyperglycemia in ischemic stroke (THIS): a randomized pilot trial. *Stroke*. 2008;39:384–9.

43. Bellolio MF, Gilmore RM, Ganti L. Insulin for glycaemic control in acute ischaemic stroke. *Cochrane Database Syst Rev*. 2014;1:CD005346.

44. Kirkman MA, Citerio G, Smith M. The intensive care management of acute ischemic stroke: an overview. *Intensive Care Med*. 2014;40:640–53.

45. Bruno A, Durkalski VL, Hall CE, Juneja R, Barsan WG, Janis S, et al. The Stroke Hyperglycemia Insulin Network Effort (SHINE) trial protocol: a randomized, blinded, efficacy trial of standard vs. intensive hyperglycemia management in acute stroke. *Int J Stroke*. 2014;9:246–51.

46. Jauch EC, Saver JL, Adams HP, Bruno A, Connors JJ, Demaerschalk BM, et al. Guidelines for the early management of patients with acute ischemic stroke: a guideline for healthcare professionals from the American Heart Association/American Stroke Association. *Stroke*. 2013;44:870–947.

47. Passero S, Ciacci G, Ulivelli M. The influence of diabetes and hyperglycemia on clinical course after intracerebral hemorrhage. *Neurology*. 2003;61:1351–6.

48. Kruyt ND, Biessels GJ, de Haan RJ, Vermeulen M, Rinkel GJ, Coert B, et al. Hyperglycemia and clinical outcome in aneurysmal subarachnoid hemorrhage: a meta-analysis. *Stroke*. 2009;40:e424–e430.

49. Barletta JF, Figueroa BE, DeShane R, Blau SA, McAllen KJ. High glucose variability increases cerebral infarction in patients with spontaneous subarachnoid hemorrhage. *J Crit Care*. 2013;28:798–803.

50. Wright WL. Sodium and fluid management in acute brain injury. *Curr Neurol Neurosci Rep*. 2012;12:466–73.

51. Bhardwaj A. Neurological impact of vasopressin dysregulation and hyponatremia. *Ann Neurol*. 2006;59:229–36.

52. Verbalis JG. Vasopressin V2 receptor antagonists. *J Mol Endocrinol*. 2002;29:1–9.

53. Levin ER, Gardner DG, Samson WK. Natriuretic peptides. *N Engl J Med*. 1998;339:321–8.

54. Rabinstein AA, Wijdicks EF. Hyponatremia in critically ill neurological patients. *Neurologist*. 2003;9:290–300.

55. Robertson GL, Aycinena P, Zerbe RL. Neurogenic disorders of osmoregulation. *Am J Med*. 1982;72:339–53.

56. Rahman M, Friedman WA. Hyponatremia in neurosurgical patients: clinical guidelines development. *Neurosurgery*. 2009;65:925–35.

57. Diringer MN, Zazulia AR. Hyponatremia in neurologic patients: consequences and approaches to treatment. *Neurologist*. 2006;12:117–26.

58. Palmer BF. Hyponatremia in patients with central nervous system disease: SIADH versus CSW. *Trends Endocrinol Metab*. 2003;14:182–7.

59. Tisdall M, Crocker M, Watkiss J, Smith M. Disturbances of sodium in critically ill adult neurologic patients: a clinical review. *J Neurosurg Anesthesiol*. 2006;18:57–63.

60. Moritz ML, Ayus JC. Hospital-acquired hyponatremia—why are hypotonic parenteral fluids still being used? *Nat Clin Pract Nephrol*. 2007;3:374–82.

61. Biswas M, Davies JS. Hyponatraemia in clinical practice. *Postgrad Med J*. 2007;83:373–8.

62. Pasantes-Morales H, Franco R, Ordaz B, Ochoa LD. Mechanisms counteracting swelling in brain cells during hyponatremia. *Arch Med Res*. 2002;33:237–44.

63. Adrogue HJ, Madias NE. Hyponatremia. *N Engl J Med*. 2000;342:1581–9.

64. Palmer BF, Gates JR, Lader M. Causes and management of hyponatremia. *Ann Pharmacother*. 2003;37:1694–702.

65. Nathan BR. Cerebral correlates of hyponatremia. *Neurocrit Care*. 2007;6:72–8.

66. Lampl C, Yazdi K. Central pontine myelinolysis. *Eur Neurol*. 2002;47:3–10.

67. Ayus JC, Krothapalli RK, Arieff AI. Treatment of symptomatic hyponatremia and its relation to brain damage. A prospective study. *N Engl J Med*. 1987;317:1190–5.

68. Martin RJ. Central pontine and extrapontine myelinolysis: the osmotic demyelination syndromes. *J Neurol Neurosurg Psychiatry*. 2004;75 (Suppl 3):iii22–iii28.

69. Sterns RH, Riggs JE, Schochet SS, Jr. Osmotic demyelination syndrome following correction of hyponatremia. *N Engl J Med*. 1986;314:1535–42.

70. Reynolds RM, Seckl JR. Hyponatraemia for the clinical endocrinologist. *Clin Endocrinol*. 2005;63:366–74.

71. Kirkman MA, Albert AF, Ibrahim A, Doberenz D. Hyponatremia and brain injury: historical and contemporary perspectives. *Neurocrit Care*. 2013;18:406–16.

72. Singh S, Bohn D, Carlotti AP, Cusimano M, Rutka JT, Halperin ML. Cerebral salt wasting: truths, fallacies, theories, and challenges. *Crit Care Med*. 2002;30:2575–9.

73. Kirkman MA. Managing hyponatremia in neurosurgical patients. *Minerva Endocrinol*. 2014;39:13–26.

74. Verbalis JG, Grossman A, Hoybye C, Runkle I. Review and analysis of differing regulatory indications and expert panel guidelines for the treatment of hyponatremia. *Curr Med Res Opin*. 2014;30:1201–7.

75. Ellis SJ. Severe hyponatraemia: complications and treatment. *QJM*. 1995;88:905–9.

76. Van AT, Bakshi R, Devaux CB, Schwabe S. Hyponatremia associated with carbamazepine and oxcarbazepine therapy: a review. *Epilepsia*. 1994;35:181–8.

77. Mewasingh L, Aylett S, Kirkham F, Stanhope R. Hyponatraemia associated with lamotrigine in cranial diabetes insipidus. *Lancet*. 2000;356:656.

78. Hasan D, Wijdicks EF, Vermeulen M. Hyponatremia is associated with cerebral ischemia in patients with aneurysmal subarachnoid hemorrhage. *Ann Neurol*. 1990;27:106–8.

79. Qureshi AI, Suri MF, Sung GY, Straw RN, Yahia AM, Saad M, et al. Prognostic significance of hypernatremia and hyponatremia among patients with aneurysmal subarachnoid hemorrhage. *Neurosurgery*. 2002;50:749–55.

80. Brimioulle S, Orellana-Jimenez C, Aminian A, Vincent JL. Hyponatremia in neurological patients: cerebral salt wasting versus inappropriate antidiuretic hormone secretion. *Intensive Care Med.* 2008;34:125–31.

81. Sterns RH, Silver SM. Cerebral salt wasting versus SIADH: what difference? *J Am Soc Nephrol.* 2008;19:194–6.

82. Schwartz WB, Bennett W, Curelop S, Bartter FC. A syndrome of renal sodium loss and hyponatremia probably resulting from inappropriate secretion of antidiuretic hormone. *Am J Med.* 1957;23:529–42.

83. Robertson GL.Regulation of arginine vasopressin in the syndrome of inappropriate antidiuresis. *Am J Med.* 2006;119:S36–S42.

84. Ellison DH, Berl T. Clinical practice. The syndrome of inappropriate antidiuresis. *N Engl J Med.* 2007;356:2064–72.

85. Janicic N, Verbalis JG. Evaluation and management of hypo-osmolality in hospitalized patients. *Endocrinol Metab Clin North Am.* 2003;32:459–81.

86. Taplin CE, Cowell CT, Silink M, Ambler GR. Fludrocortisone therapy in cerebral salt wasting. *Pediatrics.* 2006;118:e1904–e1908.

87. Ghali JK, Koren MJ, Taylor JR, Brooks-Asplund E, Fan K, Long WA, et al. Efficacy and safety of oral conivaptan: a V1A/V2 vasopressin receptor antagonist, assessed in a randomized, placebo-controlled trial in patients with euvolemic or hypervolemic hyponatremia. *J Clin Endocrinol Metab.* 2006;91:2145–52.

88. Wright WL, Asbury WH, Gilmore JL, Samuels OB. Conivaptan for hyponatremia in the neurocritical care unit. *Neurocrit Care.* 2009;11:6–13.

89. Moritz ML. Syndrome of inappropriate antidiuresis and cerebral salt wasting syndrome: are they different and does it matter? *Pediatr Nephrol.* 2012;27:689–93.

90. Adler SM, Verbalis JG. Disorders of body water homeostasis in critical illness. *Endocrinol Metab Clin North Am.* 2006;35:873–94.

91. Adrogue HJ, Madias NE. Hypernatremia. *N Engl J Med.* 2000;342:1493–9.

92. Li M, Hu YH, Chen G. Hypernatremia severity and the risk of death after traumatic brain injury. *Injury.* 2013;44:1213–8.

93. Kraft MD, Btaiche IF, Sacks GS, Kudsk KA. Treatment of electrolyte disorders in adult patients in the intensive care unit. *Am J Health Syst Pharm.* 2005;62:1663–82.

94. Espay AJ.Neurologic complications of electrolyte disturbances and acid-base balance. *Handb Clin Neurol.* 2014;119:365–82.

95. Powner DJ, Boccalandro C, Alp MS, Vollmer DG. Endocrine failure after traumatic brain injury in adults. *Neurocrit Care.* 2006;5:61–70.

96. Schneider HJ, Kreitschmann-Andermahr I, Ghigo E, Stalla GK, Agha A. Hypothalamopituitary dysfunction following traumatic brain injury and aneurysmal subarachnoid hemorrhage: a systematic review. *JAMA.* 2007;298:1429–38.

97. Crompton MR. Hypothalamic lesions following closed head injury. *Brain.* 1971;94:165–72.

98. Benvenga S, Campenni A, Ruggeri RM, Trimarchi F. Clinical review 113: Hypopituitarism secondary to head trauma. *J Clin Endocrinol Metab.* 2000;85:1353–61.

99. Vespa PM. Hormonal dysfunction in neurocritical patients. *Curr Opin Crit Care.* 2013;19:107–12.

100. Hackl JM, Gottardis M, Wieser C, Rumpl E, Stadler C, Schwarz S, et al. Endocrine abnormalities in severe traumatic brain injury—a cue to prognosis in severe craniocerebral trauma? *Intensive Care Med.* 1991;17:25–9.

101. Woolf PD, Lee LA, Hamill RW, McDonald JV. Thyroid test abnormalities in traumatic brain injury: correlation with neurologic impairment and sympathetic nervous system activation. *Am J Med.* 1988;84:201–8.

102. Schneider M, Schneider HJ, Yassouridis A, Saller B, von RF, Stalla GK. Predictors of anterior pituitary insufficiency after traumatic brain injury. *Clin Endocrinol.* 2008;68:206–12.

103. Dimopoulou I, Alevizopoulou P, Dafni U, Orfanos S, Livaditi O, Tzanela M, et al. Pituitary-adrenal responses to human corticotropin-releasing hormone in critically ill patients. *Intensive Care Med.* 2007;33:454–9.

104. Morganti-Kossmann MC, Rancan M, Stahel PF, Kossmann T. Inflammatory response in acute traumatic brain injury: a double-edged sword. *Curr Opin Crit Care.* 2002;8:101–5.

105. Aimaretti G, Ambrosio MR, Di SC, Gasperi M, Cannavò S, Scaroni C, et al. Residual pituitary function after brain injury-induced hypopituitarism: a prospective 12-month study. *J Clin Endocrinol Metab.* 2005;90:6085–92.

106. Bondanelli M, De ML, Ambrosio MR, Monesi M, Valle D, Zatelli MC, et al. Occurrence of pituitary dysfunction following traumatic brain injury. *J Neurotrauma.* 2004;21:685–96.

107. Parenti G, Cecchi PC, Ragghianti B, Schwarz A, Ammannati F, Mennonna P, et al. Evaluation of the anterior pituitary function in the acute phase after spontaneous subarachnoid hemorrhage. *J Endocrinol Invest.* 2011;34:361–5.

108. Agha A, Sherlock M, Phillips J, Tormey W, Thompson CJ. The natural history of post-traumatic neurohypophysial dysfunction. *Eur J Endocrinol.* 2005;152:371–7.

109. Agha A, Thornton E, O'Kelly P, Tormey W, Phillips J, Thompson CJ. Posterior pituitary dysfunction after traumatic brain injury. *J Clin Endocrinol Metab.* 2004;89:5987–92.

110. Gasco V, Prodam F, Pagano L, Grottoli S, Belcastro S, Marzullo P, et al. Hypopituitarism following brain injury: when does it occur and how best to test? *Pituitary.* 2012;15:20–4.

111. Agha A, Thompson CJ. Anterior pituitary dysfunction following traumatic brain injury (TBI). *Clin Endocrinol.* 2006;64:481–8.

112. Ghigo E, Masel B, Aimaretti G, Léon-Carrión J, Casanueva FF, Dominguez-Morales MR, et al. Consensus guidelines on screening for hypopituitarism following traumatic brain injury. *Brain Inj.* 2005;19:711–24.

113. Schneider HJ, Stalla GK, Buchfelder M. Expert meeting: hypopituitarism after traumatic brain injury and subarachnoid haemorrhage. *Acta Neurochir (Wien).* 2006;148:449–56.

114. Cohan P, Wang C, McArthur DL, Cook SW, Dusick JR, Armin B, et al. Acute secondary adrenal insufficiency after traumatic brain injury: a prospective study. *Crit Care Med.* 2005;33:2358–66.

115. Park KD, Kim DY, Lee JK, Nam HS, Park YG. Anterior pituitary dysfunction in moderate-to-severe chronic traumatic brain injury patients and the influence on functional outcome. *Brain Inj.* 2010;24:1330–5.

116. Kopczak A, Kilimann I, von Rosen F, Krewer C, Schneider HJ, Stalla GK, et al. Screening for hypopituitarism in 509 patients with traumatic brain injury or subarachnoid hemorrhage. *J Neurotrauma.* 2014;31:99–107.

117. Hannon MJ, Crowley RK, Behan LA, O'Sullivan EP, O'Brien MM, Sherlock M, et al. Acute glucocorticoid deficiency and diabetes insipidus are common after acute traumatic brain injury and predict mortality. *J Clin Endocrinol Metab.* 2013;98:3229–37.

118. Schneider HJ, Schneider M, Saller B, Petersenn S, Uhr M, Husemann B, et al. Prevalence of anterior pituitary insufficiency 3 and 12 months after traumatic brain injury. *Eur J Endocrinol.* 2006;154:259–65.

119. Aimaretti G, Ambrosio MR, Di Somma C, Fusco A, Cannavò S, Gasperi M, et al. Traumatic brain injury and subarachnoid haemorrhage are conditions at high risk for hypopituitarism: screening study at 3 months after the brain injury. *Clin Endocrinol.* 2004;61:320–6.

120. Bernard F, Outtrim J, Menon DK, Matta BF. Incidence of adrenal insufficiency after severe traumatic brain injury varies according to definition used: clinical implications. *Br J Anaesth.* 2006;96:72–6.

121. Powner DJ, Boccalandro C. Adrenal insufficiency following traumatic brain injury in adults. *Curr Opin Crit Care.* 2008;14:163–6.

122. Alderson P, Roberts I. Corticosteroids for acute traumatic brain injury. *Cochrane Database Syst Rev.* 2005;1:CD000196.

123. Schneider HJ, Aimaretti G, Kreitschmann-Andermahr I, Stalla GK, Ghigo E. Hypopituitarism. *Lancet.* 2007;369:1461–70.

124. Fleischer AS, Rudman DR, Payne NS, Tindall GT. Hypothalamic hypothyroidism and hypogonadism in prolonged traumatic coma. *J Neurosurg.* 1978;49:650–7.

125. Ulfarsson T, Arnar GG, Rosen T, Blomstrand C, Sunnerhagen KS, Lundgren-Nilsson A, et al. Pituitary function and functional outcome in adults after severe traumatic brain injury: the long-term perspective. *J Neurotrauma*. 2013;30:271–80.

126. Munoz A, Urban R. Neuroendocrine consequences of traumatic brain injury. *Curr Opin Endocrinol Diabetes Obes*. 2013;20:354–8.

127. Agha A, Rogers B, Mylotte D, Taleb F, Tormey W, Phillips J, et al. Neuroendocrine dysfunction in the acute phase of traumatic brain injury. *Clin Endocrinol*. 2004;60:584–91.

128. Bavisetty S, Bavisetty S, McArthur DL, Dusick JR, Wang C, Cohan P, et al. Chronic hypopituitarism after traumatic brain injury: risk assessment and relationship to outcome. *Neurosurgery*. 2008;62:1080–93.

129. High WM, Jr., Briones-Galang M, Clark JA, Gilkison C, Mossberg KA, Zgaljardic DJ, et al. Effect of growth hormone replacement therapy on cognition after traumatic brain injury. *J Neurotrauma*. 2010;27:1565–75.

130. Hwang JJ, Hwang DY. Treatment of endocrine disorders in the neuroscience intensive care unit. *Curr Treat Options Neurol*. 2014;16:271.

131. Vargas G, Gonzalez B, Guinto G, Mendoza VI, López-Félix B4, Zepeda E, et al. Pituitary apoplexy in non-functioning pituitary macroadenomas: a case-control study. *Endocr Pract*. 2014;20(12):1274–80.

132. Ranasinghe AM, Bonser RS. Endocrine changes in brain death and transplantation. *Best Pract Res Clin Endocrinol Metab*. 2011;25:799–812.

133. Novitzky D, Cooper DK, Rosendale JD, Kauffman HM. Hormonal therapy of the brain-dead organ donor: experimental and clinical studies. *Transplantation*. 2006;82:1396–401.

134. Rech TH, Moraes RB, Crispim D, Czepielewski MA, Leitão CB. Management of the brain-dead organ donor: a systematic review and meta-analysis. *Transplantation*. 2013;95:966–74.

CHAPTER 29

Brain death

Jeanne Teitelbaum and Sam Shemie

Death determined by neurological criteria, or brain death, is better considered as brain arrest, or the final clinical expression of complete and irreversible neurological failure. A review of the history of brain death has been published by Baron et al. (1). Despite widespread national, international, and legal acceptance of the concept of brain death, substantial variation exists in the definition of terms, as well as in the standards for diagnosis and their application (2–6).

In 2002, a survey conducted by Wijdicks (2) explored the international practices for diagnosing brain death and found stunning, often troubling differences. Whilst there is relative consistency in the requirement for examination of brainstem reflexes, there is surprising variation in the performance, methods, and targets of the apnoea test, in the number of physicians required to complete the tests, and in the type and requirement for confirmatory tests. In leading US hospitals, variations have also been found in the prerequisites for the diagnosis of brain death, including acceptable core temperature and the number of required examinations, amongst others (7). Chart audits have also revealed incomplete documentation of the findings during the confirmation of brain death (8). In an attempt to address this considerable practice variation, the United Kingdom, Canada, Australia, and the United States have issued national guidelines and checklists in order to standardize practice (9,10–13). Yet, despite this, considerable practice variation remains. The current evidence base for the existing guidelines on the determination of death by neurological criteria is inadequate, but clear medical standards, in association with clarification of the required qualifications of physicians making the diagnosis, will improve the quality and rigor of its determination.

In this chapter, we will review the history of death determined by neurological criteria, and the specific criteria and requirements for the diagnosis of brain death, paying special attention to areas of controversy and practice inconsistency.

Terminology

There remains a need to clarify and standardize terminology. Even widely applied terms, such as brain death or the neurological determination of death (NDD), are often used loosely and mean different things to different people.

Brain death

Brain death is ubiquitous in the medical, nursing, and lay literature, and is based on the concept of the complete and irreversible loss of brain function. Brain death is equivalent to the death of the individual, even though the heart may continue to beat and spinal cord function may persist. The Canadian Neurocritical Care guidelines define brain death as 'the irreversible loss of the capacity for consciousness combined with the irreversible loss of all brainstem functions, including the capacity to breathe' (10). Whether whole-brain or only brainstem destruction is required is not addressed in this guidance, and both are accepted if they fulfil the clinical criteria of brain death. In the United States, the President's Commission for the Study of Ethical Problems in Medicine and Biomedical and Behavioral Research defines brain death as 'irreversible cessation of all functions of the entire brain, including the brainstem' (14).

Neurological death

Neurological death is a term that is similar to brain death, but is not now commonly used.

Brainstem death

Brainstem death is the irreversible loss of brainstem function through the irremediable damage of all brainstem structures. It is used as the standard for the determination of brain death in some countries, including the United Kingdom.

Neurological determination of death

The NDD is the process and procedure for determining the death of an individual using neurological criteria. NDD is not a new definition of death, but represents a clarification and standardization of the processes for the determination of death based on neurological, or brain-based, criteria.

History of brain death

With the advent of mechanical ventilation and the evolution of resuscitative measures came the ability to artificially maintain patients with severe brain injury long after brain function had ceased. In 1959, Mollaret and Goulon coined the term 'coma dépassé', meaning 'a state beyond coma', to describe this condition which is characterized by loss of consciousness, brainstem areflexia and the absence of spontaneous respiration, in association with absent encephalographic activity (15). The original intent of this work was to describe the futility of care in such cases. However, the introduction of organ transplantation later led to an inexorable linking of the issues of brain death, organ procurement, and transplantation which has continued to this day.

In 1968, the ad hoc Committee of the Harvard Medical School to Examine the Definition of Brain Death undertook to define irreversible coma and brain death (16). The committee deliberations focused on a whole-brain formulation of brain death which, to this day, serves as the foundation of the concept of brain death in the United States. In 1971, Mohandas and Chou emphasized the importance of the irreversible loss of brainstem function in brain death (17), and this primordial importance of the brainstem subsequently became the focus of a published statement in 1976 by the Conference of Medical Royal Colleges and their Faculties in the United Kingdom (18). Championed by Pallis and Harley, the brainstem formulation of brain death was formally adopted by the United Kingdom (19).

In 1981, the President's Commission for the Study of Ethical Problems in Medicine and Biomedical and Behavioral Research reaffirmed the application of a whole-brain definition of brain death in the United States, and addressed the use of ancillary diagnostic testing in the NDD (14). The Commission also made recommendations regarding the length of the observation period required before brain death assessment could be undertaken. Amongst their decisions was the recommendation that patients suffering from hypoxic brain injury should be observed for no less than 24 hours prior to the determination of brain death.

Since the 1980s, multiple guidelines (and revisions) on the diagnosis of brain death have been published in many jurisdictions. A 2002 survey by Wijdicks explored the international practices for diagnosing brain death and found important variations in the performance, methods and targets of apnoea testing, the number of physicians required to make the diagnosis, and the type and requirement for ancillary or confirmatory tests (2).

Concept of the neurological determination of death

Of interest in the international context are the differences between 'whole brain'- and 'brainstem'-based definitions of brain death. In most jurisdictions, brain death remains principally a clinical, bedside determination based on the confirmation of the absence of brainstem function. In Canada, neurologically determined death is defined as the irreversible loss of the capacity for consciousness combined with the irreversible loss of all brainstem functions, including the capacity to breathe (11). There is no insistence on whole-brain death and no explicit brainstem death because of the view that brain death is the permanent cessation of brain function as a whole, rather than a destruction of the whole brain. In the United States, the Uniform Determination of Death Act (UDDA) defines brain death as the irreversible cessation of all functions of the entire brain, including the brainstem (13). The important difference between the United States and Canada is that the US definition of brain death requires the death of all areas of the brain, whereas the Canadian definition is a clinical one that can be met either by whole-brain or brainstem death, and which may therefore result as a consequence of intracranial hypertension, primary direct brainstem injury, or both. Unlike in Pallis's original description, the hypothalamus is not specifically identified as being an integral part of the brainstem in any Canadian guidance. There are currently no satisfactory ancillary tests for the confirmation of death in instances of isolated primary brainstem injury, hence the reliance on a clinical diagnosis.

In the United Kingdom, a brainstem-based definition of brain death is applied, and this approach is supported by the 1976 statement from the Conference of Medical Royal Colleges and their Faculties that permanent functional death in the brainstem constitutes brain death (18). Although irreversible loss of brainstem function is defined as the irremediable damage of all brainstem structures, it is determined

in clinical terms with the caveat that reversible causes of brainstem dysfunction have been excluded. The argument is that loss of ascending reticular activating system function will lead to loss of consciousness, and that supplemental testing is therefore not required. As noted earlier, although Pallis included the hypothalamus and interruption of the corticothalamic tract as an extended brainstem in his original diagrams, these areas cannot be tested using the clinical criteria for the determination of brainstem death, and the UK Code of Practice also does not require evidence that the brainstem (medullary) centres controlling heart rate and blood pressure have ceased to function (13). Proponents of the brainstem formulation of brain death have no difficulty with the whole-brain criteria because the clinical determinants are fundamentally similar.

In most countries, the concept of brain death is legally accepted as death, when its determination is made according to accepted medical standards.

Determination of death by neurological criteria

The determination of death by neurological criteria is summarized in Box 29.1, and there are several components that are worthy of specific consideration.

Timing of the initial assessment

There are two key timing issues in the declaration of brain death. One relates to the timing of the first examination relative to the primary injury, and the other to the time interval between examinations if more than one is required.

Pallis and Harley in the United Kingdom defined the time of the first assessment for brain death as the first point at which the pre-conditions for the determination of brain death had been met. These are the presence of unresponsive apnoeic coma, a cause of coma capable of producing brain death, a determination that the neurological damage is irremediable, and the absence of confounding factors (19). Most countries support this approach. The most difficult aspect to determine is the irremediable nature of the event, especially when the damage is hypoxic/ischaemic in nature or due to a severe metabolic condition, such as insulin overdose with extreme and prolonged hypoglycaemia, or severe electrolyte abnormalities. For this reason, many countries' guidelines recommend a minimum observation period, although with a time frame that varies widely, in addition to the presence of the aforementioned pre-conditions.

In the United Kingdom, the Academy of Medical Royal Colleges recommends that 'brain-stem testing should be undertaken only if, after continuing clinical observation and investigation, there is no possibility of a reversible or treatable underlying cause being present' (13). The 1998 guidelines from the Australian and New Zealand Intensive Care Society (ANZICS) are more specific and recommend that no fewer than 4 hours of documented coma should precede the first examination for brain death; edition 3.2 of the guidance, published in 2013, clarifies that, in cases of acute hypoxic/ischaemic brain injury including cardiac arrest, the clinical testing for brain death should be delayed for 24 hours following the injury or arrest (12). In the United States, the 1995 American Academy of Neurology (AAN) guidelines, and its 2010 update, concludes that there is insufficient evidence to determine a minimally acceptable period of observation to ensure that neurological

---

Box 29.1 Key aspects of the neurological determination of death

Minimum clinical criteria

◆ *Established cause*—capable of causing neurological death, with definite clinical or neuroimaging evidence of an acute CNS event that is consistent with the irreversible loss of neurological function.

◆ *Presence of deep unresponsive coma*—absence of spontaneous movements originating in the CNS, such as cranial nerve function, CNS-mediated motor response to pain in any distribution, seizures, and decorticate and decerebrate responses.

◆ *Absence of confounding factors:*
  • unresuscitated shock
  • hypothermia
  • severe metabolic disturbance
  • clinically significant drug intoxications
  • peripheral nerve or muscle dysfunction or neuromuscular blockade.

◆ *Brainstem areflexia*—defined by the absence of:
  • corneal responses bilaterally
  • pupillary responses to light, with pupils at midsize or greater bilaterally
  • gag reflex
  • cough reflex
  • vestibulo-ocular responses bilaterally.

◆ *Absent respiratory effort*—confirmed by the apnoea test.

Ancillary tests

◆ Ancillary tests should be performed when minimum clinical criteria cannot be completed or confounding factors cannot be corrected, or as a routine part of the assessment in some jurisdictions.

◆ Demonstration of the global absence of intracerebral blood flow, with four-vessel cerebral angiography or radionuclide cerebral blood flow imaging, is the gold standard for determination of death by ancillary testing.

◆ Newer imaging modalities, such as CT and MRI angiography, hold promise but have not been sufficiently validated at this time.

◆ EEG is no longer recommended as an ancillary test.

Country-dependent overarching principles

◆ The assessment for brain death can be made when the pre-conditions for its determination have been met.

◆ There is no evidence that a second examination enhances the diagnostic accuracy of brain death, but two assessments are required in some countries.

◆ In many countries, existing law states that for the purposes of postmortem donation, the fact of death shall be determined by two physicians.

◆ The required qualifications of the physicians declaring neurological death varies between countries and jurisdictions.

◆ The legal time of death is marked by the first determination of death in Canada and the United Kingdom, and after the second assessment in the United States and Australia.

functions have ceased irreversibly (9). Their recommendation is therefore vague, stating that 'a certain period of time must have passed' (usually several hours) between the initial insult and the clinical examination for brain death.

The Canadian forum addresses this issue at length and offers the most clarity. For the timing of the first examination, even though there was no compelling evidence, several practical factors were taken into consideration in developing the recommendations. First, neurological assessment may be unreliable in the acute (up to 24 hours) post-resuscitation phase after cardiorespiratory arrest (20). Indeed, restoration of initially absent pupillary and motor responses has been reported in the first 24 hours after cardiac arrest (21). In addition, there are case reports in which brain death was confirmed 6 hours after a cardiac arrest but with return of some brainstem function by 24 hours; there were however several confounders in these reports (22). Second, after severe metabolic or pure hypoxic injury (e.g. hypoglycaemia, asphyxia, or hypernatraemia), it may be very difficult to determine at what time the neurological status can be deemed irreversible. With these factors in mind, the Canadian recommendations are as follows:

◆ In cases of acute hypoxic-ischaemic brain injury, clinical evaluation for the NDD should be delayed for 24 hours after the cardiorespiratory arrest, or an ancillary test performed.

◆ In the situation of hypothermia post cardiac arrest there are insufficient data to make a firm recommendation. Twenty-four hours after re-warming to 36°C is insufficient (20), and 72 hours after restoration of normothermia and discontinuation of sedation may be reasonable (21–23).

◆ In cases of extreme metabolic insult, sufficient time should have passed for the clinician to believe that the insult is permanent, and, in addition, there should be evidence of diffuse cerebral insult on imaging (e.g. magnetic resonance imaging (MRI)). If irreversibility remains an issue, an ancillary test should be performed in addition to the clinical examination.

Number of examinations

Although there is no scientific evidence that a second examination enhances the diagnostic accuracy of brain death, most jurisdictions require a second assessment for the purposes of organ donation. In the United Kingdom, two assessments are always required and two physicians must be present at each assessment (13). If two assessments are required, the recommended time interval between them varies widely. In Canada, the assessments can be performed concurrently except in children under 1 year of age. In the United Kingdom and Australia, they must be performed separately, with a full clinical examination, including the apnoea test, being performed on each occasion, but with no fixed examination interval regardless of the primary cause. In the United Kingdom, the 2008 guidance from the Academy of Medical Royal Colleges states that the interval can be quite short, although always long enough to allow recovery of stable arterial blood gases after the first apnoea test (13). The initial ANZICS guidelines (1998) recommended that the interval between the two assessments should be no less than 2 hours, although the 2010 update requires no fixed interval between assessments except where age-related criteria apply (12). The two independent and complete assessments can be performed consecutively, but not simultaneously, and each by separate physicians.

The legal time of death is marked by the first determination of death in Canada and the United Kingdom, and after the second assessment in the United States and Australia. The timings and findings of the examinations to determine brain death must be clearly documented (Figure 29.1).

Qualifications of the physicians performing the assessment

The required qualifications of the physicians performing the clinical assessment of brain death are extremely variable. Canadian practitioners need full and current licensure for independent medical practice in the relevant Canadian jurisdiction, skill and knowledge in the management of patients with severe brain injury and in the NDD, and no association with a proposed transplant recipient that might influence their judgement in the case of potential organ donors (11). In the United States, the required expertise varies by state and sometimes by individual institution. The United

Documentation form for adults and children aged 1 year and older (UK example)

Diagnos is is to be made by two doctors who have been registered for more than five years and are competent in the procedure. At least one should be a consultant. Testing should be undertaken by the doctors together and must always be performed completely and successfully on two occasions in total.

Patient name and unit number:

Pre-conditions: Does the patient have a condition that can and has led to irreversible brain damage?
Time of observation adequate?

Have potentially reversible causes been ruled out?

Physician	Dr A	Dr B
Depressant Rx		
Neuromuscular blockade		
Endocrine / electrolyte disturbance		
Shock or hypothermia		

Clinical Criteria

	Dr A set 1	Dr B set 1	Dr A set 2	Dr B set 2
BP and T°				
Deep unresponsive coma				
Bilateral absence of motor response?				
Absent cough?				
Absent gag?				
Bilateral absence of comeal reflex?				
Absence of Vestibulo-ocular reflex?				
Absent pupillary response to light?				
Apnea?				
pCO_2, pre-test (35-45 mm Hg)				
pCO_2, pH post-test (> 50 mm Hg)				
pH ost test (< 7.3)				
pCO_2 rise (> 20)				

Date and time of first set of tests: Dr A Signature:

Date and time of second set of tests: Dr B Singature:

Fig. 29.1 Documentation form for adults and children aged 1 year and older (example from the United Kingdom).

Kingdom requires two medical practitioners who have been registered for more than 5 years with a licence to practice, and who are competent in the conduct and interpretation of brainstem testing; at least one of the doctors must be a consultant (13). Those carrying out the tests must have no clinical conflict of interest, and neither doctor should be a member of a transplant team. The ANZICS guidance states that the 'NDD should be performed by two medical practitioners whose expertise is defined by local legislation' (12). However, it goes on to say that 'care of the donor and family must be provided by an intensivist with specific expertise that may be acquired through specialized education, reference documents and ongoing clinical experience'.

Despite some international differences, all would agree that the physician diagnosing brain death should be a licensed experienced practitioner with skill and knowledge in the management of patients with severe brain injury as well as specific expertise in the neurological determination of death.

Clinical evaluation

The requirements for the confirmation of brain death are quite uniform across guidelines and are cautious to exclude any potential diagnostic error or reversible conditions. The prerequisites for the clinical assessment for the NDD usually include normal blood pressure and temperature although exact values are not always stipulated and vary between guidelines (see below).

The minimum clinical criteria for the NDD in adults (Box 29.1) include:

◆ *An established cause* capable of causing neurological death, with definite clinical or neuroimaging evidence of an acute central nervous system (CNS) event that is consistent with the irreversible loss of neurological function, and the absence of reversible conditions capable of mimicking neurological death. Neurological death may occur as a consequence of intracranial hypertension, primary direct brainstem injury (United Kingdom, Canada), or both.

◆ *The presence of deep unresponsive coma* with bilateral absence of motor responses (excluding spinal reflexes), which implies a lack of spontaneous movements, and an absence of movement originating in the CNS, including cranial nerve function, CNS-mediated motor response to pain in any distribution, seizures, and decorticate and decerebrate responses. Spinal reflexes confined to spinal distribution may persist, and have been reported in up to 75% of patients progressing to brain death (22). Several spinal-originating movements have been documented and described in brain-dead patients, and should not confuse the determination of brain death (24).

◆ *Absence of confounding factor* (see below).

◆ *Brainstem areflexia* defined by the absence of:
  • bilateral corneal responses
  • bilateral pupillary responses to light, with pupils at midsize or greater
  • gag reflex
  • cough reflex
  • bilateral vestibulo-ocular responses (Box 29.2).

◆ *Absent respiratory effort* confirmed by the apnoea test (see below).

> **Box 29.2** Oculocephalic reflex (caloric) testing
>
> ◆ Place the head of the bed at 30°.
> ◆ Confirm the patency of the external auditory canal and remove excess wax and debris.
> ◆ Check that there is a clear view of both tympanic membranes and rule out tears or perforation.
> ◆ Prepare ice-cold water in a kidney basin.
> ◆ Hold the eyes open.
> ◆ Irrigate one ear at a time with ice-cold saline using a 50 or 60 mL syringe and a 20-gauge, short intravenous catheter.
> ◆ Observe the eyes during and after irrigation for a full minute.
> ◆ Allow 5 minutes between ears.
> ◆ Full inhibition of the vestibular system requires 20 seconds of contact with a temperature of 0°C, and the inhibition takes a minimum of 2 minutes to wear off after ice-water irrigation.

There are different requirements in neonates and infants as follows:

◆ For infants aged 30 days to 1 year (corrected for gestational age) the criteria include the oculocephalic reflex instead of the vestibulo-ocular reflex because of the unique anatomy of the external auditory canal.

◆ For neonates from term (36 weeks of gestation) to 30 days, clinical criteria have primacy, as they do in the child and adult. Minimum clinical criteria include the absence of oculocephalic reflex and suck reflex.

Confounding factors

All guidelines place the achievement of normal blood pressure and temperature in the prerequisites for clinical evaluation but the acceptable threshold values differ. The list of possible confounding factors is otherwise identical and shown in Box 29.3.

When assessing for neurological death, examiners are cautioned to review these confounding factors in the context of the cause of the neurological injury and their clinical assessment. If physicians are confounded by any finding or investigation, either absolutely or from their own perspective, they should not proceed with the NDD. Clinical judgement is always the deciding factor.

There are key considerations that must be specifically addressed in the neurological determination of death.

Unresuscitated shock

The AAN guidelines in the United States require a systolic blood pressure above 100 mmHg before brain death assessment, whereas Canadian, UK, and Australian guidelines require systolic pressures greater than 90 mmHg.

Hypothermia

Canadian guidelines require that core temperature is measured through central blood, rectal, or oesophageal-gastric routes, whereas methods of temperature measurement are not specified by the AAN. The accepted temperature for performing the clinical examination of brain death varies in different guidelines between 34°C and 36°C. There is no evidence to favour a particular temperature

---

Box 29.3 Confounding factors

- Conditions that can mimic brain death.

- Hypotensive shock—systolic blood pressure too low to assure brain perfusion (variably defined as systolic blood pressure > 90 or 100 mmHg).

- Hypothermia (core temperature < 34°C).

- Peripheral nerve or muscle dysfunction or neuromuscular blockade.

- Brainstem ischaemia causing a locked-in syndrome.

- Drug effects—paralysing agents, barbiturate or benzodiazepine overdose, anaesthetic agents.

- Conditions that affect the ability to confirm irreversibility.

- Severe metabolic disorders capable of causing a potentially reversible coma.

- Severe metabolic abnormalities—glucose; electrolytes, including potassium, phosphate, calcium, and magnesium; inborn errors of metabolism; liver and renal dysfunction may play a role in clinical presentation.

---

within this range, but 34°C is the minimum at which the tests are accepted as valid; there are no reports of hypothermia-related loss of brainstem reflexes above 34°C. Further, increasing hypothermic patients' temperature to 34°C does not pose significant risk to the patient or difficulty for the treating physician. Canadian and UK guidelines require the core temperature to be 34°C or higher, the ANZICS guidance states 35°C or higher, and the AAN guidelines stipulate a minimum temperature of 36°C. Ideally temperature should be as close to normal as possible prior to performing the assessment for brain death, although this is not always achievable.

Drug intoxication

Although clinically significant drug intoxications (e.g. alcohol, barbiturates, sedatives, or hypnotics) are confounders that must be addressed before clinical assessment for brain death, therapeutic levels, or therapeutic dosing of anticonvulsants, sedatives, and analgesics do not preclude the diagnosis of brain death. The administration of paralytic or anaesthetic medication is a major confounder and these agents must be discontinued and eliminated from the system prior to any clinical assessment of brain death.

The approach to the presence of medications (e.g. sedation, analgesia, or barbiturates) that may depress CNS function varies throughout the world. Issues to consider when assessing the potential to confound the clinical evaluation of brain death include drug type, dose, duration of administration, and hepatorenal function. If uncertainty exists, drugs should be discontinued and adequate time allowed for elimination, drug levels should be monitored, specific antagonists administered, the absence of neuromuscular blockade be confirmed, or an ancillary test performed.

Severe metabolic disturbance

Severe metabolic disorders capable of causing a potentially reversible coma should be excluded. If the primary cause does not fully explain the clinical picture, and/or if the treating physician's judgement is that a metabolic abnormality may play a role in the coma, it should be corrected or an ancillary test performed.

Apnoea testing

Demonstration of the failure to breathe must be assessed in a reliable and consistent manner, and is an integral part of the assessment for brain death. This is achieved by confirming the absence of a breathing drive in response to an increase in $PaCO_2$ to higher than normal levels, with clear documentation of the test. Apnoea testing requires the presence of normotension, normothermia, euvolaemia, adequate oxygenation, and eucapnia ($PaCO_2$ 4.67–6 kPa (35–45 mmHg)) at the start of the test, and the absence of prior CO_2 retention (i.e. chronic obstructive pulmonary disease or severe obesity). Canadian guidelines recommend that the thresholds at the completion of the apnoea test be a $PaCO_2$ of 8 kPa (60 mmHg) or higher, and 2.67 kPa (20 mmHg) higher than the pre-apnoea test level, with a pH of 7.28 or lower (11). The United States also requires a CO_2 rise of at least 2.67 kPa (20 mmHg) but has no threshold for the pH (9), whereas ANZICS requires a pH threshold of 7.3 (12). The UK code requires that the $PaCO_2$ should be 6.0 kPa (45 mmHg) or higher at the start of the apnoea test and that it should rise by at least 0.5 kPa (3.75 mmHg) to above 6.5 kPa (48.8 mmHg) at the conclusion of the test (13). In cases of chronic carbon dioxide retention, the $PaCO_2$ should be adjusted to ensure that the pH is lower than 7.4 at the completion of the test. All guidelines agree that these thresholds must be documented by arterial blood gas measurement at the start and end of the apnoea test.

To interpret an apnoea test correctly, the certifying physician must continuously observe the patient for respiratory effort, and ensure that adequate oxygenation and blood pressure is maintained, throughout the test. For patients with severe lung disease, caution must be exercised in considering the validity of the apnoea test. If there is a history of chronic respiratory insufficiency and responsiveness to only supranormal levels of carbon dioxide, or if the patient depends on a hypoxic drive, the validity of the apnoea test might be in doubt. In such circumstances an ancillary test should be administered. The conduct of the apnoea test is described in detail in Box 29.4.

In potential organ donors, the application of continuous airway pressure between 8 and 10 cmH$_2$O during the apnoea test is associated with an increase in the number of eligible and retrieved lungs suitable for transplantation (25).

Ancillary tests

Sometimes clinical criteria for the determination of brain death cannot be applied reliably. This includes situations where the cranial nerves cannot be adequately examined, when neuromuscular paralysis or drug intoxication is present, in patients in whom the apnoea test is precluded (e.g. respiratory instability or high cervical spine injury) or invalid (high CO_2 retainers), and when confounding factors remain unresolved. In these situations, ancillary tests, sometimes called supplementary or confirmatory tests, may be helpful.

Different guidelines specify when ancillary testing should be performed, and the requirements that must still be met prior to testing. Unresuscitated shock and hypothermia must be corrected as a minimum before ancillary tests are performed, and, as with the clinical determination of brain death, specific clinical criteria must be met. An established cause of neurological injury capable of causing neurological death must be present, the patient must be in a deep unresponsive coma, and reversible conditions capable of mimicking neurological death must be excluded.

Box 29.4 Apnoea testing

- Maintain systolic blood pressure greater than or equal to 90 (or 100) mmHg.

- Preoxygenate for at least 10 minutes with 100% O_2.

- Reduce ventilator frequency to obtain normocarbia (10 breaths per minute).

- Baseline blood gas should have $PaCO_2$ of 35–45 mmHg, O_2 greater than or equal to 200 mmHg, and pH greater than or equal to 7.3.

- Disconnect the ventilator.

- Deliver 100% O_2 at 2–6 L/min through a catheter placed through the endotracheal tube to the level of the carina, or via bulk flow using a Mapleson C type re-breathing circuit with continuous positive airway pressure.

- Observe for respiratory movements for 8–10 minutes.

- Abort if systolic pressure is less than 90 mmHg or SpO_2 less than 85%.

- Draw second blood gas after the 8–10 minutes of apnoea and confirm sufficient rise in $PaCO_2$.

- Reconnect the ventilator and return FiO_2 to baseline level.

In 2006, Young and colleagues published a critical review of the various ancillary tests that are used to support the NDD (26). Tests of brain perfusion are the only tests to satisfy standard criteria for suitability, with electrophysiological and other tests considered inadequate. The demonstration of the global absence of intracranial blood flow using established imaging modalities is presently considered the standard for the NDD by ancillary testing. Although many guidelines still require an electroencephalogram (EEG) as part of the NDD (2,3), it is no longer recommended by others because of its substantial limitations. The AAN guideline update lists four acceptable tests, including EEG, but requires only one for validation (9). The UK guidance highlights the pros and cons of various ancillary tests, but does not stipulate the use of any (13).

Recommended ancillary tests

Four-vessel cerebral angiography (12) and radionuclide tests of brain blood flow/perfusion (20) are accepted as valid confirmatory tests of brain death.

Cerebral angiography

A selective radiocontrast four-vessel angiogram visualizing both the anterior and posterior cerebral circulation should be obtained. Cerebral-circulatory arrest is confirmed when intracerebral pressure exceeds arterial inflow pressure. Provided the patient has an adequate blood pressure, absence of blood flow above the level of the carotid siphon in the anterior circulation and above the foramen magnum in the posterior circulation is considered diagnostic of brain death (27). External carotid circulation should be evident and filling of the superior sinus may be present. Angiography requires technical expertise and is performed in the radiology department, necessitating transport of potentially unstable patients. Arterial puncture and catheter-related complications are described and

radiocontrast can produce idiosyncratic reactions and end-organ damage, such as renal dysfunction, which can be an issue in potential organ donors.

Radionuclide imaging techniques

Radionuclide angiography (perfusion scintigraphy) has been widely accepted for the confirmation of brain death for several years. In the last decade, radiopharmaceuticals, especially Tc99m hexamethylpropylene-amine oxime (Tc99m HMPAO), have been studied extensively and provide enhanced detection of intracerebral, posterior fossa, and brainstem blood flow (21,23). Tc99m HMPAO is lipid soluble, crossing the blood–brain barrier, and provides information on cerebral blood flow and uptake of tracer within perfused brain tissue. The traditional gamma cameras used in this technique are immobile, necessitating patient transfer for the study, but newer technologies are portable allowing studies to be performed at the bedside.

Newer imaging modalities

Computed tomography (CT) angiography holds future promise because it is a non-invasive, easily accessible, operator-independent, and inexpensive way to measure cerebral perfusion (28). However, it remains insufficiently validated for the confirmation of brain death at this time. MRI-based angiography and imaging also hold future promise but are not easily available and have likewise been insufficiently validated at this time.

Transcranial Doppler ultrasonography

Using a pulse Doppler instrument, the intracerebral arteries, including the vertebral or basilar arteries, are insonated bilaterally. Brain-dead patients display either absent or reversed diastolic flow or small systolic spikes. The non-invasiveness and portability of this technique are advantageous but it requires substantial clinical expertise for proper application and interpretation, and is not widely available. The absence of acoustic windows makes it inapplicable in certain patients, and its interpretation is operator dependent (29). TCD has not been sufficiently validated for the confirmation of brain death at this time and should only be used as a bedside screening tool prior to a definitive investigation of CBF (12).

Electroencephalography

EEG is readily available in most tertiary medical centres worldwide. It has long been used as a supplementary test for brain death, and can be performed at the bedside. However, it has significant limitations (3,26). The EEG detects only cortical electrical activity and is unable to detect deep cerebral or brainstem function. The high sensitivity requirement for EEG recording may result in the detection of electric interference from many of the devices that are commonplace in the intensive care unit. EEG is also significantly affected by hypothermia, drug administration, and metabolic disturbances, diminishing its clinical utility in the circumstances when ancillary tests are most often required. It is therefore no longer recommended as an ancillary test to confirm brain death.

Children

Regardless of age, clinical examination remains paramount in the determination of neurological death. However, the clinical determination of brain death in children, specifically in the young infant, is more problematic than in adults because of the difficulties in performing the examination, the presence of open cranial sutures and fontanelles, and the relative immaturity of some brainstem reflexes. In most guidelines, the recommendations established for adults are applicable to children older than 1 year, although in the United Kingdom adult guidelines apply to children older than 2 months. The uncertainty surrounding the determination of brain death in those under 36 weeks of gestation is such that no international guidelines currently address this problem.

Canadian forum recommendations

In infants aged less than 1 year, and term newborns (36 weeks of gestation), a full clinical examination, including apnoea test, must be performed by two physicians at two different times; the absence of the suck reflex is added to the brainstem examination in this age group (11). For infants there is no fixed interval between examinations, whereas in newborns the first examination should be delayed until 48 hours after birth, and the interval between examinations should be a minimum of 24 hours.

The ANZICS guidelines for diagnosis of brain death in children have been modelled on the recommendations of the Canadian Forum, and are therefore very similar.

UK guidelines

A 1991 working party of the British Paediatric Association (BPA) produced guidelines for the diagnosis of brain death in infants and children and this is used as the basis for the paediatric section of the Academy of Medical Royal Colleges 2008 guidance on the diagnosis of death (13). This notes that it is rarely possible to diagnose brainstem death confidently in term newborns (from 37 weeks of gestation) to 2 months of age, and that the concept of brainstem death is inappropriate for infants below 37 weeks of gestation. In this age group, decisions on whether or not to continue intensive care should be based on an assessment of the likely outcome of the underlying condition, after close discussion with the family.

US guidelines

The American Academy of Pediatrics has published guidance on the determination of brain death in children (30). In term newborns (37 weeks of gestation) to 30 days of age, two examinations including an apnoea test with each examination, separated by an observation period of 24 hours, are required. In children aged from 30 days to 18 years, two examinations, also including an apnoea test with each examination, separated by an observation period of 12 hours are required. Assessment of neurological function following cardiopulmonary resuscitation or other severe acute brain injuries should be deferred for 24 hours or longer if there are concerns or inconsistencies in the examination.

Conclusion

The accurate and reliable determination of brain death currently has variability in many of its elements, with significant international variation (1–3,5). The one constant is the absolute certainty that must attend the diagnosis of brain death. Meticulous attention to detail and strict adherence to local protocols are the essential elements of every diagnosis of brain death. In this way the infallible nature of the confirmation of death by neurological criteria can be assured.

References

1. Baron L, Shemie SD, Teitelbaum J, Doig CJ. Brief review: history, concepts and controversies in the neurological determination of death. *Can J Anesth*. 2006;53:602–8.
2. Wijdicks EF. Brain death worldwide: accepted fact but no global consensus in diagnostic criteria. *Neurology*. 2002;58:20–5.
3. Shemie SD. Variability of brain death practices. *Crit Care Med*. 2004;32:2564–5.
4. Powner DJ, Hernandez M, Rives TE. Variability among hospital policies for determining brain death in adults. *Crit Care Med*. 2004;32:1284–8.
5. Mejia RE, Pollack MM. Variability in brain death determination practices in children. *JAMA*. 1995;274:550–3.
6. Hornby K, Shemie SD, Teitelbaum J, Doig C. Variability in hospital-based brain death guidelines in Canada. *Can J Anaesth*. 2006;53:613–19.
7. Greer DM, Varelas PN, Haque S, Wijdicks EF. Variability of brain death determination guidelines in leading US neurologic institutions. *Neurology*. 2008;70:284–9.
8. Wang M, Wallace P, Gruen JP. Brain death documentation: analysis and issues. *Neurosurgery*. 2002;51:731–6.
9. Wijdicks EF, Varelas PN, Gronseth GS, Greer DM, American Academy of Neurology. American Academy of Neurology evidence-based guideline update: determining brain death in adults: report of the Quality Standards Subcommittee of the American Academy of Neurology. *Neurology*. 2010;74:1911–18.
10. Canadian Neurocritical Care Group. Guidelines for the diagnosis of brain death. *Can J Neurol Sci*. 1999;26:64–6.
11. Shemie SD, Doig C, Dickens B,Byrne P, Wheelock B, Rocker G, *et al*. Severe brain injury to neurologic determination of death: Canadian forum recommendations. *CMAJ*. 2006;174:S1–13.
12. Australian and New Zealand intensive Care Society (ANZICS). *The ANZICS Statement on Death and Organ Donation* (Edition 3.2). Melbourne: ANZICS, 2013.
13. Academy of the Medical Royal Colleges. *A Code of Practice for the Diagnosis and Confirmation of Death*. London: Academy of the Medical Royal Colleges; 2008. http://www.aomrc.org.uk/reports-guidance.html
14. Guidelines for the determination of death. Report of the medical consultants on the diagnosis of death to the President's Commission for the Study of Ethical Problems in Medicine and Biomedical and Behavioral Research. *JAMA*. 1981;246:2184–6.
15. Mollaret P, Goulon M. The depassed coma (preliminary memoir). *Rev Neurol (Paris)*. 1959;101:3–15
16. A definition of irreversible coma. Report of the Ad Hoc committee of the Harvard medical school to examine the definition of brain death. *JAMA*. 1968;205:337–40.
17. Mohandas A, Chou SN. Brain death. A clinical and pathological study. *J Neurosurg*. 1971;35:211–18.
18. Diagnosis of brain death. Statement issued by the honorary secretary of the conference of Medical Royal Colleges and their Faculties in the United Kingdom on 11 October 1976. *Br Med J*. 1976;2:1187–8.
19. Pallis C, Harley DH. *ABC of Brainstem Death* (2nd edn). London: BMJ Publishing Group; 1996.
20. Booth CM, Boone RH, Tomlinson G, Detsky AS. Is this patient dead, vegetative, or severely neurologically impaired? Assessing outcome for comatose survivors of cardiac arrest. *JAMA*. 2004;291:870–9.
21. Zanbergen EG, DeHaan RI, Stoutenbeck CP, Hijdra A. Systematic review of early prediction of poor outcome in anoxic-ischemic coma. *Lancet*. 1998:352:1808–12.
22. Shemie SD, Langevin S, Farrell C. Therapeutic hypothermia after cardiac arrest, another confounding factor in brain-death testing. *Pediatr Neurol*. 2010;42:304.
23. Webb AC, Samuels OB. Reversible brain death after cardiopulmonary arrest and induced hypothermia. *Crit Care Med*. 2011;39:1538–42.
24. Saposnick G, Basile VS, Young GB. Movements in brain death: a systematic review. *Can J Neurol Sci*. 2009;26:154–60.

25. Mascia L, Pasero D, Slutsky A, Arguis MJ, Berardino M, Grasso S, *et al.* Effect of a lung protective strategy for organ donors on eligibility and availability of lungs for transplantation: a randomized controlled trial. *JAMA.* 2010;304:2620–7.

26. Young GB, Shemie SD, Doig CG, Teitelbaum J. Brief review: the role of ancillary tests in the neurological determination of death. *Can J Anaesth.* 2006;53:620–7.

27. Rosenklint A, Jorgensen PB. Evaluation of angiographic methods in the diagnosis of brain death. Correlation with local and systemic arterial pressure and intracranial pressure. *Neuroradiology.* 1974;7:215–19.

28. Quesnel C, Fulgencio J-P, Adrie C, Marro B, Payen L, Lembert N, *et al.* Limitations of computed tomographic angiography in the diagnosis of brain death. *Intensive Care Med.* 2007;33:2129–35.

29. Kalanuria A, Nyquist PA, Armonda RA, Razumovsky A. Use of transcranial Doppler (TCD) ultrasound in the neurocritical care unit. *Neurosurg Clin N Am.* 2013;24:441–56.

30. Nakagawa TA, Ashwal S, Mathur M, Mysore M, Society of Critical Care Medicine, Section on Critical Care and Section on Neurology of American Academy of Pediatrics, *et al.* Clinical report—Guidelines for the determination of brain death in infants and children: an update of the 1987 task force recommendations. *Pediatrics.* 2011;128:e720–40.

CHAPTER 30

Principles of organ donation

Ivan Rocha Ferreira da Silva and Jennifer A. Frontera

Transplant medicine is an ever growing specialty, but the gap between organ donors and those awaiting a transplant remains a problem worldwide. According to the United Network for Organ Sharing (UNOS), a private, non-profit organization that helps manage the organ transplantation system in the United States, there were 117,064 patients on the waiting list for a transplant in 2012 but only 10,535 donors (1). A similar situation pertains in Europe. For example, in the United Kingdom in 2012, there were 2912 transplants (using organs from just over 1000 deceased donors) but more than 7600 patients on the transplant waiting list. Data from the US Department of Health and Human Services show that an average of 79 people received organ transplants each day in 2009, whilst 18 died each day waiting for a transplant (2). Organ transplantation is a life-saving and life-changing event; as of May 2009, the percentage 5-year survival after specific organ transplantation in the United States was 69.3% for kidneys, 74.9% for hearts, 73.8% for livers, and 54.4% for lungs (2).

Around the world, most organ donations come after brain death, also known as donation after neurological death (DND), but donation after cardiac death (DCD) is rapidly becoming an option to increase deceased donation in some countries. Tissue donation, including cornea, bone, musculoskeletal tissue, and skin, are also possible.

Donation after neurological death

A major challenge in the field of organ donation is the regional and worldwide variability in the definition of brain death (see Chapter 29). Many countries require two neurological examinations to confirm brain death, with a specified time between them depending on the patient's age (from 6 hours for adults to 48 hours for newborns), and this delay reduces to potential for organ donation. However, several states in the United States have moved to a single neurological examination for those aged over 1 year, as there is evidence to suggest that a second examinations does not add sensitivity or specificity to the diagnosis of brain death but decreases organ donation consent rates and organ viability (3). Similarly, eligibility for organ donation is highly variable depending on the local organ procurement organization and transplant team.

Identifying potential organ donors

Although the exact details of communication with the local organ donor network vary, there should always be a low threshold for reporting a potential organ donor. Indeed, in many states in the United States, notification of potential organ donors is mandated by law and required by The Joint Commission. In countries where

there is no legal mandate, notification is often recommended by professional, consensus guidance. In general, the criteria to trigger notification as a potential organ donor are catastrophic brain injury and impending brain death (with clinical signs of brain herniation or a Glasgow Coma Scale score ≤ 4) and planned withdrawal of life-sustaining measures (for DCD), as well as all deaths (usually within 1 hour) for tissue donation. Any medical caregiver may report a potential donor to a local organ donor network.

The critical care team should contact the organ donor network regardless of the age of the patient, medical history, or aetiology of death, as physicians are not expected to screen for eligibility for potential donation. Additionally, it is important for the organ donor network to have an understanding of the volume of patients that are brain dead or who undergo withdrawal of life-sustaining therapy (even if ineligible to donate) to calculate the donor potential and evaluate strategies to improve donation. Thus, even if the healthcare provider believes that the patient will be ineligible for, or medically ruled out of, donation, the potential donor should still be reported to the local organ donor network.

Table 30.1 shows some of the generally accepted contraindications to donation. Some previously accepted impediments to donation have been demystified by recent studies. Bacteraemia or fungaemia without sepsis do not preclude donation, as some data suggest that infections are rarely transmitted and outcomes of recipients are not significantly different from those receiving organs from uninfected donors (4,5). Patients with past history of cancer with long cancer-free intervals are also generally able to be potential donors because the risk of cancer transmission is considered to be very low (6,7). However, patients with active carcinoma of the lung, breast, kidney, or colon, melanoma, choriocarcinoma, or lymphoma at the time of donation are ineligible to donate as there is a 43% rate of cancer recurrence after transplantation and associated immunosuppression (8,9). Patients with isolated central nervous systems neoplasms can be potential donors, with the potential exception of high-grade tumours (mainly glioblastoma and medulloblastoma), as there are reports of cancer transmission from such donors (10). Most systemic viral infections are considered contraindications, but there is evidence that routine prophylaxis against cytomegalovirus is very effective in reducing the associated morbidity and mortality (11,12). Additionally, hepatitis B or C donors can be transplanted into similarly positive recipients.

Consent and family approach

The first step in caring for a patient and family is communication. Before any approach for organ donation can be made, families must understand the medical prognosis for the patient. In the

Table 30.1 Contraindications to organ donation

Contraindications to organ donation	Comments
Multisystem organ failure secondary to sepsis	Most bacterial infections without sepsis are not a contraindication
Bacterial infections	Tuberculosis, intra-abdominal sepsis
Fungal infections	Active *Cryptococcus, Aspergillus, Histoplasma, Coccidioides*, candidaemia and invasive yeast infections
Viral infections	HIV, HTLV I and II, rabies, reactive HBsAg, measles, West Nile virus, SARS, adenovirus, enterovirus, parvovirus, active HSV, VZV, EBV, viral encephalitis/meningitis
Parasitic infections	Leishmania, trypanosome (Chagas), *Strongyloides*, malaria
Prion disease	CJD, vCJD, fatal familial insomnia, Gerstmann–Straussler Scheinker
Cancer	No active cancer, no history of previously treated cancer (refer to possible exceptions in the text). May be eligible to donate: skin cancer (other than melanoma), certain primary brain tumours, remote prostate cancer

CJD, Creutzfeldt–Jakob disease; EBV, Epstein–Barr virus; HIV, human immunodeficiency virus; HSV, herpes simplex virus; HTLV, human T-lymphotropic virus; HbSAg, surface antigen of the hepatitis B virus; SARS, severe acute respiratory syndrome virus; VZV, varicella zoster virus; vCJD, variant Creutzfeldt–Jakob disease.

case of brain death, it is incumbent on the treating physician to explain to the family that brain death is an irreversible process as well as a legal determination of death, clearly separating this from withdrawal of care and subsequent potential for organ donation. Families that better understand the physiological process of brain death are more likely to agree to organ donation (13).

Typically, the organ donor network team approaches the family for consent for organ or tissue donation, since maintaining a clear distinction between the treating team and organ donation network can avoid or minimize any perceived conflicts of interest. Certainly, members of the transplant team should not be involved in the consent process. The separation of the consent approach from the treating team is known as decoupling. However, intensive care unit (ICU) physicians have a crucial role in caring for patients and families in these circumstances, and the care they provide is enhanced through training, attention to the specific issues, and collaboration with organ procurement organization personnel (14). There is also some evidence that the presence of an ICU physician during the approach for organ donation (known as coupling) may have a beneficial impact on consent rates. More data examining different methods of approach for consent are therefore needed. Religious, cultural, and ethical issues often arise during the consent process and offering as much support as possible, including palliative care, and support from social workers and faith leaders, can assist with accompanying end-of-life discussions. It is also advisable to mention that organ donation does not disfigure the donor's body, nor preclude funeral arrangements that incorporate viewing of the deceased's body. A rare exception to this would be a planned face or hand transplant, which would require additional education and discussion with family.

It should be clearly documented if donation is refused because of a living will or by a family that does not wish to pursue donation.

In many countries, families now have the right to be appropriately counselled by an organ donor network representative, regardless of any previously manifested comments during the patient's hospital admission.

Critical care management of the brain dead organ donor

The intensivist has a key role, not only in promptly identifying potential organ donors and contacting the local organ procurement service, but also in adequately managing the profound physiological changes associated with catastrophic brain injuries, in order to maximize the potential for donation (15) The progression from brain death to somatic death can result in the loss of 10–20% of potential donors (16) and a single donor can save up to eight lives (2), so optimal donor management is crucial.

Physiological changes after brain death

Brain death culminates in a cascade of events leading to severe cardiovascular instability. It is the result of a rostral-to-caudal brain ischaemic process, precipitated by overwhelmingly high intracranial pressure. At first, a sympathetic surge occurs to maintain cerebral perfusion pressure, with an associated massive release of catecholamines leading to hypertension (secondary to elevated systemic vascular resistance), left ventricular dysfunction (with cardiac stunning), arrhythmias, and neurogenic pulmonary oedema (17). These clinical findings are corroborated by animal models and post-mortem studies in humans showing that brainstem ischaemia is associated with the development of contraction band necrosis, mostly concentrated in the subendocardium of the left ventricle (18,19). Subsequently, herniation following brain death results in high spinal cord ischaemia and infarction, leading to a 'clinical decapitation' and deafferentation. In a controlled animal model of brain death, this deafferentation resulted in loss of sympathetic tone, with associated vasodilation, low levels of serum catecholamines, and loss of cardiac stimulation (20).

Finally, with diencephalic destruction, pituitary hormonal secretion ceases, leading to a severe panhypopituitarism. This state is characterized by very low levels of thyroid hormones, cortisol, antidiuretic hormone, and insulin, leading to further hypotension (21, 22). Furthermore, this hypotensive state is aggravated with volume depletion, generally secondary to ensuing diabetes insipidus (DI).

Immediately after haemodynamic and endocrine changes occur, a massive release of serum and tissue inflammatory mediators, such as interleukin (IL)-1, IL-6, tumour necrosis factor, and adhesion molecules (E-selectin, intercellular adhesion molecule 1 (ICAM-1), vascular cell adhesion molecule 1 (VCAM-1)), take place as observed in animal and human studies (22). The significance of this phenomenon is unclear, but it has been suggested that the presence of these inflammatory mediators may be associated with accelerated graft rejection (23).

Managing haemodynamic instability

Hypotension may initially be present in up to 80% of potential donors (24) and conventional management of hypotension is often inadequate; persistent haemodynamic instability is observed in 34–45% (25–27). Most of the current data regarding haemodynamic management is derived from trials in non-brain dead septic or trauma patients, without the characteristic hormonal deficiencies and low sympathetic tone usually seen in brain dead donors. Moreover, brain dead patients can be extremely volume depleted as a result of osmotic diuretics used to treat high intracranial pressure prior to brain death, and the DI that occurs secondary to diencephalic injury at the time of brain death.

The approach to haemodynamic management of the brain dead organ donor is variable in the literature. Some authors advocate a more conventional, step-wise approach, using a combination of fluid resuscitation and vasopressors, usually norepinephrine, epinephrine, phenylephrine, or dopamine, followed by standard inotropes such as dobutamine and milrinone, as first-line therapy, with hormone replacement therapy for refractory cases (16,28). However, a growing number of centres (including that of the authors) favour a more physiologically rational approach, with adequate fluid resuscitation and hormonal replacement as first-line therapy (15).

Fluid therapy

As most donors are volume depleted, the first step in resuscitation is fluid replacement with crystalloid solutions. Packed red blood cell units are used to maintain adequate tissue oxygenation only if active bleeding is occurring and/or the haemoglobin concentration is less than 70 g/L. A recent study showed that a more conservative protocol of red blood cell transfusion in patients with gastrointestinal haemorrhages (threshold of 70 g/L) leads to better clinical outcomes, when compared to a more liberal approach (90 g/L) (29). Of note, patients with acute coronary syndrome, symptomatic peripheral vasculopathy, and recent stroke were excluded in this study. In patients with extremely elevated serum sodium concentration (> 155 mg/dL) due to DI, hypo-osmolar solutions (0.45% saline) can be used temporarily until specific treatment is initiated. Dextrose-based solutions should be avoided; not only can they precipitate hyperglycaemia, with consequent further osmotic diuresis, but they also tend to extravasate to the third space. It is controversial whether hydroxyethyl starch (HES) can induce renal injury and compromise renal graft function (30–32), but it is not recommended as a first-line volume expander. Additionally, HES has been shown to increase mortality and the need for renal replacement therapy in sepsis and is now not a preferred resuscitative fluid (33,34). As brain dead donors tend to become hypothermic, it is generally recommended that infused fluids should be warmed to 37°C. It is worth noting that a minimally positive fluid balance may increase rates of lung procurement in potential lung donors (16).

Hormonal replacement therapy

Hormonal replacement therapy (HRT) should be started promptly, as hormonally deficient brain dead patients tend to respond less effectively to vasopressors and fluid repletion. HRT has been shown to minimize electrocardiographic changes, acid–base abnormalities, and cardiovascular instability in brain dead patients (30,35–37). A prospective study of 19 haemodynamically unstable brain dead patients demonstrated that the addition of levothyroxine and methylprednisolone resulted in significant decreases in vasopressor requirement, with 53% of patients completely weaned off traditional pressors (38). In a large retrospective study, donors who received HRT (insulin, triiodothyronine, and vasopressin) had a 22.5% higher organ yield, with a significant increase of kidney, pancreas, heart, liver, and lung donation (39). Similarly, in a study of 4543 heart transplant

recipients, donor organs exposed to HRT have significantly less graft loss or dysfunction, with an associated 46% reduction in the odds of 30-day recipient death (40).

Metabolic abnormalities also occur as a consequence of hormone deficiency. Studies in animal models of brain death show a marked reduction in anaerobic metabolism, with decreased utilization of glucose, palmitate, and pyruvate, and consequent accumulation of lactate and free fatty acids, which were fully reversed with the administration of intravenous triiodothyronine (41). Exogenous replacement of antidiuretic hormone has been associated with higher organ yield (27,39) as well as with successful maintenance of haemodynamic stability, without impairment of graft function (30,42,43). Vasopressin also enhances vascular sensitivity to catecholamines (44), and is now recommended by the American College of Cardiology as the initial vasopressor of choice in potential organ donors (45). Vasopressin is also recommended as the standard treatment for DI even in haemodynamically stable donors (see Figure 30.1 for monitoring and titration).

It is not necessary to complete the confirmation of brain death or obtain consent for organ donation to initiate HRT, since it is the most physiological medical therapy to thwart haemodynamic instability in this patient population, and has been shown to be superior to conventional pressors. Levothyroxine is an inotrope and vasopressin has vasopressor characteristics. In centres that require two examinations, it may take on average 19 hours to declare a patient brain dead and intervening multisystem organ failure can ensue without HRT (3). The authors advocate that intensivists take an early and proactive role in initiating organ-sparing therapy, while awaiting guidance from their local organ donor network or organ procurement organization. The authors' practice is to initiate volume resuscitation in association with intravenous levothyroxine and vasopressin in hypotensive patients with suspected or confirmed brain death (15). Some centres advocate starting all four hormone replacements even in haemodynamically stable donors to achieve improved physiological stability. Recently, a prospective study comparing high doses of methylprednisolone versus a lower-dose protocol using hydrocortisone showed no differences in donor pulmonary, haemodynamic, or cardiac function and similar transplant success rates between the two groups, but a decrease in insulin requirements and improved glycaemic control in the lower-dose group (46). Clinical doses, titration, and side effects of HRT are described in Figure 30.1 and Table 30.2.

By using organ-sparing therapy, the physician is preserving the option to donate, which gives many patients' families great solace during an otherwise difficult time. It is the authors' ethical belief that if a physician chooses not to aggressively implement organ-sparing therapy (including volume resuscitation and HRT) in a potential donor, that physician is effectively allowing for organ failure and thereby limiting the family and patient's options for donation.

Vasopressors/inotropes

In patients who are hypotensive, despite generous fluid repletion and HRT, additional conventional vasopressors or inotropes may be needed. Dopamine was used in older studies and publications but despite its possible immunomodulatory effects (47) dopamine may suppress the function of the anterior pituitary gland (48). In patients with associated cardiac dysfunction, the addition of an inotrope (dobutamine, milrinone, low dose of epinephrine) is therefore recommended (Figure 30.1).

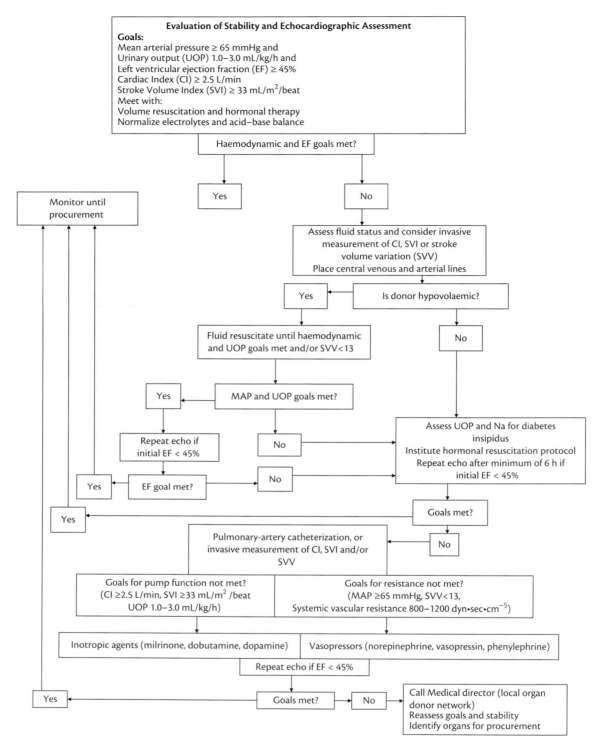

Fig. 30.1 Algorithm for management of the potential brain dead donor.

Monitoring

As with any unstable critically ill patient on the ICU, placement of a central venous catheter and arterial line to guide cardiovascular resuscitation is highly recommended for optimal donor management. Though very commonly cited in older publications, the routine use of a pulmonary artery catheter (PAC) is no longer recommended. Less invasive methods of haemodynamic monitoring, such as transpulmonary thermodilution, pulse-contour analysis,

stroke volume variation, oesophageal Doppler monitoring, and bedside transthoracic echocardiogram are now preferred. The PAC is now reserved for very exceptional cases, such as severe right ventricular dysfunction, severe pulmonary artery hypertension, congenital heart disease, and uncontrollable tachyarrhythmia.

Although there are no controlled studies identifying the monitoring goals for the optimal resuscitation of a brain dead organ donor, standardization of donor management, using well-defined

Table 30.2 Organ-sparing hormone replacement therapy

Drug	Suggested dosage	Notes
Vasopressin	0.5–6 units/h, IV	Titrate to mean arterial pressure > 65 mmHg
		Serum sodium < 155 mg/dL
		Urine specific gravity > 1.005
		Urine output 1–3 mL/kg/h
		May cause digit ischaemia
		DDAVP can be an alternative for haemodynamically stable donors with DI
Steroids	Hydrocortisone 100 mg 8-hourly IV or methylprednisolone 15 mg/kg daily, IV	Closely monitor systolic blood pressure and serum glucose during infusion
Insulin	1 unit/h, continuous intravenous infusion, titrate to maintain serum glucose 100–140 mg/dL	
Thyroxine (T4)	20 mcg T4 intravenous bolus (optional) followed by 10 mcg/h of T4 intravenous infusion, maximum dose 20 mcg/h	Bolus dosing has been associated with tachyarrhythmias
		T4 may trigger hyperkalaemia during infusion
		Consider administration of insulin and glucose solution prior to bolus
		Titrate T4 infusion to haemodynamic state (inotropic effects)

clinical parameters as resuscitation goals, has improved the transplant outcome of potential donors in some studies (30,49–51). The authors consider acceptable targets to be mean arterial pressure of at least 65 mmHg, heart rate 60–100 bpm, and urine output of 1–3 mL/kg/h. We do not routinely measure central venous pressure as it has been shown to have an extremely poor relationship with volume status (52). High requirements of vasopressors were previously considered exclusion criteria for organ donation, but a series of studies demonstrated limited or no association between intensity of vasoactive support and outcomes after transplantation (53–55). Figure 30.1 shows a suggested algorithm for haemodynamic management in brain dead donors.

Ventilator management and lung preservation

Lung preservation for donation is probably the most challenging part of the critical care management of the potential organ donor. As such, lung donation is only achieved in 15–25% of potential donors (56,57). It is particularly limited by very strict donation criteria, including PaO_2 to FiO_2 ratio (P/F ratio) of 300 or higher, bronchoalveolar lavage free of bacteria or fungus, morphologically normal bronchoscopy demonstrating no unexpected lesions or masses, and a normal chest radiograph (58). Though stringent, these criteria have been shown to predict poorly early graft outcome (59,60). Further, their relevance as criteria for lung donation has been disputed following studies demonstrating that recipients of lungs procured using extended donation criteria (e.g. infiltrates on chest radiograph, P/F ratio 300, purulent sputum on bronchoscopy, or tobacco use of > 50 packs/year) had the same clinical outcomes, including allograft dysfunction, length of ICU stay and mortality, as recipients of organs donated according to the traditional criteria (61–66). Moreover, the use of extended donation criteria resulted in more transplants and an expanded donor pool (62,63,66).

The onset of brain death can be detrimental to the lungs for several reasons. First the sympathetic surge associated with the onset of brain death can lead to significant cardiac dysfunction with consequent pulmonary oedema, as well as neurogenic pulmonary oedema secondary to extreme vasoconstriction of the pulmonary vein and increased capillary leakage. Later an inflammatory state develops, with systemic and local release of proinflammatory cytokines that has sometimes been associated with early graft failure and mortality after lung transplantation (67,68). This proinflammatory state is less common in DCD, suggesting that it is triggered by the central nervous system (69,70). Other factors, such as prolonged mechanical ventilation and associated ventilator-induced lung injury, broncho-aspiration, atelectasis, transfusion-related acute lung injury (ALI), fluid overload, and systemic inflammation, can also contribute to lung damage.

Ventilation strategies

As adequate gas exchange and good oxygenation have been used as the more important criteria for lung donation so far, many centres worldwide have adopted ventilation strategies aiming for lung recruitment using high tidal volume and high positive end-expiratory pressure (PEEP) in an attempt to increase organ procurement. An observational survey conducted in 2006 showed that the average tidal volume in brain dead donors was 9.7 mL/kg of ideal body weight, with PEEP ranging from 0 to 8 cmH_2O, and that 97% of donors had no further adjustments to ventilator settings after brain death was officially declared (71). It is well known from the sepsis and acute respiratory distress syndrome (ARDS) literature that high tidal volume ventilation exacerbates pulmonary and systemic inflammation, as well as worsening existing ALI or ARDS (72,73). Furthermore, a ventilator regimen with high tidal volumes has recently been shown to be associated with the development of ALI development in patients with traumatic brain injury (74). The seminal Acute Respiratory Distress Syndrome Network Trial demonstrated more than a decade ago that in patients with ALI/ARDS, mechanical ventilation with a lower tidal volume results in decreased mortality and increased number of days without ventilator use (30). Moreover, recent studies replicated the same findings using lung protective ventilation in patients without ALI/ARDS (75).

Improved oxygenation has not been shown to correlate with better outcome in trials in living patients with ALI/ARDS. For example, numerous trials using prone posture, nitric oxide, direct measurement of transpulmonary pressures, and recruitment manoeuvres with high levels of PEEP did not show mortality benefit, despite very successful improvement of gas exchange (76–81). Additionally, hyperoxia can be detrimental in critically ill patients (82). Improved oxygenation alone is therefore probably not the best surrogate to determine if a brain dead patient could be a potential lung donor.

A recent study corroborated the current trend of using lung protective ventilator strategies in organ donors. This study enrolled 118 patients, equally divided into a group ventilated with low tidal volumes and the other ventilated with the conventional strategies (high tidal volumes) used in brain dead patients. The percentage of patients who met lung donor eligibility was 54% in the conventional strategy group and 95% in the protective strategy group (P < 0.001). The number of patients in whom lungs were retrieved was also significantly higher in the protective strategy group, and 6-month recipient survival rates did not differ between the groups (83). The authors recommend using lung protective strategies, including limiting tidal volumes to 6 mL/kg of ideal body weight and plateau pressures equal to or less than 30 cm H_2O, in potential organ donors.

Airway pressure release ventilation (APRV) has been evaluated as an alternative ventilation mode for lung donors. Studies have demonstrated only that this method of ventilation improves oxygenation, and further donation outcomes were not analysed (84,85). The authors believe that APRV poses the same problems as high tidal volume ventilatory modes, that is, improved oxygenation but at the cost of further inflammatory damage, ventilator-induced lung injury, and haemodynamic compromise. Also, most of the haemodynamic and pulmonary benefits previously described with APRV in living patients are highly dependent on the capacity of spontaneous breaths over the high continuous pressure gradient applied (86,87), which is clearly not relevant in brain dead patients. Finally, studies comparing APRV with more traditional modes of ventilation in living patients have never demonstrated better clinical outcomes other than improved oxygenation (88–92).

Other strategies

Data exist suggesting that high-dose steroids (methylprednisolone 15 mg/kg daily) might improve oxygenation and lung procurement rates (93). Animal and human *ex vivo* studies have shown that terbutaline, a beta-adrenergic aerosol, might increase alveolar fluid clearance (94,95). A large randomized multicentre trial (the BOLD trial) is being conducted to verify the hypothesis that albuterol improves oxygenation and lung procurement rates in brain dead donors (96). Additionally, a protocol of aggressive lung management including intense chest therapy, optimal ventilator management, early bronchoscopy, and judicious fluid management has been shown to improve lung donation rates (97).

Recently, *ex vivo* lung perfusion (EVLP) has emerged as an effective tool for increasing the number of lungs accepted for transplantation. EVLP provides the opportunity to evaluate donor lungs under physiological conditions and allows optimization of these lungs for donation (98,99). Multiple small, non-randomized studies have shown that EVLP increases lung procurement and makes lungs initially rejected by traditional criteria transplantable (100–105). The

first prospective clinical trial reporting the use of *ex vivo* perfusion for the re-evaluation of high-risk donor lungs before transplantation showed promising results (101). In this study, high-risk donor lungs were defined by specific criteria, including the presence of pulmonary oedema and a P/F ratio less than 300 mmHg, and the incidence of primary graft dysfunction 72 hours after transplantation was 15% in the EVLP group and 30% in the control group (P = 0.11). There was a dramatic improvement of oxygenation in the high-risk lungs after commencement on EVLP, with a median P/F ratio increase from 335 mmHg to 414 mmHg and 443 mmHg at 1 and 4 hours of perfusion respectively (P < 0.001).

Cardiac management and preservation

A great number of donors exhibit early cardiac dysfunction after brain death, secondary to catecholamine surge (with cardiac stunning), hormone deficiency, and haemodynamic instability. An early transthoracic echocardiogram should be performed, and patients with an ejection fraction of 45% or less should be optimized with prompt treatment with levothyroxine because of its inotropic properties. Cardiac donation should not be excluded on the basis of the first ejection fraction, as a considerable number of hearts can recover left ventricular function pre or post transplantation (106,107). Some authors defend the use of PAC for better optimization of the potential donor with heart dysfunction (108,109), but no controlled trials support its use. Small studies have demonstrated that dipyridamole stress-test echocardiography can be an interesting tool to extend donor criteria in heart transplantation (110–112).

Arrhythmias are frequently seen in brain dead donors and may be highly resistant to treatment (113). Lidocaine or amiodarone are first-line treatments for ventricular arrhythmias, and amiodarone is also effective for supraventricular arrhythmias (17). In bradyarrhythmias, isoproterenol and epinephrine are preferred; atropine is usually ineffective because of vagal nucleus disruption after brain death (17).

If the patient is a potential cardiac donor, organ procurement should be expedited because prolonged intensive care is associated with a lower yield of cardiac allografts (114). Some organ procurement organizations require cardiac catheterization prior to transplant, and this should be considered an emergency procedure and expedited to maximize the possibility of cardiac transplantation.

Renal preservation

The main target for renal preservation after brain death is the avoidance of severe haemodynamic instability and subsequent acute tubular necrosis. To this end, the authors recommend maintenance of a mean arterial pressure of at least 65 mmHg and urine output of 1.0–3.0 mL/kg/h. HRT also improves donation rates and renal allograft function (39). Nephrotoxic agents, including radiological contrast agents, should be avoided if possible (115). Interestingly, some studies suggest that there is a beneficial immunomodulatory effect of catecholamines on the kidneys (47,55). As with other organs, *ex vivo* perfusion techniques, which are now commonly used, have been studied with promising results (116,117).

Other supportive care measures

Because of the complex pathophysiological changes that accompany brain death, multiple other systems require intensive support.

Diabetes insipidus

Central DI, secondary to posterior pituitary insufficiency, is observed in up to 90% of brain dead donors (118–120). It is characterized by an increased urine output (> 5 mL/kg/h for > 2 hours), hypernatraemia, low urine specific gravity (< 1.005), and increased serum osmolality (> 300 mOsm/kg) with a disproportionately low urine osmolality (< 200 mOsm/kg), denoting incapacity of the renal system to concentrate urine in response to increased serum osmolality. Volume repletion, with isotonic or modestly hypotonic solutions, is required to compensate for the loss of free water, but the standard therapy is hormone replacement with antidiuretic hormone, desmopressin, or vasopressin. Vasopressin is usually preferred as it is easier to titrate and also provides vasoactive support. The goal should be a urine output of 1–3 mL/kg/h and serum sodium of less than 150 meq/L. Serum sodium values should be checked at least every 6 hours. Potential side effects of vasopressin include hyponatraemia and severe vasoconstriction with the possibility of digital and bowel ischaemia.

Hepatic preservation

The liver is usually very resistant to ischaemic insults, but it is controversial whether hypernatraemia can be harmful. It is hypothesized that a hyperosmolar state could lead to the accumulation of idiogenic osmoles within the liver cells, with consequent intracellular water accumulation after the organ is transplanted into a recipient with normal or low serum sodium (118). Hypernatraemia was associated with a primary non-functioning graft after liver transplantation in some retrospective series (121–123), but more recent studies have not reproduced these findings (124,125). Similarly to lungs and kidneys, there is growing interest in the use of *ex vivo* perfusion devices to optimize liver donation (126–128). Liver defatting has also been recommended as an approach to facilitate steatotic liver transplantation (129,130).

Hyperglycaemia

Hyperglycaemia is often seen in brain dead donors, in part due to the development of insulin resistance (131). Hyperglycaemia can also occur secondary to catecholamine release, previously diagnosed diabetes mellitus, steroid use, and infusion of dextrose-containing fluids. It is theorized that hyperglycaemia could be detrimental to pancreatic beta cells (132). Glucose levels of greater than 11 mmol/L were associated with pancreas allograft loss in a multivariate analysis (133), so the authors strongly suggest aggressive glycaemic control (5.5–7.8 mmol/L), with early use of insulin infusions, in brain dead donors.

Coagulation

Disseminated intravascular coagulation can occur in brain dead donors, probably as a consequence of brain injury-related release of thromboplastin, cerebral gangliosides, and plasminogen (134). Although some literature has suggested coagulation goals of an international normalized ratio (INR) less than 2, and platelet count greater than 80,000/μL(16), there is no conclusive evidence available to support these goals-based data. The authors typically opt for a target INR lower than 1.5, platelet count greater than 50,000/μL, fibrinogen greater than 100 mg/dL, and normal partial thromboplastin time.

Temperature

Loss of hypothalamic regulation, associated with peripheral vasodilation and an inability to shiver, leads to thermal instability and poikilothermia (135). Hypothermia is extremely common after brain death and can result in cardiac dysfunction, arrhythmias, electrolyte abnormalities, coagulopathy, cold diuresis, pancreatitis, and a leftward shift of the oxyhaemoglobin dissociation curve. The core temperature should be maintained above 35°C, by means of the warming of replacement fluids, use of convective warming blankets, and heating of inhaled gases (16).

Donation after cardiac death

In recent years there has been increasing interest in DCD as a means of addressing the gap between the number of donor organs available and the number of patients awaiting transplantation. Before the definition of brain death in 1968 by the Ad Hoc Committee of Harvard Medical School, all organs for transplant were derived from donors who had suffered cardiopulmonary demise. However, as higher rates of successful transplantation were achieved from brain dead donors, DCD fell out of vogue and is only now being reconsidered to accommodate the growing need for donor organs. More recently, DCD usually occurs in patients on mechanical ventilation as the consequence of devastating and irreversible brain injuries, typically secondary to trauma or intracranial haemorrhage, but may also take place in those with high spinal cord injury or end-stage musculoskeletal disease who are considering withdrawal of life-sustaining therapy, and whose death is considered imminent after withdrawal or withholding of such therapy (136). It is worth mentioning that the first successfully transplanted heart in history, performed by Christiaan Barnard, was retrieved from a DCD donor (137).

Studies demonstrating that kidneys retrieved from DCD donors have the same long-term outcome as those from DND (138–140) have prompted many countries to support the development of DCD programmes (141–144). Moreover, while DCD programmes initially focused on kidney retrieval, other organs with a lower tolerance for warm ischaemia, such as the liver, pancreas, and lungs, are increasingly being retrieved and successfully transplanted (145–147). Some authors believe that, with the current advances in neurocritical care and acceptance of the notion of withdrawal of support in hopeless situations, fewer patients will evolve to brain death and that DCD will gain more importance in maintaining and improving organ procurement rates worldwide (148).

DCD is directly influenced by local legislation, difference in medical practices and resources, public attitudes, as well as religious beliefs. In the United Kingdom, Switzerland, Japan, United States, and the Netherlands, DCD accounts for a substantial proportion of donations, but is non-existent in other countries such as Germany and Portugal (140,142,149,150). In Spain, DCD accounts for 10% of all organ donation but is limited to uncontrolled DCD (see 'Controlled and uncontrolled donation after cardiac death') (142). In South America and Asia, DCD policies are currently undergoing intense debate, with the confrontation of organ shortage and cultural beliefs (151,152). Table 30.3 summarizes the characteristics and main differences of DCD protocols worldwide (148,151–167).

Despite the endorsement and support of DCD in many countries, the practice is still viewed as controversial by some, raising ethical and legal dilemmas (168–170). Some studies show that some healthcare providers remain uncomfortable with the practice (170–172), usually in centres where it is not routine or a policy is not well structured.

Table 30.3 Worldwide differences in standards for donation after cardiac death

Country	Year the programme started	Time after loss of pulse to start organ retrieval (minutes)	Procedures allowed for organ procurement	Prevailing type of donor in 2008 (Maastricht classification)	Comments
Austria	1994	10		II	1 centre, local allocation of organs
Australia	2008	2–5	Femoral arterial and venous cannulation (for perfusion with cold solution)		May need consent from coroner, discourage ECG monitoring in the OT
Belgium	1994	5	Super-rapid laparotomy with direct arterial cannulation	III	National programme
Canada	2005	5	Aorta and IVC cannulation, with *in situ* cold perfusion of the kidneys and liver with Custodiol® histidine tryptophan ketoglutarate solution		Allowed to wait up to 2 h in the OT for loss of pulse
Czech Republic	1972	10	ECMO/double balloon (one balloon infra-diaphragmatic and another infrarenal to allow flow to intra-abdominal organs only)	III	
France	2006	5	ECMO/double balloon	I	Only uncontrolled DCD, some centres
Italy	2005	20	ECMO	II	Local allocation of organs
Japan	First DCD transplant in 1956		CPR/cannulation for perfusion with cold solution	II/III	DNC only approved since 1997. Cultural resistance to brain death led to large DCD programme
Latvia	1992	15	ECMO/double balloon	III	
The Netherlands	1981	5	Super-rapid laparotomy with direct arterial cannulation	III	National programme, controlled and uncontrolled DCD
Spain	1994	5	ECMO/double balloon	I	Local allocation, uncontrolled DCD only. Legislation with presumed organ donation
Switzerland	1993	10			Local centres only
United Kingdom	1989	5	Super-rapid laparotomy with direct arterial cannulation	III	National programme with local allocation. Largest programme in Europe
United States	First kidney transplant from DCD in 1964. Policy reinforced by the IOM in 1997	5 (protocols may vary within states and hospitals)	ECMO ± double balloon femoral cannulation for perfusion with cold solution. (Protocols may vary within states and hospitals.)	III	No uncontrolled DCD. IOM and JCAHO support development of local protocols.
Countries currently discussing DCD policies	Brazil, Cyprus, Estonia, Israel, Luxembourg, Norway, Poland, Portugal, Romania, Slovak Republic, Slovenia, and Sweden China (before 2007 allowed in executed prisoners) Middle East and Gulf Region: some kidney transplants performed in Jordan with organs retrieved after cardiac death. Some Arabic countries currently discussing DCD in South Africa is limited to 1 centre (kidney transplant), and mostly from brain-dead donors who suffered a cardiac arrest. Transplant legislation approved in 2012 not clear about brain-death criteria				
Countries where DCD is forbidden by law	As of 2011 in Europe: Finland, Germany, Greece, Poland, Portugal, and Luxembourg				

CPR, cardiopulmonary resuscitation; ECG, electrocardiogram; ECMO, extracorporeal membrane oxygenation; IOM, Institute of Medicine; IVC, inferior vena cava; JCAHO, Joint Commission on Accreditation of Healthcare Organizations; OT, operating theatre.

Controlled and uncontrolled donation after cardiac death

DCD can be categorized as controlled or uncontrolled. Controlled DCD is usually seen in patients in the ICU or emergency department (ED) where a cardiac arrest is anticipated, usually after withdrawal of life support or because of severe instability in a brain dead patient. Uncontrolled DCD can occur after an unexpected cardiac arrest, death on arrival at hospital, unsuccessful resuscitation, or unexpected arrest in the ED/ICU, and it is usually limited to kidney donation in a centre capable of performing immediate *ex vivo* perfusion. The modified Maastricht classification is widely used to categorize DCD donors (173). Categories I, II, and V describe organ retrieval following unexpected and irreversible cardiac arrest, while categories III and IV refer to retrieval that follows death resulting from planned withdrawal of life support (142). Table 30.4 shows the modified Maastricht classification.

Identifying potential donors after cardiac death

Usually, patients younger than 60 years of age who are expected to die within 1 hour of withdrawal of life-sustaining therapies are potential candidates for DCD. Normally, continued ischaemia and hypoxia for more than 60 minutes would render organs unusable for donation. The justification for using 60 minutes as the time limit to pursue organ retrieval is derived from the concept of functional warm ischaemic time (WIT). This is loosely defined as the time starting when the donor's systolic blood pressure decreases to less than 50 mmHg (or 60 mmHg, depending on local criteria), arterial oxygenation drops to less than 70% (not considered in some protocols), or both, and ending when cold perfusion is started (or lung expansion in the case of the lungs) (174,175). The WIT threshold for kidney donation is normally 120 minutes, 60 minutes (time to re-inflation) for lung, and 30 minutes for liver and pancreas (142).

Reliably predicting which patients are likely to die within a 60-minute timeframe from withdrawal of life-sustaining therapy is challenging. Two numerical tools, the UNOS and the University of Wisconsin DCD tools, have been developed to identify such patients (1,175,176). Both use clinical criteria, such as apnoea when ventilatory support is withheld, the presence of vasoactive or cardiac support, age, and lung oxygenation

Table 30.4 Modified Maastricht classification of donation after cardiac death

Category	Clinical description	Type
I	Dead on arrival	Uncontrolled
II	Unsuccessful resuscitation	Uncontrolled
III	Anticipated cardiac arrest	Controlled
IV	Cardiac arrest in a brain-dead donor	Controlled
V	Unexpected arrest in ICU patient	Uncontrolled

The typification of a DCD as controlled or uncontrolled refers to the ability of the ICU/ED and transplant teams to minimize and tightly control warm ischaemic time after cardiac arrest.

This article was published in *Transplant Proceedings*, 27, 5, Kootstra G, Daemen JH, Oomen AP, 'Categories of non-heart-beating donors', pp. 2893–2894, Copyright Elsevier 1995.

Box 30.1 UNOS criteria for predicting asystole after withdrawal of life-sustaining therapy

Respiratory pattern after spontaneous breathing trial (10 minutes):
  Apnoea, RR < 8 or > 30
  Presence of LVAD
  Presence of RVAD
  V-A ECMO or V-V ECMO
  Pacemaker-unassisted heart rate < 30 bpm
  PEEP ≥ 10 cmH$_2$O and SaO$_2$ ≤ 92%
  FiO$_2$ ≥ 0.5 and SaO$_2$ ≤ 92%
  Norepinephrine or phenylephrine ≥ 0.2 mcg/kg/min
  Dopamine ≥15 mcg/kg/min
  IABP 1:1 or (dobutamine or dopamine ≥ 10 mcg/kg/min and CI ≤ 2.2)
  IABP 1:1 and CI ≤ 1.5
Number of UNOS criteria present: percentage with death < 60 minutes
  • 0: 29%
  • 1: 52%
  • 2: 65%
  • 3: 82%
  • 4–5: 76%

IABP, intra-aortic balloon pump; LVAD, left ventricular assist device; PEEP, positive end-expiratory pressure; RR, respiratory rate; RVAD, right ventricular assist device; V-A ECMO, venous-arterial extracorporeal membrane oxygenation; V-V ECMO, venous-venous extracorporeal membrane oxygenation.

---

capacity. Box 30.1 and Table 30.5 show the UNOS and Wisconsin criteria in details.

Consent and family approach

In the case of DCD, the decision to withdraw life-sustaining treatment should be made prior to, and independently, from any discussions regarding organ donation. The decision to withhold life-sustaining therapy is typically determined based on the patient's known wishes or implied wishes as best understood by the legal next of kin or designated decision-maker. Despite different legislations such decisions should always be informed by a patient-centred discussion, giving the patient and family the autonomy to decide. Adequate time should be provided to allow the family (or patient) to reach a decision, and the intensive care team should be sensitive to religious, moral, cultural, and ethical dilemmas as well as questions brought by family members. The decision regarding goals of care should be well documented by the healthcare provider and, if a decision to withdraw life sustaining measures is made, the organ donor network should be contacted. The initial approach for consent for DCD should be performed by a member of the organ donor network, to avoid any perceived conflict of interests.

Critical care management of donation after cardiac death

As with DND, the intensivist's role in managing the potential DCD donor is critical (156). The withdrawal of life-supportive therapies

Table 30.5 Wisconsin criteria for predicting asystole after withdrawal of life-sustaining therapy

Criteria	Assigned points
Spontaneous respirations after 10 min:	1
◆ rate > 12	3
◆ rate < 12	
Tidal volume > 200 mL	1
Tidal volume < 200 mL	3
Negative inspiratory force > 20 mmHg	1
Negative inspiratory force < 20 mmHg	3
No spontaneous respirations	9
Body mass index:	1
◆ < 25	2
◆ 25–29	3
◆ > 30	
Vasopressors:	1
◆ no vasopressors	2
◆ single vasopressor	3
◆ multiple vasopressors	
Patient age:	1
◆ 0–30	2
◆ 31–50	3
◆ > 51	
Intubation:	3
◆ endotracheal tube	1
◆ tracheostomy	
Oxygenation after 10 min:	1
◆ oxygen saturation > 90%	2
◆ oxygen saturation 80–89%	3
◆ oxygen saturation < 80%	

Scoring:
- ◆ 8–12 high risk for continuing to breathe after extubation
- ◆ 13–18 moderate risk for continuing to breathe after extubation
- ◆ 19–24 low risk for continuing to breathe after extubation

Reprinted with permission from Lewis, J et al., 'Development of the University of Wisconsin Donation after Cardiac Death Evaluation Tool. *Progress in Transplantation* 2003;13:265–273.

should ideally happen near to or in the operating theatre to minimize WIT. Some protocols even include prepping and draping the patient prior to extubation so that the retrieval process can be expedited once cardiopulmonary death is declared. Whichever approach is taken, the retrieval team should not be present during withdrawal of care to avoid any conflict of interests.

After terminal extubation, all subsequent care is focused on comfort measures, and the coordination of comfort care remains the responsibility of the intensive care team. Opiates are normally used to mitigate pain and respiratory distress, and benzodiazepines are commonly used for anxiolysis and sedation. Antipsychotics may be used for agitation, and anticholinergic drugs (glycopyrronium) for secretion and sputum control. The titration of medication for comfort care is the most controversial part of the DCD process. Some of

the normally used medications to ease pain and dyspnoea can also depress the respiratory drive and decrease the donor's blood pressure. The concept of 'double effect' ethically addresses the notion that medications intended for one purpose (comfort care) may shorten a patient's life and this principle clearly distinguishes palliative care from euthanasia, since the treatment is primarily intended to alleviate pain and severe discomfort not to cause death. Some providers may not be comfortable with this concept and if so, may refrain from participation in the DCD process.

Cardiopulmonary arrest is defined by the irreversible cessation of circulation and respiration. Most DCD protocols recommend waiting a minimum of 2 minutes and a maximal of 5 minutes after cessation of the pulse before the patient is declared dead, based on the observation that autoresuscitation has never been reported after 65 seconds of cardiopulmonary arrest (177). The donor may still have cardiac electrical activity, but this should be interpreted as pulseless electrical activity and does not preclude the determination of death. After the confirmation of death the patient should be rapidly transferred to the operating theatre if this was not the location of treatment withdrawal. The critical care provider may then leave the patient, and the surgical team is allowed to proceed with organ retrieval. If the donor does not expire within 60 minutes, the DCD process should be cancelled and the patient transferred back to the location of their previous care. In most centres, family members are allowed to stay with the patient until death is pronounced.

The use of medications and devices during the DCD process to optimize organ procurement is controversial. Although many centres administer heparin before the DCD process is started to minimize the risk of the development of microthrombi that might lead to further ischaemic injury (174), the use of vasodilators to improve organ perfusion (178) is not widely accepted because it could in theory precipitate death by decreasing the donor's blood pressure and offers no benefit in terms of comfort care. Pre-mortem femoral arterial and venous cannulation prior to withdrawal of life-sustaining measures to allow rapid infusion of cold preservation solutions is performed in some centres, but any procedures performed before declaration of death must be thoroughly discussed with family members and written consent obtained. Some selected centres have been using extracorporeal membrane oxygenation (ECMO) after certification of death, with improved outcomes in liver, pancreas, and kidney recipients (179–182). However, the ethical dilemma with ECMO is that minimal brain function could potentially be restored, signifying resuscitation (183). In order to mitigate against this risk, some authors suggest blocking the circulation to the central nervous system, using intravascular balloons to occlude the thoracic aorta, before ECMO is started; blood flow above the diaphragm is blocked whilst abdominal organs remain perfused with oxygenated blood (182). As with DND, *ex vivo* perfusion research is growing exponentially and is likely to expand organ procurement rates in DCD (30,99,117,184–186).

Conclusion

The persistent gap between organ donors and those awaiting transplants has stimulated an expanding role for the intensivist in the process of identifying and managing potential donors, with a trend towards a more proactive approach. The management of the donor for DND and DCD involves skills frequently dominated by the intensivist, and the lack of this specific knowledge can lead to a loss of donor potential and salvageable lives in awaiting recipients. Prompt and effective communication with the organ donor network is essential, as well as an understanding of all the steps involved in organ donation.

References

1. United Network for Organ Sharing. *Transplant Trends, 2012*. UNOS. [Online] http://www.unos.org/data

2. The Organ Procurement and Transplantation Network. *Data*. OPTN. [Online] http://optn.transplant.hrsa.gov/converge/data/

3. Lustbader D, O'Hara D, Wijdicks EF, MacLean L, Tajik W, Ying A, et al. Second brain death examination may negatively affect organ donation. *Neurology*. 2011;76(2):119–24.

4. Angelis M, Cooper JT, Freeman RB. Impact of donor infections on outcome of orthotopic liver transplantation. *Liver Transpl*. 2003;9(5):451–62.

5. Freeman RB, Giatras I, Falagas ME, Supran S, O'Connor K, Bradley J, et al. Outcome of transplantation of organs procured from bacteremic donors. *Transplantation*. 1999;68(8):1107–11.

6. Kauffman HM, McBride MA, Delmonico FL. First report of the United Network for Organ Sharing Transplant Tumor Registry: donors with a history of cancer. *Transplantation*. 2000;70(12):1747–51.

7. Myron Kauffman H, McBride MA, Cherikh WS, Spain PC, Marks WH, Roza AM. Transplant tumor registry: donor related malignancies. *Transplantation*. 2002;74(3):358–62.

8. Buell JF, Beebe TM, Trofe J, Gross TG, Alloway RR, Hanaway MJ, et al. Donor transmitted malignancies. *Ann Transplant*. 2004;9(1):53–6.

9. Gandhi MJ, Strong DM. Donor derived malignancy following transplantation: a review. *Cell Tissue Bank*. 2007;8(4):267–86.

10. Buell JF, Trofe J, Sethuraman G, Hanaway MJ, Beebe TM, Gross TG, et al. Donors with central nervous system malignancies: are they truly safe? *Transplantation*. 2003;76(2):340–3.

11. Beam E, Razonable RR. Cytomegalovirus in solid organ transplantation: epidemiology, prevention, and treatment. *Curr Infect Dis Rep*. 2012;14(6):633–41.

12. Sund F, Tufveson G, Döhler B, Opelz G, Eriksson BM. Clinical outcome with low-dose valacyclovir in high-risk renal transplant recipients: a 10-year experience. *Nephrol Dial Transplant*. 2013;28(3):758–65.

13. DeJong W, Franz HG, Wolfe SM, Nathan H, Payne D, Reitsma W, et al. Requesting organ donation: an interview study of donor and nondonor families. *Am J Crit Care*. 1998;7(1):13–23.

14. Williams MA, Lipsett PA, Rushton CH, Grochowski EC, Berkowitz ID, Mann SL, et al. The physician's role in discussing organ donation with families. *Crit Care Med*. 2003;31(5):1568–73.

15. Frontera JA, Kalb T. How I manage the adult potential organ donor: donation after neurological death (part 1). *Neurocrit Care*. 2010;12(1):103–10.

16. Wood KE, Becker BN, McCartney JG, D'Alessandro AM, Coursin DB. Care of the potential organ donor. *N Engl J Med*. 2004;351(26):2730–9.

17. Wilhelm MJ, Pratschke J, Laskowski IA, Paz DM, Tilney NL. Brain death and its impact on the donor heart-lessons from animal models. *J Heart Lung Transplant*. 2000;19(5):414–8.

18. Baroldi G, Di Pasquale G, Silver MD, Pinelli G, Lusa AM, Fineschi V. Type and extent of myocardial injury related to brain damage and its significance in heart transplantation: a morphometric study. *J Heart Lung Transplant*. 1997;16(10):994–1000.

19. Novitzky D, Horak A, Cooper DK, Rose AG. Electrocardiographic and histopathologic changes developing during experimental brain death in the baboon. *Transplant Proc*. 1989;21(1 Pt 3):2567–9.

20. Shivalkar B, Van Loon J, Wieland W, Tjandra-Maga TB, Borgers M, Plets C, et al. Variable effects of explosive or gradual increase of intracranial pressure on myocardial structure and function. *Circulation*. 1993;87(1):230–9.

21. Cooper DK. Hormonal resuscitation therapy in the management of the brain-dead potential organ donor. *Int J Surg*. 2008;6(1):3–4.

22. Novitzky D, Cooper DK, Rosendale JD, Kauffman HM. Hormonal therapy of the brain-dead organ donor: experimental and clinical studies. *Transplantation*. 2006;82(11):1396–401.

23. Pratschke J, Wilhelm MJ, Kusaka M, Beato F, Milford EL, Hancock WW, et al. Accelerated rejection of renal allografts from brain-dead donors. *Ann Surg*. 2000;232(2):263–71.

24. Nygaard CE, Townsend RN, Diamond DL. Organ donor management and organ outcome: a 6-year review from a Level I trauma center. *J Trauma*. 1990;30(6):728–32.

25. Chen JM, Cullinane S, Spanier TB, Artrip JH, John R, Edwards NM, et al. Vasopressin deficiency and pressor hypersensitivity in hemodynamically unstable organ donors. *Circulation*. 1999;100(19 Suppl):II244–6.

26. Riou B, Dreux S, Roche S, Arthaud M, Goarin JP, Léger P, et al. Circulating cardiac troponin T in potential heart transplant donors. *Circulation*. 1995;92(3):409–14.

27. Wheeldon DR, Potter CD, Oduro A, Wallwork J, Large SR. Transforming the "unacceptable" donor: outcomes from the adoption of a standardized donor management technique. *J Heart Lung Transplant*. 1995;14(4):734–42.

28. Shemie SD, Ross H, Pagliarello J, Baker AJ, Greig PD, Brand T, et al. Organ donor management in Canada: recommendations of the forum on Medical Management to Optimize Donor Organ Potential. *CMAJ*. 2006;174(6):S13–32.

29. Villanueva C, Colomo A, Bosch A, Concepción M, Hernandez-Gea V, Aracil C, et al. Transfusion strategies for acute upper gastrointestinal bleeding. *N Engl J Med*. 2013;368(1):11–21.

30. The Acute Respiratory Distress Syndrome Network. Ventilation with lower tidal volumes as compared with traditional tidal volumes for acute lung injury and the acute respiratory distress syndrome. *N Engl J Med*. 2000;342(18):1301–8.

31. Cittanova ML, Leblanc I, Legendre C, Mouquet C, Riou B, Coriat P. Effect of hydroxyethylstarch in brain-dead kidney donors on renal function in kidney-transplant recipients. *Lancet*. 1996;348(9042):1620–2.

32. Deman A, Peeters P, Sennesael J. Hydroxyethyl starch does not impair immediate renal function in kidney transplant recipients: a retrospective, multicentre analysis. *Nephrol Dial Transplant*. 1999;14(6):1517–20.

33. Myburgh JA, Finfer S, Bellomo R, Billot L, Cass A, Gattas D, et al. Hydroxyethyl starch or saline for fluid resuscitation in intensive care. *N Engl J Med*. 2012;367(20):1901–11.

34. Perner A, Haase N, Guttormsen AB, Tenhunen J, Klemenzson G, Åneman A, et al. Hydroxyethyl starch 130/0.42 versus Ringer's acetate in severe sepsis. *N Engl J Med*. 2012;367(2):124–34.

35. Novitzky D, Cooper DK. Results of hormonal therapy in human brain-dead potential organ donors. *Transplant Proc*. 1988;20(5 Suppl 7):59–62.

36. Novitzky D, Cooper DK, Human PA, Reichart B, Zuhdi N. Triiodothyronine therapy for heart donor and recipient. *J Heart Transplant*. 1988;7(5):370–6.

37. Novitzky D, Cooper DK, Reichart B. Hemodynamic and metabolic responses to hormonal therapy in brain-dead potential organ donors. *Transplantation*. 1987;43(6):852–4.

38. Salim A, Vassiliu P, Velmahos GC, Sava J, Murray JA, Belzberg H, et al. The role of thyroid hormone administration in potential organ donors. *Arch Surg*. 2001;136(12):1377–80.

39. Rosendale JD, Kauffman HM, McBride MA, Chabalewski FL, Zaroff JG, Garrity ER, et al. Aggressive pharmacologic donor management results in more transplanted organs. *Transplantation*. 2003;75(4):482–7.

40. Rosendale JD, Kauffman HM, McBride MA, Chabalewski FL, Zaroff JG, Garrity ER, et al. Hormonal resuscitation yields more transplanted hearts, with improved early function. *Transplantation*. 2003;75(8):1336–41.

41. Novitzky D, Cooper DK, Morrell D, Isaacs S. Change from aerobic to anaerobic metabolism after brain death, and reversal following triiodothyronine therapy. *Transplantation*. 1988;45(1):32–6.

42. Katz K, Lawler J, Wax J, O'Connor R, Nadkarni V. Vasopressin pressor effects in critically ill children during evaluation for brain death and organ recovery. *Resuscitation*. 2000;47(1):33–40.

43. Pennefather SH, Bullock RE, Mantle D, Dark JH. Use of low dose arginine vasopressin to support brain-dead organ donors. *Transplantation*. 1995;59(1):58–62.

44. Iwai A, Sakano T, Uenishi M, Sugimoto H, Yoshioka T, Sugimoto T. Effects of vasopressin and catecholamines on the maintenance of circulatory stability in brain-dead patients. *Transplantation*. 1989;48(4):613–7.

45. Hunt SA, Baldwin J, Baumgartner W, Bricker JT, Costanzo MR, Miller L, *et al*. Cardiovascular management of a potential heart donor: a statement from the Transplantation Committee of the American College of Cardiology. *Crit Care Med*. 1996;24(9):1599–601.

46. Dhar R, Cotton C, Coleman J, Brockmeier D, Kappel D, Marklin G, *et al*. Comparison of high- and low-dose corticosteroid regimens for organ donor management. *J Crit Care*. 2013;28(1):111 e1–7.

47. Schnuelle P, Berger S, de Boer J, Persijn G, van der Woude FJ. Effects of catecholamine application to brain-dead donors on graft survival in solid organ transplantation. *Transplantation*. 2001;72(3):455–63.

48. Debaveye YA, Van den Berghe GH. Is there still a place for dopamine in the modern intensive care unit? *Anesth Analg*. 2004;98(2):461–8.

49. Grossman MD, Reilly PM, McMahon D, Hawthorne RV, Kauder DR, Schwab CW. Who pays for failed organ procurement and what is the cost of altruism? *Transplantation*. 1996;62(12):1828–31.

50. Hagan ME, McClean D, Falcone CA, Arrington J, Matthews D, Summe C. Attaining specific donor management goals increases number of organs transplanted per donor: a quality improvement project. *Prog Transplant*. 2009;19(3):227–31.

51. Lopez-Navidad A, Caballero F. For a rational approach to the critical points of the cadaveric donation process. *Transplant Proc*. 2001;33(1-2):795–805.

52. Marik PE, Baram M, Vahid B. Does central venous pressure predict fluid responsiveness? A systematic review of the literature and the tale of seven mares. *Chest*. 2008;134(1):172–8.

53. Finfer S, Bohn D, Colpitts D, Cox P, Fleming F, Barker G. Intensive care management of paediatric organ donors and its effect on post-transplant organ function. *Intensive Care Med*. 1996;22(12):1424–32.

54. Koning OH, Ploeg RJ, van Bockel JH, Groenewegen M, van der Woude FJ, Persijn GG, *et al*. Risk factors for delayed graft function in cadaveric kidney transplantation: a prospective study of renal function and graft survival after preservation with University of Wisconsin solution in multi-organ donors. European Multicenter Study Group. *Transplantation*. 1997;63(11):1620–8.

55. Schnuelle P, Lorenz D, Mueller A, Trede M, Van Der Woude FJ. Donor catecholamine use reduces acute allograft rejection and improves graft survival after cadaveric renal transplantation. *Kidney Int*. 1999;56(2):738–46.

56. Hornby K, Ross H, Keshavjee S, Rao V, Shemie SD. Non-utilization of hearts and lungs after consent for donation: a Canadian multicentre study. *Can J Anaesth*. 2006;53(8):831–7.

57. Van Raemdonck D, Neyrinck A, Verleden GM, Dupont L, Coosemans W, Decaluwé H, *et al*. Lung donor selection and management. *Proc Am Thorac Soc*. 2009;6(1):28–38.

58. Frost AE. Donor criteria and evaluation. *Clin Chest Med*. 1997;18(2):231–7.

59. Fisher AJ, Dark JH, Corris PA. Improving donor lung evaluation: a new approach to increase organ supply for lung transplantation. *Thorax*. 1998;53(10):818–20.

60. Fisher AJ, Donnelly SC, Pritchard G, Dark JH, Corris PA. Objective assessment of criteria for selection of donor lungs suitable for transplantation. *Thorax*. 2004;59(5):434–7.

61. Aigner C, Winkler G, Jaksch P, Seebacher G, Lang G, Taghavi S, *et al*. Extended donor criteria for lung transplantation—a clinical reality. *Eur J Cardiothorac Surg*. 2005;27(5):757–61.

62. Bhorade SM, Vigneswaran W, McCabe MA, Garrity ER. Liberalization of donor criteria may expand the donor pool without adverse consequence in lung transplantation. *J Heart Lung Transplant*. 2000;19(12):1199–204.

63. Kron IL, Tribble CG, Kern JA, Daniel TM, Rose CE, Truwit JD, *et al*. Successful transplantation of marginally acceptable thoracic organs. *Ann Surg*. 1993;217(5):518–22.

64. Lardinois D, Banysch M, Korom S, Hillinger S, Rousson V, Boehler A, *et al*. Extended donor lungs: eleven years experience in a consecutive series. *Eur J Cardiothorac Surg*. 2005;27(5):762–7.

65. Schiavon M, Falcoz PE, Santelmo N, Massard G. Does the use of extended criteria donors influence early and long-term results of lung transplantation? *Interact Cardiovasc Thorac Surg*. 2012;14(2):183–7.

66. Whiting D, Banerji A, Ross D, Levine M, Shpiner R, Lackey S, *et al*. Liberalization of donor criteria in lung transplantation. *Am Surg*. 2003;69(10):909–12.

67. Fisher AJ, Donnelly SC, Hirani N, Burdick MD, Strieter RM, Dark JH, *et al*. Enhanced pulmonary inflammation in organ donors following fatal non-traumatic brain injury. *Lancet*. 1999;353(9162):1412–3.

68. Fisher AJ, Donnelly SC, Hirani N, Haslett C, Strieter RM, Dark JH, *et al*. Elevated levels of interleukin-8 in donor lungs is associated with early graft failure after lung transplantation. *Am J Respir Crit Care Med*. 2001;163(1):259–65.

69. Kang CH, Anraku M, Cypel M, Sato M, Yeung J, Gharib SA, *et al*. Transcriptional signatures in donor lungs from donation after cardiac death vs after brain death: a functional pathway analysis. *J Heart Lung Transplant*. 2011;30(3):289–98.

70. Neyrinck AP, Van De Wauwer C, Geudens N, Rega FR, Verleden GM, Wouters P, *et al*. Comparative study of donor lung injury in heart-beating versus non-heart-beating donors. *Eur J Cardiothorac Surg*. 2006;30(4):628–36.

71. Mascia L, Bosma K, Pasero D, Galli T, Cortese G, Donadio P, *et al*. Ventilatory and hemodynamic management of potential organ donors: an observational survey. *Crit Care Med*. 2006;34(2):321–7; quiz 328.

72. Ranieri VM, Suter PM, Tortorella C, De Tullio R, Dayer JM, Brienza A, *et al*. Effect of mechanical ventilation on inflammatory mediators in patients with acute respiratory distress syndrome: a randomized controlled trial. *JAMA*. 1999;282(1):54–61.

73. Tremblay L, Valenza F, Ribeiro SP, Li J, Slutsky AS. Injurious ventilatory strategies increase cytokines and c-fos m-RNA expression in an isolated rat lung model. *J Clin Invest*. 1997;99(5):944–52.

74. Mascia, L, Zavala E, Bosma K, Pasero D, Decaroli D, Andrews P, *et al*. High tidal volume is associated with the development of acute lung injury after severe brain injury: an international observational study. *Crit Care Med*. 2007;35(8):1815–20.

75. Schultz MJ, Haitsma JJ, Slutsky AS, Gajic O. What tidal volumes should be used in patients without acute lung injury? *Anesthesiology*. 2007;106(6):1226–31.

76. Brower RG, Lanken PN, MacIntyre N, Matthay MA, Morris A, Ancukiewicz M, *et al*. Higher versus lower positive end-expiratory pressures in patients with the acute respiratory distress syndrome. *N Engl J Med*. 2004;351(4):327–36.

77. Brower RG, Morris A, MacIntyre N, Matthay MA, Hayden D, Thompson T, *et al*. Effects of recruitment maneuvers in patients with acute lung injury and acute respiratory distress syndrome ventilated with high positive end-expiratory pressure. *Crit Care Med*. 2003;31(11):2592–7.

78. Guerin C, Gaillard S, Lemasson S, Ayzac L, Girard R, Beuret P, *et al*. Effects of systematic prone positioning in hypoxemic acute respiratory failure: a randomized controlled trial. *JAMA*. 2004;292(19):2379–87.

79. Meade MO, Cook DJ, Guyatt GH, Slutsky AS, Arabi YM, Cooper DJ, *et al*. Ventilation strategy using low tidal volumes, recruitment maneuvers, and high positive end-expiratory pressure for acute lung injury and acute respiratory distress syndrome: a randomized controlled trial. *JAMA*. 2008;299(6):637–45.

80. Taylor RW, Zimmerman JL, Dellinger RP, Straube RC, Criner GJ, Davis K Jr, *et al*. Low-dose inhaled nitric oxide in patients with acute lung injury: a randomized controlled trial. *JAMA*. 2004;291(13):1603–9.

81. Wheeler AP, Bernard GR, Thompson BT, Schoenfeld D, Wiedemann HP, deBoisblanc B, et al. Pulmonary-artery versus central venous catheter to guide treatment of acute lung injury. *N Engl J Med*. 2006;354(21):2213–24.

82. Martin DS, Grocott MP. Oxygen therapy in critical illness: precise control of arterial oxygenation and permissive hypoxemia. *Crit Care Med*, 2013 41(2):423–32.

83. Mascia L, Pasero D, Slutsky AS, Arguis MJ, Berardino M, Grasso S, et al. Effect of a lung protective strategy for organ donors on eligibility and availability of lungs for transplantation: a randomized controlled trial. *JAMA*. 2010;304(23):2620–7.

84. Hanna K, Seder CW, Weinberger JB, Sills PA, Hagan M, Janczyk RJ. Airway pressure release ventilation and successful lung donation. *Arch Surg*. 2011;146(3):325–8.

85. Powner DJ, Graham R. Airway pressure release ventilation during adult donor care. *Prog Transplant*. 2010;20(3):269–73.

86. Hering R, Viehöfer A, Zinserling J, Wrigge H, Kreyer S, Berg A, et al. Effects of spontaneous breathing during airway pressure release ventilation on intestinal blood flow in experimental lung injury. *Anesthesiology*. 2003;99(5):1137–44.

87. Kreyer S, Putensen C, Berg A, Soehle M, Muders T, Wrigge H, et al. Effects of spontaneous breathing during airway pressure release ventilation on cerebral and spinal cord perfusion in experimental acute lung injury. *J Neurosurg Anesthesiol*. 2010;22(4):323–9.

88. Gonzalez M, Arroliga AC, Frutos-Vivar F, Raymondos K, Esteban A, Putensen C, et al. Airway pressure release ventilation versus assist-control ventilation: a comparative propensity score and international cohort study. *Intensive Care Med*. 2010;36(5):817–27.

89. Liu L, Tanigawa K, Ota K, Tamura T, Yamaga S, Kida Y, et al. Practical use of airway pressure release ventilation for severe ARDS—a preliminary report in comparison with a conventional ventilatory support. *Hiroshima J Med Sci*. 2009;58(4):83–8.

90. Maung AA, Kaplan LJ. Airway pressure release ventilation in acute respiratory distress syndrome. *Crit Care Clin*. 2011;27(3):501–9.

91. Maung AA, Schuster KM, Kaplan LJ, Ditillo MF, Piper GL, Maerz LL, et al. Compared to conventional ventilation, airway pressure release ventilation may increase ventilator days in trauma patients. *J Trauma Acute Care Surg*. 2012;73(2):507–10.

92. Maxwell RA, Green JM, Waldrop J, Dart BW, Smith PW, Brooks D, et al. A randomized prospective trial of airway pressure release ventilation and low tidal volume ventilation in adult trauma patients with acute respiratory failure. *J Trauma*. 2010;69(3):501–10; discussion 511.

93. Follette DM, Rudich SM, Babcock WD. Improved oxygenation and increased lung donor recovery with high-dose steroid administration after brain death. *J Heart Lung Transplant*. 1998;17(4):423–9.

94. Matthay MA, Folkesson HG, Clerici C. Lung epithelial fluid transport and the resolution of pulmonary edema. *Physiol Rev*. 2002;82(3):569–600.

95. Ware LB, Fang X, Wang Y, Sakuma T, Hall TS, Matthay MA. Selected contribution: mechanisms that may stimulate the resolution of alveolar edema in the transplanted human lung. *J Appl Physiol*. 2002;93(5):1869–74.

96. Ware LB, Koyama T, Billheimer D, Landeck M, Johnson E, Brady S, et al. Advancing donor management research: design and implementation of a large, randomized, placebo-controlled trial. *Ann Intensive Care*. 2011;1(1):20.

97. Gabbay E, Williams TJ, Griffiths AP, Macfarlane LM, Kotsimbos TC, Esmore DS, et al. Maximizing the utilization of donor organs offered for lung transplantation. *Am J Respir Crit Care Med*. 1999;160(1):265–71.

98. Sanchez PG, Bittle GJ, Burdorf L, Pierson RN 3rd, Griffith BP. State of art: clinical ex vivo lung perfusion: rationale, current status, and future directions. *J Heart Lung Transplant*. 2012;31(4):339–48.

99. Sanchez PG, D'Ovidio F. Ex-vivo lung perfusion. *Curr Opin Organ Transplant*. 2012;17(5):490–5.

100. Aigner C, Slama A, Hötzenecker K, Scheed A, Urbanek B, Schmid W, et al. Clinical ex vivo lung perfusion—pushing the limits. *Am J Transplant*. 2012;12(7):1839–47.

101. Cypel M, Yeung JC, Liu M, Anraku M, Chen F, Karolak W, et al. Normothermic ex vivo lung perfusion in clinical lung transplantation. *N Engl J Med*. 2011;364(15):1431–40.

102. Cypel M, Yeung JC, Machuca T, Chen M, Singer LG, Yasufuku K, et al. Experience with the first 50 ex vivo lung perfusions in clinical transplantation. *J Thorac Cardiovasc Surg*. 2012;144(5):1200–6.

103. Wallinder A, Ricksten SE, Hansson C, Riise GC, Silverborn M, Liden H, et al. Transplantation of initially rejected donor lungs after ex vivo lung perfusion. *J Thorac Cardiovasc Surg*. 2012;144(5):1222–8.

104. Wigfield CH, Cypel M, Yeung J, Waddell T, Alex C, Johnson C, et al. Successful emergent lung transplantation after remote ex vivo perfusion optimization and transportation of donor lungs. *Am J Transplant*. 2012;12(10):2838–44.

105. Valenza F, Rosso L, Gatti S, Coppola S, Froio S, Colombo J, et al. Extracorporeal lung perfusion and ventilation to improve donor lung function and increase the number of organs available for transplantation. *Transplant Proc*. 2012;44(7):1826–9.

106. Kono T, Nishina T, Morita H, Hirota Y, Kawamura K, Fujiwara A. Usefulness of low-dose dobutamine stress echocardiography for evaluating reversibility of brain death-induced myocardial dysfunction. *Am J Cardiol*. 1999;84(5):578–82.

107. Milano A, Livi U, Casula R, Bortolotti U, Gambino A, Zenati M, et al. Influence of marginal donors on early results after heart transplantation. *Transplant Proc*. 1993;25(6):3158–9.

108. Jenkins DH, Reilly PM, McMahon DJ, Hawthorne RV. Minimizing charges associated with the determination of brain death. *Crit Care*. 1997;1(2):65–70.

109. Potter CD, Wheeldon DR, Wallwork J. Functional assessment and management of heart donors: a rationale for characterization and a guide to therapy. *J Heart Lung Transplant*. 1995;14(1 Pt 1):59–65.

110. Arpesella G, Gherardi S, Bombardini T, Picano E. Recruitment of aged donor heart with pharmacological stress echo. A case report. *Cardiovasc Ultrasound*. 2006;4:3.

111. Leone O, Gherardi S, Targa L, Pasanisi E, Mikus P, Tanganelli P, et al. Stress echocardiography as a gatekeeper to donation in aged marginal donor hearts: anatomic and pathologic correlations of abnormal stress echocardiography results. *J Heart Lung Transplant*. 2009;28(11):1141–9.

112. Stabile D, Pretagostini R, Fiaschetti P, Peritore D, Oliveti A, Gabbrielli F. Strategies to increase heart transplantation in centre-sud transplant organization. *Transplant Proc*. 2012;44(7):1835–6.

113. Power BM, Van Heerden PV. The physiological changes associated with brain death—current concepts and implications for treatment of the brain dead organ donor. *Anaesth Intensive Care*. 1995;23(1):26–36.

114. Cantin B, Kwok BW, Chan MC, Valantine HA, Oyer PE, Robbins RC, et al. The impact of brain death on survival after heart transplantation: time is of the essence. *Transplantation*. 2003;76(9):1275–9.

115. Shah VR. Aggressive management of multiorgan donor. *Transplant Proc*. 2008;40(4):1087–90.

116. Henry SD, Guarrera JV. Protective effects of hypothermic ex vivo perfusion on ischemia/reperfusion injury and transplant outcomes. *Transplant Rev (Orlando)*. 2012;26(2):163–75.

117. Hosgood SA, Nicholson ML. Normothermic kidney preservation. *Curr Opin Organ Transplant*. 2011;16(2):169–73.

118. Dictus C, Vienenkoetter B, Esmaeilzadeh M, Unterberg A, Ahmadi R. Critical care management of potential organ donors: our current standard. *Clin Transplant*. 2009;23 Suppl 21:2–9.

119. Gramm HJ, Meinhold H, Bickel U, Zimmermann J, von Hammerstein B, Keller F, et al. Acute endocrine failure after brain death? *Transplantation*. 1992;54(5):851–7.

120. Howlett TA, Keogh AM, Perry L, Touzel R, Rees LH. Anterior and posterior pituitary function in brain-stem-dead donors. A possible role for hormonal replacement therapy. *Transplantation*. 1989;47(5):828–34.

121. Gonzalez FX, Rimola A, Grande L, Antolin M, Garcia-Valdecasas JC, Fuster J, et al. Predictive factors of early postoperative graft function in human liver transplantation. *Hepatology*. 1994;20(3):565–73.

122. Totsuka E, Dodson F, Urakami A, Moras N, Ishii T, Lee MC, *et al.* Influence of high donor serum sodium levels on early postoperative graft function in human liver transplantation: effect of correction of donor hypernatremia. *Liver Transpl Surg.* 1999;5(5):421–8.

123. Avolio AW, Agnes S, Magalini SC, Foco M, Castagneto M. Importance of donor blood chemistry data (AST, serum sodium) in predicting liver transplant outcome. *Transplant Proc.* 1991;23(5):2451–2.

124. Mangus RS, Fridell JA, Vianna RM, Milgrom ML, Chestovich P, Vandenboom C, *et al.* Severe hypernatremia in deceased liver donors does not impact early transplant outcome. *Transplantation.* 2010;90(4):438–43.

125. Tector AJ, Mangus RS, Chestovich P, Vianna R, Fridell JA, Milgrom ML, *et al.* Use of extended criteria livers decreases wait time for liver transplantation without adversely impacting posttransplant survival. *Ann Surg.* 2006;244(3):439–50.

126. Bae C, Henry SD, Guarrera JV. Is extracorporeal hypothermic machine perfusion of the liver better than the 'good old icebox'? *Curr Opin Organ Transplant.* 2012;17(2):137–42.

127. Bellomo R, Suzuki S, Marino B, Starkey GK, Chambers B, Fink MA, *et al.* Normothermic extracorporeal perfusion of isolated porcine liver after warm ischaemia: a preliminary report. *Crit Care Resusc.* 2012;14(3):173–6.

128. Chung WY, Gravante G, Al-Leswas D, Alzaraa A, Sorge R, Ong SL, *et al.* The autologous normothermic ex vivo perfused porcine liver-kidney model: improving the circuit's biochemical and acid-base environment. *Am J Surg.* 2012;204(4):518–26.

129. Nativ NI, Maguire TJ, Yarmush G, Brasaemle DL, Henry SD, Guarrera JV, *et al.* Liver defatting: an alternative approach to enable steatotic liver transplantation. *Am J Transplant.* 2012;12(12):3176–83.

130. Perkins JD. Defatting the fatty liver with normothermic perfusion of the liver allograft. *Liver Transpl.* 2009;15(10):1366–7.

131. Masson F, Thicoipe M, Gin H, de Mascarel A, Angibeau RM, Favarel-Garrigues JF, *et al.* The endocrine pancreas in brain-dead donors. A prospective study in 25 patients. *Transplantation.* 1993;56(2):363–7.

132. Powner DJ. Donor care before pancreatic tissue transplantation. *Prog Transplant.* 2005;15(2):129–36.

133. Gores PF, Gillingham KJ, Dunn DL, Moudry-Munns KC, Najarian JS, Sutherland DE. Donor hyperglycemia as a minor risk factor and immunologic variables as major risk factors for pancreas allograft loss in a multivariate analysis of a single institution's experience. *Ann Surg.* 1992;215(3):217–30.

134. Hefty TR, Cotterell LW, Fraser SC, Goodnight SH, Hatch TR. Disseminated intravascular coagulation in cadaveric organ donors. Incidence and effect on renal transplantation. *Transplantation.* 1993;55(2):442–3.

135. Smith M. Physiologic changes during brain stem death—lessons for management of the organ donor. *J Heart Lung Transplant.* 2004;23(9 Suppl):S217–22.

136. Steinbrook R. Organ donation after cardiac death. *N Engl J Med.* 2007;357(3):209–13.

137. Toledo-Pereyra LH. Heart transplantation. *J Invest Surg.* 2010;23(1):1–5.

138. Akoh JA, Denton MD, Bradshaw SB, Rana TA, Walker MB. Early results of a controlled non-heart-beating kidney donor programme. *Nephrol Dial Transplant.* 2009;24(6):1992–6.

139. Summers DM, Johnson RJ, Allen J, Fuggle SV, Collett D, Watson CJ, *et al.* Analysis of factors that affect outcome after transplantation of kidneys donated after cardiac death in the UK: a cohort study. *Lancet.* 2010;376(9749):1303–11.

140. Weber M, Dindo D, Demartines N, Ambühl PM, Clavien PA. Kidney transplantation from donors without a heartbeat. *N Engl J Med.* 2002;347(4):248–55.

141. Recommendations for nonheartbeating organ donation. A position paper by the Ethics Committee, American College of Critical Care Medicine, Society of Critical Care Medicine. *Crit Care Med.* 2001;29(9):1826–31.

142. Manara AR, Murphy PG, O'Callaghan G. Donation after circulatory death. *Br J Anaesth.* 2012;108 Suppl 1:i108–21.

143. Ridley S, Bonner S, Bray K, Falvey S, Mackay J, Manara A, *et al.* UK guidance for non-heart-beating donation. *Br J Anaesth.* 2005;95(5):592–5.

144. Lamy FX, Atinault A, Thuong M. (Organ procurement in France: New challenges). *Presse Med.* 2013;42(3):295–308.

145. Muthusamy AS, Mumford L, Hudson A, Fuggle SV, Friend PJ. Pancreas transplantation from donors after circulatory death from the United Kingdom. *Am J Transplant.* 2012;12(8):2150–6.

146. White SA, Prasad KR. Liver transplantation from non-heart beating donors. *BMJ.* 2006;332(7538):376–7.

147. Wigfield CH, Love RB. Donation after cardiac death lung transplantation outcomes. *Curr Opin Organ Transplant.* 2011;16(5):462–8.

148. Dominguez-Gil B, Haase-Kromwijk B, Van Leiden H, Neuberger J, Coene L, Morel P, *et al.* Current situation of donation after circulatory death in European countries. *Transpl Int.* 2011;24(7):676–86.

149. Daemen JH, de Wit RJ, Bronkhorst MW, Yin M, Heineman E, Kootstra G. Non-heart-beating donor program contributes 40% of kidneys for transplantation. *Transplant Proc.* 1996;28(1):105–6.

150. Yoshida K, Endo T, Saito T, Iwamura M, Ikeda M, Kamata K, *et al.* Factors contributing to long graft survival in non-heart-beating cadaveric renal transplantation in Japan: a single-center study at Kitasato University. *Clin Transplant.* 2002;16(6):397–404.

151. Chaib E, Massad E. The potential impact of using donations after cardiac death on the liver transplantation program and waiting list in the state of Sao Paulo, Brazil. *Liver Transpl.* 2008;14(12):1732–6.

152. Huang J, Millis JM, Mao Y, Millis MA, Sang X, Zhong S. A pilot programme of organ donation after cardiac death in China. *Lancet.* 2012;379(9818):862–5.

153. Aita K. New organ transplant policies in Japan, including the family-oriented priority donation clause. *Transplantation.* 2011;91(5):489–91.

154. Arbour R, AlGhamdi HM, Peters L. Islam, brain death, and transplantation: culture, faith, and jurisprudence. *AACN Adv Crit Care.* 2012;23(4):381–94.

155. Faraj W, Fakih H, Mukherji D, Khalife M. Organ donation after cardiac death in the Middle East. *Transplant Proc.* 2010;42(3):713–5.

156. Frontera JA. How I manage the adult potential organ donor: donation after cardiac death (part 2). *Neurocrit Care.* 2010;12(1):111–6.

157. Hernandez-Alejandro R, Caumartin Y, Chent C, Levstik MA, Quan D, Muirhead N, *et al.* Kidney and liver transplants from donors after cardiac death: initial experience at the London Health Sciences Centre. *Can J Surg.* 2010;53(2):93–102.

158. McQuoid-Mason D. Human tissue and organ transplant provisions: chapter 8 of the National Health Act and its Regulations, in effect from March 2012—what doctors must know. *S Afr Med J.* 2012;102(9):733–5.

159. Mizraji R, Alvarez I, Palacios RI, Fajardo C, Berrios C, Morales F, Luna E, *et al.* Organ donation in Latin America. *Transplant Proc.* 2007;39(2):333–5.

160. Muller EM, Barday Z, McCurdie F, Kahn D. Deceased donor organ transplantation: A single center experience from Cape Town, South Africa. *Indian J Nephrol.* 2012;22(2):86–7.

161. Oto T. Lung transplantation from donation after cardiac death (non-heart-beating) donors. *Gen Thorac Cardiovasc Surg.* 2008;56(11):533–8.

162. Quigley M, Wright L, Ravitsky V. Organ donation and priority points in Israel: an ethical analysis. *Transplantation.* 2012;93(10):970–3.

163. Roberts KJ, Bramhall S, Mayer D, Muiesan P. Uncontrolled organ donation following prehospital cardiac arrest: a potential solution to the shortage of organ donors in the United Kingdom? *Transpl Int.* 2011;24(5):477–81.

164. Yoshimura N, Okajima H, Ushigome H, Sakamoto S, Fujiki M, Okamoto M. Current status of organ transplantation in Japan and worldwide. *Surg Today.* 2010;40(6):514–25.

165. Organ and Tissue Authority. *DonateLife Network, Australia.* [Online] http://www.donatelife.gov.au

166. Institute of Medicine. *Non-Heart-Beating Organ Transplantation: Practice and Protocols.* Washington, DC: National Academy Press; 2000.

167. Starzl TE, Marchioro TL, Brittain RS, Holmes JH, Waddell WR. Problems in renal homotransplantation. *JAMA.* 1964;187:734–40.

168. Bell MD. Non-heart beating organ donation: old procurement strategy—new ethical problems. *J Med Ethics.* 2003;29(3):176–81.

169. Gardiner D, Riley B. Non-heart-beating organ donation—solution or a step too far? *Anaesthesia.* 2007;62(5):431–3.

170. Motta ED. The ethics of heparin administration to the potential non-heart-beating organ donor. *J Prof Nurs.* 2005;21(2):97–102.

171. DuBois JM, Anderson EE. Attitudes toward death criteria and organ donation among healthcare personnel and the general public. *Prog Transplant.* 2006;16(1):65–73.

172. St Ledger U, Begley A, Reid J, Prior L, McAuley D, Blackwood B. Moral distress in end-of-life care in the intensive care unit. *J Adv Nurs.* 2013;69(8):1869–80.

173. Kootstra G, Daemen JH, Oomen AP. Categories of non-heart-beating donors. *Transplant Proc.* 1995;27(5):2893–4.

174. Bernat JL, D'Alessandro AM, Port FK, Bleck TP, Heard SO, Medina J, *et al.* Report of a National Conference on Donation after cardiac death. *Am J Transplant.* 2006;6(2):281–91.

175. DeVita MA, Brooks MM, Zawistowski C, Rudich S, Daly B, Chaitin E. Donors after cardiac death: validation of identification criteria (DVIC) study for predictors of rapid death. *Am J Transplant.* 2008;8(2):432–41.

176. Lewis J, Peltier J, Nelson H, Snyder W, Schneider K, Steinberger D, Anderson M, *et al.* Development of the University of Wisconsin donation After Cardiac Death Evaluation Tool. *Prog Transplant.* 2003;13(4):265–73.

177. Bernat JL. Point: are donors after circulatory death really dead, and does it matter? Yes and yes. *Chest.* 2010;138(1):13–6.

178. Polyak MM, Arrington BO, Kapur S, Stubenbord WT, Kinkhabwala M. Donor treatment with phentolamine mesylate improves machine preservation dynamics and early renal allograft function. *Transplantation.* 2000;69(1):184–6.

179. Fondevila C, Hessheimer AJ, Ruiz A, Calatayud D, Ferrer J, Charco R, *et al.* Liver transplant using donors after unexpected cardiac death: novel preservation protocol and acceptance criteria. *Am J Transplant.* 2007;7(7):1849–55.

180. Gravel MT, Arenas JD, Chenault R 2nd, Magee JC, Rudich S, Maraschio M, *et al.* Kidney transplantation from organ donors following cardiopulmonary death using extracorporeal membrane oxygenation support. *Ann Transplant.* 2004;9(1):57–8.

181. Ko WJ, Chen YS, Tsai PR, Lee PH. Extracorporeal membrane oxygenation support of donor abdominal organs in non-heart-beating donors. *Clin Transplant.* 2000;14(2):152–6.

182. Magliocca JF, Magee JC, Rowe SA, Gravel MT, Chenault RH 2nd, Merion RM, *et al.* Extracorporeal support for organ donation after cardiac death effectively expands the donor pool. *J Trauma.* 2005;58(6):1095–101.

183. Bernat JL. The boundaries of organ donation after circulatory death. *N Engl J Med.* 2008;359(7):669–71.

184. Fondevila C, Hessheimer AJ, Maathuis MH, Muñoz J, Taurá P, Calatayud D, *et al.* Superior preservation of DCD livers with continuous normothermic perfusion. *Ann Surg.* 2011;254(6):1000–7.

185. Nakajima D, Chen F, Yamada T, Sakamoto J, Ohsumi A, Bando T, *et al.* Reconditioning of lungs donated after circulatory death with normothermic ex vivo lung perfusion. *J Heart Lung Transplant.* 2012;31(2):187–93.

186. Sanchez PG, Bittle GJ, Williams K, Pasrija C, Xu K, Wei X, *et al.* Ex vivo lung evaluation of prearrest heparinization in donation after cardiac death. *Ann Surg,* 2013;257(3):534–41.

CHAPTER 31

Outcome after neurointensive care

Lakshmi P. Chelluri and Jayaram Chelluri

In the past few decades there has been increasing provision of specialized neurological critical care units following evidence that outcomes are better when patients are managed in units focused on providing care for critically ill neurological patients (see Chapter 1) (1,2). Although mortality and functional status after critical illness in general are well studied, outcomes after neuro-critical care are less so. This chapter will review the outcome of patients receiving care in a neurocritical care unit (NCCU) and focus on the following:

◆ General and disease-specific risk adjustment models in intensive care

◆ Risk factors, mortality, and long-term outcomes after neurocritical care

◆ Mechanical ventilation and outcome in patients with neurological injury

◆ Quality of life (QOL) in patients surviving neurological injury after intensive care, and caregiver needs and burdens.

General risk adjustment models

Risk adjustment models are designed to allow outcome assessment in patients with different levels of illness severity (3–9). The Acute Physiology And Chronic Health Evaluation (APACHE), Mortality Prediction Model (MPM), Severity of Illness And Physiology Score (SAPS), Sequential Organ Failure Score (SOFA), and Multiple Organ Dysfunction Score (MODS) are the major models used in general intensive care. One of the initial goals of such models was to apply their prognostications to guide bedside decision-making but the accuracy of such predictions has proved inadequate for this purpose. However, the models are useful for risk adjustment in research and for comparing performance between different intensive care units (ICUs) for quality assessment and administrative purposes. Although use of risk-adjusted outcomes may identify areas for improvement in individual ICUs, the models do not capture some of the important factors impacting performance such as care prior to NCCU or hospital admission, limitations of life-sustaining therapy, and early transfers to other clinical areas or nursing homes.

Accurate data collection for model input, data acquisition from diverse ICU diagnoses, and model recalibration based on validated outcomes are crucial for maximizing the utility of risk adjustment models. The differences and reliability of the various models depend on model development and case-mix. Thus general risk adjustment models are not applicable to patients with specific diseases or to ICUs focusing on the management of such patients either because the sample sizes are inadequate or the models have not been validated for the specific disease population. Model development and validation has been comprehensively reviewed by Iezzoni in *Risk Adjustment for Measuring Health Outcomes* (10).

Model performance is primarily evaluated by discrimination and calibration with regard to expected and observed outcomes. Discrimination evaluates a binary outcome (e.g. mortality) by calculating model sensitivity and specificity, plotting specificity and 1 – specificity, and calculating the area under the receiver-operating characteristic (AUROC) curve. Good model performance is indicated by an AUROC greater than 0.8. Calibration measures model performance over a range of probabilities, usually arranged in ascending deciles. The Hosmer–Lemeshow goodness-of-fit test is the most commonly used method of assessing calibration. In this, a chi-square is calculated for each decile and overall, and a P value greater than 0.05 is considered adequate model performance indicating that there is no significant difference between expected and observed outcomes (11).

Key aspects of APACHE, MPM, and SAPS are discussed below and are summarized in Table 31.1 (5–7).

Acute physiology and chronic health evaluation

APACHE was developed by Knaus et al., and has been revised four times (APACHE I–IV) over the last 30 years (3,5). It is the most commonly used risk adjustment model and has two components—acute physiology and chronic health evaluation scores. The physiology score includes variables reflecting pulmonary, cardiac, renal, and neurological function, the latter assessed by the Glasgow Coma Scale (GCS). Because some of the variables in the GCS are affected by sedation and intubation, there can be substantial variation in the GCS input to the model and therefore in the resulting APACHE score calculated. APACHE IV, the latest version, includes mechanical ventilation, inability to assess GCS, and initiation of thrombolytic therapy for acute myocardial infarction as additional predictor variables. Acute physiology score, disease group, and age are variables with most explanatory power in prediction using APACHE. The APACHE IV model performs well, with an AUROC of 0.88 and Hosmer–Lemeshow chi-square of 16.8 (P = 0.8) (5).

Table 31.1 Comparison of three risk adjustment models—Acute Physiology And Chronic Health Evaluation (APACHE), Mortality Prediction Model (MPM), and Severity of illness And Physiology Score (SAPS)

	APACHE IV	MPM III	SAPS III
Population	USA	USA	35 countries; mostly European
Time of data collection	First 24 hours in ICU	1st hour in ICU	1st hour in ICU
Total number of variables	142	16	20
Physiological variables	17	3	10
Model development—variable selection	Expert	Statistical	Expert
Outcome	Mortality—ICU/hospital	Mortality—ICU/hospital	Mortality—hospital
	Length of stay—ICU/hospital		
Data collection burden (4) (minutes)	37.3 (less if data collection is automated)	11.1	19.6
ROC (discrimination)	0.88	0.823	0.848
Hosmer–Lemeshaw C statistic (calibration)	16.9 P = 0.08	11.62 P = 0.31	10.56 P = 0.39
Missing data (assumption)	Normal	Normal	Normal

Data from various sources (see References).

Mortality prediction model

The MPM is a statistically driven model that has been revised three times (MPM I–III) (3,6). The model was based on a North American patient population and the variables include physiology (coma/deep stupor, heart rate > 150/min, systolic blood pressure ≤ 90 mmHg), chronic diagnoses (chronic renal insufficiency, cirrhosis, metastatic neoplasm), acute diagnoses (acute kidney injury, cardiac dysrhythmia, cerebrovascular incident, gastrointestinal bleed, intracranial mass effect) and other factors (age, cardiopulmonary resuscitation, mechanical ventilation within 1 hour of admission, resuscitation status, medical or unscheduled surgical admission). MPM III performs adequately with an AUROC of 0.823 and Hosmer–Lemeshow chi-square of 11.62 (P = 0.31) (6).

Severity of illness and physiology score

The SAPS is a model developed in Europe that has been revised three times (SAPS 1–3) (3,7). Its constituent variables include renal, cardiac, and pulmonary function, white blood cell count, GCS score, bilirubin, and temperature, recorded within 1 hour of ICU admission and reflect acute physiological derangements. The outcome variable of interest is hospital survival. SAPS 3 has an AUROC of 0.848 and Hossemer–Lemeshow chi-square 14.29 (P = 0.16) (7).

Sequential organ failure score and multiple organ dysfunction score

The SOFA and MODS are designed to evaluate hospital outcome based on organ dysfunction over time and include respiratory, circulatory, coagulation, hepatic, neurological, and renal function variables. Both assess increasing weights of derangement from normal. They are useful in monitoring organ dysfunction but their predictive accuracy is lower than more general risk adjustment models.

SOFA and MODS have not been evaluated in patient populations with different case-mix indexes, and this limits their utility (8,9).

Neurological disease-specific risk adjustment models

General risk adjustment models do not perform well in patients with specific diseases, including neurological disease. They were created from heterogonous case mixes and do not have adequate samples of patients with specific diseases, such as traumatic brain injury (TBI), to develop disease specific models. There are, however, many neurological-specific risk adjustment models including those for TBI, subarachnoid haemorrhage (SAH), intracerebral haemorrhage (ICH), and acute ischaemic stroke (AIS). Some, such as the GCS and the Hunt and Hess Scale and World Federation of Neurologic Societies scale for SAH, precede the development of general risk adjustment models.

Neurological-specific models include clinical, radiological, and laboratory data and, similar to general models, are useful for making group predictions and research studies, but insufficiently accurate to guide individual decision-making. Some disease-specific models include patients with mild or moderate disease who do not require admission to an ICU, so the predicted mortality and functional outcomes may not be similar to those reported in studies of patients admitted to an NCCU. These prognostic models/scores have specific advantages and limitations, and inadequate validation in external samples limits their widespread use.

Traumatic brain injury

TBI is a major cause of mortality and morbidity worldwide, particularly in young males. Mortality after TBI increases with age and, although many patients regain their pre-injury functional status, others develop significant cognitive and functional deficits (12).

Several models have been developed to aid prognostication after TBI.

Glasgow Coma Scale and extended Glasgow Coma Scale

The GCS and extended GCS evaluate neurological function after injury (13). They have three components (eye opening, verbal response, and motor response) and a minimum score of 3 and maximum score of 15. A higher score indicates better neurological status and predicted outcome (see Chapter 26). The extended GCS includes an assessment of post-traumatic amnesia (PTA) and its duration (14). As the GCS has a ceiling effect (at 15) and does not identify patients with mild neurological injury and long-term effects, the inclusion of PTA provides an assessment of cognitive dysfunction post injury. Inability to adequately evaluate verbal response and motor response in patients who are intubated or sedated is a limitation of GCS.

Full Outline of UnResponsiveness Score

The Full Outline of UnResponsiveness (FOUR) score was developed to address the shortcomings of the GCS, particularly with respect to the verbal component which is difficult to assess in sedated or intubated patients. The components of the FOUR score are brainstem reflexes, eye response, motor response, breathing pattern, and respiratory drive (see Chapter 26). The score ranges from 0 to 16 with a higher score predictive of better outcome. Iyer and colleagues evaluated the FOUR score in a group of medical ICU patients and reported good inter-rater reliability (15). Performance of the model to predict hospital mortality and neurological outcome is also good, with AUROC for in-hospital mortality and poor neurological outcome (Rankin score 3–6) of 0.86 and 0.75 respectively.

Corticosteroid Randomization after Significant Head injury model

The Corticosteroid Randomization after Significant Head injury (CRASH) model was developed from a multinational study of TBI in patients with a GCS score of 14 or less (16). Clinical (age, GCS score, pupillary reaction, and major extracranial trauma) and radiological (petechial haemorrhages, obliteration of third ventricle, SAH, midline shift, and non-evacuated haematoma) variables at admission were included in the model, and mortality was assessed at 14 days and disability at 6 months after injury. Discrimination is good for mortality and functional outcomes, and calibration is also good. However, there are differences in model prediction between high- and low-income countries. The CRASH model calculator is available at http://www.trialscoordinatingcentre.lshtm.ac.uk/Risk%20calculator/index.html.

International Mission for Prognosis and Analysis of Clinical Trials in TBI model

The International Mission for Prognosis and Analysis of Clinical Trials in TBI (IMPACT) model was developed from data collected from 11 studies of moderate and severe TBI in patients with a GCS score less than 12 (17). Clinical (age, motor component of GCS, pupillary reaction hypoxia, and hypotension), radiological (traumatic SAH and epidural haematoma) and laboratory values (haemoglobin and blood glucose) were included, and outcomes assessed at 6 months. Three models were created incorporating increasing number of variables and complexity. The basic model, which includes only age, GCS motor score, and pupillary reaction, has an AUROC of 0.66 and 0.84 for the construction and validation data sets respectively. Inclusion of radiological and laboratory

data, generating the extended and lab models respectively, slightly improve the performance. The IMPACT model under-predicts poor outcomes in both high- and low-income countries, but less so in high-income countries (18). The IMPACT calculator is available at http://www.tbi-impact.org/?p=impact/calc.

Risk Adjustment In Neurocritical Care

The Risk Adjustment In Neurocritical Care (RAIN) study externally validated three established risk adjustment models—the CRASH (16) and IMPACT (17) databases and the study by Hukkelhoven and colleagues (19). The RAIN study included 3221 TBI patients with GCS score less than 15 admitted to participating critical care units in the United Kingdom (20). Actual mortality at 6 months was 26%, 30% of survivors had moderate disability at 6 months, and 26% were independent, but the models under-predicted unfavourable outcome. RAIN also compared treatment in dedicated NCCUs with treatment in combined NCCU/general ICUs. Six-month mortality was similar in both types of unit but functional outcome was slightly better in patients managed in specialized NCCUs.

Tasaki prognostic indicators and outcome prediction model

Tasaki et al. also reported outcomes and a risk adjustment model in patients with severe TBI (GCS score < 9) (21). Prediction variables were age, pupillary light reflex, traumatic SAH, midline shift, and increased intracranial pressure (ICP), and the outcome variables were mortality and Glasgow outcome score (GOS) at 6 months. AUROC was 0.977 and the Hosmer–Lemeshow goodness-of-fit 0.86. However, the sample size is this study was small, and the model has not been externally validated.

Subarachnoid haemorrhage

Hunt and Hess developed a grading scale for SAH based on clinical criteria at the time of admission (22). It is commonly used with other clinical and radiological criteria to assess SAH severity, but the subjectivity in assessing grades 1 and 2 is one of the limitations of the Hunt and Hess score. In 1988, the World Federation of Neurologic Surgeons (WFNS) developed another scale to assess SAH severity, and this was modified by Rosen and colleagues who added clinical factors—age, history of hypertension, systolic blood pressure at the time of admission, aneurysm size/location, thickness of blood clot, and vasospasm (23–25). Although the modified scale performs slightly better than the standard WFNS scale, it is more complex and therefore more difficult to use. Oshiro et al. compared the ability of the Hunt and Hess, WFNS and GCS scales to predict mortality, length of hospital stay and GOS, and found the Hunt and Hess scale to be the best predictor of mortality and GCS of GOS (23). A literature review of prediction models after SAH concluded that the Hunt and Hess and WFNS scales are not reliable because of poor inter- and intra-rater reliability (26). Intracerebral haemorrhage, fever, and vasospasm are also reported to be independent predictors of both mortality and disability after SAH (27–29).

Intracerebral haemorrhage

Clinical (age, GCS score, and resuscitation status) and radiological (haemorrhage volume, location, and ventricular extension) are risk factors for mortality after ICH. A 'do not resuscitate' order in the first 48 hours after ICH has also been reported to be a crucial factor in determining outcome, with multiple authors expressing concern about a 'self-fulfilling prophecy' for increased mortality because of a potentially unreliable prediction of poor outcome and avoidance of aggressive therapy early after the ictus (30,31).

ICH score

Hemphill and colleagues developed an ICH score which includes GCS, ICH volume (≤ 30 mL or > 30 mL), intraventricular haemorrhage (yes/no), infratentorial haemorrhage location (yes/no), and age up to and including 80 or older than 80 years (32). The score ranges from 0 to 6 and a higher score indicates increased severity of ICH. Calibration is good and the score has been validated in an external sample (33).

FUNC score

The FUNC score is a functional outcome risk stratification scale developed to predict mortality and functional status after ICH (34). FUNC is an 11-point score and includes age, ICH location and volume, GCS score, and the presence of pre-ICH cognitive impairment as predictor variables. Survival at 90 days and functional neurological status at discharge are outcome variables, and a score of 4 or less is associated with poor outcome. In one study, a FUNC score of 4 or less in patients with supratentorial ICH was associated with a 100% incidence of poor outcome (35). The FUNC score calculator can be found at http://www2.massgeneral.org/stopstroke/funcCalculator.aspx.

Acute ischaemic stroke (AIS)

The National Institutes of Health Stroke Scale (NIHSS) is the most commonly used scale to predict outcome after AIS. NIHSS is a 15-item scale with a score ranging from 0 to 42, with a higher score indicating worse neurological function. In a study of 373 patients, Muir et al. evaluated the prediction of outcomes at 2, 3, 6, and 12 months after AIS using NIHSS, and reported accuracy, sensitivity and specificity for poor outcome (care in a nursing home or death) of 0.83, 0.71, and 0.9 respectively (36). A cut off of NIHSS 13 at baseline discriminated outcomes well. Adams developed a model based on NIHSS using data from Trial of Org 10172 in Acute Stroke Treatment (TOAST) based on outcomes defined as GOS and Barthel Index (BI) at 7 days and 3 months (37). An NIHSS score of less than 3 at 7 days after AIS was predictive of good outcome, and a score of greater than 15 at 3 months was predictive of poor outcome. Using a German stroke database, Weimar and colleagues developed a model to predict disability at 100 days after AIS (38). Age, lower extremity paresis, NIHSS score, gender, history of stroke, diabetes, fever, and complications were identified as risk factors. This model correctly predicted functional status in 80.7% of cases and mortality in 90.4%. Ntaios and colleagues developed the ASTRAL (Age, Severity, onset to admission Time, Range of visual fields, Acute glucose and Level of consciousness) score to predict poor outcome at 3 months after AIS (39). AUROC was 0.85 and the model performed well in derivation and validation samples. A clinical score, the A^2DS^2 (Age > 75 years, Atrial fibrillation; Dysphagia; male Sex, Stroke severity) score, was developed by Hoffman et al. to predict the development of pneumonia after AIS and has good discrimination and calibration (40).

Neurocritical care and outcome

The increasing trend towards the management of critically ill neurological patients in specialized NCCUs has been driven by positive evaluations of such specialty delivered care on outcome (41–55).

Although there are follow-up studies evaluating outcomes in specific diseases such as AIS, TBI, and SAH, there are only a few evaluating outcomes of NCCU patient populations overall (Table 31.2). Kramer reviewed studies comparing the impact of specialized NCCU provision and found a positive impact on mortality and favourable outcomes (41).

Impact of neurocritical care teams

In an observational study, Veralas et al. evaluated outcome in a semi-closed NCCU before and after the introduction of a dedicated and specialized neurocritical care team (46). There was a 42% reduction in the risk of death in the initial 3 days after NCCU admission and a decrease in unadjusted length of stay (LOS) following the introduction of the team. There was also an increase in the number of patients discharged home and associated reduction in discharges to a nursing home. In another study, the outcome of patients with ICH admitted to a neuroscience or a general ICU was assessed, and the risk of in-hospital death was higher in a general compared to a specialist unit (47). The presence of an intensivist in both types of unit was associated with lower mortality but, in this study, LOS was higher in patients managed in an NCCU. Importantly, the decreased LOS after the introduction of specialized neurocritical care teams occurred without a change in the number of readmissions (48). In a study of 1155 patients admitted to an NCCU, more than half of whom had a diagnosis of SAH, ICH, or AIS, the overall ICU mortality was 18%, with admission severity of illness being the primary prognostic factor (49). Other outcome predictors included admission diagnosis, age, and ICU LOS.

These observational studies indicate that hospital outcomes are improved when critically ill neurological patients are cared for in an NCCU by a dedicated neurocritical care team, although some reported higher resource use (50,51). Long-term outcome benefits, including QOL and interventions to improve QOL, require further evaluation in prospective studies.

Mechanical ventilation and tracheal extubation

Mechanical ventilation is a common intervention in the NCCU, and weaning and extubation attempts are often complicated and sometimes delayed because of the patient's neurological status (see Chapter 4). Table 31.3 summarizes the available data on outcomes after mechanical ventilation and factors influencing extubation decision in neurological patients (56–63).

In a prospective cohort study, Coplin and colleagues investigated the impact of extubation delay in brain-injured patients meeting standard weaning criteria (56). Neurological function, haemodynamic status, arterial oxygenation, ventilator mechanics, and absence of specific indications for continued support (e.g. scheduled surgery), were reviewed daily and used to determine readiness for extubation. Ninety nine of 136 patients (73%) were extubated within 48 hours of meeting the defined readiness criteria, whereas extubation was delayed beyond 48 hours in 37 (27%) because of concerns over neurological status. Patients with delayed extubation had a higher incidence of pneumonia (38% versus 21%), longer ICU and hospital LOS and mortality, and higher hospitals costs, but reintubation rate was similar in the two groups. The need for airway care was evaluated daily using a six-part semi-quantitative airway care score (ACS) based on assessment of spontaneous cough, gag, suctioning frequency, and sputum quantity, character, and viscosity. Although higher ACS, indicating poorer airway function, was

Table 31.2 Summary of selected studies of outcome after neurocritical care

Authors	Primary diagnosis	Intervention/ comparison	Age (years, mean)	LOS (days, mean)	Outcome (%)	Risk factors
Mirski et al. (45)	ICH	General ICU vs neuro ICU	62.8 vs 65.7		Mortality (36% vs 19%) Discharge home (48% vs 69%)	Large bleed, Intraventricular extension, brain stem haemorrhage
Varelas et al. (46)	Head trauma (30%), tumour (18%), spine injury (14%), SAH/ICH (25%)	Before and after introduction of neurointensivist	51.8 vs 51.6	ICU: 3.5 vs 2.9 Hospital: 7.9 vs 7.32	Hospital mortality (10.1% vs 9.1%) Increased discharges to home and decreased discharges to nursing home after introduction of neurointensivist	
Diringer et al. (47)	ICH	General ICU vs neuro ICU	62.6 vs 56	ICU: 4.5 vs 7.8 Hospital: 11.4 vs 15.5	Lower mortality in patients with admission to neuro ICU	GCS, age, full time intensivist, neuro ICU
Suarez et al. (48)	Acute ischaemic stroke, ICH/SAH, trauma, neoplasm	No neuro team vs Neuro team	59.3 vs 60.2	Hospital Neurosurgical: 9.8 vs 8.4 Neurological: 10 vs 8.4	Mortality ICU (5.2 vs 4.3%) Hospital (10.6% vs 8.0%)	Gender, APACHE III, disability prior to admission, admission from another ICU
Broessner et al. (49)	SAH, ICH, stroke		55	ICU 9.1	ICU mortality (18%)	Admission diagnosis, age, TISS 28, LOS
Ziai et al. (50)	Postoperative brain tumour surgery	LOS in NCCU ≤ 24 h vs > 24 h	49 vs 52	NCCU: 1 vs 6 Hospital: 7 vs 15	Hospital mortality (0% vs 4%) Discharged home (93% vs 52%)	Mechanical ventilation, Intraoperative factors
Diringer et al. (51)	ICH, ischaemic stroke, trauma	Effect of fever on outcome No fever vs > 39°C	58 vs 53	ICU: 1.7 vs 11.9	Hospital mortality (9.1% vs 28.7%)	complications higher in patients with fever > 39° C compared to no fever
Flores-Cordero et al. (52)	Community-acquired bacterial meningitis		45.5	ICU/Hospital: 4/17 (median)	Hospital mortality (10.9%)	APACHE II score
Kiphuth et al. (53)	Neuro ICU 61.4% on MV		67	Median ICU 4 MV duration 3	Hospital mortality (27.7% 1 year 45%) Good functional recovery: 28.4%	Admission diagnosis, day 1 TISS 28, age, MV duration
Varelas et al. (54)	Status epileptics, management in neuro vs MICU	NICU 46 MICU 122	NICU 58.3 vs MICU 51.5			No difference in mortality, length of stay and mRS Increased continuous EEG monitoring in NICU
Golestanian et al. (55)	31,000 patients with ischaemic stroke	26% admitted to ICU	80.7	Hospital 7.3	1 month: 21% 1 year: 40%	PEG, MV, aspiration; ICU admission plus MV—5-fold increase in mortality

Data from various sources (see References).

Table 31.3 Summary of selected studies of neuro patients requiring mechanical ventilation and outcomes

Author	Diagnoses	Intervention	Age (years, mean)	Duration of MV (days, mean)	LOS (days, mean)	Outcome (%)	Risk factors/comments
Coplin et al., 2000 (56)	TBI, ICH, AIS	No delay in extubation vs Delay because of concern for neurological dysfunction	42 vs 53		ICU: 3 vs 8 Hospital: 11 vs 17	Hospital mortality (12 vs 27)	Standard weaning criteria are adequate for extubation success
Namen et al., 2001 (57)	TBI, SAH, ICH	Routine care vs ventilator management protocol	64 vs 55	6 vs 6	ICU: 14 vs 15 Hospital: 32 vs 40	Hospital mortality (31 vs 41)	GCS > 8, ratio of PaO_2 and FiO_2
Navalesi et al., 2008 (58)	SAH, TBI, brain tumour	Routine care vs weaning protocol	50 vs 50	5 vs 5	ICU: 8.8/8.1	ICU mortality: 1 vs 4	Higher SAPS II and inclusion in control group increased reintubation rate
Malmivaara et al., 2009 (60)	SAH/ ICH,TBI, SDH, tumour	None	Median 58		ICU: 5 Hospital: 14	Mortality 30 days: 27 1 year: 45 5 years: 59	
Pelosi et al., 2011 (61)	ICH AIS TBI	None	60 64 46	5 4 6	Hospital: 11 13 16	Hospital mortality: 53 45 33	Stroke, GCS on day 1, severity of illness
Karanjia et al., 2011 (62)	Neuro ICU and received MV	None	56		ICU 7		Successfully extubation 67% Reintubation 6.1% Tracheostomy 14% Extubation for comfort 23% care
Roquilly et al., 2013 (59)	Neuro ICU and received MV	Evidence-based weaning bundle. Comparison of pre and post implementation		Pre 14.9 Post 12.6 P = 0.02	ICU Pre 20 Post 18 P = 0.48	90-day mortality Pre 28.4 Post 23.5 P = 0.22	Decrease in MV duration and ventilator-free days and unplanned extubation

AIS, acute ischaemic stroke; ICH, intracerebral haemorrhage; MV, mechanical ventilation; SAH, subarachnoid haemorrhage; SDH, subdural haematoma; TBI, traumatic brain injury.

Data from various sources (see References).

associated with extubation delay, many patients were extubated without delay despite poor markers of airway function and clearance. This study suggests that there is no justification for delaying extubation in patients in whom the only indication for continued intubation is a depressed level of consciousness and that timely extubation of brain-injured patients who meet standard weaning criteria is associated with a lower incidence of pneumonia.

Weaning protocols, incorporating daily screens of multiple variables and spontaneous breathing trials (SBTs), have been associated with superior outcomes in mechanically ventilated medical patients, but validated primarily in patients with coronary and respiratory disease. Multiple studies have attempted to address whether such protocols are relevant to patients with acute brain injury, but with mixed results. In one, extubation was delayed for 2 days in 82% of patients who met pre-determined criteria for weaning because of concerns about decreased level of consciousness (57). PaO_2/FiO_2 ratio and GCS score were independently associated with successful extubation. Seventy-five per cent of patients with a GCS score

of 8 or above were successfully extubated compared to only 33% of those with a GCS score less than 8. In another study, a systematic approach to weaning and extubation was compared to standard care in 318 mixed neuroscience patients requiring mechanical ventilation for longer than 12 hours (58). The rate of reintubation was lower in the systematic compared to standard care group (5% versus 12.5%), but there was no difference in ICU mortality, need for tracheostomy, duration of mechanical ventilation, or ICU LOS. Patients who were reintubated had higher mortality than those who remained extubated (18.5%). Thus, a systematic approach to weaning and extubation appears to reduce the rate of extubation failure without increasing the duration of mechanical ventilation. The impact of the introduction of an evidence-based weaning bundle, including lung protective ventilation, nutritional support, empirical antibiotic therapy for hospital-acquired pneumonia, and a systematic approach to extubation, on duration of mechanical ventilation and mortality was investigated by Roquilly and colleagues (59). Compliance with elements of the bundle varied from

42% to 83% and the complete bundle was delivered in only 21% of patients. However, the duration of mechanical ventilation was lower after introduction of the bundle (12.6 days versus 14.9 days), and 90-day mortality was also lower but not statistically significant (23.5% versus 28.4%).

Long-term outcomes after mechanical ventilation have been reported in 346 patients with intracranial pathology (60). Thirty-day, 1-month, and 1-year mortality was 27%, 45%, and 59% respectively, and 49% of survivors (70/143) had a good recovery at 5 years. Sixty-nine per cent of survivors (98/143) were living at home and 22% (32/143) in a nursing home. One-third of the survivors were still in hospital at 6 months but only 2% remained hospitalized at 5 years, emphasizing the importance of long-term follow-up in brain injury studies. Pelosi et al. compared 552 patients with haemorrhagic/ischaemic stroke and brain trauma requiring mechanical ventilation for longer than 12 hours from a large group of 4030 of patients admitted to ICU for non-neurological reasons (61). Overall, neurological patients had longer duration of mechanical ventilation and higher rates of tracheostomy than those with non-neurological illness, although they developed fewer complications during mechanical ventilation with the exception of a higher rate of ventilator-associated pneumonia in the brain trauma cohort. Fewer patients with stroke met the 'ready-to-wean' criteria within 28 days compared with non-neurological or brain trauma patients, and neurological patients could be extubated less frequently after passing the first SBT. Cough, peak flow, volume and quality of secretions, and ability to complete four tasks (open eyes, follow with eyes, grasp hand, and stick out tongue) were predictors of successful extubation.

In summary, extubation is often delayed in neurological patients even when traditional extubation criteria are met, and delayed extubation is associated with an increased incidence of ventilator-acquired pneumonia and higher ICU LOS. Cough, gag, quality and quantity of secretions, and neurological function are the primary factors determining extubation success.

Withdrawal of life-sustaining therapy

Withdrawal of life-sustaining therapy (WLST) is appropriate in some NCCU patients with severe brain injury. Yee et al. reviewed factors impacting time to death after WLST in comatose patients and found that about 50% (75/149) developed cardiac arrest within 60 minutes (64). Absence of corneal and cough reflexes, extensor or absent motor response, and poor oxygenation were predictors of early death. In another study, WLST in an NCCU was reviewed over a 3-year period (65). Thirty-two of the 74 (43%) non-brain dead patients had therapy withdrawn, primarily by cessation of mechanical ventilation and extubation. Of these, 69% died within 24 hours and the median survival time after extubation of 7.5 hours. Depth of coma did not predict the duration of survival after extubation. The most frequent symptoms after extubation were agonal or laboured breathing (59%) and tachypnoea (34%), and symptomatic treatment was successful in alleviating these. Eighty-eight per cent of surrogates were satisfied with the overall process of WLST, although 75% felt the patient had suffered minimally before death. However, all but one would make the same decision again with regard to WLST.

Rabinstein et al. developed a model to predict death within 60 minutes after WLST in an attempt to identify appropriate patients for organ donation after cardiac death (66). The model included absent corneal reflex and cough reflex, best motor response, and oxygenation index as predictor variables. The score ranges from 0 to 5, with higher scores associated with higher likelihood of death within 60 minutes. A score of 3 or greater is associated with a 74% chance of dying within 60 minutes and a score of 2 or less with a 77% chance of survival beyond 60 minutes.

Quality of life and functional outcomes

In the past few decades there has been an increased focus on evaluating long-term outcomes, particularly functional status, in addition to mortality. Evaluation of health-related QOL and functional status is important to allow assessment of the value of medical care in general and, because of its high cost, of critical care in particular. A variety of instruments have been designed to evaluate different domains of QOL, and integrate costs and QOL into an assessment of quality-adjusted life years (QALYs) (67–80). The National Institute of Neurologic Disorders and Stroke (NINDS) commissioned the Quality of Life in Neurologic Disorders project to develop a health-related QOL tool appropriate for neurological disease, and this evaluates both physical and psychological domains (67). Although the use of QOL tools provides consistency across studies, caution is required in interpreting small changes which may be statistically but not clinically significant (68).

Instruments for measuring quality of life and functional status

Table 31.4 summarizes the frequently used instruments to assess QOL and functional status in neurological outcome studies.

Activities of daily living and instrumental activities of daily living

As the name suggests, activities of daily living (ADLs) measure basic functions necessary for daily life, and describe dependency (69). Although an individual may be independent in all ADLs, he/she may have significant deficits with higher level functions because ADL has a floor effect and does not measure higher level function. The instrumental activities of daily living (IADL) measurement captures more complex activities such as shopping, managing finances and cooking (70).

Barthel index

The BI is similar to ADL but measures activity level and self-care (71). It is commonly used in outcome studies in neurological patients because of its relative simplicity.

Modified Rankin Score

The Modified Rankin Score (mRS) grades disability on a scale of 0 (no disability or symptoms) to 6 (death) (72). A score of 3 or less indicates independence and 5 or greater indicates poor outcome (severe disability/death) (73). Although commonly used to assess disability after neurological injury, the mRS has a ceiling effect because a zero score does not correspond to normal function.

Functional independent measure

The functional independent measure assesses functional status in five domains (self-care, sphincter control, mobility, locomotion, communication and social and cognitive skills) on a 7-point scale (1 = total assistance required; 7 = complete independence) (74). Higher scores indicate better function.

Table 31.4 Summary of instruments for quality of life and functional status

Activities of Daily Living (69) Range 0–6 Higher score—independent	Barthel Index (71) Range 0–100 Higher score—independent	Instrumental Activities of Daily Living (70) Range 0–8 Higher score—independent	Functional Independence Measure (74)	Short Form 36 (80) Range 0–100 High score better	EuroQoL (79)	Glasgow Outcome Scale (GOS) (77,78)
Bathing	Bathing	Ability to use phone	Self-care	Physical health	Mobility	Good Recovery
Feeding	Feeding	Shopping	Sphincter control	Physical functioning (PF)	Self-care	Moderate disability
Toileting	Grooming	Food preparation	Mobility	Role physical (RP)	Usual activities	Severe Disability
Dressing	Dressing	Housekeeping	Locomotion	Body pain (BP)	Pain/discomfort	Vegetative state
Continence	Bowels	Laundry	Communication	General health (GH)	Anxiety/depression	
Transferring	Bladder	Medication	Social and cognitive skills	Mental health	How good is your health today 0–100	
	Toilet use	Transportation		Vitality (VT)		
	Transfer (bed to chair)	Managing Finances		Social function (SF)		
	Mobility			Role emotional (RE)		
	Stairs			Mental health (MH)		

Data from various sources (see References).

Disability Rating Scale

The Disability Rating Scale (DRS) was developed to assess disability in patients with moderate to severe TBI and tracks an individual's short- and long-term disability (75,76). The DRS includes eight items—eye opening, communication ability, motor response, cognitive state, ability to feed, toilet, and groom, overall level of functioning, and employability—and the score ranges from 0 to 30, with 30 indicative of death. The DRS is used in multiple settings but it is insensitive to small changes, particularly in patients with mild TBI.

Glasgow Outcome Scale and Extended Glasgow Outcome Scale

The GOS was originally developed for the evaluation of disability after TBI but is now used to evaluate disability after non-traumatic brain injury (77,78). The GOS evaluation comprises a structured interview that includes the following domains—consciousness, independence inside and outside the home, work, social, and leisure activities, family and friendships, and return to normal life. Outcome in survivors, based on a summary of the responses, is described as vegetative state, severe disability, moderate disability, or good recovery. Similar to other scales, the GOS has a ceiling effect. The extended GOS (GOSE) adds additional subcategories to better define need for assistance and return to normal life (78).

EuroQol-5D (EQ-5D)

The EuroQol is a QOL instrument designed to measure self-reported health status in five domains—mobility, self-care, usual activities, pain and discomfort, anxiety and depression—and a general health score (79). Each domain is reported on a five-level scale with 1 indicating 'no problem' and 5 an 'extreme problem'. The general health scale is a visual analogue scale with 0 indicating 'worst health you can imagine', and 100 the 'best health you can imagine'.

Short Form 36 (SF 36)

The Short Form 36 evaluates QOL in physical and mental health domains and in terms of general health. The score ranges from 0 to 100, with a higher score indicting better outcomes (80).

Studies on functional outcomes in neurological patients

Although there are many studies evaluating functional outcome in individual disease states, there are only a few focused on NCCU patient population overall (Table 31.5). The instruments used in these studies are variable and, unsurprisingly, the results vary (49,53,81–97). BI, mRS, DRS, and GOSE are the most commonly score used to assess disability.

All studies show that large numbers of patients have residual disability after discharge from an NCCU and need a prolonged period of time to reach pre-illness functional status (if they ever do). Functional outcomes are often variable and difficult to predict. Cognitive dysfunction and impairment of executive functions are frequent in patients with brain injury, and older age, more severe injury, and worse socioeconomic status are some of the factors that adversely impact on post-discharge QOL and functional status. Depression and post-traumatic stress disorder (PTSD) is reported in many patients surviving critical illness. Although the exact risk factors are poorly understood, interventions to prevent development of PTSD and early recognition and treatment may ameliorate the symptoms and subsequent disability (98–100).

Neurorehabilitation

Rehabilitation after neurocritical care is an important intervention that impacts positively on long-term outcome. Neurorehabilitation encompasses many factors including reacquisition of mobility skills,

Table 31.5 Summary of selected studies on quality of life and functional status after neurocritical care and specific diseases

Author	Patients/disease	Age (years mean)	Follow-up/ method	Instrument	Results	Risk factors
Broessner et al., 2007 (49)	Neuro ICU	55 > 50	2.7 years Telephone	Glasgow Outcome Score (GOS) mRS	GOS 1–3 in 48% (422/875) of survivors mRS 2–6 in 41.5% (361/875) of survivors	Age, TISS 28, Admission diagnosis
Kiphuth et al., 2010 (53)	Neuro ICU	67	1 year Mail, phone	mRS	mRS 0–2 2in 8.4% of survivors	Age, MV duration, TISS 28, diagnosis
Ronne-Engstrom 2011 (81)	SAH	55	9 months Self-report	ED-5D	Older: worse mobility, self-care, usual activities Younger: increased anxiety depression	Age, severity of disease, volume of blood in the brain
Greebe et al., 2010 (83)	SAH	51	4 months, 5 and 12.5 years Phone	mRS SF-36	Improved from 4 months to 5 years, minimal change from 5 to 12.5 years	
Malmivaara et al., 2011 (84)	Decompressive craniectomy 3-year mortality 53%	48	2.8 years (median)	EQ-5D	EQ-5D poor: SAH 0.15 Other 0.62 Living at home: SAH 73% Other 89%	Cost/QALY SAH: €11,000 Other: €2,000
Paul et al., 2005 (85)	Stroke	75.5	5 years 45% alive	Assessment of QOL	Poor QOL 20%	Older age, low socioeconomic status, severity of stroke
Legriel et al., 2010 (86)	Convulsive status epilepticus Mechanical ventilation—85% Hospital mortality 15%	53	90 days	Glasgow Outcome Scale	Poor (GOS 1–3) 34.8% Good (GOS 4,5) 67.2%	Older age, seizure duration, refractory status, neurological symptoms on site, cerebral insult
Kouloulas et al., 2013 (89)	TBI GCS score < 8	35.8	12 months	GOS, FIM	61% independent 39% dependent	GCS day 15, motor response is better predictor
Kelley et al., 2012 (90)	Moderate/ severe TBI	57	5 years	Satisfaction with life scale, caregiver burden	Impaired self-awareness. Patients overstate functional capability	Greater self-awareness of cognitive deficits associated with increased employment
Haug et al., 2010 (92)	SAH Hunt & Hess grade V and aggressively treated	52	1 year	GOS, mRS	14/26 good cognitive/motor function	Age (older), lower education level, hydrocephalus, shunt
Von Vogelsang et al., 2013 (93)	SAH	60.7	10 years	GOS, depression, EQ-5D	GOS 4,5 at discharge 76% Higher score on functional scales and lower scores on pain/psychological scores	QOL low—decreased functional status, lower GOS scores, comorbidities, perceived lack of improvement
Christensen et al., 2009 (94)	ICH	64	3 months	EQ, Utility Score	13% Utility Score 1 (good outcome)	Age (older), SBP (higher), ICH volume, location, neurological deficits
Roch et al., 2003 (95)	ICH Mechanical ventilation	64	1 year	BI, mRS	42% independent 21% dependent	Age > 65, GCS
Haacke et al., 2006 (96)	Ischaemic stroke	77	4 years	BI, mRS, HAD	BI 80% independent mRS 60% independent	Age, depression, incontinence, mRS, and physical dependence
Hong et al., 2010 (97)	Ischaemic stroke	66.5	3 months	DALY, mRS	mRS 0 28% 5–6 14%	Pneumonia, complications

BI, Barthel Index; DALY, disability adjusted life years; mRS, modified Rankin Scale; QALY, quality adjusted life-years.

Data from various sources (see References).

communication, and other ADLs, as well as nutritional and psychological elements of post-NCCU recovery (101,102). Although early mobilization has been shown to be of benefit in general ICU patients, discomfort of the caregivers about the safety of early physiotherapy is perceived (incorrectly) to be a barrier to its implementation in patients in the NCCU (103). Roth et al. evaluated the effect of early physiotherapy using passive range of motion on intracranial pressure and cerebral perfusion pressure and confirmed that it was safe (104). Importantly, there were no therapy-related complications that required interruption of therapy. Notwithstanding these findings, the feasibility and safety of physiotherapy in the NCCU requires detailed evaluation. Indeed advances in this field may affect many of the predictive models described earlier in the chapter, and their performance may require re-evaluation if advances in acute neurorehabilitation results in improved functional outcomes.

Although current data are sparse, neurorehabilitation incorporating a multidisciplinary and multifaceted approach is believed to have a positive impact on functional outcome after AIS, TBI, spinal cord injury, and likely other types of brain injury (105–108). Early initiation of rehabilitation with high intensity and specific goals delivered by a multidisciplinary team has been shown to be associated with improved outcome in patients with TBI, stroke, and other neurological injuries (106–108). Neurorehabilitation has progressed from one based on teaching NCCU survivors to compensate for their new deficits to a speciality focused on advances in knowledge of neuroplasticity (106,109–111). MacDonald and others have provided good examples of the potential effects of neuroplasticity in enhancing recovery after spinal cord injury (105,106,114), and similar approaches are being developed after stroke and TBI. Surviving anatomical and neurophysiological functions are identified and neurorehabiltiation procedures that will enhance plasticity and neural reorganization devised such that new abilities can be developed (107,108,112–115). Notably neuroplasticity potential is greater in younger than older patients, and seems to be related to the volume of white matter (110). Mosenthal et al. demonstrated that older TBI patients required more inpatient rehabilitation than younger patients, but that significant improvement could be identified 6 months after injury (116).

Early mobilization and evaluation of its efficacy in patients with stroke are the goals of an ongoing study—A Very Early Rehabilitation Trial (AVERT) Phase 2. Preliminary results indicate that early mobilization and intensive physiotherapy are feasible and safe (117). Constraint-induced therapy, ambulation with body weight support treadmill training, virtual reality, transcranial magnetic stimulation, and improvement in orthotics are investigational therapies which may contribute to improved outcomes.

Caregiver needs and burden

Survivors of critical illness may have a prolonged period of disability and remain dependent on caregivers in the long term. Family caregivers provide significant support during hospitalization and in the post-discharge recovery period, and the personal impact of providing such care is substantially affected by the level of provision of professional care (118–121). The demands of caregiving may result in depression and other psychological problems, neglect of self-care, restriction of lifestyle including the ability to work, as well as a substantial financial burden. Although caregiver needs and burdens are not well studied in survivors of patients receiving neurological critical care generally, they are relatively

well documented in specific neurological disease states, particularly after stroke. Hickenbottom and colleagues reported that 74% of stroke patients had more than one ADL/IADL disability and 57% had residual health problems directly attributable to the stroke (119). Sixty nine per cent of those with stroke-related problems were receiving informal (usually family) caregiver support and required between 8.6 and 18.6 hours of care per week. The authors estimated that the annual cost of such care provision was around $6.1 billion in the United States in 1999. In another study, caregiver burden persisted beyond 1 year after stroke, and older patient age, caregiver factors (age, gender, and training), and social support were identified as variables affecting caregiver burden (120). Disruption to interpersonal relationships is the most stressful aspect of caregiving (121). Larach et al. provide a personal view of the lifelong burden on patient and family caregivers and highlight the critical importance of QOL and need for intensive rehabilitation after massive stroke (122). They also recommend reconsideration of the strong bias healthcare providers generally show regarding life-and-death decisions based on their own biases regarding QOL in survivors.

Evaluations of function status and QOL over time, as well as caregiver needs and burdens, should be standardized so that interventions to improve QOL of both patients and caregivers can be better evaluated. In view of the increased focus on the value and effectiveness of healthcare, accurate information on long-term outcomes will assist both clinical decision making and the development of healthcare policy.

References

1. Sung GY. Outcomes of neurocritical care. *Curr Neurol Neurosci Rep.* 2001;1:593–8.
2. Rincon F, Mayer SA. Neurocritical care: a distinct discipline. *Curr Opin Crit Care.* 2007;13:115–21.
3. Breslow MJ, Badawi O. Severity scoring in the critically ill. Part 1 – interpretation and accuracy of outcome prediction scoring systems. *Chest.* 2012;141:245–52
4. Keegan MT, Gajic O, Afessa B. Comparison of APACHE III, APACHE IV, SAPS 3, and MPM_0- III and influence of resuscitation status on model performance. *Chest.* 2012;142:851–85.
5. Zimmerman JE, Kramer AA, McNair DS, Malia FM. Acute Physiology and Chronic Health Evaluation (APACHE) IV: hospital mortality assessment for today's critically ill patients. *Crit Care Med.* 2006;34:1297–310.
6. Higgins TL, Teres D, Copes WS, Nathanson BH, Stark M, Kramer AA. Assessing contemporary intensive care unit outcome: an updated mortality probability admission model (MPM_0-III). *Crit Care Med.* 2007;35:827–35.
7. Moreno RP, Metnitz PGH, Almeida E. SAPS 3—From evaluation of the patient to evaluation of the intensive care unit. Part 2: Development of a prognostic model for hospital mortality at ICU admission. *Intensive Care Med.* 2005;31:1345–55.
8. Kajdacsy-Balla Amaral AC, Andrade FM, Moreno R, Artigas A, Cantraine F, Vincent JL. Use of sequential organ failure assessment score as a severity score *Intensive Care Med.* 2005;31:243–9.
9. Heyland DK, Muscedere J, Drover J, Jiang X, Day AG. Persistent organ dysfunction plus death: a novel composite outcome measure for critical care trials. *Crit Care.* 2011;15(2):R98.
10. Iezzoni LI. *Risk Adjustment for Measuring Health Outcomes* (3rd edn). Chicago, IL: Health Administration Press; 2003.
11. Nathanson BH, Higgins TL. An introduction to statistical methods used in binary outcome modeling. *Semin Cardiothorac Vasc Anesth.* 2008;12:153–66.

12. Corrigan JD, Selassie AW, Orman JA. The epidemiology of traumatic brain injury. *J Head Trauma Rehabil.* 2010;25:72–80.

13. Jennett B. Development of Glasgow Coma and Outcome Scales. *Nepal J Neuroscience.* 2005;2:24–8.

14. Drake AI, McDonald EC, Magnus NE, Gray N, Gottshall K. Utility of Glasgow Coma Scale—extended in symptom prediction following mild traumatic brain injury. *Brain Inj.* 2006;20:469–75.

15. Iyer VN, Mandrekar JN, Danielson RD, Zubkov AY, Elmer JL, Wijdicks EFM. Validity of the FOUR score coma scale in the medical intensive care unit. *Mayo Clin Proc.* 2009;84:694–701.

16. MRC CRASH Trial Collaborators. Predicting outcome after traumatic brain injury: practical prognostic models based on large cohort of international patients. *BMJ.* 2008;336:425–9.

17. Steyerberg EW, Mushkudiani N, Perel P, Butcher I, Lu J, McHugh G, et al. Predicting outcome after traumatic brain injury: development and international validation of prognostic scores based on admission characteristics. *PLoS Med.* 2008;5:1251–61.

18. Roozenbeek B, Lingsma HF, Lecky FE, Lu J, Weir J, Butcher I, et al. Prediction of outcome after moderate and severe traumatic brain injury: external validation of the International Mission on Prognosis and Analysis of Clinical Trials (IMPACT) and Corticoid Randomization After Significant Heat Injury (CRASH) prognostic models. *Crit Care Med.* 2012;40:1609–17.

19. Hukkelhoven C, Steyerberg EW, Habbema JD, Farace E, Marmarou A, Murray GD, et al. Predicting outcome after traumatic brain injury: development and validation of a prognostic score based on admission characteristics. *J Neurotrauma.* 2005;22:1025–39.

20. Harrison DA, Prabhu G, Grieve R, Harvey SE, Sadique MZ, Gomes M, et al. Risk Adjustment In Neurocritical Care (RAIN)—prospective validation of risk prediction models for adult patients with acute traumatic brain injury to use to evaluate the optimum location and comparative costs of neurocritical care: a cohort study. Executive Summary. *Health Technol Assess.* 2013;17(23):vii–viii, 1–350.

21. Tasaki O, Shiozaki T, Hamasaki T, Kajino K, Nakae H, Tanaka H, et al. Prognostic indicators and outcome prediction model for severe traumatic brain injury. *J Trauma.* 2009;66:304–8.

22. Hunt WE, Hess RM. Surgical risks as related to time of intervention in the repair of intracranial aneurysms. *J Neurosurg.* 1968;28:14–20.

23. Oshiro EM, Walter KA, Piantadosi S, Witham T, Tamargo RJ. A new subarachnoid hemorrhage grading system based on the Glasgow Coma Scale: a comparison with the Hunt and Hess and World Federation of Neurological Surgeons scales in a clinical series. *Neurosurgery.* 1997;41:140–8.

24. Drake CG. Report of World Federation of Neurological Surgeons Committee on a universal subarachnoid hemorrhage grading scale. *Neurosurgery.* 1988;68:985–6.

25. Rosen DS, Macdonald RL. Grading of subarachnoid hemorrhage: modification of the World Federation of Neurosurgical Societies Scale on the basis of data for a large series of patients. *Neurosurgery.* 2004;54:566–576.

26. Jaja BNR, Cusimano MD, Etminan N, Hanggi D, Hasan D, Ilodigwe D, et al. Clinical prediction models for aneurysmal subarachnoid hemorrhage: a systematic review. *Neurocrit Care.* 2013;18:143–53.

27. De Rooij NK, Greving JP, Rinkel GJ, Frigns CJ. Early prediction of delayed cerebral ischemia after subarachnoid hemorrhage: development and validation of a practical risk chart. *Stroke.* 2013;44:1288–94.

28. Fernandez A, Schmidt JM, Claassen J, Pavlicova M, Huddleston D, Kreiter KT, et al. Fever after subarachnoid hemorrhage: risk factors and impact on outcome. *Neurology.* 2007;68:1013–19.

29. Güresir E, Beck J, Vatter H, Setzer M, Gerlack R, Seifert V, Raabe A. Subarachnoid hemorrhage and intracerebral hematoma: incidence, prognostic factors, and outcome. *Neurosurgery.* 2008;63:1088–94.

30. Hemphill JC, Newman J, Zhao S, Johnston SC. Hospital usage of early do-not-resuscitate orders and outcome after intracerebral hemorrhage. *Stroke.* 2004;35:1130–4.

31. Zahuranec DB, Brown DL, Lisabeth LD, Gonzales NR, Longwell PJ, Smith MA, et al. Early care limitations independently predict mortality after intracerebral hemorrhage. *Neurology.* 2007;68:1651–7.

32. Hemphill JC, Bonovich DC, Besmertis L, Manley GT, Johnston SC. The ICH score: a simple, reliable grading scale for intracerebral hemorrhage. *Stroke.* 2001;32:891–7.

33. Clarke JL, Johnston SC, Farrant M, Bernstein R, Tong D, Hemphill JC. External validation of the ICH score. *Neurocrit Care.* 2004;1:53–60.

34. Rost NS, Smith EE, Chang Y, Snider RW, Chanderraj R, Schwab K, et al. Prediction of functional outcome in patient with primary intracerebral hemorrhage. The FUNC score. *Stroke.* 2008;39:2304–9.

35. Garret JS, Zarghouni M, Layton KF, Graybeal D, Daoud YA. Validation of clinical prediction scores in patients with primary intra cerebral hemorrhage. *Neurocrit Care.* 2013;19:329–35.

36. Muir KW, Weir CJ, Murray GD, Povey C, Lees KR. Comparison of neurological scales and scoring systems for acute stroke prognosis. *Stroke.* 1996;27:1817–20.

37. Adams HP, Davis PH, Leira EC, Chang KC, Bendixen BH, Clarke WR, et al. Baseline NIH stroke scale score strongly predicts outcome after stroke: a report of the Trial of Org 10172 in Acute Stroke Treatment (TOAST). *Neurology.* 1999;53:126–31.

38. Weimar C, Ziegler A, König I, Diener H, on behalf of the German Stroke Study Collaborators. Predicting functional outcome and survival after acute ischemic stroke. *J Neurol.* 2002;249:888–95.

39. Ntaios G, Faouzi M, Ferrari J, Lang W, Vemmos K, Michel P. An integer-based score to predict functional outcome in acute ischemic stroke. The ASTRAL score. *Neurology.* 2012;78:1916–22.

40. Hoffmann S, Malzahn U, Harms H, Koennecke H, Berger K, Kalic M, et al. Development of a clinical score (A^2DS^2) to predict pneumonia in acute ischemic stroke. *Stroke.* 2012;43:2617–23.

41. Kramer AH, Zygun DA. Do neurocritical care units save lives? Measuring the impact of specialized ICUs. *Neurocrit Care.* 2011;14:329–33.

42. Kurtz P, Fitts V, Sumer Z, Jalon H, Cooke J, Kvetan V, et al. How does care differ for neurological patients admitted to a neurocritical care unit versus a general ICU? *Neurocrit Care.* 2011;15:477–80.

43. Burns JD, Green DM, Lau H, Winter M, Koyfman F, DeFusco CM, et al. The effect of a neurocritical care service without a dedicated neuro-ICU on quality of care in intracerebral hemorrhage. *Neurocrit Care.* 2013;18:305–12.

44. Samuels O, Webb A, Culler S, Martin K, Barrow D. Impact of a dedicated neurocritical care team in treating patients with aneurysmal subarachnoid hemorrhage. *Neurocrit Care.* 2011;14:334–40.

45. Mirski MA, Chang CWJ, Cowan R. Impact of a neuroscience intensive care unit on neurosurgical patient outcomes and cost of care. *J Neurosurg Anesthesiol.* 2001;13:83–92.

46. Varelas PN, Conti MM, Spanaki MV, Potts E, Bradford D, Sunstrom C, et al. The impact of a neurointensivist-led team on a semi closed neurosciences intensive care unit. *Crit Care Med.* 2004;32:2191–8.

47. Diringer MN, Edwards DF. Admission to a neurologic/neurosurgical intensive care unit is associated with reduced mortality rate after intracerebral hemorrhage. *Crit Care Med.* 2001;29:635–40.

48. Suarez JI, Zaidt OO, Suri MF, Feen ES, Lynch G, Hickman J, et al. Length of stay and mortality in neurocritically ill patients: impact of a specialized neurocritical care team. *Crit Care Med.* 2004;32:2311–17.

49. Broessner G, Helbok R, Lackner P, Mitterberger M, Beer R, Engelhardt K, et al. Survival and long-term functional outcome in 1,155 consecutive neurocritical care patients. *Crit Care Med.* 2007;35:2025–30.

50. Ziai WC, Varelas PN, Zeger SL, Mirski MA, Ulatowski JA. Neurologic intensive care resource use after brain tumor surgery: an analysis of indications and alternative strategies. *Crit Care Med.* 2003;31:2782–7.

51. Diringer MN, Reaven NL, Funk SE, Urman GC. Elevated body temperature independently contributes to increased length of stay in neurologic intensive care unit patients. *Crit Care Med.* 2004;32:1489–95.

52. Flores-Cordero JM, Amaya-Villar R, Rincon-Ferrari MD et al. Acute community-acquired bacterial meningitis in adults admitted to the intensive care unit: clinical manifestations, management and prognostic factors. *Intensive Care Med.* 2003;29:1967–73.

53. Kiphuth IC, Schellinger PD, Kohrmann M, Bardutzky J, Lücking H, Kloska S, et al. Predictors for good functional outcome after neurocritical care. *Crit Care.* 2010;14: R136.

54. Varelas PN, Corry J, Rehman M, Abdelhak T, Schultz L, Spanaki M, Bartscher J. Management of status epilepticus in neurological versus medical intensive care unit: does it matter? *Neurocrit Care.* 2013;19:4–9.

55. Golestanian E, Liou J, Smith M. Long-term survival in older critically ill patients with acute ischemic stroke. *Crit Care Med.* 2009;37:3107–13.

56. Coplin, WM, Pierson, DJ, Cooley, KD, Newell DW, Rubenfeld GD. Implications of extubation delay in brain injured patients meeting standard weaning criteria. *Am J Respir Crit Care Med.* 2000;161:1530–6.

57. Namen AM, Ely EW, Tatter S, Case LD, Lucia MA, Smith A, et al. Predictors of successful extubation in neurosurgical patients. *Am J Respir Crit Care Med.* 2001;163:658–64.

58. Navalesi P, Frigerio P, Moretti MP, Sommariva M, Vesconi S, Baiardi P, et al. Rate of reintubation in mechanically ventilated neurosurgical and neurologic patient: evaluation of a systematic approach to waning and extubation. *Crit Care Med.* 2008;36:2986–92.

59. Roquilly A, Cinotti R, Jaber S, Vourc'h M, Pengam F, Mahe JP, et al. Implementation of an evidence- based extubation readiness bundle in 499 brain injured patients—a before-after evaluation of a quality improvement project. *Am J Resp Crit Care Med.* 2013;188(8):958–66.

60. Malmivaara KJ, Hernesniemi R, Samenpera J, Ohman RP, Roine J. Siironen, Survival and outcome of neurosurgical patients requiring ventilatory support after intensive care unit stay. *Neurosurgery.* 2009;65:530–7.

61. Pelosi P, Ferguson ND, Frutos-Vivar F, Anzueto A, Putensen C, Raymondos K, et al. Management and outcome of mechanically ventilated neurologic patients. *Crit Care Med.* 2011;39:1482–92.

62. Karanjia N, Nordquist D, Stevens R, Nyquist P. A clinical description of extubation failure in patients with primary brain injury. *Neurocrit Care.* 2011;15:4–12.

63. Salam A, Tilluckdharry L, Amoateng-Adjepong Y, Manthous CA. Neurologic status, cough, secretions and extubation outcome. *Intensive Care Med.* 2004;30:1334–9.

64. Yee AH, Rabinstein AA, Thapa P, Mandrekar J, Wijdicks EFM. Factors influencing time to death after withdrawal of life support in neurocritical care patients. *Neurology.* 2010;74:1380–5.

65. Mayer SA, Kossof S. Withdrawal of life support in the neurologic intensive care unit. *Neurology.* 1999;52:1602–9.

66. Rabinstein AA, Yee AH, Mandrekar J, Yee AH, Mandrekar J, Fugate JE, et al. Prediction of potential for organ donation after cardiac death in patient in neurocritical care: a prospective observational study. *Lancet Neurol.* 2012;11:414–19.

67. Cella D, Nowinski C, Peterman A, Nowinski C, Peterman A, Victorson D, et al. The neurology quality-of- life measurement initiative. *Arch Phys Med Rehab.* 2011;92(10 Suppl 1):S28–S36.

68. De Vet HC, Terwee CB, Ostelo RW, Beckerman H, Knol DL, Bouter LM. Minimal changes in health status questionnaires: distinction between minimally detectable change and minimally important change. *Health Qual Life Outcomes.* 2006;4:54.

69. Shelkey M, Wallace M. *Katz Index of Independence in Activities of Daily Living (ADL).* The Hartford Institute for Geriatric Nursing. [Online] http://hartfordign.org

70. Lawton MP, Brody EM. *Instrumental Activities of Daily Living (IADL).* Abramsom Center for Jewish Life, 2012. [Online] http://www.abramsoncenter.org/pri/documents/iadl.pdf

71. The Internet Stroke Center. *The Barthel Index.* http://www.strokecenter.org/wp-content/uploads/2011/08/barthel.pdf

72. The Internet Stroke Center. *Modified Rankin Scale.* http://www.strokecenter.org/wp-content/uploads/2011/08/modified_rankin.pdf

73. Banks JL, Marotta CA. Outcomes validity and reliability of the Modified Rankin Scale: implication for stroke clinical trials. A literature review and synthesis. *Stroke.* 2007;38:1091–6.

74. Masedo AL, Jensen HM, Ehde D, Cardenas DD. Reliability and validity of a self-report FIM™ (FIM-SR) in persons with amputation or spinal cord injury and chronic pain. *Am J Phys Med Rehabil.* 2005;84:167–76.

75. Bellon K, Wright J, Jamison L, Kolakowsky-Hayner S. Disability Rating Scale. *J Head Trauma Rehabil.* 2012;27:449–51.

76. Center for Outcome Measurement in Brain Injury. *Disability Rating Scale.* [Online] http://www.tbims.org/combi/drs/DRS%20Form.pdf

77. Jennett B, Bond M. Assessment of outcome after severe brain damage. A practical scale. *Lancet.* 1975;1:285–93.

78. Wilson LJT, Pettigrew LEL, Teasdale GM. Structured interview for the Glasgow Outcome Scale and the Extended Glasgow Outcome Scale: guidelines for their use. *J Neurotrauma.* 1998;15:573585.

79. EuroQol Research Foundation. EQ-5D-5L Health Questionnaire. [Online] http://www.euroqol.org

80. Ware JE Jr. *SF-36® Health Survey Update.* The SF Community. [Online] http://www.sf-36.org/tools/sf36.shtml

81. Ronne-Engstrom E, Enbald P, Lundstrom E. Outcome after spontaneous subarachnoid hemorrhage measured with the EQ-5D. *Stroke.* 2011;42:3284–6.

82. Wong GKC, Poon WS, Boet R, Chan MT, Gin T, Ng SC, et al. Health-related quality of life after aneurysmal subarachnoid hemorrhage: profile and clinical factors. *Neurosurgery.* 2011;68:1556–61.

83. Greebe P, Rinkel GJE, Hop JW, Visser-Miley JMA, Algra A. Functional outcome and quality of life 5 and 12.5 years after aneurismal subarachnoid haemorrhage. *J Neurol.* 2010;257:2059–64.

84. Malmivaara K, Ohman J, Kivissari R, Hernesniemi, Siironen J. Cost-effectiveness of decompressive craniectomy in non-traumatic neurologic emergencies. *Eur J Neurol.* 2011;18:402–9.

85. Paul SL, Strum JW, Dewey HM, Donnan GA, Macdonell RA, Thrift AG. Long-term outcome in the North East Melbourne Stroke Incidence Study. Predictors of quality of life at 5 years after stroke. *Stroke.* 2005;36;2082–6.

86. Legriel S, Azoulay E, Resche-Region M, Lemiale V, Mourvillier B, Kouatchet A, et al. Functional outcome after convulsive status epilepticus. *Crit Care Med.* 2010;38:2295–303.

87. Al-Khinidi T, Macdonald RL, Schweizer TA. Cognitive and functional outcome after aneurysmal subarachnoid hemorrhage. *Stroke.* 2010;41:e519–e536.

88. Van Asch CJJ, Luitse MJA, Rinkel GJE, van der Tweel I, Algra A, Klijn CJ. Incidence, case fatality, and functional outcome of intracerebral haemorrhage over time according to age, sex, and ethnic origin: a systematic review and meta-analysis. *Lancet Neurol.* 2010;9:167–76.

89. Kouloulas EJ, Papadeas AG, Michail X, Sakas DE, Boviatsis EJ. Prognostic value of time-related Glasgow Coma Scale components in severe traumatic brain injury: a prospective evaluation with respect to 1-year survival and functional outcome. *Int J Rehabil Res.* 2013;35:260–7.

90. Kelley E, Sullivan C, Loughlin JK, Hutson L, Dahdah MN, Long MK, et al. Self-awareness and neurobehavioral outcomes, 5 years or more after moderate to severe brain injury. *J Head Trauma Rehabil.* 2012;27:1–6.

91. Stevens RD, Sutter R. Prognosis in severe brain injury. *Crit Care Med.* 2013;41:1104–23.

92. Haug T, Sorteberg A, Finset A, Lindegaard K, Lundar T, Sorteberg W. Cognitive functional and health-related quality of life 1 year after aneurysmal subarachnoid hemorrhage in preoperative comatose patients (Hunt and Hess grade V patients). *Neurosurgery.* 2010;66:475–85.

93. Von Vogelsang A, Burström K, Wengström Y, Svensson M, Forsberg C. Health- related quality of life 10 years after intracranial aneurysm rupture: a retrospective cohort study using EQ-5D. *Neurosurgery.* 2013;72:397–406.

94. Christensen MC, Mayer SA, Ferran J. Quality of life after intracerebral hemorrhage: results of the Factor Seven for Acute Hemorrhagic Stroke (FAST) Trial. *Stroke.* 2009;40:1677–82.

95. Roch A, Mihelet P, Jullien AC, Thirion X, Bregeon F, Papazian L, et al. Long-term outcome in intensive care unit survivors after mechanical ventilation for intracerebral hemorrhage. *Crit Care Med.* 2003;31:2651–6.

96. Haacke C, Althaus A, Spottke A, Seibert U, Back T, Dodel R. Long-term outcome after stroke: evaluating health-related quality of life using utility measurements. *Stroke.* 2006;37:193–8.

97. Hong KS, Saver JL, Kang DW, Bae HJ, Yu K, Koo J, et al. Years of optimum health lost due to complication after acute ischemic stroke: disability-adjusted life-years analysis. *Stroke*. 2010;41:1758–65.

98. Cuthbertson BH, Hull A, Strachan M, Scott J. Post-traumatic stress disorder after critical illness requiring intensive care. *Intensive Care Med*. 2004;30:450–5.

99. Peris A, Bonizzoli M, Iozzelli D, Migliaccio ML, Zagli G, Bacchereti A, et al. Early intra-intensive care unit psychological intervention promotes recovery from post-traumatic stress disorders and depression symptoms in critically ill patients. *Crit Care*. 2001;15:R41.

100. Hatch R, McKechnie S, Griffiths J. Psychological intervention to prevent ICU-related PTSD: who, when and how far long? *Crit Care*. 2011;15:141.

101. Greenwald BD, Rigg JL, Greenwald BD, Rigg JL. Neurorehabilitation in traumatic brain injury: does it make a difference? *Mt Sinai J Med*. 2009;76:182–9.

102. Ifejika-Jones NL, Barrett AM. Rehabilitation—emerging technologies, innovative therapies, and future objectives. *Neurotherapeutics*. 2011;8:452–62.

103. Mendez-Tellez PA, Nusr R, Feldman D, Needham DM. Early physical rehabilitation in the ICU: a review for Neurohospitalist. *Neurohopsitalist*. 2012;2:96–105.

104. Roth C, Stitz H, Kalhout A, Kleffmann, Deinsberger W, Ferbert A. Effect of early physiotherapy on intracranial pressure and cerebral perfusion pressure. *Neurocrit Care*. 2013;18:33–8.

105. McDonald JW. Repairing the damaged spinal cord. *Sci Am*. 1999;281:64–73.

106. Sadowsky CL, McDonald JW. Activity-based restorative therapies: concepts and applications in spinal cord injury-related neurorehabilitation. *Dev Disabil Res Rev*. 2009;15:112–16.

107. Albert SJ, Kesselring J, Albert SJ, Kesselring J. Neurorehabilitation of stroke. *J Neurol*. 2012;259:817–32.

108. Berthier ML, Pulvermuller F, Berthier ML, Pulvermuller F. Neuroscience insights improve neurorehabilitation of post stroke aphasia. *Nat Rev Neurol*. 2011;7:86–97.

109. Warraich Z, Kleim JA. Neural plasticity: the biological substrate for neurorehabilitation. *PM R*. 2010;2:S208–19.

110. Berlucchi G, Berlucchi G. Brain plasticity and cognitive neurorehabilitation. *Neuropsychol Rehabil*. 2011;21:560–78.

111. Gillick BT, Zirpel L. Neuroplasticity: an appreciation from synapse to system. *Arch Phys Med Rehabil*. 2012;93;1846–55.

112. Brainin M, Zorowitz RD. Advances in stroke recovery and rehabilitation. *Stroke*. 2013;44:311–13.

113. Becker D, Sadowsky CL, McDonald JW, Becker D, Sadowsky CL, McDonald JW. Restoring function after spinal cord injury. *Neurologist*. 2003; 9:1–15.

114. Pekna M, Pekny M, Nilsson M. Modulation of neural plasticity as a basis for stroke rehabilitation. *Stroke*. 2012;43:2819–28.

115. Labruyere R, Agarwala A, Curt A. Rehabilitation in spine and spinal cord trauma. *Spine*. 2010;35:S259–62.

116. Mosenthal AC, Livingston DH, Lavery RF, Knudson MM, Lee S, Morabito D, et al. The effect of age on functional outcome in mild traumatic brain injury: 6-month report of a prospective multicenter trial. *J Trauma*. 2004;56:1042–8.

117. Van Wijk R, Cumming T, Chrilov L, Donnan G, Bernhardt J. An early mobilization protocol successfully delvers more and earlier therapy to acute stroke patients: further results from phase II of AVERT. *Neurorehabil Neural Repair*. 2012;26:20–6.

118. Van Pelt DC, Milbrandt EB, Qin L, Weissfeld LA, Rotondi AJ, Schulz R, et al. Informal caregiver burden among survivors of prolonged mechanical ventilation, *Am J Respir Crit Care Med*. 2007;175:167–73.

119. Hickenbottom SL, Fendrick AM, Kutcher JS, Kabeto MU, Katz SJ, Langa KM. A national study of the quantity and cost of informal caregiving for the elderly with stroke. *Neurology*. 2002;58:1754–9.

120. McCullagh E, Brigstocke G, Donaldson N, Karla L. Determinants of caregiving burden and quality of life in caregivers of stroke patients. *Stroke*. 2005;36:2181–6.

121. King RB, Ainsworth CR, Ronen M, Hartke RJ. Stroke caregivers: pressing problems reported during the first months of caregiving. *J Neurosci Nurs*. 2010;42:3.

122. Larach DR, Larach DB, Larach MG. A life worth living: seven years after craniectomy. *Neurocrit Care*. 2009;11:106–111.

Index

Note: Entries appear in their unabbreviated form. A list of abbreviations appears on pp. xi–xiii